EDITION 11

EXPLORING MEDICAL LANGUAGE

A STUDENT-DIRECTED APPROACH

AF856247

Danielle LaFleur Brooks, MEd, MA
Faculty, Allied Health Science
Community College of Vermont
Montpelier, Vermont

Myrna LaFleur Brooks, RN, BEd
Founding President, National Association of Health Unit Coordinators
Faculty Emeritus, Maricopa County Community Colleges
Phoenix, Arizona

Dale Levinsky, MD
Clinical Associate Professor, Family, Community, & Preventative Medicine
University of Arizona College of Medicine
Phoenix, Arizona
Clinical Associate Professor, Family and Community Medicine
University of Arizona College of Medicine
Tucson, Arizona
Clinical Instructor, Pharmacy Practice-Science
University of Arizona College of Pharmacy
Tucson, Arizona

ELSEVIER

Elsevier
3251 Riverport Lane
St. Louis, Missouri 63043

EXPLORING MEDICAL LANGUAGE, A STUDENT-DIRECTED APPROACH, ELEVENTH EDITION
978-0-323-67649-6
Set ISBN: 978-0-323-71156-2
Copyright © 2022, Elsevier Inc. All rights reserved.

No part of this publication may be reproduced or transmitted in any form or by any means, electronic or mechanical, including photocopying, recording, or any information storage and retrieval system, without permission in writing from the publisher. Details on how to seek permission, further information about the Publisher's permissions policies and our arrangements with organizations such as the Copyright Clearance Center and the Copyright Licensing Agency, can be found at our website: www.elsevier.com/permissions.

This book and the individual contributions contained in it are protected under copyright by the Publisher (other than as may be noted herein).

Although for mechanical reasons some pages of this publication are perforated, only those pages imprinted with an Elsevier Inc. copyright notice are intended for removal.

Notice

Practitioners and researchers must always rely on their own experience and knowledge in evaluating and using any information, methods, compounds or experiments described herein. Because of rapid advances in the medical sciences, in particular, independent verification of diagnoses and drug dosages should be made. To the fullest extent of the law, no responsibility is assumed by Elsevier, authors, editors or contributors for any injury and/or damage to persons or property as a matter of products liability, negligence or otherwise, or from any use or operation of any methods, products, instructions, or ideas contained in the material herein.

Previous editions copyrighted 2018, 2014, 2012, 2009, 2005, 2002, 1998, 1994, 1989, and 1985.

Library of Congress Control Number: 2020943819

Director, Content Development: Laurie Gower
Senior Content Strategist: Linda Woodard
Content Development Specialist: Elizabeth McCormac
Publishing Services Manager: Julie Eddy
Senior Project Manager: Abigail Bradberry
Design Direction: Renee Duenow

Printed in Canada

Last digit is the print number: 9 8 7 6 5 4 3 2 1

ELSEVIER Book Aid International
Working together to grow libraries in developing countries
www.elsevier.com • www.bookaid.org

For our students,
who continue to inspire us with their dedication
to learning while balancing life's other demands.
Every page is for you.

Contents

Preface

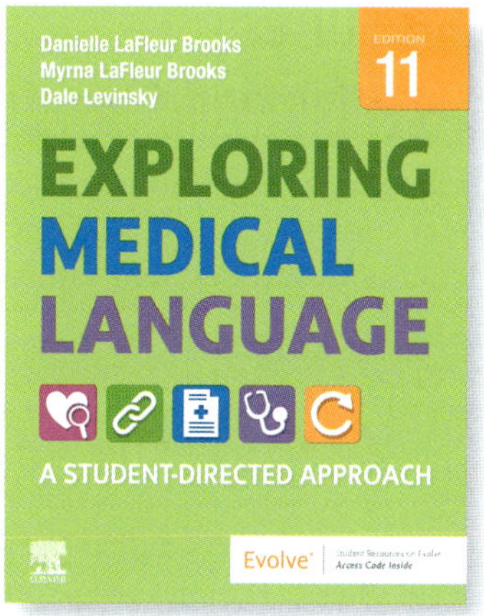

WELCOME TO THE ELEVENTH EDITION OF *EXPLORING MEDICAL LANGUAGE*

We are excited to share the new edition of *Exploring Medical Language* with you! The eleventh edition reflects knowledge we have gained through clinical practice and working alongside medical terminology students and instructors. In addition to updating content to reflect current use, we have cross-referenced terms with ICD-10 diagnosis and procedure codes to make sure terms studied are relevant. We have also continued to refine the learning system to more fully utilize learning styles and to support long-term memory. Here is an overview of new and sustaining features:

New Content

- Illustration exercises for word parts and terms
- Narrative introductions on Laboratory Tests, Diagnostic Imaging, and Endoscopy
- New term lists, including Laboratory Terms and Diagnostic Imaging Terms
- Expanded abbreviation sections grouped by categories
- More Chapter Content Quiz questions
- Chapter at a Glance content summaries
- Online Audio Glossary aligned with pronunciation exercises
- Online, gradable Practice Exams and Activities

New Instructional Strategies

- Medical terms aligned with ICD-10 diagnosis and procedure codes
- Historical and informational boxes placed within tables, closer to corresponding word parts, terms, and abbreviations
- Comprehensive Word Parts Tables that include all word parts used to analyze terms, including those presented in previous chapters
- Combined pronunciation and spelling exercises to practice similar skills
- Complementary Terms and Abbreviations categorized by topic, including Signs and Symptoms, Treatments, Equipment, and Medical Specialties
- Former Exercise Figures grouped into standalone Label exercises for streamlined practice of Terms Built from Word Parts
- Reorganized Cardiovascular, Lymphatic, Immune Systems, and Blood content in Chapter 10 for easier delivery of instruction

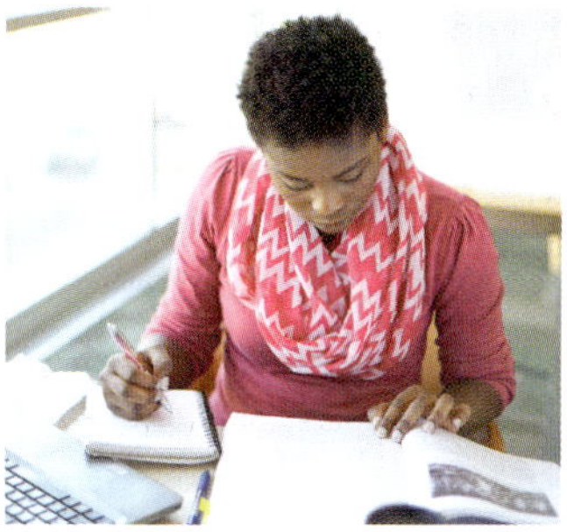

Cornerstone Features

- Paper flashcards
- Illustrations conveying medical concepts
- Word-part learning system used to analyze, define, and build terms
- Body-system organization of content
- Term lists categorized by Terms Built from Word Parts and Terms NOT Built from Word Parts
- Subcategories of terms grouped by topic: Disease and Disorder, Surgical, Diagnostic and Complementary Terms
- Application of terms in medical documents and online EHR Modules
- Online learning opportunities aligned with the chapter objectives and exercises

Exploring Medical Language provides an effective introduction to medical language for those entering health professions as well as those in related fields, including software development, computer applications and support, insurance, law, equipment supply, pharmaceutical sales, and medical writing. Its hybrid approach of print and electronic learning tools provides a balance of hands-on and virtual experiences. The wide-array of materials available provide a variety of ways to practice and to demonstrate learning, making the textbook and companion website a useful resource for a range of learning styles and classroom formats.

We remain dedicated to supporting instructors and students and invite you to contact us at:

danielle.lafleurbrooks@ccv.edu
myrnabrooks@comcast.net
dale.levinsky@gmail.com

You are also welcome to follow Myrna's educational blog at medicalterminologyblog.com.

Warm regards,
Danielle, Myrna, and Dale

FEATURES

Outline and Objectives

Chapter introductions list sections with page numbers and student learning objectives aligned with chapter content, exercises, and assessments.

PART 2 BODY SYSTEMS

Chapter 5

Respiratory System

Outline

Objectives

Upon completion of this chapter, you will be able to:

1. Pronounce organs and anatomic structures of the respiratory system.
2. Define and spell word parts related to the respiratory system.
3. Define, pronounce, and spell disease and disorder terms related to the respiratory system.
4. Define, pronounce, and spell surgical terms related to the respiratory system.

Anatomy

PRONOUNCE ANATOMIC STRUCTURES

Practice saying aloud each of the organs and specific structures on the previous pages.

To hear the terms, go to Evolve Resources at www.evolve.elsevier.com and select: Student Resources > **Audio Glossary** > Chapter 5 > Anatomic Structures

❏ Check the box when complete.

Body-system chapters introduce related anatomy and physiology (A&P). **Pronunciation of organs and anatomical structures** can be practiced using phonetic spelling in the textbook and audio available online.

NEW—**Pronunciation of anatomic structures** using the Evolve Resources Audio Glossary.

Organs and Anatomic Structures of the Respiratory System

TERM	DEFINITION
nose (nōz)	lined with mucous membrane and fine hairs; it acts as a filter to moisten and warm the entering air
nasal septum (NĀS-el) (SEP-tum)	partition separating the right and left nasal cavities
paranasal sinuses (*par*-a-NĀ-sel) (SĪ-nus-es)	air cavities within the cranial bones that open into the nasal cavities
pharynx	serves as a food and air passageway. Air enters from the nasal cavities and/or mouth

Word Parts

Word Part Tables present combining forms, suffixes, and prefixes related to chapter content. Textbook exercises, **paper** and **electronic flashcards,** and online activities reinforce learning.

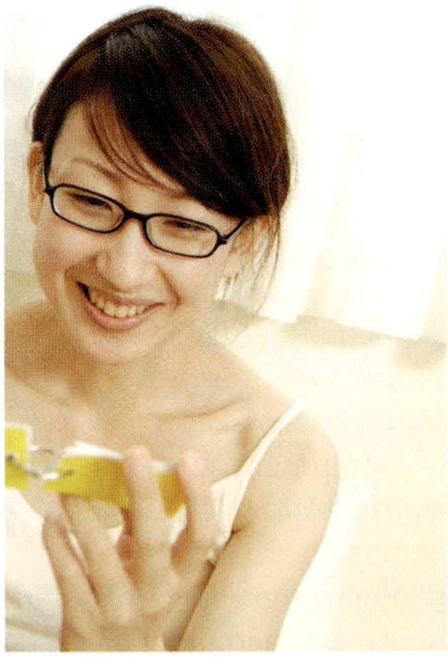

NEW—Comprehensive Word Parts Tables that include all combining forms, prefixes, and suffixes used to build terms in the chapter.

1 ▪ Respiratory System Combining Forms

COMBINING FORM	DEFINITION
adenoid/o	adenoids
alveol/o	alveolus *(s.)*, alveoli *(pl.)*
bronch/o	bronchus *(s.)*, bronchi *(pl.)*
bronchi/o	bronchus *(s.)*, bronchi *(pl.)*
diaphragmat/o	diaphragm
epiglott/o	epiglottis
laryng/o	larynx
lob/o	lobe(s)

LOBE literally means **the part that hangs down**, although it comes from the Greek **lobos**, meaning **capsule** or **pod**. **Lob/o** can also describe lobes in other areas of the body, including the ear, liver, and brain.

COMBINING FORM	DEFINITION
mediastin/o	mediastinum
nas/o	nose
pharyng/o	pharynx
pleur/o	pleura
pneum/o	lung, air
pneumon/o	lung, air
pulmon/o	lung
rhin/o	nose
sept/o	septum

SEPTUM comes from the Latin word **saeptum** meaning to **fence** or **wall off** and refers to a structure dividing cavities or tissues. **Sept/o** can also describe septa in other areas of the body, including the heart and brain.

COMBINING FORM	DEFINITION
sinus/o	sinus(es)
thorac/o	thorax, chest, chest cavity
tonsill/o	tonsil(s) *(Note: tonsil has one l, and the combining form has two ls.)*
trache/o	trachea

2 ▪ Combining Forms Used with Respiratory System Terms

COMBINING FORM	DEFINITION	COMBINING FORM	DEFINITION
atel/o	imperfect, incomplete	**orth/o**	straight
capn/o	carbon dioxide	**ox/i**	oxygen

Label Exercises

NEW—Interactive illustration exercises help students form connections between word parts and anatomic structures, apply the meaning of word parts, and recall term definitions.

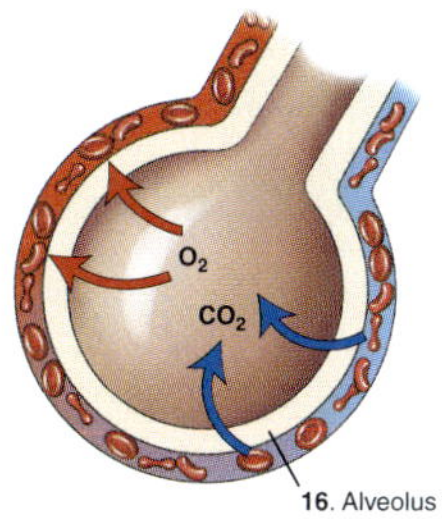

16. Alveolus

CF: ____________________

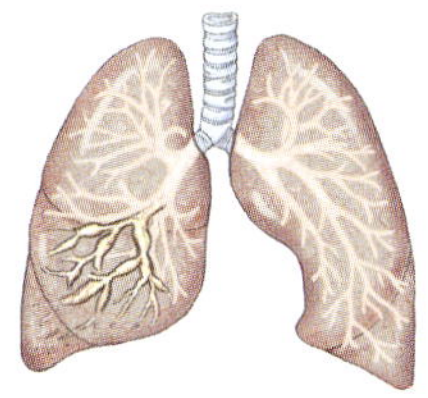

____________ / ____________

bronchi dilation

Medical Terms Built from Word Parts

Students **analyze, define,** and **build** medical terms using the meaning of word parts. Learning may be extended through practice with Evolve Student Resources, including online exercises, practice quizzes, and games.

EXERCISE 6 ■ Analyze and Define

Analyze and define the following terms by drawing slashes between word parts, writing word part abbreviations above the term, underlining combining forms, and writing combining form abbreviations below the term.

EXAMPLE: WR CV S
diaphragmat / o / cele
CF
hernia of the diaphragm

1. tracheitis

____

____

3. alveolitis

____

____

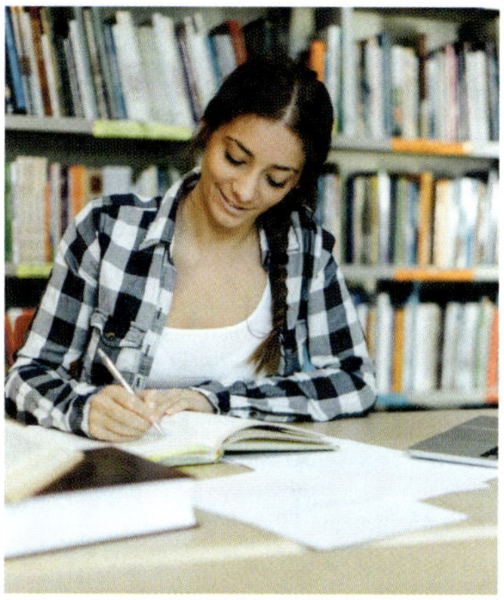

B Fill In

Build disease and disorder terms for the following definitions with the word parts you have learned.

EXAMPLE: inflammation of the tonsils tonsill / itis
WR / S

1. inflammation of the pharynx ____________ / ____________
WR / S

2. cancerous tumor originating in a bronchus ____________ / / ____________
WR / CV / S

3. pertaining to the lobe(s); diseased state of the lung ______ / ______ ______ / ______
WR / S WR / S

Medical Terms NOT Built from Word Parts

Chapters present tables of Terms NOT Built from Word Parts followed by exercises designed to facilitate memorization. Label exercises match illustrations with terms to form connections between terms and medical concepts.

B Label

Write the medical terms pictured and defined.

1. ____________________
matter foreign to the circulation, carried to the pulmonary artery and its branches, where it blocks circulation to the lungs

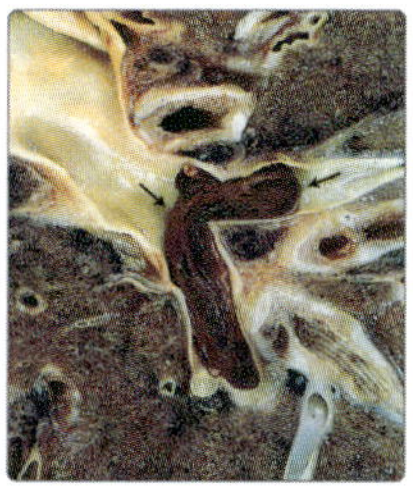

2. ____________________
repetitive pharyngeal collapse during sleep, which leads to transient periods of apnea

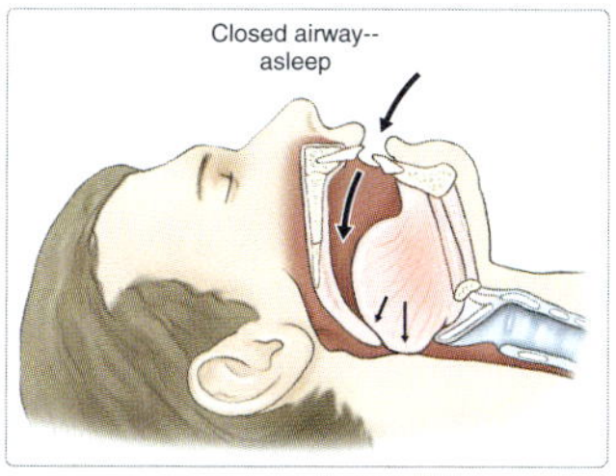

Pronunciation and Spelling

Pronunciation and spelling exercises may be completed on paper or online. Students may hear terms pronounced and practice spelling online using Evolve Resources.

NEW—Audio Glossary providing pronunciation of anatomic structures and medical terms.

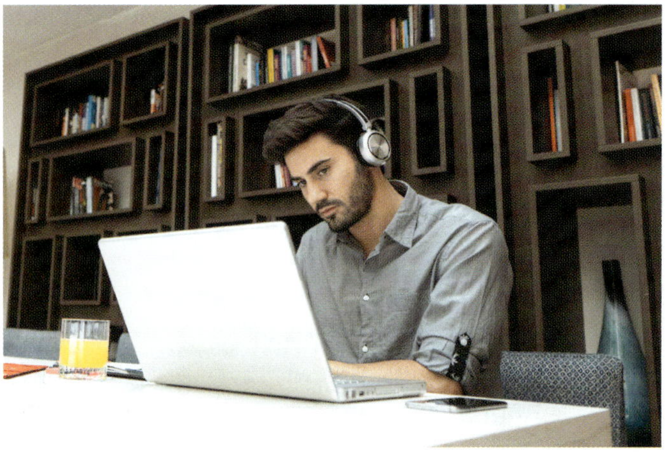

Clinical Categories and Appendices

Body-system chapters present term lists grouped by the categories of **Disease and Disorder, Surgical, Diagnostic,** and **Complementary**. With use of additional appendices in the textbook and online, students may increase their vocabulary in the areas of Pharmacology, Health Care Delivery, Integrative Medicine, Behavioral Health, Clinical Research, Nutrition, Dentistry, and Health Information Technology.

NEW—Complementary Terms categorized by topics, including Signs and Symptoms, Treatments, Equipment, Medical Specialties, and Descriptive Terms.

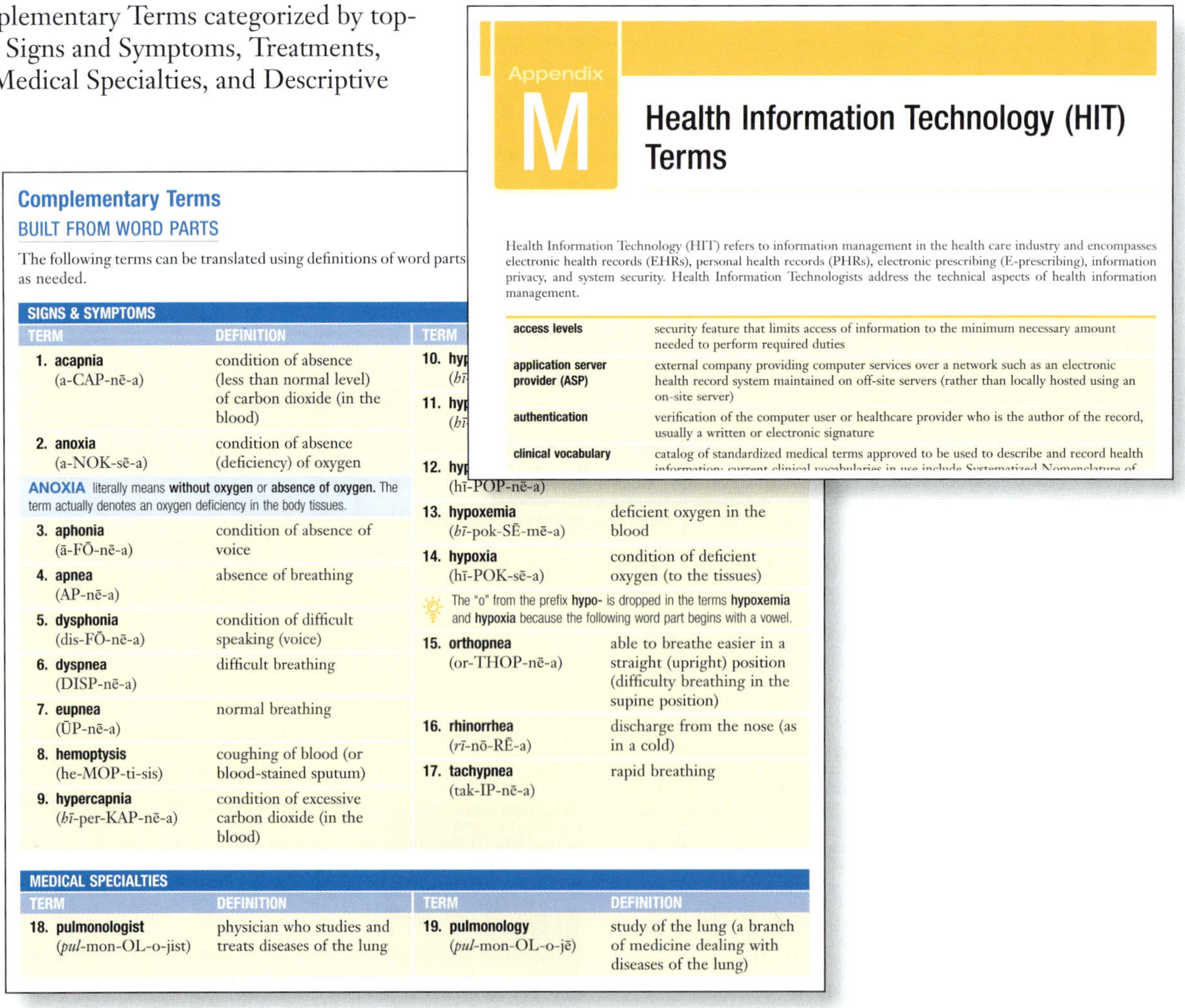

Appendix M

Health Information Technology (HIT) Terms

Health Information Technology (HIT) refers to information management in the health care industry and encompasses electronic health records (EHRs), personal health records (PHRs), electronic prescribing (E-prescribing), information privacy, and system security. Health Information Technologists address the technical aspects of health information management.

access levels	security feature that limits access of information to the minimum necessary amount needed to perform required duties
application server provider (ASP)	external company providing computer services over a network such as an electronic health record system maintained on off-site servers (rather than locally hosted using an on-site server)
authentication	verification of the computer user or healthcare provider who is the author of the record, usually a written or electronic signature
clinical vocabulary	catalog of standardized medical terms approved to be used to describe and record health

Complementary Terms

BUILT FROM WORD PARTS

The following terms can be translated using definitions of word parts as needed.

SIGNS & SYMPTOMS

TERM	DEFINITION	TERM	DEFINITION
1. **acapnia** (a-CAP-nē-a)	condition of absence (less than normal level) of carbon dioxide (in the blood)	10. hyp…	
2. **anoxia** (a-NOK-sē-a)	condition of absence (deficiency) of oxygen	11. hyp…	
		12. hyp… (hī-POP-nē-a)	
3. **aphonia** (ā-FŌ-nē-a)	condition of absence of voice	13. **hypoxemia** (*hī*-pok-SĒ-mē-a)	deficient oxygen in the blood
4. **apnea** (AP-nē-a)	absence of breathing	14. **hypoxia** (hī-POK-sē-a)	condition of deficient oxygen (to the tissues)
5. **dysphonia** (dis-FŌ-nē-a)	condition of difficult speaking (voice)	15. **orthopnea** (or-THOP-nē-a)	able to breathe easier in a straight (upright) position (difficulty breathing in the supine position)
6. **dyspnea** (DISP-nē-a)	difficult breathing	16. **rhinorrhea** (*rī*-nō-RĒ-a)	discharge from the nose (as in a cold)
7. **eupnea** (ŪP-nē-a)	normal breathing	17. **tachypnea** (tak-IP-nē-a)	rapid breathing
8. **hemoptysis** (he-MOP-ti-sis)	coughing of blood (or blood-stained sputum)		
9. **hypercapnia** (*hī*-per-KAP-nē-a)	condition of excessive carbon dioxide (in the blood)		

ANOXIA literally means **without oxygen** or **absence of oxygen.** The term actually denotes an oxygen deficiency in the body tissues.

The "o" from the prefix **hypo-** is dropped in the terms **hypoxemia** and **hypoxia** because the following word part begins with a vowel.

MEDICAL SPECIALTIES

TERM	DEFINITION	TERM	DEFINITION
18. **pulmonologist** (*pul*-mon-OL-o-jist)	physician who studies and treats diseases of the lung	19. **pulmonology** (*pul*-mon-OL-o-jē)	study of the lung (a branch of medicine dealing with diseases of the lung)

Historical Perspective and Current Use

Informational boxes anchor medical language in a **historical perspective** and provide details on the **current use of terms.**

ATELECTASIS is derived from the Greek **ateles**, meaning **not perfect**, and **ektasis**, meaning **expansion**. It denotes an incomplete expansion of the lungs.

REACTIVE AIRWAY DISEASE (RAD) is a general term and not a specific diagnosis. It is used to describe a history of wheezing, coughing, and shortness of breath. In some people RAD may lead to **asthma**.

Abbreviations

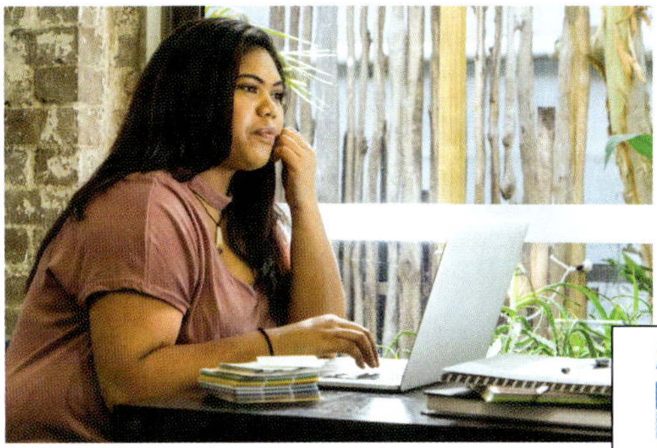

Tables introduce abbreviated medical terms related to chapter content. Textbook exercises, electronic flashcards, online exercises, and practice quizzes provide practice for new learning. Students may supplement learning with additional abbreviations and error-prone abbreviations listed in Appendix D.

NEW—Abbreviations grouped by category.

Abbreviations

DISEASE AND DISORDERS

ABBREVIATION	TERM	ABBREVIATION	TERM
ARDS	acute respiratory distress syndrome	IPF	idiopathic pulmonary fibrosis
CAP	community-acquired pneumonia	LTB	laryngotracheobronchitis
CF	cystic fibrosis	OSA	obstructive sleep apnea
COPD	chronic obstructive pulmonary disease	PE	pulmonary embolism
COVID-19	coronavirus disease	PE also abbreviates **physical examination**.	
flu	influenza	TB	tuberculosis
HAP	hospital-acquired pneumonia	URI	upper respiratory infection

SIGNS & SYMPTOMS

ABBREVIATION	TERM
SOB	shortness of breath

Practical Application

Students apply medical terms to case studies and medical records.

EXERCISE 34 ■ Interact with Medical Documents

A

Read the report and complete it by writing medical terms on answer lines within the document. Definitions of terms to be written appear after the document.

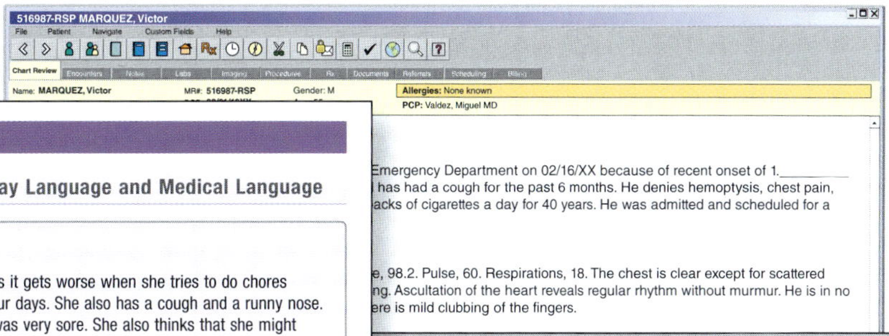

PRACTICAL APPLICATION

EXERCISE 33 ■ Case Study: Translate Between Everyday Language and Medical Language

CASE STUDY: Roberta Pawlaski

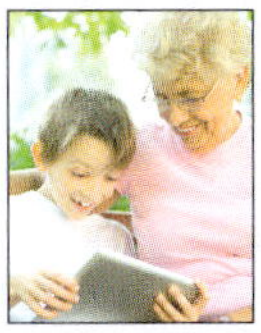

Roberta is experiencing difficulty breathing. She notices it gets worse when she tries to do chores around the house. This has been going on for about four days. She also has a cough and a runny nose. Today when she woke up she noticed that her throat was very sore. She also thinks that she might have a fever because she feels hot all over. She tried taking some over-the-counter cough medicine but this didn't seem to help. She notices when she coughs that a thick yellow mucus comes out. She hasn't had a cough like this since before she quit smoking about 10 years ago. She remembers that her grandson who stays with her after school has missed school because of a cold. She decides to call her doctor to schedule an appointment.

Now that you have worked through Chapter 5, on the respiratory system, consider the medical terms that might be used to describe Roberta's experience. See the Chapter at a Glance section at the end of the chapter for a list of terms that might apply.

Electronic Health Records (EHR)

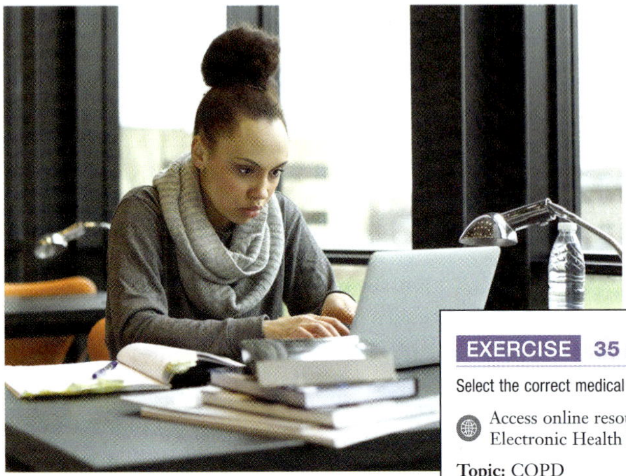

EHR Modules in Practice Student Resources on the Evolve website provide three related medical records for one patient. Students identify medical terms in context while gaining a familiarity with computer applications used in the field.

EXERCISE 35 ■ Use Medical Language in Online Electronic Health Records

Select the correct medical terms to complete three medical records in one patient's electronic file.

Access online resources at evolve.elsevier.com > Evolve Resources > Student Resources > Activities > Chapter 5 > Electronic Health Records

Topic: COPD
Record 1: Progress Note
Record 2: Radiology Report
Record 3: Pulmonary Function Department Note

❑ Check the box when complete.

Healthcare records are stored and used in an electronic system called **Electronic Health Records (EHR)**. Electronic health records contain a collection of health information of an individual patient; the digitally formatted record can be shared through computer networks with patients, physicians, and other healthcare providers.

Chapter Content Quiz

Designed as formative assessments, Chapter Content Quizzes allow students to test their knowledge by identifying medical terms and abbreviations used in context.

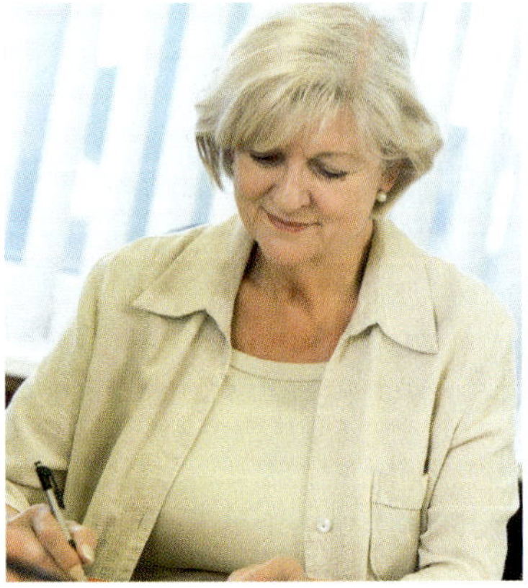

C CHAPTER REVIEW

EXERCISE 37 ■ Chapter Content Quiz

Test your understanding of terms and abbreviations introduced in this chapter. Circle the letter for the medical term or abbreviation related to the words in italics

1. The patient was admitted to the emergency department with a *severe nosebleed.*
   a. rhinomycosis
   b. epistaxis
   c. nasopharyngitis
2. The accident caused damage to the *larynx*, necessitating a *surgical repair.*
   a. laryngectomy
   b. laryngostomy
   c. laryngoplasty
3. Mr. Garcia was *able to breathe easier in an upright position*, so the nurse recorded that he had:
   a. orthopnea
   b. eupnea
   c. dyspnea
4. The *test on arterial blood to determine oxygen, carbon dioxide, and pH levels* indicated that the patient was *deficient in oxygen*, or had:
   a. pulse oximetry, dysphonia
   b. pulmonary functions tests, hypocapnia
   c. arterial blood gas, hypoxia
5. The physician informed the patient that her *coughing of blood* might be due to tuberculosis.
   a. hemoptysis
   b. pneumothorax
   c. thoracentesis
6. The patient reported dizziness brought on by *ventilation of the lungs beyond normal bodily needs.*
   a. hyperventilation
   b. hypoventilation
9. After surgery, the patient had *foreign matter causing a block in the circulation to the pulmonary artery.*
   a. pleural effusion
   b. pulmonary edema
   c. pulmonary embolism
10. The patient was diagnosed as having *a fungal disease affecting the lung.*
    a. obstructive sleep apnea
    b. coccidioidomycosis
    c. tuberculosis
11. The physician ordered a *radiographic image of the chest* because he suspected *community-acquired pneumonia.*
    a. chest radiograph, CAP
    b. chest CT scan, CPAP
    c. bronchoscopy, HAP
12. The patient received an *intradermal injection* to determine if she had been exposed to TB.
    a. AFB
    b. ABG
    c. PPD skin test
13. The patient was experiencing *rapid breathing.*
    a. hypopnea
    b. tachypnea
    c. eupnea
14. The nurse practitioner heard *discontinuous sounds during respiration that resembled the sound of the rustling of cellophane.*
    a. stridor
    b. rhonchi
    c. crackles

Review of Content

NEW—Review of Terms exercises appear throughout the chapter providing pauses to reflect on new learning and to consider all of the terms from a section, such as Disease and Disorder.

EXERCISE 12 ▪ Review Disease and Disorder Terms

Can you define, pronounce, and spell the following terms?

acute respiratory distress syndrome (ARDS)	coccidioidomycosis	laryngospasm	pulmonary edema
adenoiditis	coronavirus disease	laryngotracheobronchitis (LTB)	pulmonary embolism (PE)
alveolitis	croup	lobar pneumonia	pulmonary neoplasm
atelectasis	cystic fibrosis (CF)	nasopharyngitis	pyothorax
asphyxia	deviated septum	obstructive sleep apnea (OSA)	rhinitis
asthma	diaphragmatocele	pertussis	rhinomycosis
bronchiectasis	diphtheria	pharyngitis	rhinorrhagia
bronchitis	emphysema	pleural effusion	sinusitis
bronchogenic carcinoma	epiglottitis		tonsillitis
	epistaxis		

NEW—Chapter at a Glance provides a summary of word parts new to the chapter and terms presented.

CHAPTER AT A GLANCE Word Parts New to this Chapter

COMBINING FORMS
adenoid/o, alveol/o, atel/o, bronch/o, bronchi/o, capn/o, coni/o
lob/o, mediastin/o, muc/o, nas/o, orth/o, ox/i, phary…
pulmon/o, py/o, rhin/o

PREFIXES
a-, an-, endo-

SUFFIXES
-ar, -ary, -cele
-pnea, -ptysis, -rrhagia

CHAPTER AT A GLANCE Respiratory System Terms Built from Word Parts

DISEASE AND DISORDER
adenoiditis, alveolitis, atelectasis, bronchiectasis, bronchitis, bronchogenic carcinoma, bronchopneumonia, bronchospasm
nasopharyngitis, pharyngitis, pleuritis, pneumoconiosis

SURGICAL
adenoidectomy, bronchoplasty, laryngectomy

DIAGNOSTIC
bronchoscope, bronchoscopy, capnometer

CHAPTER AT A GLANCE Respiratory System Terms NOT Built from Word Parts

DISEASE AND DISORDER
acute respiratory distress syndrome (ARDS), asphyxia, asthma, chronic obstructive pulmonary disease (COPD), coccidioidomycosis, coronavirus disease, croup, cystic fibrosis (CF), deviated septum, diphtheria, emphysema
influenza (flu), obstructive sleep apnea (OSA), pertussis, pleural effusion, pulmonary edema, pulmonary embolism (PE), tuberculosis (TB), upper respiratory infection (URI)

DIAGNOSTIC
acid-fast bacilli (AFB) smear
chest computed tomography (CT) scan, chest radiograph (CXR), lung ventilation/perfusion scan (V/Q scan), peak flow meter (PFM), percussion, PPD skin test, pulmonary function tests (PFTs), pulse oximetry, stethoscope

COMPLIMENTARY
bronchoconstrictor, bronchodilator, crackles, effusion, hyperventilation, hypoventilation, mucopurulent, nebulizer, nosocomial infection, paroxysm, patent, rhonchi, sputum, stridor, ventilator

Online Evolve Resources

Evolve Resources provide multiple ways to practice and assess learning.

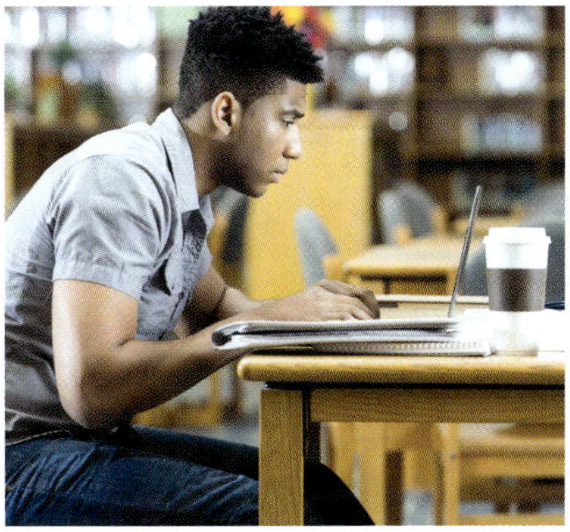

Student Resources

- Audio Glossary
- Word Part and Abbreviation Flashcards
- Spelling Exercises
- Games
- Electronic Health Records
- Practice Quizzes

Mobile Resources

- Flashcards
- Practice Quizzes

Gradable Student Resources

- Match the Word Parts
- Terms Built from Word Parts Activity
- Practice Exams

Instructor Resources

- TEACH Handouts
- TEACH Lesson Plans
- TEACH PowerPoints
- Test Bank
- Image Collection
- Sample Course Syllabus and Outline

ORGANIZATION OF THE TEXTBOOK

Chapters 1 through 3 provide a foundation for building medical vocabulary. Chapters 4 through 16 organize content by body systems, presenting related word parts, terms, and abbreviations. The textbook concludes with a series of appendices designed to extend student learning as desired.

Introductory Chapters

Chapter 1… may be the most important chapter in the text, because you will apply the knowledge acquired here in the rest of the chapters to learn terms in an easy, quick fashion. The chapter introduces the two categories of terms—those built from word parts and those which are not; each category is accompanied by different types of exercises. Also introduced in this chapter are the **four word parts**—word root, suffix, prefix, and combining vowel, which are the basis of terms built from word parts category.

EXAMPLE **INTRAVENOUS**	WORD PART	MEANING
prefix	intra-	within
word root	ven	vein
suffix	-ous	pertaining to
term = p + wr + s	intra/ven/ous	pertaining to within a vein

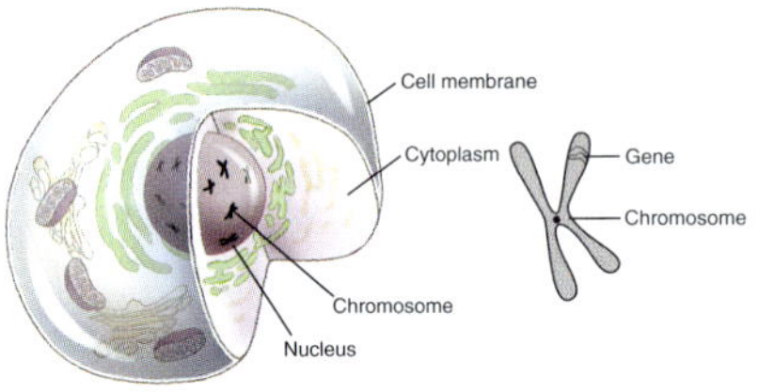

Chapter 2… introduces body structure, oncology, and laboratory tests, while providing immediate practice in recognizing the two categories of terms along with corresponding exercises for each. You will likely be surprised at how fast you learn the meaning and spelling of many medical terms.

Chapter 3… introduces directional terms, positioning, and diagnostic imaging, all of which are relevant to subsequent body systems chapters and their specific medical terms.

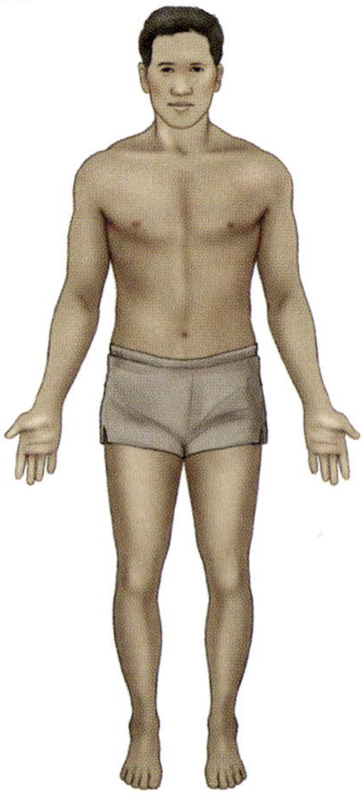

Body System Chapters

Chapters 4 through 16… introduce specific body systems with related word parts, terms, and abbreviations and follow a consistent format.

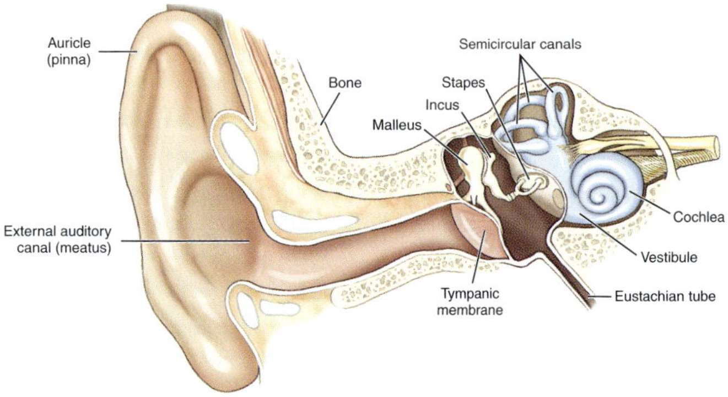

Appendices

Appendices A-E… appear in the textbook and provide an answer key for chapter exercises, comprehensive lists of word parts and abbreviations, a list of error-prone abbreviations, and pharmacology terms.

Appendices F-M… in Practice Student Resources on the Evolve website provide lists of additional word parts, Health Care Delivery Terms, Integrative Medicine Terms, Behavioral Health Terms, Nutrition Terms, Dental Terms, and Health Information Technology Terms. Online appendices may be found by clicking on the Extra Content tab from the main menu.

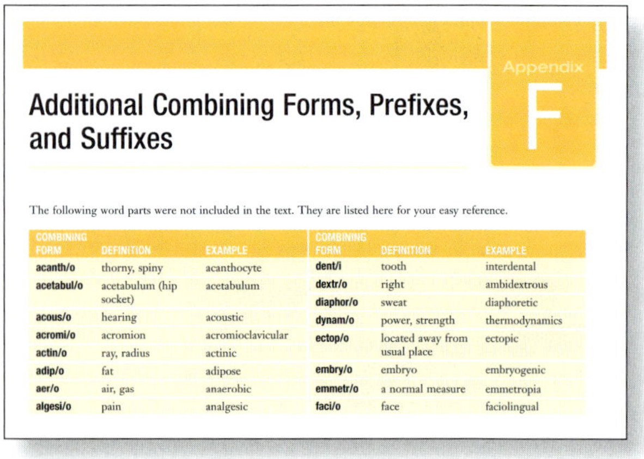

Appendix F

Additional Combining Forms, Prefixes, and Suffixes

The following word parts were not included in the text. They are listed here for your easy reference.

COMBINING FORM	DEFINITION	EXAMPLE	COMBINING FORM	DEFINITION	EXAMPLE
acanth/o	thorny, spiny	acanthocyte	**dent/i**	tooth	interdental
acetabul/o	acetabulum (hip socket)	acetabulum	**dextr/o**	right	ambidextrous
			diaphor/o	sweat	diaphoretic
acous/o	hearing	acoustic	**dynam/o**	power, strength	thermodynamics
acromi/o	acromion	acromioclavicular	**ectop/o**	located away from usual place	ectopic
actin/o	ray, radius	actinic			
adip/o	fat	adipose	**embry/o**	embryo	embryogenic
aer/o	air, gas	anaerobic	**emmetr/o**	a normal measure	emmetropia
algesi/o	pain	analgesic	**faci/o**	face	faciolingual

ANATOMY OF A CHAPTER

Let's take a look at the structure of a body system chapter using Chapter 5 on the respiratory system as an example.

Objectives and Chapter Outline

↓

ANATOMY →

↓

WORD PARTS →

↓

MEDICAL TERMS →

↓

PRACTICAL APPLICATION →

↓

CHAPTER REVIEW →

DEAR STUDENT

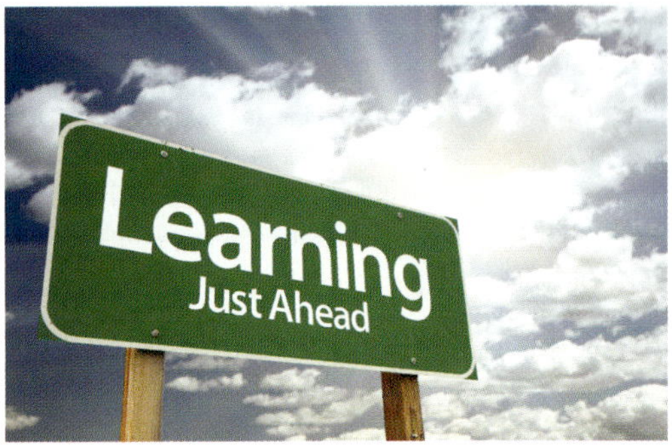

If you are reading this, you are most likely enrolled in a medical terminology course and preparing for your journey of learning medical language using this textbook. As you flip through the pages of *Exploring Medical Language* you may be thinking, "There is so much to learn. How will I do it?" or "Why are there so many exercises?"

Let us assure you that you will acquire the language in a quick and easy manner by completing chapter exercises. While it may seem daunting at first, we encourage you to be as active as possible as you read and work through each chapter.

The exercises approach the terms from all angles: pronunciation, writing, defining, spelling, and application. Chapter content flows from one chapter to the next in a repetitive manner, making the best use of your time. You may build a foundational medical vocabulary by using the textbook alone or you may choose to extend your learning by utilizing Evolve Resources, which provide supplemental materials online. To register for the *Exploring Medical Language* 11e Evolve Resources, please, visit evolve.elsevier.com or call 1-800-222-9570.

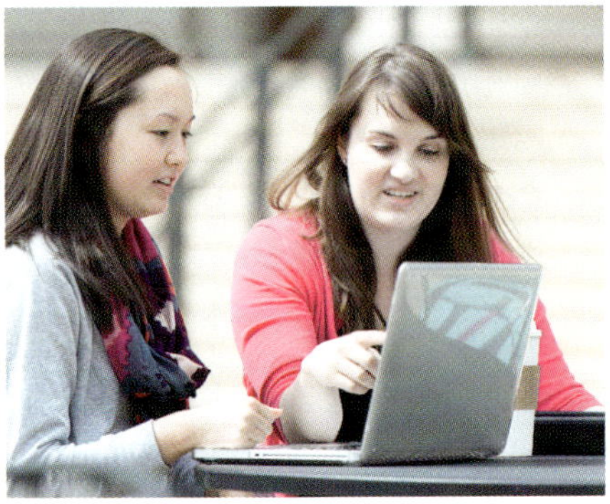

We wish you the best as you embark on this journey. You will join a select group of students who have used *Exploring Medical Language* as a textbook for over 35 years. We would like to hear of your experience with *Exploring Medical Language*, including exercises that were most useful, suggestions for improvement, and so forth. Reach us by e-mail at the following addresses:

danielle.lafleurbrooks@ccv.edu
myrnabrooks@comcast.net
dale.levinsky@gmail.com

We also invite you to visit Myrna's educational blog at **medicalterminologyblog.com**. Follow the blog while you are a student and after you finish your course to help you build on your vocabulary in a fun and engaging way. Posts include quizzes, crosswords, videos, word scrambles, and introduction to emerging medical terms.

Sincerely,
Danielle, Myrna, and Dale

ONLINE STUDENT RESOURCES evolve.elsevier.com

Evolve Resources provide practice activities, gradable exercises and exams, and mobile resources that can be accessed from a portable device.

Student Resources
- Audio Glossary
- Word Part and Abbreviation Flashcards
- Spelling Exercises
- Electronic Health Record Modules
- Games
- Practice Quizzes
- Career Videos
- Additional Appendices with Term Lists by Medical Specialty

Mobile Resources
- Word Part and Abbreviation Flashcards
- Practice Quizzes

Gradable Student Resources
- Exercises: Match the Word Parts and Terms Built from Word Parts
- Practice Exams

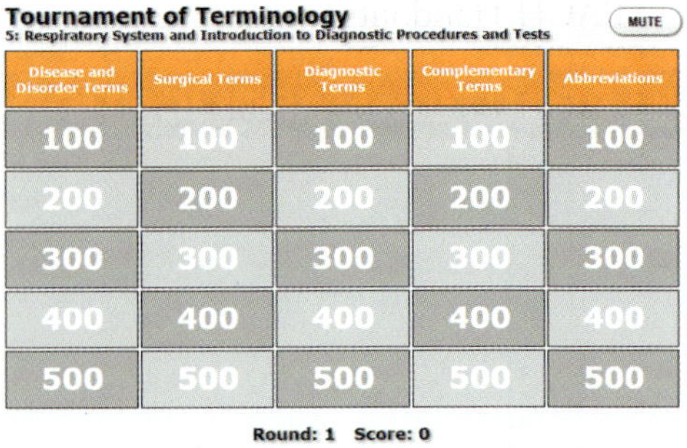

For assistance in registering for Evolve Resources,
call **1-800-222-9570** or visit **evolvesupport.elsevier.com**

DEAR INSTRUCTOR

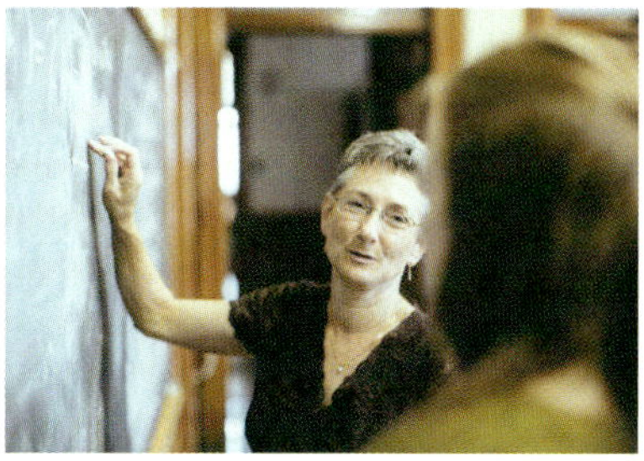

Thank you for choosing *Exploring Medical Language!* We hope you find this learning system supportive of your teaching methods and effective for your students' learning styles. With the purchase of a new textbook, students receive paper flashcards for word parts and pincode access to Evolve Resources for students. You may find the flashcards and online resources, such as pronunciation for term lists and games, useful for class activities and exam preparation.

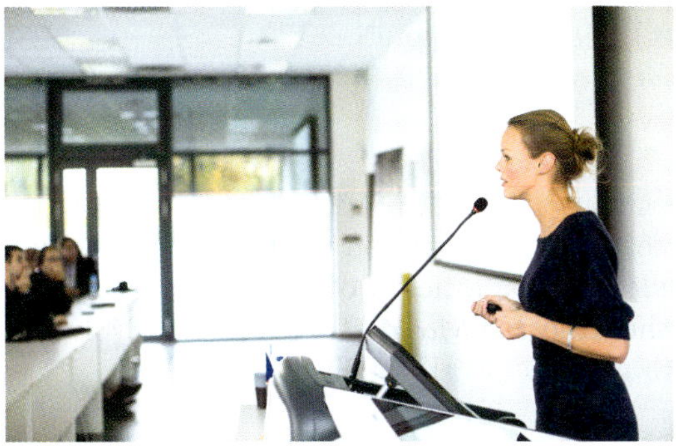

Additional teaching materials are available online using Evolve Resources for Instructors. All resources are objective based, and we recommend beginning with the TEACH Lesson Plans for an overview of how to use the various teaching tools. The first step in accessing teaching materials is to register for the *Exploring Medical Language* 11e Evolve Resources. Please, visit evolve.elsevier.com or call 1-800-222-9570 to register.

We welcome your comments and questions by email. Danielle, who teaches medical terminology in the traditional classroom, online, and in hybrid formats, is also happy to share ideas and materials. Contact us at:

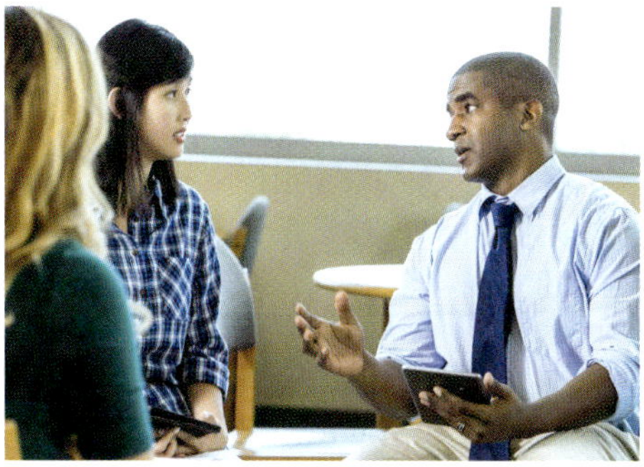

danielle.lafleurbrooks@ccv.edu
myrnabrooks@comcast.net
dale.levinsky@gmail.com

We also invite you to visit Myrna's educational blog at **medicalterminologyblog.com** to keep up with trends in teaching medical terminology and emerging medical language.

Looking forward to hearing from you,
Danielle, Myrna, and Dale

ONLINE INSTRUCTOR RESOURCES evolve.elsevier.com

Instructor Resources
- Image Collection
- Sample Course Syllabus and Outline
- TEACH Handouts
- TEACH Lesson Plans
- TEACH PowerPoint Slides
- Test Bank

Assessment
- Formative and summative assessment plan for each lesson, TEACH Lesson Plans in Evolve Instructor Resources
- Pretest TEACH Lesson Plans, in Evolve Instructor Resources
- Gradable Practice Exams, Evolve Student Resources
- Test Bank to build quizzes and exams, Evolve Instructor Resources

Course Tools
- Grades
- Grading Que
- Roster & Teams
- Question Bank
- Course Calendar
- Login Report
- Search

Access to online course management tools, such as a gradebook and a discussion board, is included.

For assistance in registering for Evolve Resources and Course Tools, call **1-800-222-9570** or visit **evolvesupport.elsevier.com**

Contributors, Reviewers, and Advisors

Contributors

Melanie Meyer, ND, MS
Faculty, Allied Health Science
Community College of Vermont
Montpelier, Vermont
Appendix G Introducing Healthcare Delivery
Appendix H Integrative Medicine
Appendix K Nutrition Terms

Erinn Kao, PharmD, RPh
Pharmacist
Rx Outreach, Inc
St. Louis, Missouri
Appendix E Pharmacology

Reviewers and Advisors

Charo E. Bautista, B.S.N.
Adjunct Faculty
Health Unit Coordinating/Patient Care Associate
GateWay Community College
Maricopa Community Colleges
Phoenix, Arizona

Ashleigh du Plessis
Student, STEM Studies
Community College of Vermont
Montpelier, Vermont

Erin Hayes, MS, MAT
Overland Park, KS

Gregory Labenz, MD
Diagnostic Radiologist, Catalina Radiology, PLC
Nuclear Medicine Medical Director, Northwest Medical Center
Tucson, Arizona

Elyse Levinsky, MD, MHSc, FRCSC
Assistant Professor, Obstetrics and Gynaecology
University of Toronto
Toronto, Ontario, Canada

Lynnae Lockett, RN, RMA, CMRS, MSN
Allied Health Program Director
Bryant & Stratton College
Parma, Ohio

Melanie Meyer, ND, MS
Faculty, Allied Health Science
Community College of Vermont
Montpelier, Vermont

Past Reviewers and Advisors

Delena Kay Austin, BTIS, CMA (AAMA)
Health Science Technology Faculty
Macomb Community College
Warren, Michigan

Cynthia Ann Bjerklie, BS
Faculty, Allied Health Science
Community College of Vermont
Montpelier, Vermont

William Bohnert, MD
Past President, American Urological Association
CDI Consultant, Dignity Health
St. Joseph's Hospital
Phoenix, Arizona

Julene Bredeson, CMA (AAMA), PHN, BSN, RN
Medical Assistant Instructor
Ridgewater College
Willmar, Minnesota

Richard K. Brooks, MD, FACP, FACG
Internal Medicine and Gastroenterology
Mayo Clinic (retired)
Clinical Instructor
Geisel School of Medicine
Dartmouth College
Quechee, Vermont

Sharon A. Brooks, MSN, BA, RN
Practical Nursing Program Director
Sumner College
Portland, Oregon

Ruth Buchner, MEd
Family and Consumer Science / Health Science Educator
Chippewa Falls High School
Chippewa Falls, Wisconsin

Christine Costa, BS, GCM, HUC
Geriatric Care Manager
Tempe, Arizona

Angela Dawson-Walker, CMA, LVN
Apple Valley Unified School District
Apple Valley, California

Christopher Fields, OD
Optometrist
Fields of Vision Eye Care, Inc.
Lebanon, New Hampshire

Robert L. Fortune, MD
Cardiovascular Surgery (retired)
Scottsdale, Arizona

Janet Funk, MD
Associate Professor of Medicine & Nutritional Sciences
The University of Arizona Cancer Center
Phoenix, Arizona

Deborah Greer, MEd, RT(R)(M)
Program Director-RT Education
Penn Medicine
Philadelphia, Pennsylvania

Jane A. Hlopko, MA, RHIA
Department Chairman, Associate Professor, Health Information Technology
SUNY Broome Community College
Binghamton, New York

Colleen Horan, MD
Gynecologist and Obstetrician
Central Vermont Medical Center
Berlin, Vermont

Marjorie "Meg" Holloway, MS, RN, APRN
Instructor, Foundations of Medicine and Leader, Medicine & Healthcare Strand
Blue Valley CAPS
Overland Park, Kansas

Bradley D. Johnson, MEd, RT(R)(ARRT)
Faculty, Medical Radiography
Gateway Community College
Phoenix, Arizona

Sheri Lavadour, RN, BSN, HTP
Sumner College of Nursing, Instructor
Portland, Oregon

Kara Stuart Lewis, MD
Phoenix Children's Hospital
Phoenix, Arizona

Charles Machia
Billing Customer Service
University of Vermont Medical Center
Burlington, Vermont

Melody Miller, LPN
Medical Assistant Instructor
Lancaster County Career and Technology Center
Willow Street, Philadelphia

Veronique M. Parker, MBA (Healthcare Management)
Faculty
Maricopa Community Colleges
Phoenix, Arizona

Stephen M. Picca, MD
Mandl School: The College of Applied Health
New York, New York

Maynard D. Poland, MD
Internal Medicine Board—Certified
Retired:
Medical Practice & Medical Director,
Milwaukee Medical Clinic and Columbia—St. Mary's Hospitals, Milwaukee, Wisconsin
Assistant Clinical Professor, Medical College of Wisconsin
Adjunct Faculty, Edison State College, Ft. Myers, Florida

Toni L. Rodriguez, EdD, RRT, FAARC
Program Director
Respiratory Care Program
GateWay Community College
Phoenix, Arizona

Patricia L. Shinn, PhD, RN
Chair, Nursing Department
River Valley Community College
Claremont, New Hampshire

Charlene Thiessen, MEd, CMT, AHDI-F
Program Director, Medical Transcription
GateWay Community College
Phoenix, Arizona

Ann Vadala, BA
Professor, Office Administration
St. Lawrence College
Kingston, Ontario

Kari Williams, BS, DC
Program Director
Front Range Community College
Longmont, Colorado

Dokagari Woods, RN, PhD
Assistant Professor of Nursing, Undergraduate Program Director
Tarleton State University
Stephenville, Texas

Acknowledgments

We are incredibly lucky to be supported by a team of skilled professionals who worked tirelessly in creating the 11th edition of *Exploring Medical Language*. We are grateful for the time, effort, and talents of the following individuals:

Luke Held, Content Development Manager, who guided us through the initial stages of the revision. He expertly facilitated communication between teams working on the project and set us off on a productive path. His work with *Exploring Medical Language* over the years has been tremendously helpful and has made a lasting impact.

Elizabeth McCormac, Content Development Specialist, who gracefully stepped in to guide the editorial portion of the project. Her organizational skills were a tremendous asset, and we greatly appreciated her steady presence.

Linda Woodard, Content Strategist, who led the development of textbook ancillaries, including Evolve Resources and TEACH. She has nurtured our work over many years, and we treasure her insight and guidance.

Renee Duenow, Book Designer, who created the beautiful design of the 11th edition. Her work was instrumental in creating a welcoming and effective learning system. We are grateful for her attention to detail and the ability to translate our vision to what appears on the page.

Julie Eddy, Publishing Services Manager, who has been a proactive leader in the publishing phase of the project and shown tremendous adaptability in working with an anomalous process. It has been a privilege to work with Julie's team.

Abigail Bradberry, Senior Project Manager, who guided us through the production phase of the project. Her competence and calm demeanor were much appreciated. Moreover, her steady dedication to the project was instrumental in creating a high-quality product.

Mahalakshmi Subramaniam, Digital Media Producer, who facilitated the development of electronic companions to the textbook.

Carolyn Kruse, for using her linguistic knowledge and pleasing voice for updating pronunciation, both in print and audio.

Jeanne Robertson, Medical Illustrator, whose art has brought to life many medical concepts. We have the greatest respect for her attention to detail and ability to bring beauty to technical images.

Winifred K. Starr (1921-1993), who was Myrna's first coauthor and whose creative contributions remain in the text today.

Contributors, Reviewers, and **Advisors** listed on the previous pages who shared their expertise and knowledge.

Faculty, who have adopted the text to teach medical language and have used their valuable time to give us feedback.

Students, who over the years have worn thin the pages of previous editions. Your pursuit of knowledge has been truly inspirational.

Each page of the 11th Edition is better because of your collective contributions.

Thank you.

Chapter 1

Introduction to Medical Language

Outline

Objectives

Upon completion of this chapter, you will be able to:

1. Describe the origins of medical language.
2. Define two categories of medical terms.
3. Identify and define the four word parts and the combining form.
4. Analyze and define medical terms using the meaning of word parts.
5. Build medical terms using the meaning of word parts.

INTRODUCTION TO MEDICAL TERMS AND MEDICAL LANGUAGE

Medical terms are words used to describe disease, as well as aspects of medicine and health care. Terms built from Greek and Latin word parts, eponyms, acronyms, and modern language are types of medical terms.

Medical language or terminology is the use of medical terms to attain a standardized means of communication within the practice of medicine and in the healthcare industry. The need for fluency in medical language cannot be exaggerated.

Why are many medical terms different than words we use in everyday life? Medical language allows for clear, concise and consistent communication locally, nationally, and internationally. It enables everyone involved in medicine and health care to perform more accurately and efficiently for the patient's benefit. For example, using the medical term **osteoarthritis** (Fig. 1.1), which means **inflammation of the bone and joint,** offers a clear and concise written or verbal communication using one word instead of six. No matter the national language used, the meaning of the medical term does not change.

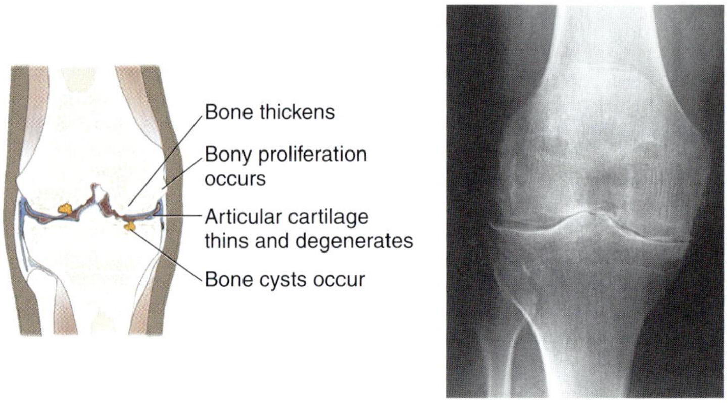

FIG. 1.1 Osteoarthritis of the knee joint, illustration and radiograph.

Origins of Medical Language

The vocabulary of medical language reflects its development over time beginning with the ancient Greeks. More than 2,000 years ago, Hippocrates and Aristotle were among the first to study and write about medicine. The Romans continued the practice, adopting elements of the Greek language to use alongside Latin. The majority of terms in use today are **built from Greek and Latin word parts**. For learning purposes, these terms are categorized as **Terms Built from Word Parts** in this textbook.

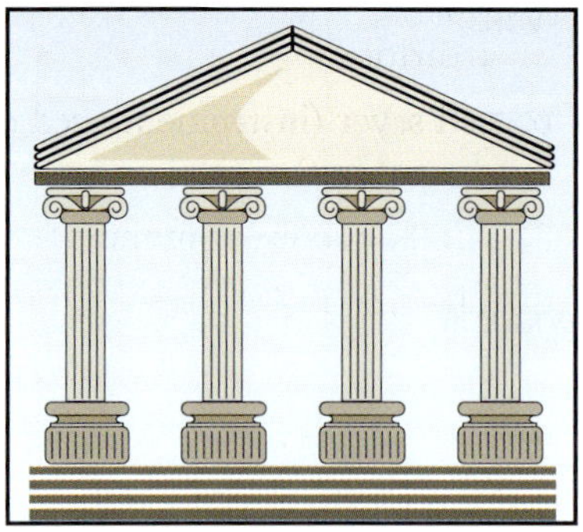

Terms Built from Word Parts, such as arthritis, are of Greek and Latin origin.

As scientific knowledge, medical technology, and medical practice evolved, so did the language of medicine, which now also includes **eponyms, acronyms, and terms from modern language**. Eponyms are terms derived from a name or place. Acronyms are terms formed from the first letters of a phrase. Modern language refers to terms from the English language, which are often descriptive of technology and procedures. For learning purposes, these terms are categorized as **Terms NOT Built from Word Parts** in this textbook.

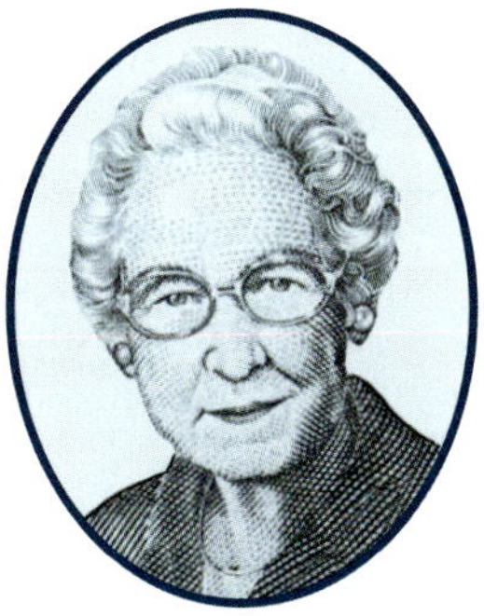

Eponyms are terms derived from the name of a person or place. Examples include **Apgar score**, named after the person who developed it, and **West Nile virus**, named after the first geographical location the virus was identified.

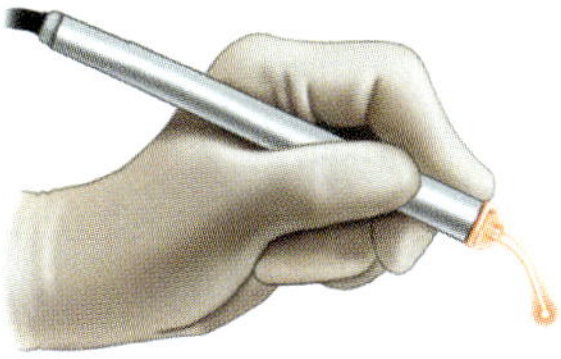

Acronyms, such as **laser** (light amplification by stimulated emission of radiation), are terms formed from the first letters of words in a phrase. Acronyms usually contain a vowel and are spoken as a whole word.

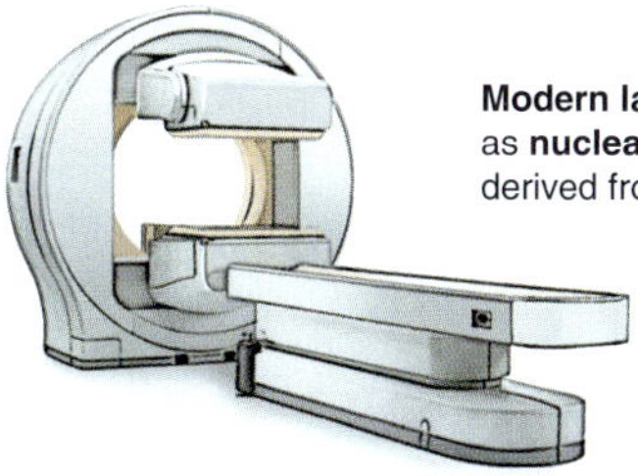

Modern language terms**,** such as **nuclear medicine scanner,** are derived from the English language.

VIRGINIA APGAR an obstetric anesthesiologist born in New Jersey, developed the Apgar score in 1952 to measure the physical condition of the newborn.

EXERCISE 1 ■ Origins of Medical Language

Place the letter from the first column to identify the origin of the term in the second column. You may use an answer more than once. *To check your answers to the exercises in this chapter, go to Appendix A at the back of the textbook.*

a. Greek and Latin word parts
b. eponym
c. acronym
d. modern language

_____ 1. Middle Eastern respiratory syndrome
_____ 2. hepatitis
_____ 3. MRSA (methicillin-resistant *Staphylococcus aureus*)
_____ 4. posttraumatic stress disorder
_____ 5. arthritis
_____ 6. cell saver (instrument used during surgery to recover blood lost from the patient)
_____ 7. AIDS (acquired immunodeficiency syndrome)
_____ 8. Alzheimer disease

ALZHEIMER DISEASE VS. ALZHEIMER'S DISEASE The need for clarity and consistency in medical language has resulted in the **modern trend to eliminate the possessive form of eponyms and use instead the non-possessive form**. The non-possessive form is observed by the Association for Healthcare Documentation Integrity, the American Medical Association's Manual of Style, in most medical dictionaries, and is the style used throughout this textbook. With either use, the noun that follows is not capitalized.

Categories of Medical Terms and Learning Methods

For the purposes of our studies, medical terms are categorized as *Built from Word Parts* and *NOT Built from Word Parts*. Specific learning methods will be used for each category as noted in Table 1.1.

EXERCISE 2 ■ Categories of Medical Terms

Complete the following. *To check your answers, go to Appendix A.*

Medical terms ________ ________ ________ ________ can be translated to find their meanings, whereas medical terms ________ ________ ________ ________ ________ cannot be easily translated to find their meanings.

TABLE 1.1 Categories of Medical Terms and Learning Methods

CATEGORY	ORIGIN	EXAMPLE	LEARNING METHODS
Terms Built from Word Parts (can be translated to find their meanings)	1. Word parts of Greek and Latin origin placed together to form terms that can be translated literally to find their meanings	1. arthr/itis	1. Analyzing terms 2. Defining terms 3. Building terms
Terms NOT Built from Word Parts (cannot be easily translated to find their meanings)	1. Eponyms, terms derived from the name of a person or place 2. Acronyms, terms formed from the first letters of a phrase that can be spoken as a whole word and usually contains a vowel 3. Modern language, terms derived from the English language 4. Terms of Greek and Latin word parts that cannot be easily translated to find their meanings	1. Alzheimer disease 2. MRSA (methicillin-resistant *Staphylococcus aureus*) 3. complete blood count with differential 4. orthopedics	1. Recalling terms 2. Matching terms 3. Defining terms

MEDICAL TERMS BUILT FROM WORD PARTS

Medical terms categorized as Built from Word Parts are composed of Greek and Latin **word roots, prefixes,** and **suffixes** and can be translated to find their meanings. A **combining vowel** is often added to ease pronunciation (Table 1.2 and Table 1.3). Techniques to learn these terms are **analyzing, defining,** and **building** medical terms.

Four Word Parts

Most medical terms categorized as Built from Word Parts consist of some or all of the following components:

1. Word root
2. Suffix
3. Prefix
4. Combining vowel

WORD ROOT

The word root is the word part that is the core of the word. The word root contains the fundamental meaning of the word.

EXAMPLES

In the word	play/er, *play* is the word root.
In the medical term	arthr/itis, *arthr* (which means *joint*) is the word root.
In the medical term	hepat/itis, *hepat* (which means *liver*) is the word root.

The word root is the core of the word. All medical terms have at least one word root.

SUFFIX

The suffix is a word part attached to the end of the word root to modify its meaning.

EXAMPLES

In the word	play/er, *-er* is the suffix.
In the medical term	hepat/ic, *-ic* (which means *pertaining to*) is the suffix and *hepat* is the word root for *liver;* therefore, *hepatic* means *pertaining to the liver.*
In the medical term	hepat/itis, *-itis* (which means *inflammation*) is the suffix. The medical term *hepatitis* means *inflammation of the liver.*

The suffix is used to modify the meaning of a word. Most medical terms have a suffix.

SUFFIXES frequently indicate:

- **procedures,** such as -scopy, meaning visual examination, or -tomy, meaning incision
- **conditions,** such as -itis, meaning inflammation
- **diseases,** such as -oma, meaning tumor

PREFIX

The prefix is a word part attached to the beginning of a word root to modify its meaning.

EXAMPLES

In the word	re/play, *re-* is the prefix.
In the medical term	sub/hepat/ic, *sub-* (which means *under*) is the prefix, *hepat* is the word root for *liver,* and *-ic* is the suffix for *pertaining to.* The medical term *subhepatic* means *pertaining to under the liver.*
In the medical term	intra/ven/ous, *intra-* (which means *within*) is the prefix, *ven* (which means *vein*) is the word root, and *-ous* (which means *pertaining to*) is the suffix. The medical term *intravenous* means *pertaining to within the vein.*

A prefix can be used to modify the meaning of a word. Many medical terms do not have a prefix.

PREFIXES often indicate:

- **number,** such as bi-, meaning two
- **position,** such as sub-, meaning under
- **direction,** such as intra-, meaning within
- **time,** such as brady-, meaning slow
- **negation,** such as a-, meaning without

EXERCISE 3 ■ Define

Complete the following sentences. *To check your answers, go to Appendix A.*

1. The word root is ______________________________.
2. The suffix is ______________________________.
3. The prefix is ______________________________.

COMBINING VOWEL

The combining vowel is a word part, usually an o, used to ease pronunciation.
The combining vowel is:

- Placed to connect two word roots
- Placed to connect a word root and a suffix
- **Not** placed to connect a prefix and a word root

EXAMPLES:

In the medical term oste/o/arthr/itis,
o is the combining vowel used between two word roots *oste* (which means *bone*) and *arthr* (which means *joint*).

In the medical term arthr/o/pathy,
o is the combining vowel used between the word root *arthr* and the suffix *-pathy* (which means *disease*).

In the medical term sub/hepat/ic,
the combining vowel is not used between the prefix *sub-* (which means *under*) and the word root *hepat* (which means *liver*).

VOWELS are speech sounds represented by the letters a, e, i, o, u, and sometimes y.

The combining vowel is used to ease pronunciation; therefore, not all medical terms have combining vowels. Medical terms introduced throughout the text that have combining vowels other than o are highlighted at their introduction.

Four Guidelines for Using Combining Vowels

Learning the four guidelines for using combining vowels will assist you in correctly spelling medical terms categorized as Built from Word Parts. Refer to Table 1.2, as you build terms in the following chapters until the guidelines are second nature to you.

Guideline One

When connecting a word root and a suffix, a combining vowel is used if the suffix does not begin with a vowel.

EXAMPLE

In the medical term arthr/o/pathy,
the suffix *-pathy* does not begin with a vowel; therefore, a combining vowel is used.

TABLE 1.2 Guidelines for Using Combining Vowels

COMBINING VOWEL GUIDELINES	EXAMPLE
1. When connecting a word root and a suffix, a combining vowel is **used** if the suffix **does not begin** with a vowel.	arthr/**o**/pathy
2. When connecting a word root and a suffix, a combining vowel is **usually not used** if the suffix **begins** with a vowel.	hepat/ic
3. When connecting two word roots, a combining vowel is **usually used** even if vowels are present at the junction.	oste/**o**/arthr/itis
4. When connecting a prefix and a word root, a combining vowel is **not used.**	sub/hepat/ic

Guideline Two

When connecting a word root and a suffix, a combining vowel is usually not used if the suffix begins with a vowel.

EXAMPLE

In the medical term hepat/ic,
the suffix *-ic* begins with the vowel *i;* therefore, a combining vowel is not used.

Guideline Three

When connecting two word roots, a combining vowel is usually used even if vowels are present at the junction.

EXAMPLE

In the medical term oste/o/arthr/itis,
o is the combining vowel used, even though the word root *oste* ends with the vowel *e,* and the word root *arthr* begins with the vowel *a.*

Guideline Four

When connecting a prefix and a word root, a combining vowel is not used.

EXAMPLE

In the medical term sub/hepat/ic,
the combining vowel is not used between the prefix *sub-* and the word root *hepat.*

EXERCISE 4 ■ Combining Vowel

Complete the following. *To check your answers, go to Appendix A.*

1. A combining vowel is ____
____.
2. When connecting a word root and a suffix, a combining vowel is __________ if the suffix does not begin with a vowel.
3. When connecting a word root and a suffix, a combining vowel is usually not used if the suffix begins with a ______________.
4. When connecting two ______________, a combining vowel is usually used, even if vowels are present at the junction.
5. When connecting a prefix and a word root, a combining vowel is __________ used.

Combining Form

A combining form is a word root with the combining vowel attached, separated by a slash. The combining form is not a word part per se; rather it is the word root and the combining vowel. *For learning purposes, word roots are presented with their combining vowels as* ***combining forms.***

EXAMPLES

arthr/o
oste/o
ven/o

Word roots are presented as combining forms throughout the text.

EXERCISE 5 ■ Define

Complete the following. *To check your answers, go to Appendix A.*

A combining form is ____
____
____.

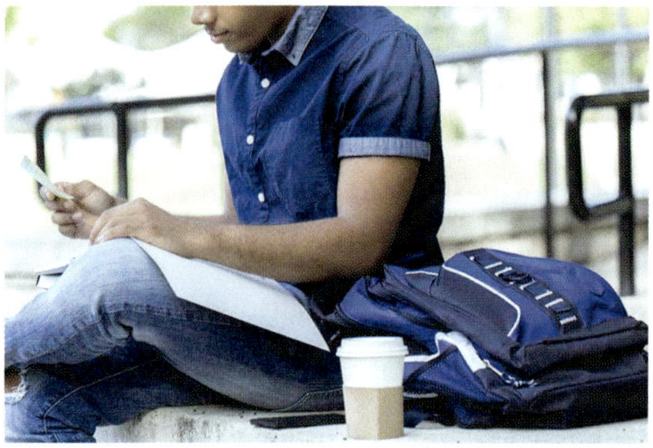

EXERCISE 6 ■ Match

Match the phrases in the first column with the correct terms in the second column. *To check your answers, go to Appendix A.*

_____ 1. attached to the beginning of a word root	a. combining vowel
_____ 2. usually an *o*	b. prefix
_____ 3. all medical terms built from word parts contain at least one	c. combining form
_____ 4. attached to the end of a word root	d. word root
_____ 5. word root with combining vowel attached	e. suffix

EXERCISE 7 ■ True/False

Answer **T** for true and **F** for false. *To check your answers, go to Appendix A.*

_____ 1. There are always prefixes at the beginning of medical terms.

_____ 2. A combining vowel is always used when connecting a word root and a suffix that begins with the letter *o*.

_____ 3. A prefix modifies the meaning of the word.

_____ 4. A combining vowel is used to ease pronunciation.

_____ 5. *I* is the most commonly used combining vowel.

_____ 6. The word root is the core of a medical term.

_____ 7. A combining vowel is used between a prefix and a word root.

_____ 8. A combining form is a word part.

_____ 9. A combining vowel is used when connecting a word root and a suffix if the suffix begins with the letter *g*.

TABLE 1.3 Word Parts and Combining Form

WORD PARTS, COMBINING FORM	DEFINITION	EXAMPLE
Word root	The core of the word	**hepat**/itis
Suffix	Attached to the end of a word root to modify its meaning	hepat/**itis**
Prefix	Attached to the beginning of a word root to modify its meaning	**sub**/hepa/tic
Combining vowel	Usually an o used to ease pronunciation	hepat/**o**/megaly
Combining form	Word root with a combining vowel attached, separated by a slash	**hepat/o**

Techniques for Learning Medical Terms Built from Word Parts

Analyzing, defining, and **building** medical terms are used in this text to learn medical terms categorized as Built from Word Parts. You will use them many times to complete exercises in the following chapters. Refer to **Table 1.4** as often as needed, until you become familiar with these techniques.

ANALYZING MEDICAL TERMS

To analyze a medical term, divide it into word parts, and label each word part and each combining form. Follow the procedure below:

1. **Divide the term** into word parts with slashes.

   EXAMPLE: oste / o / arthr / o / pathy

2. **Label each word part** by using the following abbreviations.
   WR Word Root
   P Prefix
   S Suffix
   CV Combining Vowel

   WR CV WR CV S
   EXAMPLE: oste / o /arthr / o / pathy

3. **Identify each combining form by underlining the word root and combining vowel, and then writing the abbreviation CF below the combining form.**

   WR CV WR CV S
   EXAMPLE: oste / o / arthr / o / pathy
   CF CF

EXERCISE 8 ■ Analyzing Medical Terms

A

Complete the following. *To check your answers, go to Appendix A.*

Three steps to analyze medical terms are:

1. ______________________________
2. ______________________________
3. ______________________________

B

Analyze the following medical term using the three step-procedure. Use the Word Part List on p. 10 as a reference. *To check your answers, go to Appendix A.*

o s t e o p a t h y

DEFINING MEDICAL TERMS

To define medical terms, apply the meaning of each word part.

Once a term has been analyzed, it is defined using the meanings of word parts identified. Usually, a term's definition starts with the meaning of the suffix, if present, and then shifts to the beginning of the term with the meanings of the word parts and combining forms in the order they appear. Often definitions of terms built from word parts contain additional words, such as articles (the), conjunctions (and), and prepositions (of).

WORD PART LIST

WORD ROOTS	DEFINITIONS	SUFFIXES	DEFINITIONS	PREFIXES	DEFINITIONS	COMBINING VOWEL
arthr	joint	-itis	inflammation	intra-	within	o
hepat	liver	-ic	pertaining to	sub-	under	
ven	vein	-ous	pertaining to			
oste	bone	-pathy	disease			
		-megaly	enlargement			

EXERCISE 9 ■ Defining Medical Terms

A

Complete the following. *To check your answers, go to Appendix A.*

To define medical terms categorized as Built from Word Parts, ______________________________

____

B

Define the following medical term. Use the Word Part List as a reference. *To check your answers, go to Appendix A.*

EXAMPLE: oste/o/arthr/o/pathy

1. Begin by defining the suffix, *-pathy*. Write the definition on the line below.
2. Move to the beginning of the term; define the word roots *oste* and *arthr*. Write the definitions on the line below, continuing the definition of the term.

oste/o/arthr/o/pathy means ____________ of the ____________ and ____________
-pathy oste arthr

Most medical terms categorized as Built from Word Parts can be defined by beginning with the meaning of the suffix.

EXERCISE 10 ■ Analyze and Define

Using the Word Part List, analyze and define the following terms. Underline the combining forms. *To check your answers, go to Appendix A.*

EXAMPLE:
WR CV WR CV S
oste / o / arthr / o / pathy
CF CF
disease of the bone and joint

1. arthritis

____

____

2. hepatitis

____

____

3. subhepatic

____

____

4. intravenous

____

____

5. arthropathy

____

____

6. osteitis

____

____

7. hepatomegaly

____

____

8. hepatic

____

____

BUILDING MEDICAL TERMS

To build medical terms, place word parts together to form terms.

Building medical terms is a learning technique used to practice the meaning of word parts and to learn definitions of terms built from word parts. In this text, we will build commonly accepted medical terms used in healthcare professions.

EXERCISE 11 ■ Building Medical Terms

A

Complete the following. *To check your answers, go to Appendix A.*

To build medical terms means ____

____.

Keep in mind that the beginning of the definition usually indicates the suffix.

B

Build the medical term for **disease of a joint.** Use the Word Part List on p. 10 as a reference, and follow the instructions below. *To check your answers, go to Appendix A.*

1. Find the word part for *disease*. Write the word part in the correct space below.
2. Find the word part for *joint*. Write the word part in the correct space below.
3. Insert the combining vowel *o* in the correct space below. (*A combining vowel is needed because the suffix does not begin with a vowel.*)

______________ / ____ / ______________

WR / CV / S

TABLE 1.4 Techniques to Learn Medical Terms Built from Word Parts

• **Analyzing**	1. Divide medical terms into word parts	oste / o / arthr / o / pathy
	2. Label each word part	WR CV WR CV S oste / o / arthr / o / pathy
	3. Underline and label each combining form	WR CV WR CV S oste / o / arthr / o / pathy CF CF
• **Defining**	1. Apply the meaning of each word part contained in the term	WR CV WR CV S oste / o / arthr / o / pathy
	2. Begin by defining the suffix, then move to the beginning of the term	**disease** of the **bone** and **joint**
• **Building**	1. Place word parts together to form terms; the beginning of the definition usually indicates the suffix	**disease** of the **bone** and **joint** oste / / arthr / / pathy WR / CV / WR / CV / S
	2. Add combining vowels	oste / o / arthr / o / pathy WR / CV / WR / CV / S

EXERCISE 12 ■ Build

Using the Word Part List on p. 10 as a reference, complete A and B. *To check your answers, go to Appendix A.*

A

Fill in the blanks with word parts defined to label the illustration.

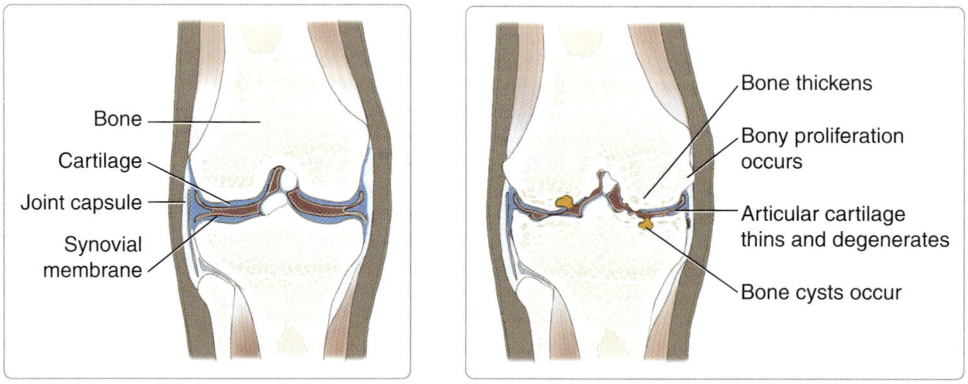

Normal knee joint

Knee joint showing
_______ / _____ / _______ / ___________
bone cv joint inflammation

B

Build medical terms for the following definitions.

EXAMPLE: **disease of a joint** arthr / o / pathy (WR / CV / S)

At this time, do not be concerned about which word root goes first when building a term that contains two word roots. The order is usually dictated by common practice; for surgical or diagnostic terms, word roots are sometimes arranged by the order of function or by the order in which an instrument may encounter a structure. As you practice and learn, you will become accustomed to the accepted order.

1. inflammation of a joint ______ / ______ (WR / S)
2. pertaining to the liver ______ / ______ (WR / S)
3. pertaining to under the liver ______ / ______ / ______ (P / WR / S)
4. pertaining to within the vein ______ / ______ / ______ (P / WR / S)
5. inflammation of the bone ______ / ______ (WR / S)
6. inflammation of the liver ______ / ______ (WR / S)
7. disease of the bone and joint ______ / ___ / ______ / ___ / ______ (WR / CV / WR / CV / S)
8. enlargement of the liver ______ / ___ / ______ (WR / CV / S)

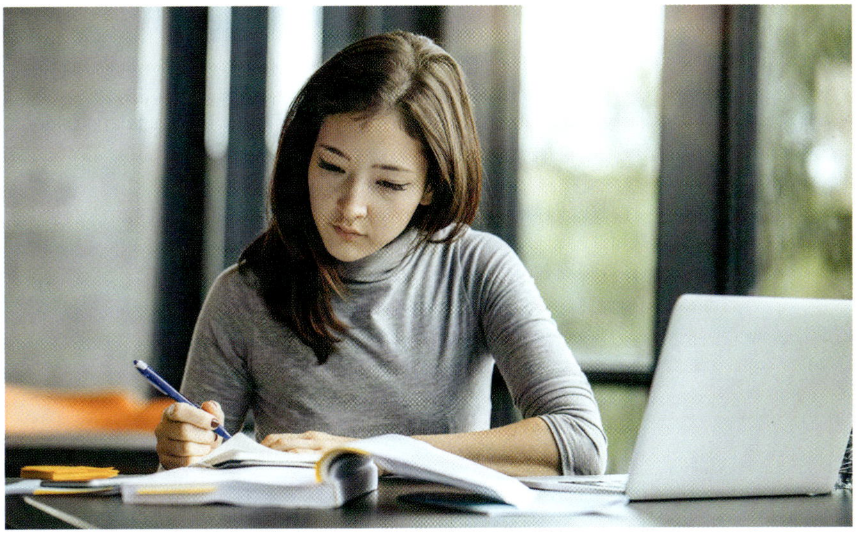

MEDICAL TERMS *NOT* BUILT FROM WORD PARTS

Medical terms categorized as NOT Built from Word Parts are terms that cannot be easily translated to find their meanings. Memorization is the primary method for learning these terms. Many varied exercises are presented in each chapter to assist with memorization. Origins of terms NOT Built from Word Parts are:

1. **Eponyms,** terms derived from the name of a person or place, such as Apgar score and West Nile virus.
2. **Acronyms,** terms formed from the first letter of words in a phrase that can be spoken as a whole word and usually contains a vowel, such as MRSA (methicillin-resistant *Staphylococcus aureus*).
3. **Modern language,** terms derived from the English language such as complete blood count with differential.
4. **Terms made up of Greek and Latin word parts that cannot be easily translated to find their meaning,** such as orthopedic. Orth/o/ped/ic is made up of three word parts: orth/o meaning straight, ped/o meaning child or foot, and -ic meaning pertaining to. Translated literally, **orthopedic** means **pertaining to a straight child or foot,** whereas its meaning as used today is a **branch of medicine dealing with the study and treatment of diseases and abnormalities of the musculoskeletal system.** Because it cannot be translated from word parts to understand its meaning, the term orthopedic is categorized as NOT Built from Word Parts in this textbook.

Some terms containing recognizable word parts are categorized as NOT Built from Word Parts because they are difficult to translate for an understanding of their current meanings.

EXERCISE 13 ▪ Identify

Place a check mark in the space provided to identify terms NOT Built from Word Parts. This may be the first time you have seen some of these terms. Apply your newly acquired knowledge and see how you do. *To check your answers, go to Appendix A.*

1. ______ arthritis
2. ______ upper respiratory infection
3. ______ Lyme disease
4. ______ AIDS
5. ______ macular degeneration
6. ______ hepatitis
7. ______ nuclear medicine scanner
8. ______ malignant
9. ______ osteopathy
10. ______ Alzheimer disease

CHAPTER REVIEW

REVIEW OF CATEGORIES OF MEDICAL TERMS

Terms Built from Word Parts—can be translated to find their meaning

Terms NOT Built from Word Parts—cannot be translated easily to find their meaning

REVIEW OF MEDICAL TERMS BUILT FROM WORD PARTS

Word root—core of a word; example, **hepat**

Suffix—attached to the end of a word root to modify its meaning; example, **-ic**

Prefix—attached to the beginning of a word root to modify its meaning; example, **sub-**

Combining vowel—usually an o used between two word roots or a word root and suffix to ease pronunciation; example, hepat **o** pathy

Combining form—word root plus combining vowel separated by a slash; example, **hepat/o**

Analyzing—dividing medical terms into word parts, then labeling each word part and combining form

Defining—applying the meaning of each word part contained in the medical term to derive its meaning

Building—placing word parts together to form terms

REVIEW OF MEDICAL TERMS *NOT* BUILT FROM WORD PARTS

Eponyms—name of a person or place; examples, Apgar score and West Nile virus

Acronyms—from first letter of words, example, MRSA

Modern language—terms derived from the English language, example, complete blood count with differential

Terms made up of Greek and Latin word parts not easily translated—example, orthopedic

REVIEW OF OBJECTIVES

To complete this chapter successfully, you do not need to know what the word parts, such as *arthr*, mean. You will learn these in subsequent chapters. **It is important that you have met these objectives:**

1. Can you describe the origins of medical language? yes ☐ no ☐
2. Can you define two categories of medical terms? yes ☐ no ☐
3. Can you identify and define the four word parts and combining form? yes ☐ no ☐
4. Can you use word parts to analyze and define medical terms? yes ☐ no ☐
5. Can you use word parts to build medical terms for a given definition? yes ☐ no ☐

If you answered yes to these questions, you need no further practice because you will be using these concepts repeatedly as you work your way through this text. Refer to this chapter to refresh your memory as needed. Move on to Chapter 2 and begin to build your medical vocabulary.

Chapter 2

Body Structure, Oncology, and Laboratory Tests

Objectives

Upon completion of this chapter, you will be able to:

1 Pronounce anatomic structures of the human body.

2 Define and spell word parts related to body structure, color, oncology, and laboratory tests.

3 Define, pronounce, and spell body structure terms.

4 Define, pronounce, and spell oncology terms.

5 Define, pronounce, and spell laboratory terms.

6 Define, pronounce, and spell complementary terms related to body structure, color, oncology, and laboratory tests.

7 Identify and use singular and plural endings.

8 Interpret the meaning of abbreviations related to body structure, oncology, and laboratory tests.

9 Apply medical language in clinical contexts.

Outline

ANATOMY

Organization of the Body

The structure of the human body falls into the following four categories: cells, tissues, organs, and systems. Each structure is a highly organized unit of smaller structures.

TERM	DEFINITION
cell (sel)	basic unit of all living things (Fig. 2.1). The human body is composed of trillions of cells, which vary in size and shape according to function.
cell membrane (sel) (MEM-brān)	forms the boundary of the cell
cytoplasm (SĪ-tō-*plas*-em)	gel-like fluid inside the cell
nucleus (NŪ-klē-us)	largest structure within the cell, usually spherical and centrally located. It contains chromosomes for cellular reproduction and is the control center for cellular activity.
chromosomes (KRŌ-ma-sōms)	located in the nucleus of the cell. There are 46 chromosomes in all normal human cells, with the exception of mature sex cells, which have 23.
genes (JĒNS)	regions within the chromosome. Each chromosome has several thousand genes that determine hereditary characteristics.
DNA (D-N-A)	comprises each gene; is a genetic material that regulates the activities of the cell. DNA abbreviates deoxyribonucleic acid.
tissue (TISH-ū)	group of similar cells that performs a specific function
muscle tissue (MUS-el) (TISH-ū)	composed of cells that have a special ability to contract, usually producing movement
nervous tissue (NURV-us) (TISH-ū)	similarly specialized cells united in the performance of a particular function; found in the nerves, spinal cord, and brain. It is responsible for coordinating and controlling body activities.
connective tissue (ke-NEK-tiv) (TISH-ū)	connects, supports, penetrates, and encases various body structures. Adipose (fat), osseous (bone) tissues, and blood are types of connective tissue. Fibrous tissue is a type of connective tissue that provides strength and stability such as in ligaments and tendons.
epithelial tissue (*ep*-i-THĒ-lē-al) (TISH-ū)	the major covering of the external surface of the body; forms membranes that line body cavities and organs; and is the major tissue in glands. Glandular tissue is designed to secrete substances such as digestive enzymes.

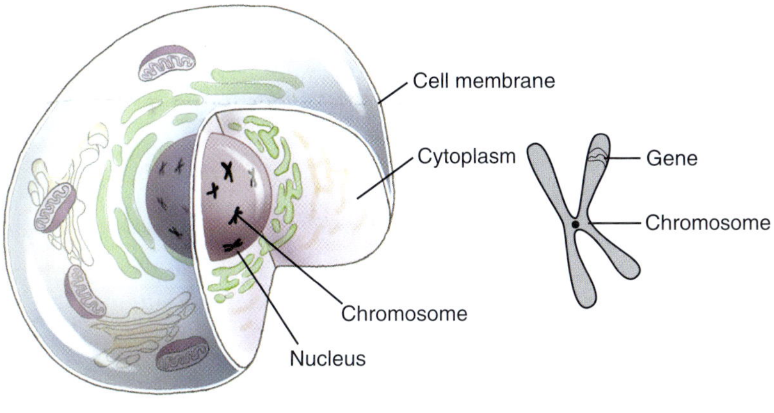

FIG. 2.1 Body cell.

CHROMOSOME is derived from the Greek **chromos**, meaning **color**, and **soma**, meaning **body**. German anatomist Waldeyer first used the term in 1888.

Organization of the Body—cont'd

TERM	DEFINITION
organ (OR-gen)	two or more types of tissues that together perform special body functions. For example, the skin is an organ composed of epithelial, connective, muscle, and nervous tissue.
viscera (VIS-er-a)	large internal organs contained in the body cavities, especially in the abdominal cavity
system (SIS-tem)	group of organs that work together to perform complex body functions. For example, the cardiovascular system consists of the heart, blood vessels, and blood. Its function is to transport nutrients and oxygen to the cells and remove carbon dioxide and other waste products (Table 2.1).

MEDICAL GENOMICS

A **genome** is the complete set of information in the DNA of a specific organism. Experts in **genomics** study the genome to determine its DNA sequences and perform genetic mapping to help understand disease. **Medical genomics** is an emerging discipline that uses a person's individual genome as part of their clinical care. Genomic Medicine is being used in areas such as oncology, pharmacology, and infectious disease.

Gene therapy is an experimental procedure to treat or prevent disease. Possible treatments may include replacing a mutated gene with a healthy one, inactivating a mutated gene that doesn't function properly, or introducing a new gene into the body to help fight a disease. The technique remains risky and is currently being tested only for diseases that have no other cures.

TABLE 2.1 **Body Systems**

BODY SYSTEMS	ORGANS AND FUNCTION
INTEGUMENTARY SYSTEM	Composed of skin, nails, and glands. Forms a protective covering for the body, regulates body temperature, and helps manufacture vitamin D.
RESPIRATORY SYSTEM	Composed of nose, pharynx (throat), larynx (voice box), trachea (windpipe), bronchial tubes, and lungs. Performs respiration, which provides for the exchange of oxygen and carbon dioxide within the body.
URINARY SYSTEM	Composed of kidneys, ureters, bladder, and urethra. Removes waste material (urine) from the body, regulates fluid volume, and maintains electrolyte concentration.
REPRODUCTIVE SYSTEM	Female reproductive system is composed of ovaries, uterine tubes, uterus, vagina, and mammary glands. Male reproductive system is composed of testes, urethra, penis, prostate gland, and associated tubes. Responsible for heredity and reproduction.
CARDIOVASCULAR SYSTEM	Composed of the heart and blood vessels. Pumps and transports blood throughout the body.
LYMPHATIC/IMMUNE SYSTEM	Composed of a network of vessels, ducts, nodes, and organs. Provides for defense against infection and drainage of extracellular fluid.
DIGESTIVE SYSTEM	Composed of the gastrointestinal tract, which includes the mouth, esophagus, stomach, small and large intestines, and anus, plus accessory organs, liver, gallbladder, and pancreas. Prepares food for use by the body cells and eliminates waste.
MUSCULOSKELETAL SYSTEM	Composed of muscle, bones, and joints. Provides movement and framework for the body, protects vital organs such as the brain, stores calcium, and produces red blood cells.
NERVOUS SYSTEM	Composed of the brain, spinal cord, nerves, and sensory organs. Regulates specific body activities by sending and receiving messages. Sensory organs, such as the eye and ear, are also part of the nervous system.
ENDOCRINE SYSTEM	Composed of glands that secrete hormones. Hormones regulate many specific body activities.

Body Cavities

The body is not a solid structure as it appears on the outside, but has five cavities (Fig. 2.2), each containing an orderly arrangement of the internal organs.

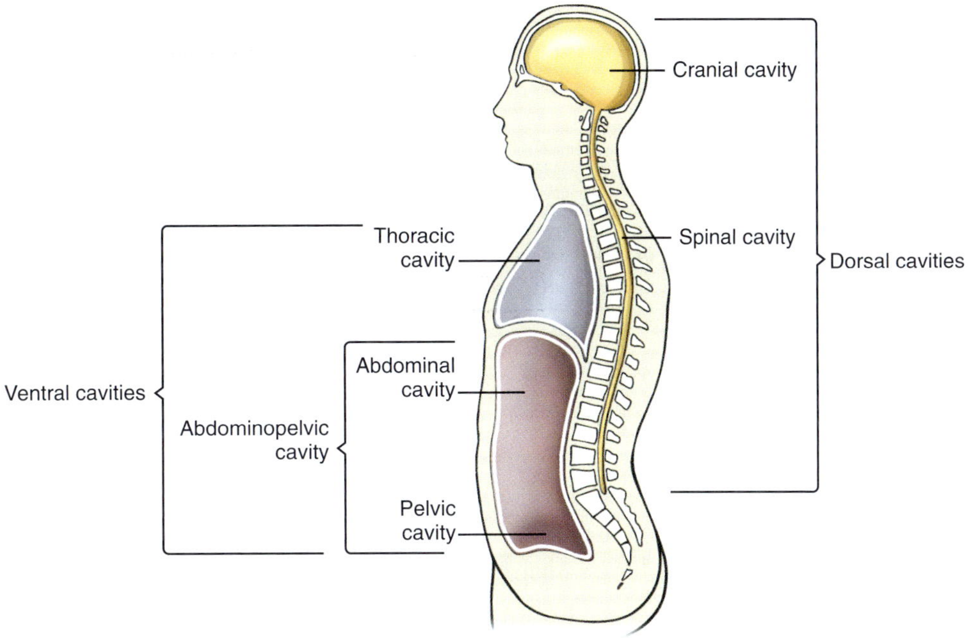

FIG. 2.2 Body cavities.

TERM	DEFINITION
cranial cavity (KRĀ-nē-al) (KAV-i-tē)	space inside the skull (cranium) containing the brain
spinal cavity (SPĪ-nal) (KAV-i-tē)	space inside the spinal column containing the spinal cord
thoracic cavity (thō-RAS-ic) (KAV-i-tē)	space containing the heart, aorta, lungs, esophagus, trachea, bronchi, and mediastinal area
abdominal cavity (ab-DOM-i-nal) (KAV-i-tē)	space containing the stomach, intestines, kidneys, adrenal glands, liver, gallbladder, pancreas, spleen, and ureters
pelvic cavity (PEL-vik) (KAV-i-tē)	space containing the urinary bladder, certain reproductive organs, parts of the small and large intestine, and the anus
abdominopelvic cavity (ab-*dom*-i-nō-PEL-vik) (KAV-i-tē)	both the pelvic and abdominal cavities

PRONOUNCE ANATOMIC STRUCTURES

Practice saying aloud each of the Organization of the Body Terms on the previous pages.

To hear the terms, go to Evolve Resources at www.evolve.elsevier.com and select:
Student Resources > Audio Glossary > Chapter 2 > **Anatomic Structures**

❑ Check the box when complete.

TABLE 2.2 Pronunciation Key

GUIDELINES	EXAMPLES	
1. Words are distorted minimally to indicate proper phonetic sound.	doctor (dok-tor)	
2. The macron (¯) indicates the long vowel sound.	donate (dō-nāte)	
	ā as in say	**ō** as in no
	ē as in me	**ū** as in cute
	ī as in spine	
3. Vowels with no markings should have a short sound.	medical (med-i-cal)	
	a as in sad	**o** as in top
	e as in get	**u** as in cut
	i as in sit	
4. Primary accents are indicated by capital letters; the secondary accent (which is stressed, but not as strongly as the primary accent) is indicated by italics. *There may be geographical variations in pronunciation.*	altogether (*all*-tū-GETH-er)	
	pancreatitis (*pan*-krē-a-TĪ-tis)	

WORD PARTS

Use paper flashcards or electronic flashcards on Evolve to assist with memorization of word parts used to analyze, define, and build terms presented in this chapter. To reinforce learning, study one section of the Word Part Table at a time, and then complete the corresponding exercise on the following pages.

1 ■ Body Structure Combining Forms

COMBINING FORM	DEFINITION	COMBINING FORM	DEFINITION
aden/o	gland	**my/o**	muscle
cyt/o	cell	**neur/o**	nerve
epitheli/o	epithelium	**organ/o**	organ
fibr/o	fiber	**sarc/o**	flesh, connective tissue
hemat/o	blood	**system/o**	system
hist/o	tissue	**viscer/o**	internal organs
lip/o	fat		

2 ■ Combining Forms Used with Body Structure Terms

COMBINING FORM	DEFINITION
aut/o	self
bi/o	life
cancer/o	cancer
carcin/o	cancer

CANCER is a disease characterized by the unregulated, abnormal growth of new cells

COMBINING FORM	DEFINITION
crypt/o	hidden
necr/o	death (cells, body)
eti/o	cause (of disease)
gno/o	knowledge
iatr/o	physician, medicine (also means treatment)
lei/o	smooth
onc/o	tumor, mass
path/o	disease
rhabd/o	rod-shaped, striated
somat/o	body
vir/o	virus

3 ■ Color Combining Forms

COMBINING FORM	DEFINITION
cyan/o	blue
erythr/o	red
leuk/o	white
melan/o	black
xanth/o	yellow

4 ■ Prefixes

PREFIX	DEFINITION
dia-	through, complete
dys-	painful, abnormal, difficult, labored
hyper-	above, excessive
hypo-	below, incomplete, deficient, under
meta-	after, beyond, change
micro-	small
neo-	new
pro-	before

5 ■ Suffixes

SUFFIX	DEFINITION
-al, -ic, -ous	pertaining to
-cyte	cell (NOTE: the combining form for cell is cyt/o; the suffix for cell is -cyte, ending with an e.)
-gen	substance or agent that produces or causes
-genic	producing, originating, causing
-logist	one who studies and treats (specialist, physician)
-logy	study of
-megaly	enlargement
-oid	resembling
-oma	tumor, swelling
-opsy	view of, viewing
-osis	abnormal condition (means *increase* when used with blood cell word roots)
-pathy	disease
-plasia	condition of formation, development, growth
-plasm	growth, substance, formation
-sarcoma	malignant tumor
-sis	state of
-stasis	control, stop, standing

Refer to **Appendix B** and **Appendix C** for alphabetical lists of word parts and their meanings.

EXERCISE 1 ■ Body Structure Combining Forms

Refer to the first section of the word parts table.

Reminder: the word root is the core of the word. The combining form is the word root with the combining vowel attached, separated by a vertical slash.

A Label

Fill in the blanks with combining forms in this diagram of types of tissues. *To check your answers, go to Appendix A at the back of the textbook.*

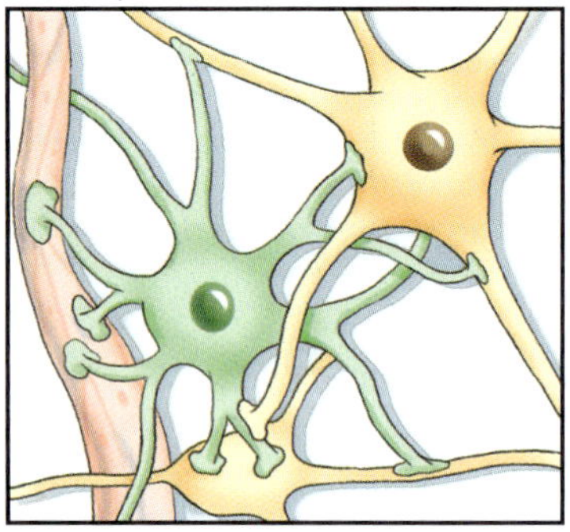

1. Nerve

CF: ____________________

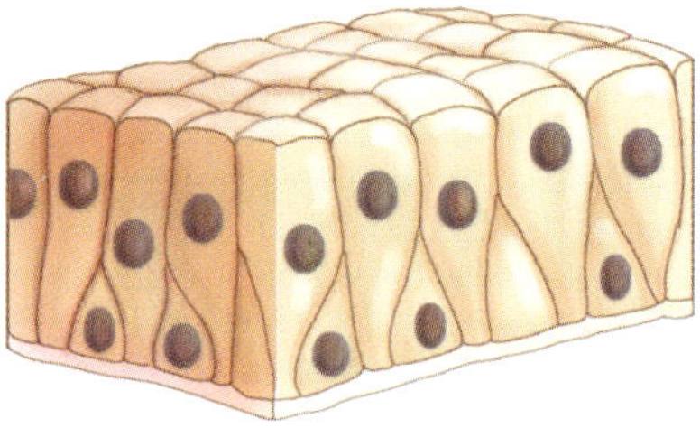

2. Epithelium

CF: ____________________

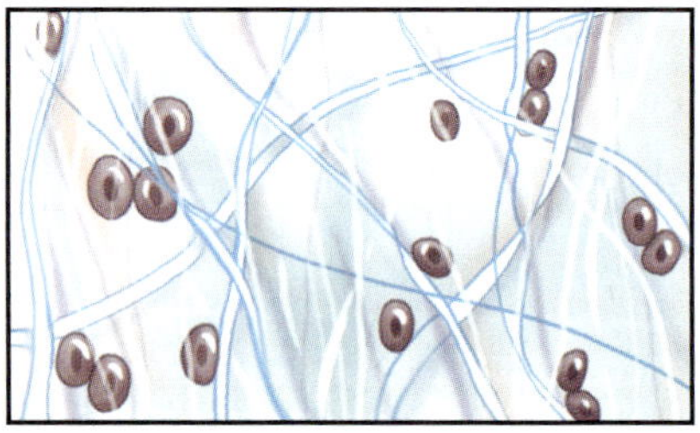

3. Connective

CF: ____________________

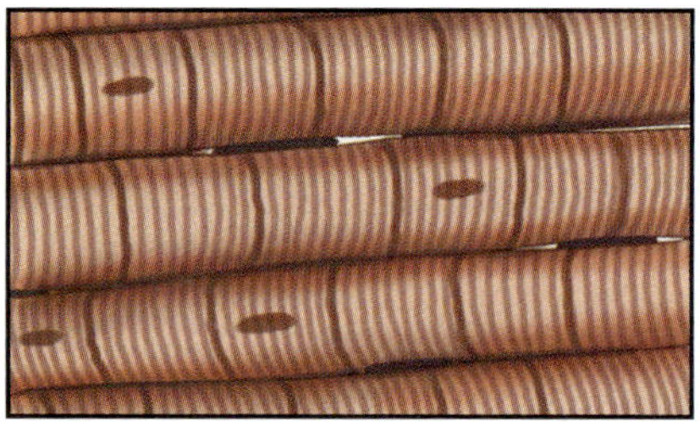

4. Muscle

CF: ____________________

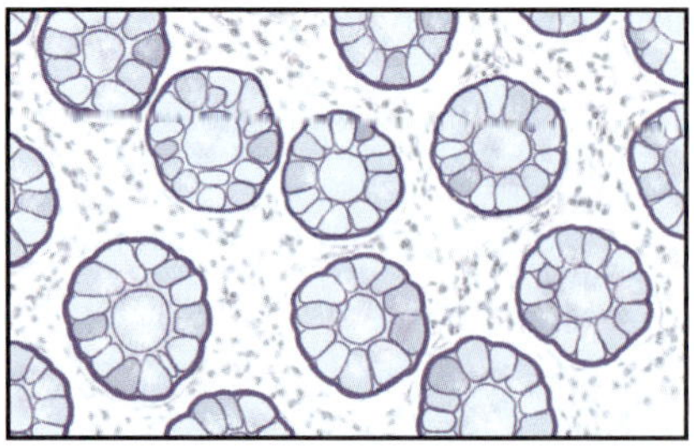

5. Gland

CF: ____________________

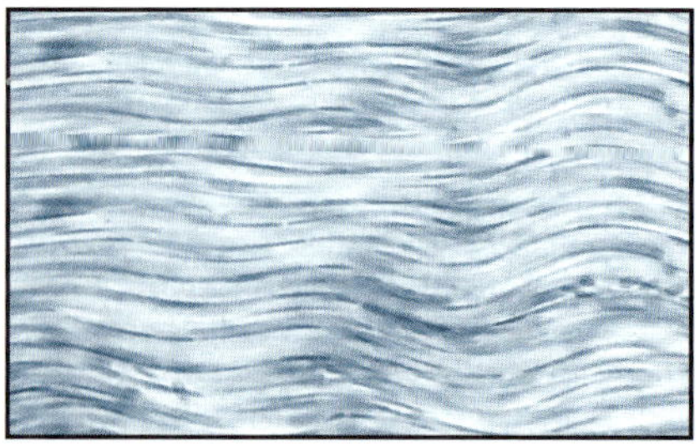

6. Fiber

CF: ____________________

B Label

Fill in the blanks with combining forms in this diagram of the organization of the body.

1. Tissue
CF: ______________

2. Cell
CF: ______________

4. System
CF: ______________

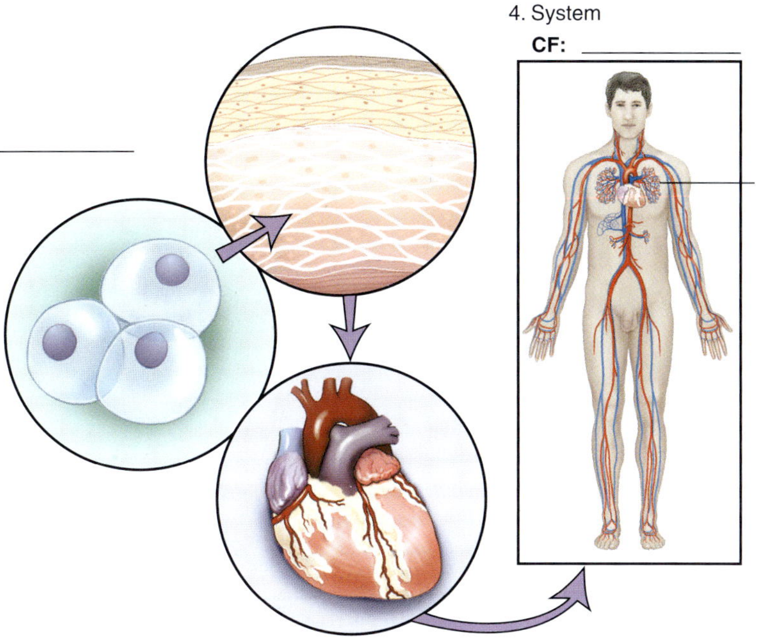

5. Internal organs
CF: ______________

3. Organ
CF: ______________

C Define and Match

Step 1: Write the definitions after the following combining forms.
Step 2: Match the descriptions on the right with the combining forms and definitions.

d	1. sarc/o, flesh, connective tissue	a. produces movement
d	2. lip/o, Fat	b. group of similar cells
c	3. viscer/o, viscera	c. contained in body cavities
f	4. cyt/o, cel	d. type of connective tissue
b	5. hist/o, tissue	e. tissue that encases various structures
a	6. my/o, Muscle	f. basic unit of all living things

D Define and Match

Step 1: Write the definitions after the following combining forms.
Step 2: Match the descriptions on the right with the combining forms and definitions.

c 1. neur/o, nerve	a. major tissue in glands
f 2. organ/o, organ	b. connective tissue found in ligaments
d 3. system/o, system	c. responsible for coordinating and controlling body activities
a 4. epitheli/o, epithelium	d. group of organs working together
b 5. fibr/o, Fiber	e. tissue designed to secrete something
e 6. aden/o, Gland	f. made up of at least two kinds of tissues
g 7. hemat/o, blood	g. type of connective tissue

EXERCISE 2 ■ Combining Forms Used with Body Structure Terms

Refer to the second section of the word parts table.

A Define

Write the definitions of the following combining forms. *To check your answers, go to Appendix A at the back of the textbook.*

1. onc/o Tumor
2. carcin/o Cancer
3. eti/o origin of disease
4. path/o desease
5. somat/o body
6. cancer/o Cancer
7. rhabd/o rod
8. lei/o Smooth
9. gno/o know
10. iatr/o Physician
11. bi/o life
12. vir/o Viros
13. aut/o self
14. necr/o death

CANCER

Carcin and **cancer** are derived from Latin and Greek words meaning **crab**. They originated before the nature of malignant growth was understood. One explanation was that the swollen blood vessels around the diseased area looked like the claws of a crab.

B Identify

Write the combining form for each of the following.

1. disease ______
2. tumor, mass ______
3. cause (of disease) ______
4. cancer a. ______
   b. ______
5. body ______
6. smooth ______
7. rod-shaped, striated ______
8. knowledge ______
9. physician, medicine ______
10. self ______
11. virus ______
12. life ______
13. death ______

EXERCISE 3 ■ Color Combining Forms

Refer to the third section of the word parts table.

A Define

Write the definitions of the following combining forms. *To check your answers, go to Appendix A at the back of the textbook.*

1. cyan/o ____ blue ____
2. erythr/o ____ Red ____
3. leuk/o ____ white ____
4. xanth/o ____ Yelow ____
5. melan/o ____ Black ____

ERYTHR/O Aristotle noted "two colors of blood" and applied the term **erythros** to the dark red blood.

B Identify

Write the combining form for each of the following.

1. blue ____________
2. red ____________
3. white ____________
4. black ____________
5. yellow ____________

EXERCISE 4 ■ Prefixes

Refer to the fourth section of the word parts table.

Reminder: prefixes are placed at the beginning of word roots to modify their meanings.

A Define

Write the definitions of the following prefixes. *To check your answers, go to Appendix A at the back of the textbook.*

1. neo- ____ new ____
2. hyper- ____ 2 much excresive ____
3. meta- ____ After change ____
4. hypo- ____ 2 low deficient ____
5. dys- ____ pain ____
6. dia- ____ through ____
7. pro- ____ before ____
8. micro- ____ small ____

B Identify

Write the prefix for each of the following.

1. new ____________
2. above, excessive ____________
3. below, incomplete, deficient, under ____________
4. after, beyond, change ____________
5. painful, abnormal, difficult, labored ____________
6. through, complete ____________
7. before ____________
8. small ____________

EXERCISE 5 ■ Suffixes

Refer to the fifth section of the word parts table.

Reminder: suffixes are placed at the end of word roots to modify their meanings.

A Label

Write the suffixes pictured and defined. *To check your answers, go to Appendix A at the back of the textbook.*

1. ______________________
cell

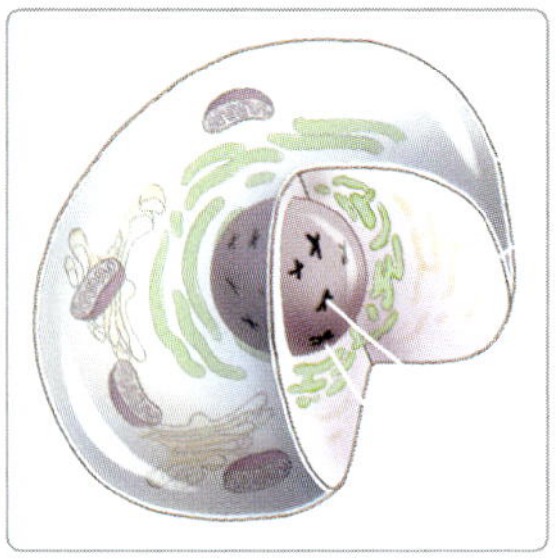

2. ______________________
condition of formation, development, growth

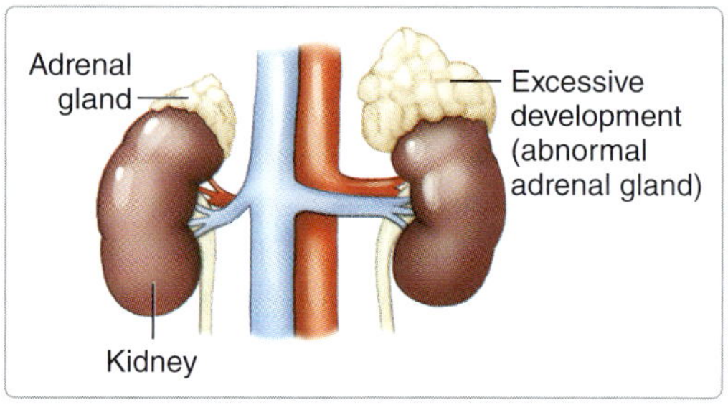

3. ______________________
one who studies and treats (specialist, physician)

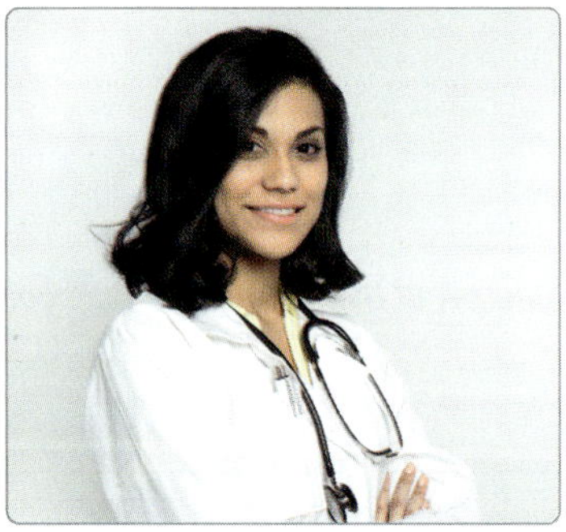

4. ______________________
study of

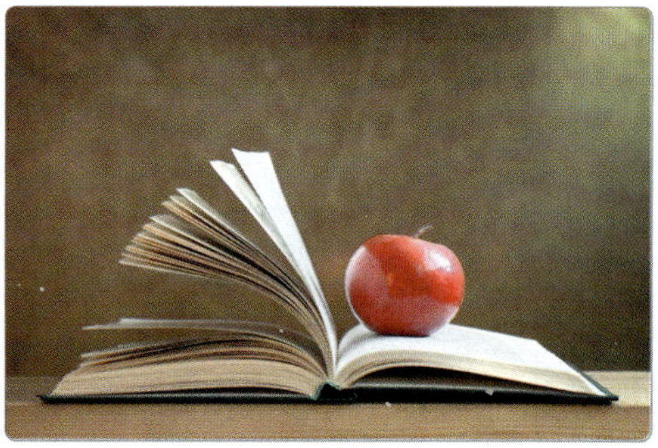

5. ______________________
enlargement

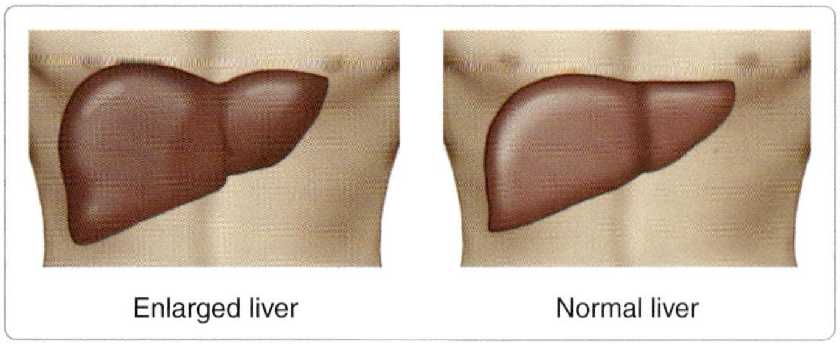

6. ______________________
tumor, swelling

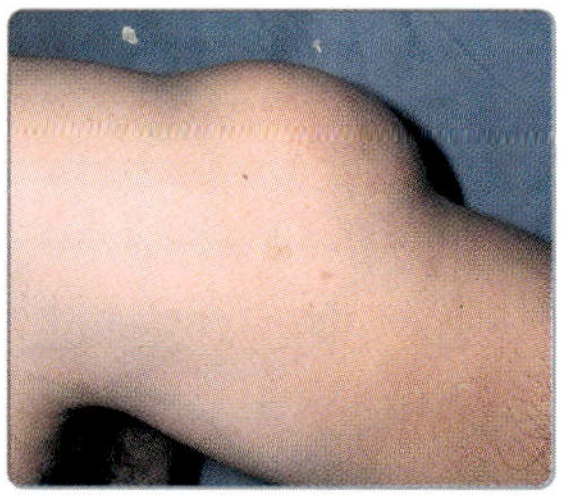

B Match

Match the suffixes in the first column with their correct definitions in the second column.

g	1. -osis	a. producing, originating, causing
j	2. -pathy	b. growth, substance, formation
b	3. -plasm	c. pertaining to
c	4. -al, -ic, -ous	d. resembling
e	5. -stasis	e. control, stop, standing
d	6. -oid	f. substance that produces
f	7. -gen	g. abnormal condition
i	8. -sarcoma	h. state of
a	9. -genic	i. malignant tumor
h	10. -sis	j. disease
k	11. -opsy	k. view of, viewing

Some suffixes are made of a word root plus a suffix; they are presented as suffixes for ease of learning. For example, **-pathy** is made up of the word root **path** and the noun ending **-y**. When analyzing a medical term, divide the suffixes as learned. For example, **somatopathy** will be divided as somat/o/pathy and **not** somat/o/path/y.

C Define

Write the definitions of the following suffixes.

1. -logist ____________
2. -pathy ____________
3. -logy ____________
4. -ic ____________
5. -stasis ____________
6. -cyte ____________
7. -osis ____________
8. -ous ____________
9. -plasm ____________
10. -al ____________
11. -plasia ____________
12. -oid ____________
13. -gen ____________
14. -genic ____________
15. -oma ____________
16. -sarcoma ____________
17. -sis ____________
18. –megaly ____________
19. -opsy ____________

The suffix -**logist** may indicate a specialist such as in **psychologist who is not a physician**, or a specialist such as in **oncologist who is a physician**. For learning purposes in the text, if the specialist is a physician, it will be indicated in the definition such as **oncologist** . . . a **physician who studies and treats (malignant) tumors**. Also, some physicians, such as pathologists, do not treat. The definition of -logist will vary.

Practice two things in your dealings with disease: either help or do not harm the patient.—**Hippocrates** 460–375 BC

MEDICAL TERMS

Medical terms relevant to this chapter have been grouped by topics, such as Body Structure, and are listed in tables designated as Built from Word Parts or NOT Built from Word Parts. The exercises following each table assist with learning term definitions, pronunciations, and spellings.

Body Structure Terms

BUILT FROM WORD PARTS

The following terms can be translated using definitions of word parts. Further explanation is provided within parentheses as needed.

TERM	DEFINITION
1. cytogenic (*sī*-tō-JEN-ik)	producing cells
2. cytology (*sī*-TOL-o-jē)	study of cells
3. dysplasia (dis-PLĀ-zha)	abnormal development (See Fig. 2.4)
4. epithelial (*ep*-i-THĒ-lē-al)	pertaining to epithelium
5. erythrocyte (RBC) (e-RITH-rō-sīt)	red (blood) cell
6. erythrocytosis (e-*rith*-rō-sī-TŌ-sis)	increase in the number of red (blood) cells
7. histology (his-TOL-o-jē)	study of tissue
8. hyperplasia (*hī*-per-PLĀ-zha)	excessive development (number of cells) (See Fig. 2.4)
9. hypoplasia (hī-pō-PLĀ-zha)	incomplete development (of an organ or tissues)
10. leukocyte (WBC) (LŪ-kō-sīt)	white (blood) cell
11. leukocytosis (*lū*-kō-sī-TŌ-sis)	increase in the number of white (blood) cells
12. lipoid (LIP-oid)	resembling fat
13. myopathy (mī-OP-a-thē)	disease of the muscle
14. necrosis (ne-KRŌ-sis)	condition of cell death (cells and tissue die because of disease)
15. neuropathy (nū-ROP-a-thē)	disease of the nerves
16. organomegaly (*or*-ga-nō-MEG-a-lē)	enlargement of an organ
17. somatic (sō-MAT-ik)	pertaining to the body
18. somatogenic (*sō*-ma-tō-JEN-ik)	originating in the body (organic as opposed to originating in the mind)
19. systemic (sis-TEM-ik)	pertaining to a (body) system (or the body as a whole)
20. visceral (VIS-er-al)	pertaining to the internal organs

Ellipsis is the practice of omitting an essential part of a word by common consent. Note this practice in the terms **erythrocyte** (red **blood** cell) and **leukocyte** (white **blood** cell). The word root for blood is omitted.

EXERCISE 6 ■ Pronounce and Spell

Practice pronunciation and spelling on paper and online.

1. Practice on Paper

a. **Pronounce:** Read the phonetic spelling and say aloud the terms listed in the previous table. Refer to the pronunciation key on p. 20 as necessary.

b. **Spell:** Have a study partner read the terms aloud. Write the spelling of the terms on a separate sheet of paper.

2. Practice Online

a. **Access** online learning resources. Go to evolve.elsevier.com > Evolve Resources > Student Resources.
b. **Pronounce:** Select Audio Glossary > Chapter 2 > Exercise 6. Select a term to hear its pronunciation and repeat aloud.
c. **Spell:** Select Activities > Chapter 2 > Spell Terms > Exercise 6. Select the audio icon and type the correct spelling of the term.

❑ Check the box when complete.

EXERCISE 7 ■ Analyze and Define

Analyze and define the following body structure terms by drawing slashes between word parts, writing word part abbreviations above the term, underlining combining forms, and writing combining form abbreviations below the term. Refer to Chapter 1 to review analyzing and defining techniques. **This is an important exercise; do not skip any portion of it.** *To check your answers, go to Appendix A at the back of the textbook.*

WR CV S

EXAMPLE: cyt / o / genic

CF

producing cells

1. cytology

2. histology

3. visceral

4. hypoplasia

5. neuropathy

6. systemic

7. somatic

8. somatogenic

9. epithelial

10. erythrocytosis

11. leukocytosis

12. myopathy

13. erythrocyte

____

____

14. leukocyte

____

____

EXERCISE 8 ■ Build

A Fill In

Build medical terms for the following body structure definitions by using the word parts you have learned. Refer to Chapter 1 to review medical term building techniques. **This is an integral part of the learning process; do not skip any part of this exercise.**

EXAMPLE: Example: producing cells cyt / o / genic (WR / CV / S)

1. disease of the nerves ______ / ______ / ______ (WR / CV / S)

2. study of cells ______ / ______ / ______ (WR / CV / S)

3. pertaining to the body ______ / ______ (WR / S)

4. disease of the muscle ______ / ______ / ______ (WR / CV / S)

5. abnormal development ______ / ______ (P / S(WR))

When analyzing medical terms that have a suffix containing a word root, it may appear, as in the word **dysplasia,** that the term is composed of only a prefix and a suffix. Keep in mind that the word root is embedded in the suffix and is indicated in the *Building Medical Terms* exercises by S(WR).

6. pertaining to the internal organs ______ / ______ (WR / S)

7. originating in the body ______ / ______ / ______ (WR / CV / S)

8. enlargement of an organ ______ / ______ / ______ (WR / CV / S)

9. resembling fat ______ / ______ (WR / S)

10. pertaining to a (body) system ______ / ______ (WR / S)

B Label

Build terms pictured by writing word parts above the definitions.

1.

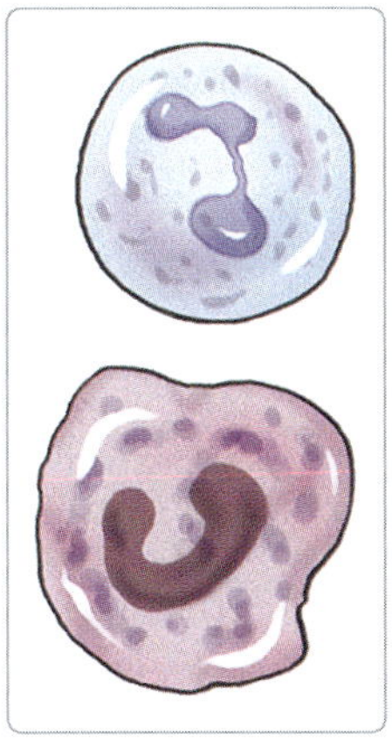

_______ / ___ / _______
white CV cell(s)

2.

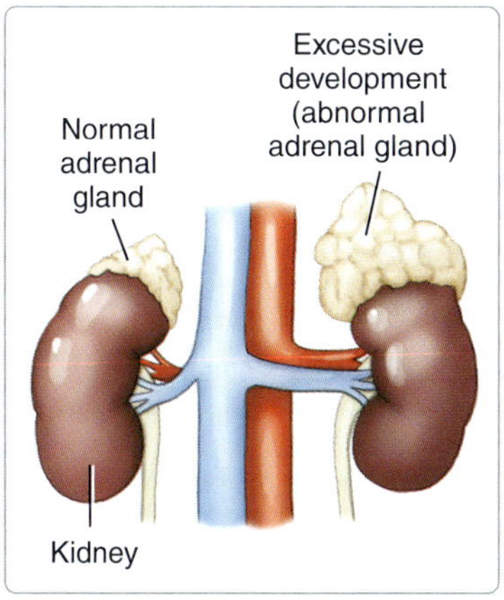

_______ / _______
excessive development

3.

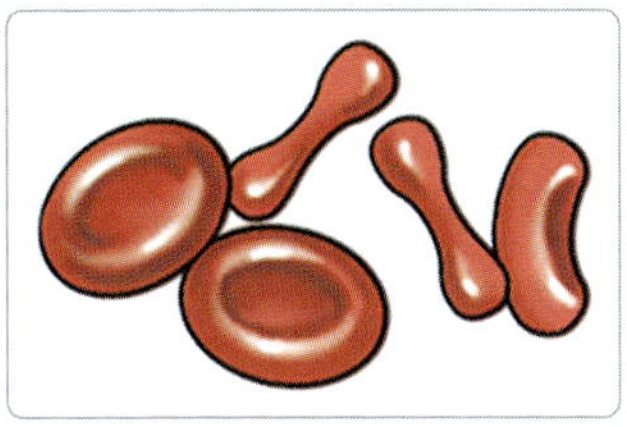

_______ / ___ / _______
red CV cell(s)

4.

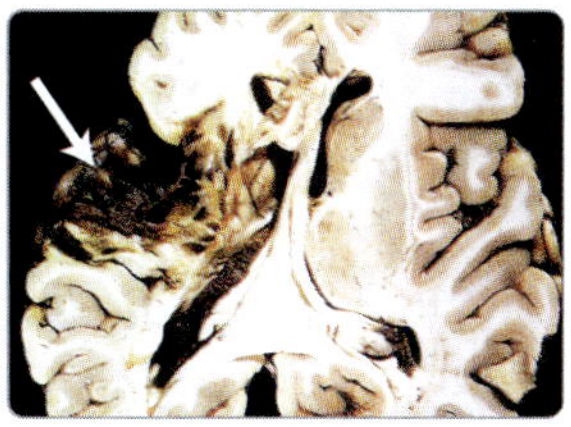

_______ / _______
death abnormal condition

EXERCISE 9 ■ Review of Body Structure Terms

Can you define, pronounce, and spell the following body structure terms?

cytogenic	erythrocytosis	leukocytosis	organomegaly
cytology	histology	lipoid	somatic
dysplasia	hyperplasia	myopathy	somatogenic
epithelial	hypoplasia	necrosis	systemic
erythrocyte (RBC)	leukocyte (WBC)	neuropathy	visceral

Oncology

Oncology is the study of tumors. Tumors can develop from excessive growth of cells. Tumors, or masses, can be benign (noncancerous) or malignant (cancerous). The names of tumors often include the word root for the body part and the suffix **-oma,** as in the term *my/oma*, which means "tumor composed of muscle." Oncology terms are introduced in this chapter because of their relation to cells and cell abnormalities. This is an introductory list only. **More oncology terms appear in subsequent chapters and are presented with the introduction of the related body systems.**

Oncology Terms

BUILT FROM WORD PARTS

The following terms can be translated using definitions of word parts. Further explanation is provided within parentheses as needed. *At first the list of terms may seem long to you; however, many of the word parts are repeated in many of the terms. You will soon find that knowing parts of the terms makes learning the words easy.* ***Analyzing, defining,*** *and* ***building exercises*** *are used to learn these terms.*

TERM	DEFINITION
1. **adenocarcinoma** (*ad*-e-nō-*kar*-si-NŌ-ma)	cancerous tumor of glandular tissue
2. **adenoma** (ad-e-NŌ-ma)	tumor composed of glandular tissue (benign)
3. **carcinoma (CA)** (*kar*-si-NŌ-ma)	cancerous tumor (malignant) (See Fig. 2.3)
4. **epithelioma** (*ep*-i-*thē*-lē-Ō-ma)	tumor composed of epithelium (may be benign or malignant)
5. **fibroma** (fī-BRŌ-ma)	tumor composed of fiber (fibrous tissue) (benign)
6. **fibrosarcoma** (fī-brō-sar-KŌ-ma)	malignant tumor composed of fiber (fibrous tissue)
7. **leiomyoma** (*lī*-ō-mī-Ō-ma)	tumor composed of smooth muscle (benign)
8. **leiomyosarcoma** (*lī*-ō-*mī*-ō-sar-KŌ-ma)	malignant tumor of smooth muscle
9. **lipoma** (li-PŌ-ma)	tumor composed of fat (benign tumor)
10. **liposarcoma** (*lip*-ō-sar-KŌ-ma)	malignant tumor of fat
11. **melanocarcinoma** (*mel*-a-nō-*kar*-si-NŌ-ma)	cancerous black tumor (malignant)
12. **melanoma** (mel-a-NŌ-ma)	black tumor (primarily of the skin)
13. **metastasis (*pl.* metastases) (METS)** (me-TAS-ta-sis) (me-TAS-ta-sēz	beyond control (transfer of cells from one organ to another, as in malignant tumors) (Fig. 2.3)
14. **myoma** (mī-Ō-ma)	tumor composed of muscle (benign)
15. **neoplasm** (NĒ-ō-plazm)	new growth (of abnormal tissue, benign or malignant)
16. **neuroma** (nū-RŌ-ma)	tumor composed of nerve (benign)
17. **rhabdomyoma** (*rab*-dō-mī-Ō-ma)	tumor composed of striated muscle (benign)
18. **rhabdomyosarcoma** (*rab*-dō-*mī*-ō-sar-KŌ-ma)	malignant tumor of striated muscle
19. **sarcoma** (sar-KŌ-ma)	tumor of connective tissue (such as bone or cartilage; highly malignant)

SARCOMA has been used since the time of ancient Greece to describe any fleshy tumor. Since the introduction of cellular pathology, the meaning has become **malignant connective tissue tumor**. Often, an additional word root is used to denote the type of tissue involved, such as **oste** in **osteosarcoma**, which refers to a malignant tumor of the bone.

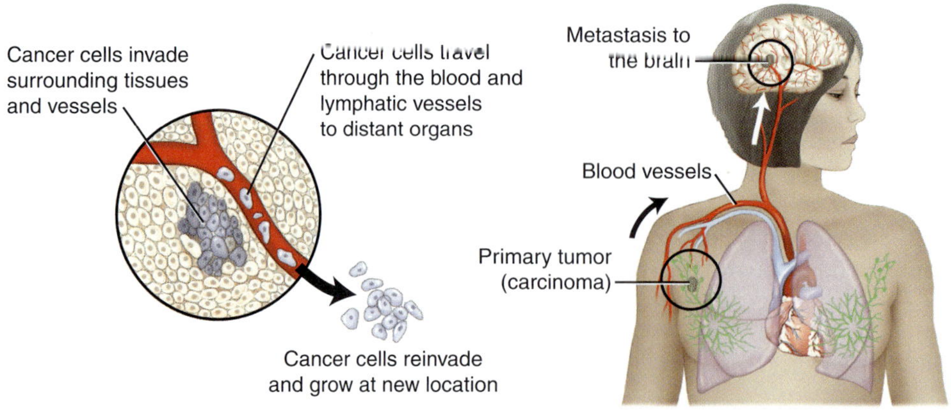

FIG. 2.3 Metastasis.

TNM STAGING SYSTEM OF CANCER

AJCC (American Joint Committee on Cancer) has devised a classification widely used to stage certain types of cancer properly.

T refers to size and the extent of the primary tumor (ranked 0-4).

N denotes the involvement of the lymph nodes (ranked 0-4).

M defines whether there is metastasis (0 = none; 1 = present).

For example, T_2 N_1 M_0

T_2 refers to the primary tumor of 2 cm.

N_1 means spread of tumor to ipsilateral (same side) lymph nodes.

M_0 means no distant metastasis.

This system helps communicate the extent of cancer and is frequently cited by oncologists, surgeons, and radiation oncologists.

EXERCISE 10 ■ Pronounce and Spell

Practice pronunciation and spelling on paper and online.

1. Practice on Paper

a. **Pronounce:** Read the phonetic spelling and say aloud the terms listed in the previous table. Refer to the pronunciation key on p. 20 as necessary.

b. **Spell:** Have a study partner read the terms aloud. Write the spelling of the terms on a separate sheet of paper.

2. Practice Online

a. **Access** the online learning resources. Go to evolve.elsevier.com > Evolve Resources > Student Resources.

b. **Pronounce:** Select Audio Glossary > Chapter 2 > Exercise 10. Select a term to hear its pronunciation and repeat aloud.

c. **Spell:** Select Activities > Chapter 2 > Spell Terms > Exercise 10. Select the audio icon and type the correct spelling of the term.

❑ Check the box when complete.

EXERCISE 11 ■ Analyze and Define

Analyze and define the following oncology terms by drawing slashes between word parts, writing word part abbreviations above the term, underlining combining forms, and writing combining form abbreviations below the term. *To check your answers, go to Appendix A at the back of the textbook.*

	WR CV	WR CV	S
EXAMPLE:	lei / o /	my / o /	sarcoma
	CF	CF	

malignant tumor of smooth muscle

1. sarcoma

____

____

2. melanoma

____

____

3. epithelioma

____

____

4. lipoma

____

____

5. neoplasm

____

____

6. myoma

____

____

7. neuroma

____

____

8. carcinoma

____

____

9. melanocarcinoma

____

____

10. rhabdomyosarcoma

____

____

11. adenoma

____

____

12. rhabdomyoma

____

____

13. fibroma

____

____

14. liposarcoma

____

____

15. fibrosarcoma

____

____

16. metastasis

____

____

EXERCISE 12 ■ Build

A Label

Build terms pictured by writing word parts above the definitions.

1.

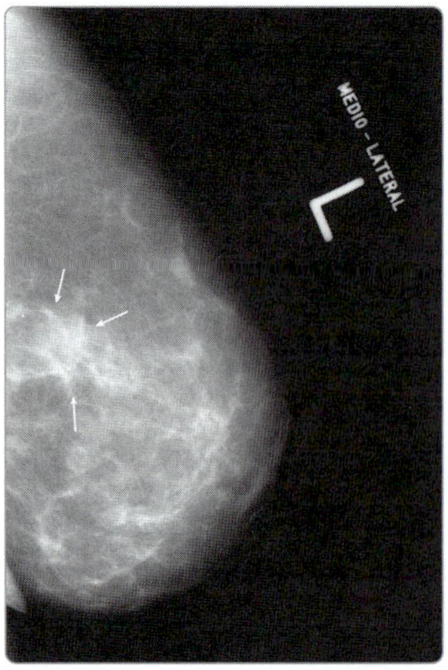

_______ / _______ of the breast
cancer tumor

2.

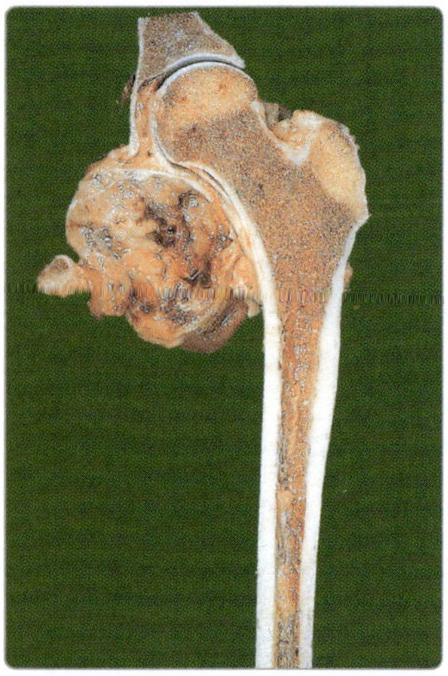

_______ / _______ of the femur
connective tissue tumor

3.

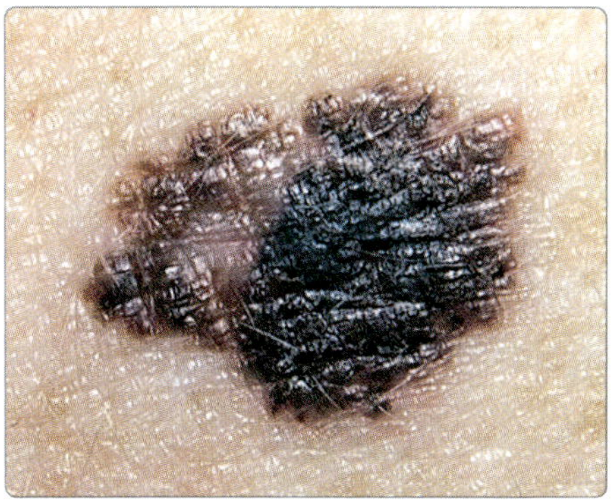

_____ / _____
black tumor

4.

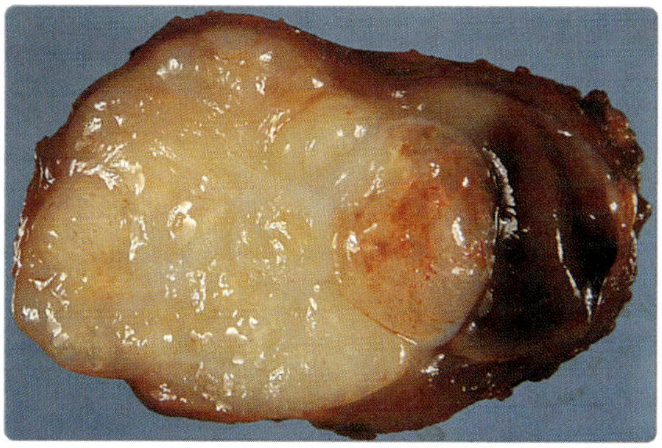

_____ / _____ / _____ / _____ / _____
striated CV muscle CV malignant tumor

5.

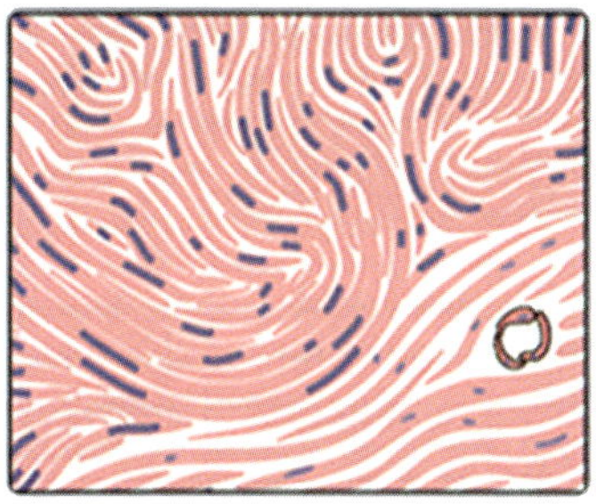

_____ / _____ / _____ / _____
smooth CV muscle tumor

6.

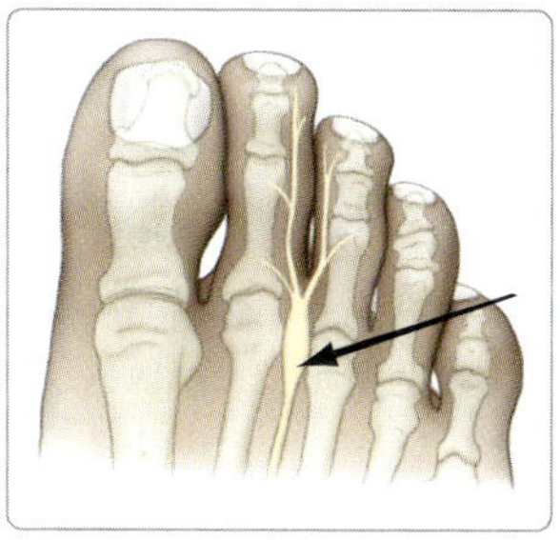

_____ / _____
nerve tumor

B Fill In

Build oncology terms for the following definitions by using the word parts you have learned.

EXAMPLE: tumor composed of fat lip / oma
WR / S

1. tumor composed of striated muscle (benign) _____ / _____ / _____ / _____
WR / CV / WR / S

2. malignant tumor of fat _____ / _____ / _____
WR / CV / S

3. new growth _____ / _____
P / S(WR)

4. tumor composed of epithelium _____ / _____
WR / S

5. tumor composed of fibrous tissue _____ / _____
WR / S

6. cancerous black tumor _____ / _____ / _____ / _____
WR / CV / WR / S

7. beyond control ______ P / ______ S(WR)

8. tumor composed of muscle ______ WR / ______ S

9. malignant tumor composed of fibrous tissue ______ WR / CV / ______ S

10. cancerous tumor of glandular tissue ______ WR / CV / ______ WR / ______ S

INCIDENTALOMA refers to a lesion that is discovered unexpectedly during diagnostic imaging and has nothing to do with the patient's symptoms or primary diagnosis. The most common organs involved are the adrenal glands; they may also be noted in the pituitary and thyroid glands, as well as the lungs, liver, kidneys, pancreas, and ovaries.

Oncology Terms

NOT BUILT FROM WORD PARTS

Though word parts may be present in terms categorized as NOT Built from Word Parts, their meanings are not clear from the definition of word parts. New knowledge may have changed the term's meaning, or the term may be from a Greek or Latin word not easily divided into parts. Others are eponyms, acronyms, modern language, and some have no apparent explanation for their names.

Medical terms NOT built from word parts cannot be easily translated to find their meanings. The terms are learned by memorizing the whole word and by using recall and spelling exercises.

TERM	DEFINITION
1. **benign** (be-NĪN)	not malignant, nonrecurrent, favorable for recovery (See Fig. 2.5)
2. **biological therapy** (bī-ō-LOJ-i-kel) (THER-a-pē)	treatment of cancer with biological response modifiers (BRM) that work with the immune system (also called **biotherapy** or **immunotherapy**) (Table 2.3)
3. **carcinoma in situ** (kar-si-NŌ-ma) (in) (SĪ-too)	cancer in the early stage before invading surrounding tissue (Fig. 2.4)
SITU is from the Latin term **situs**, which means **position** or **place**. Think of **in situ** as meaning "in place" or "not wandering around."	
4. **chemotherapy (chemo)** (kē-mō-THER-a-pē)	treatment of cancer with drugs
5. **encapsulated** (en-KAP-sū-lā-ted)	enclosed within a capsule, as with benign or malignant tumors that have not spread beyond the capsule of the organ in which it originated
6. **hospice** (HOS-pis)	provides palliative or supportive care for terminally ill patients and their families. Usually offered to those who have a prognosis of approximately 6 months or less, when curative forms of treatment are no longer possible or desired. A team-based approach delivers care in a variety of settings, most often in the patient's home.
7. **malignant** (ma-LIG-nant)	tending to become progressively worse and to cause death, as in cancer (Fig. 2.5)
8. **palliative** (PAL-ē-a-tiv)	providing relief but not cure. Symptom management is provided to relieve suffering in all stages of disease, and is not limited to care at the end of life. It can be given with curative or life-prolonging treatment, or with end-of-life (hospice) care. While hospice care includes palliative care, not all of palliative care is hospice care.

TERM	DEFINITION
9. radiation therapy (XRT) (*rā*-dē-Ā-shun) (THER-a-pē)	treatment of cancer with a radioactive substance, x-ray, or radiation (also called **radiation oncology** and **radiotherapy**)
10. remission (rē-MISH-un)	improvement or absence of signs of disease

TABLE 2.3 Cancer Therapies

THERAPY	DESCRIPTION
Neoadjuvant therapy	a cancer treatment that precedes other treatment, such as administering chemotherapy or radiation therapy to a patient before surgery.
Adjuvant chemotherapy	the use of chemotherapy after or in combination with another form of cancer treatment such as administering chemotherapy after surgery or with radiation therapy.
Brachytherapy 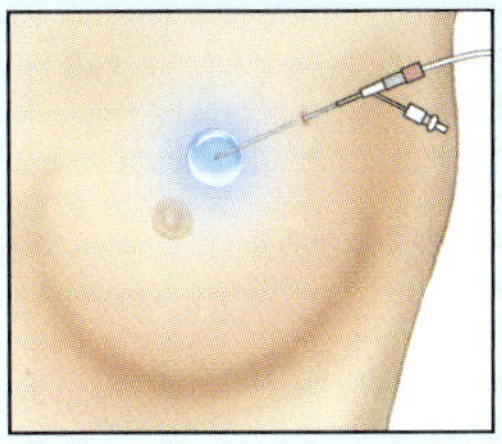	the use of radiotherapy, where the source of radiation is placed within or close to the area being treated, such as implantation of radiation sources into the breast to treat cancer (as shown in the illustration).
Biological therapy	the treatment of cancer with the use of man-made biological response modifiers (BRM) that occur naturally in the body. They alter the immune system's interaction with cancer cells to restore, direct, or boost the body's ability to fight disease. For example, an agent called **rituximab (Rituxan),** a monoclonal antibody, is used to treat some lymphomas. Other biological agents are **thalidomide,** which is used to treat multiple myeloma, and **interferon,** which is used in the treatment of lymphomas.

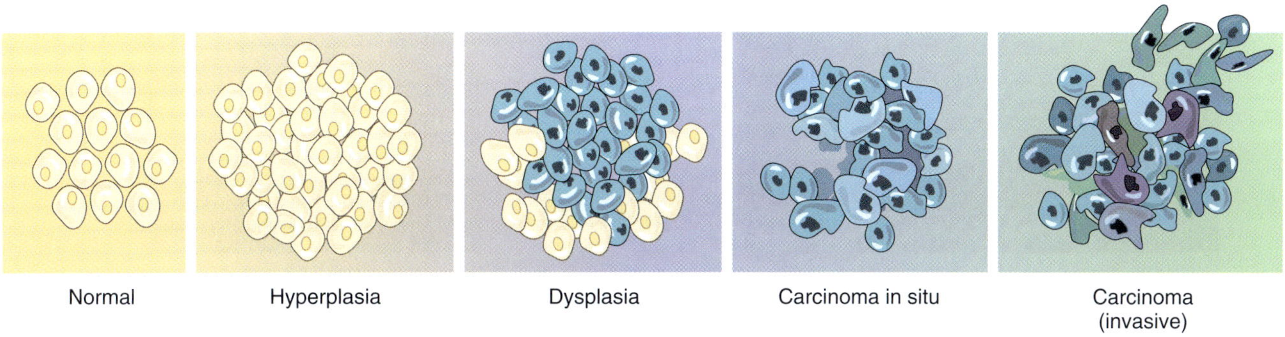

FIG. 2.4 Progression of cell growth.

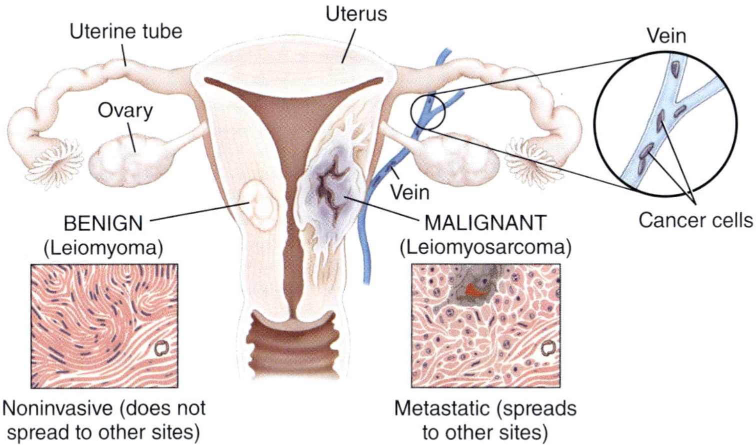

FIG. 2.5 Examples of benign and malignant tumors.

BENIGN AND MALIGNANT

Benign is derived from the Latin word root **bene**, meaning **well** or **good**, as used in **benefit** or **benefactor**. **Malignant** is derived from the Latin word root **mal** meaning **bad**, as used in **malicious**, **malaise**, **malady**, and **malign**.

EXERCISE 13 ■ Pronounce and Spell

Practice pronunciation and spelling on paper and online.

1. Practice on Paper

a. **Pronounce:** Read the phonetic spelling and say aloud the terms listed in the previous table. Refer to the pronunciation key on p. 20 as necessary.
b. **Spell:** Have a study partner read the terms aloud. Write the spelling of the terms on a separate sheet of paper.

2. Practice Online

a. **Access** online learning resources. Go to evolve.elsevier.com > Evolve Resources > Student Resources.
b. **Pronounce:** Select Audio Glossary > Chapter 2 > Exercise 13. Select a term to hear its pronunciation and repeat aloud.
c. **Spell:** Select Activities > Chapter 2 > Spell Terms > Exercise 13. Select the audio icon and type the correct spelling of the term.

❑ Check the box when complete.

EXERCISE 14 ■ Fill In

A Label

Write the medical terms pictured and defined. *To check your answers, go to Appendix A at the back of the textbook.*

1. ______________________
enclosed within a capsule

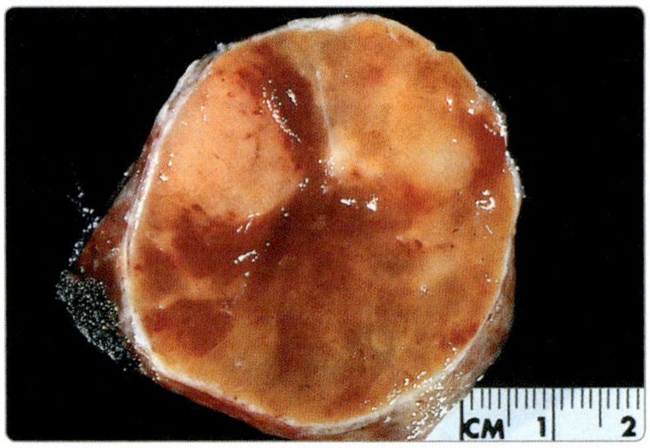

2. ______________________
treatment of cancer with a radioactive substance, x-ray, or radiation

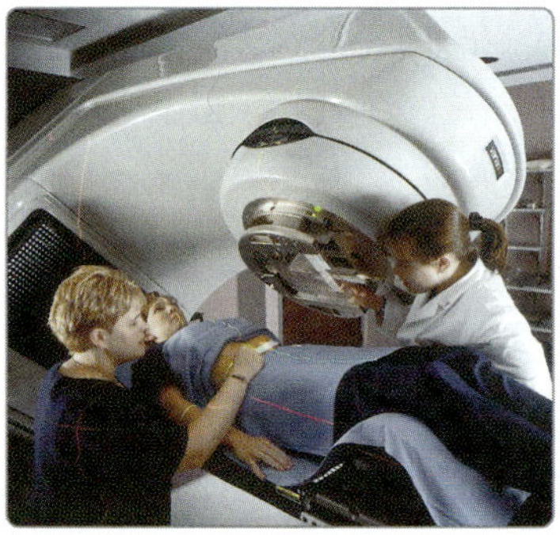

3. ______________________
not malignant, nonrecurrent, favorable for recovery

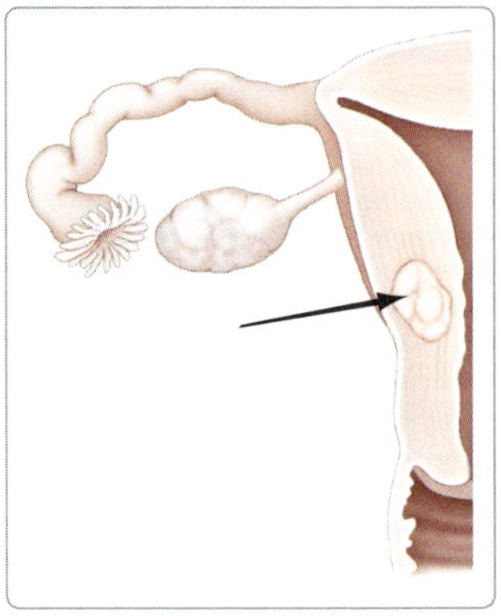

4. ______________________
tending to become progressively worse and to cause death

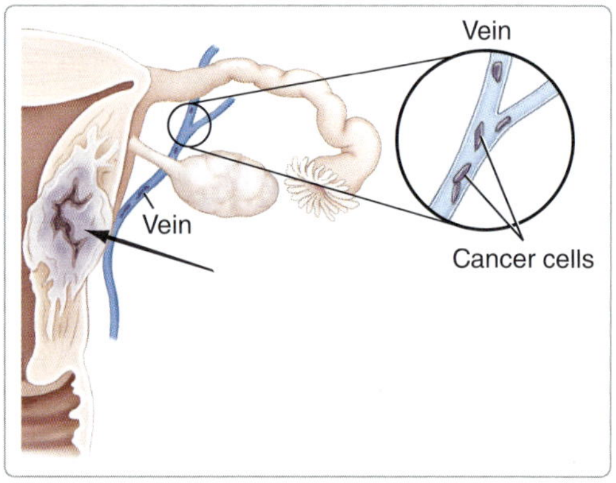

5. ______________________
treatment of cancer with drugs

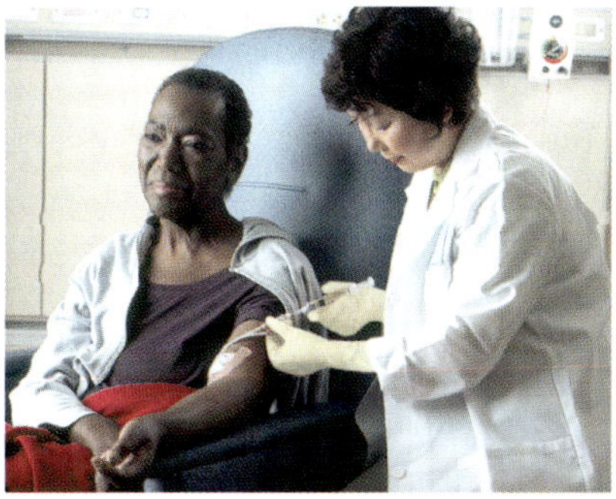

6. ______________________
cancer in the early stage before invading surrounding tissue

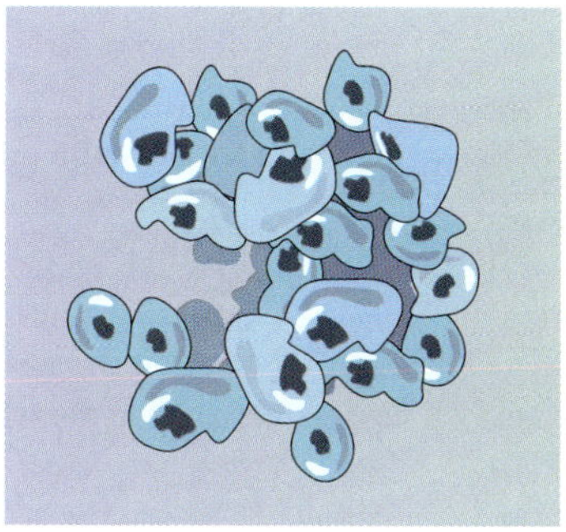

B Identify

Fill in the blanks with the correct terms.

1. **Treatment of cancer with agents that work with the immune system** ______________________ may be used to treat diseases such as lymphoma and myeloma.
2. **Providing relief but not cure** ______________ care may be used at any time during the course of a disease.
3. **Improvement or absence of signs of disease** ______________________ may last from days to years, or may not occur at all.
4. Although frequently associated with end-of-life treatment for cancer patients, **provides palliative or supportive care for terminally ill patients and their families** ______________________ can be offered to a person with any type of disease that has a life expectancy of 6 months or less.

C Match

Match the terms in the first column with their correct definitions in the second column.

__h__ 1. malignant	a. provides palliative or supportive care for terminally ill patients and their families
__i__ 2. remission	b. not malignant, nonrecurrent, favorable for recovery
__g__ 3. carcinoma in situ	c. enclosed within a capsule
__b__ 4. benign	d. providing relief but not cure
__d__ 5. hospice	e. treatment of cancer with drugs
__j__ 6. radiation therapy	f. treatment of cancer with biological response modifiers (BRM) that work with the immune systems
__c__ 7. encapsulated	g. cancer in the early stage before invading surrounding tissue
__d__ 8. palliative	h. tending to become progressively worse and to cause death, as in cancer
__e__ 9. chemotherapy	i. improvement or absence of signs of disease
__f__ 10. biological therapy	j. treatment of cancer with a radioactive substance, x-ray, or radiation

EXERCISE 15 ■ Review of Oncology Terms

Can you define, pronounce, and spell the following oncology terms?

adenocarcinoma	epithelioma	malignant	palliative
adenoma	fibroma	melanocarcinoma	radiation therapy (XRT)
benign	fibrosarcoma	melanoma	remission
biological therapy	hospice	myoma	rhabdomyoma
carcinoma (CA)	leiomyoma	metastasis (*pl.* metastases) (METS)	rhabdomyosarcoma
carcinoma in situ	leiomyosarcoma	neoplasm	sarcoma
chemotherapy (chemo)	lipoma	neuroma	
encapsulated	liposarcoma		

Refer to Appendix E for pharmacology terms related to oncology.

Laboratory Tests

Laboratory tests are performed to establish a diagnosis and/or prognosis, and to monitor and evaluate treatment. Specimens that are studied include blood (most common), urine, stool, sputum, sweat, and wound drainage or discharge from body openings, washings, and tissue. General categories are hematology studies, blood chemistry studies, urine studies, and microbiology studies (See Table 2.4). Diagnostic laboratories, or labs, are located in hospitals, provider's offices, and in stand-alone facilities. These physical labs are divided into sections according to specialization, such as cytology for the study of cells.

The abbreviation **lab**, short for laboratory, can refer to the physical location of the laboratory where specimens are analyzed and for the resulting report providing information on findings.

TABLE 2.4 Types of Laboratory Tests

Hematology studies relate to the physical properties of blood, such as the number of blood cells in the specimen or the clotting and bleeding factors.

Blood chemistry studies measure the amount of certain substances in the body, including electrolytes (such as sodium, potassium, and chloride), fats, proteins, glucose (sugar), and enzymes.

Urine studies are performed on urine specimens to diagnose and monitor urinary tract disease. They are also used to detect and monitor diseases related to the kidney, such as diabetic nephropathy, kidney stones, or lupus.

Microbiology studies identify the microorganisms that cause disease and infection, and can be divided into traditional and modern methods.

Traditional microbiology studies include:

Culture and sensitivity, a common study performed on almost any specimen. Other microbiology studies include **staining and microscopy** (looking at a sample under a microscope after applying a stain that highlights the suspected microorganism), and **biochemical testing** (using enzymes or other compounds that will cause reactions in a specific pathogen).

Modern microbiology studies include:

Polymerase chain reactions (PCR) work with tiny amounts of DNA from an unknown pathogen in a sample and match it against the DNA of known pathogens, including viruses, bacteria, and parasites. This can be done very quickly (within hours) compared to cultures, which can take days to weeks.

Serology tests depend on antibody/antigen reactions. Antibodies are substances produced by a person's immune system to help defend against infection. Antigens are substances produced by microorganisms that can trigger an immune response in the body. Serology tests are especially helpful for microorganisms that cannot be cultured, including the bacteria that cause syphilis.

Laboratory Terms

BUILT FROM WORD PARTS AND *NOT* BUILT FROM WORD PARTS

The first portion of the table contains laboratory terms that can be translated using definitions of word parts. The second portion of the table contains laboratory terms that cannot be fully understood using the definitions of word parts.

Built from Word Parts

TERM	DEFINITION
1. **autopsy** (AW-top-sē)	view of self (postmortem examination to determine the cause of death or obtain evidence)
2. **biopsy (Bx)** (BĪ-op-sē)	view of life (the removal of living tissue from the body to be viewed under the microscope)
3. **cytopathology** (*sī*-tō-pa-THOL-o-jē)	study of (changes in) cells in disease
4. **hematology** (hē-ma-TOL-o-jē)	study of blood (branch of medicine that deals with diseases of the blood)
5. **histopathology** (his-to-pa-THOL-o-jē)	study of tissue in disease (study of tissue samples taken from patients)
6. **microbiology** (*mī*-krō-bī-OL-o-jē)	study of small life (study of microorganisms, such as bacteria, fungi, viruses and parasites)
7. **pathology** (pa-THOL-o-jē)	study of disease (a branch of medicine dealing with the study of the causes of disease and death)
8. **virology** (vi-ROL-o-jē)	study of viruses (branch of microbiology that is concerned with viruses and viral diseases)

NOT Built from Word Parts

TERM	DEFINITION
1. **chemistry panel** (KEM-is-trē) (PAN-el)	a series of tests performed on a blood sample that give information regarding multiple systems including the kidneys, liver, and lungs; these also provide glucose and protein levels. (also called **comprehensive metabolic panel**)
2. **complete blood count with differential (CBC with diff)** (com-PLĒT) (blud) (kownt) (with) (dif-er-EN-shal)	laboratory test for basic blood screening that measures various aspects of erythrocytes (red blood cells), leukocytes (white blood cells), and thrombocytes (platelets); this automated test quickly provides a tremendous amount of information about the blood.
3. **culture and sensitivity (C&S)** (KUL-cher) (and) (sen-si-TIV-i-tē)	test performed on a sample to determine the presence of pathogenic bacteria. The specimen is placed on a medium for growth (culture) and if pathogenic bacteria grow, is then tested for antibiotic sensitivity to identify an antibiotic that will provide the most effective treatment. C&S is used to identify the pathogen present and causing the infection.
4. **genetic testing** (je-NET-ik) (TEST-ing)	examines DNA, the chemical database that carries instructions for the body's functions; can reveal changes in genes that may cause illness or disease.
5. **specimen** (SPES-i-men)	sample of blood, urine, or body tissue that is taken for medical testing (also called **collection sample**)

EXERCISE 16 ■ Pronounce and Spell

Practice pronunciation and spelling on paper and online.

1. Practice on Paper

a. **Pronounce:** Read the phonetic spelling and say aloud the terms listed in the previous table. Refer to the pronunciation key on p. 20 as necessary.
b. **Spell:** Have a study partner read the terms aloud. Write the spelling of the terms on a separate sheet of paper.

2. Practice Online

a. **Access** online learning resources. Go to evolve.elsevier.com > Evolve Resources > Student Resources.
b. **Pronounce:** Select Audio Glossary > Chapter 2 > Exercise 16. Select a term to hear its pronunciation and repeat aloud.
c. **Spell:** Select Activities > Chapter 2 > Spell Terms > Exercise 16. Select the audio icon and type the correct spelling of the term.

❑ Check the box when complete.

EXERCISE 17 ■ Laboratory Terms Built from Word Parts

A Analyze and Define

Analyze and define the following laboratory terms by drawing slashes between word parts, writing word part abbreviations above the term, underlining combining forms, and writing combining form abbreviations below the term. *To check your answers, go to Appendix A.*

WR CV S
EXAMPLE: hemat / o / logy
CF
study of blood

1. cytopathology
____
____

2. histopathology
____
____

3. virology
____
____

4. microbiology
____
____

5. autopsy
____
____

6. biopsy
____
____

B Fill In

Build laboratory terms for the following definitions by using the word parts you have learned.

1. study of tissue in disease ______ / ______ / ______ / ______ / ______
WR / CV / WR / CV / S

2. study of viruses

_____ / _____ / _____
WR / CV / S

3. study of (changes in) cells in disease

_____ / _____ / _____ / _____ / _____
WR / CV / WR / CV / S

C Label

Build terms pictured by writing word parts above the definitions.

1.

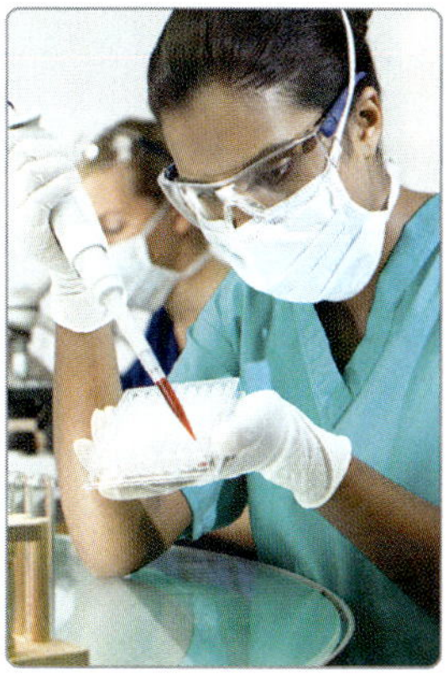

_____ / _____ / _____
blood / CV / study of

2.

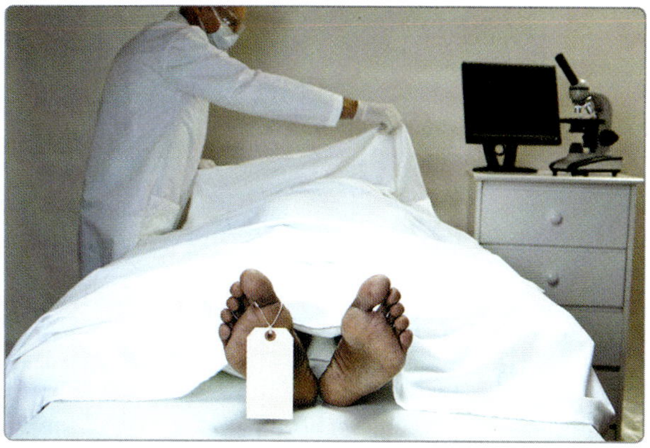

_____ / _____
self / view

3.

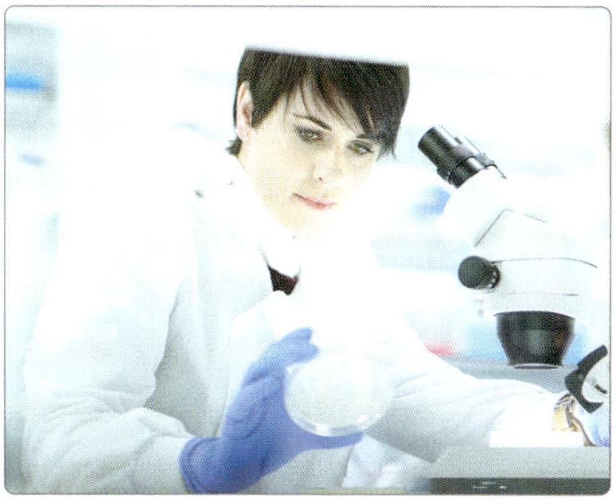

_____ / _____ / _____
small life / CV / study of

4.

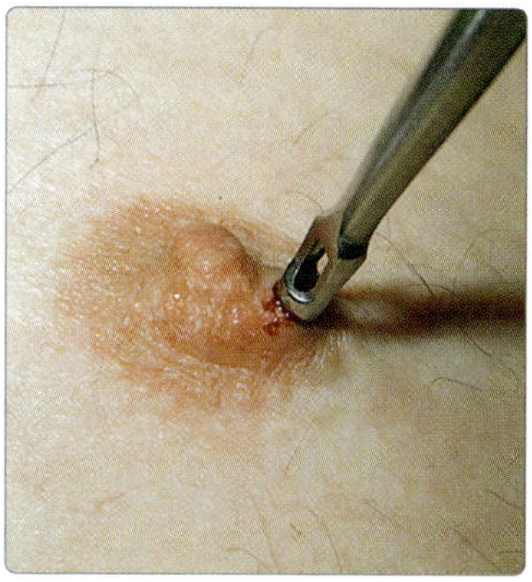

_____ / _____
life / view

EXERCISE 18 ■ Laboratory Terms NOT Built from Word Parts

A Identify

Fill in the blanks with the correct terms.

1. A test that examines DNA, the chemical database that carries instructions for the body's functions, is known as _____________________.

2. _____________________ is a series of tests performed on a blood sample that gives information regarding multiple systems including the kidneys, liver, and lungs.

3. A laboratory test for basic blood screening that measures various aspects of erythrocytes, leukocytes, and thrombocytes is a ______________________________

4. ______________________ is also called a collection sample.

5. The test that places a specimen on a growth medium to check for bacteria and determine the most effective antibiotic is called ______________________ and ______________________.

B Label

Write the medical terms pictured and defined.

1. ______________________________
sample of blood, urine, or body tissue that is taken for medical testing

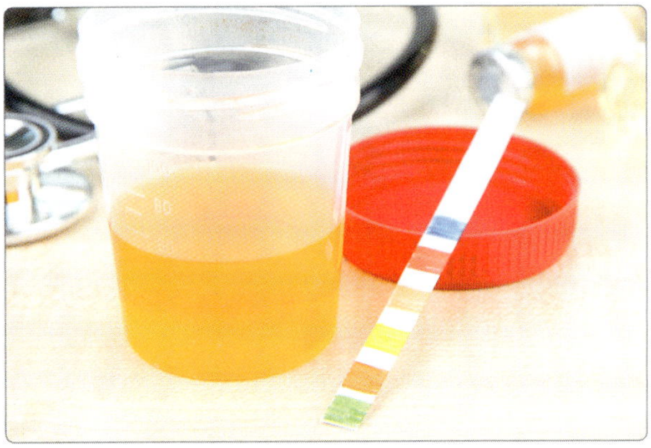

2. ______________________________
series of tests performed on a blood sample that gives information regarding multiple systems

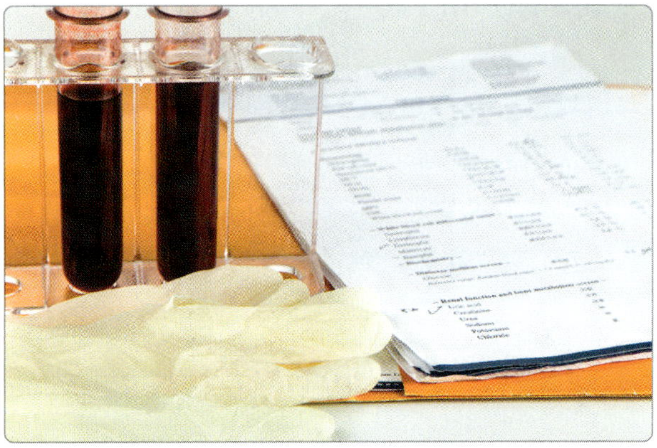

3. ______________________________
can reveal changes in DNA that may cause illness or disease

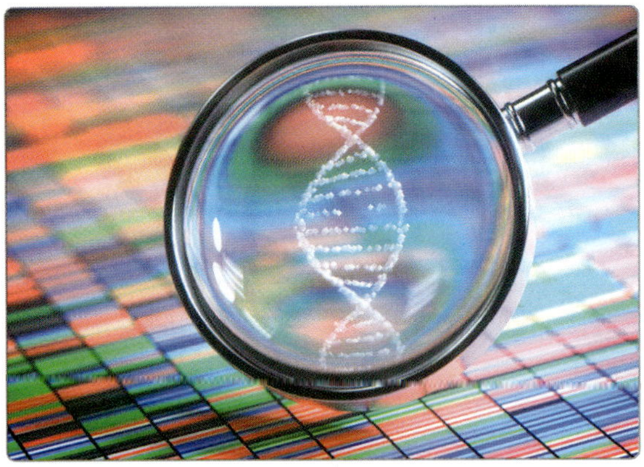

4. ______________________________
test performed on a sample to determine the presence of pathogenic bacteria

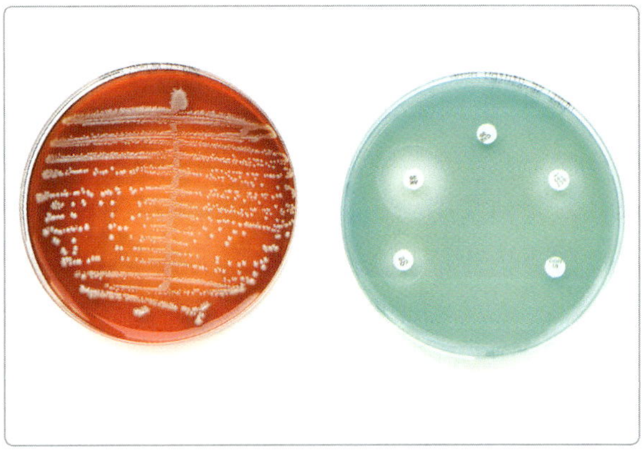

EXERCISE 19 ■ Review of Laboratory Terms

Can you define, pronounce, and spell the following laboratory terms?

autopsy
biopsy (Bx)
chemistry panel
complete blood count with differential (CBC with diff)
culture and sensitivity (C&S)
cytopathology
genetic testing
hematology
histopathology
microbiology
specimen
virology

Complementary Terms

Complementary terms complete the vocabulary presented in the chapter by describing signs, symptoms, medical specialties, specialists, and related words. A **sign** is objective information and is detected on physical examination such as observation that the patient has cyanosis of the nail beds. A **symptom** is subjective and is evidence of disease perceived by the patient, such as stating the feeling of pain in the chest while walking.

Built from Word Parts

The following terms can be translated using definitions of word parts. Further explanation is provided within parentheses as needed.

SIGNS & SYMPTOMS

TERM	DEFINITION	TERM	DEFINITION
1. **cyanosis** (*sī*-a-NŌ-sis)	abnormal condition of blue (bluish discoloration, especially of the skin, caused by inadequate supply of oxygen in the blood)	2. **xanthosis** (zan-THŌ-sis)	abnormal condition of yellow (discoloration)

MEDICAL SPECIALTIES AND PROFESSIONS

TERM	DEFINITION	TERM	DEFINITION
3. **oncologist** (ong-KOL-o-jist)	physician who studies and treats (malignant) tumors	5. **pathologist** (pa-THOL-o-jist)	physician who studies diseases (examines biopsies and performs autopsies to determine the cause of disease or death)
4. **oncology** (ong-KOL-o-jē)	study of tumors (a branch of medicine concerned with the study of malignant tumors)	6. **pathology** (pa-THOL-o-jē)	study of disease (a branch of medicine dealing with the study of the causes of disease and death)

DESCRIPTIVE TERMS

TERM	DEFINITION	TERM	DEFINITION
7. **cancerous** (KAN-ser-us)	pertaining to cancer	13. **iatrogenic** (ī-*at*-rō-JEN-ik)	produced by a physician (the unexpected results from a treatment prescribed by a physician)
8. **carcinogen** (kar-SIN-o-jen)	substance that causes cancer	14. **oncogenic** (*ong*-kō-JEN-ik)	causing tumors
9. **carcinogenic** (*kar*-sin-ō-JEN-ik)	producing cancer	15. **pathogenic** (path-ō-JEN-ik)	producing disease
10. **carcinoid** (KAR-si-noyd)	resembling cancer	16. **prognosis (Px)** (prog-NŌ-sis)	state of before knowledge (prediction of the outcome of disease based on the patient's signs, symptoms, and test results)
11. **diagnosis (Dx)** (*dī*-ag-NŌ-sis)	state of complete knowledge (the art of identifying a disease based on the patient's signs, symptoms, and test results)		
12. **etiology** (*ē*-tē-OL-o-jē)	study of causes (of diseases)		

PROGNOSIS was used by Hippocrates to mean the same then as now: **to foretell the course of a disease**.

EXERCISE 20 ■ Pronounce and Spell

Practice pronunciation and spelling on paper and online.

1. Practice on Paper

a. **Pronounce:** Read the phonetic spelling and say aloud the terms listed in the previous table. Refer to the pronunciation key on p. 20 as necessary.
b. **Spell:** Have a study partner read the terms aloud. Write the spelling of the terms on a separate sheet of paper.

2. Practice Online

a. **Access** online learning resources. Go to evolve.elsevier.com > Evolve Resources > Student Resources.
b. **Pronounce:** Select Audio Glossary > Chapter 2 > Exercise 20. Select a term to hear its pronunciation and repeat aloud.
c. **Spell:** Select Activities > Chapter 2 > Spell Terms > Exercise 20. Select the audio icon and type the correct spelling of the term.

❑ Check the box when complete.

EXERCISE 21 ■ Analyze and Define

Analyze and define the following complementary terms by drawing slashes between word parts, writing word part abbreviations above the term, underlining combining forms, and writing combining form abbreviations below the term. *To check your answers, go to Appendix A at the back of the textbook.*

EXAMPLE:

WR CV S
path / o / genic
CF
producing disease

1. pathology

____
____

2. pathologist

____
____

3. diagnosis

____
____

4. oncogenic

____
____

5. oncology

____
____

6. cancerous

____
____

7. carcinogenic

____
____

8. cyanosis

____
____

9. etiology

____
____

10. xanthosis

____
____

11. carcinoid

____
____

12. carcinogen

____
____

13. oncologist

____
____

14. prognosis

____
____

EXERCISE 22 ■ Build

A Label

Build terms pictured by writing word parts above the definitions.

1.

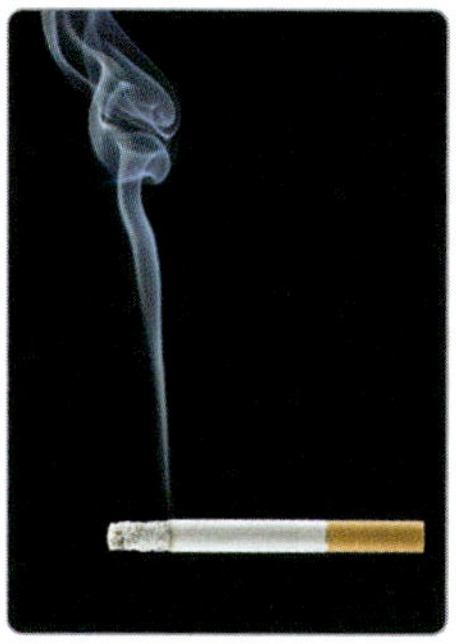

_______ / _____ / _______
cancer / CV / substance that causes

2.

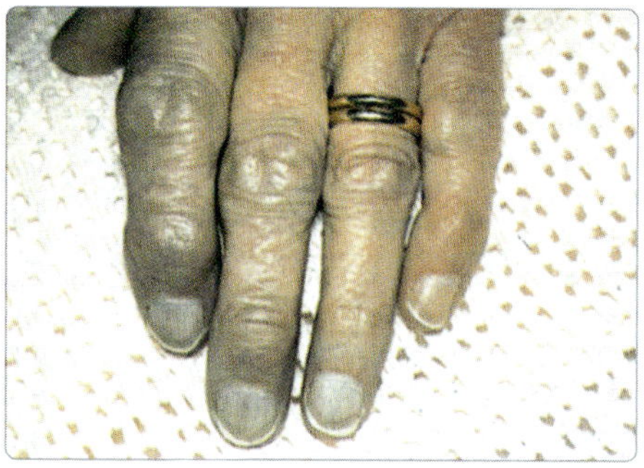

_______ / _______
blue / abnormal condition

3.

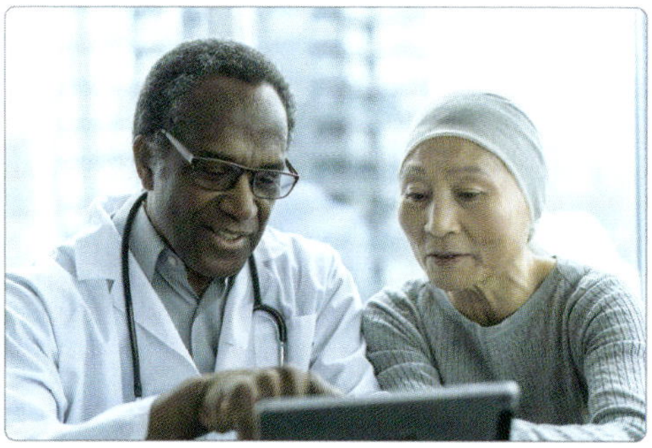

_______ / _____ / _______
(malignant) tumors / CV / physician who studies

4.

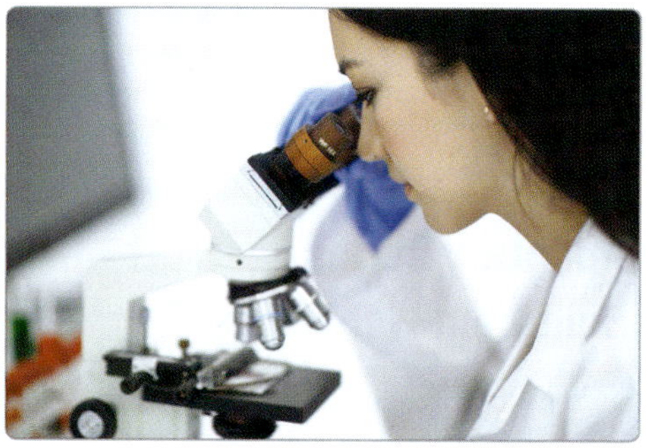

_______ / _____ / _______
diseases / CV / physician who studies

B Fill In

Build complementary terms for the following definitions by using the word parts you have learned.

EXAMPLE: producing disease path / o / genic (WR / CV / S)

1. state of complete knowledge ____ P / ____ WR / ____ S
2. produced by a physician ____ WR / ____ CV / ____ S
3. study of causes (of diseases) ____ WR / ____ CV / ____ S
4. study of tumors ____ WR / ____ CV / ____ S
5. study of disease ____ WR / ____ CV / ____ S
6. producing cancer ____ WR / ____ CV / ____ S
7. abnormal condition of yellow ____ WR / ____ S
8. causing tumors ____ WR / ____ CV / ____ S
9. pertaining to cancer ____ WR / ____ S
10. state of before knowledge ____ P / ____ WR / ____ S

Complementary Terms

■ *NOT* Built from Word Parts

Word parts may be present in the following terms; however, their full meanings cannot be translated using definitions of word parts alone.

SIGNS & SYMPTOMS

TERM	DEFINITION
1. afebrile (ā-FEB-ril)	without fever
2. erythema (*er*-i-THĒ-ma)	redness
3. febrile (FEB-ril)	having a fever
4. inflammation (in-fla-MĀ-shun)	localized protective response to injury or tissue destruction characterized by redness, swelling, heat, and pain

DESCRIPTIVE TERMS

TERM	DEFINITION	TERM	DEFINITION
5. exacerbation (eg-zas-er-BĀ-shun)	increase in the severity of a disease or its symptoms	**7. morbidity** (mor-BID-i-tē)	state of being diseased; incidence of illness in a population
6. idiopathic (id-ē-ō-PATH-ik)	pertaining to disease of unknown origin	**8. mortality** (mor-TAL-i-tē)	state of being mortal (death); incidence of the number of deaths in a population

OTHER TERMS

TERM	DEFINITION
9. bacteria (*s.* bacterium) (bak-TĒR-ē-a) (bak-TĒR-ē-um)	single-celled microorganisms that reproduce by cell division and may cause infection by invading body tissue
10. fungus (*pl.* fungi) (FUN-gus) (FUN-jī)	organism that feeds by absorbing organic molecules from its surroundings and may cause infection by invading body tissue; single-celled fungi (yeast) reproduce by budding; multi-celled fungi (mold) reproduce by spore formation
11. infection (in-FEK-shun)	invasion of pathogens in body tissue. Types of infection include bacterial, viral, and fungal. An **acute** infection may remain localized if the body's defense mechanisms are effective or may persist to become **subacute** or **chronic**. A **systemic** infection occurs when the pathogen causing a local infection gains access to the vascular or lymphatic system and becomes disseminated throughout the body.
12. microorganism (mī-krō-OR-gan-iz-um)	a form of life that is too small to be seen without a microscope; includes bacteria, fungi, and viruses
13. virus (*pl.* viruses) (VĪ-ras) (VĪ-ras-uz)	minute microorganism, much smaller than a bacterium, characterized by a lack of independent metabolism and the ability to replicate only within living host cells; these may cause infection by invading body tissue.

EXERCISE 23 ■ Pronounce and Spell

Practice pronunciation and spelling on paper and online.

1. Practice on Paper

a. **Pronounce:** Read the phonetic spelling and say aloud the terms listed in the previous table. Refer to the pronunciation key on p. 20 as necessary.
b. **Spell:** Have a study partner read the terms aloud. Write the spelling of the terms on a separate sheet of paper.

2. Practice Online

a. **Access** online learning resources. Go to evolve.elsevier.com > Evolve Resources > Student Resources.
b. **Pronounce:** Select Audio Glossary > Chapter 2 > Exercise 23. Select a term to hear its pronunciation and repeat aloud.
c. **Spell:** Select Activities > Chapter 2 > Spell Terms > Exercise 23. Select the audio icon and type the correct spelling of the term.

❑ Check the box when complete.

EXERCISE 24 ■ Fill In

A Label

Write the medical terms pictured and defined. *To check your answers, go to Appendix A at the back of the textbook.*

1. ______________________________
having a fever

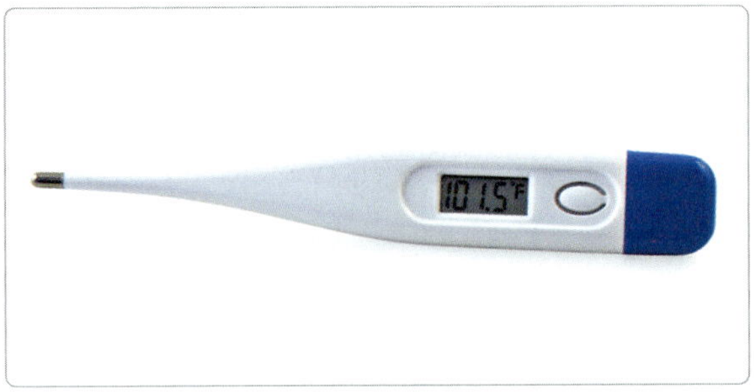

2. ______________________________
minute microorganism characterized by a lack of independent metabolism

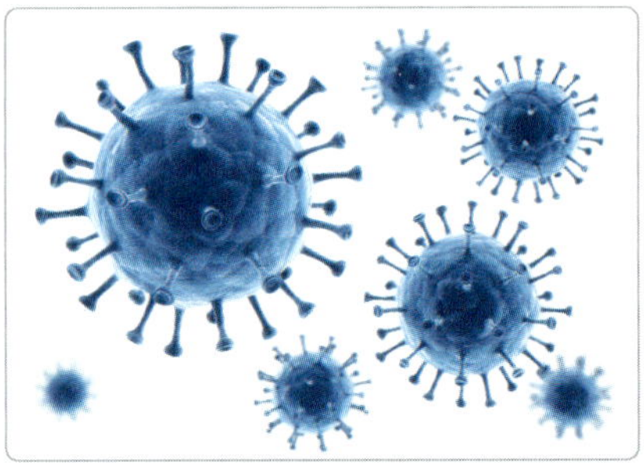

3. ______________________________
localized protective response characterized by redness, swelling, heat, and pain

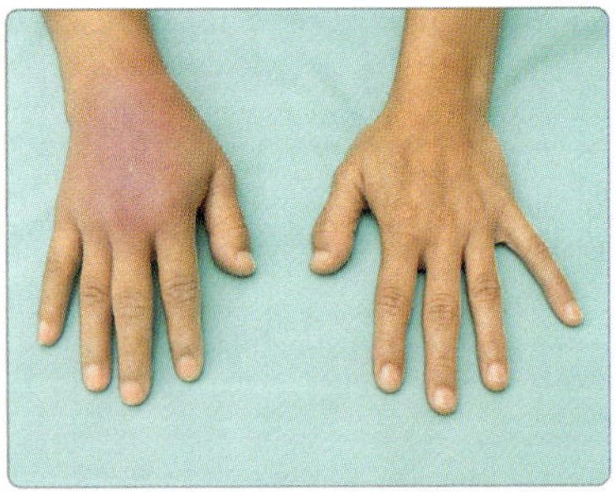

4. ______________________________
single-celled microorganisms that reproduce by cell division and may cause infection by invading body tissue

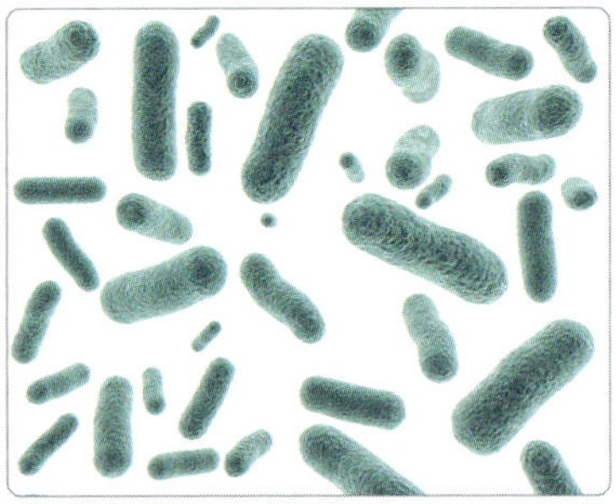

B Identify

Write the definitions for the following terms.

1. morbidity ______________________________
2. fungus ______________________________
3. afebrile ______________________________
4. microorganism ______________________________
5. erythema ______________________________
6. infection ______________________________
7. mortality ______________________________
8. idiopathic ______________________________
9. exacerbation ______________________________

EXERCISE 25 ■ Match

A

Match the complementary terms in the first column with the correct definitions in the second column.

_____ 1. inflammation
_____ 2. morbidity
_____ 3. bacteria
_____ 4. microorganism
_____ 5. exacerbation
_____ 6. febrile
_____ 7. fungus

a. single-celled microorganisms that reproduce by cell division and may cause infection by invading body tissue
b. increase in the severity of a disease or its symptoms
c. a form of life that is too small to be seen without a microscope; includes bacteria, fungi, and viruses.
d. having a fever
e. state of being diseased; incidence of illness in a population
f. localized protective response to injury or tissue destruction characterized by redness, swelling, heat, and pain
g. organism that feeds by absorbing organic molecules from its surroundings; may be single-celled or multi-celled.

B

Match the complementary terms in the first column with the correct definitions in the second column.

_____ 1. infection
_____ 2. erythema
_____ 3. mortality
_____ 4. afebrile
_____ 5. idiopathic
_____ 6. virus

a. pertaining to disease of unknown origin
b. minute microorganism, characterized by a lack of independent metabolism and the ability to replicate only within living host cells
c. without fever
d. redness
e. state of being mortal (death); incidence of the number of deaths in a population
f. invasion of pathogens in body tissue

EXERCISE 26 ■ Review of Complementary Terms

Can you define, pronounce, and spell the following complementary terms?

afebrile	erythema	inflammation	oncology
bacteria (*s.* bacterium)	etiology	infection	pathogenic
cancerous	exacerbation	microorganism	pathologist
carcinogen	febrile	morbidity	pathology
carcinogenic	fungus (*pl.* fungi)	mortality	prognosis (Px)
carcinoid	iatrogenic	oncogenic	virus (*pl.* viruses)
cyanosis	idiopathic	oncologist	xanthosis
diagnosis (Dx)			

Plural Endings for Medical Terms

In the English language plurals are formed by simply adding an "s" or "es" to the end of a word. For example, hand becomes plural by adding an "s" to form hands. Likewise, box becomes boxes by adding "es." In the language of medicine, many terms have Latin or Greek suffixes, and forming plurals for these terms is not quite as easy. Table 2.5, Common Plural Endings for Medical Terms, lists the most common singular and plural endings used in medical terminology. When appropriate, both singular and plural endings are included in the word lists throughout the text, such as metastasis/metastases.

TABLE 2.5 Common Plural Endings for Medical Terms

SINGULAR ENDINGS	SINGULAR FORMS		PLURAL ENDINGS	PLURAL FORMS	
-a	vertebr**a**	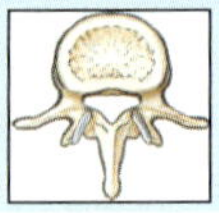	-ae	vertebr**ae**	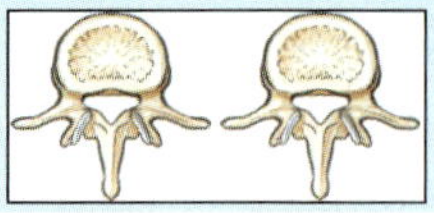
-ax	thor**ax**	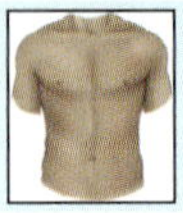	-aces	thor**aces**	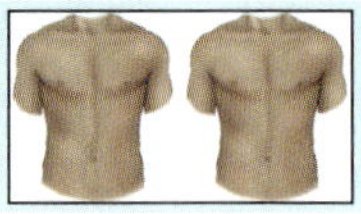
-is	test**is**	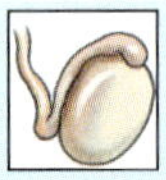	-es	test**es**	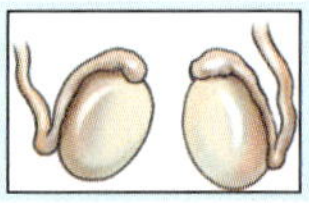
-ix	append**ix**	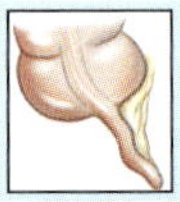	-ices	append**ices**	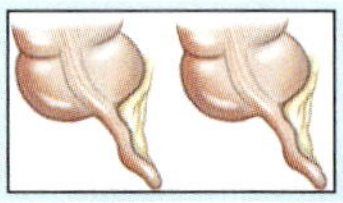
-ma	carcino**ma**	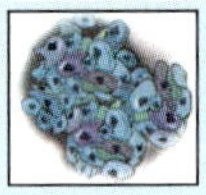	-mata	carcino**mata**	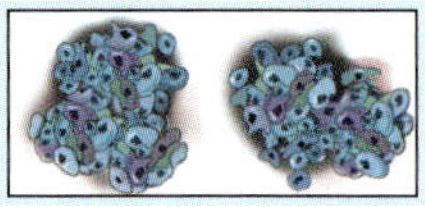
-nx	lary**nx**	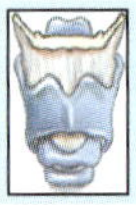	-nges	lary**nges**	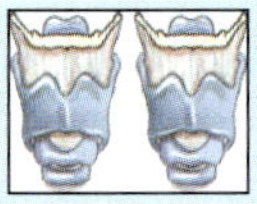
-on	gangli**on**	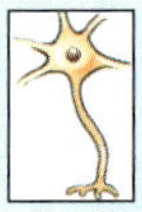	-a	gangli**a**	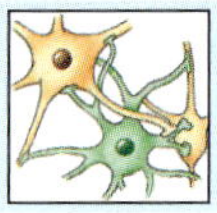
-sis	metasta**sis**	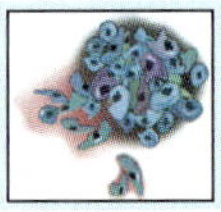	-ses	metasta**ses**	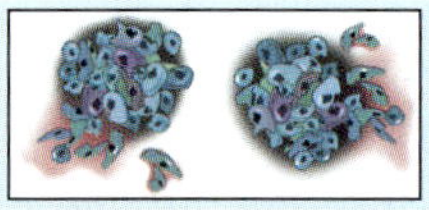
-um	ov**um**	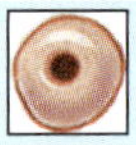	-a	ov**a**	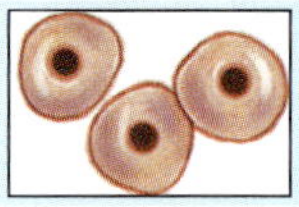
-us	fung**us**	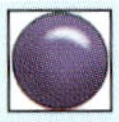	-i	fung**i**	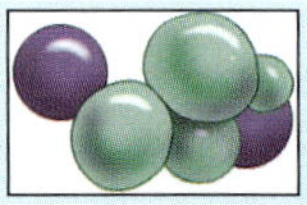
-y	biops**y**	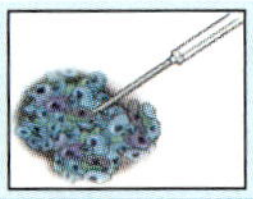	-ies	biops**ies**	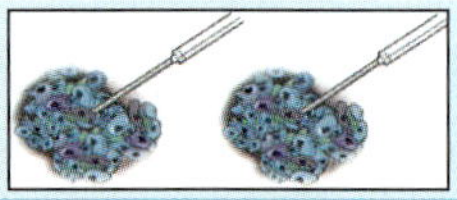

Because of common usage, some plural forms of medical terms will add an "s" rather than use Greek or Latin plural endings. **Carcinomas** rather than **carcinomata** is frequently seen in medical literature.

EXERCISE 27 ■ Plural Endings

Convert each of the following terms from singular to plural. Refer to Table 2.5 for guidance. Do not be concerned about the meaning of these terms; concentrate only on the plural endings. *To check your answers, go to Appendix A.*

1. etiology ______________________
2. staphylococcus ______________________
3. cyanosis ______________________
4. bacterium ______________________
5. nucleus ______________________
6. pharynx ______________________
7. sarcoma ______________________
8. carcinoma ______________________
9. anastomosis ______________________
10. pubis ______________________
11. prognosis ______________________
12. spermatozoon ______________________
13. fimbria ______________________
14. thorax ______________________
15. appendix ______________________

EXERCISE 28 ■ Identify

Circle the correct singular or plural form in each sentence.

1. During a colonoscopy the gastroenterologist noted that the patient had several (**diverticula, diverticulum**) in his transverse colon.
2. Bronchogenic carcinoma was diagnosed in the patient's left (**bronchus, bronchi**).
3. Bilateral (two sides) orchiditis is inflammation of the (**testes, testis**).
4. The light brown mole with notched borders turned out to be a (**melanomata, melanoma**).
5. Multiple (**embolus, emboli**) were observed on the lung scan.
6. Many (**diagnosis, diagnoses**) of benign tumors are picked up during whole-body scanning.
7. Diagnostic studies have shown (**metastasis, metastases**) of the patient's carcinoma of the breast to both her lungs and brain.

Abbreviations

Abbreviations are frequently used verbally and in writing to communicate in the medical and healthcare setting. Abbreviations that are easily misinterpreted and may lead to medication errors are reported to the Institute for Safe Medication Practices. See **Appendix D** for The Joint Commission's "Do Not Use" list of abbreviations. Abbreviations of the terms included in the chapter are listed in the following table.

BODY STRUCTURE

ABBREVIATION	TERM	ABBREVIATION	TERM
RBC	red blood cell (erythrocyte)	**WBC**	white blood cell (leukocyte)

ONCOLOGY

ABBREVIATION	TERM	ABBREVIATION	TERM
CA	carcinoma	**METS**	metastases

LABORATORY

ABBREVIATION	TERM	ABBREVIATION	TERM
Bx	biopsy	**C&S**	culture and sensitivity
CBC with diff	complete blood count with differential		

TREATMENTS

ABBREVIATION	TERM	ABBREVIATION	TERM
chemo	chemotherapy	**XRT**	radiation therapy

DESCRIPTIVE

ABBREVIATION	TERM	ABBREVIATION	TERM
Dx	diagnosis	**Px**	prognosis

EXERCISE 29 ■ Abbreviations

Write the term for each of the abbreviations in the following paragraph.

A 55-year-old woman was admitted to the oncology unit after a **Bx** ______________ revealed a **Dx** ______________ of **CA** ______________. She was noted to have **METS** ______________ to the lungs and brain. Her **Px** ______________ was guarded. Laboratory tests, including **RBC** ______________ ______________ ______________ and **WBC** ______________ ______________ ______________ counts, were ordered. She will receive both **chemo** ______________ and **XRT** ______________ ______________. Her **CBC with diff** ______________ ______________ ______________ with ______________ will be monitored to check for any signs of bone marrow suppression. **C&S** ______________ and ______________ will be obtained if she develops any signs of infection.

PRACTICAL APPLICATION

EXERCISE 30 ■ Case Study: Translate Between Everyday Language and Medical Language

CASE STUDY: Tova Smelkinson

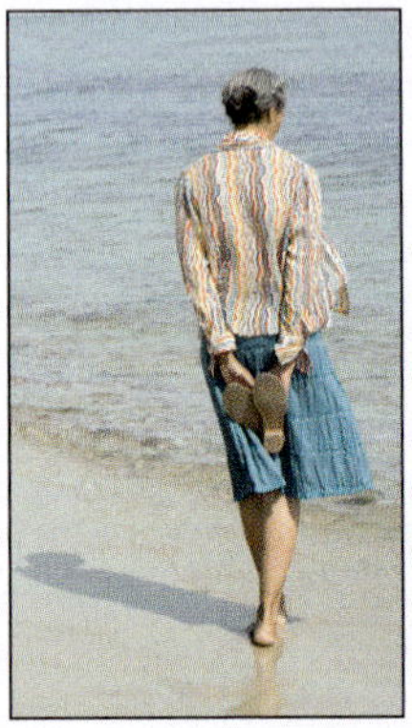

Tova has been having diarrhea. Even worse, she notices blood in it. She had this before when she was younger—and the disease was identified—but she couldn't remember the name. She recalls it was not a cancerous tumor and noted she did not have a fever. She was put on medicine and got better. It looked like a positive outcome. Now it's been going on for 3 weeks. She has pain in her belly with cramps and feels kind of full all the time. She notices she is losing weight, even though she isn't trying. She also feels more tired than usual. Tova makes an appointment with her family doctor to see if she needs to go back on medicine.

Now that you have worked through Chapter 2 on body structure, color, and oncology consider the medical terms that might be used to describe Tova's experience. See the Chapter at a Glance at the end of the chapter for a list of terms that might apply.

A. *Underline phrases in the case study that could be substituted with medical terms.*

B. *Write the medical term and its definition for three of the phrases you underlined.*

MEDICAL TERM	DEFINITION
1. ____________________	____________________
2. ____________________	____________________
3. ____________________	____________________

DOCUMENTATION: Excerpt from Clinical Notation

Tova was able to see her family doctor. The following is a portion of what was noted in her clinical electronic health record (EHR):

A 54-year-old woman presented to the office with 3-week history of bloody diarrhea. She had been diagnosed with ulcerative colitis at the age of 25 years. She was referred for a colonoscopy. The examination revealed a suspicious lesion on the transverse colon. A biopsy was performed and a cytology specimen was obtained. Advanced dysplasia and inflammation were present. The pathologist made a diagnosis of carcinoma of the colon.

C. *Underline medical terms presented in Chapter 2 in the previous excerpt from Tova's medical record (EHR).*

D. *Select and define three of the medical terms you underlined.*

MEDICAL TERM	DEFINITION
1. ____________________	____________________
2. ____________________	____________________
3. ____________________	____________________

EXERCISE 31 ■ Interact with Medical Documents

A

Read the report and complete it by writing medical terms on answer lines within the document. Definitions of terms to be written appear after the document.

830293-ONC GREELEY, Morris

File Patient Navigate Custom Fields Help

Chart Review | Encounters | Notes | Labs | Imaging | Procedures | Rx | Documents | Referrals | Scheduling | Billing

Name: **GREELEY, Morris** MR#: **830293-ONC** DOB: **08/03/19XX** Gender: M Age: 67 **Allergies:** Codeine **PCP:** Seth Barkley MD

Progress Note
Encounter Date: 11/12/20XX
Subjective: Mr. Greeley arrives today for a 1.______________________ treatment for 2.______________________ ____ of the sigmoid colon. He had an anterior sigmoid resection in October. 3.______________________ report revealed 4.______________________ tumor cells in two of six lymph nodes. The 5FU/Leucovorin protocol is being administered weekly for 6 weeks. Today is his sixth infusion. We plan to start 5.______________ ______________ after a 2-week hiatus from chemotherapy. The patient continues to do well and is receiving significant support from his family. He has had no hair loss, oral ulcerations, abdominal pain, nausea, or diarrhea.

Objective: Vital signs: Temperature of 98°F. Pulse is 60 beats per minute. Respirations 20. Blood pressure 108/65 mm Hg. His current weight is 183 pounds. HEENT: Tongue and pharynx are normal. PULMONARY: Clear to auscultation. HEART: Regular rate and rhythm without a murmur, rub, or gallop. ABDOMEN: Soft and nontender. No masses or 6.______________________. Extremities: No edema or 7.______________________.

Assessment: 1. Adenocarcinoma of the sigmoid colon with 8.______________________ to regional lymph nodes.

Plan: 1. 5FU/Leucovorin protocol as outlined above, treatment six of six today, followed by radiation therapy after a 2-week period of rest.

Electronically signed: Brian Smith MD 11/12/20XX 16:30

Start | Log On/Off | Print | Edit

Definitions of Medical Terms to Complete the Document

Write the medical terms defined on corresponding answer lines in the document.

1. Treatment of cancer by using drugs
2. Cancerous tumor of glandular tissue
3. Study of disease
4. Tending to become progressively worse
5. Treatment of cancer by using radioactive substance, x-rays, or radiation
6. Enlargement of an organ
7. Abnormal condition of blue
8. Beyond control

B

Read the medical report, and answer the questions below it.

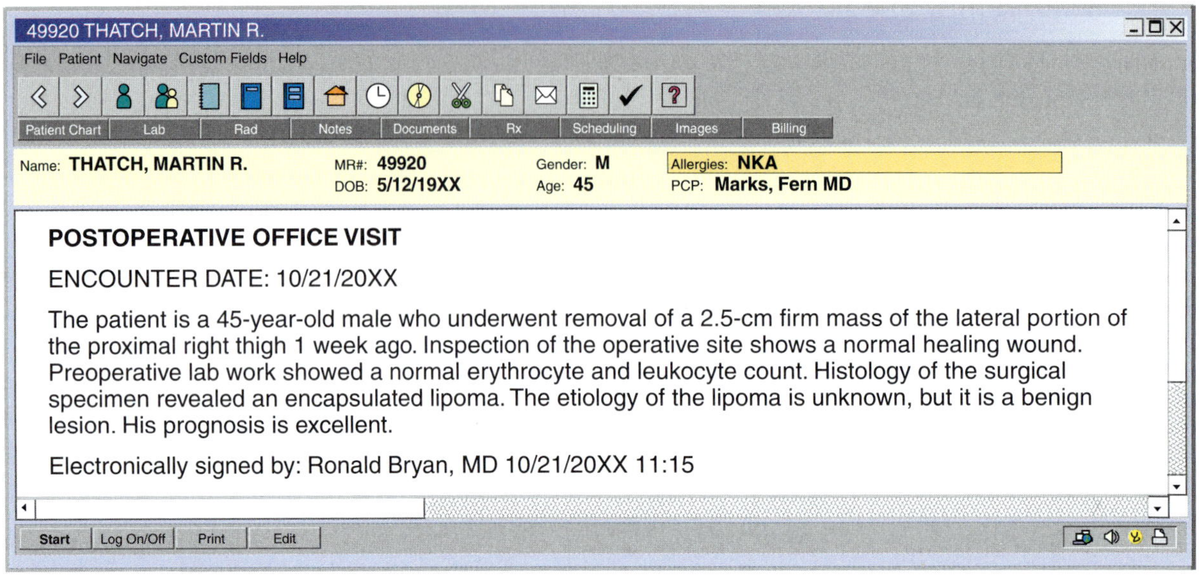
49920 THATCH, MARTIN R.

File Patient Navigate Custom Fields Help

Patient Chart | Lab | Rad | Notes | Documents | Rx | Scheduling | Images | Billing

Name: **THATCH, MARTIN R.** MR#: **49920** DOB: **5/12/19XX** Gender: **M** Age: **45** Allergies: **NKA** PCP: **Marks, Fern MD**

POSTOPERATIVE OFFICE VISIT

ENCOUNTER DATE: 10/21/20XX

The patient is a 45-year-old male who underwent removal of a 2.5-cm firm mass of the lateral portion of the proximal right thigh 1 week ago. Inspection of the operative site shows a normal healing wound. Preoperative lab work showed a normal erythrocyte and leukocyte count. Histology of the surgical specimen revealed an encapsulated lipoma. The etiology of the lipoma is unknown, but it is a benign lesion. His prognosis is excellent.

Electronically signed by: Ronald Bryan, MD 10/21/20XX 11:15

Start | Log On/Off | Print | Edit

Use the medical report above to answer the questions.

1. The firm mass was confirmed as a lipoma from the surgical specimen in which area of study?
   a. cell
   b. tissue
   c. blood
   d. plasma
2. The lipoma was
   a. spreading.
   b. enclosed in a capsule.
   c. inflamed.
   d. blue in color.
3. Erythr/o and leuk/o refer to the ________ of cells.
   a. size
   b. shape
   c. amount
   d. color
4. Write the plural form of
   a. prognosis ________________
   b. lipoma ________________
   c. histology ________________

EXERCISE 32 ■ Pronounce Medical Terms in Use

Practice pronunciation of terms by reading aloud the following paragraph. Use the phonetic spellings to assist with pronunciation. The script also contains medical terms not presented in the chapter. If interested, research their meanings using a medical dictionary and reliable online sources.

A 54-year-old woman presented to the office with a 3-week history of bloody diarrhea. She had been diagnosed with ulcerative colitis at age 25 years. She was referred for a colonoscopy. The examination revealed a suspicious lesion in the transverse colon. A **biopsy** (BĪ-op-sē) was performed and a **cytology** (sī-TOL-o-jē) specimen was obtained. The **pathologist** (pa-THOL-o-jist) made a **diagnosis** (dī-ag-NŌ-sis) of **carcinoma** (kar-si-NŌ-ma) of the colon. Advanced **dysplasia** (dis-PLĀ-zha) and **inflammation** (in-fla-MĀ-shun) existed in the **specimen** (SPES-i-men). The patient underwent surgery and was found to have no evidence of **metastasis** (me-TAS-ta-sis). Her entire colon was removed because of a high risk for developing a **malignant** (ma-LIG-nant) lesion in the remaining colon. She made an uneventful recovery and was referred to an **oncologist** (ong-KOL-o-jist) for consideration of **chemotherapy** (kē-mō-THER-a-pē). Her **prognosis** (prog-NŌ-sis) is generally positive. **Radiation therapy** (rā-dē-Ā-shun) (THER-a-pē) or **biological therapy** (bī-ō-LOJ-i-kel) (THER-a-pē) were not indicated in this case.

CHAPTER REVIEW

EXERCISE 33 ■ Chapter Content Quiz

Test your understanding of terms and abbreviations introduced in this chapter. Circle the letter for the medical term or abbreviation related to the words in italics. *To check your answers, go to Appendix A.*

1. Mr. Roberts was diagnosed as having a *cancerous tumor of connective tissue* or:
   a. sarcoma
   b. melanoma
   c. lipoma
2. The doctor said the tumor was *becoming progressively worse*; that is, it was:
   a. benign
   b. malignant
   c. pathogenic
3. The blood test showed an *increased amount of red blood cells*, or:
   a. erythrocytosis
   b. leukocytosis
   c. cyanosis
4. A *sample of blood, urine, or body tissue that is taken for medical testing* is a:
   a. biopsy
   b. specimen
   c. autopsy
5. The patient was diagnosed with a *tumor composed of fat*, or:
   a. neuroma
   b. carcinoma
   c. lipoma
6. The fatty tumor was *benign*, or:
   a. cancerous
   b. nonrecurrent
   c. recurrent
7. Substances thought to *cause cancer* are called:
   a. carcinoma
   b. carcinogenic
   c. cancerous
8. *Etiology* is the study of:
   a. causes of disease
   b. tissue disease
   c. causes of tumors
9. A *tumor* may be called:
   a. cytoplasm
   b. neoplasm
   c. karyoplasm
10. A *test performed on a sample to determine the presence of pathogenic bacteria* is:
    a. chemistry panel
    b. complete blood count
    c. culture and sensitivity
11. Any *disease of a muscle* is called:
    a. myoma
    b. myopathy
    c. somatopathy
12. The ultrasound revealed marked *abnormal development* on the right kidney or:
    a. hypoplasia
    b. dysplasia
    c. hyperplasia
13. The term that means *produced by a physician* is:
    a. diagnosis
    b. iatrogenic
    c. prognosis
14. The incidence of *black tumor (primarily of the skin)* is increasing.
    a. fibrosarcoma
    b. fibroma
    c. melanoma
15. The *study of tissue in disease* is:
    a. microbiology
    b. histopathology
    c. cytopathology
16. Which of the following is a *malignant tumor*?
    a. sarcoma
    b. fibroma
    c. myoma
17. A *minute microorganism, characterized by a lack of independent metabolism and the ability to replicate only within living host cells* is a:
    a. bacteria
    b. fungus
    c. virus
18. Which of the following provides *palliative and supportive care for the terminally ill* and their families?
    a. hospice
    b. palliative care
    c. therapy
19. The overall survival and acceptable *state of being diseased* justifies performing a therapeutic lymphadenectomy for nodal metastatic melanoma.
    a. mortality
    b. morbidity
    c. prognosis
20. A laboratory test was ordered for a *leukocyte* count or:
    a. WBC
    b. RBC
    c. XRT

CHAPTER AT A GLANCE Word Parts New to This Chapter

COMBINING FORMS

aden/o
aut/o
bi/o
cancer/o
carcin/o
cyan/o
cyt/o
epitheli/o
erythr/o
eti/o
fibr/o
gno/o
hemat/o
hist/o
iatr/o
lei/o
leuk/o
lip/o
melan/o
my/o
necr/o
neur/o
onc/o
organ/o
path/o
rhabd/o
sarc/o
somat/o
system/o
vir/o
viscer/o
xanth/o

PREFIXES

dia-
dys-
hyper-
hypo-
meta-
micro-
neo-
pro-

SUFFIXES

-al,
-cyte
-gen
-genic
-ic
-logist
-logy
-megaly
-oid
-oma
-opsy
-osis
-ous
-pathy
-plasia
-plasm
-sarcoma
-sis
-stasis

CHAPTER AT A GLANCE Medical Terms Built from Word Parts

BODY STRUCTURE

cytogenic
cytology
dysplasia
epithelial
erythrocyte (RBC)
erythrocytosis
histology
hyperplasia
hypoplasia
leukocyte (WBC)
leukocytosis
lipoid
necrosis
myopathy
neuropathy
organomegaly
somatic
somatogenic
systemic
visceral

ONCOLOGY

adenocarcinoma
adenoma
carcinoma (CA)
epithelioma
fibroma
fibrosarcoma
leiomyoma
leiomyosarcoma
lipoma
liposarcoma
melanocarcinoma
melanoma
myoma
metastasis (*pl.* metastases) (METS)
neoplasm
neuroma
rhabdomyoma
rhabdomyosarcoma
sarcoma

LABORATORY

autopsy
biopsy
cytopathology
hematology
histopathology
microbiology
virology

COMPLEMENTARY

autopsy
biopsy
cancerous
carcinogen
carcinogenic
carcinoid
cyanosis
cytopathology
diagnosis (Dx)
etiology
hematology
histopathology
iatrogenic
microbiology
oncogenic
oncologist
oncology
pathogenic
pathologist
pathology
prognosis (Px)
virology
xanthosis

CHAPTER AT A GLANCE Medical Terms *NOT* Built from Word Parts

ONCOLOGY

benign
biological therapy
carcinoma in situ
chemotherapy (chemo)
encapsulated
hospice
malignant
palliative
radiation therapy (XRT)
remission

LABORATORY

chemistry panel
complete blood count with differential (CBC with diff)
culture and sensitivity (C&S)
genetic testing
specimen

COMPLEMENTARY

afebrile
bacteria (*s.* bacterium)
erythema
exacerbation
febrile
fungus (*pl.* fungi)
idiopathic
infection
inflammation
microorganism
morbidity
mortality
virus (*pl.* viruses)

Chapter 3

Directional Terms, Positions, and Imaging

Outline

Objectives

Upon completion of this chapter, you will be able to:

1. Define and spell word parts related to directional terms and diagnostic imaging.
2. Define, pronounce, and spell directional terms.
3. Define, pronounce, and spell terms used to describe abdominopelvic regions.
4. Define, pronounce, and spell terms used to describe anatomic planes.
5. Define, pronounce, and spell terms used to describe body positions.
6. Define, pronounce, and spell diagnostic imaging terms.
7. Interpret the meaning of abbreviations presented in this chapter.
8. Apply medical language in clinical contexts.

Types of body movement are presented in Chapter 14, Musculoskeletal System. Terms related to body movement are: *abduction, adduction, inversion, eversion, extension, flexion, pronation, supination,* and *rotation.*

ANATOMIC POSITION

When using directional terms, the body is assumed to be in the standard, neutral position of reference, called the **anatomic position** (Fig. 3.1). In this position, the body is viewed as standing erect, arms at the side, palms of the hands facing forward, and feet side by side. The directional terms are the same whether the person is standing or supine (lying face up).

WORD PARTS

Use paper flashcards or electronic flashcards on Evolve to assist with memorization of word parts used to analyze, define, and build terms presented in this chapter. To reinforce learning, study one section of the Word Parts Table at a time, and then complete the corresponding exercise on the following pages.

1 ■ Directional Combining Forms

COMBINING FORM	DEFINITION	COMBINING FORM	DEFINITION
anter/o	front	**later/o**	side
caud/o	tail (downward)	**medi/o**	middle
cephal/o	head (upward)	**poster/o**	back, behind
dist/o	away (from the point of attachment)	**proxim/o**	near (the point of attachment)
dors/o	back	**super/o**	above
infer/o	below	**ventr/o**	belly (front)

2 ■ Diagnostic Imaging Combining Forms

COMBINING FORM	DEFINITION	COMBINING FORM	DEFINITION
radi/o	x-rays, ionizing radiation	**tom/o**	to cut, section, or slice
son/o	sound		

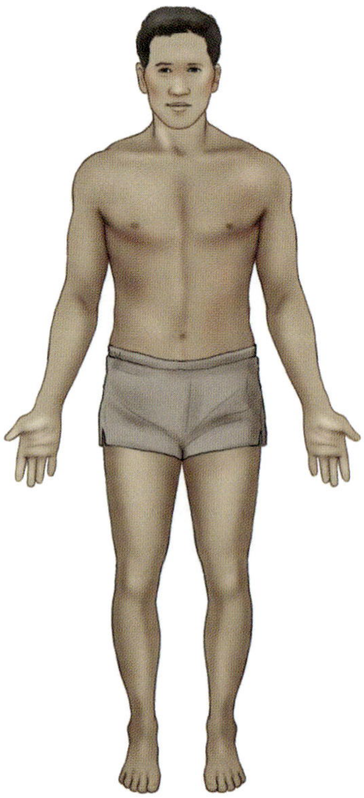

FIG. 3.1 Anatomic position.

3 ■ Prefixes

PREFIX	DEFINITION	PREFIX	DEFINITION
bi-	two	**uni-**	one

4 ■ Suffixes

SUFFIX	DEFINITION	SUFFIX	DEFINITION
-ad	toward	**-graphy**	process of recording, radiographic imaging
-al	pertaining to	**-ic**	pertaining to
-gram	the record, radiographic image	**-ior**	pertaining to
-graph	instrument used to record, the record	**-logist**	one who studies and treats (specialist, physician)
		-logy	study of

Many suffixes mean **pertaining to**. Three were introduced in Chapter 2: **-al, -ic,** and **-ous.** More will be introduced in subsequent chapters. With practice, you will learn which suffix is most commonly used with a particular word root or combining form.

Refer to **Appendix B** and **Appendix C** for alphabetical lists of word parts and their meanings.

EXERCISE 1 ■ Directional Combining Forms

Refer to the first section of the word parts table.

A Define

Write the definitions for the following combining forms. *To check your answers to the exercises in this chapter, go to Appendix A at the back of the textbook.*

1. ventr/o ______
2. cephal/o ______
3. later/o ______
4. medi/o ______
5. infer/o ______
6. proxim/o ______
7. super/o ______
8. dist/o ______
9. dors/o ______
10. caud/o ______
11. anter/o ______
12. poster/o ______

Do not be concerned about which combining form to use for front or back. As you continue to study and use medical terms, you will become familiar with common usage of each word part.

B Label

Fill in the blanks with directional combining forms. *To check your answers, go to Appendix A.*

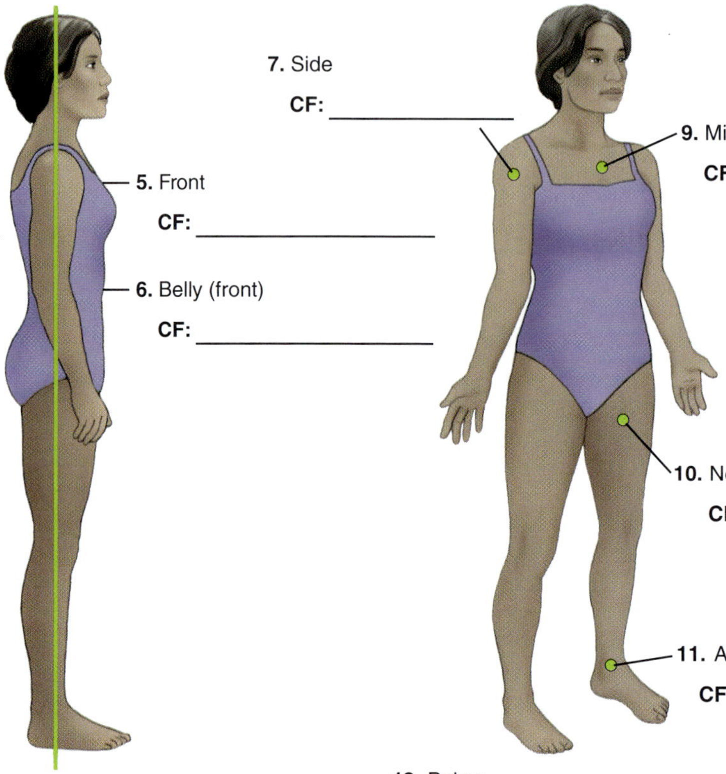

HEAD AND TRUNK ONLY Terms built from the combining forms **cephal/o** and **caud/o** are used to describe locations in the head and the trunk of the body.

EXERCISE 2 ■ Diagnostic Imaging Combining Forms

Refer to the second section of the word parts table.

A Match

Match the combining forms in the first column with their correct definitions in the second column. *To check your answers to the exercises in this chapter, go to Appendix A*

______	1. tom/o	a. x-rays, ionizing radiation
______	2. radi/o	b. sound
______	3. son/o	c. to cut, section, or slice

B Label

Write the combining forms pictured and defined.

1. ______________________
to cut, section, or slice

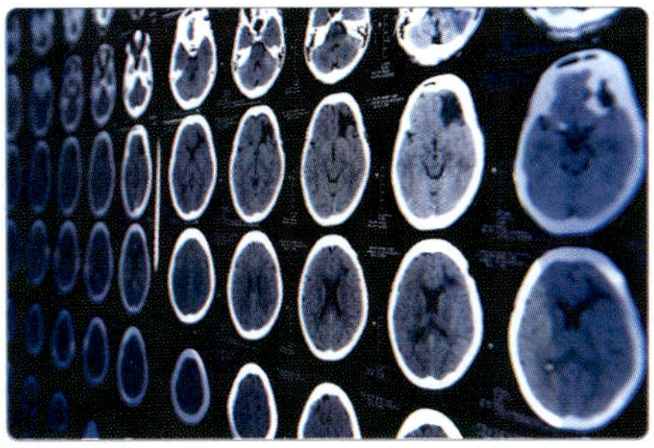

2. ______________________
x-rays, ionizing radiation

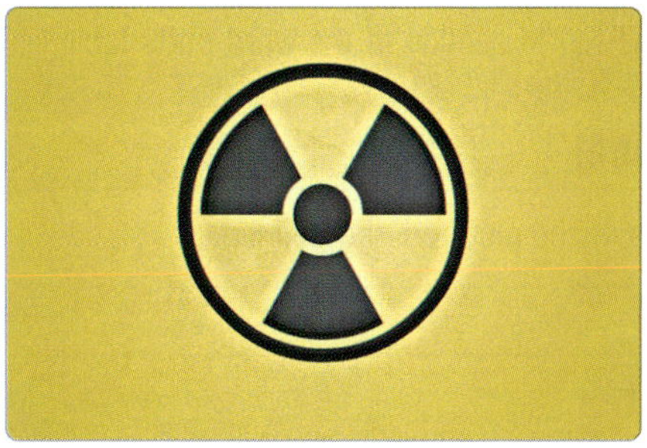

3. ______________________
sound

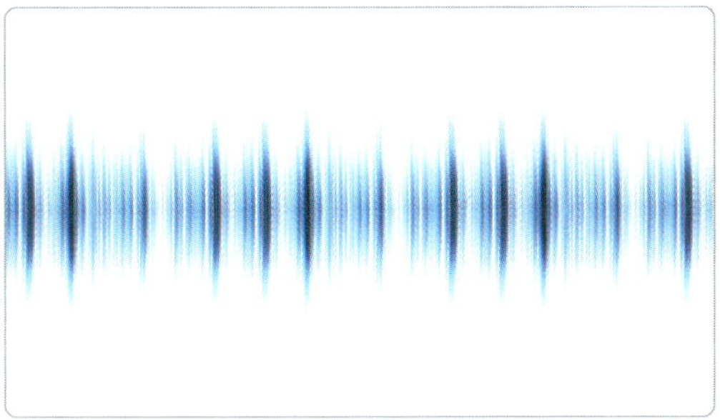

EXERCISE 3 ■ Prefixes

Refer to the third section of the word parts table.

A Label

Write the prefixes pictured and defined.

1. ______________________
one

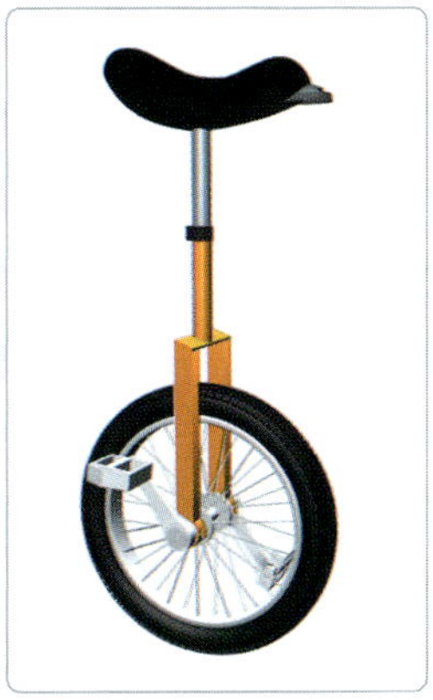

2. ______________________
two

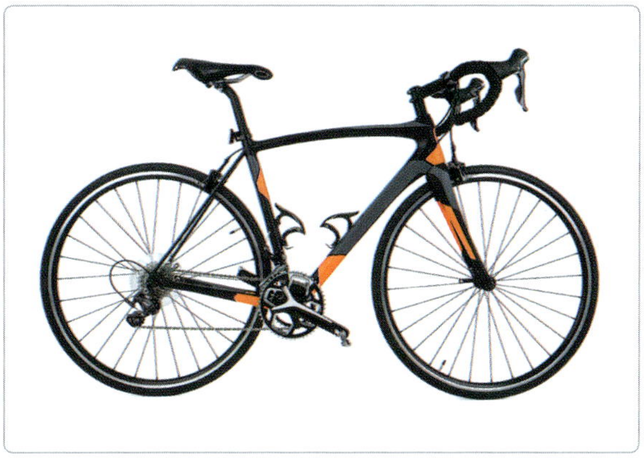

B Define

Write the definitions of the following prefixes.

1. bi- ______________________ 2. uni- ______________________

EXERCISE 4 ■ Suffixes

Refer to the fourth section of the word parts table.

A Label

Write the suffixes pictured and defined.

1. ______________________
toward

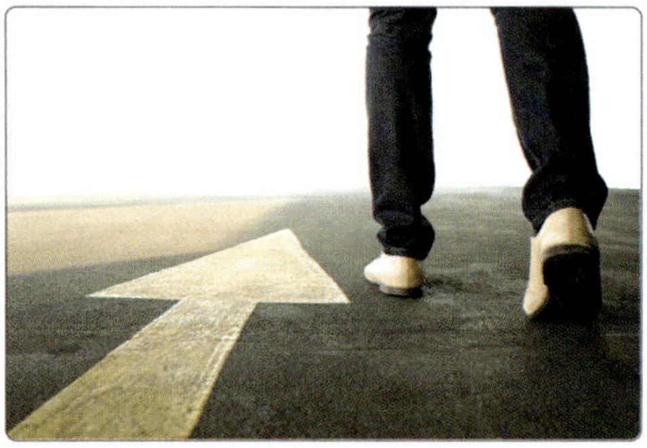

2. ______________________
process of recording, radiographic imaging

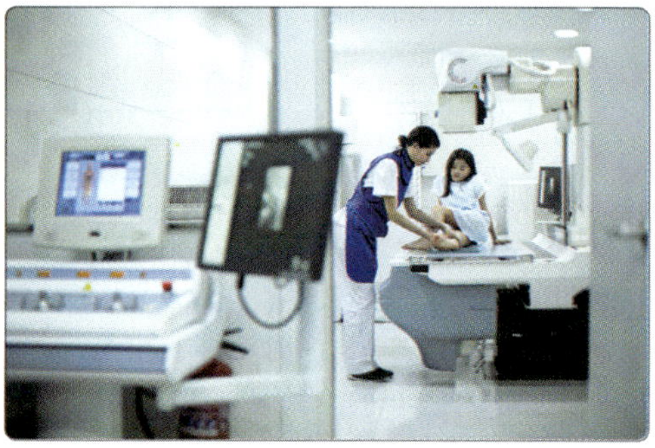

3. ______________________
A. instruction used to record, or B. the record

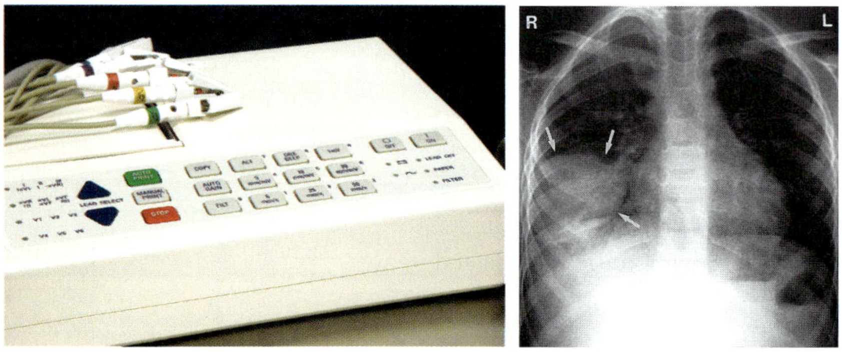

A B

4. ______________________
A. the record, or B. radiographic image

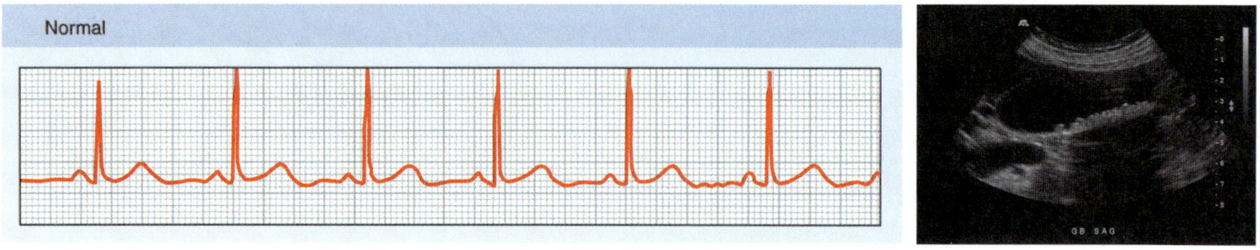

A B

B Define

Write the definitions of the following suffixes.

1. -graphy ______
2. -graph ______
3. -gram ______
4. -ior ______
5. -ad ______
6. -logist ______
7. -logy ______
8. -al, -ic ______

MOVEMENT The suffix -ad, used in directional terms, refers to movement in a specific direction. For example, **cephal/ad** indicates movement toward the head.

MEDICAL TERMS

Directional Terms

The following terms are built from word parts and can be translated using the definitions of word parts. Further explanation is provided within parentheses as needed.

TERM	DEFINITION
1. caudad (KAW-dad)	toward the tail (or the inferior portion of the trunk; downward)
2. cephalad (SEF-a-lad)	toward the head (upward)
3. lateral (lat) (LAT-er-al)	pertaining to the side
4. medial (med) (MĒ-dē-al)	pertaining to the middle
5. unilateral (ū-ni-LAT-er-al)	pertaining to one side (only)
6. bilateral (bī-LAT-er-al)	pertaining to two sides
7. mediolateral (*mē*-dē-Ō-LAT-er-al)	pertaining to the middle and to the side
8. distal (DIS-tal)	pertaining to away (from the point of attachment of a body part)
9. proximal (PROK-si-mal)	pertaining to near (to the point of attachment of a body part)
10. inferior (inf) (in-FĒR-ē-or)	pertaining to below (Fig. 3.2)
11. superior (sup) (sū-PĒR-ē-or)	pertaining to above (Fig. 3.2)
12. caudal (KAW-dal)	pertaining to the tail (synonymous with **inferior** in human anatomy when specifying location on the trunk of the body) (Fig. 3.2)
13. cephalic (se-FAL-ik)	pertaining to the head (Fig. 3.2)
14. anterior (ant) (an-TĒR-ē-or)	pertaining to the front (Fig. 3.2)
15. posterior (pos-TĒR-ē-or)	pertaining to the back (Fig. 3.2)
16. dorsal (DOR-sal)	pertaining to the back (Fig. 3.2)
17. ventral (VEN-tral)	pertaining to the belly (front) (Fig. 3.2)
18. anteroposterior (AP) (*an*-ter-ō-pos-TĒR-ē-or)	pertaining to the front and to the back
19. posteroanterior (PA) (*pos*-ter-ō-an-TĒR-ē-or)	pertaining to the back and to the front

EXERCISE 5 ■ Pronounce and Spell

Practice pronunciation and spelling on paper and online.

1. Practice on Paper

a. **Pronounce:** Read the phonetic spelling and say aloud the terms listed in the previous table. Refer to the pronunciation key on p. 20 as necessary.
b. **Spell:** Have a study partner read the terms aloud. Write the spelling of the terms on a separate sheet of paper.

2. Practice Online

a. **Access** the online learning resources. Go to evolve.elsevier.com > Evolve Resources > Student Resources.
b. **Pronounce:** Select Audio Glossary > Chapter 3 > Exercise 5. Select a term to hear its pronunciation and repeat aloud.
c. **Spell:** Select Activities > Chapter 3 > Spell Terms > Exercise 5. Select the audio icon and type the correct spelling of the term.

❑ Check the box when complete.

EXERCISE 6 ■ Analyze and Define

Analyze and define the following directional terms by drawing slashes between word parts, writing word part abbreviations above the term, underlining combining forms, and writing combining form abbreviations below the term. *To check your answers, go to Appendix A.*

WR CV WR S
EXAMPLE: medi / o / later / al
CF
pertaining to the middle and to the side

1. cephalad

____

____

2. proximal

____

____

3. lateral

____

____

4. unilateral

____

____

5. anteroposterior

____

____

6. cephalic

____

____

7. superior

____

____

8. anterior

____

____

9. caudad

___

___

10. distal

___

___

11. medial

___

___

12. bilateral

___

___

13. posteroanterior

___

___

14. caudal

___

___

15. inferior

___

___

16. posterior

___

___

17. dorsal

___

___

18. ventral

___

___

TABLE 3.1 Usage of Terms with Similar Meanings

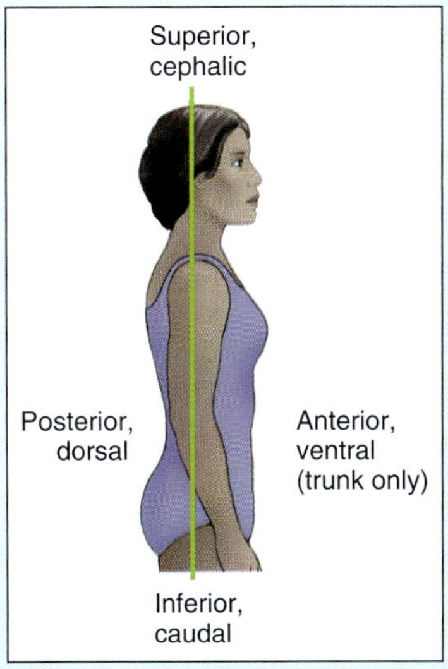

FIG. 3.2 Superior and inferior, cephalic and caudal, posterior and anterior, dorsal, and ventral.

SAME

When describing anatomic structures in the *head* and *trunk* of the body, the following terms are **similar** in meaning and are used interchangeably:

- **Superior** and **cephalic** describe above.
- **Inferior** and **caudal** describe below.
- **Posterior** and **dorsal** describe the back.
- **Anterior** and **ventral** (trunk only) describe the front.

DIFFERENT

Differences in uses of terms include:

- Directional terms ending with **-ior** can indicate spatial relationships of body parts to each other throughout the body. The nose is **anterior** to the ear, and the ear is **posterior** to the nose. The eye is **superior** to the mouth, and the mouth is **inferior** to the eye.
- **Ventral** describes the trunk of the body. The **ventral** cavity is located toward the belly and is made up of the thoracic and abdominopelvic cavities. Ventral may also denote a relationship to the anterior abdominal wall. A **ventral** hernia is a hernia in the anterior abdominal wall.
- **Dorsal** describes the back of the head and trunk. The **dorsal** cavity is located in the posterior portion of the body and is made up of the cranial and spinal cavities. Dorsal also describes the surface of the hand opposite the palm and the top of the foot. The pulse palpable on the **dorsal** surface of the foot is called dorsalis pedis pulse.
- **Cephalic** and **caudal** apply to the head and trunk of the body only, whereas **superior** and **inferior** also apply to limbs. The ankle is **inferior** to the knee.

EXERCISE 7 ■ Build

A Label

Build terms pictured by writing word parts above definitions.

1.

a. ______ / ______
above / pertaining to

b. ______ / ______
head / pertaining to

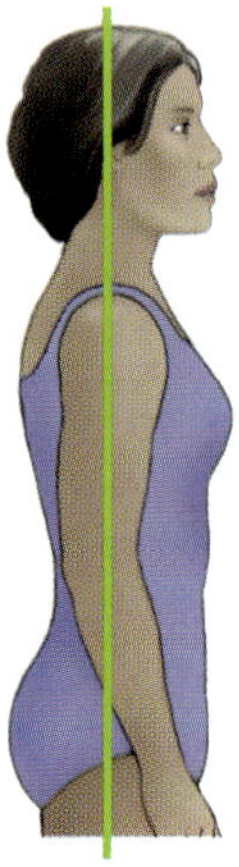

c. ______ / ______
back / pertaining to

______ / ______
back / pertaining to

f. ______ / ______
front / pertaining to

g. ______ / ______
belly (front) / pertaining to

d. ______ / ______
below / pertaining to

e. ______ / ______
tail / pertaining to

2.

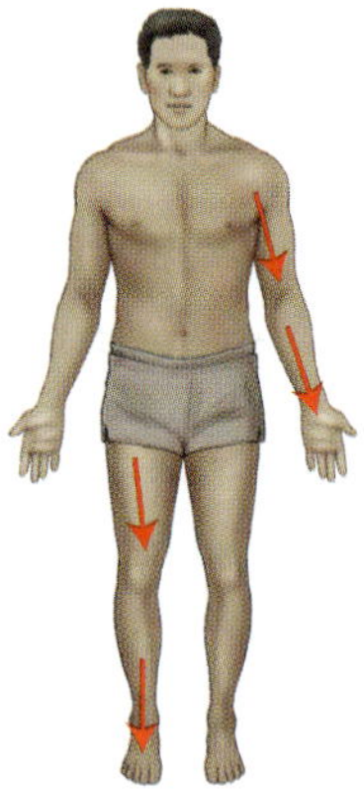

______ / ______
away from the point of attachment / pertaining to

3.

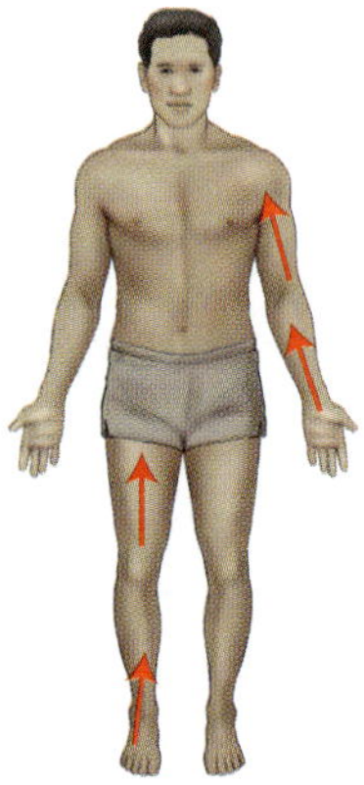

______ / ______
near the point of attachment / pertaining to

4.

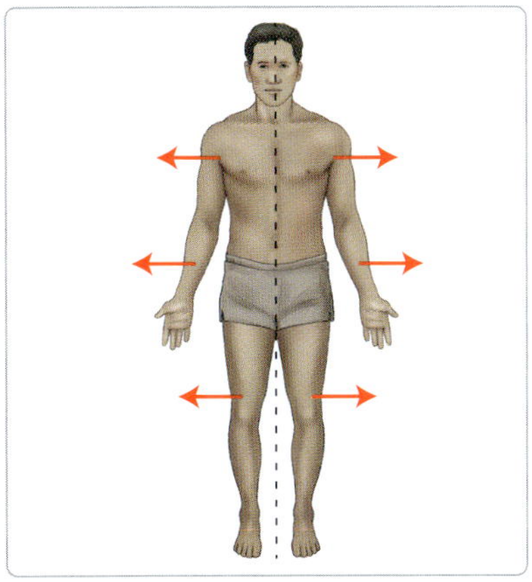

______________ / ______________
side pertaining to

5.

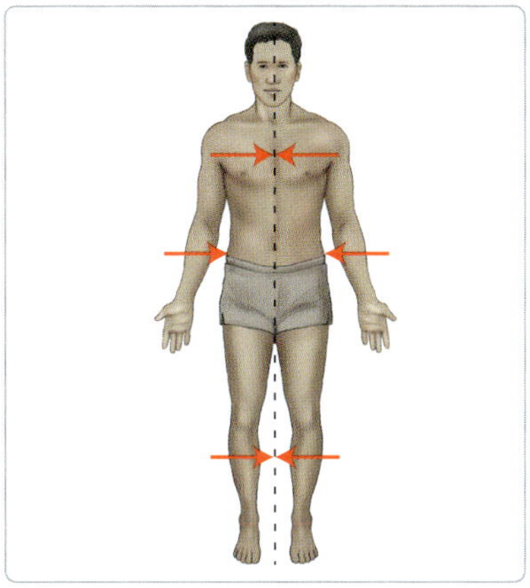

______________ / ______________
middle pertaining to

6.

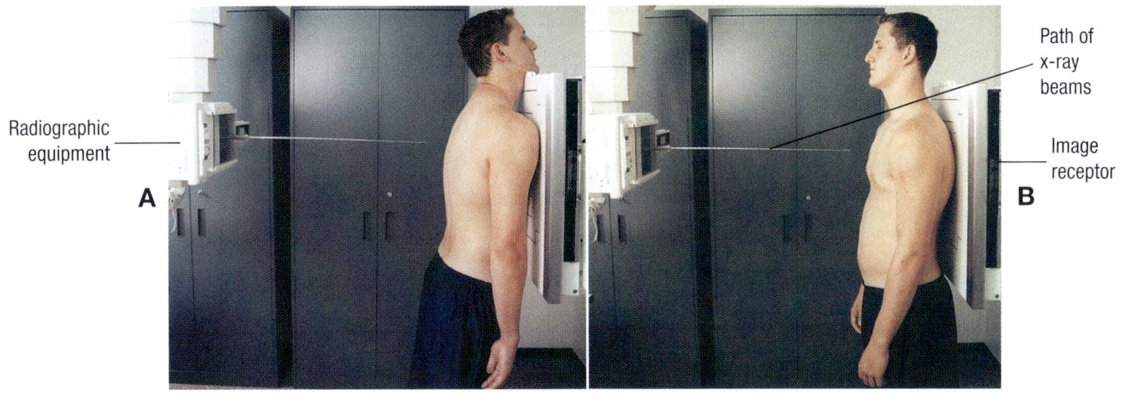

a. ______________ / ______ / ____________ / ______________ projection
back CV front pertaining to

b. ______________ / ______ / ____________ / ______________ projection
front CV back pertaining to

Organs and anatomy of interest closest to the image receptor are more accurately imaged. For example, a PA projection is used when the heart or other anterior structures are the focus of the study. An AP projection is used when the spine or other posterior structures are the primary focus.

B Fill In

Build directional terms for the following definitions by using the word parts you have learned.

1. toward the head (upward) ______________ / ______________
WR S

2. pertaining to near ______________ / ______________
WR S

3. pertaining to away ______________ / ______________
WR S

4. pertaining to two sides

______ / ______ / ______
P WR S

5. pertaining to the middle

______ / ______
WR S

6. toward the tail (downward)

______ / ______
WR S

7. pertaining to the back and to the front

______ / ___ / ______ / ______
WR CV WR S

8. pertaining to the middle and to the side

______ / ___ / ______ / ______
WR CV WR S

9. pertaining to one side (only)

______ / ______ / ______
P WR S

10. pertaining to the front and to the back

______ / ___ / ______ / ______
WR CV WR S

EXERCISE 8 ■ Review of Directional Terms

Can you define, pronounce, and spell the following directional terms?

anterior (ant)	cephalad	lateral (lat)	proximal
anteroposterior (AP)	cephalic	medial (med)	superior (sup)
bilateral	distal	mediolateral	unilateral
caudad	dorsal	posterior	ventral
caudal	inferior (inf)	posteroanterior (PA)	

Abdominopelvic Regions

To assist in locating medical problems with greater accuracy and for identification purposes, the abdomen and pelvis are divided into nine regions (Fig. 3.3). Abdominopelvic regions are often used to document the physical examination and medical history to describe signs and symptoms. The number in parentheses indicates the number of regions.

TERM	DEFINITION
1. umbilical region (1) (um-BIL-i-kal) (RĒ-jun)	around the navel (umbilicus)

UMBILICUS is a term derived from the Latin **umbo**, which denoted the boss, or protuberant part, of a shield. Around the first century, the term was used to designate either a raised or a depressed spot in the middle of anything.

TERM	DEFINITION
2. lumbar regions (2) (LUM-bar) (RĒ-junz)	to the right and left of the umbilical region, near the waist
3. epigastric region (1) (*ep*-i-GAS-trik) (RĒ-jun)	superior to the umbilical region
4. hypochondriac regions (2) (*hī*-pō-KON-drē-ak) (RĒ-junz)	to the right and left of the epigastric region

HYPOCHONDRIAC from the Greek **hypo** (meaning under), and **chondros** (meaning cartilage), was used by Hippocrates to refer to the region below rib cartilage. In 1765, it was used to refer to people who had discomfort in this area with no organic findings. Eventually, hypochondriac referred to a person who falsely believed they were ill. More recently, **cyberchondria** emerged as a term describing a pattern of using Internet research to self-diagnose symptoms, causing worry.

TERM	DEFINITION
5. hypogastric region (1) (*hī*-pō-GAS-trik) (RĒ-jun)	inferior to the umbilical region
6. iliac regions (2) (IL-ē-ak) (RĒ-junz)	to the right and left of the hypogastric region, near the groin (also called **inguinal regions**)

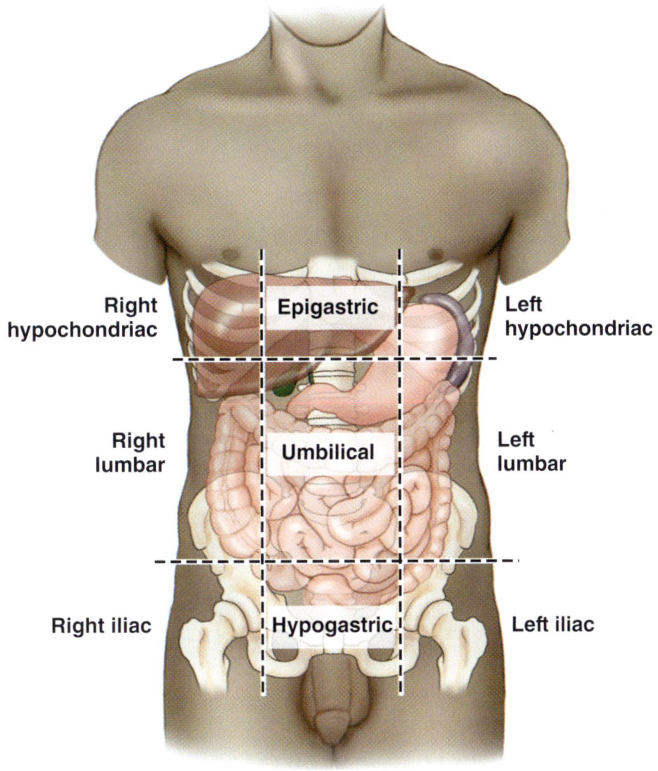

FIG. 3.3 Abdominopelvic regions. References to right and left indicate the right and left of the patient's body.

PREVENTING WRONG-SIDE ERRORS When facing the patient, your right and left will be opposite of the patient's right and left. Confusing the patient's right and left with the provider's right and left can lead to significant errors such as **wrong-sided surgery**.

Tips for preventing wrong-sided errors:

- Remember **"right"** and **"left"** pertain to the right and left of the patient's body.
- Avoid saying **"right"** when **"correct"** is meant.
- When a patient indicates the side choice is **"right,"** confirm the response meant **"correct."**

EXERCISE 9 ■ Pronounce and Spell

Practice pronunciation and spelling on paper and online.

1. Practice on Paper

a. **Pronounce:** Read the phonetic spelling and say aloud the terms listed in the previous table. Refer to the pronunciation key on p. 20 as necessary.
b. **Spell:** Have a study partner read the terms aloud. Write the spelling of the terms on a separate sheet of paper.

2. Practice Online

a. **Access** online learning resources. Go to evolve.elsevier.com > Evolve Resources > Student Resources.
b. **Pronounce:** Select Audio Glossary > Chapter 3 > Exercise 9. Select a term to hear its pronunciation and repeat aloud.
c. **Spell:** Select Activities > Chapter 3 > Spell Terms > Exercise 9. Select the audio icon and type the correct spelling of the term.

❑ Check the box when complete.

EXERCISE 10 ■ Abdominopelvic Regions

A Label

Fill in the blanks with abdominopelvic regions to label the diagram. *To check your answers, go to Appendix A.*

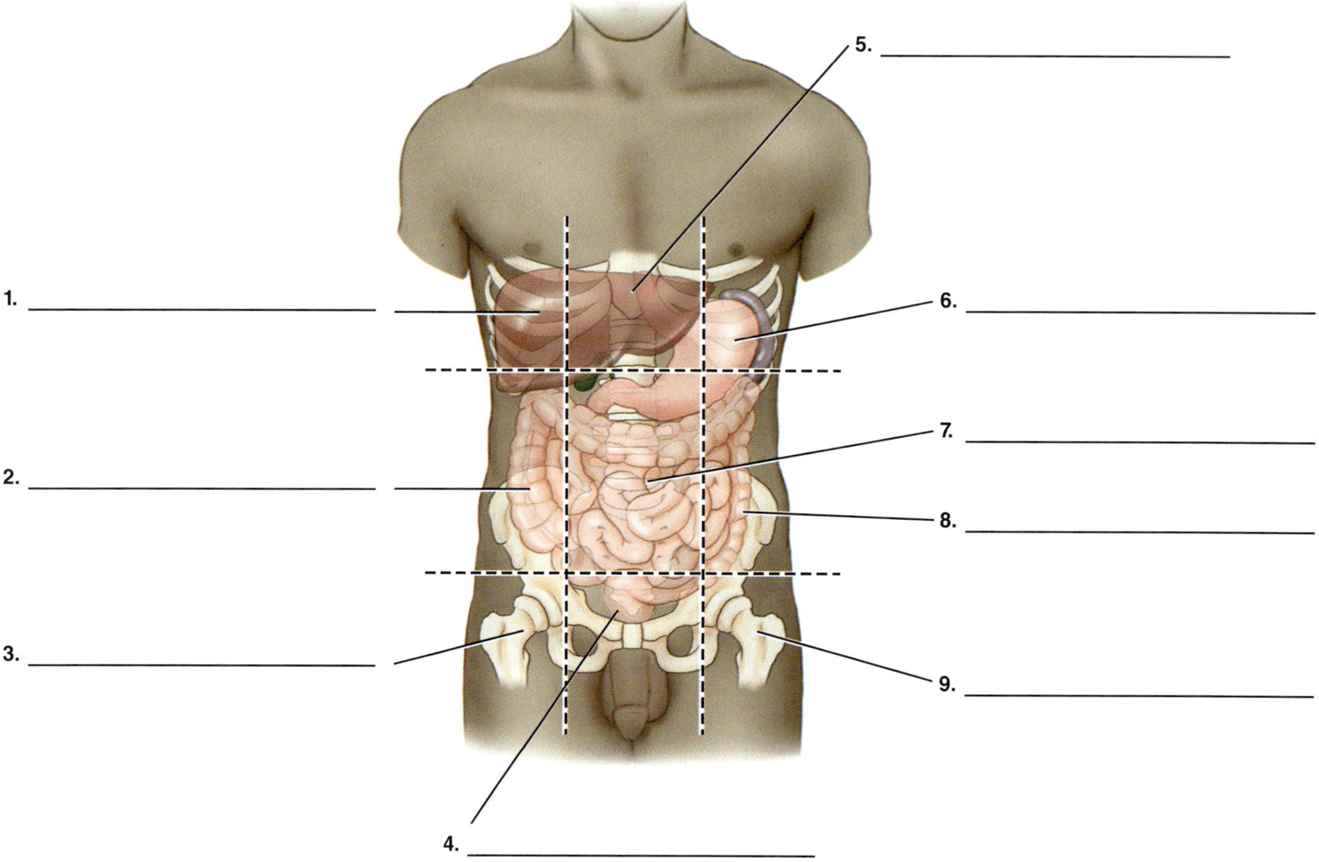

B Match

Match the terms in the first column with their correct definitions in the second column.

_____	1. epigastric	a. inferior to the umbilical region
_____	2. hypochondriac	b. superior to the umbilical region
_____	3. hypogastric	c. right and left of the umbilical region, near the waist
_____	4. iliac	d. right and left of the epigastric region
_____	5. lumbar	e. right and left of the hypogastric region, near the groin
_____	6. umbilical	f. inferior to the epigastric region

EXERCISE 11 ■ Review of Abdominopelvic Regions Terms

Can you define, pronounce, and spell the following abdominopelvic regions?

epigastric region	hypogastric region	lumbar regions
hypochondriac regions	iliac regions	umbilical region

Anatomic Planes

Planes are imaginary flat fields used as points of reference to identify or view the location of organs and anatomic structures. Anatomic planes are frequently used in diagnostic imaging and surgery. The body is assumed to be in the anatomic position unless specified otherwise (Table 3.2).

TERM	DEFINITION
1. axial (AK-see-uh-l)	horizontal plane dividing the body into superior and inferior portions (also called **transverse plane** and **horizontal plane**)
2. coronal (ko-RŌN-al)	vertical plane passing through the body from side to side, dividing the body into anterior and posterior portions (also called **frontal plane**)
3. midsagittal (mid-SAJ-i-tal)	vertical plane passing through the body from front to back at the midline, dividing the body equally into right and left halves
MIDLINE is an imaginary line that separates the body, or body parts, into halves. In medical language, midline is used as a common reference point.	
4. parasagittal (*par*-a-SAJ-i-tal)	vertical plane passing through the body from front to back, dividing the body into unequal left and right sides
5. sagittal (SAJ-i-tal)	vertical plane passing through the body from front to back, dividing the body into right and left sides (any plane parallel to the midsagittal plane)

TABLE 3.2 Anatomic Planes and Diagnostic Images

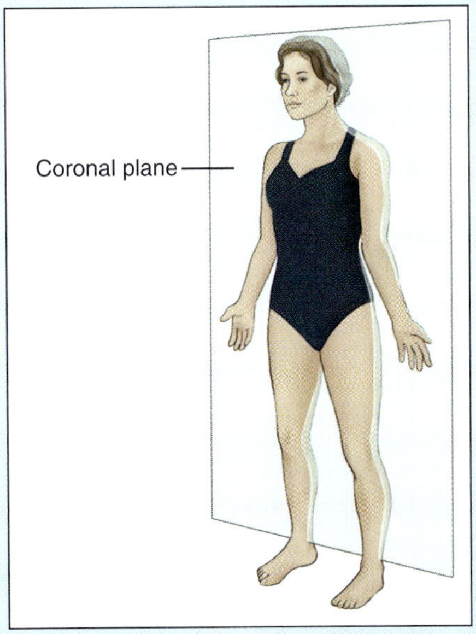

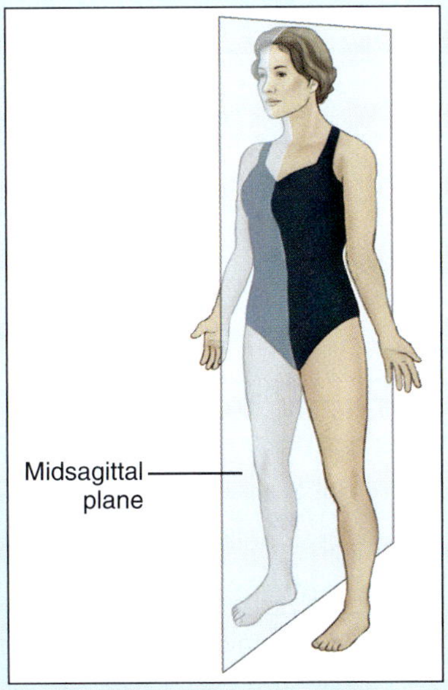

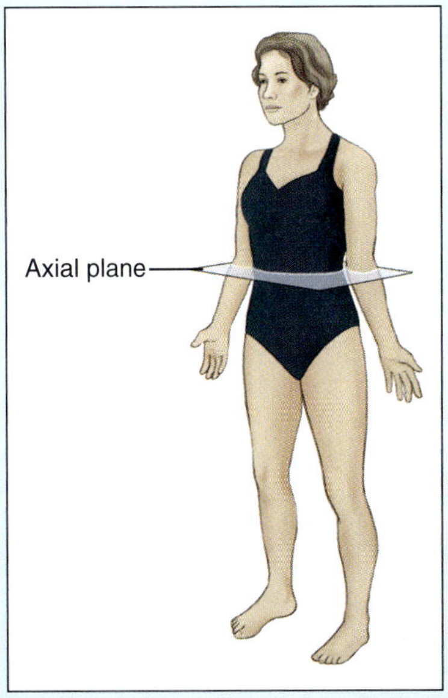

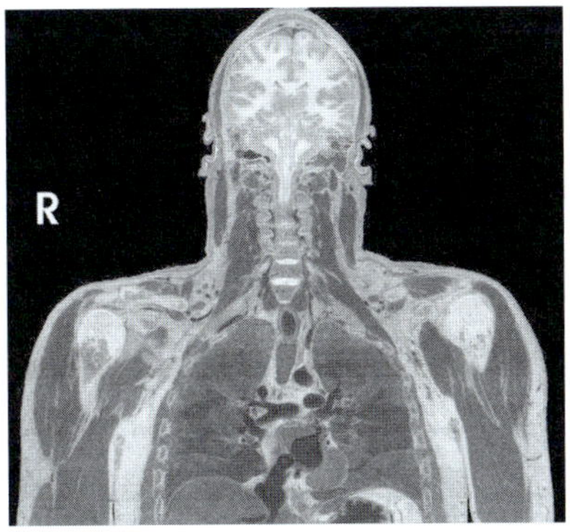

Coronal diagnostic image (MRI*)

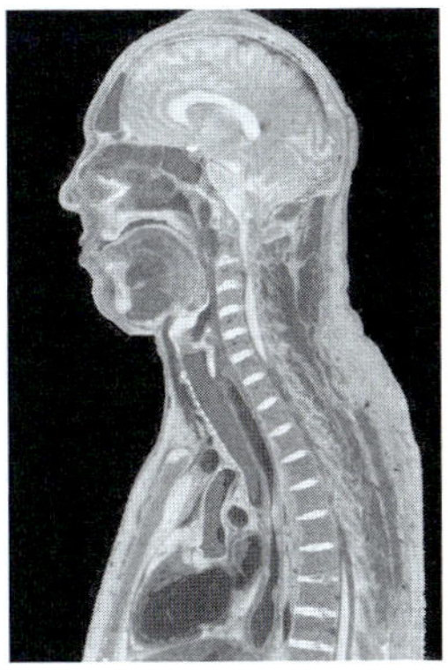
Midsagittal diagnostic image (MRI*)

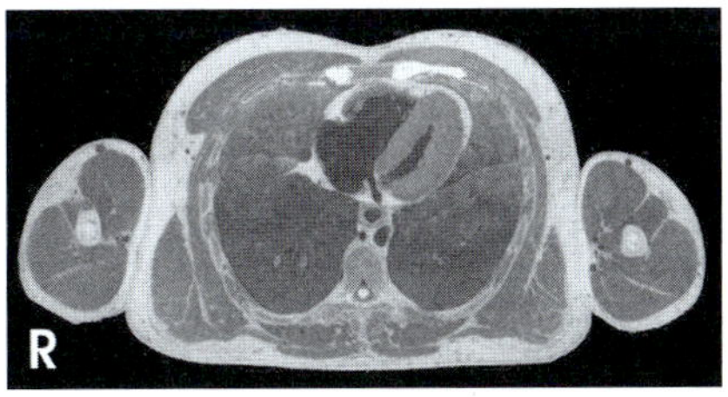

Axial diagnostic image (MRI*)

* MRI abbreviates **magnetic resonance imaging**

Sagittal describes vertical planes dividing the body into right and left sides. **Midsagittal** and **parasagittal** planes are both sagittal planes with the midsagittal plane dividing the body equally into halves and the parasagittal plane dividing the body into unequal sides.

EXERCISE 12 ■ Pronounce and Spell

Practice pronunciation and spelling on paper and online.

1. Practice on Paper

a. **Pronounce:** Read the phonetic spelling and say aloud the terms listed in the previous table. Refer to the pronunciation key on p. 20 as necessary.
b. **Spell:** Have a study partner read the terms aloud. Write the spelling of the terms on a separate sheet of paper.

2. Practice Online

a. **Access** online learning resources. Go to evolve.elsevier.com > Evolve Resources > Student Resources.
b. **Pronounce:** Select Audio Glossary > Chapter 3 > Exercise 12. Select a term to hear its pronunciation and repeat aloud.
c. **Spell:** Select Activities > Chapter 3 > Spell Terms > Exercise 12. Select the audio icon and type the correct spelling of the term.

❑ Check the box when complete.

EXERCISE 13 ■ Anatomic Planes

A Label

Fill in the blanks with anatomic planes to label the diagram.

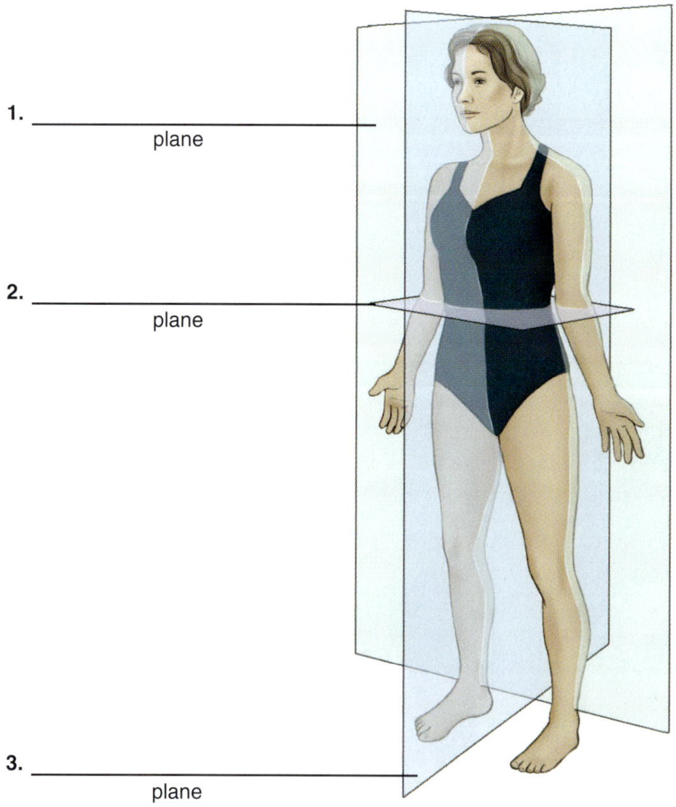

B Fill In

Fill in the blanks with the correct terms.

1. The plane that divides the body into superior and inferior portions is the ______________ plane.
2. The plane that divides the body **equally** into right and left halves is the ______________ plane.
3. The plane that divides the body into anterior and posterior portions is referred to as the ______________ plane.
4. Any plane that divides the body into right and left sides is referred to as a(n) ______________ plane.
5. The plane that divides the body into **unequal** right and left sides is the ______________ plane.

EXERCISE 14 ■ Review of Anatomic Planes Terms

Can you define, pronounce, and spell the following anatomic planes?

axial plane	parasagittal plane
coronal plane	sagittal plane
midsagittal plane	

Body Positions

Position terms are used in health care settings to communicate how the patient's body is placed for physical examination, diagnostic procedures, surgery, treatment, and recovery.

TERM	DEFINITION
1. Fowler position (FOW-ler) (pe-ZISH-en)	semi-sitting position with slight elevation of the knees

FOWLER POSITION indicates the patient is in a sitting position with the head of the bed raised between 15° and 90°. Variations in the angle are denoted by **high Fowler**, indicating an upright position at approximately 90°; **Fowler** indicating an angle between 45° and 60°; **semi-Fowler**, 30° to 45°; and **low Fowler**, where the head is slightly elevated between 15° and 30°.

TERM	DEFINITION
2. lateral recumbent position (LAT-er-al) (re-KUM-bent) (pe-ZISH-en)	lying on side; right and left precede the term to indicate the patient's side
3. lithotomy position (lith-OT-o-mē) (pe-ZISH-en)	lying on back with legs raised and feet in stirrups, hips and knees flexed, and thighs abducted (away from body) and externally rotated
4. orthopnea position (or-THOP-nē-a) (pe-ZISH-en)	sitting upright in a chair or in bed supported by pillows behind the back. Sometimes the patient tilts forward, resting on a pillow supported by an overbed table. (also called **orthopneic position**)

ORTHOPNEA POSITION **Orthopnea** is built from the combining form **orth/o** meaning straight and the suffix **-pnea** meaning breathing. Patients who need to sit up straight to breathe are placed in the **orthopnea position**.

TERM	DEFINITION
5. prone position (prōn) (pe-ZISH-en)	lying on abdomen, facing downward; head may be turned to one side; also called **ventral recumbent position**
6. recumbent position (rē-KUM-bent) (pe-ZISH-en)	lying down in any position (also called **decubitus position**) (Table 3.3)
7. Sims position (simz) (pe-ZISH-en)	lying on side in a semi-prone position with the knee drawn up toward the chest and the arm drawn behind parallel to the back. Right and left precede the term to indicate the patient's right or left side. Originally, the term specifically indicated the patient's left side; therefore, if the term Sims position is used without a description of right or left, it is assumed the patient is to be placed on the left side.

TABLE 3.3 Recumbent Positions

Recumbent position (also called **decubitus position**) is a general term indicating the patient is lying down in any position, such as supine, prone, or on one side. The specific position is indicated by additional terms.

dorsal recumbent position... lying on back; the patient is lying down facing upwards (also called **supine position**)	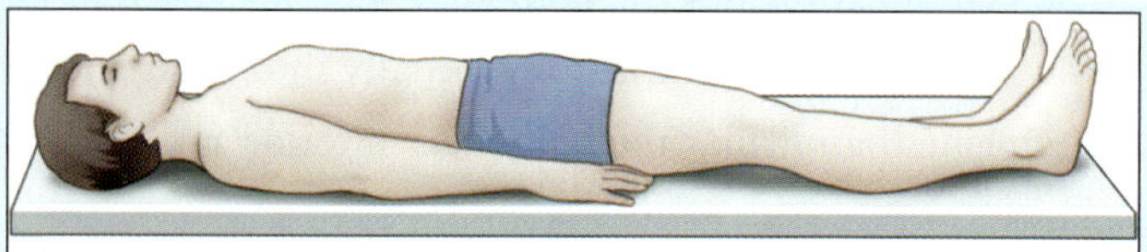 Supine
ventral recumbent position... lying face down; the patient is lying down on the belly. The face may be turned to the right or left (also called **prone position**).	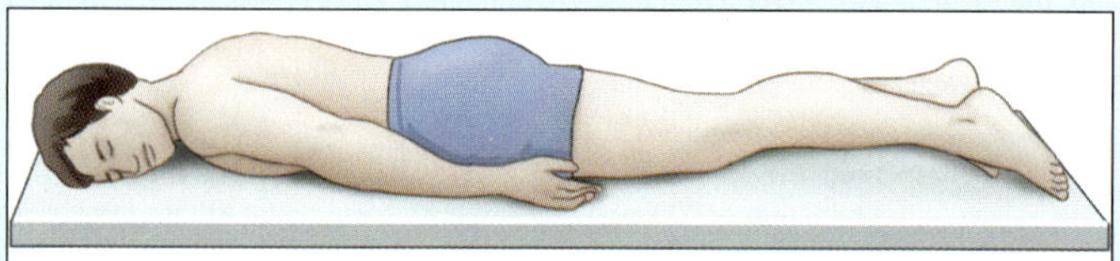 Prone
left lateral recumbent position... lying on the patient's left side (also called **left lateral decubitus position**); right knee may be drawn upward (also called **Sims position** and **left Sims position**)	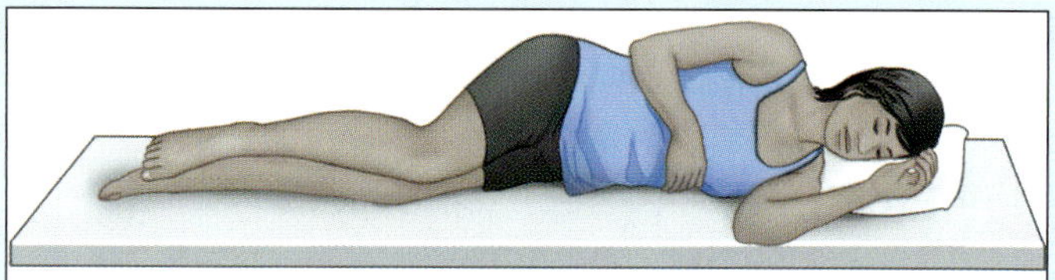 Left lateral recumbent
right lateral recumbent position... lying on the patient's right side; left knee may be drawn upward (also called **right lateral decubitus position** and **right Sims position** when knee is drawn upward)	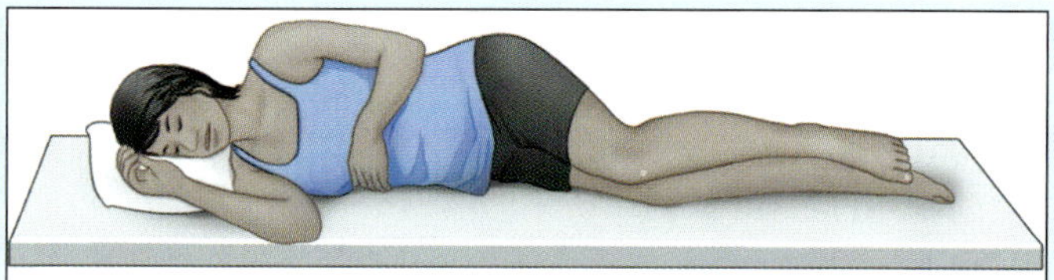 Right lateral recumbent

Body Positions—cont'd

TERM	DEFINITION	TERM	DEFINITION
8. supine position (SOO-pine) (pe-ZISH-en)	lying on back, facing upward (also called **dorsal recumbent position**)	**9. Trendelenburg position** (tren-DEL-en-berg) (pe-ZISH-en)	lying on back with body tilted so that the head is lower than the feet

EXERCISE 15 ■ Pronounce and Spell

Practice pronunciation and spelling on paper and online.

1. Practice on Paper

a. **Pronounce:** Read the phonetic spelling and say aloud the terms listed in the previous table. Refer to the pronunciation key on p. 20 as necessary.
b. **Spell:** Have a study partner read the terms aloud. Write the spelling of the terms on a separate sheet of paper.

2. Practice Online

a. **Access** online learning resources. Go to evolve.elsevier.com > Evolve Resources > Student Resources.
b. **Pronounce:** Select Audio Glossary > Chapter 3 > Exercise 15. Select a term to hear its pronunciation and repeat aloud.
c. **Spell:** Select Activities > Chapter 3 > Spell Terms > Exercise 15. Select the audio icon and type the correct spelling of the term.

❑ Check the box when complete.

EXERCISE 16 ■ Body Positions

A Match

Match the body position terms in the first column with their descriptions in the second column. *To check your answers, go to Appendix A.*

d ______ 1. Fowler position
a ______ 2. lateral recumbent position
f ______ 3. prone position
c ______ 4. supine position
b ______ 5. recumbent position
e ______ 6. Sims position

a. lying on side
b. lying down in any position
c. lying on back, facing upward
d. semi-sitting position with slight elevation of the knees
e. if "right" or "left" does not appear with the term, the patient is assumed to be placed lying on left side with right knee drawn up and with left arm drawn behind, parallel to the back
f. lying on abdomen, facing downward

B Label

Write the patient positions pictured and defined.

1. ________________ position, lying on back, facing upward (also called **dorsal recumbent position**)

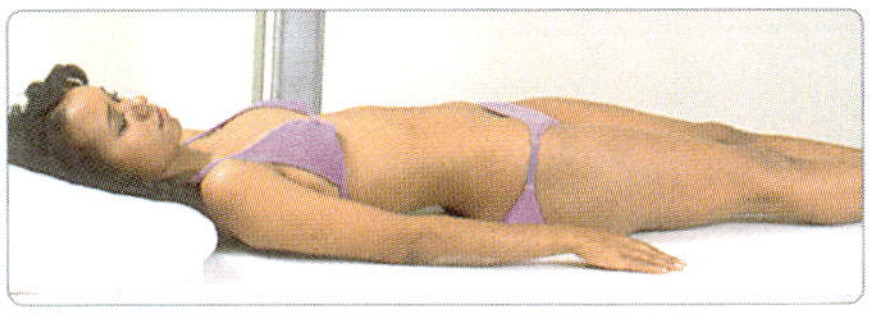

2. ________________ position, lying on abdomen, facing downward (also called **ventral recumbent position**)

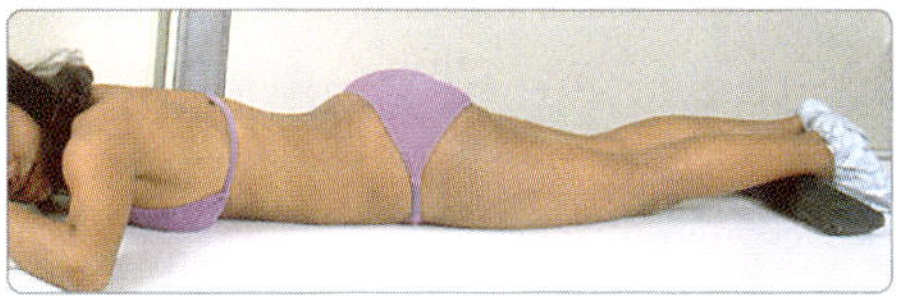

3. ________________ position, sitting upright and tilted forward resting on a pillow supported by an overbed table

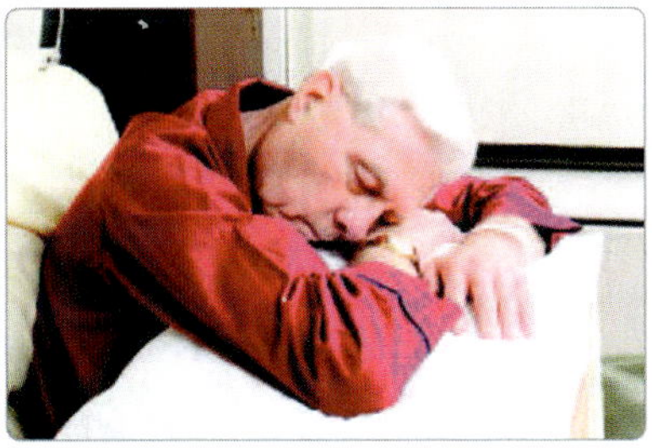

4. ________________ position, lying on back with body tilted so that the head is lower than the feet

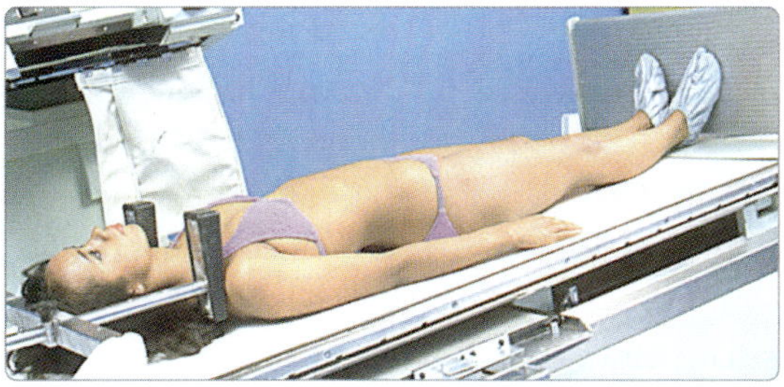

5. Modified ________________ position, lying on back with legs raised (notice legs are supported under the knees, rather than having the feet in stirrups)

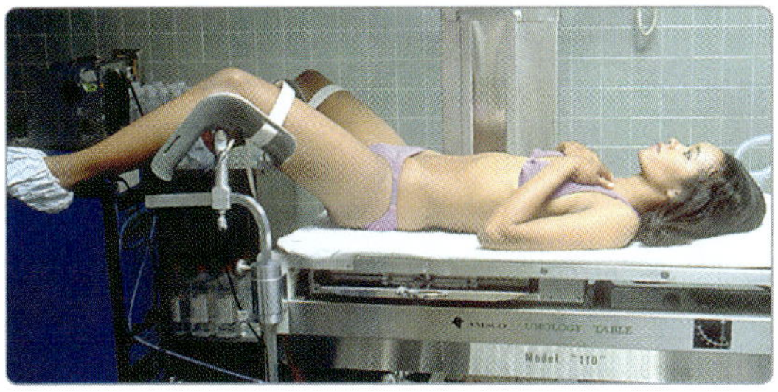

6. Modified ________________ position, lying on left side with right knee drawn up (notice the arm is placed in front, rather than behind the body)

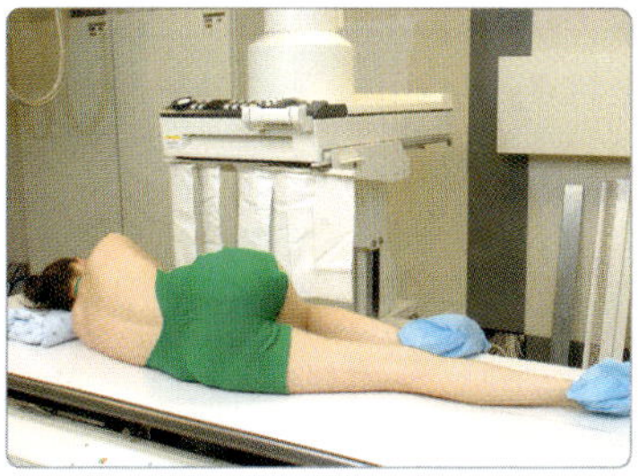

EXERCISE 17 ■ Review of Body Position Terms

Can you define, pronounce, and spell the following body position terms?

Fowler position
lateral recumbent position
lithotomy position
orthopnea position
prone position
recumbent position
Sims position
supine position
Trendelenburg position

Diagnostic Imaging

Diagnostic imaging is an important part of the evaluation of patients with a variety of signs and symptoms. The information obtained from imaging generally reveals the presence or absence of abnormalities in the area being studied.

Radiography, or the use of x-rays, was the first form of diagnostic imaging. The process as we know it was discovered in 1895 by Wilhelm Conrad Roentgen in Germany. Because he did not understand the nature of the rays, he named them "x" rays. Today we understand that radiography produces images of internal structures using ionizing radiation emitted from an x-ray tube. An image receptor catches the radiant energy that has been transmitted through the patient. The captured energy is digitally processed to form an image called a **radiograph**, which is stored electronically and displayed on a monitor. Since Roentgen's time, many forms of diagnostic imaging have been developed and are in use today. **Radiology** is the medical specialty dedicated to the use of imaging technology to diagnose and treat disease. See Table 3.4 for an overview of current diagnostic imaging procedures.

Directional terms, abdominopelvic regions, anatomic planes, and body positioning are all important aspects of diagnostic imaging. They are used to ensure that the maximum amount of information is recorded on the image, while unnecessary radiation is minimized. For example, anatomic planes are used in **computed tomography**, **magnetic resonance imaging**, and **sonography** to identify the direction of "cuts" or "slices" demonstrated in the procedure.

TABLE 3.4 Overview of Diagnostic Imaging Procedures

PROCEDURE	VISUALIZES	OFTEN USED TO EXAMINE	USED TO DETECT
Radiography	Dense structures	Bones, lungs	Fractures, tumors, lesions
Fluoroscopy	Deep tissues and hollow structures	Gastrointestinal tract, heart, urinary system, and reproductive systems	Reflux, obstruction, ulcers
Sonography	Soft tissue structures, plus movement of blood, denseness of tissue	Heart, blood vessels, eyes, thyroid, brain, breast, abdominal organs, skin, and muscle	Cysts, tumors, gallstones, vessel blockages, prenatal abnormalities
Magnetic resonance (MR)	Internal organs, spine, joints, blood vessels	Brain, spine, joints, biliary system (gallbladder and bile ducts)	Tumors, torn ligaments, gallstones
Computed tomography (CT)	Internal organs, movement of blood, denseness of tissue	Bones, heart, lungs, vessels, abdominal organs	Disease, injuries, fractures, clots, internal bleeding, tumors
Positron emission tomography (PET)	Cellular and tissue activity	Brain, heart, vessels	Cancer, flow of blood to heart
Single photon emission computed tomography (SPECT)	Blood flow, cellular and tissue activity	Heart, brain, bones	Infection, tumors, blockages

Diagnostic Imaging Terms

BUILT FROM WORD PARTS AND *NOT* BUILT FROM WORD PARTS

The first portion of the table contains Diagnostic Imaging Terms that can be translated using definitions of word parts. The second portion of the table contains Diagnostic Imaging Terms that cannot be fully understood using the definitions of word parts.

Built from Word Parts

TERM	DEFINITION
1. radiograph (RĀ-dē-ō-*graph*)	record of x-rays
2. radiography (*rā*-dē-OG-rah-fē)	process of recording x-rays
X-RAY Radiography, the procedure (the procedure) and radiograph (the resulting image) are both also called x-ray.	
3. radiologist (*rā*-dē-OL-o-jist)	physician who specializes in x-rays (specifically the diagnosis and treatment of disease using medical imaging such as x-rays, computed tomography [CT], magnetic resonance imaging [MRI], nuclear medicine [NM], and sonography)
INTERVENTIONAL RADIOLOGISTS guide targeted treatment of disease, including cancer, vascular abnormalities, and reproductive conditions, using diagnostic imaging. Interventional radiologists (IRs) are board-certified physicians who work closely with other medical specialists.	
4. radiology (*ra*-dē-OL-o-jē)	study of x-rays (a branch of medicine concerned with the study and application of imaging technology, including x-ray, computed tomography [CT], magnetic resonance imaging [MRI], nuclear medicine [NM], and sonography to diagnose and treat disease)
5. sonogram (SON-ō-gram)	record of sound
6. sonography (so-NOG-rah-fē)	process of recording sound (also called **ultrasonography [US]**)
7. tomography (to-MOG-rah-fē)	process of recording slices (anatomical cross sections)
TYPES OF TOMOGRAPHY include computed tomography (CT), positron emission tomography (PET), and single photon emission tomography (SPECT).	

NOT Built from Word Parts

TERM	DEFINITION
1. computed tomography (CT) (kom-PŪ-ted) (to-MOG-rah-fē)	imaging modality that combines x-rays with computer technology to produce detailed, cross sectional images of the body, called "slices." Oral or intravenous contrast agent may be given to highlight specific regions in the body, resulting in clearer images.
2. fluoroscopy (flōr-OS-ka-pē)	imaging of moving body structures, like an x-ray movie. An x-ray beam is passed through the body part being studied, and then the image is transmitted to a monitor in real time so that movement can be seen in detail. Contrast agent is often used to help identify and assess the function of different structures.
3. nuclear medicine (NM) (NOO-klē-er) (MED-i-sin)	imaging of internal structures by using a Gamma camera to detect radiation from different parts of the body after a radioactive material (radioisotope) has been given to the patient. Computer software assembles data into images called scans.
4. magnetic resonance imaging (MRI) (mag-NET-ik) (REZ-ō-nans) (IM-a-jing)	high strength, computer-controlled magnetic fields producing a series of sectional images (slices) that visualize abnormalities such as swelling, infections, tumors, and herniated disks
5. scan (skan)	image obtained from diagnostic imaging procedures using sensing devices and (most often) radioisotopes
SCAN also refers to diagnostic images created by the combination of data from several different angles or sections, such as CT scan or MRI scan, which may be generated without the use of radioactive contrast material.	

EXERCISE 18 ■ Pronounce and Spell

Practice pronunciation and spelling on paper and online.

1. Practice on Paper

a. **Pronounce:** Read the phonetic spelling and say aloud the terms listed in the previous table. Refer to the pronunciation key on p. 20 as necessary.
b. **Spell:** Have a study partner read the terms aloud. Write the spelling of the terms on a separate sheet of paper.

2. Practice Online

a. **Access** online learning resources. Go to evolve.elsevier.com > Evolve Resources > Student Resources.
b. **Pronounce:** Select Audio Glossary > Chapter 3 > Exercise 18. Select a term to hear its pronunciation and repeat aloud.
c. **Spell:** Select Activities > Chapter 3 > Spell Terms > Exercise 18. Select the audio icon and type the correct spelling of the term.

❑ Check the box when complete.

EXERCISE 19 ■ Diagnostic Terms Built from Word Parts

A Analyze and Define

Analyze and define the following diagnostic imaging terms by drawing slashes between word parts, writing word part abbreviations above the term, underlining combining forms, and writing combining form abbreviations below the term. *To check your answers, go to Appendix A.*

WR CV S
EXAMPLE: radi / o / logy
CF
study of x-rays

1. tomography

____

____

2. sonogram

____

____

3. radiography

____

____

4. sonography

____

____

5. radiograph

____

____

6. radiologist

____

____

B Label

Build diagnostic imaging terms pictured by writing word parts above definitions.

1.

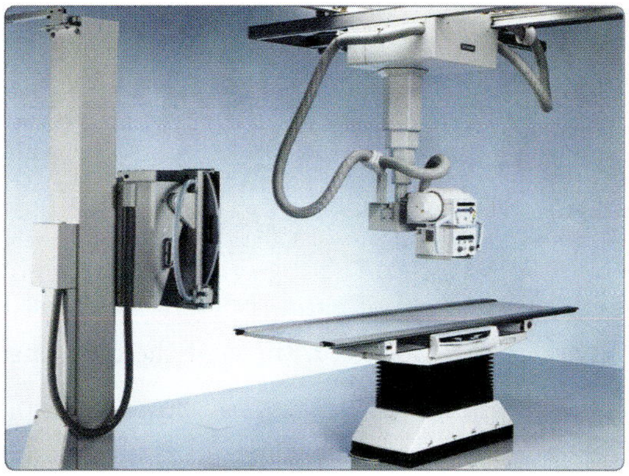

_______ / _______ / _______

x-ray CV process of recording

2.

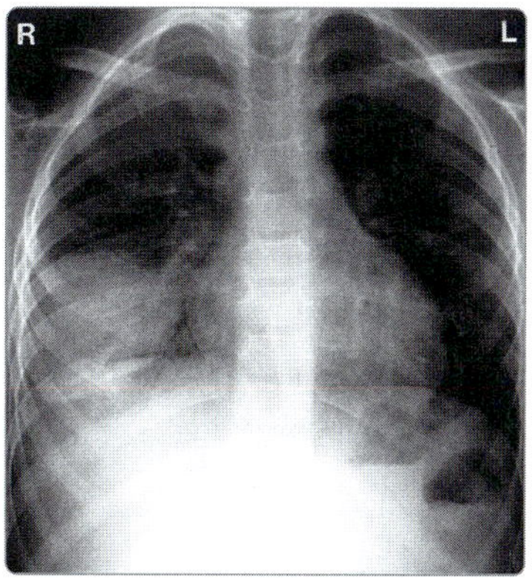

_______ / _______ / _______

x-rays CV record

3.

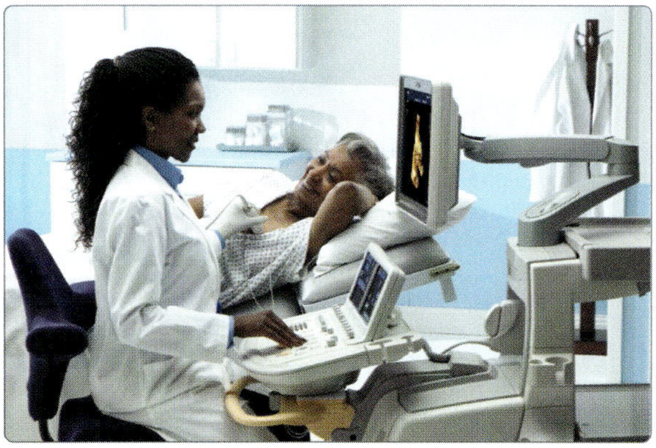

_______ / _______ / _______

sound CV process of recording

4.

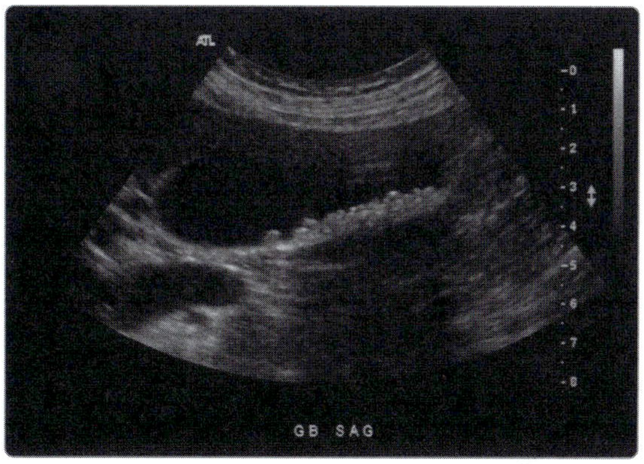

_______ / _______ / _______

sound CV record

C Fill In

Build diagnostic imaging terms for the following definitions by using the word parts you have learned.

1. process of recording slices _______ / _______ / _______
WR CV S

2. physician who specializes in x-rays _______ / _______ / _______
WR CV S

3. study of x-rays _______ / _______ / _______
WR CV S

EXERCISE 20 ■ Diagnostic Imaging Terms NOT Built from Word Parts

A Identify

Fill in the blanks with the correct terms.

1. The image obtained from sensing devices and radioisotopes is called a(n) ______________________.
2. ______________________ produces images of internal structures by using a Gamma camera to detect radiation from different parts of the body after a radioactive material has been given to the patient.
3. Moving x-ray images are produced by ______________________.
4. The procedure using high strength, computer-controlled magnetic fields to produce a series of sectional images (slices) is called ______________________.
5. ______________________ is the imaging modality combining x-rays with computer technology to produce detailed, cross sectional images of the body, called "slices."

B Label

Write the diagnostic imaging terms pictured and defined.

1. ______________________
imaging of moving body structures, like an x-ray movie; an x-ray beam is passed through the body part being studied, then the image is transmitted to a monitor in real time so that movement can be seen in detail

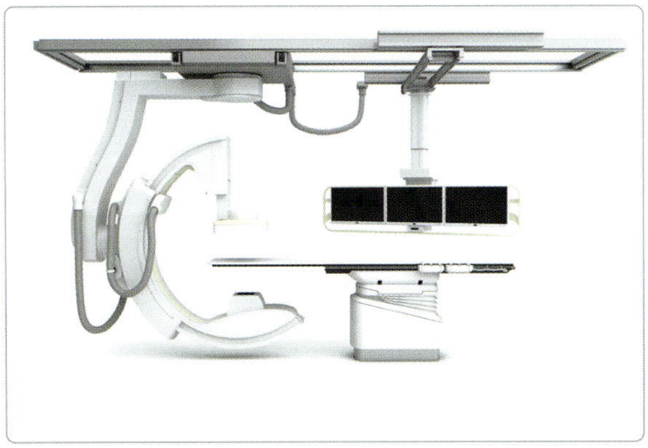

2. ______________________
imaging modality that combines x-rays with computer technology to produce detailed, cross sectional images of the body, called "slices"

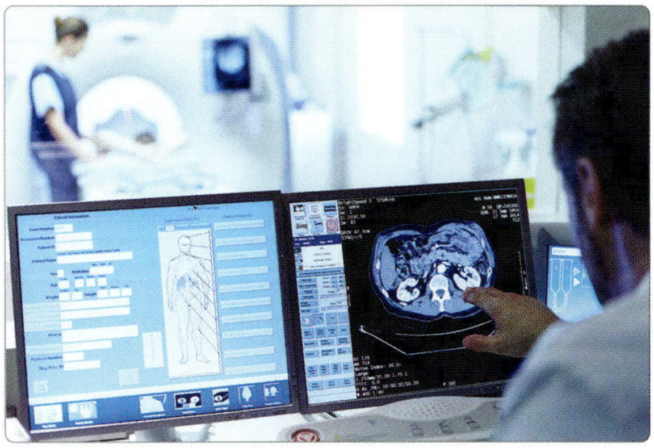

3. ______________________
imaging of internal structures by using a Gamma camera to detect radiation from different parts of the body after a radioactive material has been given to the patient

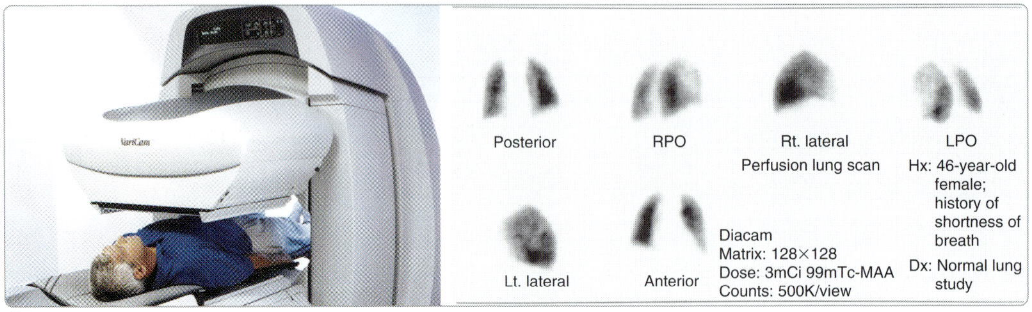

4. ______________________________
high strength, computer-controlled magnetic fields producing a series of sectional images (slices) that visualize abnormalities such as swelling, infections, tumors, and herniated disks

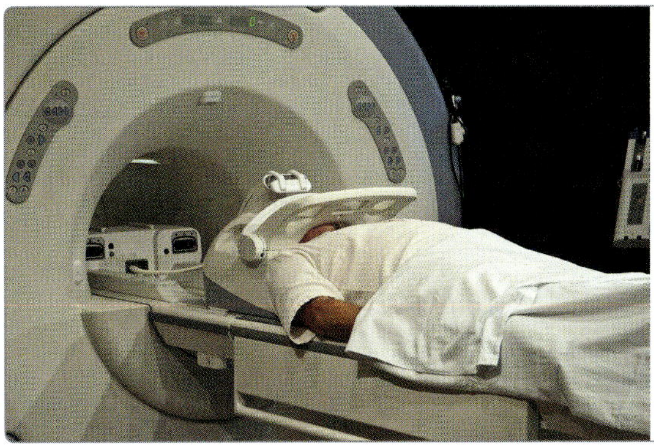

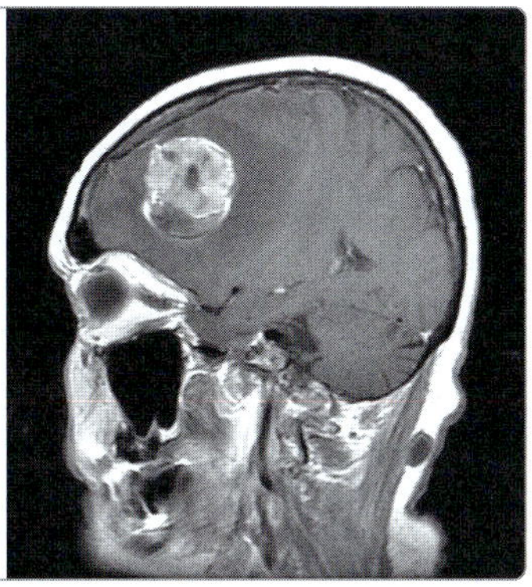

EXERCISE 21 ■ Review of Diagnostic Imaging Terms

Can you define, pronounce, and spell the following diagnostic imaging terms?

computed tomography (CT)
fluoroscopy
magnetic resonance imaging (MRI)
nuclear medicine (NM)
radiograph
radiography
radiologist
radiology
scan
sonogram
sonography
tomography

Abbreviations

DIRECTIONAL TERMS

ABBREVIATION	TERM	ABBREVIATION	TERM
ant	anterior	**med**	medial
AP	anteroposterior	**PA**	posteroanterior
inf	inferior	**sup**	superior
lat	lateral		

DIAGNOSTIC IMAGING

ABBREVIATION	TERM	ABBREVIATION	TERM
CT	computed tomography	**NM**	nuclear medicine
MR	magnetic resonance	**US**	ultrasonography
MRI	magnetic resonance imaging		

ABDOMINOPELVIC QUADRANTS

ABBREVIATION	TERM	ABBREVIATION	TERM
LLQ	left lower quadrant	**RLQ**	right lower quadrant
LUQ	left upper quadrant	**RUQ**	right upper quadrant

Refer to **Appendix D** for a complete list of abbreviations.

ABDOMINOPELVIC QUADRANTS

The abdominopelvic area can also be divided into four quadrants by using imaginary vertical and horizontal lines that intersect at the umbilicus (Fig. 3.4). These divisions are used by healthcare professionals to specify the location of pain, incisions, markings, lesions, and so forth. The quadrants provide a more general denotation than the abdominopelvic regions, and they are used to describe the location of findings from the physical examination and medical history. The four divisions are:

1. right upper quadrant (RUQ)
2. left upper quadrant (LUQ)
3. right lower quadrant (RLQ)
4. left lower quadrant (LLQ)

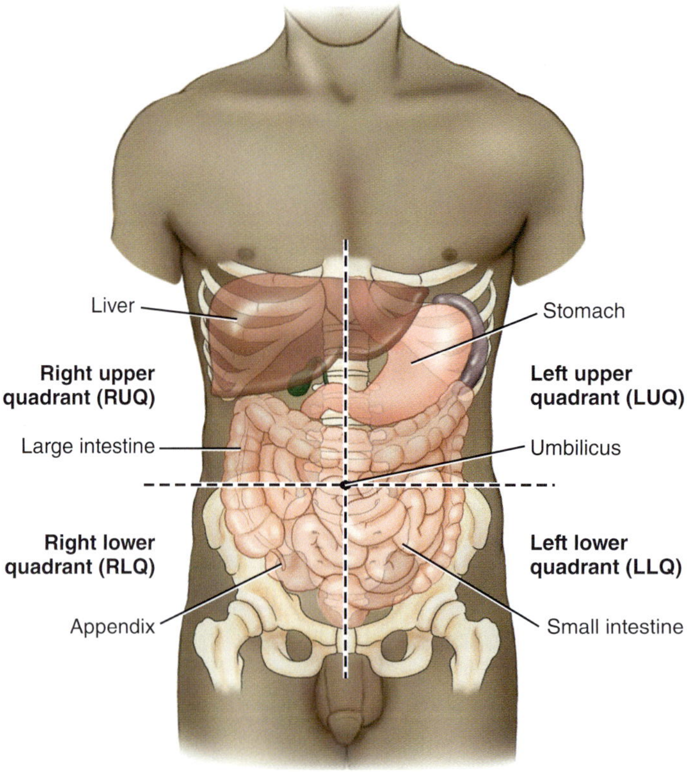

FIG. 3.4 Abdominopelvic quadrants.

EXERCISE 22 ■ Abbreviations

A Fill In

Write the terms abbreviated.

1. sup ____________________
2. ant ____________________
3. inf ____________________
4. PA ____________________
5. AP ____________________
6. med ____________________
7. lat ____________________
8. US ____________________
9. NM ____________________
10. MRI ____________________
11. CT ____________________
12. MR ____________________

B Label

Fill in the blanks with abdominopelvic quadrants and abbreviations to label the diagram.

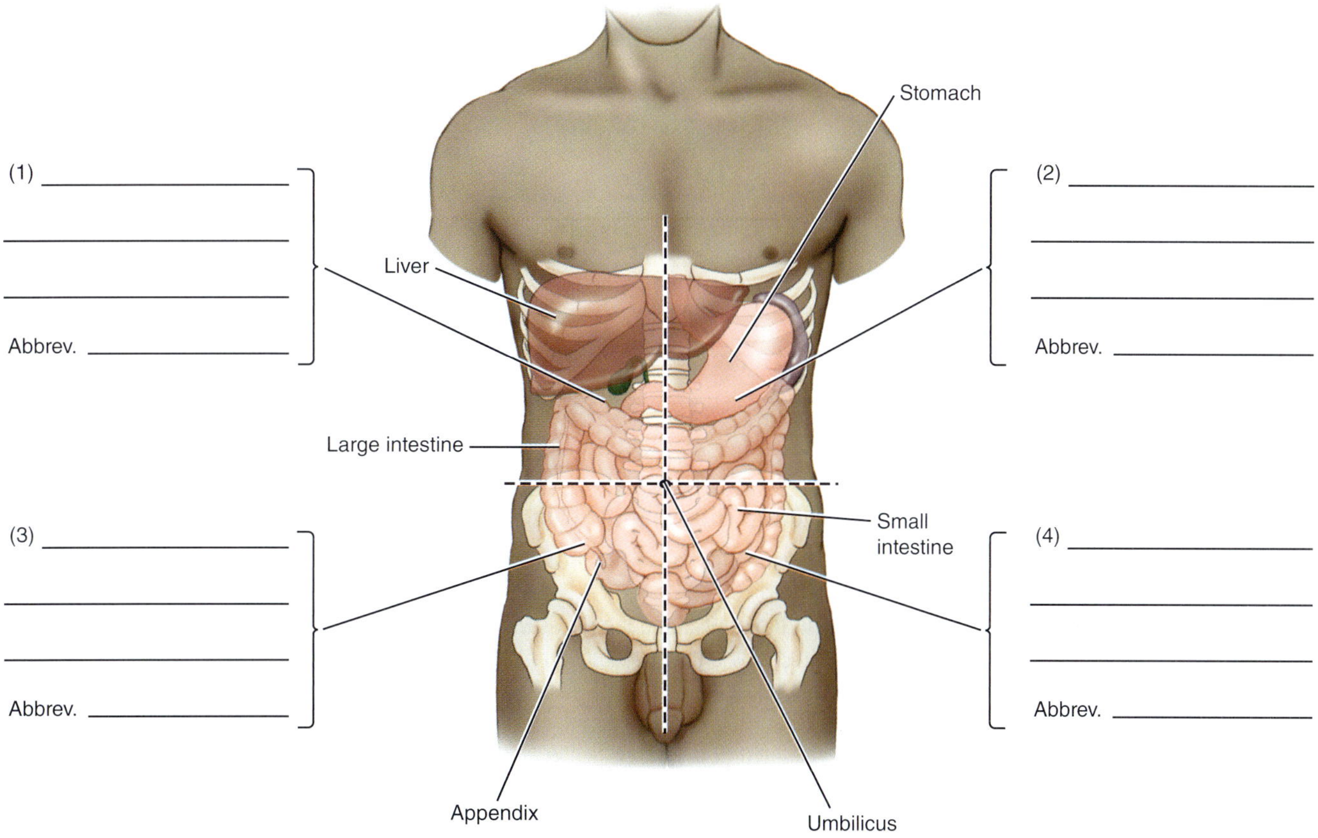

PRACTICAL APPLICATION

EXERCISE 23 ■ Case Study: Translate Between Everyday Language and Medical Language

CASE STUDY: A'idah Khalil

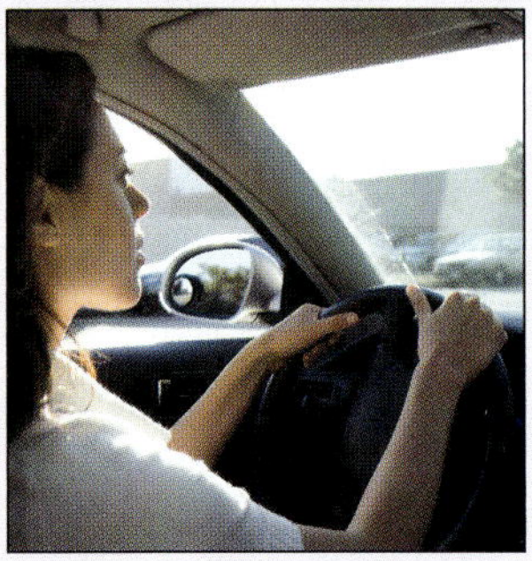

A'idah Khalil was just in a car accident, but luckily, she is awake and knows what is going on around her. The ambulance comes, and the emergency team asks her where she is hurting. Her right foot hurts the most. She has pain in her upper right arm near her shoulder and notices some bleeding there. She also has some pain in her belly near the navel and in her lower back near the waist. The paramedics put her on a hard board on her back facing upward, put some kind of collar around her neck, then load her into the ambulance and take her to the hospital. Upon arrival in the Emergency Department, she is taken to the x-ray department to have pictures taken of her foot. While there, she is also placed into a machine that allows x-ray doctors to view cross sections of her spine and the areas around it.

Now that you have worked through Chapter 3, consider the directional terms, positions, and regions that might be used to describe A'idah's experience. See the Chapter at a Glance section at the end of the chapter for a list of terms that might apply.

A. *Underline phrases in the case study that could be substituted with medical terms.*

B. *Write the medical term and its definition for two of the phrases you underlined.*

MEDICAL TERM	DEFINITION
1. ____________________	______________________________
	______________________________
2. ____________________	______________________________
	______________________________

DOCUMENTATION: Excerpt From Emergency Department Note

The following was documented in the Diagnostic Studies portion of her medical record:

Radiographs (x-rays) of the right lower extremity in the medial and lateral view identify a fracture of the calcaneus with proximal dislocation of the cuboid bone. Radiographs of the cervical spine in AP and oblique projection show no bone injury. CT scan images of the lower back reveal no significant abnormalities.

C. *Underline medical terms and abbreviations presented in Chapter 3 in the previous excerpt from A'idah's medical record. See the Chapter at a Glance section at the end of the chapter for a complete list.*

D. *Select and define two of the medical terms you underlined. To check your answers, go to Appendix A.*

MEDICAL TERM	DEFINITION
1. ____________________	______________________________
	______________________________
2. ____________________	______________________________
	______________________________

EXERCISE 24 ■ Interact with Medical Documents

A

Read the report and complete it by writing medical terms on answer lines within the document. Definitions of terms to be written appear after the document.

817254-DPQ PARKER, Zoe

File Patient Navigate Custom Fields Help

Chart Review | Encounters | Notes | Labs | Imaging | Procedures | Rx | Documents | Referrals | Scheduling | Billing

Name: PARKER, Zoe MR#: 817254-DPQ DOB: 03/27/19XX Gender: F Age: 72 Allergies: Bees PCP: Means, Robert MD

Date: 3/27/20XX
Progress Note:

Mrs. Parker is here today for follow-up on the degenerative joint disease of both knees and ankles. She arrived ambulatory with the assistance of a cane, walking slowly with a fairly steady gait.

On examination of the knees, there is marked crepitus that is palpable with pressure applied to the patellae with the knees flexed and extended, right greater than left. She has a range of motion from 10 degrees to 110 degrees in the right knee. Pain is evident at the end of extension at 10 degrees. The right knee is stable when stressed in an 1.________________________, valgus and varus manner.

On examination of the right ankle, there is some mild tenderness on palpation above the lateral malleolus. The right ankle moves from 0 degrees of dorsiflexsion to 25 degrees of plantar flexion. From the 2.________________________ joint line at the knee to the malleolus at the ankle, the right tib/fib is 1.5 cm shorter than the left. There is pigment change mainly on the 3.________________________ and 4.________________________ aspect of the right lower leg. There is a slight bony deformity over the 5.________________________ aspect of the mid-tibial area.

Diagnostic Imaging: Review of the 6. ______________ report indicates moderate arthritis of the knees and ankles, right greater than left.

Impression:
1. Degenerative joint disease of both knees and ankles, stable.

Plan:
1. Patient is to continue on current medications unchanged.

Electronically signed: Robert Means MD on 27 March 20XX 13:30

Start | Log On/Off | Print | Edit

Definitions of Medical Terms to Complete the Document

Write the medical terms defined on corresponding answer lines in the document.

1. pertaining to the front and to the back
2. pertaining to the side
3. pertaining to the back
4. pertaining to the middle
5. pertaining to the front
6. study of x-rays

B

Read the procedure documentation and answer the questions below it.

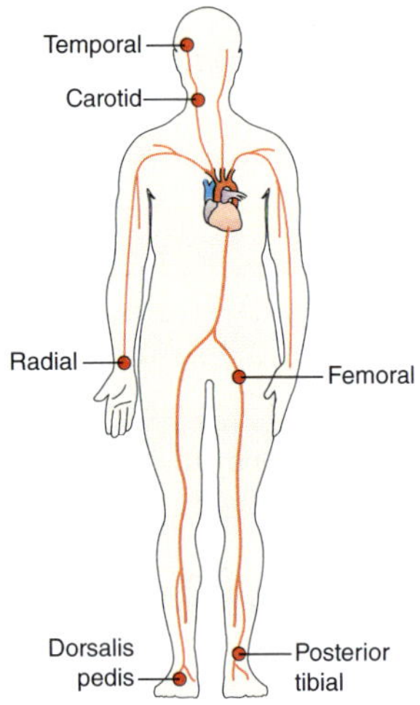

PROCEDURE FOR PALPATING ARTERIAL PULSES

Palpate arteries with the distal pads of the first two fingers. The fingertips are used because they are the most sensitive parts of the hand. Unless contraindicated, simultaneous palpation is preferred.

Temporal: Palpate over the temporal bone on each side of the head, lateral to each eyebrow.

Carotid: Palpate the anterior edge of the sternocleidomastoid muscle, just medial and inferior to the angle of the jaw. To avoid reduction of blood flow, do not palpate right and left carotid pulses simultaneously.

Radial: Palpate lateral and anterior side of wrist, proximal to the first carpal-metacarpal junction.

Femoral: This pulse is inferior to the medial inguinal ligament; the pulse is found midway between anterior superior iliac spine and pubic tubercle.

Posterior tibial: This pulse is found posterior and slightly inferior to the medial malleolus of the ankle.

Dorsalis pedis: With the foot slightly dorsiflexed, lightly palpate the dorsal surface of the foot, just lateral to the first metatarsal.

Use the procedure documentation above to answer the questions. For questions 1-3, circle the correct answer. Use a reference source to answer question 4.

1. The **temporal pulse** is palpated
   a. just above the eyebrow.
   b. to the side of the eyebrow.
   c. below the eyebrow.
   d. to the middle of the eyebrow.
2. The **radial pulse** is palpated
   a. to the side and front of the wrist.
   b. to the side and back of the wrist.
   c. to the middle and back of the wrist.
   d. to the middle and front of the wrist.
3. The **femoral pulse** is located
   a. below the medial inguinal ligament.
   b. above the medial inguinal ligament.
   c. to the front of the medial inguinal ligament.
   d. to the back of the medial inguinal ligament.
4. When used with the foot, ***dorsal*** has a different meaning. Using a medical dictionary or an online source, describe the dorsal surface of the foot. Hint: try *dorsum* and *dorsalis pedis* as search terms. The dorsal surface of the foot is ____.

EXERCISE 25 ▪ Pronounce Medical Terms in Use

Practice pronunciation of terms by reading aloud the following paragraph. Use the phonetic spellings to assist with pronunciation. The script also contains medical terms not presented in the chapter. If interested, research their meanings by using a medical dictionary or a reliable online source.

The patient presented to her physician with pain in the right **lumbar region** (LUM-bar) (RĒ-jun) and right **unilateral** (ū-ni-LAT-er-al) leg pain. The pain was felt in the **posterior** (pos-TĒR-ē -or) portion of the leg and radiated to the **distal** (DIS-tal) **lateral** (LAT-er-al) portion of the extremity. There was some **proximal** (PROK-si-mal) muscle weakness reported of the affected leg. A lumbar spine **radiograph** (RĀ-dē-ō-graph) was normal. If the pain does not respond to antiinflammatory medication, she will be referred to an orthopedist.

CHAPTER REVIEW

EXERCISE 26 ■ Chapter Content Quiz

Test your understanding of terms and abbreviations introduced in this chapter. For questions 1-19, circle the letter for the medical term or abbreviation related to the words in italics. For question 20, write medical terms for words in italics.

1. The plane that *divides the body into right and left sides* is a general term used to specify a vertical plane running through the body from the front to back.
   a. coronal plane
   b. axial plane
   c. sagittal plane
2. The *midsagittal plane* more specifically describes the sagittal plane by indicating the body is divided in:
   a. half (equal portions)
   b. unequal portions
   c. anterior and posterior portions
3. Images for computed tomography (CT) scanning can be produced from the sagittal plane, the frontal plane, and the plane *dividing the body into superior and inferior portions* called the:
   a. coronal plane
   b. parasagittal plane
   c. axial plane
4. A polyp was found in the colon *pertaining to away from the point of attachment of a body part* or ______________ to the splenic flexure.
   a. distal
   b. proximal
   c. medial
5. The drainage catheter is placed over the right *pertaining to the front* or ______________ pelvis.
   a. inferior
   b. posterior
   c. anterior
6. The incision was made at the *pertaining to above* or ______________ pole of the lesion.
   a. superior
   b. inferior
   c. lateral
7. The patient complained of *superior to umbilical region* or ______________ pain.
   a. hypochondriac region
   b. hypogastric region
   c. epigastric region
8. A *pertaining to a side* or ______________ chest radiograph displays the anatomy in the *dividing the body into right and left sides* or ______________ plane.
   a. lateral, sagittal
   b. medial, coronal
   c. bilateral, transverse
9. The patient was scheduled for an ultrasound-guided *pertaining to two (both) sides* or ______________ thoracentesis.
   a. unilateral
   b. bilateral
   c. mediolateral
10. The doctor's order indicated that the patient with dyspnea (difficulty breathing) was to be placed in the *sitting erect or upright* or ______________ position to facilitate breathing.
    a. right Sims
    b. left recumbent
    c. orthopnea
11. The patient being treated for cardiovascular shock was placed in *lying on back with the head lower than the feet* or ______________ position.
    a. Trendelenburg
    b. Fowler
    c. prone
12. Gallbladder pain is likely to be in the *abbreviated as RUQ* or ______________.
    a. lumbar region
    b. right upper quadrant
    c. upper right quadrant
13. The directional term *pertaining to the back* or ______________ is often used to describe the back of the hand or upper surface of the foot.
    a. superior
    b. anterior
    c. dorsal
14. Just before birth, the fetus shifted to a *pertaining to the head* or ______________ presentation.
    a. cephalic
    b. caudal
    c. ventral
15. A *pertaining to the tail* or ______________ epidural steroid injection may be performed to relieve chronic low back pain.
    a. dorsal
    b. caudal
    c. proximal
16. A patient who will be receiving an enema is usually placed in the left *lying on the side with the knee drawn toward the chest and the arm drawn behind* ______________ position for gravity to help the fluid flow through the sigmoid colon into the descending colon. This position may also be called left recumbent position.
    a. Fowler
    b. lithotomy
    c. Sims

17. *Imaging of moving body structures*, or __________, is frequently used to diagnose abnormalities in the gastrointestinal tract.
    a. magnetic resonance imaging
    b. fluoroscopy
    c. radiography

18. The abbreviation *CT* stands for:
    a. computed topography
    b. commuted tomography
    c. computed tomography
    d. computer tomogramy

19. An interventional *physician who specializes in x-rays*, or __________, may perform procedures such as CT-guided biopsy and radiofrequency ablation of tumors.
    a. radiologist
    b. oncologist
    c. pathologist

20. The pathology report for the patient with a palpable right breast lump included the sections listed below. Fill in the blanks with directional terms indicated by words in italics.

    Right axillary sentinel lymph node biopsy;

    a. Right breast, __________ margin biopsy (*pertaining to above*)
    b. Right breast, __________ margin biopsy (*pertaining to below*)

    Right breast, deep margin biopsy;

    c. Right breast, __________ margin biopsy (*pertaining to the middle*)
    d. Right breast, __________ margin biopsy (*pertaining to a side*)

CHAPTER AT A GLANCE Word Parts New to this Chapter

COMBINING FORMS

anter/o
caud/o
cephal/o
dist/o
dors/o
infer/o
later/o
medi/o
proxim/o
radi/o
son/o
super/o
tom/o
ventr/o

PREFIXES

bi-
uni-

SUFFIXES

-ad
-gram
-graph
-graphy
-ior

CHAPTER AT A GLANCE Medical Terms Built from Word Parts

DIRECTIONAL TERMS

anterior (ant)
anteroposterior (AP)
bilateral
caudad
caudal
cephalad
cephalic
distal
dorsal
inferior (inf)
lateral (lat)
medial (med)
mediolateral
posterior
posteroanterior (PA)
proximal
superior (sup)
unilateral
ventral

DIAGNOSTIC IMAGING

radiograph
radiography
radiologist
radiology
sonogram
sonography
tomography

CHAPTER AT A GLANCE Medical Terms NOT Built from Word Parts

ABDOMINOPELVIC REGIONS

epigastric region
hypochondriac regions
hypogastric region
iliac regions
lumbar regions
umbilical region

ANATOMIC PLANES

axial
coronal
midsagittal
parasagittal
sagittal

BODY POSITIONS

Fowler
lateral recumbent
lithotomy
orthopnea
prone
recumbent
Sims
supine
Trendelenburg

DIAGNOSTIC IMAGING

computed tomography (CT)
fluoroscopy
nuclear medicine (NM)
magnetic resonance imaging (MRI)
scan

Chapter 4

Integumentary System

Outline

Objectives

Upon completion of this chapter, you will be able to:

1. Pronounce anatomic structures of the integumentary system.
2. Define and spell word parts related to the integumentary system.
3. Define, pronounce, and spell disease and disorder terms related to the integumentary system.
4. Define, pronounce, and spell surgical terms related to the integumentary system.
5. Define, pronounce, and spell complementary terms related to the integumentary system.
6. Interpret the meaning of abbreviations related to the integumentary system.
7. Apply medical language in clinical contexts.

ANATOMY

The integumentary system is composed of the skin, glands, hair, and nails.

> **INTEGUMENTARY** is derived from the Latin word **tegere**, meaning to **cover.**

Function

The skin forms a protective covering for the body that, when unbroken, prevents entry of bacteria and other invading organisms. The skin also protects the body from water loss and the damaging effects of ultraviolet light. Other functions include regulation of body temperature and synthesis of vitamin D.

Anatomic Structures of the Integumentary System

TERM	DEFINITION
skin (skin)	organ covering the body; made up of layers (also called **cutaneous membrane**) (Fig. 4.1)

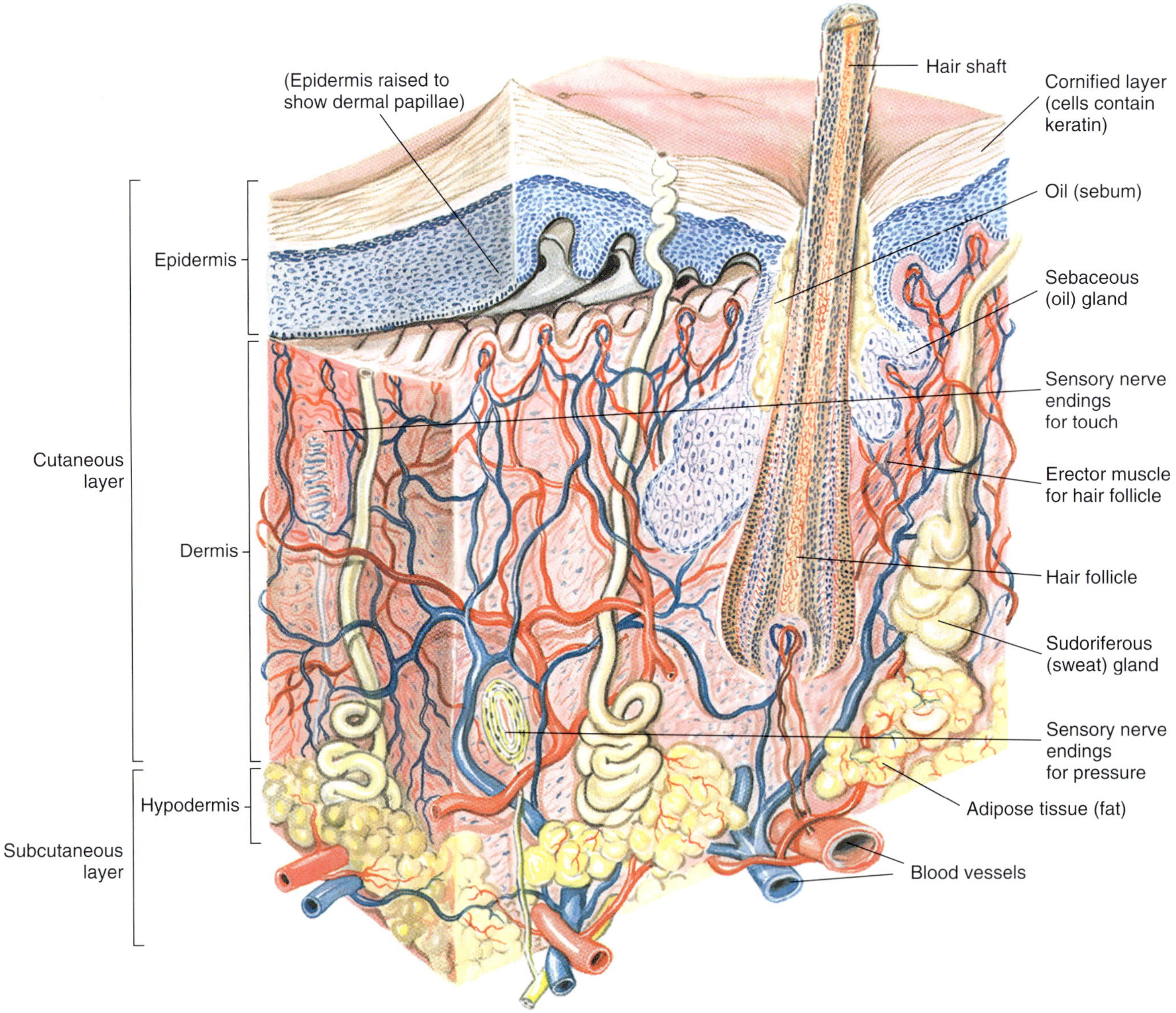

FIG. 4.1 Structure of the skin.

TERM	DEFINITION
epidermis (ep-i-DER-mis)	outer layer of skin; protects the body from the external environment
keratin (KAR-a-tin)	scleroprotein component of the horny, or cornified, layer of the epidermis. Also, the primary component of the hair and nails
melanin (MEL-a-nin)	dark pigment produced by melanocytes; amount present determines skin color
hair (hār)	compressed, keratinized cells that arise from hair follicles, the sacs that enclose the hair fibers
nails (nālz)	horny plates made from flattened epithelial cells; found on the dorsal surface of the ends of the fingers and toes
sebaceous glands (se-BĀ-shas) (glans)	secrete sebum (oil) into the hair follicles where the hair shafts pass through the dermis
sudoriferous glands (*soo*-da-RIF-er-as) (glans)	tiny, coiled, tubular structures that emerge through pores on the skin's surface and secrete sweat (also called **sweat glands**)
APPENDAGES OF THE SKIN is a common reference to hair, nails, sudoriferous glands, and sebaceous glands.	
dermis (DUR-mis)	inner layer of skin; responsible for its flexibility and mechanical strength
hypodermis (*hī*-pō-DER-mis)	layer between the dermis and the underlying tissues and organs; contains adipose tissue (fat), connective tissue, nerves, and blood vessels (also called **subcutaneous layer**)

PRONOUNCE ANATOMIC STRUCTURES

Practice saying aloud each of the organs and specific structures on the previous pages.

To hear the terms, go to Evolve Resources at www.evolve.elsevier.com and select:
Student Resources > Audio Glossary > Chapter 4 > **Anatomic Structures**

❑ Check the box when complete.

WORD PARTS

Use paper flashcards or electronic flashcards on Evolve to assist with memorization of word parts used to analyze, define, and build terms presented in this chapter. To reinforce learning, study one section of the Word Parts Table at a time, then complete the corresponding exercise on the following pages.

1 ■ Integumentary System Combining Forms

COMBINING FORM	DEFINITION	COMBINING FORM	DEFINITION
cutane/o	skin	**onych/o**	nail
derm/o	skin	**seb/o**	sebum (oil)
dermat/o	skin	**trich/o**	hair
hidr/o	sweat	**ungu/o**	nail
kerat/o	horny tissue (keratin), hard		

KERAT/O refers to the cornea of the eye when used with ophthalmology terms.

Do not be concerned about which **combining form** to use for **skin** or **nail**. As you continue to study and use medical terms, you will become familiar with common usage of each word part.

2 ■ Combining Forms Used with Integumentary System Terms

COMBINING FORM	DEFINITION	COMBINING FORM	DEFINITION
aden/o	gland	**scler/o**	hard
crypt/o	hidden	**SCLER/O** When used with ophthalmology terms, **scler/o** refers to the tough outer white portion of the eye called the sclera.	
erythr/o	red	**staphyl/o**	grapelike clusters
leuk/o	white	**strept/o**	twisted chains
myc/o	fungus	**xanth/o**	yellow
pachy/o	thick	**xer/o**	dry, dryness
rhytid/o	wrinkles		

3 ■ Prefixes

PREFIX	DEFINITION	PREFIX	DEFINITION
epi-	on, upon, over	**para-**	beside, beyond, around, abnormal
hyper-	above, excessive	**per-**	through
hypo-	below, incomplete, deficient, under	**sub-**	under, below
intra-	within	**trans-**	through, across, beyond

4 ■ Suffixes

SUFFIX	DEFINITION	SUFFIX	DEFINITION
-a	noun suffix, no meaning	**-logy**	study of
-al	pertaining to	**-malacia**	softening
-coccus (*pl.* **-cocci**)	berry-shaped (form of bacterium)	**-oma**	tumor, swelling
-ectomy	excision, surgical removal	**-osis**	abnormal condition (means increase when used with blood cell word roots)
-genic	producing, originating, causing	**-ous**	pertaining to
-ia	diseased or abnormal state, condition of	**-phagia**	eating or swallowing
-ic	pertaining to	**-plasty**	surgical repair
-itis	inflammation	**-rrhea**	flow, discharge
-logist	one who studies and treats (specialist, physician)		

Refer to **Appendix B** and **Appendix C** for alphabetical lists of word parts and their meanings.

EXERCISE 1 ■ Integumentary System Combining Forms

Refer to the first section of the word parts table.

A Label

Fill in the blanks with combining forms to label these diagrams. *To check your answers, go to Appendix A at the back of the textbook.*

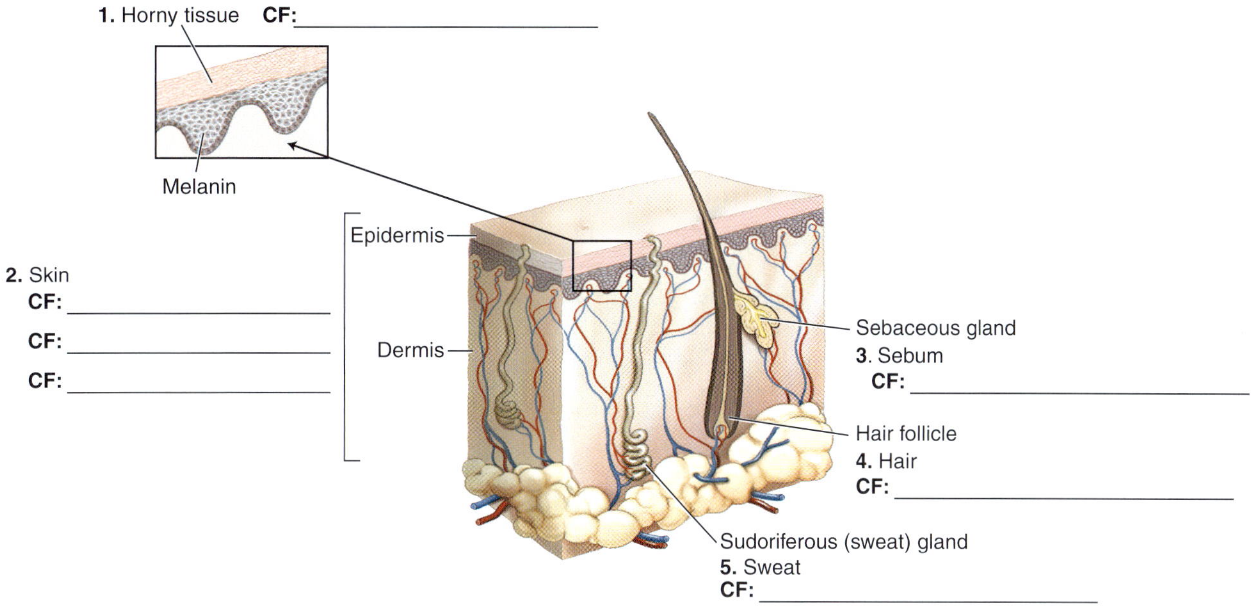

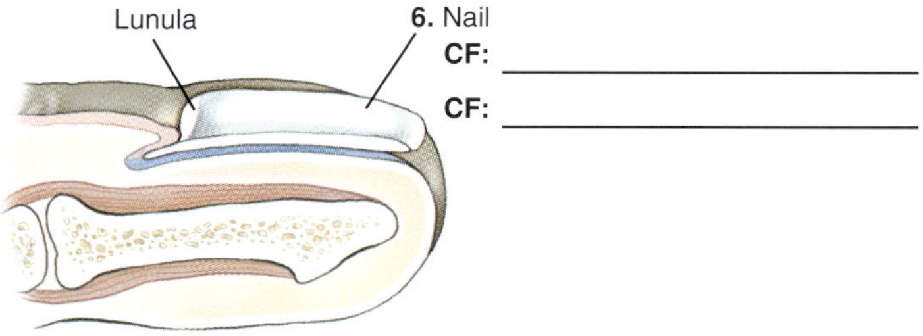

B Define and Match

Step 1: Write the definitions after the following combining forms.
Step 2: Match the descriptions on the right with the combining forms and definitions. Answers may be used more than once.

_____ 1. derm/o ____________________
_____ 2. seb/o, ____________________
_____ 3. onych/o, ____________________
_____ 4. cutane/o, ____________________
_____ 5. kerat/o, ____________________
_____ 6. ungu/o, ____________________
_____ 7. hidr/o, ____________________
_____ 8. trich/o, ____________________
_____ 9. dermat/o, ____________________

a. secreted from sudoriferous glands
b. secreted from sebaceous glands
c. horny plates made from flattened epithelial cells
d. organ covering the body; made up of layers
e. scleroprotein component of the horny, or cornified, layer of the epidermis
f. compressed, keratinized cells that arise from follicles

EXERCISE 2 ■ Combining Forms Used with Integumentary System Terms

Refer to the second section of the word parts table.

A Define

Write the definitions of the following combining forms.

1. xanth/o ______
2. staphyl/o ______
3. crypt/o ______
4. pachy/o ______
5. leuk/o ______
6. myc/o ______
7. erythr/o ______
8. scler/o ______
9. strept/o ______
10. xer/o ______
11. rhytid/o ______
12. aden/o ______

B Identify

Write the combining form for each of the following.

1. fungus ______
2. white ______
3. yellow ______
4. dry, dryness ______
5. thick ______
6. twisted chains ______
7. wrinkles ______
8. grapelike clusters ______
9. red ______
10. hidden ______
11. hard ______
12. gland ______

EXERCISE 3 ■ Prefixes

Refer to the third section of the word parts table.

A Define

Write the definitions of the following prefixes.

1. sub- ______
2. para- ______
3. epi- ______
4. intra- ______
5. per- ______
6. trans- ______
7. hypo- ______
8. hyper- ______

B Identify

Write the prefix for each of the following.

1. within ______
2. under, below ______
3. on, upon, over ______
4. beside, beyond, around, abnormal ______
5. through ______
6. through, across, beyond ______
7. above, excessive ______
8. below, incomplete, deficient, under ______

EXERCISE 4 ■ Suffixes

Refer to the fourth section of the word parts table.

A Match

Match the suffixes in the first column with their correct definitions in the second column.

______	1. -a	a. one who studies and treats (specialist, physician)
______	2. -ia	b. producing, originating, causing
______	3. -logist	c. diseased or abnormal state, condition of
______	4. -genic	d. tumor, swelling
______	5. -oma	e. noun suffix, no meaning

B Label

Write the suffixes pictured and defined.

1. ________________________
berry-shaped (form of bacterium)

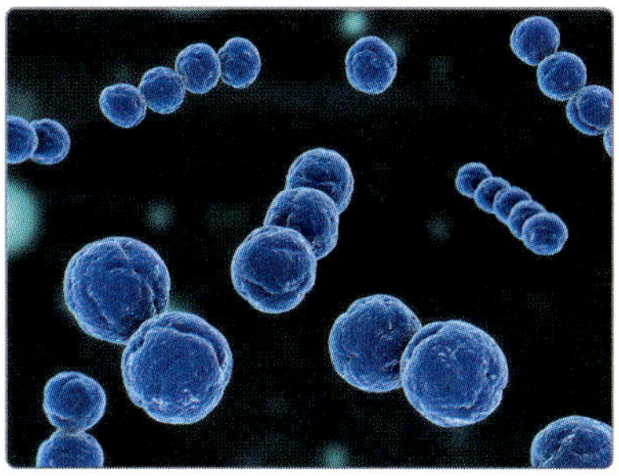

2. ________________________
flow, discharge

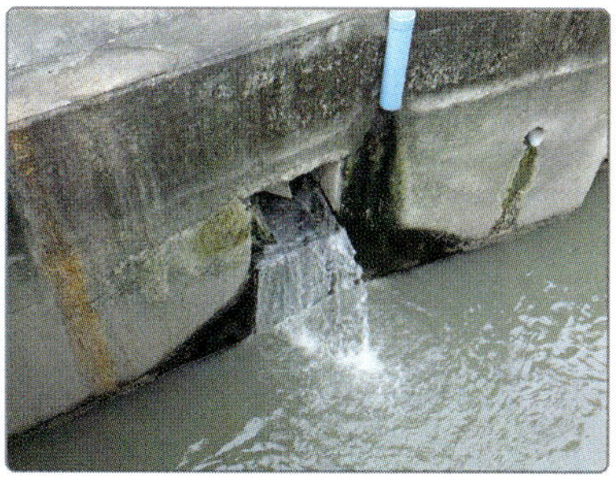

3. ________________________
softening

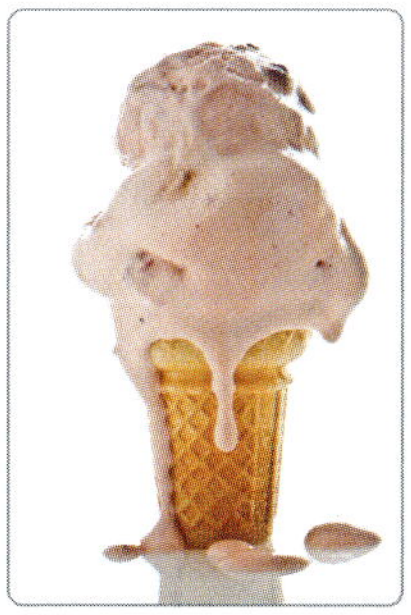

4. ________________________
inflammation

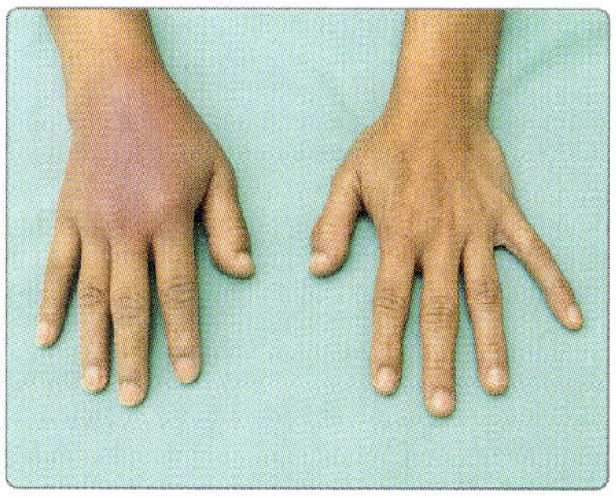

5. ________________________
surgical repair

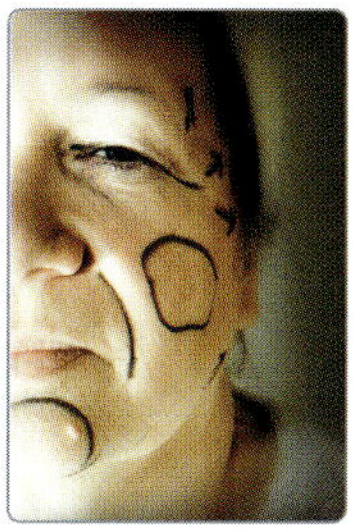

6. ________________________
eating, swallowing

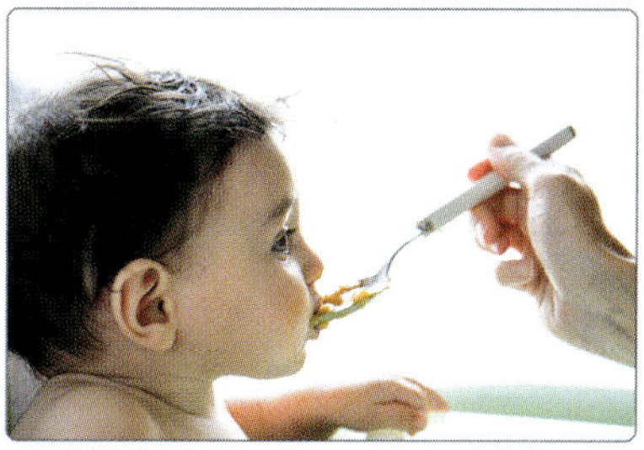

C Define

Write the definitions of the following suffixes.

1. -ous ______________________
2. -logy ______________________
3. -al ______________________
4. -osis ______________________
5. -ic ______________________
6. -ectomy ______________________

MEDICAL TERMS

Medical terms relevant to this chapter have been grouped by topics, such as Disease and Disorder, and are listed in tables designated as Built from Word Parts or *NOT* Built from Word Parts. The exercises following each table assist with learning term definitions, pronunciations, and spellings.

Disease and Disorder Terms

BUILT FROM WORD PARTS

The following terms can be translated using definitions of word parts. Further explanation is provided within parentheses as needed.

TERM	DEFINITION
1. dermatitis (*der*-ma-TĪ-tis)	inflammation of the skin (Fig. 4.2)
2. dermatofibroma (*der*-ma-tō-fī-BRŌ-ma)	fibrous tumor of the skin
3. hidradenitis (*hī*-drad-e-NĪ-tis)	inflammation of a sweat gland
4. keratosis (ker-a-TŌ-sis)	abnormal condition (growth) of horny tissue (keratin)
5. onychocryptosis (*on*-i-kō-krip-TŌ-sis)	abnormal condition of a hidden nail (also called **ingrown nail**)
6. onychomalacia (*on*-i-kō-ma-LĀ-sha)	softening of the nails
7. onychomycosis (*on*-i-kō-mī-KŌ-sis)	abnormal condition of a fungus in the nails
8. onychophagia (*on*-i-kō-FĀ-ja)	eating the nails (nail biting)
9. pachyderma (*pak*-i-DER-ma)	thickening of the skin
10. paronychia (*par*-ō-NIK-ē-a)	diseased state around the nail *(Note: the a from para- has been dropped.)*
The final vowel in a prefix may be dropped when the following word root begins with a vowel.	
11. scleroderma (skle-rō-DER-ma)	hard skin (chronic hardening or induration of the connective tissue of the skin and other organs)
12. seborrhea (seb-o-RĒ-a)	discharge of sebum (excessive)
SEBORRHEIC is the adjective form of **seborrhea** and means pertaining to excessive discharge of sebum.	
13. xanthoma (zan-THŌ-ma)	yellow tumor (benign, primarily in the skin)
14. xeroderma (*zē*-rō-DER-ma)	dry skin (a mild form of a cutaneous disorder characterized by keratinization and noninflammatory scaling)

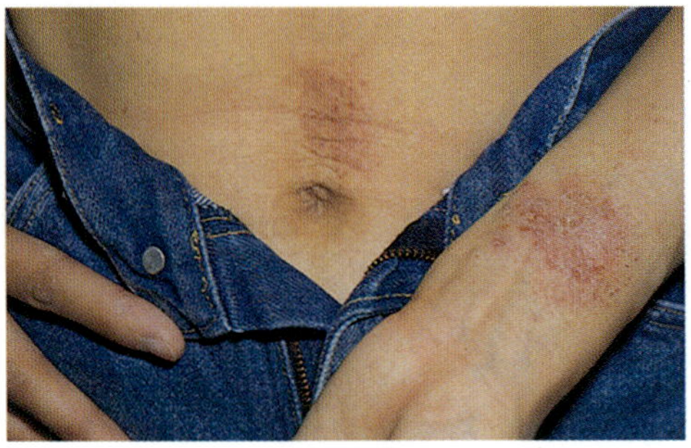

FIG. 4.2 Contact dermatitis.

EXERCISE 5 ■ Pronounce and Spell

Practice pronunciation and spelling on paper and online.

1. Practice on Paper

a. **Pronounce:** Read the phonetic spelling and say aloud the terms listed in the previous table. Refer to the pronunciation key on p. 110 as necessary.
b. **Spell:** Have a study partner read the terms aloud. Write the spelling of the terms on a separate sheet of paper.

2. Practice Online

a. **Access** online learning resources. Go to evolve.elsevier.com > Evolve Resources > Student Resources.
b. **Pronounce:** Select Audio Glossary > Chapter 4 > Exercise 5. Select a term to hear its pronunciation and repeat aloud.
c. **Spell:** Select Activities > Chapter 4 > Spell Terms > Exercise 5. Select the audio icon and type the correct spelling of the term.

❑ Check the box when complete.

EXERCISE 6 ■ Analyze and Define

Analyze and define the following Disease and Disorder Terms Built from Word Parts by drawing slashes between word parts, writing word part abbreviations above the term, underlining combining forms, and writing combining form abbreviations below the term. If needed, refer to Chapter 1 to review analyzing and defining techniques.

WR CV WR S

EXAMPLE: onych / o / myc / osis

CF

abnormal condition of a fungus in the nails

1. scleroderma
2. hidradenitis
3. dermatitis
4. pachyderma
5. onychomalacia
6. keratosis
7. dermatofibroma
8. paronychia
9. onychocryptosis
10. seborrhea

11. onychophagia

____

____

12. xeroderma

____

____

13. xanthoma

____

____

EXERCISE 7 ■ Build

A Label

Build terms pictured by writing word parts above definitions.

1.

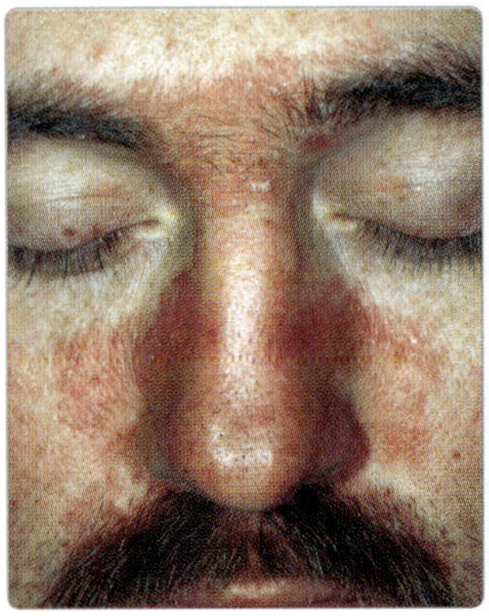

seborrheic ________ / ________
skin inflammation

2.

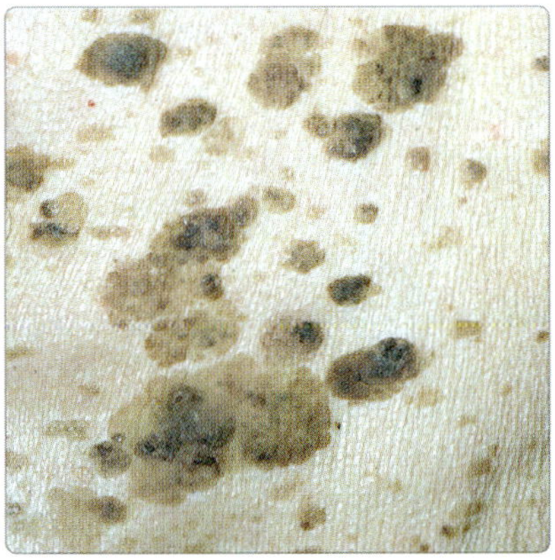

seborrheic ________ / ________
horny tissue abnormal condition

3.

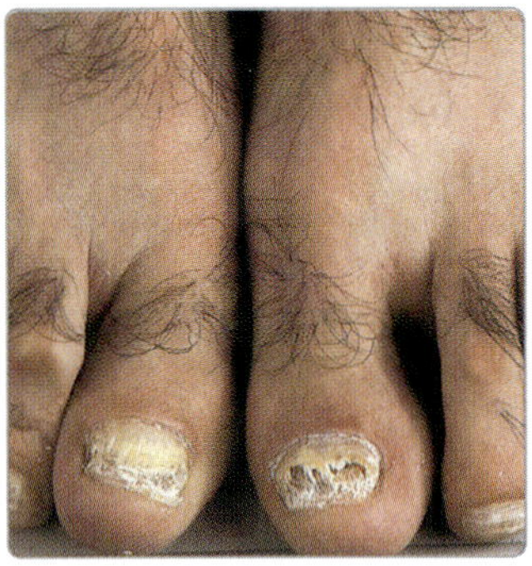

________ / ____ / ________ / ________
nail CV fungus abnormal condition

4.

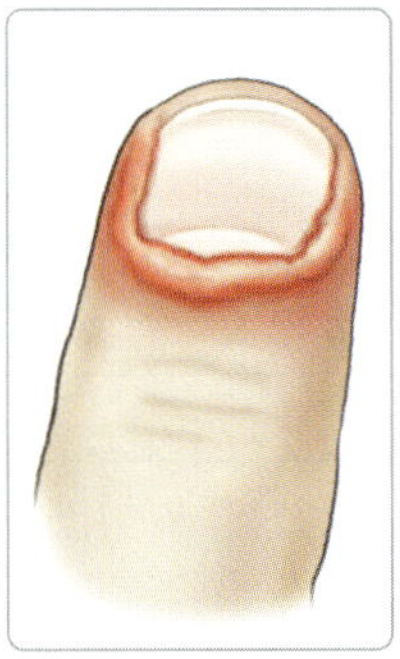

________ / ________ / ________
around nail diseased state

B Fill In

Build disease and disorder terms for the following definitions with the word parts you have learned. If you need help, refer to Chapter 1 to review term-building techniques.

EXAMPLE: abnormal condition (growth) of horny tissue (keratin) kerat / osis (WR / S)

1. thickening of the skin ______ / ______ / ______ (WR / WR / S)
2. dry skin ______ / ______ / ______ / ______ (WR / CV / WR / S)
3. discharge of sebum (excessive) ______ / ______ / ______ (WR / CV / S)
4. yellow tumor ______ / ______ (WR / S)
5. fibrous tumor of the skin ______ / ______ / ______ / ______ (WR / CV / WR / S)
6. softening of the nails ______ / ______ / ______ (WR / CV / S)
7. inflammation of a sweat gland ______ / ______ / ______ (WR / WR / S)
8. abnormal condition of a hidden nail ______ / ______ / ______ / ______ (WR / CV / WR / S)
9. hard skin ______ / ______ / ______ / ______ (WR / CV / WR / S)
10. eating the nails ______ / ______ / ______ (WR / CV / S)

Disease and Disorder Terms

NOT BUILT FROM WORD PARTS

Word parts may be present in the following terms; however, their full meanings cannot be translated using definitions of word parts alone.

TERM	DEFINITION
1. abrasion (a-BRĀ-zhun)	scraping away of the skin by mechanical process or injury
2. acne (AK-nē)	inflammatory disease of the skin involving the sebaceous glands and hair follicles
3. actinic keratosis (ack-TIN-ik) (*ker*-a-TŌ-sis)	precancerous skin condition of horny tissue formation that results from excessive exposure to sunlight. It may evolve into a squamous cell carcinoma.

Disease and Disorder Terms—cont'd

NOT BUILT FROM WORD PARTS

TERM	DEFINITION
4. albinism (AL-bi-niz-um)	congenital hereditary condition characterized by partial or total lack of pigment (melanin) in the skin, hair, and eyes

ALBINISM **Alb** is Latin word root meaning **white**. **Leuk** is the Greek word root meaning **white**.

TERM	DEFINITION
5. basal cell carcinoma (BCC) (BĀ-sal) (sel) (*kar*-si-NŌ-ma)	malignant epithelial tumor arising from the bottom layer of the epidermis called the basal layer; it seldom metastasizes, but invades local tissue and may recur in the same location. Common in individuals who have had excessive sun exposure. (Fig. 4.3)
6. candidiasis (*kan*-di-DĪ-a-sis)	infection of the skin, mouth (also called **thrush**), or vagina caused by the yeast-type fungus *Candida albicans*. *Candida* is normally present in the mucous membranes; overgrowth causes an infection. Esophageal candidiasis is often seen in patients with acquired immunodeficiency syndrome (AIDS).

CANDIDA comes from the Latin **candidus**, meaning gleaming white; **albicans** is from the Latin verb **albicare**, meaning **to make white**. The growth of the fungus is white, and the infection produces a white discharge.

TERM	DEFINITION
7. carbuncle (KAR-bung-kl)	infection of skin and subcutaneous tissue composed of a cluster of boils (furuncles, see below) caused by staphylococcal bacteria
8. cellulitis (*sel*-ū-LĪ-tis)	inflammation of the skin and subcutaneous tissue caused by infection; characterized by redness, pain, heat, and swelling
9. contusion (kon-TŪ-zhun)	injury with no break in the skin, characterized by pain, swelling, and discoloration (also called a **bruise**)
10. eczema (EK-ze-ma)	noninfectious, inflammatory skin disease characterized by redness, blisters, scabs, and itching

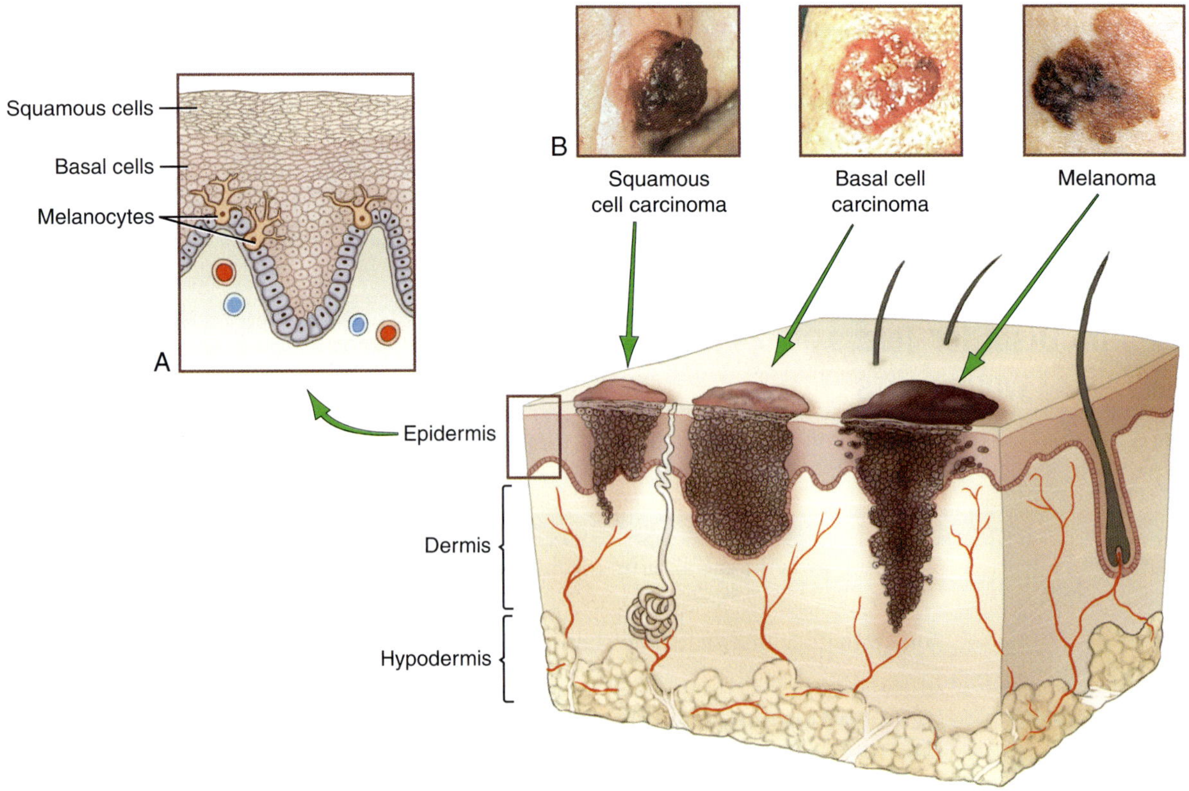

FIG. 4.3 A, Epidermal cells. B, Types of skin cancer.

TERM	DEFINITION
11. fissure (FISH-ur)	slit or cracklike sore in the skin
12. furuncle (FER-ung-kl)	painful skin nodule caused by staphylococcal bacteria in a hair follicle (also called a **boil**)
13. gangrene (GANG-grēn)	death of tissue caused by loss of blood supply followed by bacterial invasion (a form of necrosis)
14. herpes (HER-pēz)	inflammatory skin disease caused by herpes virus characterized by small blisters in clusters. Many types of herpes exist. Herpes simplex virus type 1, for example, causes fever blisters; herpes zoster, also called shingles, is characterized by painful skin eruptions that follow nerves inflamed by the virus. (see Table 4.1)
HERPES is ˜ from the Greek **herpo**, meaning to **creep along**. It is descriptive of the course and type of skin lesion.	
15. impetigo (*im*-pe-TĪ-gō)	superficial skin infection characterized by pustules and caused by either staphylococci or streptococci (see Table 4.1)
16. Kaposi sarcoma (KAP-ō-sē) (sar-KŌ-ma)	cancerous condition starting as purple or brown papules that spreads through the skin to the lymph nodes and internal organs; frequently seen with AIDS
17. keloid (KĒ-loyd)	overgrowth of scar tissue
18. laceration (*las*-er-Ā-shun)	torn, ragged-edged wound
19. measles (MĒ-zalz)	highly contagious viral disease characterized by fever, runny nose, cough, and a spreading skin rash. It is a potentially disastrous disease which can lead to pneumonia, severe bleeding, brain infections (which may cause seizures, developmental delay or chronic brain disease), and sometimes lead to death. Measles is a significant cause of death, despite the availability of a safe, effective vaccine.
MEASLES comes from the Middle English **maselen** meaning **many little spots** characteristic of the rash.	
20. MRSA infection (MER-sah) (in-FEK-shun)	invasion of body tissue by methicillin-resistant *Staphylococcus aureus*, a strain of common bacteria that has developed resistance to methicillin and other antibiotics. It can produce skin and soft tissue infections and sometimes bloodstream infections and pneumonia, which can be fatal if not treated. MRSA is quite common in hospitals and long-term care facilities but is increasingly emerging as an important infection in the general population.
21. pediculosis (pe-*dik*-ū-LŌ-sis)	invasion into the skin and hair by lice
22. pilonidal cyst (*pī*-lō-NĪ-dal) (SIST)	abnormal pocket in the skin that contains hair and skin debris. It is frequently located near the tailbone, at the top of the cleft of the buttocks. If it becomes infected, it can be severely painful and may require surgery. (Fig. 4.4)
PILONIDAL comes from the Latin words **pilus,** meaning **hair,** and **nidus,** meaning **nest. Pil/o** and **trich/o** are two combining forms for **hair**.	

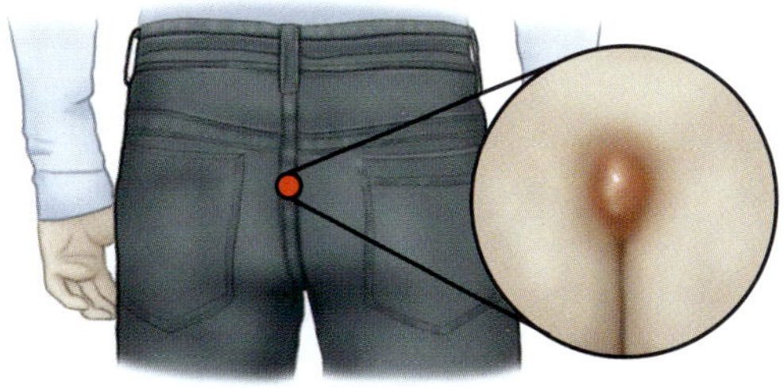

FIG. 4.4 Pilonidal Cyst.

TABLE 4.1 Common Skin Infections

Infections may be caused by a bacterium, fungus, parasite, or virus. Examples of common skin infections include the following:

TYPES	SKIN INFECTIONS	EXAMPLES
Bacterial Infections	carbuncle cellulitis furuncle impetigo MRSA paronychia	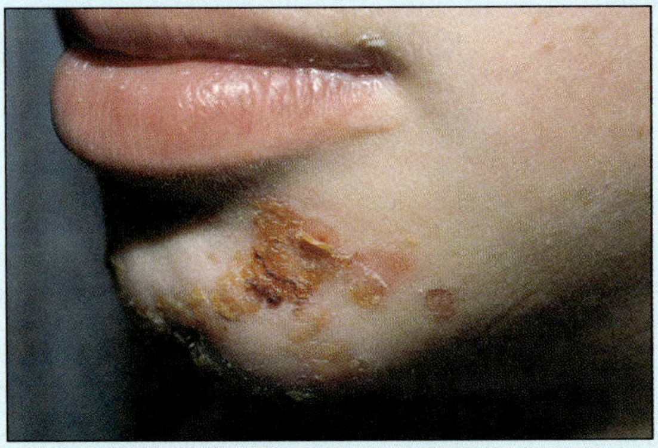 Impetigo
Fungal Infections	candidiasis tinea	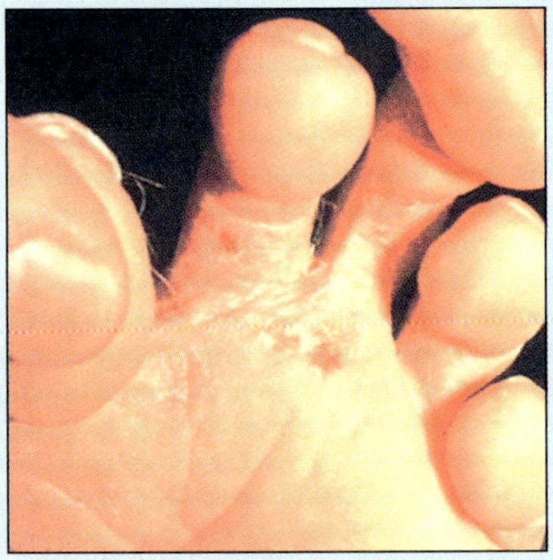 Tinea pedis (also called **athlete's foot**)
Parasitic Infections	scabies pediculosis	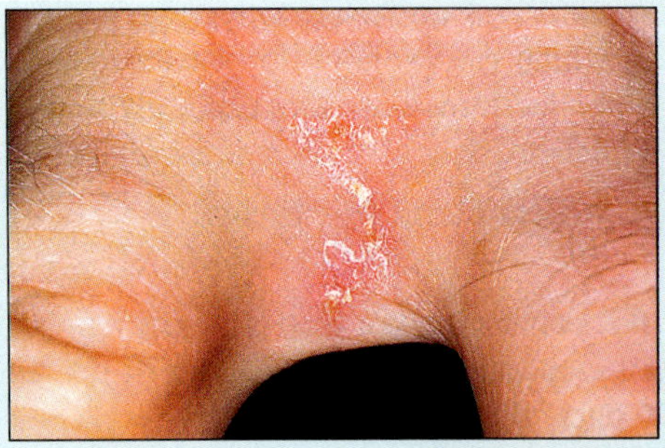 Scabies 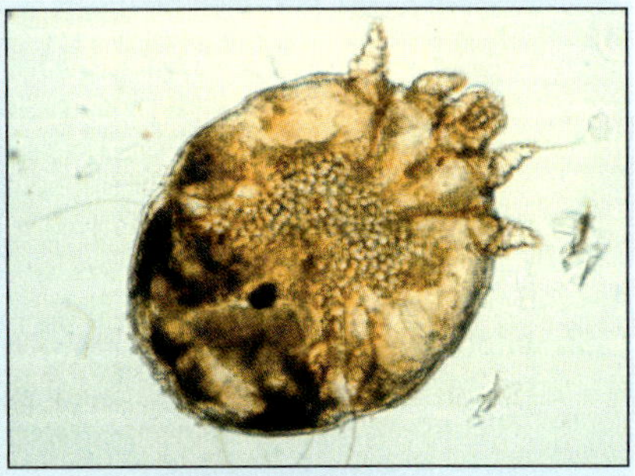 Scabies mite
Viral Infections	herpes simplex virus type 1; also called fever blister herpes zoster; also called shingles	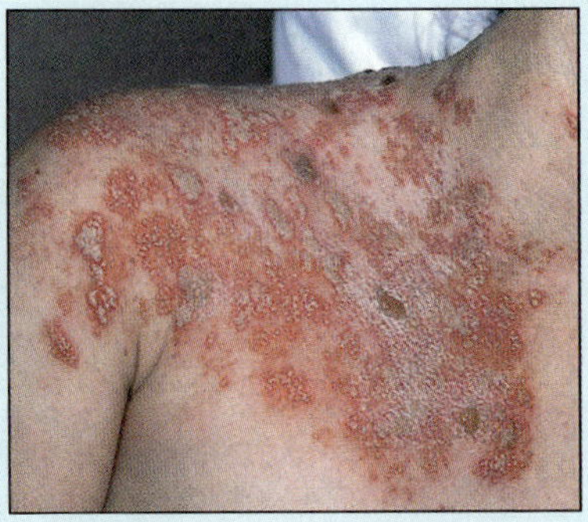 Herpes zoster, vesicles have dried and scabs have begun to form

Disease and Disorder Terms—cont'd

NOT BUILT FROM WORD PARTS

TERM	DEFINITION
23. pressure injury (PRESH-ur) (IN-ja-rē)	damage of the skin and the subcutaneous tissue caused by prolonged pressure, often occurring in bedridden patients; the injury, which may be painful, can present as intact skin or an open ulcer (also called **pressure ulcer** and **bedsore**; formerly called **decubitus ulcer**) (Fig. 4.5)
24. psoriasis (so-RĪ-a-sis)	chronic skin condition producing red lesions covered with silvery scales
25. rosacea (rō-ZĀ-shē-a)	chronic disorder of the skin that produces erythema, papules, pustules, and abnormal dilation of tiny blood vessels, usually occurring on the central area of the face in people older than 30 years
26. scabies (SKĀ-bēz)	skin infection caused by the itch mite, characterized by papule eruptions that are caused by the female burrowing into the outer layer of the skin and laying eggs. This condition is accompanied by severe itching. (Table 4.1)
27. squamous cell carcinoma (SCC) (SQWĀ-mus) (sel) (*kar*-si-NŌ-ma)	malignant growth developing from scalelike epithelial tissue of the surface layer of the epidermis; it invades local tissue and may metastasize. While most commonly appearing on the skin, SCC can occur in other parts of the body including the mouth, lips, and genitals. The most frequent cause is chronic exposure to sunlight. (Fig. 4.3)
28. systemic lupus erythematosus (SLE) (sis-TEM-ik) (LŪ-pus) (*e*-ri-*thē*-*ma*-TŌ-sus)	chronic inflammatory disease involving the skin, joints, kidneys, and nervous system. This autoimmune disease is characterized by periods of remission and exacerbations. It also may affect other organs.

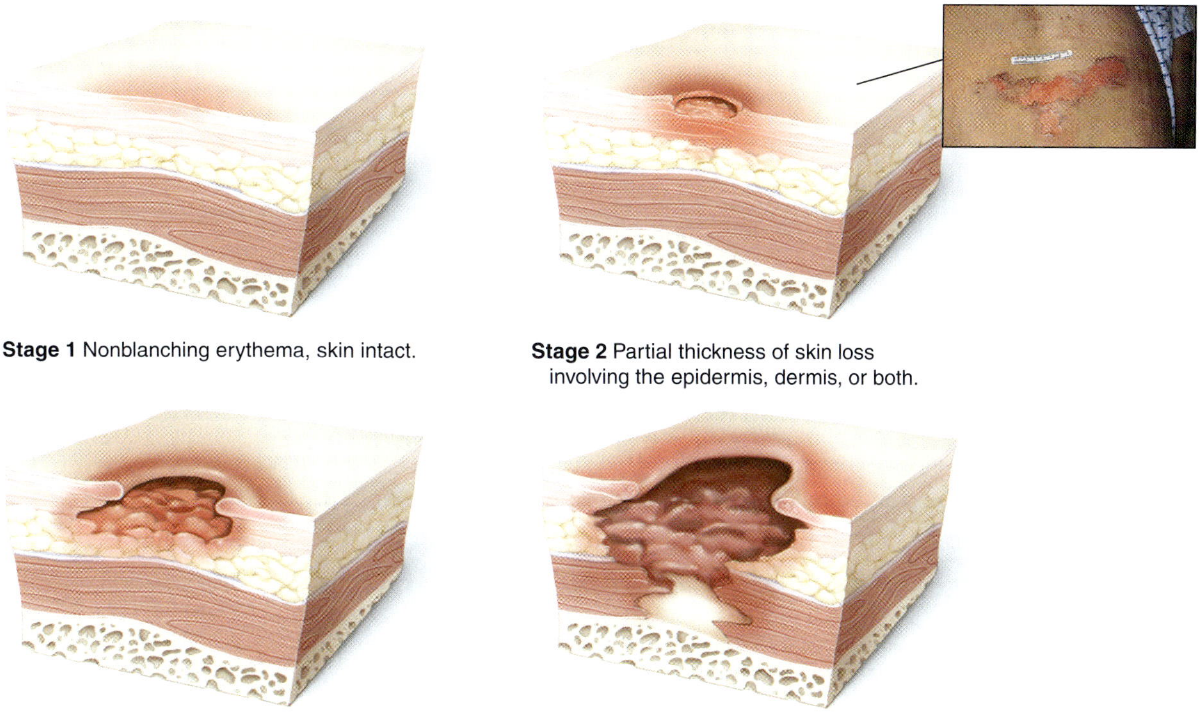

Stage 1 Nonblanching erythema, skin intact.

Stage 2 Partial thickness of skin loss involving the epidermis, dermis, or both.

Stage 3 Full thickness of skin loss involving damage or necrosis to subcutaneous tissue.

Stage 4 Full thickness of skin loss with extensive destruction, tissue necrosis, possible damage to muscle and bone tissue and other supporting structures.

FIG. 4.5 Pressure injury staging with a photograph of Stage 2.

Disease and Disorder Terms—cont'd

NOT BUILT FROM WORD PARTS

TERM	DEFINITION
29. tinea (TIN-ē-a)	fungal infection of the skin. The fungi may infect keratin of the skin, hair, and nails. Infections are classified by body regions such as *tinea capitis* (scalp), *tinea corporis* (body), and *tinea pedis* (foot). Tinea in general is also called **ringworm**, and tinea pedis specifically is also called **athlete's foot**. (Table 4.1)
30. urticaria (*ur*-ti-KAR-ē-a)	itchy skin eruption composed of wheals of varying sizes and shapes. Urticaria is sometimes associated with infections and with allergic reactions to food, medicine, or other agents. Other causes include internal disease, physical stimuli, and genetic disorders. (also called **hives**) (Table 4.2)
31. vitiligo (*vit*-i-LĪ-gō)	white patches on the skin caused by the destruction of melanocytes

EXERCISE 8 ▪ Pronounce and Spell

Practice pronunciation and spelling on paper and online.

1. Practice on Paper

a. **Pronounce:** Read the phonetic spelling and say aloud the terms listed in the previous table. Refer to the pronunciation key on p. 111 as necessary.
b. **Spell:** Have a study partner read the terms aloud. Write the spelling of the terms on a separate sheet of paper.

2. Practice Online

a. **Access** online learning resources. Go to evolve.elsevier.com > Evolve Resources > Student Resources.
b. **Pronounce:** Select Audio Glossary > Chapter 4 > Exercise 8. Select a term to hear its pronunciation and repeat aloud.
c. **Spell:** Select Activities > Chapter 4 > Spell Terms > Exercise 8. Select the audio icon and type the correct spelling of the term.

❑ Check the box when complete.

EXERCISE 9 ▪ Fill In

A Identify

Fill in the blanks with the correct disease and disorder terms.

1. A chronic inflammatory disease affecting the skin, joints, and other organs is ______________________________ ______________________________.
2. The scraping away of the skin by mechanical process or injury is called a(n) ______________.
3. ______________________________ is the name given to the invasion of the skin and hair by lice.
4. An injury with no break in the skin and characterized by pain, swelling, and discoloration is called a(n) ______________________________.
5. ______________ is the name given to tissue death caused by a loss of blood supply followed by bacterial invasion.
6. A cluster of boils caused by staphylococcal bacteria is a ______________.
7. An inflammatory skin disease that involves the oil glands and hair follicles is called ______________.
8. ______________ is the name given to a torn, ragged-edged wound.
9. A(n) ______________ ______________ is small hole or tunnel containing hair and skin that can become infected and may require surgery.

10. Damage of the skin and the subcutaneous tissue caused by prolonged pressure, often occurring in bedridden patients, is called ________________ ________________.

11. A congenital hereditary condition characterized by partial or total lack of pigment (melanin) in the skin, hair, and eyes is ________________.

12. ________________ ________________ is an invasion of methicillin-resistant *Staphylococcus aureus* in the body tissue.

B Label

Write the medical terms pictured and defined.

1. (a) ________________, cracklike sore in the skin caused by (b) ________________, a noninfectious inflammatory skin disease characterized by redness, blisters, scabs, and itching

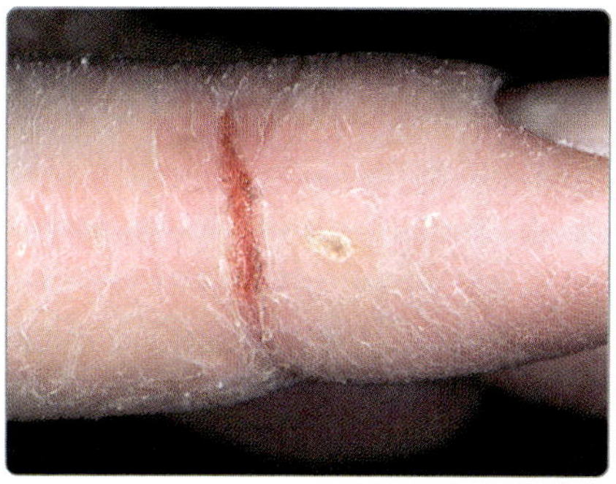

2. ________________ inflammation of the skin and subcutaneous tissue caused by infection and characterized by redness, pain, heat, and swelling

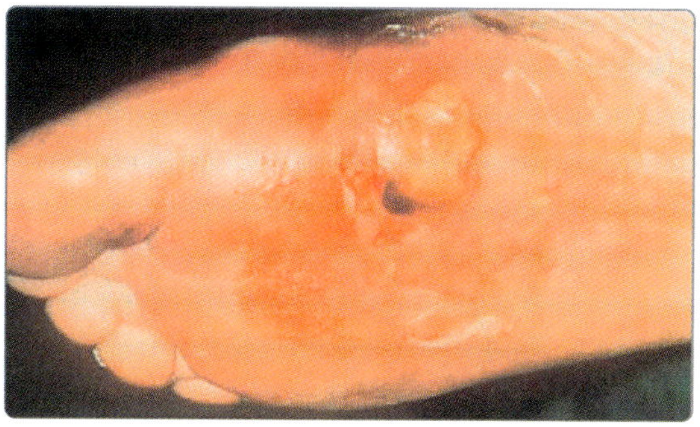

3. ________________ chronic skin condition producing red lesions covered with silvery scales

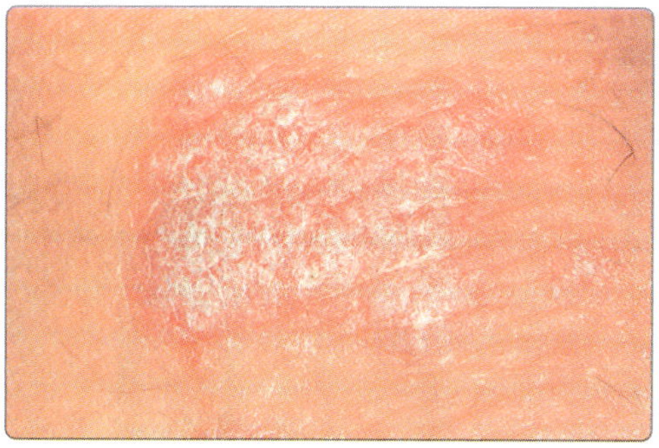

4. ________________ inflammatory skin disease caused by a virus and characterized by small blisters

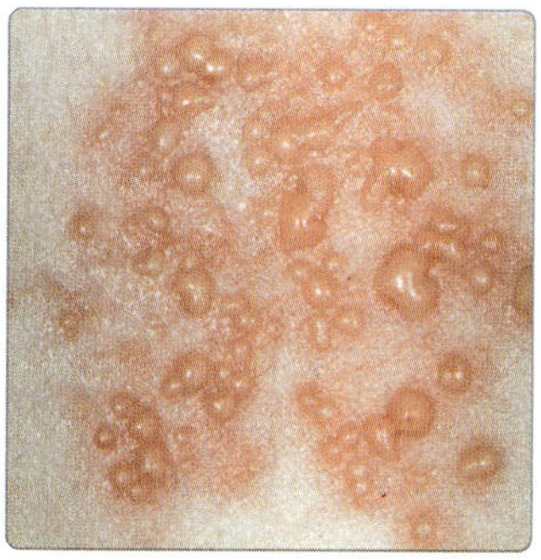

5. ________________ fungal infection of the skin, also known as *ringworm*

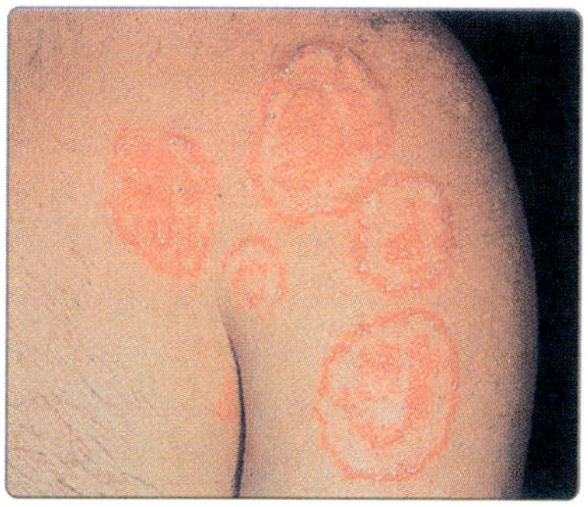

6. ________________ cancerous condition starting as purple or brown papules

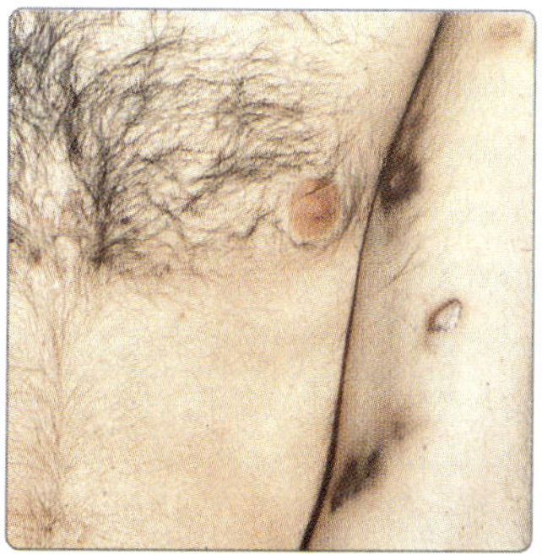

7. ______________________________
horny tissue formation that results from excessive exposure to sunlight and is precancerous

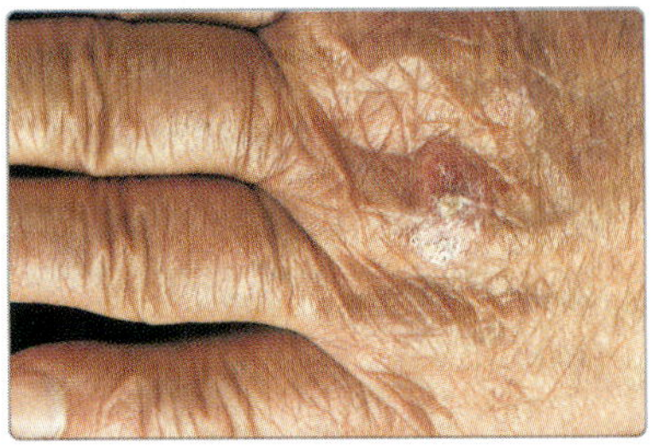

8. ______________________________
painful skin nodule caused by staphylococcal bacteria in a hair follicle

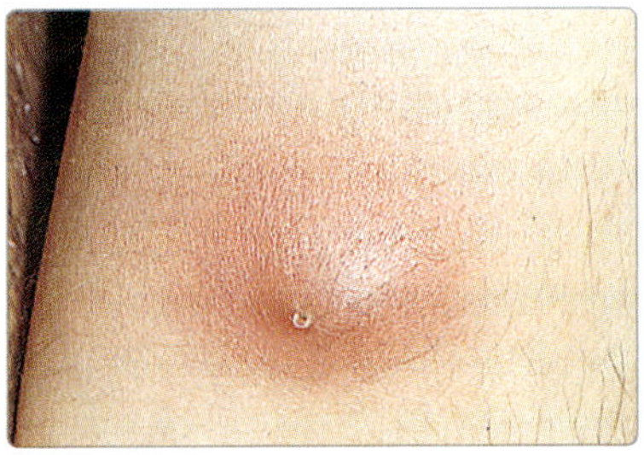

9. ______________________________
malignant growth developing from scalelike epithelial tissue of the surface layer of the epidermis; it invades local tissue and may metastasize

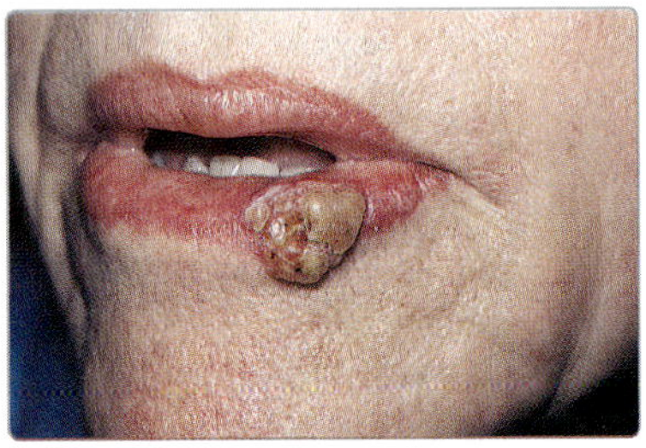

10. ______________________________
malignant epithelial tumor arising from the bottom layer of the epidermis; it seldom metastasizes, but invades local tissue and may recur in the same location

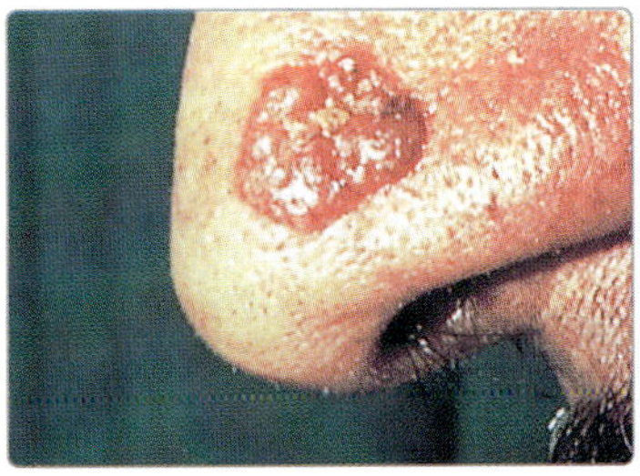

11. ______________________________
superficial skin infection characterized by pustules and caused by either staphylococci or streptococci

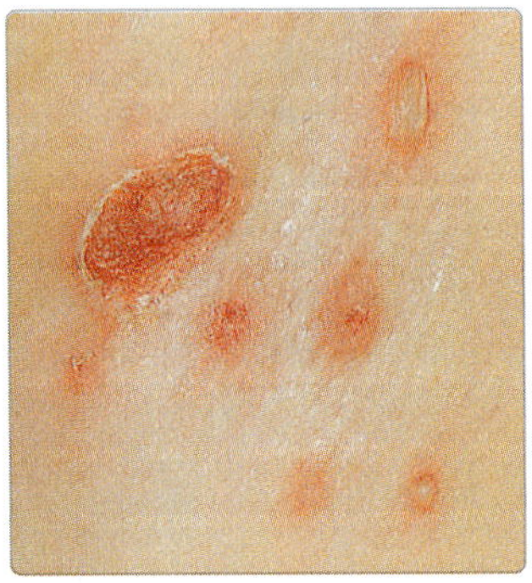

12. ______________________________
skin inflammation caused by the itch mite

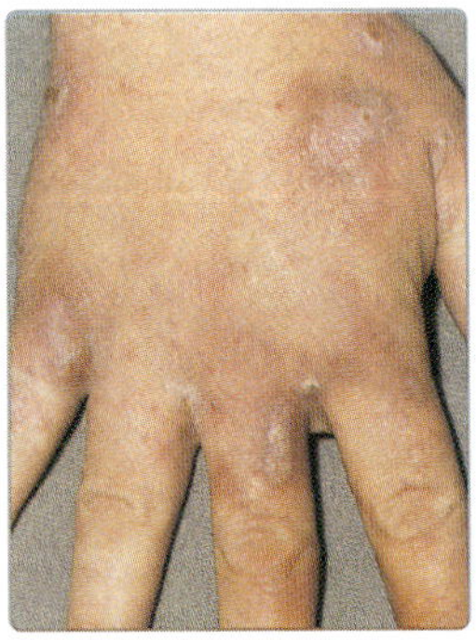

13. ______________________________
itchy skin eruption composed of wheals of varying sizes and shapes

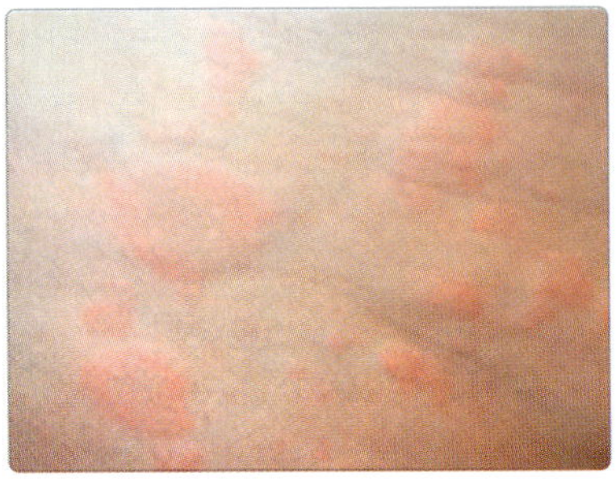

14. ______________________________
infection of the skin, mouth, or vagina caused by *Candida albicans*

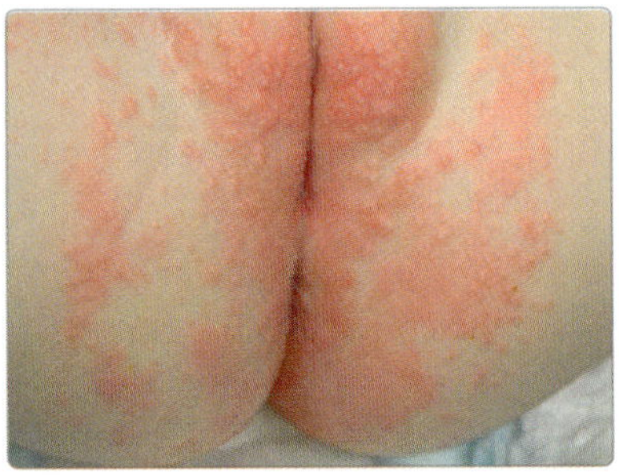

15. ____________________
white patches on the skin caused by the destruction of melanocytes

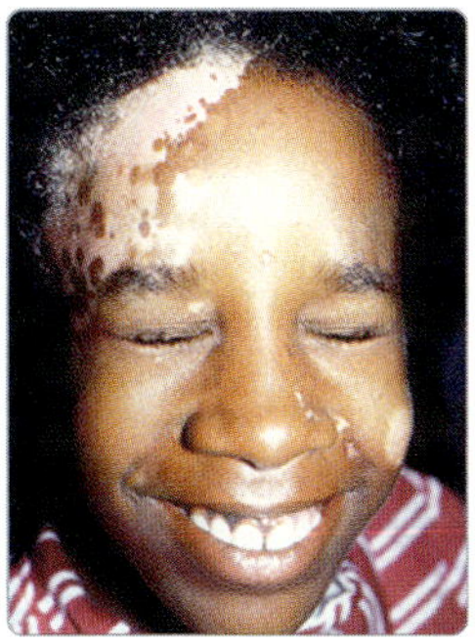

16. ____________________
chronic disorder of the skin on the central area of the face that produces erythema, papules, pustules, and abnormal dilation of tiny blood vessels

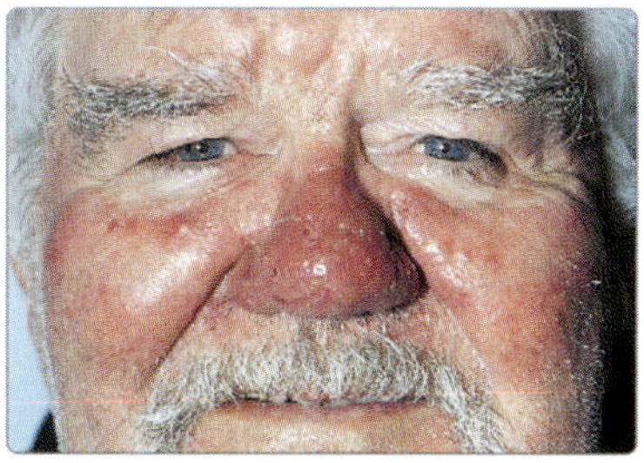

17. ____________________
a highly contagious viral disease characterized by fever, runny nose, cough, and a spreading skin rash

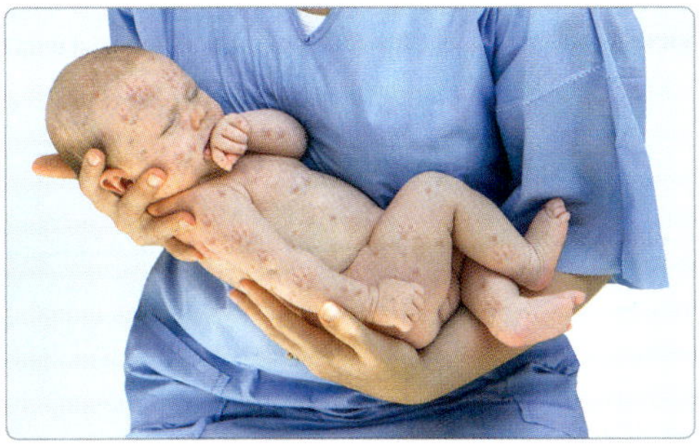

18. ____________________
overgrowth of scar tissue

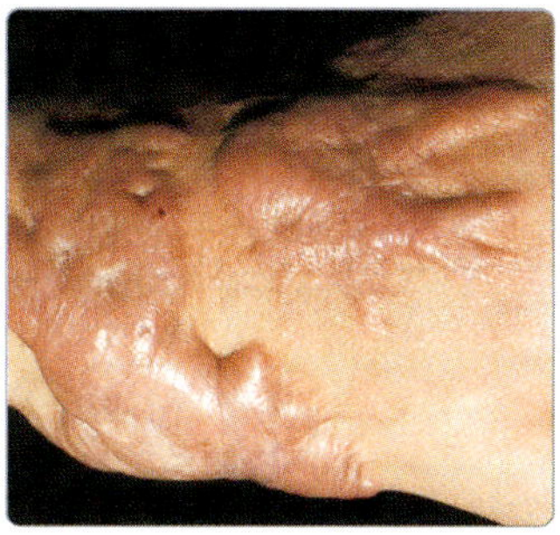

EXERCISE 10 ■ Match

Match the words in the first column with their correct definitions in the second column.

______ 1. measles	a.	death of tissue caused by loss of blood supply and entry of bacteria
______ 2. keloid	b.	cracklike sore in the skin
______ 3. furuncle	c.	cluster of boils
______ 4. actinic keratosis	d.	highly contagious viral disease characterized by fever, runny nose, cough, and a spreading skin rash
______ 5. contusion	e.	noninfectious inflammatory skin disease having redness, blisters, scabs, and itching
______ 6. carbuncle	f.	scraped-away skin
______ 7. basal cell carcinoma	g.	involves sebaceous glands and hair follicles
______ 8. fissure	h.	painful skin nodule caused by staphylococci in a hair follicle
______ 9. eczema	i.	inflammation of skin and subcutaneous tissue with redness, pain, heat, and swelling
______ 10. cellulitis	j.	overgrowth of scar tissue
______ 11. acne	k.	injury characterized by pain, swelling, and discoloration
______ 12. gangrene	l.	precancerous skin condition caused by excessive exposure to sunlight
______ 13. abrasion	m.	usually occurring in the central area of the face in people older than 30 years
______ 14. rosacea	n.	malignant epithelial tumor arising from the bottom layer of the epidermis; it seldom metastasizes, but invades local tissue and may recur in the same location
______ 15. MRSA infection	o.	potentially serious infection caused by methicillin-resistant *Staphylococcus aureus*

EXERCISE 11 ■ Match

Match the words in the first column with their correct definitions in the second column.

_____	1. herpes	a. skin inflammation caused by the itch mite
_____	2. tinea	b. fungal infection of the skin, hair, and nails
_____	3. Kaposi sarcoma	c. red lesions covered by silvery scales
_____	4. vitiligo	d. inflammatory skin disease having clusters of blisters and caused by a virus
_____	5. pressure injury	e. chronic inflammatory disease involving the skin, joints, kidney, and nervous system
_____	6. pediculosis	f. cancerous condition that starts as brown or purple papules
_____	7. pilonidal cyst	g. composed of wheals
_____	8. scabies	h. torn, ragged-edged wound
_____	9. squamous cell carcinoma	i. superficial skin condition having pustules and caused by staphylococci or streptococci
_____	10. systemic lupus erythematosus	j. characterized by lack of pigment (melanin) in the skin, hair, and eyes
		k. infection of the skin, mouth, or vagina caused by a yeast-type fungus
_____	11. impetigo	l. invasion of the hair and skin by lice
_____	12. urticaria	m. damage of the skin and the subcutaneous tissue caused by prolonged pressure
_____	13. candidiasis	n. malignant growth developing from scalelike epithelial tissue of the surface layer of the epidermis; it invades local tissue and may metastasize
_____	14. psoriasis	
_____	15. albinism	o. small hole containing hair and skin located at top of buttocks
_____	16. laceration	p. white patches on the skin caused by the destruction of melanocytes

EXERCISE 12 ■ Review of Disease and Disorder Terms

Can you define, pronounce, and spell the following terms?

abrasion
acne
actinic keratosis
albinism
basal cell carcinoma (BCC)
candidiasis
carbuncle
cellulitis
contusion
dermatitis
dermatofibroma
eczema
fissure
furuncle
gangrene
hidradenitis
herpes
impetigo
Kaposi sarcoma
keloid
keratosis
laceration
measles
MRSA infection
onychocryptosis
onychomalacia
onychomycosis
onychophagia
pachyderma
paronychia
pediculosis
pilonidal cyst
pressure injury
psoriasis
rosacea
scabies
scleroderma
seborrhea
squamous cell carcinoma (SCC)
systemic lupus erythematosus (SLE)
tinea
urticaria
vitiligo
xanthoma
xeroderma

Surgical Terms

BUILT FROM WORD PARTS AND *NOT* BUILT FROM WORD PARTS

The first portion of the table contains Integumentary System Terms that can be translated using definitions of word parts. The second portion of the table contains Integumentary System Terms that cannot be fully understood using the definitions of word parts.

■ Built from Word Parts

TERM	DEFINITION	TERM	DEFINITION
1. **dermatoplasty** (DER-ma-tō-*plas*-tē)	surgical repair of the skin	2. **rhytidectomy** (*rit*-i-DEK-to-mē)	excision of wrinkles (also called **facelift**)

NOT Built from Word Parts

TERM	DEFINITION
1. cauterization (*kaw*-tur-ī-ZĀ-shun)	destruction of tissue with a hot or cold instrument, electric current, or caustic substance (also called **cautery**)
2. cryosurgery (*krī*-ō-SER-jer-ē)	destruction of tissue by using extreme cold, often by using liquid nitrogen (Fig. 4.6)
CRYO comes from the Greek **kruos**, meaning **icy cold** or **frost**.	
3. debridement (da-BRĒD-ment)	removal of contaminated or dead tissue and foreign matter from an open wound
4. dermabrasion (*derm*-a-BRĀ-zhun)	procedure to remove skin scars with abrasive material, such as sandpaper
5. excision (ek-SIZH-en)	removal by cutting
6. incision (in-SIZH-en)	surgical cut or wound produced by a sharp instrument
7. incision and drainage (I&D) (in-SIZH-en) and (DRĀ-nij)	surgical cut made to allow the free flow or withdrawal of fluids from a lesion, wound, or cavity
8. laser surgery (LĀ-zer) (SER-jer-ē)	procedure using an instrument that emits a high-powered beam of light used to cut, burn, vaporize, or destroy tissue
9. Mohs surgery (mōz) (SER-jer-ē)	technique of microscopically controlled serial excisions of a skin cancer
MOHS SURGERY allows for complete tumor removal while sparing as much normal tissue as possible. Excised tissue is examined for tumor cells during the procedure. Tissue is removed until the biopsy margins are cancer free. The procedure is named after **Dr. Frederic E. Mohs**, Wisconsin, who first used the concept in 1936.	
10. skin graft (skin) (graft)	skin transplanted to replace a lost portion of the body skin surface; it may be a full-thickness or split-thickness graft.
11. suturing (SOO-cher-ing)	to stitch edges of a wound surgically (Fig. 4.7)

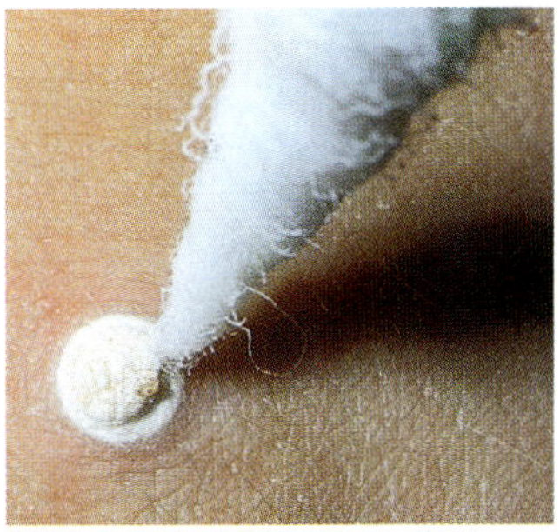

FIG. 4.6 Cryosurgery performed with a nitrogen-soaked, cotton-tipped applicator.

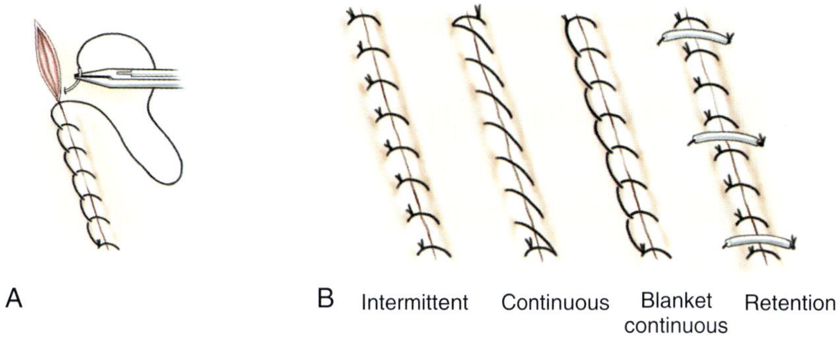

FIG. 4.7 A, Suturing. **B,** Suturing methods.

EXERCISE 13 ■ Pronounce and Spell

Practice pronunciation and spelling on paper and online.

1. Practice on Paper

a. **Pronounce:** Read the phonetic spelling and say aloud the terms listed in the previous table. Refer to the pronunciation key on p. 110 as necessary.

b. **Spell:** Have a study partner read the terms aloud. Write the spelling of the terms on a separate sheet of paper.

2. Practice Online

a. **Access** online learning resources. Go to evolve.elsevier.com > Evolve Resources > Student Resources.
b. **Pronounce:** Select Audio Glossary > Chapter 4 > Exercise 13. Select a term to hear its pronunciation and repeat aloud.
c. **Spell:** Select Activities > Chapter 4 > Spell Terms > Exercise 13. Select the audio icon and type the correct spelling of the term.

❑ Check the box when complete.

EXERCISE 14 ■ Surgical Terms Built from Word Parts

A Analyze and Define

Analyze and define the following Surgical Terms Built from Word Parts by drawing slashes between word parts, writing word part abbreviations above the term, underlining combining forms, and writing combining form abbreviations below the term. *Check your answers in Appendix A.*

1. rhytidectomy
____
____

2. dermatoplasty
____
____

B Build

Build surgical terms for the following definitions with the word parts you have learned.

1. excision of wrinkles ______ / ______
WR / S

2. surgical repair of the skin ______ / ______ / ______
WR / CV / S

EXERCISE 15 ■ Surgical Terms NOT Built from Word Parts

A Identify

Fill in the blanks with the correct surgical terms.

1. ______________ ______________ is a technique of microscopically controlled serial excisions used for treatment of many skin cancers.
2. A surgical cut or wound produced by a sharp instrument is called a(n) ______________________.
3. Destruction of tissue with a hot or cold instrument, electric current, or caustic substance is called ______________.
4. ______________ is to stitch the edges of a wound surgically.
5. A surgical cut made to allow the free flow or withdrawal of fluids from a lesion, wound, or cavity is called ______________ ______________ ______________.
6. ______________________________ is the removal of contaminated or dead tissue and foreign matter from an open wound.
7. Removal by cutting is known as ______________________.

8. ________________ ________________ is a procedure using an instrument that emits a high-powered beam of light used to cut, burn, vaporize, or destroy tissue.
9. The destruction of tissue by using extreme cold, often by using liquid nitrogen, is called ________________.
10. ________________________________ is a procedure to remove skin scars with abrasive material.
11. A full-thickness or split-thickness ________________ ________________ is skin transplanted to replace a lost portion of the body skin surface.

B Match

Match the surgical terms in the first column with their correct definitions in the second column.

_____ 1. suturing	a. destruction of tissue with a hot or cold instrument, electric current, or caustic substance
_____ 2. dermabrasion	b. technique of microscopically controlled serial excisions of a skin cancer
_____ 3. laser surgery	c. surgical cut or wound produced by a sharp instrument
_____ 4. incision and drainage	d. surgical cut made to allow the free flow or withdrawal of fluids from a lesion, wound, or cavity
_____ 5. cauterization	e. removal by cutting
_____ 6. excision	f. removal of contaminated or dead tissue and foreign matter from an open wound
_____ 7. Mohs surgery	g. procedure using an instrument that emits a high-powered beam of light used to cut, burn, vaporize, or destroy tissue
_____ 8. debridement	h. procedure to remove skin scars with abrasive material, such as sandpaper
_____ 9. cryosurgery	i. to stitch edges of a wound surgically
_____ 10. incision	j. destruction of tissue by using extreme cold, often by using liquid nitrogen
_____ 11. skin graft	k. skin transplanted to replace a lost portion of the body skin surface

EXERCISE 16 ■ Review of Surgical Terms

Can you define, pronounce, and spell the following terms?

cauterization	dermatoplasty	incision and drainage (I&D)	rhytidectomy
cryosurgery	excision	laser surgery	skin graft
debridement	incision	Mohs surgery	suturing
dermabrasion			

Complementary Terms

BUILT FROM WORD PARTS

The following terms can be translated using definitions of word parts. Further explanation is provided within parentheses as needed.

SIGNS AND SYMPTOMS

TERM	DEFINITION	TERM	DEFINITION
1. erythroderma (e-*rith*-rō-DER-ma)	red skin (abnormal redness of the skin)	**3. leukoderma** (*lū*-kō-DER-ma)	white skin (white patches caused by depigmentation)
2. hypertrichosis (*hī*-per-tri-KŌ-sis)	abnormal condition of excessive hair (growth) (also called **hirsutism**)	**4. xanthoderma** (*zan*-thō-DER-ma)	yellow skin
		5. xerosis (zēr-Ō-sis)	abnormal condition of dryness (of skin, eye, or mouth)

Complementary Terms—cont'd

BUILT FROM WORD PARTS

MEDICAL SPECIALTIES

TERM	DEFINITION
6. dermatologist (*der*-ma-TOL-o-jist)	physician who studies and treats skin (diseases)
7. dermatology (derm) (*der*-ma-TOL-o-jē)	study of the skin (branch of medicine that deals with the diagnosis and treatment of skin diseases)

DESCRIPTIVE TERMS

TERM	DEFINITION
8. cutaneous (kū-TĀ-nē-us)	pertaining to the skin
9. epidermal (*ep*-i-DER-mal)	pertaining to upon the skin
10. hypodermic (*hī*-pō-DER-mik)	pertaining to under the skin
11. intradermal (ID) (*in*-tra-DER-mal)	pertaining to within the skin
12. keratogenic (*ker*-a-tō-JEN-ik)	producing horny tissue
13. percutaneous (*per*-kū-TĀ-nē-us)	pertaining to through the skin
14. subcutaneous (subcut) (*sub*-kū-TĀ-nē-us)	pertaining to under the skin
15. subungual (sub-UNG-gwal)	pertaining to under the nail
16. transdermal (TD) (trans-DER-mel)	pertaining to through the skin
17. ungual (UNG-gwal)	pertaining to the nail

TRANSDERMAL usually means entering through the skin and refers to the administration of a drug applied to the skin in ointment or patch form. **Percutaneous** usually means performed through the skin, as in the insertion of a needle, catheter, or probe.

OTHER TERMS

TERM	DEFINITION
18. staphylococcus (*pl.* staphylococci) (staph) (*staf*-il-ō-KOK-us) (*staf*-il-ō-KOK-sī)	berry-shaped (bacterium) in grapelike clusters (these bacteria cause many skin diseases)
19. streptococcus (*pl.* streptococci) (strep) (*strep*-tō-KOK-us) (*strep*-tō-KOK-sī)	berry-shaped (bacterium) in twisted chains

EXERCISE 17 ▪ Pronounce and Spell

Practice pronunciation and spelling on paper and online.

1. Practice on Paper

a. **Pronounce:** Read the phonetic spelling and say aloud the terms listed in the previous table. Refer to the pronunciation key on p. 110 as necessary.

b. **Spell:** Have a study partner read the terms aloud. Write the spelling of the terms on a separate sheet of paper.

2. Practice Online

a. **Access** online learning resources. Go to evolve.elsevier.com > Evolve Resources > Student Resources.

b. **Pronounce:** Select Audio Glossary > Chapter 4 > Exercise 17. Select a term to hear its pronunciation and repeat aloud.

c. **Spell:** Select Activities > Chapter 4 > Spell Terms > Exercise 17. Select the audio icon and type the correct spelling of the term.

❑ Check the box when complete.

EXERCISE 18 ■ Analyze and Define

Analyze and define the following Complementary Terms Built from Word Parts by drawing slashes between word parts, writing word part abbreviations above the term, underlining combining forms, and writing combining form abbreviations below the term. *Check your answers in Appendix A.*

P WR S

EXAMPLE: intra / derm / al

pertaining to within the skin

1. ungual

2. transdermal

3. streptococcus

4. hypodermic

5. dermatology

6. subcutaneous

7. staphylococcus

8. keratogenic

9. dermatologist

10. cutaneous

11. epidermal

12. xanthoderma

13. erythroderma

14. percutaneous

15. xerosis

16. subungual

17. leukoderma

18. hypertrichosis

EXERCISE 19 ■ Build

A Label

Build terms pictured by writing word parts above definitions.

1.

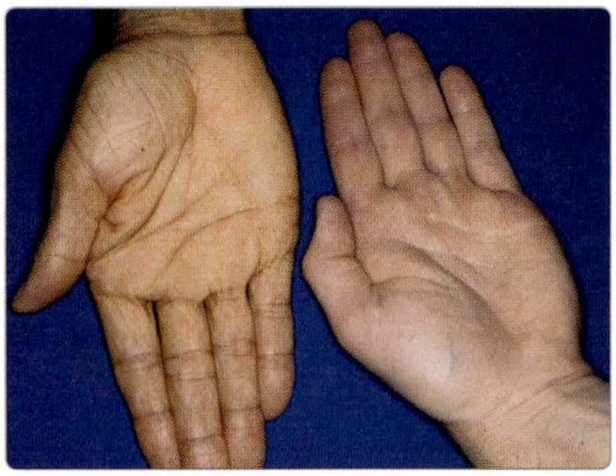

_________ /_____ /___________ /a as seen in jaundice
yellow CV skin

2.

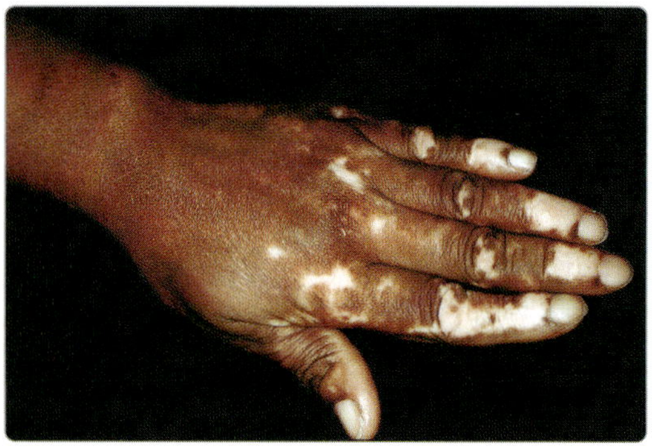

_______ /_______ /___________ /a as seen in vitiligo
white CV skin

3.

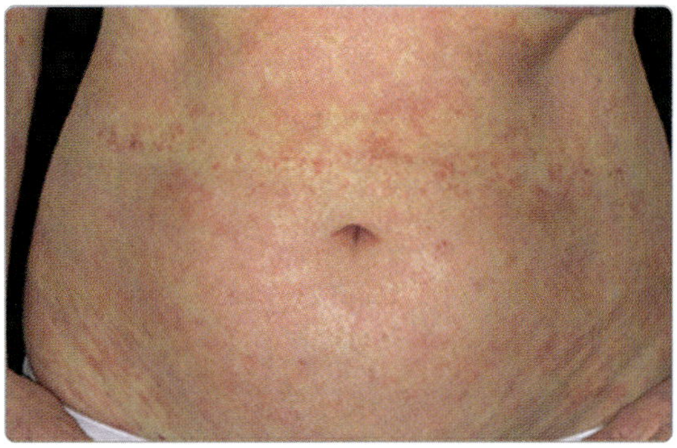

______ /___ /______ /a as seen in exfoliative dermatitis
red CV skin

4.

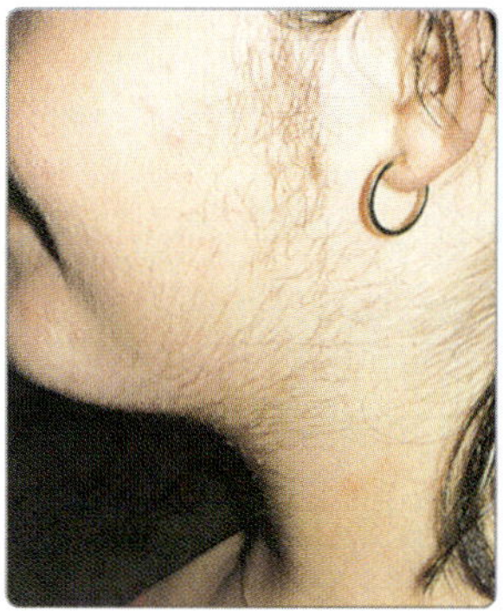

________ /________ / ________________
excessive hair abnormal condition

5.

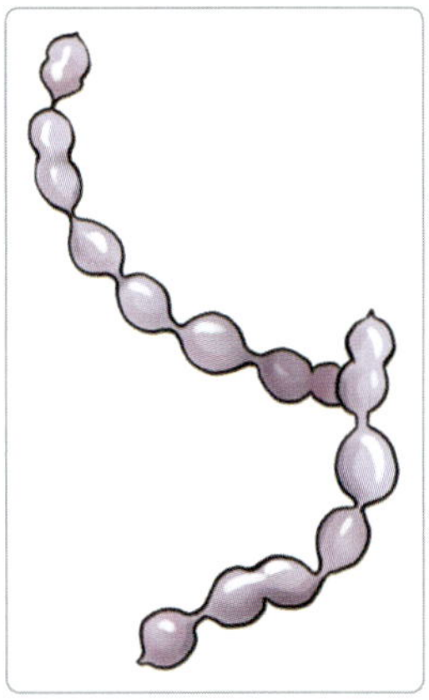

__________ /_____ /_____________
twisted CV berry-shaped chains (plural)

6.

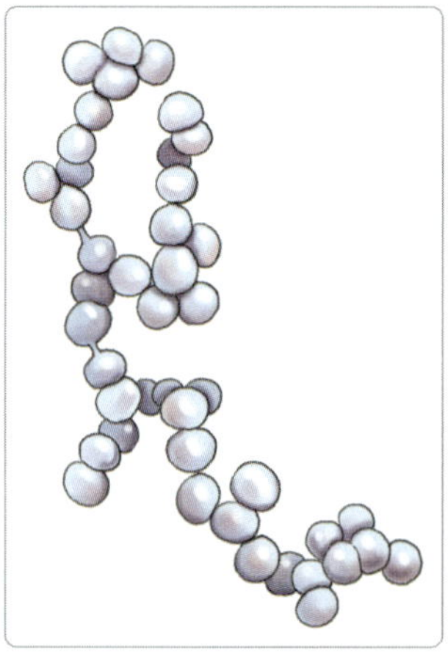

__________ /_____ /_____________
grapelike CV berry-shaped clusters (plural)

7.

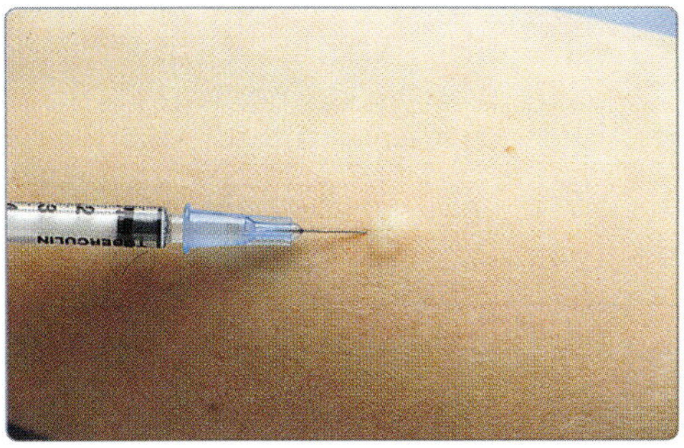

_______ / _______ / _______________ injection
within / skin / pertaining to

8.

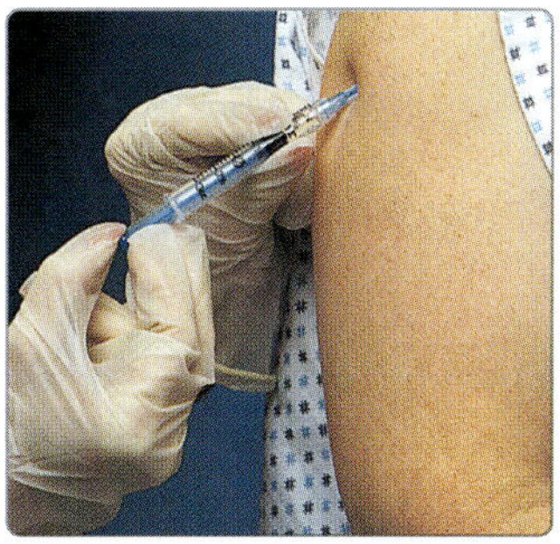

_______ / _______ / _______________ injection
under / skin / pertaining to

using a _______ / _______ / _______________ needle
under / skin / pertaining to

9.

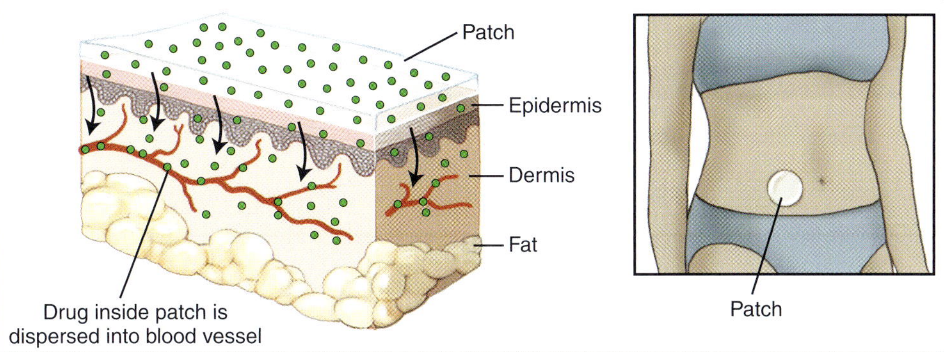

_______ / _______ / _______________ patch
through / skin / pertaining to

B Fill In

Build complementary terms with the word parts you have learned.

EXAMPLE: pertaining to under the skin hypo / derm / ic
P / WR / S

1. study of the skin _______________ / ____ / _______________
WR / CV / S

2. abnormal condition of dryness (of skin, eye, or mouth) _______________ / _______________
WR / S

3. pertaining to the nail _______________ / _______________
WR / S

4. pertaining to the skin _______________ / _______________
WR / S

5. a physician who studies and treats skin (diseases) _______________ / ____ / _______________
WR / CV / S

6. pertaining to under the nail ______ P / ______ WR / ______ S

7. pertaining to upon the skin ______ P / ______ WR / ______ S

8. pertaining to through the skin ______ P / ______ WR / ______ S

9. producing horny tissue ______ WR / ______ CV / ______ S

Complementary Terms

NOT BUILT FROM WORD PARTS

Word parts may be present in the following terms; however, their full meanings cannot be translated using definitions of word parts alone.

SIGNS AND SYMPTOMS	
TERM	**DEFINITION**
1. abscess (AB-ses)	localized collection of pus, bacteria, and other material; can occur in the skin (cutaneous abscess) or other locations within the body (internal abscess)
ABSCESS is derived from the Latin **ab**, meaning **from**, and **cedo**, meaning **to go**. The tissue dies and goes away, with the pus replacing it.	
2. alopecia (*al*-ō-PĒ-sha)	loss of hair; there are multiple types with various causes, including androgenic, areata, and traction.
ALOPECIA is derived from the Greek **alopex**, meaning **fox**. One was thought to bald like a mangy fox.	
3. cyst (sist)	closed sac containing fluid or semisolid material; can occur in the skin (cutaneous cyst) or other locations within the body (Table 4.2)
4. diaphoresis (*dī*-a-fo-RĒ-sis)	sweating
DIAPHORESIS is derived from Greek **dia**, meaning **through**, and **phoreo**, meaning **carry**. Translated, it means the carrying through of perspiration.	
5. ecchymosis (*pl.* ecchymoses) (*ek*-i-MŌ-sis) (*ek*-i-MŌ-sēz)	large (greater than 1 cm), flat, blue-purple lesion caused by escape of blood into deeper areas of the skin, as may occur when blood is withdrawn by a needle and syringe from an arm vein (Fig 4.8)
6. edema (e-DĒ-ma)	puffy swelling of tissue from the accumulation of fluid
7. induration (*in*-dū-RĀ-shun)	abnormal hard spot(s) or area of skin; may include underlying tissue
8. jaundice (JAWN-dis)	condition characterized by a yellow coloring of the skin, mucous membranes, and sclera (whites of the eyes) caused by the presence of bile (also called **icterus**)
9. lesion (LĒ-zhun)	any visible change in tissue resulting from injury or disease. It is a broad term that includes sores, wounds, ulcers, and tumors.
10. leukoplakia (*lū*-kō-PLĀ-kē-a)	condition characterized by white spots or patches on mucous membranes, which may be precancerous
11. macule (MAK-ūl)	flat, colored spot on the skin (Table 4.2)
12. nevus (*pl.* nevi) (NĒ-vus) (NĒ-vī)	circumscribed malformation of the skin, usually brown, black, or flesh colored. A congenital nevus is present at birth and is referred to as a birthmark. (also called a **mole**)

TERM	DEFINITION
13. nodule (NOD-ūl)	small, knotlike mass that can be felt by touch (Table 4.2)
14. pallor (PAL-or)	paleness
15. papule (PAP-ūl)	small, solid skin elevation (Table 4.2)

TABLE 4.2 Common Skin Lesions

LESION	DEFINITION	CUTAWAY SECTIONS	EXAMPLE
Macule	flat, colored spot on the skin	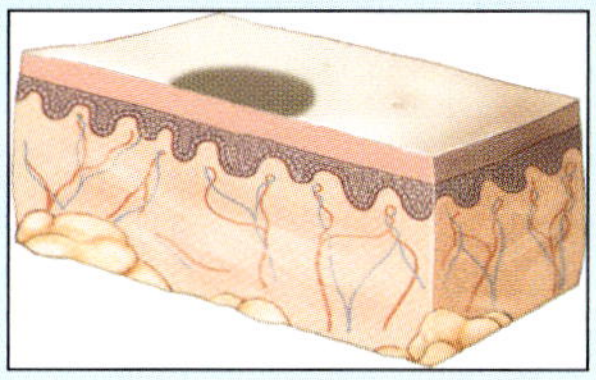	freckle
Papule	small, solid skin elevation	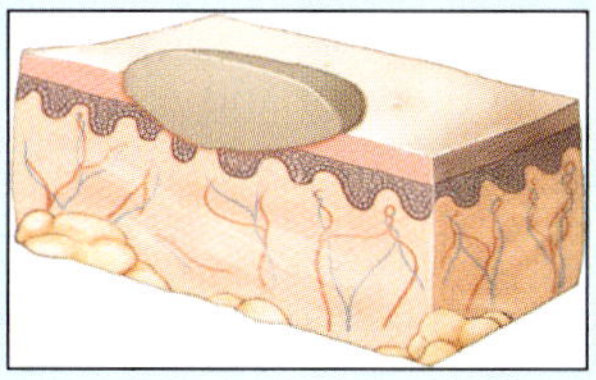	skin tag basal cell carcinoma
Nodule	small, knotlike mass	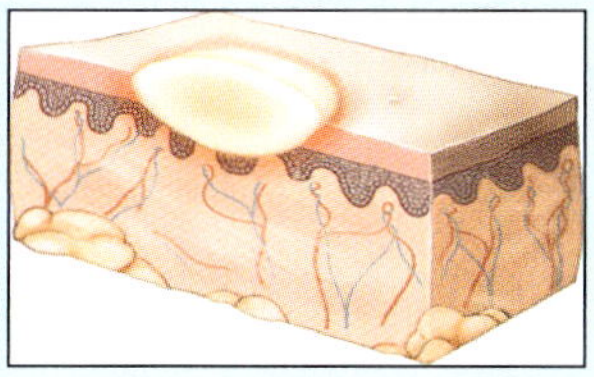	lipoma metastatic carcinoma rheumatoid nodule
Wheal	transitory, itchy elevation of the skin	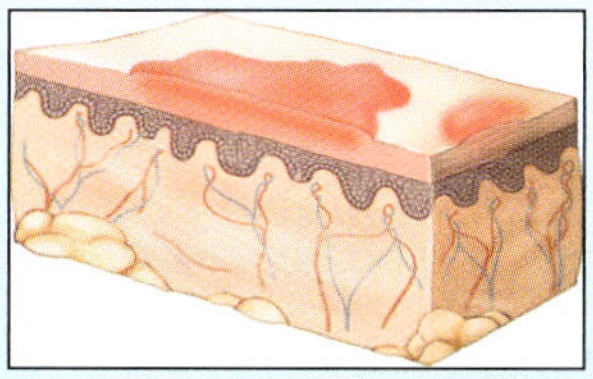	urticaria (hive)
Vesicle	small elevation of epidermis containing liquid	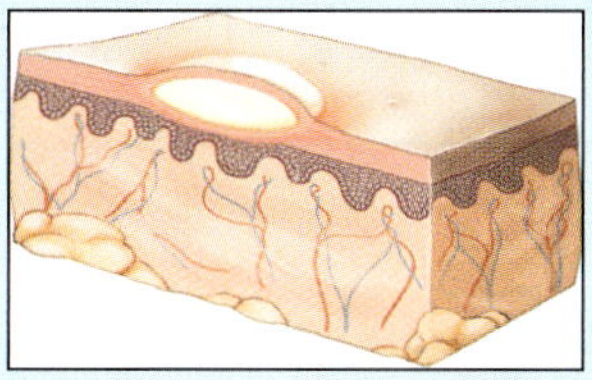	herpes zoster (shingles) herpes simplex virus type 1 contact dermatitis
Pustule	elevation of the skin containing pus	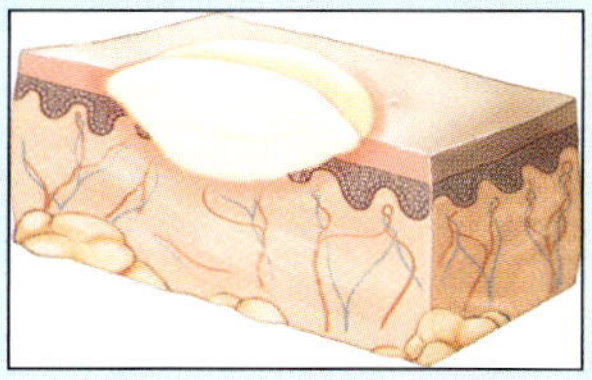	impetigo acne
Cyst	a closed sac containing fluid or semisolid material	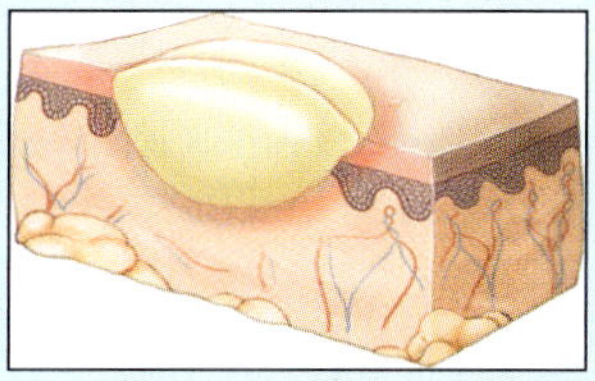	acne

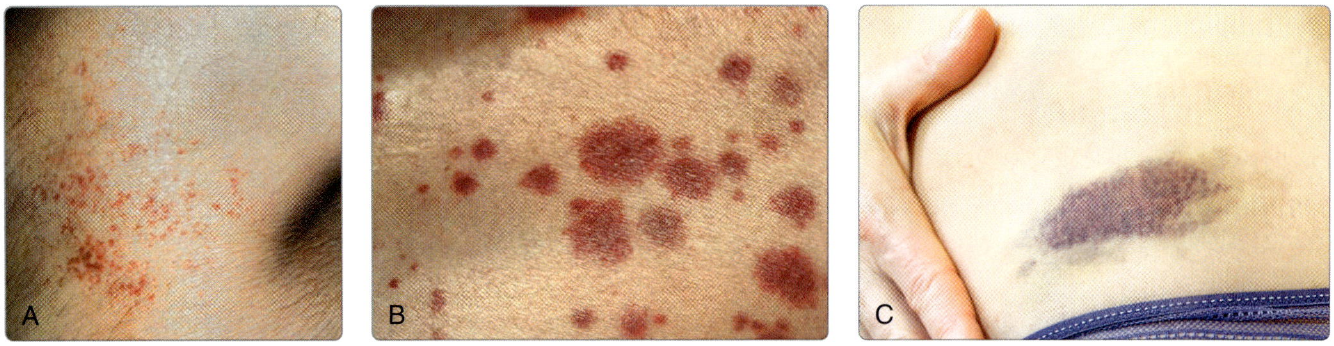

FIG. 4.8 Petechiae, purpura, and ecchymoses are related lesions caused by the escape of blood into the skin and mucous membranes. They vary in size, with petechiae being the smallest in size, up to 0.3 cm; purpura being the next largest, generally from 0.3 cm up to 1 cm; and ecchymoses being the largest, greater than 1 cm. **A,** Petechiae. **B,** Purpura. **C,** Ecchymosis.

Complementary Terms–cont'd

NOT BUILT FROM WORD PARTS

TERM	DEFINITION
16. petechiae (*s.* petechia) (pe-TĒ-kē-ē) (pe-TĒ-kē-a)	tiny (0.3 cm or smaller), pinpoint, bright red lesions that result from escape of blood into the skin and mucous membranes. (Fig 4.8)
PETECHIA is originally from the Italian **petechio**, meaning **flea bite**. The small hemorrhagic spot resembles the mark made by a flea.	
17. pruritus (prū-RĪ-tus)	itching
18. purpura (PER-pū-ra)	small (between 0.3 cm and 1 cm), reddish purple-lesions caused by escape of blood into skin and mucus membranes (Fig 4.8)
19. pustule (PUS-tūl)	elevation of skin containing pus (Table 4.2)
20. ulcer (UL-ser)	erosion of the skin or mucous membrane
21. verruca (ver-RŪ-ka)	circumscribed cutaneous elevation caused by a virus (also called **wart**)
22. vesicle (VES-i-kl)	small elevation of the epidermis containing liquid (also called **blister**) (Table 4.2)
23. wheal (hwēl)	transitory, itchy elevation of the skin with a white center and a red surrounding area; a wheal is an individual urticaria (hive) lesion (Table 4.2)

Refer to **Appendix E** for pharmacology terms related to the integumentary system.

EXERCISE 20 ▪ Pronounce and Spell

Practice pronunciation and spelling on paper and online.

1. Practice on Paper

a. **Pronounce:** Read the phonetic spelling and say aloud the terms listed in the previous table. Refer to the pronunciation key on p. 110 as necessary.

b. **Spell:** Have a study partner read the terms aloud. Write the spelling of the terms on a separate sheet of paper.

2. Practice Online

a. **Access** online learning resources. Go to evolve.elsevier.com > Evolve Resources > Student Resources.

b. **Pronounce:** Select Audio Glossary > Chapter 4 > Exercise 20. Select a term to hear its pronunciation and repeat aloud.

c. **Spell:** Select Activities > Chapter 4 > Spell Terms > Exercise 20. Select the audio icon and type the correct spelling of the term.

❑ Check the box when complete.

EXERCISE 21 ■ Fill In

A Identify

Fill in the blanks with the correct terms.

1. Sweating is called ______________________.
2. ______________________ is the name for a flat, colored skin spot.
3. A yellow coloring of the skin, mucous membranes, and sclera caused by the presence of bile is known as ______________________.
4. The condition of white spots or patches on mucous membranes is called ______________________.
5. ______________________ are tiny, pinpoint, bright-red lesions caused by escape of blood.
6. A cutaneous ______________________ is a localized collection of pus, bacteria, and other material in the skin. It may appear red and feel warm to the touch.
7. Another name for paleness is ______________________.
8. Large, flat, blue-purple lesion caused by escape of blood into deeper areas of the skin; as may occur when blood is withdrawn by a needle and syringe, is referred to as ______________________.
9. A small knotlike mass that can be felt by touch is called a(n) ______________________.
10. A closed sac containing fluid or semisolid material is called a(n) ______________________.
11. Itching is called ______________________.
12. Small (between 0.3 cm and 1 cm), reddish purple-lesions caused by escape of blood into skin and mucus membranes, are known as ______________________.
13. A small, solid skin elevation is called a(n) ______________________.
14. A transitory, itchy skin elevation with a white center and a red surrounding area is a(n) ______________________.
15. A(n) ______________________ is a skin elevation containing pus.
16. A blister is also called a(n) ______________________.
17. An abnormal hard spot(s) or area of skin is called ______________________.
18. ______________________ is the swelling of tissue.
19. ______________________ refers to any visible change in tissue resulting from injury or disease.

B Label

Write the medical terms pictured and defined.

1. ______________________
erosion of the skin or mucous membrane

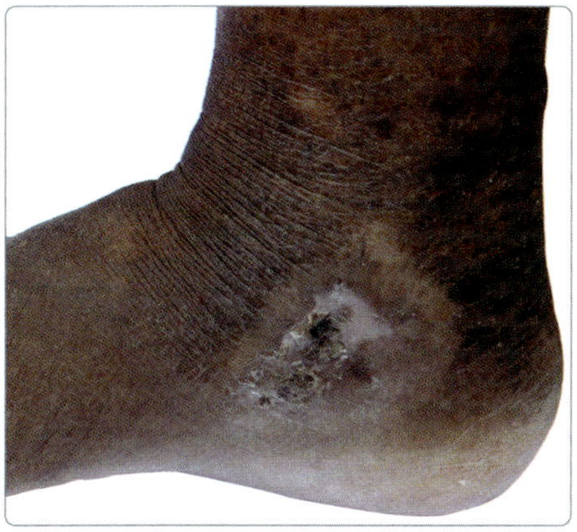

2. ______________________
circumscribed malformation of the skin, usually brown, black, or flesh colored (also called a **mole**)

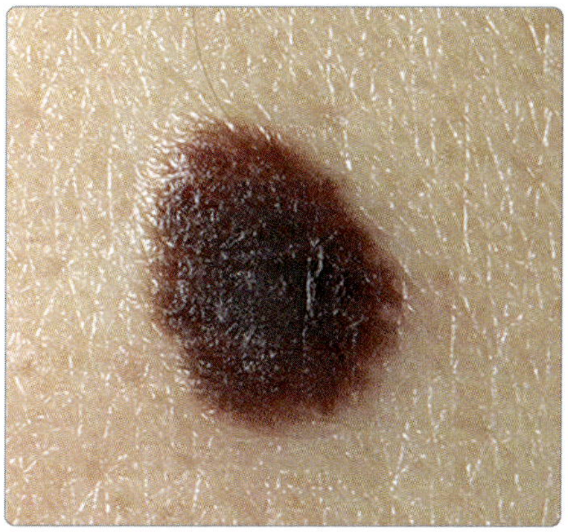

3. ______________________________
circumscribed cutaneous elevation caused by a virus (also called **wart**)

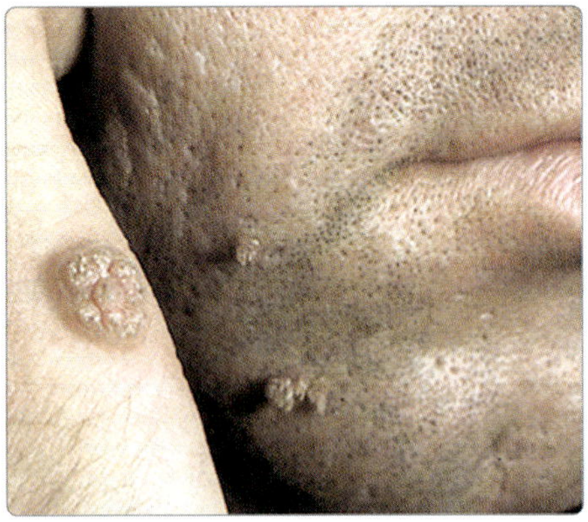

4. ______________________________
loss of hair

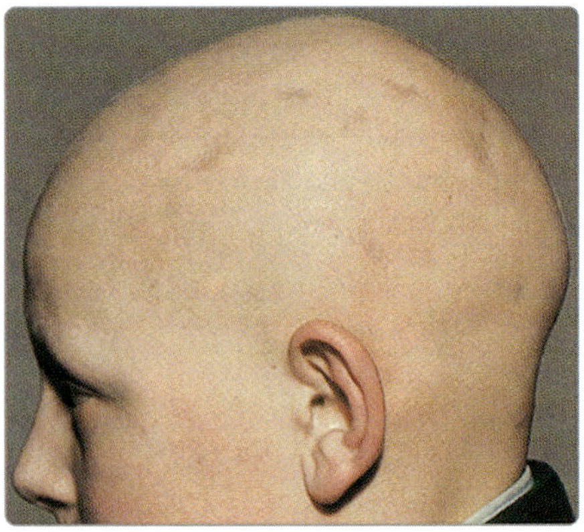

EXERCISE 22 ■ Match

Match the words in the first column with their correct definitions in the second column.

_____ 1. lesion	a. loss of hair
_____ 2. alopecia	b. large (greater than 1 cm), flat, blue-purple lesion caused by escape of blood into deeper areas of the skin
_____ 3. abscess	c. yellow color to the skin, mucous membranes, and sclera
_____ 4. nodule	d. closed sac containing fluid
_____ 5. diaphoresis	e. broad term denoting any visible change in tissue, including sores, wounds, ulcers, and tumors
_____ 6. cyst	f. small knotlike mass
_____ 7. ecchymosis	g. sweating
_____ 8. jaundice	h. swelling of tissue
_____ 9. edema	i. hard spot(s) or area of skin
_____ 10. induration	j. localized collection of pus, bacteria, and other material

EXERCISE 23 ■ Match

Match the terms in the first column with their correct definitions in the second column.

_____ 1. leukoplakia	a. mole
_____ 2. macule	b. itching
_____ 3. nevus	c. wart
_____ 4. pallor	d. condition of white spots or patches on mucous membranes
_____ 5. papule	e. small (between 0.3 cm and 1 cm), reddish purple-lesions
_____ 6. petechiae	f. skin elevation containing pus
_____ 7. pruritus	g. small elevation of epidermis containing liquid
_____ 8. purpura	h. individual urticaria lesion
_____ 9. pustule	i. flat, colored spot on skin
_____ 10. ulcer	j. small, solid skin elevation
_____ 11. verruca	k. paleness
_____ 12. vesicle	l. tiny (0.3 cm or smaller), pinpoint, bright red lesions
_____ 13. wheal	m. erosion of the skin or mucous membrane

EXERCISE 24 ■ Review of Complementary Terms

Can you define, pronounce, and spell the following terms?

abscess
alopecia
cutaneous
cyst
dermatologist
dermatology (derm)
diaphoresis
ecchymosis (*pl.* ecchymoses)
edema
epidermal
erythroderma
hypertrichosis
hypodermic
induration
intradermal (ID)
jaundice
keratogenic
lesion
leukoderma
leukoplakia
macule
nevus (*pl.* nevi)
nodule
pallor
papule
percutaneous
petechiae (*s.* petechia)
pruritus
purpura
pustule
subcutaneous (subcut)
subungual
staphylococcus (*pl.* staphylococci) (staph)
streptococcus (*pl.* streptococci) (strep)
transdermal (TD)
ulcer
ungual
verruca
vesicle
wheal
xanthoderma
xerosis

Abbreviations

DISEASE AND DISORDERS

ABBREVIATION	TERM	ABBREVIATION	TERM
BCC	basal cell carcinoma	**MRSA**	methicillin-resistant *Staphylococcus aureus*
CA-MRSA	community-associated MRSA infection	**SCC**	squamous cell carcinoma
HA-MRSA	healthcare-associated MRSA infection	**SLE**	systemic lupus erythematosus

TREATMENTS

ABBREVIATION	TERM	ABBREVIATION	TERM
FTSG	full-thickness skin graft	**STSG**	split-thickness skin graft
I&D	incision and drainage		

MEDICAL SPECIALTY

ABBREVIATION	TERM
derm	dermatology

DESCRIPTIVE

ABBREVIATION	TERM	ABBREVIATION	TERM
ID	intradermal	**TD**	transdermal
subcut	subcutaneous		

OTHER

ABBREVIATION	TERM	ABBREVIATION	TERM
staph	staphylococcus	**strep**	streptococcus

Refer to **Appendix D** for a complete list of abbreviations.

EXERCISE 25 ■ Fill In

Write the terms abbreviated.

1. The most common form of skin cancer is **BCC** ______________ ______________ ______________.
2. **STSGs** ______________-______________ ______________ ______________ involve taking the epidermis and only a top section of the dermis from the donor site; they rely on the lower dermis at the recipient site to provide nutrients for the healing skin.
3. The entire dermis, along with the epidermis, is taken from the donor site in **FTSGs** ______________-______________ ______________ ______________, which results in less scarring, but also has a higher chance of being unsuccessful.
4. Long-term exposure to sunlight is by far the most frequent cause of **SCC** ______________ ______________ ______________.
5. **SLE** ______________ ______________ ______________ is a chronic relapsing disease, often with long periods of remission.
6. The medication was administered by **subcut** ______________ injection.
7. **Staph** ______________ bacterium was cultured from the abscess.
8. The culture confirmed a **strep** ______________ infection of the throat.
9. **I&D** ______________ ______________ ______________ is used to treat cutaneous abscesses, such as a furuncle.
10. Hormone replacement therapy is available by **TD** ______________ administration.
11. The tuberculin test was administered by an **ID** ______________ injection.
12. The patient visited the **derm** ______________ clinic for a psoriasis follow-up visit.
13. **MRSA** ______________ ______________ ______________ ______________ infections originating in a healthcare setting are called **HA-MRSA** ______________-______________ ______________ ______________, whereas MRSA infections occurring in a person who has not recently been in a healthcare setting is called **CA-MRSA** ______________-______________ ______________ ______________.

PRACTICAL APPLICATION

EXERCISE 26 ■ Case Study: Translate Between Everyday Language and Medical Language

CASE STUDY: Antonne Johnson

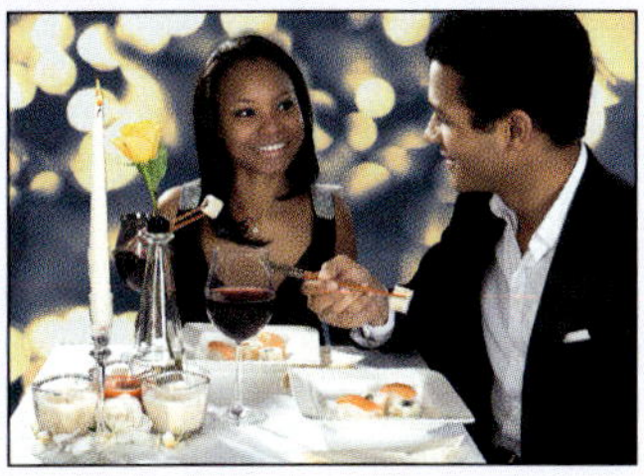

Antonne and his girlfriend were eating out when his mouth began to tingle.

"Hey, are you all right? You look pale," Sasha said.

"My stomach doesn't feel too good." This had happened before, Antonne realized, when he had eaten shellfish. Tonight he had been careful to order sushi made from fish without a shell. He signaled Sasha to call 911. In no time at all, his mouth, face, and arms felt very itchy. As she dialed, Sasha noticed his lips beginning to swell. His cheeks and arms became covered with different-sized red and white bumps. EMTs arrived just as it was becoming difficult for Antonne to breathe. Sasha quickly told them of Antonne's shellfish allergy.

Now that you have worked through Chapter 4 on the integumentary system, consider the medical terms that might be used to describe Antonne's experience. See the Chapter at a Glance section at the end of the chapter for a list of terms that might apply.

A. Underline phrases in the case study that could be substituted with medical terms.

B. Write the medical term and its definition for three of the phrases you underlined.

MEDICAL TERM	DEFINITION
1. ____________________	____
2. ____________________	____
3. ____________________	____

DOCUMENTATION: Excerpt from EMT Notes

CC: Patient says he is having trouble breathing.

History: Ambulance responded to a call from a young woman at a sushi restaurant on behalf of a 27-year-old male. Onset: Patient's symptoms were brought on suddenly while eating; he has experienced one previous episode of anaphylaxis. Medication: Patient has epinephrine injection. Allergies: Patient is allergic to shellfish.

Exam: BP: 90/60 mm Hg, Pulse: 120, O_2: 15L Non-rebreather mask. Pallor of face and hands is present; he appears to be experiencing pruritus and says he might vomit. Patient shows signs of edema around the lips and face and urticaria on his cheeks and arms. Upon auscultation of the lungs, wheezing is present. Assessment/Plan: Anaphylaxis: One dose of epinephrine was delivered by injection.

C. Underline medical terms presented in Chapter 4 in the previous excerpt from Antonne's medical record. See the Chapter at a Glance section at the end of the chapter for a complete list.

D. Select and define three of the medical terms you underlined. To check your answers, go to Appendix A.

MEDICAL TERM	DEFINITION
1. ____________________	____
2. ____________________	____
3. ____________________	____

EXERCISE 27 ■ Interact With Medical Documents

A

Read the report and complete it by writing medical terms on answer lines within the document. Definitions of terms to be written appear after the document.

76548-INT WHARTON, Sandra L.

File Patient Navigate Custom Fields Help

Chart Review | Encounters | Notes | Labs | Imaging | Procedures | Rx | Documents | Referrals | Scheduling | Billing

Name: **WHARTON, Sandra L.** MR#: **76548-INT** DOB: **10/03/19XX** Gender: F Age: 50 **Allergies:** None known **PCP:** Spring, Lincoln MD

Encounter Date: 7/27/20XX
Operative Report:

History: The patient is a 50-year-old woman presenting to the 1.______________ clinic with concerns about a 2.______________ ____________ located at the 3.______________________________aspect of her left eyebrow. The patient's medical history is also significant for 4.__________________________, primarily of the scalp and ears, as well as chronic 5.__________________________, primarily of the forearms bilaterally.

Indications for Procedure:
The 6. ____ has been present for approximately 3 months. It measures 1.5 cm x 2.0 cm and has poorly defined borders. Risks, benefits, indications and expectations were discussed with the patient regarding biopsy, and she has agreed to proceed with 7.____________________ ______________________.

Preoperative Diagnosis:
Suspicious lesion, left eyebrow.

Anesthesia: Xylocaine 1% with epinephrine.

Procedure: After written consent was obtained, the site was prepped and draped in the usual sterile fashion. Prior to the first stage, the surgical site was injected with anesthesia into the 8.__________________ layer; the site was tested for anesthesia and re-injected as needed in subsequent stages. In each stage, a(n) 9.______________________________ of a thin layer of abnormal tissue was performed, then immediately coded, cut, and stained for microscopic 10.__________________examination. The entire base and margins were examined by the 11. _____________/pathologist. 12._________________________________ was used to achieve hemostasis. 13. __________ was performed with 6-0 Vicryl, followed by 6-0 nylon for closure. Pressure dressing was applied.

The patient tolerated the procedure well, without any complications.

Postoperative Diagnosis: 14. _____________________, with clear margins.

Electronically signed: William Hickman MD on 27 July 20XX 13:30

Start | Log On/Off | Print | Edit

Definitions of Medical Terms to Complete the Document

Write the medical terms defined on corresponding answer lines in the document.

1. study of the skin
2. small, knotlike mass that can be felt by touch
3. pertaining to the middle
4. precancerous skin condition of horny tissue formation
5. noninfectious, inflammatory skin disease characterized by redness, blisters, scabs, and itching
6. any visible change in tissue resulting from injury or disease.
7. technique of microscopically controlled serial excisions of skin cancer
8. pertaining to under the skin
9. removal by cutting
10. study of disease
11. physician who studies and treats skin
12. destruction of tissue with a hot or cold instrument, electric current, or caustic substance
13. to stitch edges of a wound surgically
14. malignant epithelial tumor arising from the bottom layer of the epidermis

B

Read the medical report and answer the questions below it.

49785 LIGHT, Darla B.

File Patient Navigate Custom Fields Help

Chart Review | Encounters | Notes | Labs | Imaging | Procedures | Rx | Documents | Referrals | Scheduling | Billing

Name: **LIGHT, Darla B.** MR#: **49785** DOB: 6/15/19XX Sex: F Age: 29 **Allergies:** None known **PCP:** Papas, Aenea MD

PATHOLOGY REPORT

DATE/TIME COLL: Jun 12 20XX, 12:00

DATE RECEIVED: Jun 12 20XX, 16:00

DATE REPORTED: Jun 15 20XX

REPORT STATUS: FINAL REPORT

HISTORY: Previous incidence of melanoma and basal cell carcinoma, no metastases

PRE-OP DIAGNOSIS: Melanoma vs. compound nevus

PROCEDURE: Tissue biopsy

SPECIMEN: Skin biopsy, anterior, proximal right arm

GROSS DESCRIPTION: One container is received. Specimen in formalin labeled with the patient's name is a shave biopsy of gray-white hair-bearing skin measuring 0.4 × 0.3 cm in surface dimension and averaging 0.1 cm in thickness. The epidermal surface contains a symmetric, smooth, ordered, pigmented lesion measuring 0.3 cm in greatest diameter. The specimen is bisected and totally submitted.

MICROSCOPIC EXAMINATION: A microscopic examination has been performed.

DIAGNOSIS: Lesion, anterior, proximal right arm; benign compound nevus.

Electronically signed: J. Alvarez, MD, Pathologist, 6/15/20XX 10:48

Start | Log On/Off | Print | Edit

Use the medical report above to answer the questions.

1. Identify singular and plural forms of medical terms used in the pathology report. Write "p" for plural and "s" for singular next to the terms. Refer to Table 2.5 for plural endings.
   _____ a. melanoma
   _____ b. melanomata
   _____ c. nevi
   _____ d. nevus
   _____ e. metastasis
   _____ f. metastases
   _____ g. biopsy
   _____ h. biopsies

2. The skin biopsy was obtained from:
   a. near the shoulder on the back of the right arm
   b. near the shoulder on the front of the right arm
   c. near the wrist on the back of the right arm
   d. near the wrist on the front of the right arm

3. Use your medical dictionary or a reliable online source to find the meanings of the following terms used in the pathology report:
   a. compound ______________________________
   ____
   b. pigmented ______________________________
   ____
   c. bisected ______________________________
   ____
   d. microscopic ______________________________
   ____

EXERCISE 28 ■ Pronounce Medical Terms in Use

Practice pronunciation of terms by reading aloud the following paragraph. Use the phonetic spellings to assist with pronunciation. The script also contains medical terms not presented in the chapter. If interested, research their meanings in a medical dictionary or a reliable online source.

Emily visited the **dermatology** (*der*-ma-TOL-o-jē) clinic because of **pruritus** (prū-RĪ-tus) secondary to **dermatitis** (*der*-ma-TĪ-tis) involving her scalp and areas of her elbows and knees. A diagnosis of **psoriasis** (so-RĪ-a-sis) was made. **Eczema** (EK-ze-ma), **scabies** (SKĀ-bēz), and **tinea** (TIN-ē-a) were considered in the differential diagnosis. An emollient cream was prescribed. In addition the patient showed the **dermatologist** (der-ma-TOL-o-jist) the tender, discolored, thickened nail of her right great toe. Emily learned she had **onychomycosis** (*on*-i-kō-mī-KŌ-sis), for which she was given an additional prescription for an oral antifungal drug.

CHAPTER REVIEW

EXERCISE 29 ■ Chapter Content Quiz

Test your understanding of terms and abbreviations introduced in this chapter. Circle the letter for the medical term or abbreviation related to the words in italics.

1. *Small (between 0.3 cm and 1 cm), reddish purple-lesions caused by escape of blood into skin and mucus membranes* may be caused by blood disorders, vascular abnormalities, or trauma.
   a. pruritus
   b. purpura
   c. papule
2. The patient required incision and drainage, followed by antibiotics for his infected *abnormal pocket in the skin that contains hair and skin debris.*
   a. pressure injury
   b. pilonidal cyst
   c. pediculosis
3. A *technique of microscopically controlled serial excisions* was used to treat the patient's recurrent *malignant growth developing from scalelike epithelial tissue of the surface layer of the epidermis.*
   a. cryosurgery, STSG
   b. laser surgery, BCC
   c. Mohs surgery, SCC
4. The *localized collection of pus* was incised and drained.
   a. acne
   b. abscess
   c. cyst
5. A culture swab of the wound revealed *invasion of body tissue by methicillin-resistant Staphylococcus aureus.*
   a. MRSA infection
   b. herpes
   c. candidiasis
6. The patient newly diagnosed with a *chronic inflammatory disease involving the skin, joints, kidneys, and nervous system* experienced joint pain with swelling and stiffness, and a butterfly-shaped rash spread over her cheeks and the bridge of her nose.
   a. rosacea
   b. scleroderma
   c. systemic lupus erythematosus
7. *Abnormal condition of excessive hair growth*, also known as hirsutism, may occur in patients who have polycystic ovary syndrome.
   a. hypertrichosis
   b. alopecia
   c. furuncle
8. *Death of tissue caused by loss of blood supply followed by bacterial invasion* may be evidenced by foul-smelling discharge from the infection site.
   a. gangrene
   b. pressure injury
   c. lesion

9. The medical assisting student learned the medical term for *blister* was:
   a. verruca
   b. keloid
   c. vesicle

10. *Abnormal hard spots or areas of skin* were evident in the patient diagnosed with the *disease characterized by chronic hardening of connective tissue of the skin and other organs.*
    a. lesion, psoriasis
    b. induration, scleroderma
    c. nodule, Kaposi sarcoma

11. *Eating the nails or nail biting* can damage skin around the nails and increase chances for infection.
    a. onychophagia
    b. onychomalacia
    c. onychomycosis

12. An injection given *within the skin* is described as:
    a. subcut
    b. TD
    c. ID

13. As a result of the burn to her upper arm, the patient received *skin transplanted to replace a lost portion of the body skin surface*.
    a. laser surgery
    b. dermabrasion
    c. skin graft

14. The *transitory, itchy elevations of the skin with a white center and a red surrounding area* were distributed over the patient's entire body.
    a. nevi
    b. wheals
    c. verrucae

15. Excessive *sweating* without exertion may be a symptom of a serious condition.
    a. diaphoresis
    b. edema
    c. hidradenitis

16. The nursing assistant applied lotion to the patient exhibiting signs of *dry skin*.
    a. xanthoderma
    b. xeroderma
    c. pachyderma

17. *Surgical stitching* was performed to treat the *torn, ragged edged wound.*
    a. cryosurgery, verruca
    b. suturing, laceration
    c. dermabrasion, ulcer

18. Compression of the lateral femoral *pertaining to the skin* nerve results in sensations of aching, burning, stabbing, and/or numbness in the thigh area.
    a. epidermal
    b. cutaneous
    c. intradermal

19. *Superficial skin infection characterized by pustules and caused by either staphylococci or streptococci* is common in young children.
    a. impetigo
    b. measles
    c. herpes

20. Measles vaccine is administered via *subcut* injection, while influenza vaccine is administered via intramuscular or *ID* injection.
    a. subungual, intravasular
    b. subcutaenous, intradermal
    c. sublingual, incisional

CHAPTER AT A GLANCE Word Parts New to this Chapter

COMBINING FORMS

cutane/o
derm/o
dermat/o
hidr/o
kerat/o
myc/o
onych/o
pachy/o
rhytid/o
scler/o
seb/o
staphyl/o
strept/o
trich/o
ungu/o
xer/o

PREFIXES

epi-
intra-
para-
per-
sub-
trans-

SUFFIXES

-a
-coccus (*pl.* -cocci)
-ectomy
-ia
-itis
-malacia
-phagia
-plasty
-rrhea

CHAPTER AT A GLANCE Integumentary System Terms Built from Word Parts

DISEASE AND DISORDER
dermatitis
dermatofibroma
hidradenitis
keratosis
onychocryptosis
onychomalacia
onychomycosis
onychophagia
pachyderma
paronychia
scleroderma
seborrhea
xanthoma
xeroderma

SURGICAL
dermatoplasty
rhytidectomy

COMPLEMENTARY
cutaneous
dermatologist
dermatology (derm)
epidermal
erythroderma
hypertrichosis
hypodermic
intradermal (ID)
keratogenic
leukoderma
percutaneous
staphylococcus (*pl.* staphylococci) (staph)
streptococcus (*pl.* streptococci) (strep)
subcutaneous (subcut)
subungual
transdermal (TD)
ungual
xanthoderma
xerosis

CHAPTER AT A GLANCE Integumentary System Terms NOT Built from Word Parts

DISEASE AND DISORDER
abrasion
acne
actinic keratosis
albinism
basal cell carcinoma (BCC)
candidiasis
carbuncle
cellulitis
contusion
eczema
fissure
furuncle
gangrene
herpes
impetigo
Kaposi sarcoma
keloid
laceration
measles
MRSA infection
pediculosis
pilonidal cyst
pressure injury
psoriasis
rosacea
scabies
squamous cell carcinoma (SCC)
systemic lupus erythematosus (SLE)
tinea
urticaria
vitiligo

SURGICAL
cauterization
cryosurgery
debridement
dermabrasion
excision
incision
incision and drainage (I&D)
laser surgery
Mohs surgery
skin graft
suturing

COMPLEMENTARY
abscess
alopecia
cyst
diaphoresis
ecchymosis (*pl.* ecchymoses)
edema
induration
jaundice
lesion
leukoplakia
macule
nevus (*pl.* nevi)
nodule
pallor
papule
petechiae (*s.* petechia)
pruritus
purpura
pustule
ulcer
verruca
vesicle
wheal

Chapter 5

Respiratory System

Outline

Objectives

Upon completion of this chapter, you will be able to:

1. Pronounce organs and anatomic structures of the respiratory system.
2. Define and spell word parts related to the respiratory system.
3. Define, pronounce, and spell disease and disorder terms related to the respiratory system.
4. Define, pronounce, and spell surgical terms related to the respiratory system.
5. Define, pronounce, and spell diagnostic terms related to the respiratory system.
6. Define, pronounce, and spell complementary terms related to the respiratory system.
7. Interpret the meaning of abbreviations related to the respiratory system.
8. Apply medical language in clinical contexts.

ANATOMY

The respiratory system comprises the nose, pharynx, larynx, trachea, bronchi, and lungs. The upper respiratory tract includes the nose, pharynx, and larynx. The lower respiratory tract includes the trachea, bronchi, and lungs. (Fig. 5.1)

Function

The function of the respiratory system is the exchange of oxygen (O_2) and carbon dioxide (CO_2) between the atmosphere and body cells. This process is called **respiration** or **breathing**. During **external respiration**, air containing oxygen passes through the respiratory tract, beginning with the nose, pharynx, larynx, trachea, and, finally, bronchi to the lungs (**inhalation** or **inspiration**). There, oxygen passes from the sacs in the lungs, called **alveoli**, to the blood in tiny blood vessels called **capillaries**. At the same time, carbon dioxide passes back from the capillaries to the alveoli and is expelled through the respiratory tract (**exhalation** or **expiration**) (Fig. 5.2). During **internal respiration**, the body cells take on **oxygen** from the blood and simultaneously give back **carbon dioxide**, a waste produced when oxygen is used to extract energy from food. Carbon dioxide is transported by the blood back to the lungs for exhalation.

RESPIRATION is also called **breathing** or **ventilation.**

Organs and Anatomic Structures of the Respiratory System

TERM	DEFINITION
nose (nōz)	lined with mucous membrane and fine hairs; it acts as a filter to moisten and warm the entering air
nasal septum (NĀS-el) (SEP-tum)	partition separating the right and left nasal cavities
paranasal sinuses (*par*-a-NĀ-sel) (SĪ-nus-es)	air cavities within the cranial bones that open into the nasal cavities
pharynx (FAR-inks)	serves as a food and air passageway. Air enters from the nasal cavities and/or mouth and passes through the pharynx to the larynx. Food enters the pharynx from the mouth and passes into the esophagus. (also called the **throat**)
adenoids (AD-e-noids)	lymphoid tissue located on the posterior wall of the nasal cavity (also called **pharyngeal tonsils**)
tonsils (TON-sils)	lymphoid tissue located on the lateral wall at the junction of the oral cavity and oropharynx
larynx (LAR-inks)	location of the vocal cords. Air enters from the pharynx. (also called the **voice box**)
ADAM'S APPLE is the largest ring of cartilage in the **larynx** and is also known as the thyroid cartilage. The name came from the belief that Adam, realizing he had sinned when he ate the forbidden fruit, was unable to swallow the apple lodged in his throat.	
epiglottis (ep-i-GLOT-is)	flap of cartilage that automatically covers the opening of the larynx and keeps food from entering the larynx during swallowing
trachea (TRĀ-kē-a)	passageway for air to the bronchi from the larynx (also called the **windpipe**)
bronchus (*pl.* bronchi) (BRONG-kus) (BRONG-ki)	one of two branches from the trachea that conducts air into the lungs, where it divides and subdivides. The branchings resemble a tree; therefore, they are referred to as a **bronchial tree**.
BRONCHI originated from the Greek **brecho**, meaning **to pour** or **wet**. An ancient belief was that the esophagus carried solid food to the stomach and the bronchi carried liquids.	
bronchioles (BRONG-kē-ōlz)	smallest subdivision of the bronchial tree

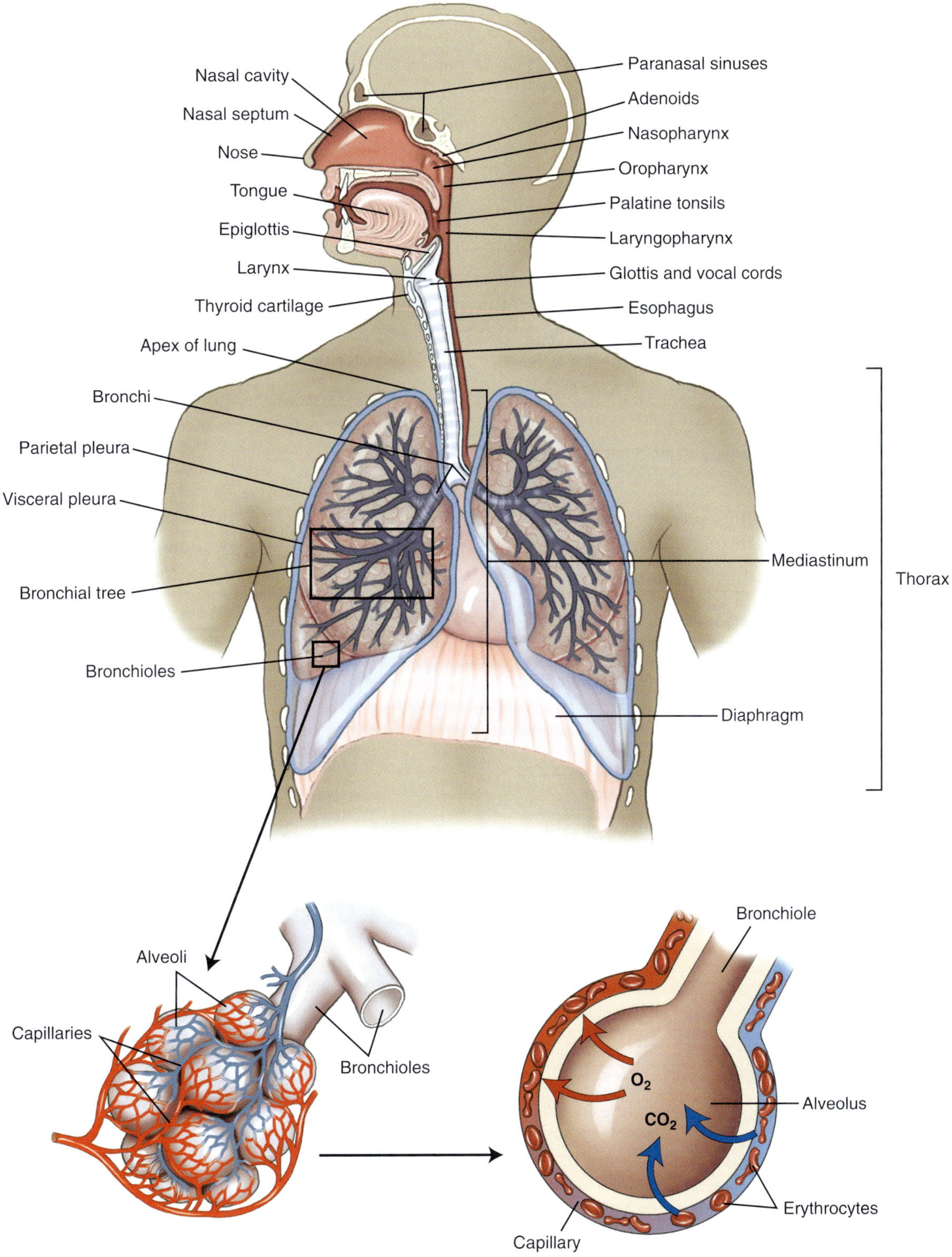

FIG. 5.1 Organs of the respiratory system.

Organs and Anatomic Structures of the Respiratory System—cont'd

TERM	DEFINITION
alveoli (*s.* alveolus) (al-VĒ-o-lī) (al-VĒ-o-lus)	air sacs at the end of the bronchioles. Oxygen and carbon dioxide are exchanged through the alveolar walls and the capillaries. (also a term for the sockets in the jaw bones into which the teeth fit)
thorax (THOR-aks)	chest, the part of the body between the neck and the diaphragm encased by the ribs. **Thoracic cavity** is the hollow space between the neck and diaphragm.
lungs (lungs)	two spongelike organs in the thoracic cavity. The right lung consists of three lobes, and the left lung has two lobes.
pleura (PLOOR-a)	double-folded, serous membrane covering each lung (visceral pleura) and lining the thoracic cavity (parietal pleura) with a small space between, called the pleural cavity, which contains serous fluid.
mediastinum (*mē*-dē-a-STĪ-num)	space between the lungs. It contains the heart, esophagus, trachea, great blood vessels, and other structures.
MEDIASTINUM literally means **to stand in the middle** because it is derived from the Latin **medius**, meaning **middle**, and **stare**, meaning **to stand**.	
diaphragm (DĪ-a-fram)	muscular partition that separates the thoracic cavity from the abdominal cavity. It aids in the breathing process by contracting and pulling air in, then relaxing and pushing air out.

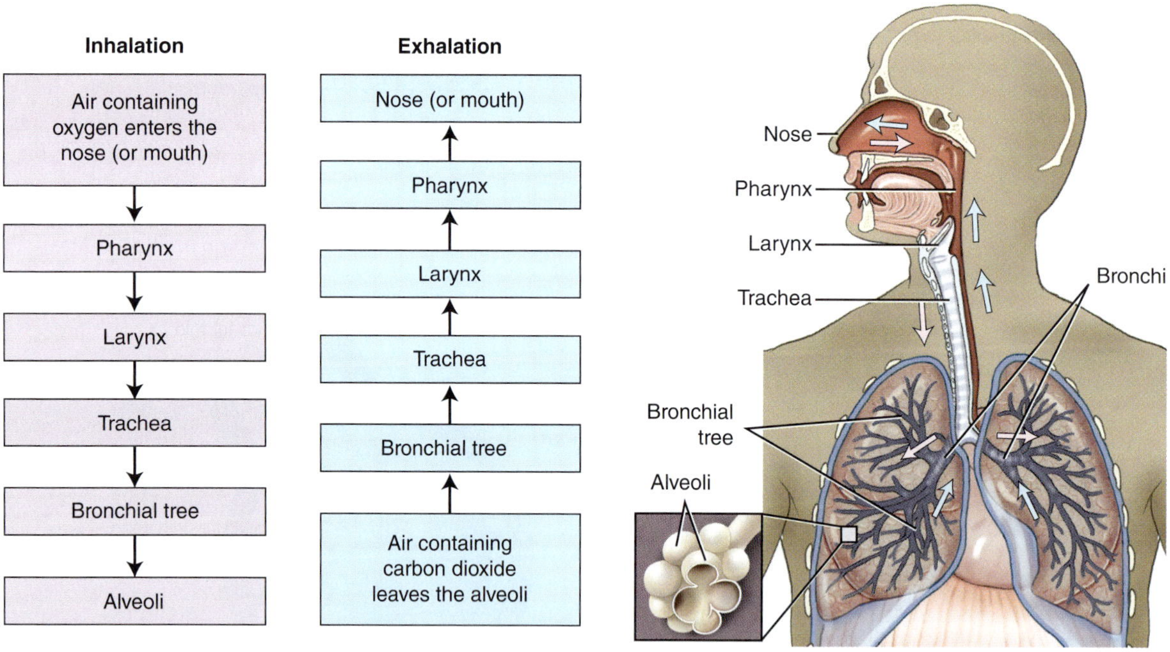

FIG. 5.2 Flow of air.

PRONOUNCE ANATOMIC STRUCTURES

Practice saying aloud each of the organs and specific structures on the previous pages.

To hear the terms, go to Evolve Resources at www.evolve.elsevier.com and select:
Student Resources > **Audio Glossary** > Chapter 5 > Anatomic Structures

❑ Check the box when complete.

WORD PARTS

Use paper flashcards or electronic flashcards on Evolve to memorize word parts used to analyze, define, and build medical terms in this chapter. To reinforce learning, study one section of the Word Parts Table at a time, then complete the corresponding exercises on the following pages.

1 ■ Respiratory System Combining Forms

COMBINING FORM	DEFINITION
adenoid/o	adenoids
alveol/o	alveolus *(s.)*, alveoli *(pl.)*
bronch/o	bronchus *(s.)*, bronchi *(pl.)*
bronchi/o	bronchus *(s.)*, bronchi *(pl.)*
diaphragmat/o	diaphragm
epiglott/o	epiglottis
laryng/o	larynx
lob/o	lobe(s)

LOBE literally means **the part that hangs down**, although it comes from the Greek **lobos**, meaning **capsule** or **pod**. **Lob/o** can also describe lobes in other areas of the body, including the ear, liver, and brain.

COMBINING FORM	DEFINITION
mediastin/o	mediastinum
nas/o	nose
pharyng/o	pharynx
pleur/o	pleura
pneum/o	lung, air
pneumon/o	lung, air
pulmon/o	lung
rhin/o	nose
sept/o	septum

SEPTUM comes from the Latin word **saeptum** meaning to **fence** or **wall off** and refers to a structure dividing cavities or tissues. **Sept/o** can also describe septa in other areas of the body, including the heart and brain.

COMBINING FORM	DEFINITION
sinus/o	sinus(es)
thorac/o	thorax, chest, chest cavity
tonsill/o	tonsil(s) *(Note: tonsil has one l, and the combining form has two ls.)*
trache/o	trachea

2 ■ Combining Forms Used with Respiratory System Terms

COMBINING FORM	DEFINITION
atel/o	imperfect, incomplete
capn/o	carbon dioxide
carcin/o	cancer
coni/o	dust
hem/o	blood
muc/o	mucus
myc/o	fungus
orth/o	straight
ox/i	oxygen
phon/o	sound, voice
py/o	pus
somn/o	sleep
spir/o	breathe, breathing

3 ■ Prefixes

PREFIX	DEFINITION
a-, an-	absence of, without *(Note: an- is used when the word root begins with a vowel.)*
dys-	painful, abnormal, difficult, labored
endo-	within
eu-	normal, good
hyper-	above, excessive
hypo-	below, incomplete, deficient, under
intra-	within
neo-	new
poly-	many, much
tachy-	fast, rapid

4 ■ Suffixes

SUFFIX	DEFINITION
-al	pertaining to
-ar, -ary	pertaining to
-cele	hernia, protrusion
HERNIA is protrusion of an organ or tissue through a membrane or cavity wall.	
-centesis	surgical puncture to aspirate fluid (with a sterile needle)
-desis	surgical fixation, fusion
-eal	pertaining to
-ectasis	stretching out, dilation, expansion
-ectomy	excision, surgical removal
-emia	in the blood
-genic	producing, originating, causing
-ia	diseased or abnormal state, condition of
-ic	pertaining to
-itis	inflammation
-logist	one who studies and treats (specialist, physician)
-logy	study of
-meter	instrument used to measure
-metry	measurement

SUFFIX	DEFINITION
-oid	resembling
-oma	tumor, swelling
-osis	abnormal condition
-ous	pertaining to
-plasm	growth, substance, formation
-plasty	surgical repair
-pnea	breathing
-ptysis	spitting, coughing
-rrhagia	excessive bleeding
The suffixes **-RRHAGIA** and **-RRHAGE** refer to excessive bleeding and come from the Greek word **rhegynai** meaning **to burst forth.**	
-rrhea	flow, discharge
-scope	instrument used for visual examination
-scopic	pertaining to visual examination
-scopy	visual examination
-spasm	sudden, involuntary muscle contraction (spasmodic contraction)
-stenosis	constriction or narrowing
-stomy	creation of an artificial opening
-thorax	chest, chest cavity
-tomy	cut into, incision

EXERCISE 1 ■ Respiratory System Combining Forms

Refer to the first section of the word parts table.

A Define and Match

Step 1: Write the definitions after the following combining forms.
Step 2: Match the descriptions on the right with the combining forms and definitions. Answers may be used more than once.

_____ 1. adenoid/o, ______________________________

_____ 2. diaphragmat/o, ______________________________

_____ 3. epiglott/o, ______________________________

_____ 4. lob/o, ______________________________

_____ 5. nas/o, ______________________________

_____ 6. pharyng/o, ______________________________

_____ 7. pneumon/o, ______________________________

_____ 8. pneum/o, ______________________________

_____ 9. rhin/o, ______________________________

_____ 10. sept/o, ______________________________

a. lined with mucous membrane and fine hairs; acts as a filter to moisten and warm the entering air
b. sections of a lung
c. spongelike organs located in the thoracic cavity
d. lymphoid tissue located on the posterior wall of the nasal cavity
e. flap of cartilage that keeps food out of the larynx
f. partition separating the right and left nasal cavities
g. passageway for food and air
h. separates the thoracic cavity from the abdominal cavity

B Label

Fill in the blanks with combining forms to label this diagram of the respiratory system. *To check your answers, go to Appendix A at the back of the textbook.*

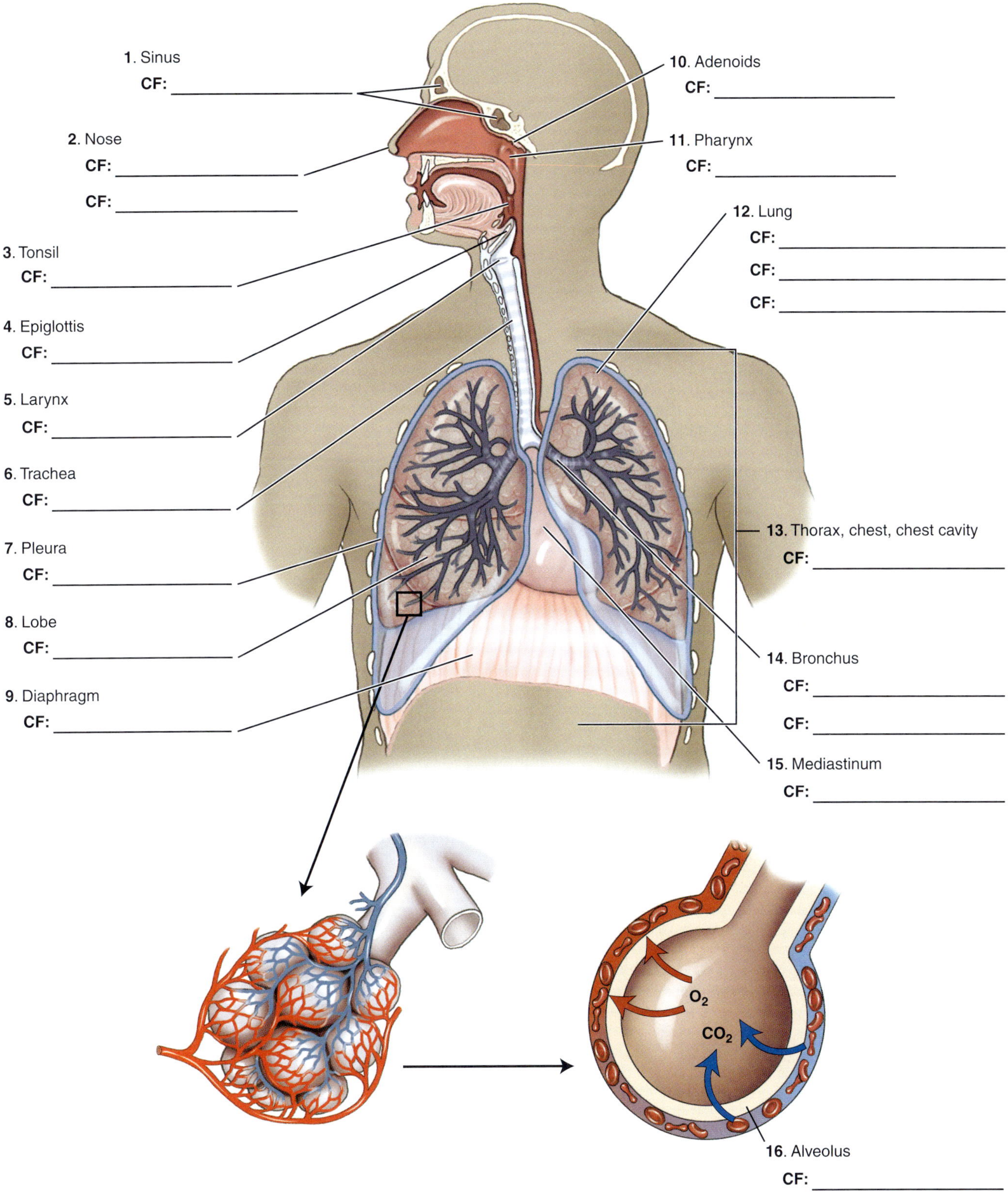

C Define and Match

Step 1: Write the definitions after the following combining forms.
Step 2: Match the descriptions on the right with the combining forms and definitions.

_____ 1. alveol/o, ____________________
_____ 2. bronch/o, bronchi/o, ____________________
_____ 3. pulmon/o, ____________________
_____ 4. laryng/o, ____________________
_____ 5. pleur/o, ____________________
_____ 6. thorac/o, ____________________
_____ 7. trache/o, ____________________
_____ 8. tonsill/o, ____________________
_____ 9. sinus/o, ____________________
_____ 10. mediastin/o, ____________________

a. space between the lungs containing heart, esophagus, trachea, and other structures
b. passageway for air to the bronchi from the larynx
c. spongelike organs located in the thoracic cavity
d. membrane covering the lung
e. lymphoid tissue located on the lateral wall at the junction of the oral cavity and oropharynx
f. air cavities within the cranial bones that open into the nasal cavities
g. location of the vocal cords
h. air sacs at the end of the bronchioles
i. the part of the body between the neck and diaphragm
j. tube carrying air between the trachea and lungs

EXERCISE 2 ■ Combining Forms Used with Respiratory System Terms

Refer to the second section of the word parts table.

A Define

Write the definition of the following combining forms.

1. ox/i ____________________
2. spir/o ____________________
3. muc/o ____________________
4. atel/o ____________________
5. orth/o ____________________
6. py/o ____________________
7. hem/o ____________________
8. somn/o ____________________
9. capn/o ____________________
10. phon/o ____________________
11. carcin/o ____________________
12. myc/o ____________________
13. coni/o ____________________

B Identify

Write the combining form for each of the following.

1. breathe, breathing ____________________
2. oxygen ____________________
3. imperfect, incomplete ____________________
4. straight ____________________
5. pus ____________________
6. mucus ____________________
7. blood ____________________
8. sleep ____________________
9. sound, voice ____________________
10. carbon dioxide ____________________
11. dust ____________________
12. cancer ____________________
13. fungus ____________________

OXYGEN was discovered in 1774 by Joseph Priestley. In 1775 Antoine-Laurent Lavoisier, a French chemist, noted that all the acids he knew contained oxygen. Because he thought it was an acid producer, he named it using the Greek **oxys**, meaning **sour**, and the suffix **gen**, meaning **to produce**.

EXERCISE 3 ■ Prefixes

Refer to the third section of the word parts table.

A Define

Write the definitions of the following prefixes.

1. endo- ______
2. a-, an- ______
3. eu- ______
4. poly- ______
5. tachy- ______
6. dys- ______
7. hypo- ______
8. intra- ______
9. hyper- ______
10. neo- ______

B Identify

Write the prefix for each of the following.

1. within a. ______
   b. ______
2. normal, good ______
3. absence of, without a. ______
   b. ______
4. many, much ______
5. fast, rapid ______
6. new ______
7. above, excessive ______
8. below, incomplete, deficient, under ______
9. painful, abnormal, difficult, labored ______

EXERCISE 4 ■ Suffixes

Refer to the fourth section of the word parts table.

A Match

Match the suffixes in the first column with their correct definitions in the second column.

______	1. -genic	a. stretching out, dilation, expansion
______	2. -ar, -ary, -eal	b. pertaining to visual examination
______	3. -cele	c. pertaining to
______	4. -desis	d. hernia, protrusion
______	5. -ectasis	e. surgical fixation, fusion
______	6. -ia	f. diseased or abnormal state, condition of
______	7. -thorax	g. producing, originating, causing
______	8. -stenosis	h. surgical puncture to aspirate fluid
______	9. -spasm	i. chest, chest cavity
______	10. -scopic	j. breathing
______	11. -centesis	k. constriction or narrowing
______	12. -itis	l. sudden, involuntary muscle contraction
______	13. -pnea	m. inflammation

B Label

Write the suffixes pictured and defined.

1. ______________________
instrument used for visual examination

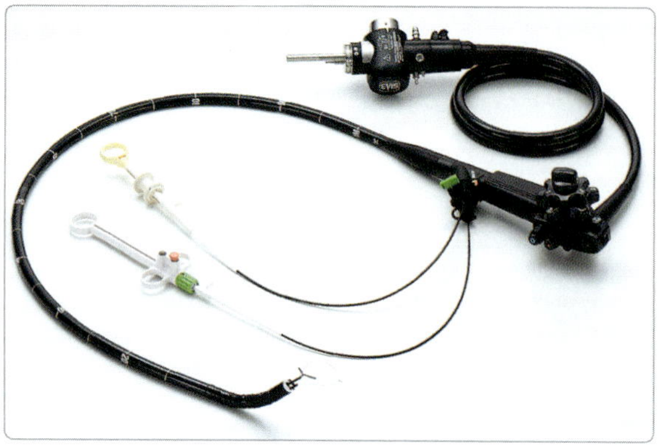

2. ______________________
visual examination

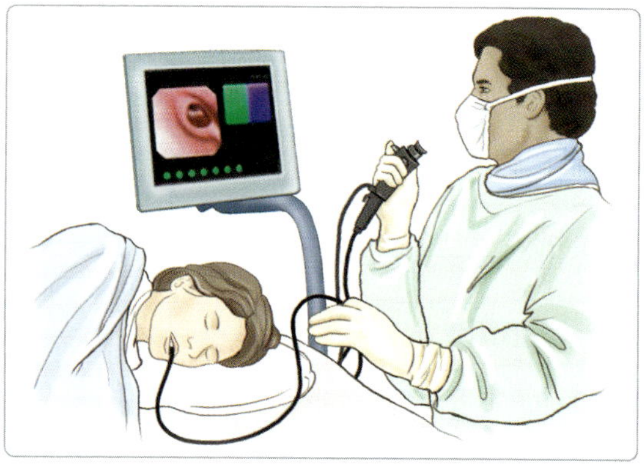

3. ______________________
cut into, incision

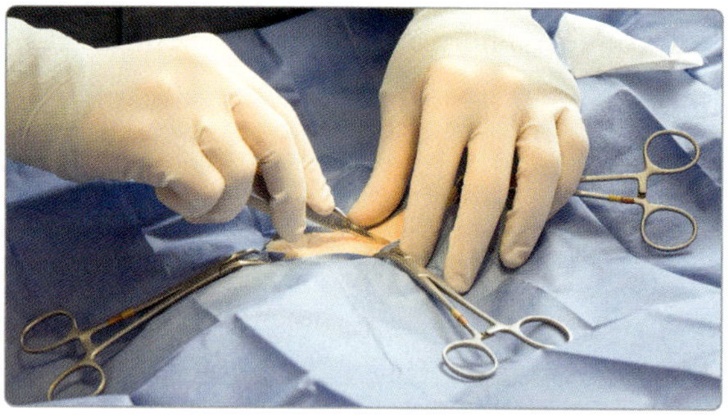

4. ______________________
creation of an artificial opening

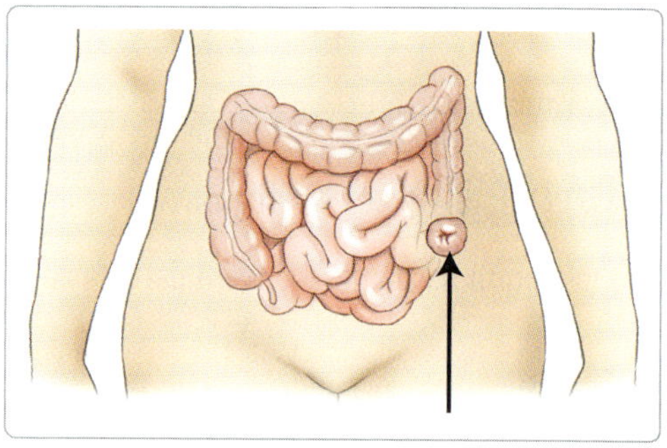

5. ______________________
instrument used to measure

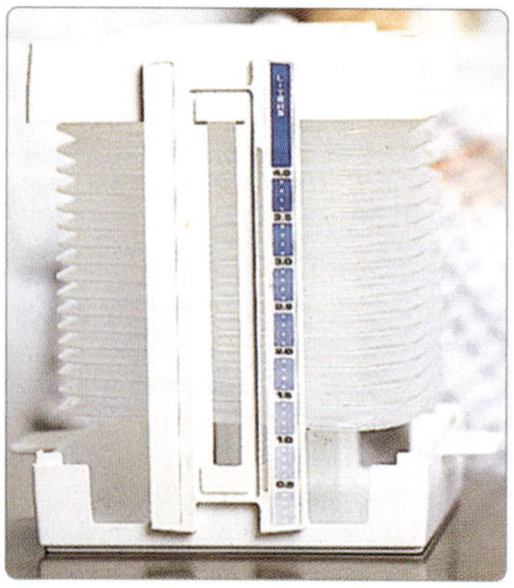

6. ______________________
measurement (use of the instrument)

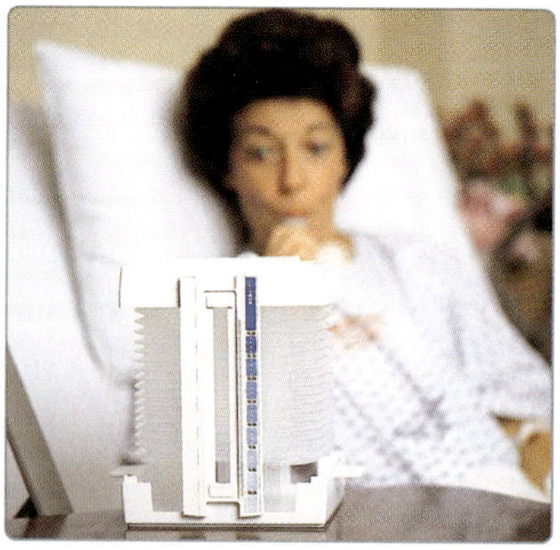

7. ______________________
excessive bleeding

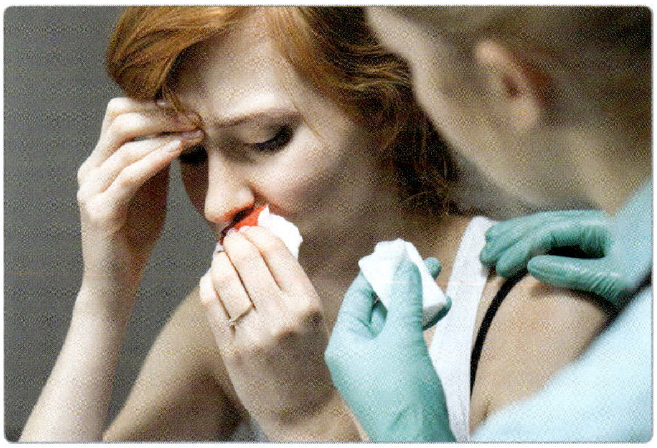

8. ______________________
spitting, coughing

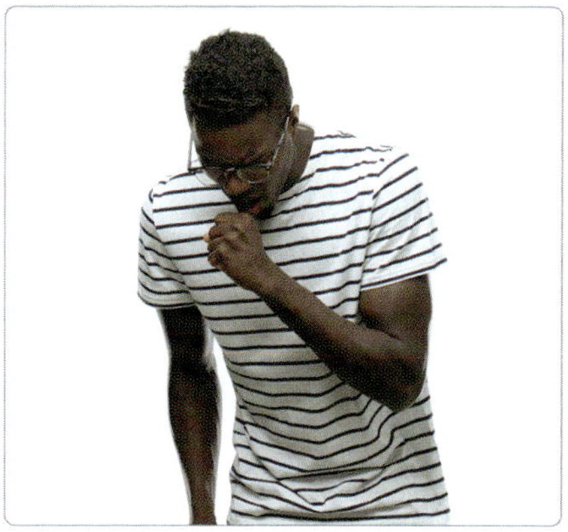

9. ______________________
excision, surgical removal

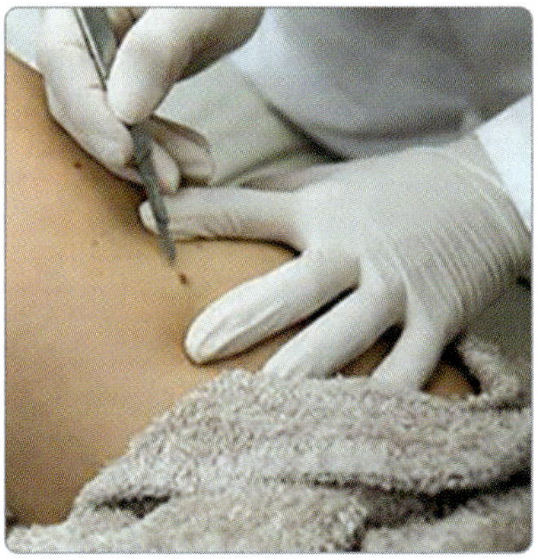

10. ______________________
in the blood

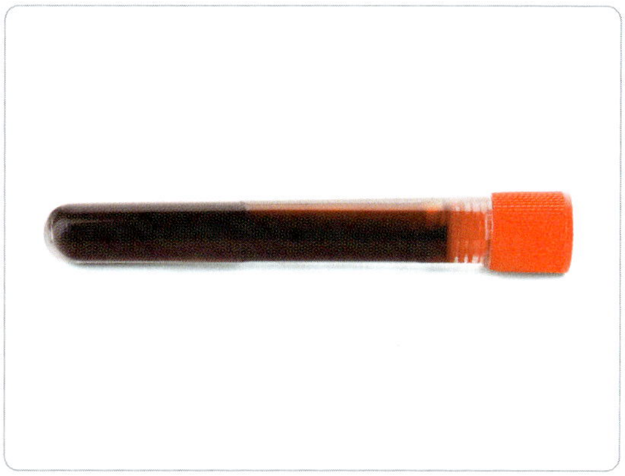

C Define

Write the definitions of the following suffixes.

1. -rrhea ______________________
2. -oid ______________________
3. -logist ______________________
4. -plasm ______________________
5. -al, -ic, -ous ______________________
6. -oma ______________________
7. -logy ______________________
8. -plasty ______________________
9. -osis ______________________

MEDICAL TERMS

Medical terms relevant to this chapter have been grouped by topics, such as Disease and Disorder, and are listed in tables designated as Built from Word Parts or *NOT* Built from Word Parts. The exercises following each table assist with learning term definitions, pronunciations, and spellings.

Disease and Disorder Terms

BUILT FROM WORD PARTS

The following terms can be translated using definitions of word parts. Further explanation is provided within parentheses as needed.

TERM	DEFINITION
1. **adenoiditis** (*ad*-e-noyd-Ī-tis)	inflammation of the adenoids
2. **alveolitis** (*al*-vē-o-LĪ-tis)	inflammation of the alveoli (pulmonary or dental)
3. **atelectasis** (*at*-e-LEK-ta-sis)	incomplete expansion (of the lung or portion of the lung) (Fig. 5.3)
ATELECTASIS is derived from the Greek **ateles**, meaning **not perfect**, and **ektasis**, meaning **expansion**. It denotes an incomplete expansion of the lungs.	
4. **bronchiectasis** (*bron*-kē-EK-ta-sis)	dilation of the bronchi
5. **bronchitis** (bron-KĪ-tis)	inflammation of the bronchi (see Fig. 5.5)
6. **bronchogenic carcinoma** (bron-kō-JEN-ik) (*kar*-si-NŌ-ma)	cancerous tumor originating in a bronchus (also referred to as **lung cancer**) (Fig. 5.4)
7. **bronchopneumonia** (*bron*-kō-nū-MŌ-nē-a)	diseased state of the bronchi and lungs (an inflammation of the lungs that begins in the terminal bronchioles)
8. **bronchospasm** (BRON-kō-*spaz*-m)	spasmodic contraction of the bronchi
9. **diaphragmatocele** (*dī*-a-frag-MAT-ō-sēl)	hernia of the diaphragm
10. **epiglottitis** (*ep*-i-glo-TĪ-tis)	inflammation of the epiglottis
11. **hemothorax** (*hē*-mō-THOR-aks)	blood in the chest cavity (pleural cavity)
12. **laryngitis** (*lar*-in-JĪ-tis)	inflammation of the larynx
13. **laryngospasm** (la-RING-gō-*spaz*-m)	spasmodic contraction of the larynx
14. **laryngotracheobronchitis (LTB)** (la-*ring*-gō-*trā*-kē-ō-bron-KĪ-tis)	inflammation of the larynx, trachea, and bronchi (the acute form is called **croup**)
15. **lobar pneumonia** (LŌ-bar) (nū-MŌ-nē-a)	pertaining to the lobe(s); diseased state of the lung (infection of one or more lobes of the lung)
16. **nasopharyngitis** (*nā*-zō-*far*-in-JĪ-tis)	inflammation of the nose and pharynx
17. **pharyngitis** (*far*-in-JĪ-tis)	inflammation of the pharynx
18. **pleuritis** (plū-RĪ-tis)	inflammation of the pleura (also called **pleurisy**)
19. **pneumoconiosis** (*nū*-mō-*kō*-nē-Ō-sis)	abnormal condition of dust in the lungs
PNEUMOCONIOSIS is the general name given for chronic inflammatory disease of the lung caused by excessive inhalation of mineral dust. When the disease is caused by a specific dust, it is named for the dust. For example, the disease caused by silica dust is called **silicosis**.	
20. **pneumonia** (nū-MŌ-nē-a)	diseased state of the lung (the infection and inflammation are caused by bacteria such as *Pneumococcus*, *Staphylococcus*, *Streptococcus*, and *Haemophilus*; viruses; and fungi)
21. **pneumonitis** (*nū*-mō-NĪ-tis)	inflammation of the lung

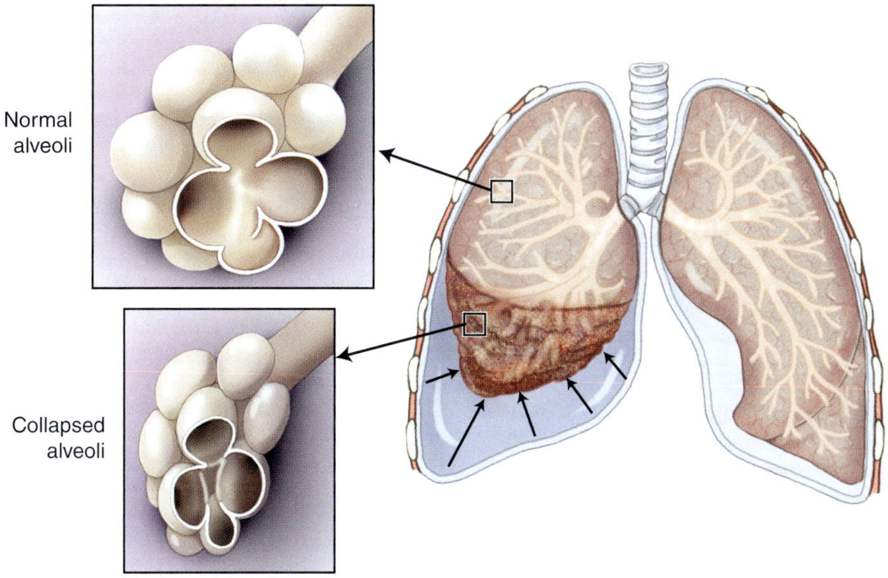

FIG. 5.3 Atelectasis showing the collapsed alveoli.

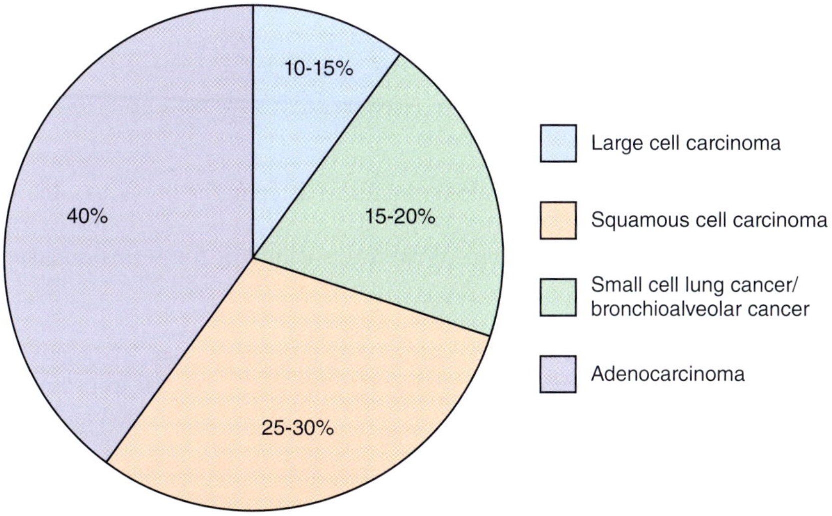

FIG. 5.4 Types of lung cancers. Lung cancer is classified as either small cell or large cell. The latter is by far the most prevalent and includes **adenocarcinoma** and **squamous cell carcinoma**. Lung cancer is one of the most common cancers in the world. It is the main cause of death due to cancer for both men and women. Smoking is the most important risk factor for the development of lung cancer. Symptoms include cough, hemoptysis, chest pain, dyspnea, fatigue, and weight loss. **Thoracentesis, bronchoscopy, chest radiograph**, **computed tomography (CT)**, and **positron emission tomography (PET)** scanning are used for diagnosis. Treatment includes **surgery, chemotherapy**, and **radiation**.

MESOTHELIOMA is a rare form of cancer most common in the pleura, the sac covering the lung, and lining the thoracic cavity, and is most often caused by inhalation exposure to asbestos. **Mesothelioma** also occurs in the lining of the abdominal cavity and in the lining of the heart.

Disease and Disorder Terms—cont'd

BUILT FROM WORD PARTS

TERM	DEFINITION
22. pneumothorax (*nū*-mō-THOR-aks)	air in the chest cavity (specifically, the pleural cavity, which causes collapse of the lung and is often a result of an open chest wound)
23. pulmonary neoplasm (PUL-mō-*nar*-ē) (NĒ-ō-*plaz*-em)	pertaining to (in) the lung, new growth (tumor)
24. pyothorax (*pī*-ō-THOR-aks)	pus in the chest cavity (pleural cavity) (also called **empyema**)
25. rhinitis (rī-NĪ-tis)	inflammation of the nose (mucous membranes)
26. rhinomycosis (*rī*-nō-mī-KŌ-sis)	abnormal condition of fungus in the nose
27. rhinorrhagia (*rī*-nō-RĀ-ja)	excessive bleeding from the nose (also called **epistaxis**)
28. sinusitis (sī-nū-SĪ-tis)	inflammation of the sinuses
29. tonsillitis (*ton*-sil-Ī-tis)	inflammation of the tonsils
30. tracheitis (*trā*-kē-Ī-tis)	inflammation of the trachea
31. tracheostenosis (*trā*-kē-ō-sten-Ō-sis)	narrowing of the trachea

EXERCISE 5 ■ Pronounce and Spell

Practice pronunciation and spelling on paper and online.

1. Practice on Paper

a. **Pronounce:** Read the phonetic spelling and say aloud the terms listed in the previous table. Refer to the pronunciation key on p. 20 as necessary.
b. **Spell:** Have a study partner read the terms aloud. Write the spelling of the terms on a separate sheet of paper.

2. Practice Online

a. **Access** online learning resources. Go to evolve.elsevier.com > Evolve Resources > Student Resources.
b. **Pronounce:** Select Audio Glossary > Chapter 5 > Exercise 5. Select a term to hear its pronunciation and repeat aloud.
c. **Spell:** Select Activities > Chapter 5 > Spell Terms > Exercise 5. Select the audio icon and type the correct spelling of the term.

❑ Check the box when complete.

EXERCISE 6 ■ Analyze and Define

Analyze and define the following terms by drawing slashes between word parts, writing word part abbreviations above the term, underlining combining forms, and writing combining form abbreviations below the term.

EXAMPLE:

WR CV S
diaphragmat / o / cele
CF
hernia of the diaphragm

1. tracheitis

____

____

2. nasopharyngitis

____

____

3. alveolitis

____

____

4. pyothorax

____

____

5. atelectasis

____
____

6. rhinomycosis

____
____

7. tracheostenosis

____
____

8. epiglottitis

____
____

9. laryngitis

____
____

10. pulmonary neoplasm

____
____

11. pneumonia

____
____

12. rhinitis

____
____

13. pneumoconiosis

____
____

14. bronchopneumonia

____
____

15. laryngotracheobronchitis

____
____

16. bronchospasm

____
____

EXERCISE 7 ■ Build

A Label

Build terms pictured by writing word parts above definitions.

1.

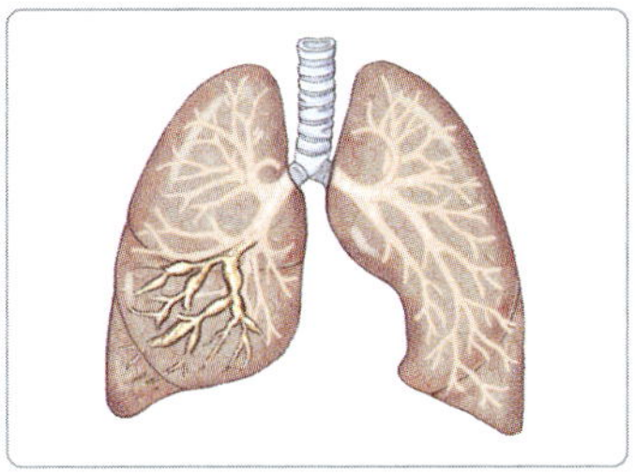

________ / ________
bronchi dilation

2.

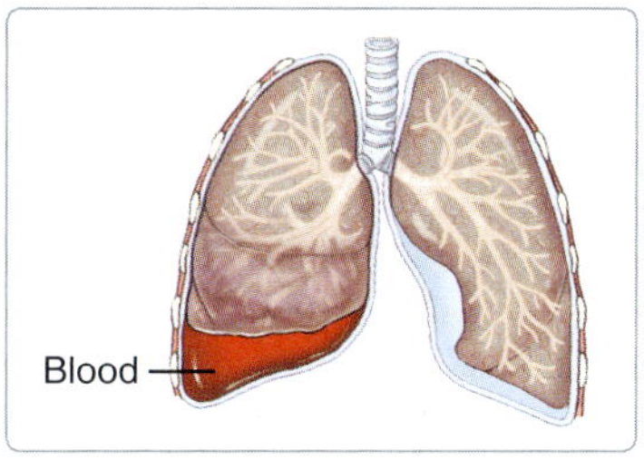

________ / ________ / ________
blood CV chest cavity

3.

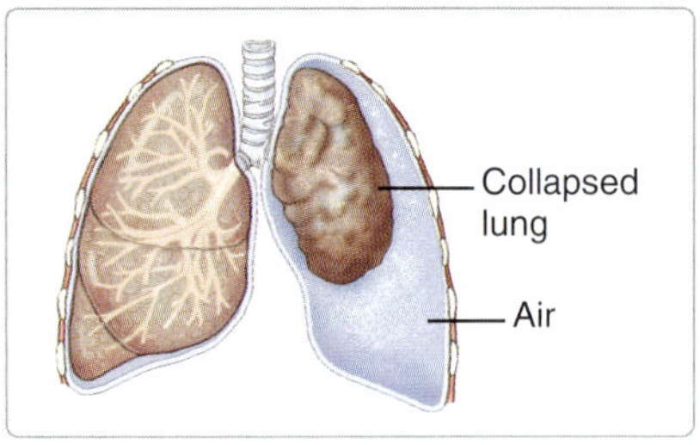

_______ / _______ / _______
air CV chest cavity

4.

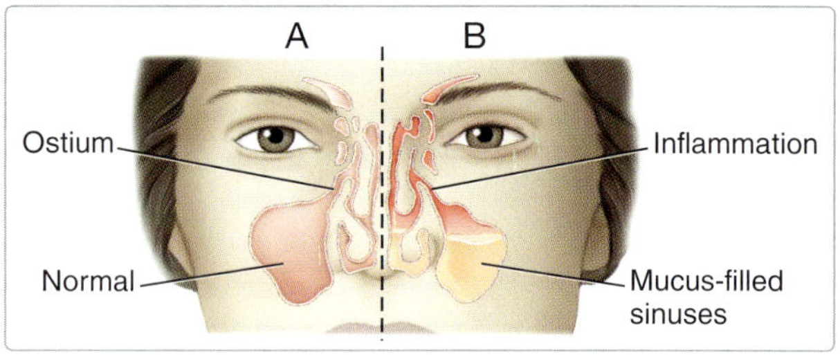

A. Normal sinuses B. _______ / _______
sinuses inflammation

5.

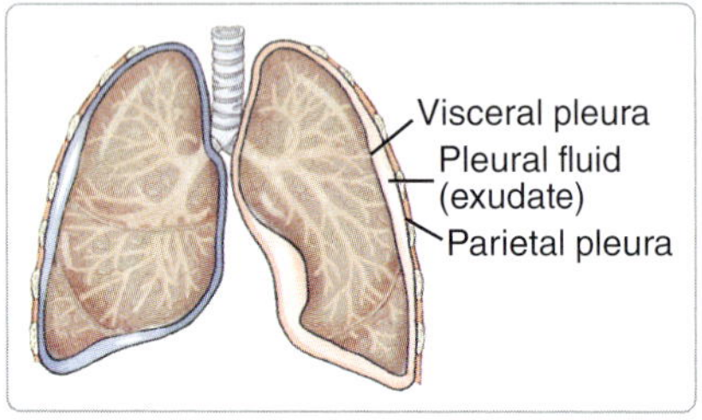

_______ / _______
pleura inflammation

6.

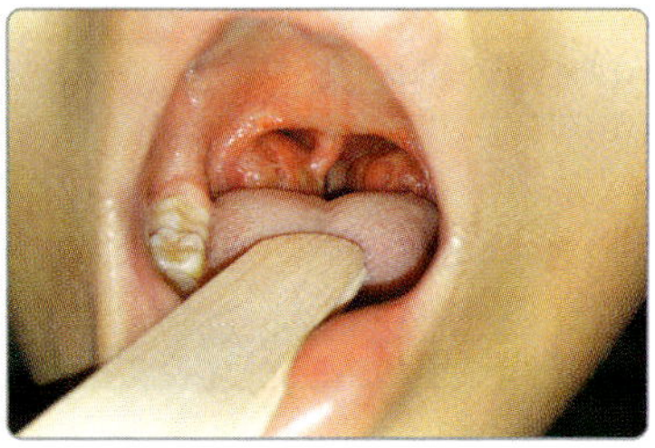

_______ / _______
tonsil inflammation

B Fill In

Build disease and disorder terms for the following definitions with the word parts you have learned.

EXAMPLE: inflammation of the tonsils tonsill / itis (WR / S)

1. inflammation of the pharynx _______ / _______ (WR / S)
2. cancerous tumor originating in a bronchus _______ / _______ / _______ (WR / CV / S) _______ / _______ (WR / S)
3. pertaining to the lobe(s); diseased state of the lung _______ / _______ (WR / S) _______ / _______ (WR / S)
4. spasmodic contraction of the larynx _______ / _______ / _______ (WR / CV / S)
5. hernia of the diaphragm _______ / _______ / _______ (WR / CV / S)
6. inflammation of the adenoids _______ / _______ (WR / S)
7. inflammation of the bronchi _______ / _______ (WR / S)

8. excessive bleeding from the nose ______ WR / CV / ______ S

9. inflammation of the lung ______ WR / ______ S

Disease and Disorder Terms

NOT BUILT FROM WORD PARTS

Word parts may be present in the following terms; however, their full meanings cannot be translated using definitions of word parts alone.

TERM	DEFINITION
1. acute respiratory distress syndrome (ARDS) (a-KŪT) (RES-pi-ra-*tor*-ē) (di-STRES) (SIN-drōm)	respiratory failure as a result of disease or injury. ARDS is respiratory failure in an adult. Symptoms include dyspnea, tachypnea, and cyanosis. (also called **adult respiratory distress syndrome**)

INSIDIOUS/ACUTE/SUBACUTE/CHRONIC are adjectives describing the onset and potential progression of a disease, condition, or syndrome.

Insidious: gradual and subtle onset of disease
Acute: sharp, sudden, short, or severe type of disease
Subacute: between acute and chronic
Chronic: disease that continues for a long time

TERM	DEFINITION
2. asphyxia (as-FIK-sē-a)	deprivation of oxygen for tissue use; suffocation
3. asthma (AZ-ma)	respiratory disease characterized by coughing, wheezing, and shortness of breath, caused by constriction and inflammation of airways that is reversible between attacks

REACTIVE AIRWAY DISEASE (RAD) is a general term and not a specific diagnosis. It is used to describe a history of wheezing, coughing, and shortness of breath. In some people RAD may lead to **asthma**.

TERM	DEFINITION
4. chronic obstructive pulmonary disease (COPD) (KRON-ik) (ob-STRUK-tiv) (PUL-mō-*nar*-ē) (di-ZĒZ)	progressive lung disease obstructing air flow, which makes breathing difficult. Chronic bronchitis and pulmonary emphysema are the two main components of COPD. Most COPD is a result of cigarette smoking. (Fig. 5.5)

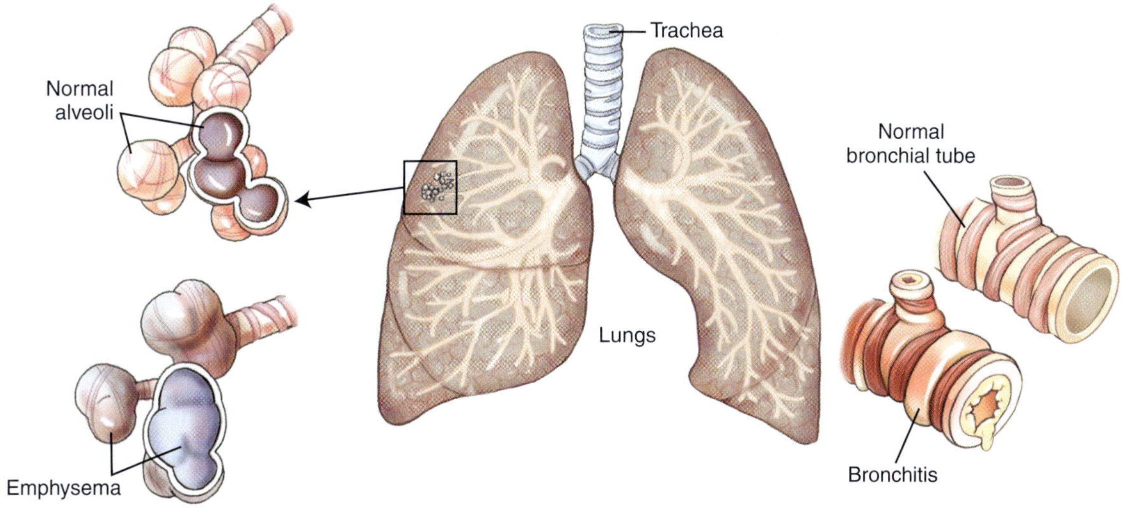

FIG. 5.5 Chronic obstructive pulmonary disease (COPD). Chronic bronchitis and emphysema are both components of COPD.

Disease and Disorder Terms—cont'd

NOT BUILT FROM WORD PARTS

TERM	DEFINITION
5. coccidioidomycosis (kok-*sid*-ē-*oy*-dō-mī-KŌ-sis)	fungal disease affecting the lungs and sometimes other organs of the body (also called **valley fever)**
6. coronavirus disease (COVID-19) (kō-RŌ-na-vī-rus) (di-ZĒZ)	respiratory infection caused by a virus with symptoms that include fever, cough, fatigue, difficulty breathing, and digestive upset; the disease course can range from mild to severe with the possibility of ARDS and multisystem organ failure

Several strains of **CORONAVIRUS** exist, including those that cause severe acute respiratory syndrome (SARS), Middle East respiratory syndrome (MERS), and coronavirus disease (COVID-19).

TERM	DEFINITION
7. croup (krūp)	condition resulting from acute obstruction of the larynx, characterized by a barking cough, hoarseness, and stridor. It may be caused by viral or bacterial infection, allergy, or foreign body. Occurs mainly in children. (also called **laryngotracheobronchitis**)
8. cystic fibrosis (CF) (SIS-tik) (fī-BRŌ-sis)	hereditary disorder of the exocrine glands characterized by excess mucus production in the respiratory tract, pancreatic deficiency, and other symptoms
9. deviated septum (DĒ-vē-*āt*-ed) (SEP-tum)	one part of the nasal cavity is smaller because of malformation or injury of the nasal septum
10. diphtheria (dif-THĒR-ē-a)	serious bacterial infection affecting the mucous membranes of the nose and throat. It creates a thick, gray sheet covering the pharynx, which can lead to difficulty breathing, heart failure, paralysis, and even death. It is rare in developed countries due to widespread vaccination against the disease.
11. emphysema (*em*-fi-SĒ-ma)	loss of elasticity of the alveoli resulting in distention causing stretching of the lung. As a result, the body does not receive enough oxygen. (component of COPD) (Fig. 5.5)
12. epistaxis (*ep*-i-STAK-sis)	nosebleed (also called **rhinorrhagia**)
13. idiopathic pulmonary fibrosis (IPF) (id-ē-ō-PATH-ik) (PUL-mō-*nar*-ē) (fī-BRŌ-sis)	chronic progressive lung disorder characterized by increasing scarring, which ultimately reduces the capacity of the lungs; etiology unknown. IPF most often affects adults over the age of 50. Smoking, pollutants, and heredity may play a role in its genesis. Symptoms include exertional dyspnea and a dry cough. Lung transplant may be indicated in severe cases; there is no cure.
14. influenza (flu) (*in*-flū-EN-za)	highly contagious and often severe viral infection of the respiratory tract

INFLUENZA PANDEMIC is the sudden outbreak of a flu that becomes widespread, affecting a region, a continent, or the world. Examples are H1N1 swine flu and H5N1 avian flu.

TERM	DEFINITION
15. obstructive sleep apnea (OSA) (ob-STRUK-tiv) (slēp) (AP-nē-a)	repetitive pharyngeal collapse during sleep, which leads to transient periods of apnea (absence of breathing); can produce daytime drowsiness and elevated blood pressure (Fig. 5.6)
16. pertussis (per-TUS-sis)	highly contagious bacterial infection of the respiratory tract characterized by a severe hacking cough, followed by an acute crowing inspiration, or whoop. It mainly affects infants too young to be vaccinated and adults whose immunity to the vaccine has faded. (also called **whooping cough**)
17. pleural effusion (PLŪ-ral) (e-FŪ-zhun)	fluid in the pleural cavity caused by a disease process or trauma
18. pulmonary edema (PUL-mō-*nar*-ē) (e-DĒ-ma)	fluid accumulation in the alveoli and bronchioles, most often a manifestation of heart failure

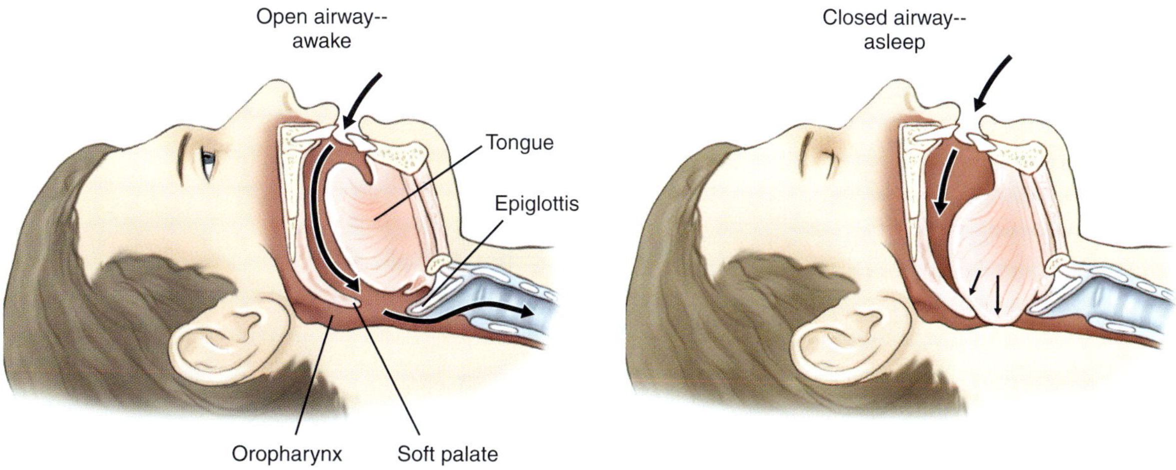

FIG. 5.6 Obstructive sleep apnea (OSA). During sleep, the absence of activity of the pharyngeal muscle structure allows the airway to close. OSA is associated with increased risk for elevated blood pressure, cardiovascular disease, diabetes, and stroke. Obesity is a major risk factor and weight loss can be an effective treatment. **Polysomnography** is used to diagnose OSA. Treatment includes the use of **CPAP (continuous positive airway pressure)** during sleep and **uvulopalatopharyngoplasty (UPPP),** a surgical procedure.

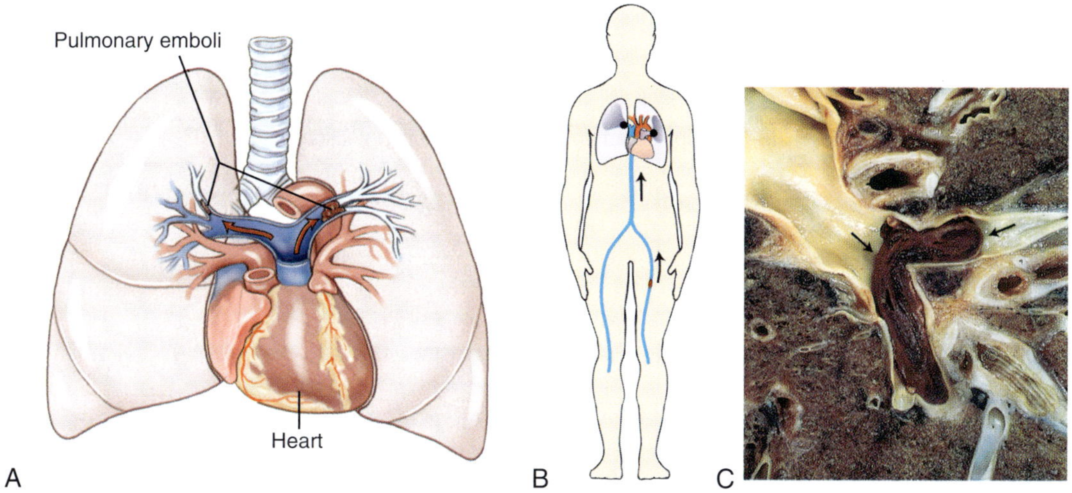

FIG. 5.7 **A,** Bilateral pulmonary emboli. **B,** Pulmonary emboli usually originate in the deep veins of the lower extremities. **C,** Necropsy specimen of the lung showing a large embolus.

TERM	DEFINITION
19. pulmonary embolism (PE) (PUL-mō-*nar*-ē) (EM-bo-liz-em)	matter foreign to the circulation, carried to the pulmonary artery and its branches, where it blocks circulation to the lungs and can be fatal if of sufficient size or number. Blood clots broken loose from the deep veins of the lower extremities are the most common cause of pulmonary embolism. (Fig. 5.7)
20. tuberculosis (TB) (tū-*ber*-kū-LŌ-sis)	infectious bacterial disease, most commonly spread by inhalation of small particles and usually affecting the lungs; may spread to other organs

TUBERCULOSIS (TB) is one of the most common causes of death worldwide from infectious disease, though it is preventable and curable. The risk for active TB is higher in HIV-infected persons and others with weakened immune systems. The development of multidrug–resistant TB is becoming a problem in treatment of the disease.

TERM	DEFINITION
21. upper respiratory infection (URI) (UP-er) (RES-pi-ra-*tor*-ē) (in-FEK-shun)	infection of the nasal cavity, pharynx, or larynx usually caused by a virus (commonly called a **cold**) (Fig. 5.8)

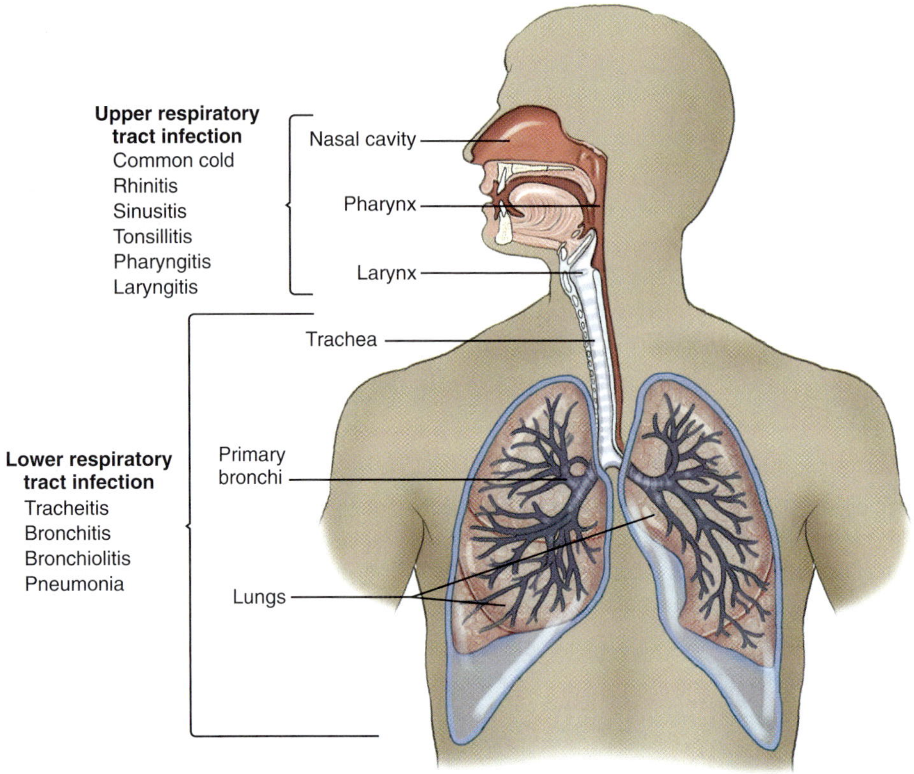

FIG. 5.8 Upper and lower respiratory tract infections.

EXERCISE 8 ■ Pronounce and Spell

Practice pronunciation and spelling on paper and online.

1. Practice on Paper

a. **Pronounce:** Read the phonetic spelling and say aloud the terms listed in the previous table. Refer to the pronunciation key on p. 20 as necessary.
b. **Spell:** Have a study partner read the terms aloud. Write the spelling of the terms on a separate sheet of paper.

2. Practice Online

a. **Access** online learning resources. Go to evolve.elsevier.com > Evolve Resources > Student Resources.
b. **Pronounce:** Select Audio Glossary > Chapter 5 > Exercise 8. Select a term to hear its pronunciation and repeat aloud.
c. **Spell:** Select Activities > Chapter 5 > Spell Terms > Exercise 8. Select the audio icon and type the correct spelling of the term.

❑ Check the box when complete.

EXERCISE 9 ■ Fill In

A Identify

Fill in the blanks with the correct terms.

1. ________________ ________________ is a hereditary disorder characterized by excess mucus production in the respiratory tract.
2. The medical name of a highly contagious respiratory infection commonly referred to as *flu* is ________________.
3. Chronic bronchitis and emphysema are two main components of ________________________________ ________________ ________________ ________________.
4. The medical name for a highly contagious bacterial infection of the respiratory tract characterized by a severe hacking cough, followed by a whoop is ________________________________.

5. ______________ is a condition resulting from an acute obstruction of the larynx characterized by a barking cough, hoarseness, and stridor.
6. A condition in which fluid accumulates in the alveoli and bronchioles is ______________ ______________.
7. ______________ is another name for nosebleed.
8. A chronic progressive lung disorder that ultimately reduces the capacity of the lungs is ______________ ______________ ______________.
9. ______________ is a serious bacterial infection affecting the mucous membranes of the nose and throat, which creates a thick gray sheet over the pharynx; it is rare in countries with high rates of vaccination.
10. Deprivation of oxygen for tissue use, or suffocation is called ______________.
11. An infectious bacterial disease usually affecting the lungs and caused by inhaling infected small particles is ______________.
12. ______________ ______________ ______________ ______________ is also called adult respiratory distress syndrome.
13. The respiratory infection with symptoms including fever, cough, fatigue, and difficulty breathing, or ______________ ______________, is caused by the virus SARS-CoV-2 and is referred to as COVID-19.

B Label

Write the medical terms pictured and defined.

1. ______________
matter foreign to the circulation, carried to the pulmonary artery and its branches, where it blocks circulation to the lungs

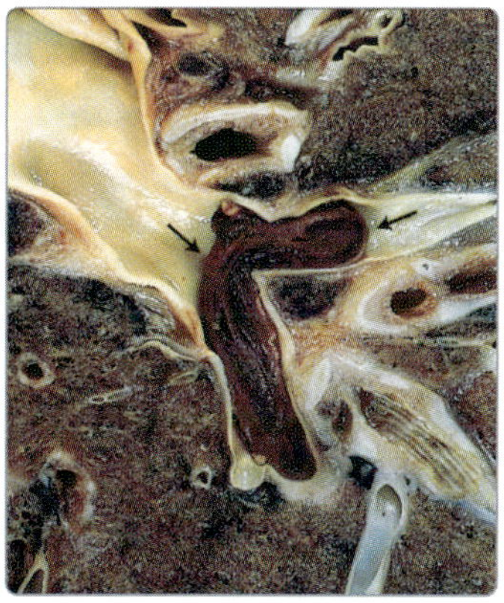

2. ______________
repetitive pharyngeal collapse during sleep, which leads to transient periods of apnea

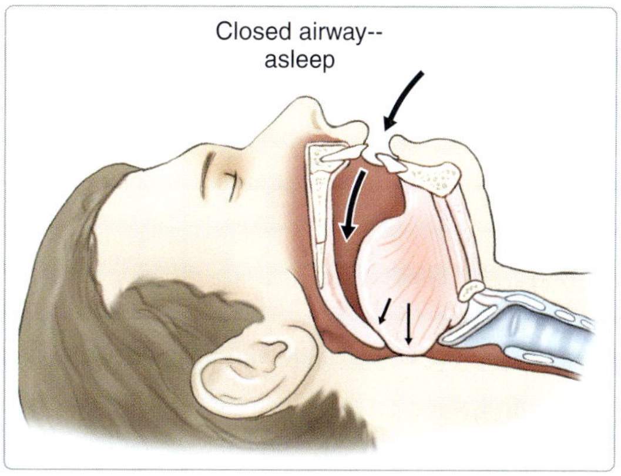

3. ______________
one part of the nasal cavity is smaller because of malformation or injury of the nasal septum

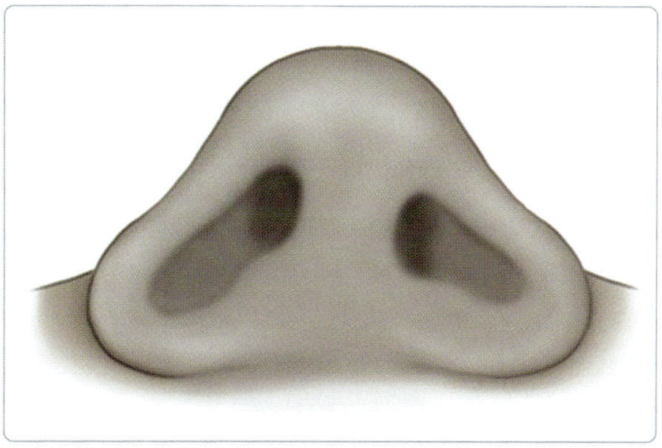

4. ______________
fluid in the pleural cavity caused by a disease process or trauma

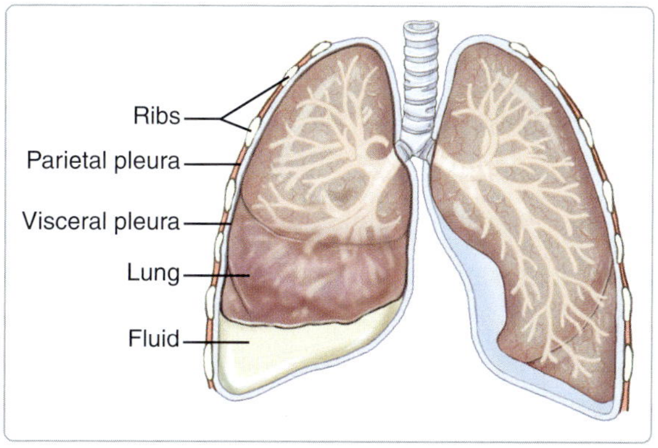

5. ______________________________
respiratory disease characterized by coughing, wheezing, and shortness of breath, caused by constriction and inflammation of airways that is reversible between attacks

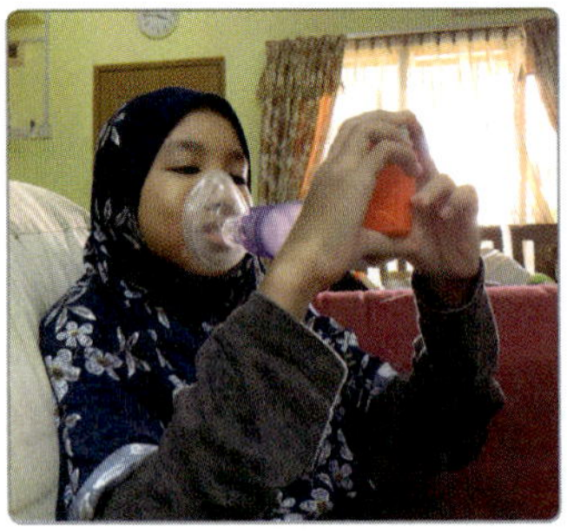

6. ______________________________
fungal disease affecting the lungs and sometimes other organs of the body

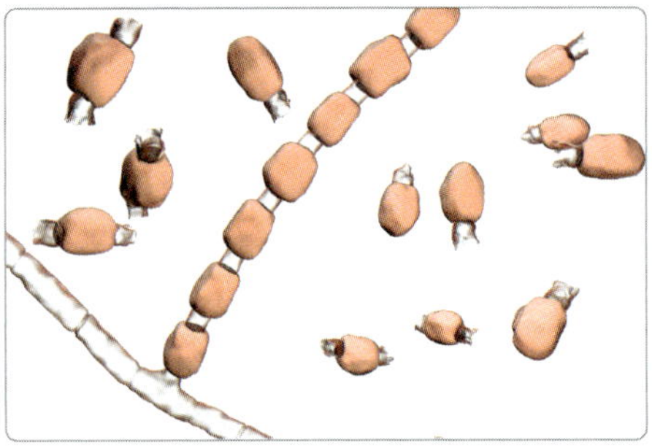

7. ______________________________
loss of elasticity of the alveoli resulting in distention causing stretching of the lung

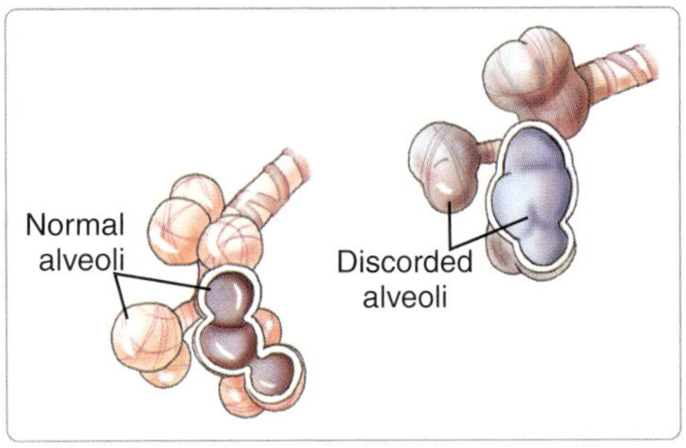

8. ______________________________
infection of the nasal cavity, pharynx, or larynx usually caused by a virus; commonly called a cold

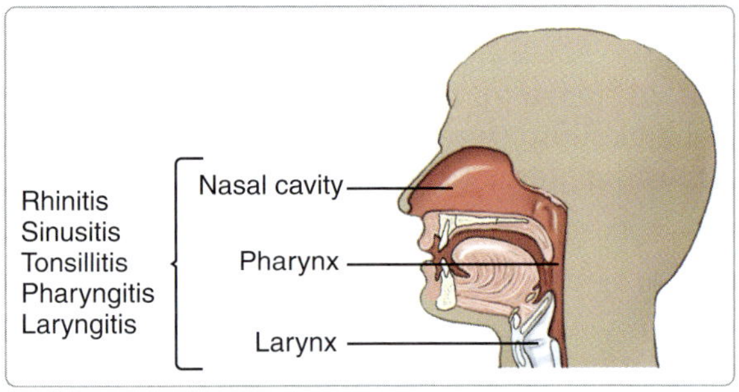

EXERCISE 10 ■ Match

Match the terms in the first column with their correct definitions in the second column.

_____ 1. diphtheria	a. loss of elasticity of alveoli resulting in stretching of the lung
_____ 2. asthma	b. caused by a virus (commonly called flu)
_____ 3. chronic obstructive pulmonary disease	c. hereditary disorder characterized by excess mucus in the respiratory system
_____ 4. coccidioidomycosis	d. most often caused by cigarette smoking
_____ 5. croup	e. nosebleed
_____ 6. cystic fibrosis	f. condition resulting from acute obstruction of the larynx
_____ 7. emphysema	g. also called valley fever
_____ 8. epistaxis	h. characterized by scarring of the lung
_____ 9. influenza	i. caused by restriction of airways that is reversible between attacks
_____ 10. idiopathic pulmonary fibrosis	j. serious bacterial infection that creates a thick gray sheet covering the pharynx

EXERCISE 11 ■ Match

Match the terms in the first column with their correct definitions in the second column.

_____ 1. pertussis
_____ 2. pleural effusion
_____ 3. pulmonary edema
_____ 4. pulmonary embolism
_____ 5. upper respiratory infection
_____ 6. deviated septum
_____ 7. obstructive sleep apnea
_____ 8. tuberculosis
_____ 9. acute respiratory distress syndrome
_____ 10. asphyxia
_____ 11. coronavirus disease

a. respiratory failure as a result of disease or injury
b. viral illness with fever, cough, fatigue, and difficulty breathing
c. fluid accumulation in alveoli and bronchioles
d. whooping cough
e. foreign material, carried to the pulmonary artery, where it blocks circulation to the lungs
f. commonly called a cold
g. unequal size of nasal cavities
h. repetitive pharyngeal collapse
i. infectious bacterial disease usually affecting the lungs
j. deprivation of oxygen for tissue use
k. fluid in the pleural cavity

EXERCISE 12 ■ Review of Disease and Disorder Terms

Can you define, pronounce, and spell the following terms?

acute respiratory distress syndrome (ARDS)
adenoiditis
alveolitis
atelectasis
asphyxia
asthma
bronchiectasis
bronchitis
bronchogenic carcinoma
bronchopneumonia
bronchospasm
chronic obstructive pulmonary disease (COPD)
coccidioidomycosis
coronavirus disease (COVID-19)
croup
cystic fibrosis (CF)
deviated septum
diaphragmatocele
diphtheria
emphysema
epiglottitis
epistaxis
hemothorax
idiopathic pulmonary fibrosis (IPF)
influenza (flu)
laryngitis
laryngospasm
laryngotracheobronchitis (LTB)
lobar pneumonia
nasopharyngitis
obstructive sleep apnea (OSA)
pertussis
pharyngitis
pleural effusion
pleuritis
pneumoconiosis
pneumonia
pneumonitis
pneumothorax
pulmonary edema
pulmonary embolism (PE)
pulmonary neoplasm
pyothorax
rhinitis
rhinomycosis
rhinorrhagia
sinusitis
tonsillitis
tracheitis
tracheostenosis
tuberculosis (TB)
upper respiratory infection (URI)

Surgical Terms

BUILT FROM WORD PARTS

The following terms can be translated using definitions of word parts. Further explanation is provided within parentheses as needed.

TERM	DEFINITION	TERM	DEFINITION
1. adenoidectomy (*ad*-e-noyd-EK-to-mē)	excision of the adenoids	**4. laryngoplasty** (la-RING-gō-*plas*-tē)	surgical repair of the larynx
2. bronchoplasty (BRON-kō-*plas*-tē)	surgical repair of a bronchus	**5. laryngostomy** (*lar*-in-GOS-to-mē)	creation of an artificial opening into the larynx
3. laryngectomy (*lār*-in-JEK-to-mē)	excision of the larynx	**6. laryngotracheotomy** (la-*ring*-gō-*trā*-kē-OT-o-mē)	incision into the larynx and trachea

Surgical Terms—cont'd

BUILT FROM WORD PARTS

TERM	DEFINITION
7. **lobectomy** (lō-BEK-to-mē)	excision of a lobe (of the lung) (Fig. 5.9)
8. **pleurodesis** (plū-rō-DĒ-sis)	fusion of the pleura (procedure to remove the space between the layers lining the lung; prevents the build up of fluid such as water, blood, or pus)
9. **pneumonectomy** (*nū*-mō-NEK-to-mē)	excision of a lung (Fig. 5.9)
10. **rhinoplasty** (RĪ-nō-*plas*-tē)	surgical repair of the nose
11. **septoplasty** (SEP-tō-*plas*-tē)	surgical repair of the (nasal) septum
12. **sinusotomy** (*sī*-nū-SOT-o-mē)	incision into a sinus
13. **thoracentesis** (thor-a-sen-TĒ-sis)	surgical puncture to aspirate fluid from the chest cavity (also called **thoracocentesis**)
The combining vowel "o" and the "c" in **thorac/o** are dropped in the term **thoracentesis**.	
14. **thoracotomy** (*thor*-a-KOT-o-mē)	incision into the chest cavity (Fig. 5.10)
15. **tonsillectomy** (*ton*-sil-EK-to-mē)	excision of the tonsils
16. **tracheoplasty** (TRĀ-kē-ō-*plas*-tē)	surgical repair of the trachea
17. **tracheostomy** (*trā*-kē-OS-to-mē)	creation of an artificial opening into the trachea (Fig. 5.11)
18. **tracheotomy** (*trā*-kē-OT-o-mē)	incision into the trachea (Fig. 5.11)

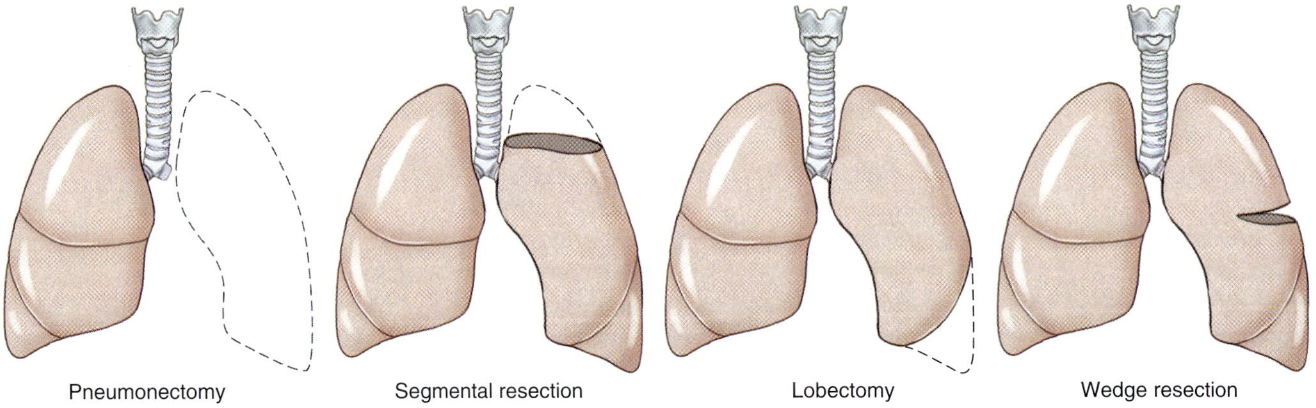

FIG. 5.9 Types of lung resection. The diagram illustrates the amount of lung tissue removed with each type of surgery.

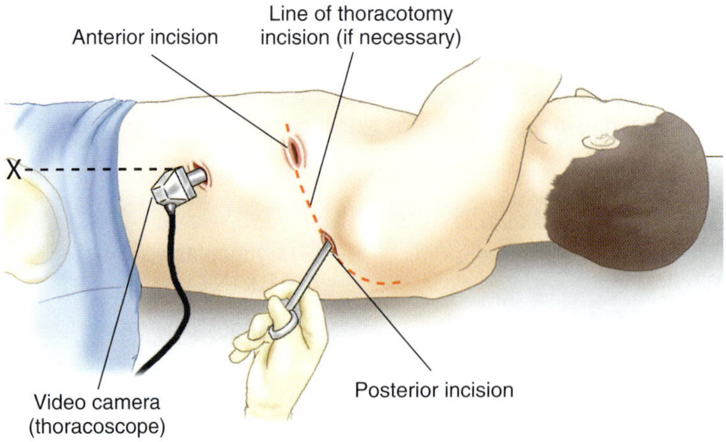

FIG. 5.10 Video-assisted thoracic surgery (VATS) is the use of a **thoracoscope** and video equipment for an endoscopic approach to diagnose and treat thoracic conditions. It often replaces the traditional **thoracotomy,** which required a large incision and greater recovery time.

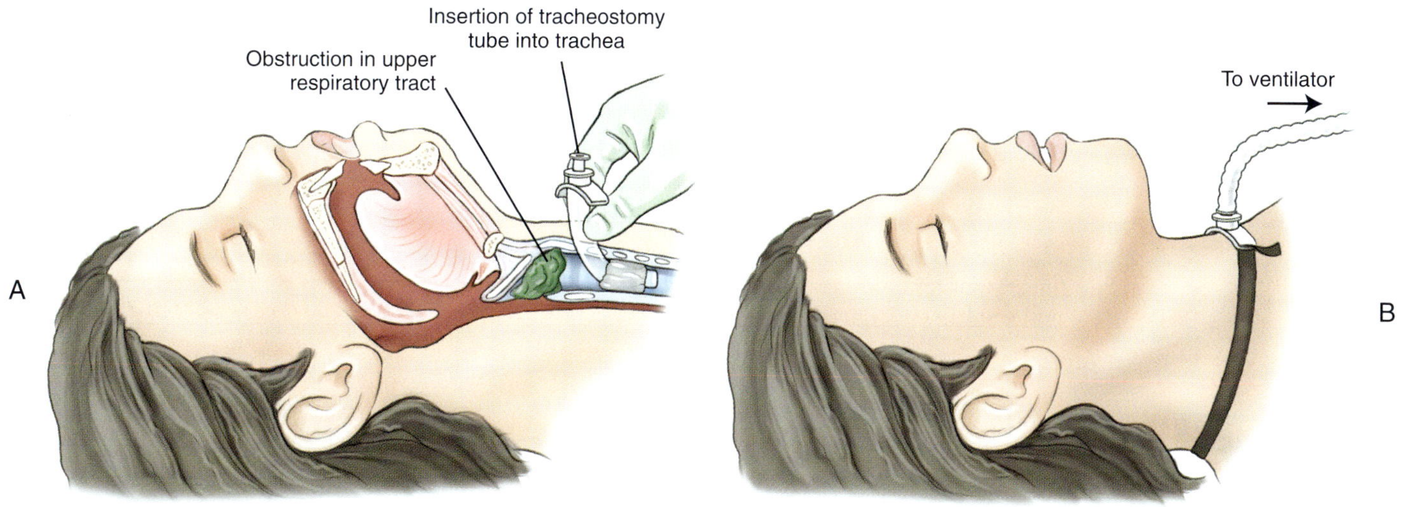

FIG. 5.11 **A,** A **tracheotomy** is performed to establish an airway when normal breathing is obstructed. If the opening needs to be maintained, a tube is inserted, creating a tracheostomy. **B,** A **tracheostomy** may be temporary, as for prolonged mechanical ventilation to support breathing or it may be permanent, as in airway reconstruction after laryngeal cancer surgery.

EXERCISE 13 ■ Pronounce and Spell

Practice pronunciation and spelling on paper and online.

1. Practice on Paper

a. **Pronounce:** Read the phonetic spelling and say aloud the terms listed in the previous table. Refer to the pronunciation key on p. 20 as necessary.
b. **Spell:** Have a study partner read the terms aloud. Write the spelling of the terms on a separate sheet of paper.

2. Practice Online

a. **Access** online learning resources. Go to evolve.elsevier.com > Evolve Resources > Student Resources.
b. **Pronounce:** Select Audio Glossary > Chapter 5 > Exercise 13. Select a term to hear its pronunciation and repeat aloud.
c. **Spell:** Select Activities > Chapter 5 > Spell Terms > Exercise 13. Select the audio icon and type the correct spelling of the term.

❏ Check the box when complete.

EXERCISE 14 ■ Analyze and Define

Analyze and define the following terms by drawing slashes between word parts, writing word part abbreviations above the term, underlining combining forms, and writing combining form abbreviations below the term.

EXAMPLE:
WR S
pneumon/ectomy
excision of a lung

1. tracheoplasty

____

____

2. septoplasty

____

____

3. laryngostomy

____

____

4. sinusotomy

____

____

5. laryngoplasty

____

____

6. thoracotomy

____

____

EXERCISE 15 ■ Build

A Label

Build terms pictured by writing word parts above definitions.

1.

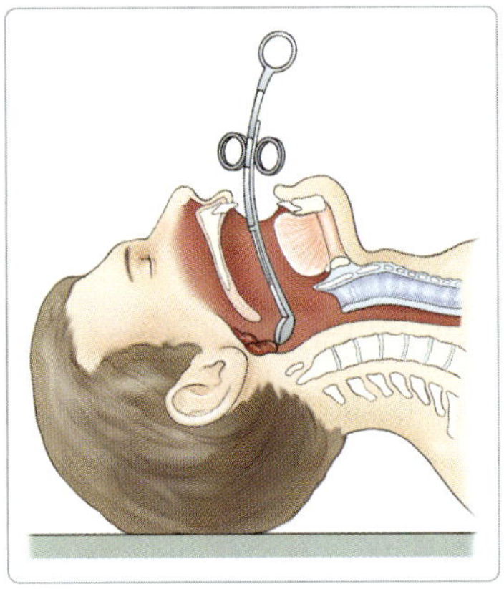

_____ / _____
adenoid / excision

2.

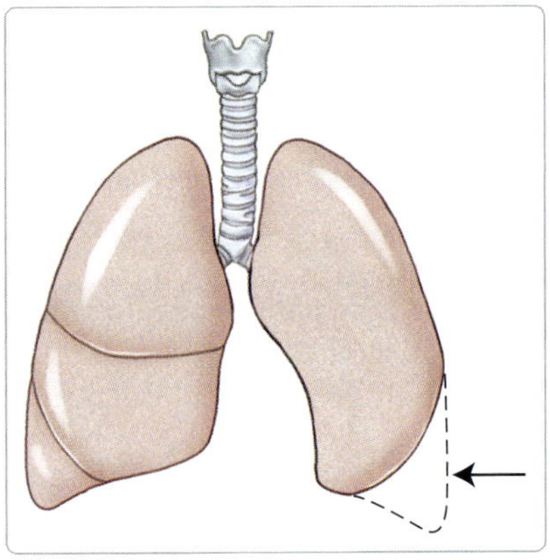

_____ / _____
lobe / excision

3.

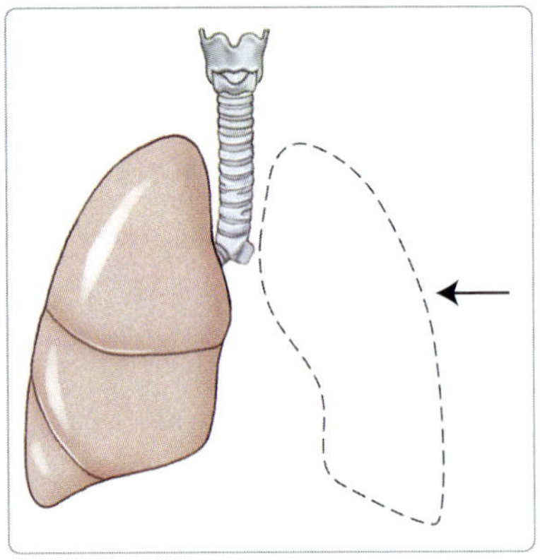

_____ / _____
lung / excision

4.

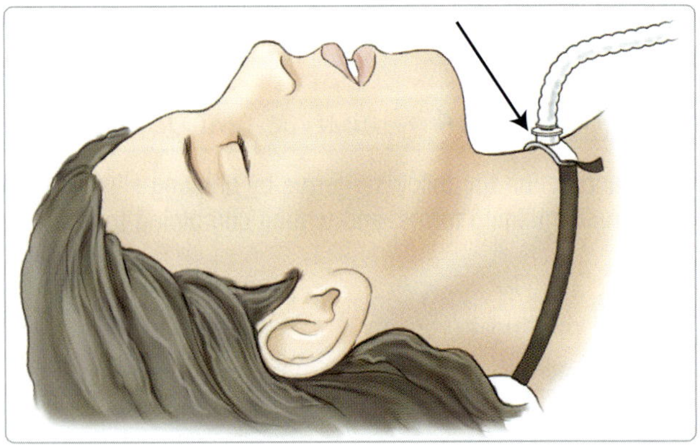

_____ / _____ / _____
trachea / CV / creation of an artificial opening

5.

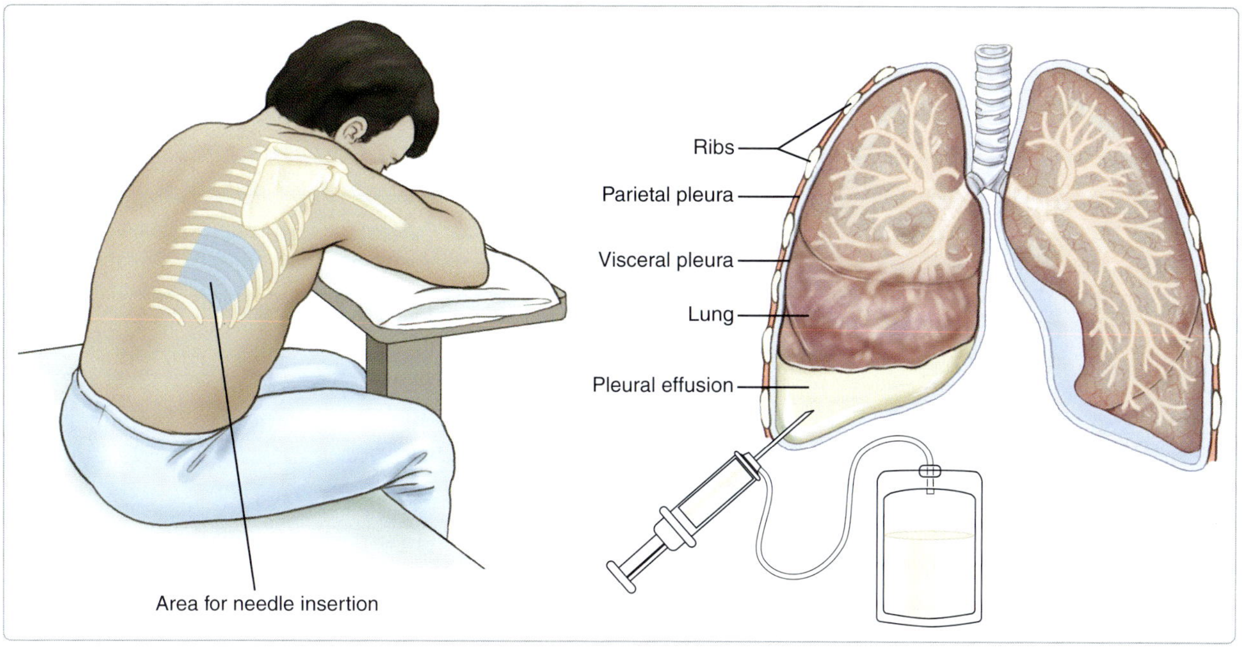

_______________ / _______________ is used for both diagnosis and treatment.
chest cavity / surgical puncture to aspirate fluid

6.

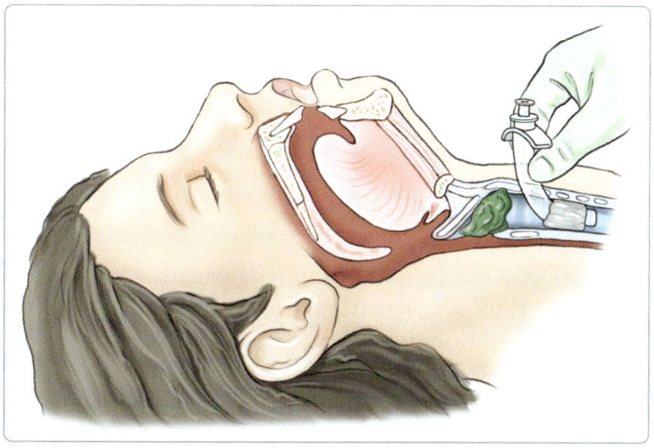

_______________ / _______ / _______________
trachea / CV / incision

B Fill In

Build surgical terms for the following definitions by using the word parts you have learned.

EXAMPLE: surgical repair of the larynx laryng / o / plasty
WR / CV / S

1. incision into the larynx and trachea _______ / _______ / _______ / _______ / _______
WR / CV / WR / CV / S

2. fusion of the pleura _______ / _______ / _______
WR / CV / S

3. excision of the tonsils ______ / ______
WR / S

4. surgical repair of a bronchus ______ / ___ / ______
WR / CV / S

5. excision of the larynx ______ / ______
WR / S

6. surgical repair of the nose ______ / ___ / ______
WR / CV / S

EXERCISE 16 ■ Review of Surgical Terms

Can you define, pronounce, and spell the following terms?

adenoidectomy	laryngotracheotomy	septoplasty	tracheoplasty
bronchoplasty	lobectomy	sinusotomy	tracheostomy
laryngectomy	pleurodesis	thoracentesis	tracheotomy
laryngoplasty	pneumonectomy	thoracotomy	
laryngostomy	rhinoplasty	tonsillectomy	

Endoscopy

Endoscopy is the general term for direct observation of a hollow body organ or cavity. Endoscopy dates to the time of Hippocrates (460-375 BC) and is translated from the Greek words **"endon"** (**within** or **inward**) and **"skopein"** (to **see** or **view**). By the end of the nineteenth century, cystoscopy, proctoscopy, and esophagoscopy were well established. The original endoscopes were rigid and used for direct observation. Adding lights and lenses to the endoscope allowed visualization of deeper structures.

Current endoscopy uses smaller, flexible, tubular instruments and incorporates fiber optics and cameras, which allows images to be viewed on a monitor. Endoscopic procedures and instruments are named after the body part visualized. For example, **bronchoscopy** means **visual examination of the bronchi**, and **bronchoscope** means **instrument used for visual examination of the bronchi** (Fig 5.12).

Endoscopes are also used in endoscopic surgery, where internal organs are reached through natural openings, such as the mouth, or through small incisions. Endoscopic surgery is considered to be **minimally invasive** when compared to the large incisions usually required for traditional surgery. The endoscope allows the surgeon to use the monitor to see inside the body, and to use very small tools at the surgical site.

Diagnostic Terms

The Diagnostic Terms section in this and subsequent chapters presents terms used for tests, labs, and procedures used to diagnose diseases and disorders. Generally, they include laboratory, diagnostic imaging, and endoscopy. In Chapter 5, additional categories have been added to include other diagnostic procedures.

BUILT FROM WORD PARTS

The following terms can be translated using definitions of word parts. Further explanation is provided within parentheses as needed.

ENDOSCOPY			
TERM	**DEFINITION**	**TERM**	**DEFINITION**
1. bronchoscope (BRON-kō-skōp)	instrument used for visual examination of the bronchi (Fig. 5.12)	**2. bronchoscopy** (bron-KOS-ko-pē)	visual examination of the bronchi (Fig. 5.12)

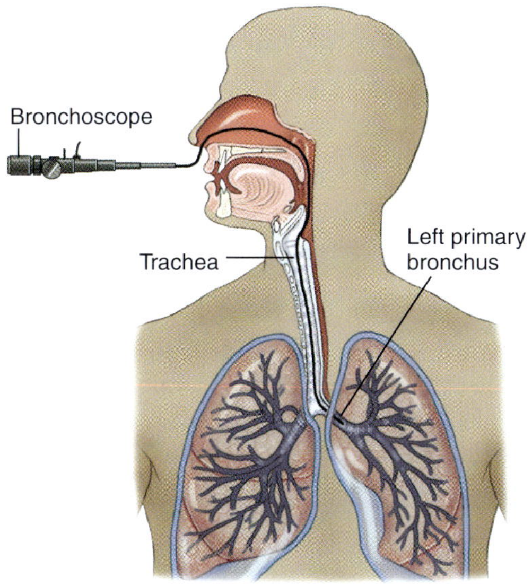

FIG. 5.12 Bronchoscopy. A bronchoscope is inserted through the nostril, pharynx, larynx, and trachea into the bronchus.

TABLE 5.1 Endoscopy Suffixes

Most often the suffixes **-scope**, **-scopy**, and **-scopic** refer to visual examination. An exception is the term **stethoscope**, which is an **instrument used for listening** to body sounds.

Suffix	Names
-scope	the instrument used to view or to examine, such as in the term endoscope; noun
-scopy	visual examination procedure, such as in the term endoscopy; noun
-scopic	means pertaining to visual examination, such as in the term endoscopic; adjective

TERM	DEFINITION
3. **endoscope** (EN-dō-skōp)	instrument used for visual examination within (a hollow organ or body cavity)
4. **endoscopic** (*en*-dō-SKOP-ik)	pertaining to visual examination within (a hollow organ or body cavity)
5. **endoscopy** (en-DOS-ko-pē)	visual examination within (a hollow organ or body cavity)
6. **laryngoscope** (la-RING-go-skōp)	instrument used for visual examination of the larynx
7. **laryngoscopy** (*lar*-in-GOS-ko-pē)	visual examination of the larynx
8. **mediastinoscopy** (*mē*-dē-*a*-sti-NOS-ko-pē)	visual examination of the mediastinum
9. **thoracoscope** (tho-RAK-ō-skōp)	instrument used for visual examination of the chest cavity (see Fig. 5.10)
10. **thoracoscopy** (*thor*-a-KOS-ko-pē)	visual examination of the chest cavity

SLEEP STUDIES

TERM	DEFINITION
11. **polysomnography (PSG)** (*pol*-ē-som-NOG-rah-fē)	process of recording many (tests) during sleep (performed to diagnose obstructive sleep apnea [see Fig. 5.6]). Tests include **electrooculography, electrocardiography, electromyography, electroencephalography, air flow monitoring,** and **oximetry**.

PULMONARY FUNCTION

TERM	DEFINITION
12. **capnometer** (kap-NOM-e-ter)	instrument used to measure carbon dioxide (levels in expired gas)
13. **oximeter** (ok-SIM-e-ter)	instrument used to measure oxygen (saturation in the blood) *(Note: the combining vowel is* i.*)*
14. **spirometer** (spī-ROM-e-ter)	instrument used to measure breathing (or lung volumes)
15. **spirometry** (spī-ROM-e-trē)	a measurement of breathing (or air flow)

EXERCISE 17 ■ Pronounce and Spell

Practice pronunciation and spelling on paper and online.

1. Practice on Paper

a. Pronounce: Read the phonetic spelling and say aloud the terms listed in the previous table. Refer to the pronunciation key on p. 20 as necessary.

b. Spell: Have a study partner read the terms aloud. Write the spelling of the terms on a separate sheet of paper.

2. Practice Online

a. Access online learning resources. Go to evolve.elsevier.com > Evolve Resources > Student Resources.

b. Pronounce: Select Audio Glossary > Chapter 5 > Exercise 17. Select a term to hear its pronunciation and repeat aloud.

c. Spell: Select Activities > Chapter 5 > Spell Terms > Exercise 17. Select the audio icon and type the correct spelling of the term.

❑ Check the box when complete.

EXERCISE 18 ■ Analyze and Define

Analyze and define the following terms by drawing slashes between word parts, writing word part abbreviations above the term, underlining combining forms, and writing combining form abbreviations below the term.

EXAMPLE:

WR CV S
bronch / o / scopy
CF
visual examination of the bronchi

1. spirometer

____

____

2. laryngoscope

____

____

3. capnometer

____

____

4. spirometry

____

____

5. oximeter

____

____

6. laryngoscopy

____

____

7. bronchoscope

____

____

8. thoracoscope

____

____

9. endoscope

____

____

10. thoracoscopy

____

____

11. endoscopic

____

____

12. endoscopy

____

____

13. polysomnography

____

____

14. mediastinoscopy

____

____

EXERCISE 19 ■ Build

A Label

Build terms pictured by writing word parts above definitions.

1.

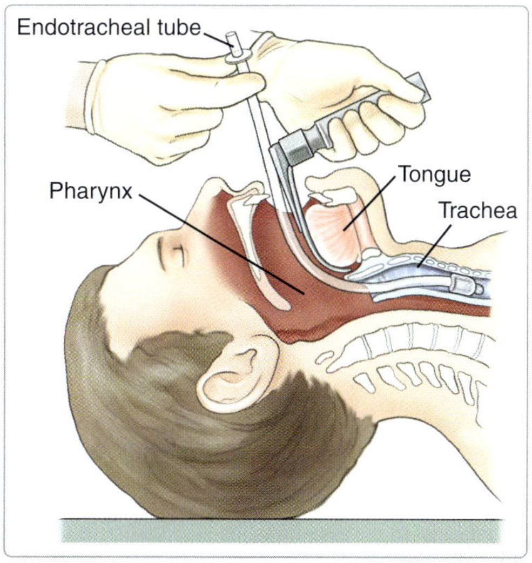

A ___________ /_______ /_______________ is used to guide the endotracheal tube into place.
larynx CV instrument used for visual examination

2.

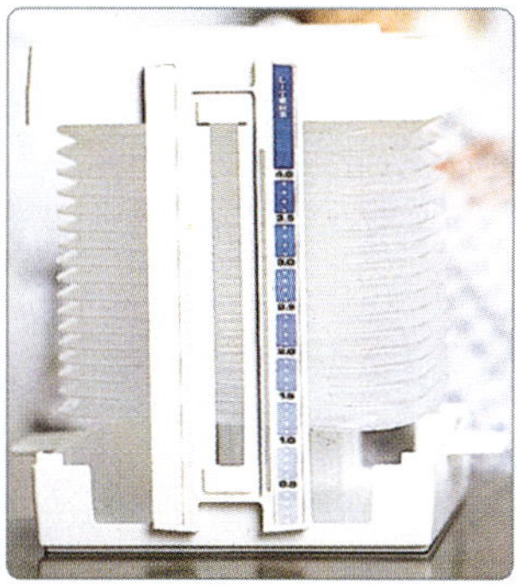

___________ /_______ /_______________
breathing CV instrument used to measure

3.

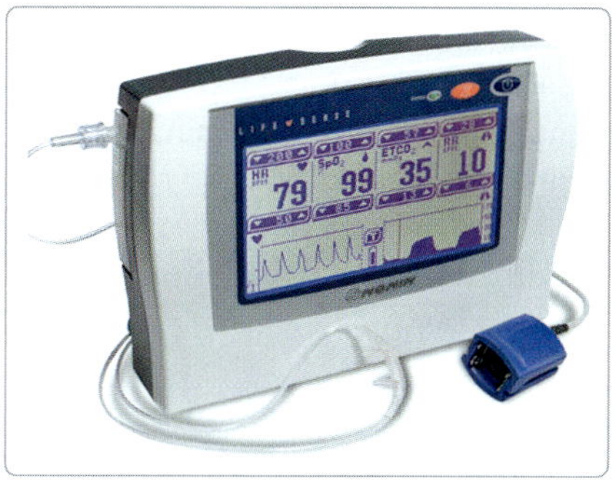

___________ /_______ /_______________
carbon dioxide CV instrument used to measure

4.

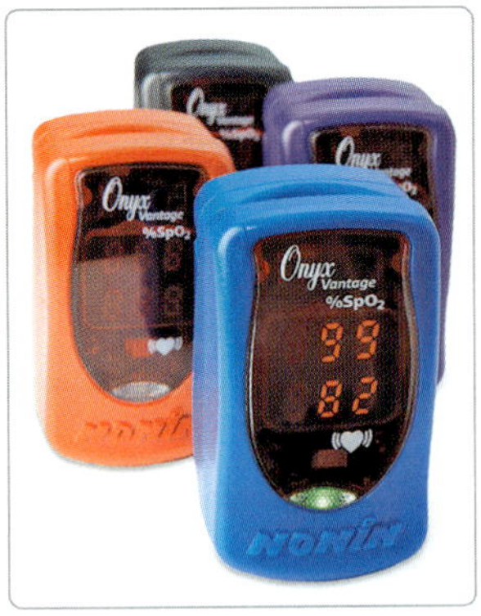

Pulse ________ / ______ / ______________

oxygen | CV | instrument used to measure

5.

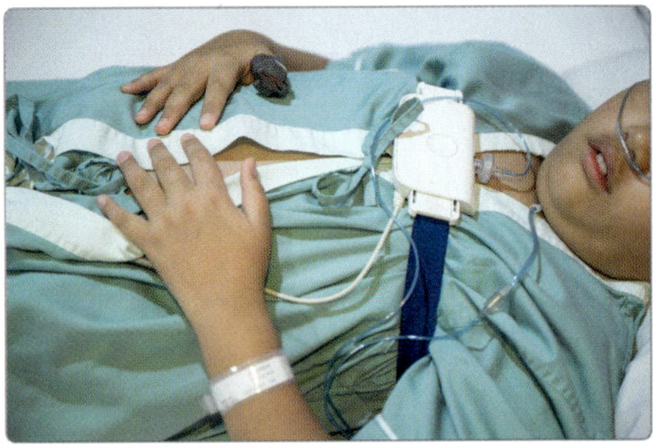

______ / ______ / ______ / ______________

many | sleep (tests) | CV | process of recording

B Fill In

Build diagnostic terms for the following definitions by using the word parts you have learned.

EXAMPLE: instrument used to measure oxygen ox / i / meter (WR / CV / S)

1. visual examination of the larynx ______ / ______ / ______ (WR / CV / S)
2. visual examination of the mediastinum ______ / ______ / ______ (WR / CV / S)
3. pertaining to visual examination within (a hollow organ or body cavity) ______ / ______ (P / S(WR))
4. visual examination of the chest cavity ______ / ______ / ______ (WR / CV / S)
5. visual examination of the bronchi ______ / ______ / ______ (WR / CV / S)
6. measurement of breathing ______ / ______ / ______ (WR / CV / S)
7. instrument used for visual examination of the bronchi ______ / ______ / ______ (WR / CV / S)
8. visual examination within (a hollow organ or body cavity ______ / ______ (P / S(WR))
9. instrument used for visual examination of the chest cavity ______ / ______ / ______ (WR / CV / S)
10. instrument used for visual examination within (a hollow organ or body cavity) ______ / ______ (P / S(WR))

Diagnostic Terms

NOT BUILT FROM WORD PARTS

Word parts may be present in the following terms; however, their full meanings cannot be translated using definitions of word parts alone.

DIAGNOSTIC IMAGING

TERM	DEFINITION
1. chest computed tomography (CT) scan (chest) (kom-PŪ-ted) (tō-MOG-ra-fē) (skan)	computerized radiographic images of the chest performed to diagnose tumors, abscesses, and pleural effusion

COMPUTED TOMOGRAPHY (CT) combines x-rays with computer technology to produce detailed, cross sectional images of the body, called "slices." Oral or intravenous contrast agents may be given to highlight specific regions in the body, resulting in clearer images.

TERM	DEFINITION
2. chest radiograph (CXR) (chest) (RĀ-dē-ō-*graf*)	radiographic image of the chest performed to evaluate the lungs and the heart (also called a **chest x-ray**)
3. lung ventilation/perfusion scan (V/Q scan) (lung) (*ven*-ti-LĀ-shun) (per-FŪ-zhun) (skan)	two nuclear scan tests, one to measure air flow throughout the lungs (ventilation), and one to measure circulation to all areas of the lungs (perfusion). A V/Q scan is used most often to help diagnose or rule out a pulmonary embolism (PE).

LABORATORY

TERM	DEFINITION
4. acid-fast bacilli (AFB) smear (AS-id-fast) (bah-SIL-ī) (smēr)	test performed on sputum to determine the presence of acid-fast bacilli, which cause tuberculosis

ACID-FAST means not easily discolored by acid after staining.

PULMONARY FUNCTION

TERM	DEFINITION
5. arterial blood gas (ABG) (ar-TĒ-rē-al) (blud) (gas)	test performed on arterial blood to determine levels of oxygen (O_2), carbon dioxide (CO_2), and pH (acidity)
6. peak flow meter (PFM) (pēk) (flō) (MĒ-ter)	portable instrument used to measure air flow early in forced exhalation; helps monitor asthma and adjust medication accordingly
7. pulmonary function tests (PFTs) (PUL-mō-*nar*-ē) (FUNK-shun) (tests)	group of tests performed to measure breathing capacity and used to determine external respiratory function; when abnormal, they are useful in distinguishing COPD from asthma. Some tests involve the use of a spirometer.
8. pulse oximetry (puls) (ok-SIM-e-trē)	noninvasive method of measuring oxygen in the blood by using a device that attaches to the fingertip

OTHER

TERM	DEFINITION
9. auscultation (*aws*-kul-TĀ-shun)	the act of listening through a stethoscope for sounds within the body which are abnormal and that suggest abnormalities or disease; used for assessing and diagnosing conditions of the lungs, pleura, heart, arteries, and abdomen
10. percussion (per-KUSH-un)	the act of tapping of a body surface to determine the density of the part beneath by the sound obtained. A dull sound where normally a hollow sound would be elicited indicates displacement of air by fluid or solid waste in a body space or cavity such as in a potential pleural space.

Diagnostic Terms—cont'd

NOT BUILT FROM WORD PARTS

OTHER	
TERM	**DEFINITION**
11. PPD skin test (P-P-D) (skin) (test)	test performed on individuals who may have been exposed to tuberculosis. PPD (purified protein derivative) of the tuberculin bacillus is injected intradermally. Positive tests indicate previous exposure, not necessarily active tuberculosis. (also called **TB skin test**)
12. stethoscope (STETH-ō-skōp)	instrument used to hear internal body sounds; used for performing auscultation and blood pressure measurement

EXERCISE 20 ▪ Pronounce and Spell

Practice pronunciation and spelling on paper and online.

1. Practice on Paper

a. **Pronounce:** Read the phonetic spelling and say aloud the terms listed in the previous table. Refer to the pronunciation key on p. 20 as necessary.
b. **Spell:** Have a study partner read the terms aloud. Write the spelling of the terms on a separate sheet of paper.

2. Practice Online

a. **Access** online learning resources. Go to evolve.elsevier.com > Evolve Resources > Student Resources.
b. **Pronounce:** Select Audio Glossary > Chapter 5 > Exercise 20. Select a term to hear its pronunciation and repeat aloud.
c. **Spell:** Select Activities > Chapter 5 > Spell Terms > Exercise 20. Select the audio icon and type the correct spelling of the term.

❑ Check the box when complete.

EXERCISE 21 ▪ Fill In

A Label

Write the medical terms pictured and defined.

1. ______________________
test performed by intradermal injection on individuals who may have been exposed to tuberculosis

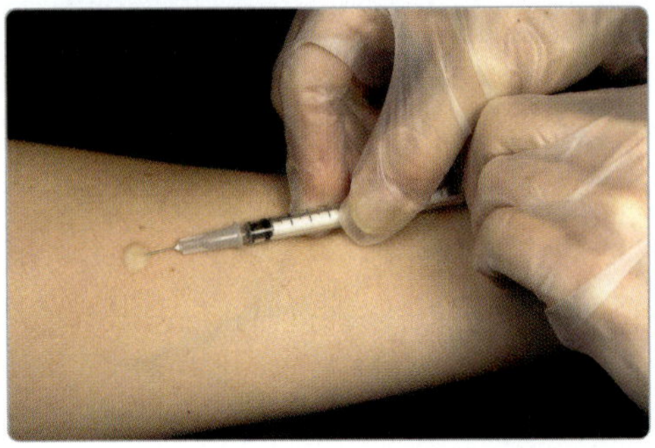

2. ______________________
portable instrument used to measure air flow in forced exhalation; helps monitor asthma and adjust medication accordingly

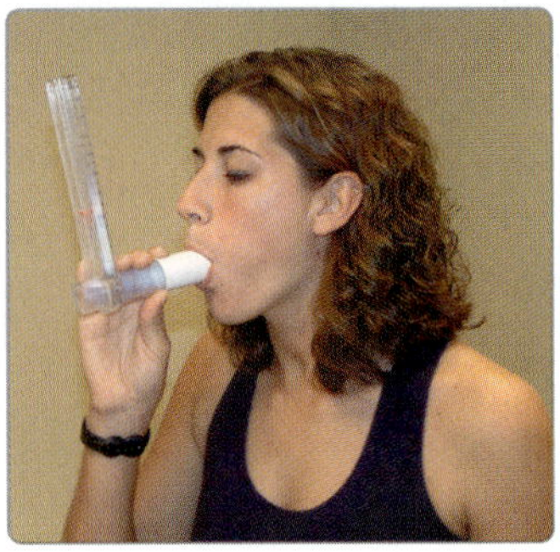

3. ______________________________

test performed on arterial blood to determine levels of oxygen (O_2), carbon dioxide (CO_2), and pH (acidity)

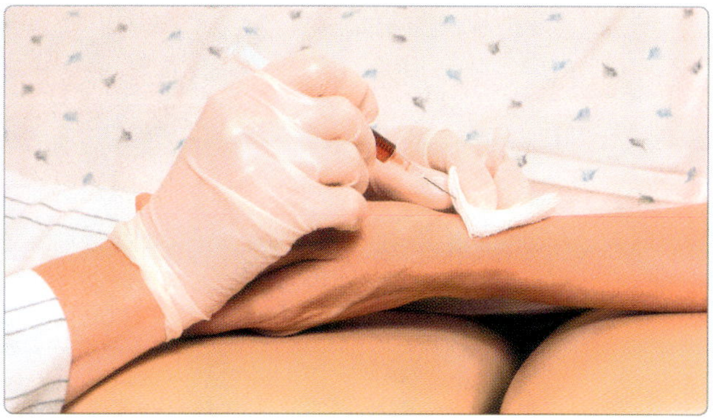

4. ______________________________

noninvasive method of measuring oxygen in the blood by using a device that attaches to the fingertip

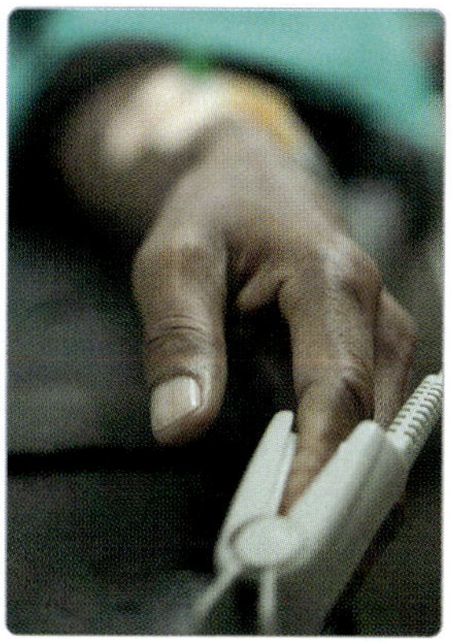

5. ______________________________

instrument used to hear internal body sounds; used for performing auscultation and blood pressure measurement

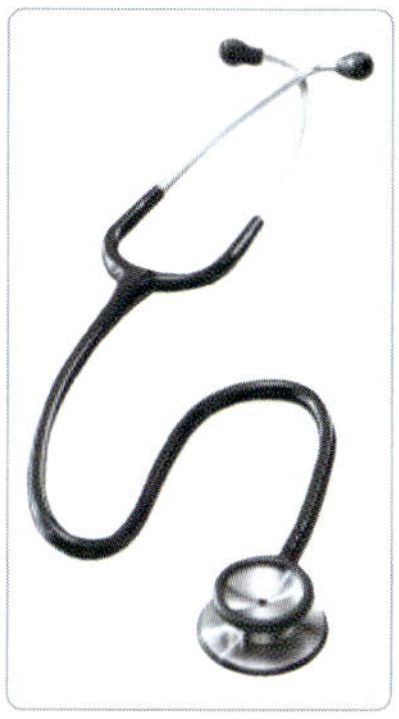

6. ______________________________

____

two nuclear scan tests used to help diagnose or rule out pulmonary embolism

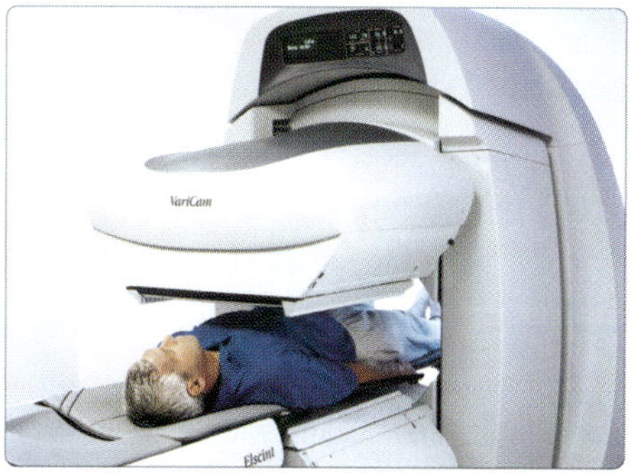

7. ______________________________

radiographic image of the chest performed to evaluate the lungs and the heart

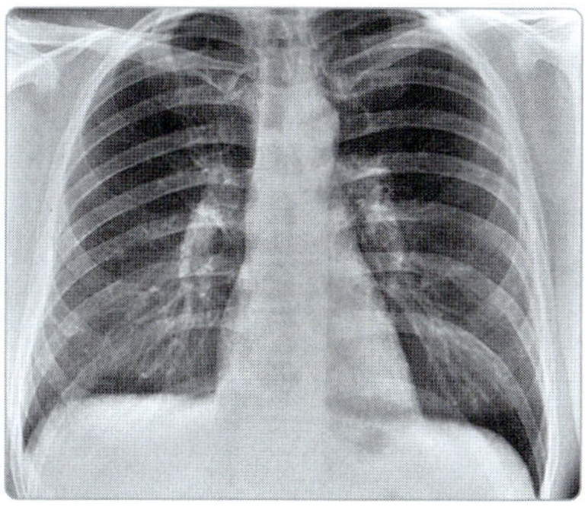

8. ______________________________

____

computerized radiographic images of the chest performed to diagnose tumors, abscesses, and pleural effusions

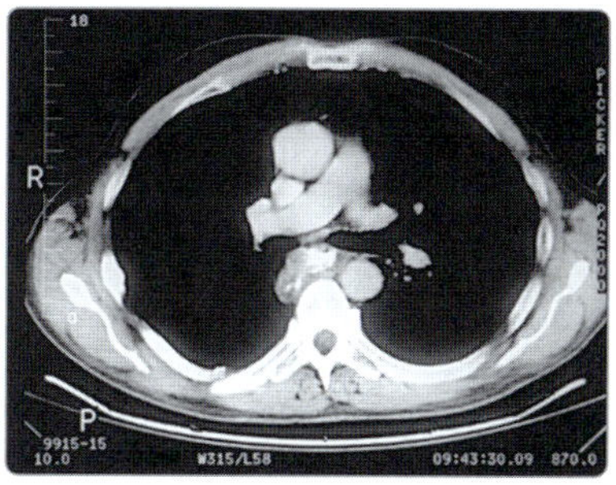

9. ______________________________
the act of listening through a stethoscope for sounds within the body which are abnormal and that suggest abnormalities or disease

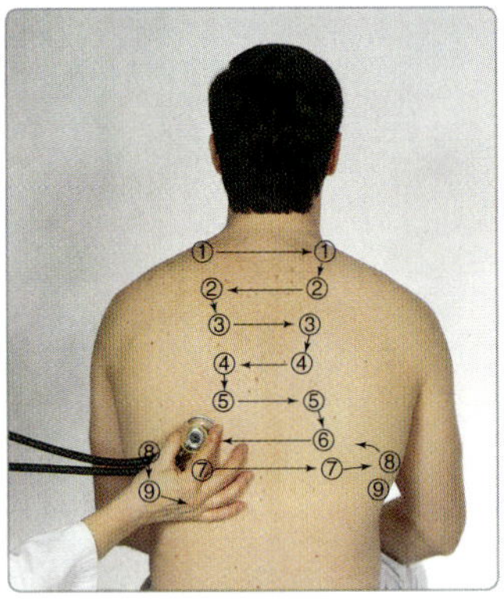

10. ______________________________
the act of tapping of a body surface to determine the density of the part beneath by the sound obtained

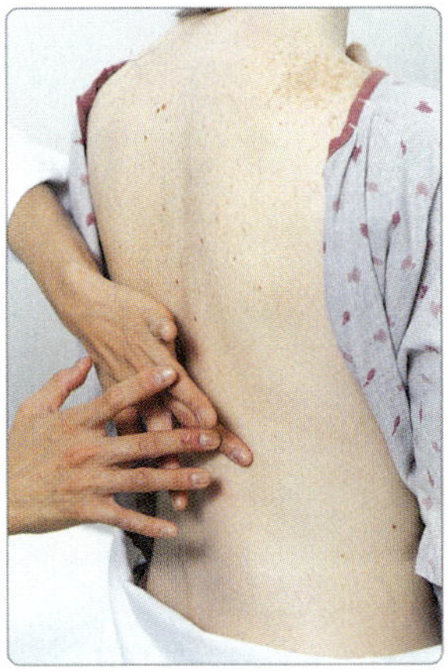

B Identify

Fill in the blanks with the correct terms.

1. A test performed on sputum to diagnose tuberculosis is called ______________________________.
2. ______________________________ is the name of a group of tests performed to measure breathing capacity and to determine external respiratory function or abnormalities.

EXERCISE 22 ■ Match

Match the terms in the first column with their correct definitions in the second column.

_____ 1. lung ventilation/perfusion scan
_____ 2. chest radiograph
_____ 3. chest CT scan
_____ 4. acid-fast bacilli smear
_____ 5. pulse oximetry
_____ 6. arterial blood gas
_____ 7. pulmonary function tests
_____ 8. PPD skin test
_____ 9. auscultation
_____ 10. stethoscope
_____ 11. peak flow meter
_____ 12. percussion

a. computerized images of the chest
b. noninvasive method used to measure oxygen in the blood
c. arterial blood test used to determine levels of oxygen, carbon dioxide, and pH
d. test on sputum for tuberculosis
e. chest x-ray
f. nuclear medicine procedure used to diagnose pulmonary embolism
g. group of tests performed to measure breathing capacity
h. test performed on individuals who may have been exposed to tuberculosis
i. instrument used for auscultation
j. used to help monitor asthma
k. the act of listening for sounds within the body through a stethoscope
l. the act of tapping a body surface to determine density

EXERCISE 23 ■ Review of Diagnostic Terms

Can you define, pronounce, and spell the following terms?

acid-fast bacilli smear (AFB)
arterial blood gas (ABG)
auscultation
bronchoscope
bronchoscopy
capnometer
chest radiograph (CXR)
chest computed tomography (CT) scan
endoscope
endoscopic
endoscopy
laryngoscope
laryngoscopy
lung ventilation/perfusion scan (V/Q scan)
mediastinoscopy
oximeter
peak flow meter (PFM)
percussion
polysomnography (PSG)
PPD skin test
pulmonary function tests (PFTs)
pulse oximetry
spirometer
spirometry
stethoscope
thoracoscope
thoracoscopy

Complementary Terms

BUILT FROM WORD PARTS

The following terms can be translated using definitions of word parts. Further explanation is provided within parentheses as needed.

SIGNS AND SYMPTOMS

TERM	DEFINITION
1. **acapnia** (a-CAP-nē-a)	condition of absence (less than normal level) of carbon dioxide (in the blood)
2. **anoxia** (a-NOK-sē-a)	condition of absence (deficiency) of oxygen

ANOXIA literally means **without oxygen** or **absence of oxygen.** The term actually denotes an oxygen deficiency in the body tissues.

TERM	DEFINITION
3. **aphonia** (ā-FŌ-nē-a)	condition of absence of voice
4. **apnea** (AP-nē-a)	absence of breathing
5. **dysphonia** (dis-FŌ-nē-a)	condition of difficult speaking (voice)
6. **dyspnea** (DISP-nē-a)	difficult breathing
7. **eupnea** (ŪP-nē-a)	normal breathing
8. **hemoptysis** (he-MOP-ti-sis)	coughing of blood (or blood-stained sputum)
9. **hypercapnia** (*hī*-per-KAP-nē-a)	condition of excessive carbon dioxide (in the blood)
10. **hyperpnea** (*hī*-perp-NĒ-a)	excessive breathing
11. **hypocapnia** (*hī*-pō-KAP-nē-a)	condition of deficient carbon dioxide (in the blood)
12. **hypopnea** (hī-POP-nē-a)	deficient breathing
13. **hypoxemia** (*hī*-pok-SĒ-mē-a)	deficient oxygen in the blood
14. **hypoxia** (hī-POK-sē-a)	condition of deficient oxygen (to the tissues)

The "o" from the prefix **hypo-** is dropped in the terms **hypoxemia** and **hypoxia** because the following word part begins with a vowel.

TERM	DEFINITION
15. **orthopnea** (or-THOP-nē-a)	breathing (more easily) in a straight (upright position) (indicates difficulty breathing in the supine position)
16. **rhinorrhea** (*rī*-nō-RĒ-a)	discharge from the nose (as in a cold)
17. **tachypnea** (tak-IP-nē-a)	rapid breathing

MEDICAL SPECIALTIES

TERM	DEFINITION
18. **pulmonologist** (*pul*-mon-OL-o-jist)	physician who studies and treats diseases of the lung
19. **pulmonology** (*pul*-mon-OL-o-jē)	study of the lung (a branch of medicine dealing with diseases of the lung)

Complementary Terms—cont'd

BUILT FROM WORD PARTS

DESCRIPTIVE TERMS

TERM	DEFINITION
20. alveolar (al-VĒ-ō-lar)	pertaining to the alveolus
21. bronchoalveolar (*bron*-kō-al-VĒ-o-lar)	pertaining to the bronchi and alveoli
22. diaphragmatic (*dī*-a-frag-MAT-ik)	pertaining to the diaphragm
23. endotracheal (*en*-dō-TRĀ-kē-al)	pertaining to within the trachea
24. intrapleural (*in*-tra-PLUR-al)	pertaining to within the pleura (space between the two pleural membranes)
25. laryngeal (lar-IN-jē-al)	pertaining to the larynx
26. mediastinal (mē-dē-a-STĪ-nel)	pertaining to the mediastinum
27. mucoid (MŪ-koyd)	resembling mucus
28. mucous (MŪ-kus)	pertaining to mucus

MUCUS is the noun that describes slimy fluid secreted by the membrane lining cavities that lead outside of the body. **Mucous** is the adjective that means pertaining to mucus. Pronunciation is the same for both terms.

TERM	DEFINITION
29. nasopharyngeal (*nā*-zō-fa-RIN-jē-al)	pertaining to the nose and pharynx
30. pulmonary (PUL-mō-*nar*-ē)	pertaining to the lungs
31. septal (SEP-tal)	pertaining to the septum
32. thoracic (thō-RAS-ik)	pertaining to the chest

EXERCISE 24 ■ Pronounce and Spell

Practice pronunciation and spelling on paper and online.

1. Practice on Paper

a. **Pronounce:** Read the phonetic spelling and say aloud the terms listed in the previous table. Refer to the pronunciation key on p. 20 as necessary.
b. **Spell:** Have a study partner read the terms aloud. Write the spelling of the terms on a separate sheet of paper.

2. Practice Online

a. **Access** online learning resources. Go to evolve.elsevier.com > Evolve Resources > Student Resources.
b. **Pronounce:** Select Audio Glossary > Chapter 5 > Exercise 24. Select a term to hear its pronunciation and repeat aloud.
c. **Spell:** Select Activities > Chapter 5 > Spell Terms > Exercise 24. Select the audio icon and type the correct spelling of the term.

❑ Check the box when complete.

EXERCISE 25 ■ Analyze and Define

Analyze and define the following terms by drawing slashes between word parts, writing word part abbreviations above the term, underlining combining forms, and writing combining form abbreviations below the term.

EXAMPLE:
P WR S
hyper / capn / ia
condition of excessive carbon dioxide (in the blood)

1. mediastinal

____

____

2. pulmonology

____

____

3. mucous

____

____

4. apnea

____

____

5. hypoxia

____

____

6. nasopharyngeal

____

____

7. intrapleural

____

____

8. acapnia

____

____

9. dysphonia

____

____

10. hypoxemia

____

____

11. thoracic

____

____

12. diaphragmatic

____

____

13. bronchoalveolar

____

____

14. hypopnea

____

____

EXERCISE 26 ■ Build

A Label

Build terms pictured by writing word parts above definitions.

1.

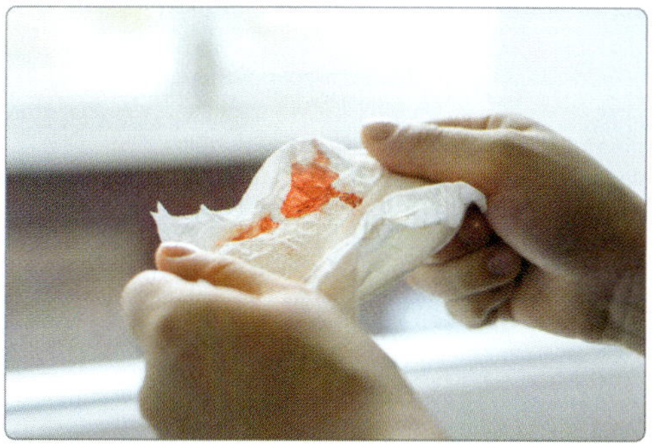

_______ / _______ / _______
blood CV coughing

2.

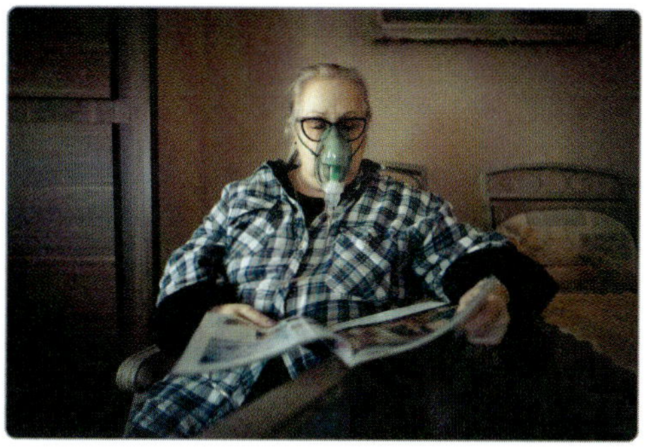

_______ / _______ / _______
straight CV breathing
(able to breathe more easily in an upright position)

3.

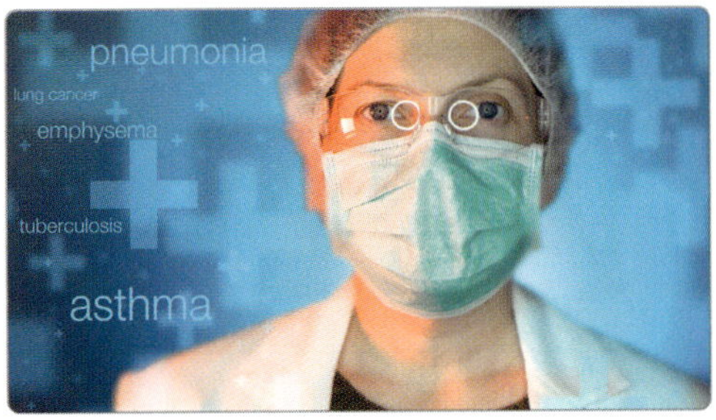

_______ / _______ / _______
lung / CV / physician who studies and treats

4.

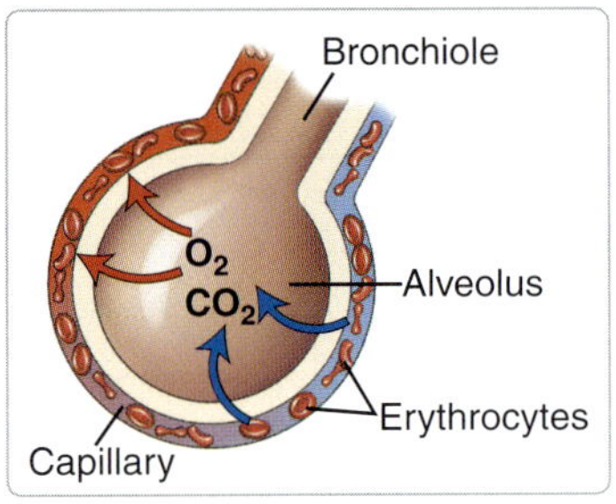

_______ / _______
alveolus / pertaining to

5.

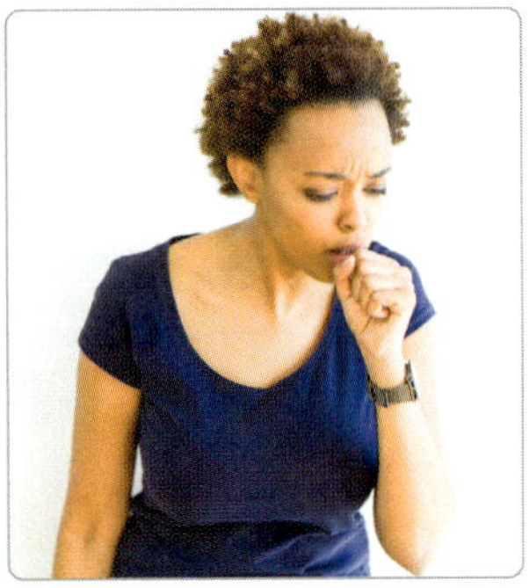

_______ / _______
difficult / breathing

6.

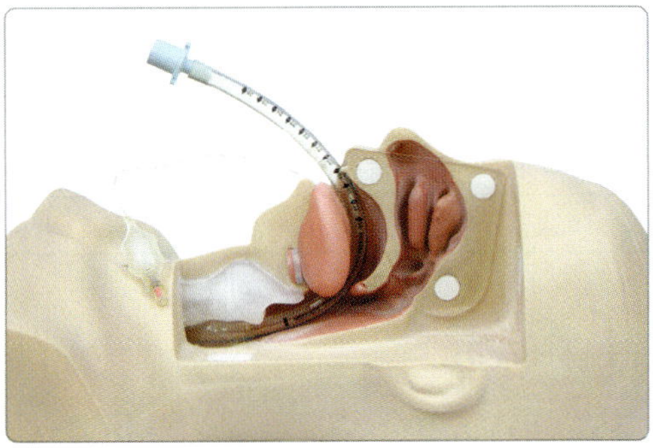

_______ / _______ / _______ tube
within / trachea / pertaining to

B Fill In

Build complementary terms for the following definitions by using the word parts you have learned.

EXAMPLE: pertaining to bronchi and alveoli bronch / o / alveol / ar
WR / CV / WR / S

1. rapid breathing _______ / _______
P / S(WR)

2. resembling mucus _______ / _______
WR / S

3. discharge from the nose _______ / _______ / _______
WR / CV / S

4. condition of excessive carbon dioxide (in the blood) _______ / _______ / _______
P / WR / S

5. condition of absence of oxygen _______ / _______ / _______
P / WR / S

6. excessive breathing _______ / _______
P / S(WR)

7. pertaining to the larynx ______ / ______
WR / S

8. condition of deficient carbon dioxide (in the blood) ______ / ______ / ______
P / WR / S

9. normal breathing ______ / ______
P / S(WR)

10. condition of absence of voice ______ / ______ / ______
P / WR / S

11. pertaining to the lungs ______ / ______
WR / S

12. pertaining to the septum ______ / ______
WR / S

Complementary Terms

NOT BUILT FROM WORD PARTS

Word parts may be present in the following terms; however, their full meanings cannot be translated using definitions of word parts alone.

SIGNS AND SYMPTOMS

TERM	DEFINITION
1. crackles (KRAK-els)	discontinuous sounds heard primarily with a stethoscope during inspiration that resemble the sound of the rustling of cellophane; often heard at the base of the lung posteriorly in heart failure, pneumonia, and pulmonary fibrosis (also called **rales**)
2. effusion (e-FŪ-zhun)	escape of fluid into tissue or body cavity
3. hyperventilation (*hī*-per-*ven*-ti-LĀ-shun)	ventilation of the lungs beyond normal body needs
4. hypoventilation (*hī*-pō-*ven*-ti-LĀ-shun)	ventilation of the lungs that does not fulfill the body's gas exchange needs
5. paroxysm (PAR-ok-siz-em)	periodic, sudden attack
6. rhonchi (RONG-kī)	low-pitched, with a snoring quality, breath sounds heard with a stethoscope suggesting secretions in the large airways
7. stridor (STRĪD-ir)	harsh, high-pitched breath sound heard on inspiration; indicates an acute laryngeal obstruction
8. wheeze (wēz)	whistling noise with a high pitch, caused by air flowing through narrowed airways. Commonly associated with asthma and chronic bronchitis.

TREATMENTS

TERM	DEFINITION
9. bronchoconstrictor (*bron*-kō-kon-STRIK-tor)	agent causing narrowing of the bronchi
10. bronchodilator (*bron*-kō-dī-LĀ-tor)	agent causing the bronchi to widen

Complementary Terms—cont'd

NOT BUILT FROM WORD PARTS

EQUIPMENT	
TERM	**DEFINITION**
11. nebulizer (NEB-ū-lī-zer)	device that creates a mist used to deliver medication for giving respiratory treatment
12. ventilator (VEN-ti-*lā*-tor)	mechanical device used to assist with or substitute for breathing (Fig. 5.13)

DESCRIPTIVE TERMS	
TERM	**DEFINITION**
13. mucopurulent (*mū*-kō-PŪR-ū-lent)	containing both mucus and pus
14. patent (PĀ-tent)	open, the opposite of closed or compromised, thus allowing passage of air, as in patent trachea and bronchi (can be applied to any tubular passageway in the body, as in a patent artery, allowing passage of blood)
15. sputum (SPŪ-tum)	mucus from the lungs, bronchi, and trachea expelled through the mouth

SPUTUM is derived from the Latin **spuere**, meaning **to spit**. In a 1693 dictionary, it is defined as a "secretion thicker than ordinary spittle."

OTHER	
TERM	**DEFINITION**
16. airway (ĀR-wā)	passageway by which air enters and leaves the lungs as well as a mechanical device used to keep the air passageway unobstructed
17. aspirate (AS-per-āt)	to withdraw fluid or suction fluid; also to draw foreign material into the respiratory tract
18. nosocomial infection (nos-ō-KŌ-mē-al) (in-FEK-shun)	an infection acquired during hospitalization

Refer to **Appendix E** for pharmacology terms related to the respiratory system.

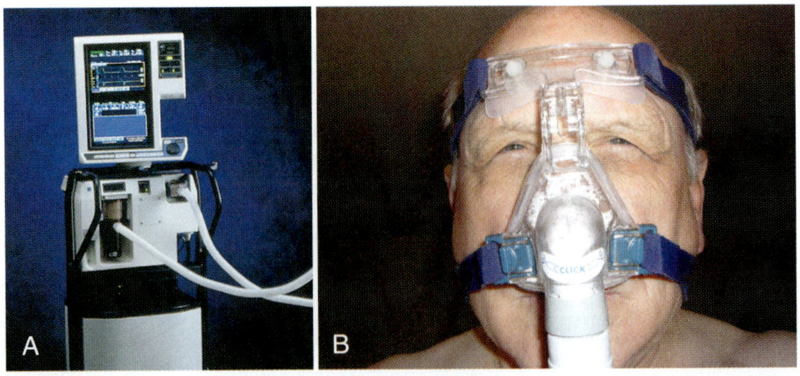

FIG. 5.13 A, Invasive ventilator. Positive pressure ventilator is applied to the patient's airway through an **endotracheal** or **tracheostomy** tube and is used when spontaneous breathing is inadequate to sustain life. **B,** CPAP (continuous positive airway pressure) is a noninvasive ventilation device used for patients who can initiate their own breathing and is often used to treat **obstructive sleep apnea**. BiPAP (bilevel positive airway pressure) not shown, is another noninvasive device that delivers two levels of pressure, one for inspiration, one for expiration whereas the CPAP machine delivers a predetermined level of pressure.

EXERCISE 27 ■ Pronounce and Spell

Practice pronunciation and spelling on paper and online.

1. Practice on Paper

a. **Pronounce:** Read the phonetic spelling and say aloud the terms listed in the previous table. Refer to the pronunciation key on p. 20 as necessary.
b. **Spell:** Have a study partner read the terms aloud. Write the spelling of the terms on a separate sheet of paper.

2. Practice Online

a. **Access** online learning resources. Go to evolve.elsevier.com > Evolve Resources > Student Resources.
b. **Pronounce:** Select Audio Glossary > Chapter 5 > Exercise 27. Select a term to hear its pronunciation and repeat aloud.
c. **Spell:** Select Activities > Chapter 5 > Spell Terms > Exercise 27. Select the audio icon and type the correct spelling of the term.

❑ Check the box when complete.

EXERCISE 28 ■ Fill In

A Label

Write the medical terms pictured and defined.

1. ______________________
passageway by which air enters and leaves the lungs as well as a mechanical device used to keep the air passageway unobstructed

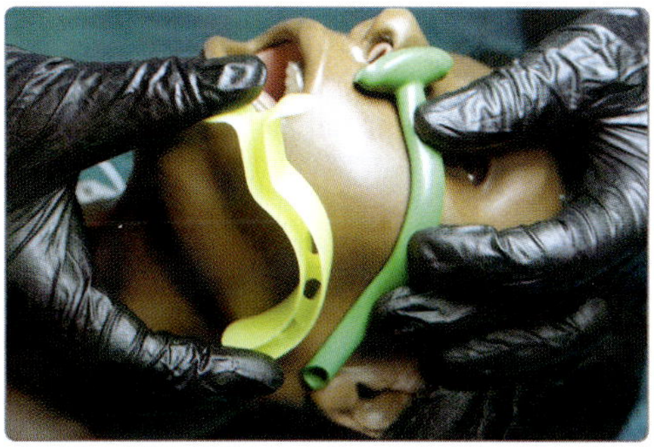

2. ______________________
agent causing the bronchi to widen

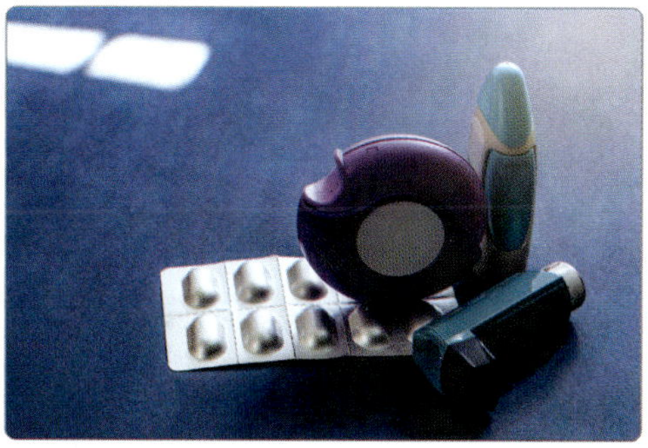

3. ______________________
device that creates a mist used to deliver medication for giving respiratory treatment

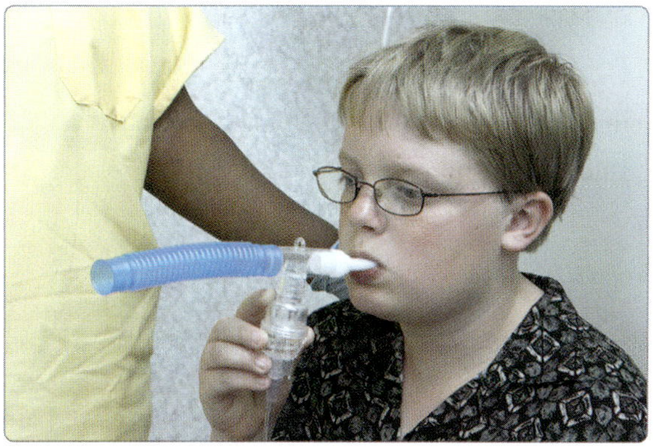

4. ______________________
mechanical device used to assist with or substitute for breathing

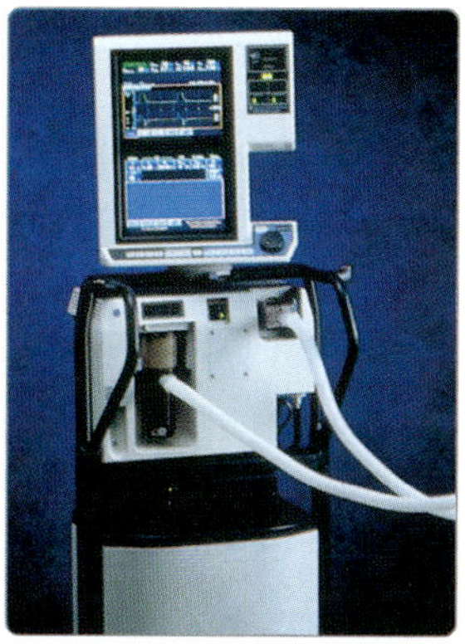

B Identify

Fill in the blanks with the correct terms.

1. Another term for ventilation of the lungs beyond normal body needs is ______________________________.
2. A whistling noise with a high pitch, commonly associated with asthma, is ______________________________.
3. Mucus from the lungs, bronchi, and trachea, expelled through the mouth, is called ______________________________.
4. To suction or withdraw fluid is to ______________________________.
5. Harsh, high pitched, breath sound heard on inspiration is called ______________________________.
6. Low-pitched breath sounds heard with a stethoscope are called ______________________________.
7. Material containing both mucus and pus is referred to as being ______________________________.
8. ______________________________ is the name given to ventilation of the lungs that does not fulfill the body's gas exchange needs.
9. An infection acquired during hospitalization is called ______________________________.
10. The term that applies to a periodic, sudden attack is ______________________________.
11. An airway must be kept ______________ (open) for the patient to breathe.
12. An agent that causes bronchi to narrow is called a(n) ______________________________.
13. ______________ is the name given to the escape of fluid into tissue or a body cavity.
14. Resembling the sound of rustling cellophane, ______________ may be a presenting sign in pneumonia.

EXERCISE 29 ■ Match

Match the terms in the first column with their correct definitions in the second column.

______ 1. airway	a. low pitched sounds that suggest secretions in the large airways
______ 2. aspirate	b. mechanical device used to keep the air passageway unobstructed
______ 3. bronchoconstrictor	c. agent that narrows the bronchi
______ 4. bronchodilator	d. discontinuous sounds heard mainly at the base of the lungs with a stethoscope during inspiration
______ 5. rhonchi	e. escape of fluid into tissue or body cavity
______ 6. crackles	f. ventilation of the lungs beyond normal body needs
______ 7. hyperventilation	g. to draw foreign material into the respiratory tract
______ 8. effusion	h. agent that widens the bronchi
______ 9. stridor	i. indicates acute laryngeal obstruction

EXERCISE 30 ■ Match

Match the terms in the first column with their correct definitions in the second column.

______ 1. hypoventilation	a. open
______ 2. mucopurulent	b. mucus from lungs, bronchi, and trachea, expelled through the mouth
______ 3. wheeze	c. respiratory treatment device that sends a mist
______ 4. nebulizer	d. mechanical breathing device
______ 5. nosocomial infection	e. ventilation of the lungs that does not fulfill the body's gas exchange needs
______ 6. patent	f. periodic, sudden attack
______ 7. sputum	g. containing both mucus and pus
______ 8. ventilator	h. whistling noise with a high pitch, caused by air flowing through narrowed airways
______ 9. paroxysm	i. hospital-acquired infection

EXERCISE 31 ■ Review of Complementary Terms

Can you define, pronounce, and spell the following terms?

acapnia	dyspnea	intrapleural	pulmonologist
airway	effusion	laryngeal	pulmonology
alveolar	endotracheal	mediastinal	rhinorrhea
anoxia	eupnea	mucoid	rhonchi
aphonia	hemoptysis	mucopurulent	septal
apnea	hypercapnia	mucous	sputum
aspirate	hyperpnea	nasopharyngeal	stridor
bronchoalveolar	hyperventilation	nebulizer	tachypnea
bronchoconstrictor	hypocapnia	nosocomial infection	thoracic
bronchodilator	hypopnea	orthopnea	ventilator
crackles	hypoxemia	paroxysm	wheeze
diaphragmatic	hypoxia	patent	
dysphonia	hypoventilation	pulmonary	

Abbreviations

DISEASE AND DISORDERS

ABBREVIATION	TERM	ABBREVIATION	TERM
ARDS	acute respiratory distress syndrome	**IPF**	idiopathic pulmonary fibrosis
CAP	community-acquired pneumonia	**LTB**	laryngotracheobronchitis
CF	cystic fibrosis	**OSA**	obstructive sleep apnea
COPD	chronic obstructive pulmonary disease	**PE**	pulmonary embolism
COVID-19	coronavirus disease	**PE** also abbreviates **physical examination**.	
flu	influenza	**TB**	tuberculosis
HAP	hospital-acquired pneumonia	**URI**	upper respiratory infection

SIGNS AND SYMPTOMS

ABBREVIATION	TERM
SOB	shortness of breath

DIAGNOSTIC

ABBREVIATION	TERM	ABBREVIATION	TERM
ABG	arterial blood gas	**PFTs**	pulmonary function tests
AFB	acid-fast bacilli	**PSG**	polysomnography
CXR	chest radiograph (chest x-ray)	**VBG**	venous blood gas
PFM	peak flow meter	**V/Q scan**	lung ventilation/perfusion scan

TREATMENTS

ABBREVIATION	TERM
CPAP	continuous positive airway pressure

DESCRIPTIVE

ABBREVIATION	TERM	ABBREVIATION	TERM
LLL	left lower lobe	**RLL**	right lower lobe
LUL	left upper lobe	**RML**	right middle lobe
		RUL	right upper lobe

Abbreviations—cont'd

OTHER			
ABBREVIATION	TERM	ABBREVIATION	TERM
CO_2	carbon dioxide	O_2	oxygen

Refer to **Appendix D** for a complete list of abbreviations.

EXERCISE 32 ■ Fill In

Write the terms abbreviated.

1. A variety of tests are used to diagnose **COPD** ________ ________ ________ ________, including:
   - **PFTs** ________ ________ ________,
   - **CXR** ________ ________,
   - **ABG** ________ ________ ________, and
   - **VBG** ________ ________ ________.
2. **SOB** ________ ________ ________ is often a symptom of COPD.
3. A. The lobes of the left lung are:
   - **LUL** ________ ________ ________
   - **LLL** ________ ________ ________

   B. The lobes of the right lung are:
   - **RUL** ________ ________ ________
   - **RML** ________ ________ ________
   - **RLL** ________ ________ ________
4. **AFB** ________-________ ________ smear is used to support the diagnosis of **TB** ________.
5. **PSG** ________ is used to confirm the diagnosis of **OSA** ________ ________ ________, which can be treated with **CPAP** ________ ________ ________ ________.
6. Respiration is the exchange of **O_2** ________ and **CO_2** ________ ________ between the atmosphere and body cells.
7. Measurements obtained from using a **PFM** ________ ________ ________ can be used to adjust medication for persons with asthma.
8. The etiology of **IPF** ________ ________ ________ is unknown.

TABLE 5.2 Other Common Abbreviations Used in Respiratory Care

ABBREVIATION	TERM	ABBREVIATION	TERM
BiPAP	bilevel positive airway pressure	**MDI**	metered-dose inhaler
CPT	chest physiotherapy	**NIPPV**	noninvasive positive-pressure ventilator
DPI	dry powder inhaler	**PEP**	positive expiratory pressure
HME	heat/moisture exchanger	**RT**	respiratory therapist
IPPB	intermittent positive-pressure breathing	**SVN**	small-volume nebulizer
		VAP	ventilator-associated pneumonia

9. The **flu** ______________ and **COVID-19** ______________ ______________ are serious systemic infections caused by viruses. **URIs** ______________ ______________ ______________s are most often caused by viruses, though they can also be caused by bacteria.
10. **HAP** ______________-______________ ______________ is one type of nosocomial infection.
11. A **V/Q scan** __________ ______________/______________ __________ was ordered to rule out **PE** ______________ ______________.
12. **ARDS** __________ __________ ______________ ______________ is a life-threatening lung condition that usually occurs after a serious illness or injury.
13. **CF** ______________ ______________ is a hereditary disorder of the exocrine glands characterized by excess mucus production in the respiratory tract, pancreatic deficiency, and other symptoms.
14. The acute form of **LTB** ______________ is called croup.
15. In **CAP** ______________-______________ ______________ the infection occurs outside of a healthcare setting.

PRACTICAL APPLICATION

EXERCISE 33 ■ Case Study: Translate Between Everyday Language and Medical Language

CASE STUDY: Roberta Pawlaski

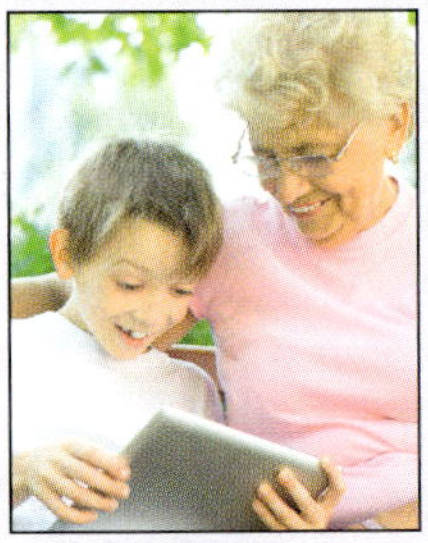

Roberta is experiencing difficulty breathing. She notices it gets worse when she tries to do chores around the house. This has been going on for about 4 days. She also has a cough and a runny nose. Today when she woke up, she noticed that her throat was very sore. She also thinks that she might have a fever because she feels hot all over. She tried taking some over-the-counter cough medicine, but this didn't seem to help. She notices when she coughs that a thick yellow mucus comes out. She hasn't had a cough like this since before she quit smoking about 10 years ago. She remembers that her grandson who stays with her after school has missed school because of a cold. She decides to call her doctor to schedule an appointment.

Now that you have worked through Chapter 5, on the respiratory system, consider the medical terms that might be used to describe Roberta's experience. See the Chapter at a Glance section at the end of the chapter for a list of terms that might apply.

A. *Underline phrases in the case study that could be substituted with medical terms.*

B. *Write the medical term and its definition for three of the phrases you underlined.*

MEDICAL TERM	DEFINITION
1. ____________________	____________________
2. ____________________	____________________
3. ____________________	____________________

DOCUMENTATION: Excerpt from Hospital Admission Report

Roberta was able to see her primary care physician later that afternoon. In her electronic health record (EHR), it was noted in the Objective section of the report:

The patient is in no acute distress but exhibits dyspnea when walking. A fair amount of grey, mucoid, sputum was produced on forced cough. HEENT exam is normal except for erythema and swelling of the pharynx without exudates. Tympanic membranes are clear. There is a moderate amount of purulent rhinorrhea. The nasal mucosa is moderately swollen. Auscultation of the heart reveals a regular rhythm without a murmur, gallop, or rub. The chest is dull to percussion at the right lower base and there are crackles and rhonchi as well.

C. *Underline medical terms presented in Chapter 5 used in the previous excerpt from Roberta's medical record. See the Chapter at a Glance section at the end of the chapter for a complete list.*

D. *Select and define three of the medical terms you underlined. To check your answers, go to Appendix A.*

MEDICAL TERM	DEFINITION
1. ____________________	____________________
2. ____________________	____________________
3. ____________________	____________________

EXERCISE 34 ■ Interact with Medical Documents

A

Read the report and complete it by writing medical terms on answer lines within the document. Definitions of terms to be written appear after the document.

516987-RSP MARQUEZ, Victor

File | Patient | Navigate | Custom Fields | Help

Chart Review | Encounters | Notes | Labs | Imaging | Procedures | Rx | Documents | Referrals | Scheduling | Billing

Name: **MARQUEZ, Victor** | MR#: **516987-RSP** | DOB: **02/01/19XX** | Gender: M | Age: 55 | **Allergies:** None known | **PCP:** Valdez, Miguel MD

Encounter Date: 02/16/20XX

History:

Victor Marquez is a 55-year-old male who came to the Emergency Department on 02/16/XX because of recent onset of 1.__________ ________________. He has also had weight loss and has had a cough for the past 6 months. He denies hemoptysis, chest pain, fever, or night sweats. He has a history of smoking two packs of cigarettes a day for 40 years. He was admitted and scheduled for a 2.______________ consultation.

Physical Examination:

Vital signs: Blood pressure, 148/82 mm Hg. Temperature, 98.2°F. Pulse, 60. Respirations, 18. The chest is clear except for scattered 3.______________________ over the left posterior lung. Ascultation of the heart reveals regular rhythm without murmur. He is in no acute distress. Pulses are full and equal throughout. There is mild clubbing of the fingers.

Diagnostic Imaging:

4.______________ ____________________ reveals a suspicious lesion in the upper left lobe of the lung with diffuse interstitial fibrotic lesions.

Procedure:

Fiberoptic 5.____________________ shows edematous vocal cords with no obvious nodules. At the entry of the left bronchus, a lesion is observed that partially obstructs the opening. A biopsy and brush cytology of the lesion were obtained. 6.______________ _________________ _______________ shows mild 7.______________________________.

Impression:

The patient has 8.__________________ _____________________.

Plan:

1. Obtain 9.______________ ________________ _______________ to include lung volumes and diffusing capacity.
2. Obtain a CT scan of the chest and a 10.________________________ surgery consultation.

Electronically signed: Miguel Valdez MD on 16 February 20XX 14:50

Start | Log On/Off | Print | Edit

Definitions of Medical Terms to Complete the Document

Write the medical terms defined on corresponding answer lines in the document.

1. difficult breathing
2. pertaining to the lungs
3. low pitched with a snoring quality breath sounds heard with a stethoscope
4. radiographic image used to evaluate the lungs and heart
5. visual examination of the bronchi
6. test performed on arterial blood to determine the presence of oxygen, carbon dioxide, and pH.
7. deficient oxygen in the blood
8. cancerous tumor originating in the bronchus
9. group of tests performed on breathing
10. pertaining to the chest

EXERCISE 34 ■ Interact with Medical Documents—cont'd

B

Read the medical report and answer the questions below it.

7463802 FRANK, Abigail

File Patient Navigate Custom Fields Help

Chart Review | Encounters | Notes | Labs | Imaging | Procedures | Rx | Documents | Referrals | Scheduling | Billing

Name: **FRANK, Abigail** MR#: **7463802** DOB: 10/15/19XX Gender: F Age: 47 **Allergies:** Penicillan **PCP:** Irene Buchanan MD

Date: 11/16/20XX
Radiology Report: CT CHEST W/CONTRAST AT 1117 HOURS
Exam: CT OF THE CHEST
History: Cervical cancer
Technique: Multiple contiguous axial images were obtained to the chest during the uneventful infusion of intravenous contrast.

Findings: There has been interval decrease in size of bilateral pulmonary metastases. Again the largest is noted within the left lower lobe and measures 4.8 x 3.9 cm compared to 6.5 x 5.0 cm previously. Multiple smaller lesions within both lungs have decreased in size.

No significant adenopathy is identified. Postsurgical changes centrally within the right lower lobe are again noted with a surgical staple in place. There has been interval development of several patchy probably interstitial opacities within both lungs. Some are located adjacent to metastases that have decreased in size.

No new masses are noted. There is no pericardial or pleural effusion. The osseous structures remain within normal limits.

A left adrenal nodule remains essentially unchanged measuring approximately 2 cm in greatest dimension.

Impression: Interval decrease in size of bilateral pulmonary metastases as described following chemotherapy and radiation therapy. Development of occasional patchy predominately interstitial opacities. Given the history of chemotherapy and radiation therapy this likely reflects a postradiation or post-therapeutic pneumonitis or hyper-sensitivity. Additional considerations are an infectious pneumonitis or hemorrhage. Continued follow-up is recommended. Stable small left adrenal nodule.

Electronically signed: Radiologist Brian Benson DO, 11/16/20XX 14:30

Start | Log On/Off | Print | Edit

Use the medical report above to answer the questions.

_____ 1. The diagnostic imaging exam performed uses
a. computerized radiographic images producing "slices"
b. ionizing radiation produced by a light source
c. mathematically constructed images and magnetic fields
d. radiopharmaceuticals

2. **T F** Fluid is present in the pleural space.

3. **T F** Following chemotherapy and radiation, metastases in one lung were decreased.

4. **T F** The patchy interstitial opacities likely reflect a postradiation or post-therapeutic inflammation of the lung.

EXERCISE 35 ■ Use Medical Language in Online Electronic Health Records

Select the correct medical terms to complete three medical records in one patient's electronic file.

Access online resources at evolve.elsevier.com > Evolve Resources > Student Resources > Activities > Chapter 5 > Electronic Health Records

Topic: COPD
Record 1: Progress Note
Record 2: Radiology Report
Record 3: Pulmonary Function Department Note

❏ Check the box when complete.

Healthcare records are stored and used in an electronic system called **Electronic Health Records (EHR)**. Electronic health records contain a collection of health information of an individual patient; the digitally formatted record can be shared through computer networks with patients, physicians, and other healthcare providers.

EXERCISE 36 ■ Pronounce Medical Terms in Use

Practice pronunciation of terms by reading aloud the following paragraph. Use the phonetic spellings to assist with pronunciation. The script also contains medical terms not presented in the chapter. If interested, research their meanings using a medical dictionary and reliable online sources.

A 24-year-old man visited the emergency department because of **dyspnea** (DISP-nē-a), **hyperpnea** (hī-perp-NĒ-a), and **paroxysms** (PAR-ok-sizms) of cough producing thick, tenacious mucus. He had a history of **asthma** (AZ-ma) since the age of 12 years. A **chest radiograph** (chest) (RĀ-dē-ō-*graf*) was negative for **pneumonia** (nū-MŌ-nē-a). **Arterial blood gas** (ar-TĒ-rē-al) (blud) (gas) showed **hypoxemia** (hī-pok-SĒ-mē-a) but no **hypercapnia** (hī-per-KAP-nē–a). **Pulmonary function tests** (PUL-mō-ner-ē) (FUNK-shun) (tests) disclosed bronchoconstriction, which was corrected by a **bronchodilator** (*bron*-kō–dī-LĀ-tor). A **nebulizer** (NEB-ū-lī-zer) was prescribed for treatment. The asthma attack was probably precipitated by an episode of **bronchitis** (bron-KĪ-tis).

CHAPTER REVIEW

EXERCISE 37 ■ Chapter Content Quiz

Test your understanding of terms and abbreviations introduced in this chapter. Circle the letter for the medical term or abbreviation related to the words in italics

1. The patient was admitted to the emergency department with a *severe nosebleed.*
   a. rhinomycosis
   b. epistaxis
   c. nasopharyngitis
2. The accident caused damage to the *larynx*, necessitating a *surgical repair.*
   a. laryngectomy
   b. laryngostomy
   c. laryngoplasty
3. Mr. Garcia was *breathing more easily in a straight, upright position*, so the nurse recorded that he had:
   a. orthopnea
   b. eupnea
   c. dyspnea
4. The *test on arterial blood to determine oxygen, carbon dioxide, and pH levels* indicated that the patient was *deficient in oxygen*, or had:
   a. pulse oximetry, dysphonia
   b. pulmonary functions tests, hypocapnia
   c. arterial blood gas, hypoxia
5. The physician informed the patient that her *coughing of blood* might be due to tuberculosis.
   a. hemoptysis
   b. pneumothorax
   c. thoracentesis
6. The patient reported dizziness brought on by *ventilation of the lungs beyond normal bodily needs.*
   a. hyperventilation
   b. hypoventilation
   c. dysphonia
7. The physician ordered a *device that delivers mist* treatment for her patient with severe asthma symptoms.
   a. airway
   b. nebulizer
   c. ventilator
8. The patient with *blood in the chest cavity* was diagnosed as having:
   a. pneumothorax
   b. pleuritis
   c. hemothorax
9. After surgery, the patient had *foreign matter causing* a *block in the circulation to the pulmonary artery.*
   a. pleural effusion
   b. pulmonary edema
   c. pulmonary embolism
10. The patient was diagnosed as having *a fungal disease affecting the lung.*
    a. obstructive sleep apnea
    b. coccidioidomycosis
    c. tuberculosis
11. The physician ordered a *radiographic image of the chest* because he suspected *community-acquired pneumonia.*
    a. chest radiograph, CAP
    b. chest CT scan, CPAP
    c. bronchoscopy, HAP
12. The patient received an *intradermal injection* to determine if she had been exposed to TB.
    a. AFB
    b. ABG
    c. PPD skin test
13. The patient was experiencing *rapid breathing.*
    a. hypopnea
    b. tachypnea
    c. eupnea
14. The nurse practitioner heard *discontinuous sounds during respiration that resembled the sound of the rustling of cellophane.*
    a. stridor
    b. rhonchi
    c. crackles
15. *Fusion of the pleura* was performed for the patient with *chronic fluid in the pleural cavity caused by a disease process or trauma* due to untreatable bronchogenic carcinoma.
    a. pneumonectomy, pulmonary edema
    b. pleurodesis, pleural effusion
    c. bronchoplasty, pneumothorax
16. *Serious bacterial infection affecting the mucous membranes of the nose and throat* is less common in developed countries where vaccines are readily available.
    a. idiopathic pulmonary fibrosis
    b. croup
    c. diphtheria

17. Patients with asthma or chronic bronchitis may experience *whistling noise with a high pitch, caused by air flowing through narrowed airways.*
    a. wheeze
    b. rhonchi
    c. crackles

18. A chest CT scan was ordered for the patient with *chronic progressive lung disorder characterized by increasing scarring, which ultimately reduces the capacity of the lungs.*
    a. PE
    b. ARDS
    c. IPF

19. *Escape of fluid into tissue or body cavity* may occur in a variety of locations including around the lungs (pleural), the heart (pericardial), or the joints.
    a. paroxysm
    b. stridor
    c. effusion

20. *Visual examination of the mediastinum* may be performed in patients with lung cancer to biopsy the lymph nodes and assist with staging of the malignancy.
    a. mediastinoscopy
    b. bronchoscopy
    c. thoracoscopy

CHAPTER AT A GLANCE Word Parts New to this Chapter

COMBINING FORMS

adenoid/o
alveol/o
atel/o
bronch/o
bronchi/o
capn/o
coni/o
diaphragmat/o
epiglott/o
hem/o
laryng/o
lob/o
mediastin/o
muc/o
nas/o
orth/o
ox/i
pharyng/o
phon/o
pleur/o
pneum/o
pneumon/o
pulmon/o
py/o
rhin/o
sept/o
sinus/o
somn/o
spir/o
thorac/o
tonsill/o
trache/o

PREFIXES

a-
an-
endo-
eu-
poly-
tachy-

SUFFIXES

-ar
-ary
-cele
-centesis
-desis
-eal
-ectasis
-ectomy
-emia
-meter
-metry
-pnea
-ptysis
-rrhagia
-scope
-scopic
-scopy
-spasm
-stenosis
-stomy
-thorax
-tomy

CHAPTER AT A GLANCE Respiratory System Terms Built from Word Parts

DISEASE AND DISORDER

adenoiditis
alveolitis
atelectasis
bronchiectasis
bronchitis
bronchogenic carcinoma
bronchopneumonia
bronchospasm
diaphragmatocele
epiglottitis
hemothorax
laryngitis
laryngospasm
laryngotracheobronchitis (LTB)
lobar pneumonia
nasopharyngitis
pharyngitis
pleuritis
pneumoconiosis
pneumonia
pneumonitis
pneumothorax
pulmonary neoplasm
pyothorax
rhinitis
rhinomycosis
rhinorrhagia
sinusitis
tonsillitis
tracheitis
tracheostenosis

SURGICAL

adenoidectomy
bronchoplasty
laryngectomy
laryngoplasty
laryngostomy
laryngotracheotomy
lobectomy
pleurodesis
pneumonectomy
rhinoplasty
septoplasty
sinusotomy
thoracentesis
thoracotomy
tonsillectomy
tracheoplasty
tracheostomy
tracheotomy

DIAGNOSTIC

bronchoscope
bronchoscopy
capnometer
endoscope
endoscopic
endoscopy
laryngoscope
laryngoscopy
mediastinoscopy
oximeter
polysomnography (PSG)
spirometer
spirometry
thoracoscope
thoracoscopy

CHAPTER AT A GLANCE Respiratory System Terms Built from Word Parts—cont'd

COMPLEMENTARY

acapnia
alveolar
anoxia
aphonia
apnea
bronchoalveolar
diaphragmatic
dysphonia
dyspnea
endotracheal
eupnea
hemoptysis
hypercapnia
hyperpnea
hypocapnia
hypopnea
hypoxemia
hypoxia
intrapleural
laryngeal
mediastinal
mucoid
mucous
nasopharyngeal
orthopnea
pulmonary
pulmonologist
pulmonology
rhinorrhea
septal
tachypnea
thoracic

CHAPTER AT A GLANCE Respiratory System Terms *NOT* Built from Word Parts

DISEASE AND DISORDER

acute respiratory distress syndrome (ARDS)
asphyxia
asthma
chronic obstructive pulmonary disease (COPD)
coccidioidomycosis
coronavirus disease (COVID-19)
croup
cystic fibrosis (CF)
deviated septum
diphtheria
emphysema
epistaxis
idiopathic pulmonary fibrosis (IPF)
influenza (flu)
obstructive sleep apnea (OSA)
pertussis
pleural effusion
pulmonary edema
pulmonary embolism (PE)
tuberculosis (TB)
upper respiratory infection (URI)

DIAGNOSTIC

acid-fast bacilli (AFB) smear
arterial blood gas (ABG)
auscultation
chest computed tomography (CT) scan
chest radiograph (CXR)
lung ventilation/perfusion scan (V/Q scan)
peak flow meter (PFM)
percussion
PPD skin test
pulmonary function tests (PFTs)
pulse oximetry
stethoscope

COMPLEMENTARY

airway
aspirate
bronchoconstrictor
bronchodilator
crackles
effusion
hyperventilation
hypoventilation
mucopurulent
nebulizer
nosocomial infection
paroxysm
patent
rhonchi
sputum
stridor
ventilator
wheeze

Chapter 6

Urinary System

Outline

Objectives

Upon completion of this chapter, you will be able to:

1 Pronounce organs and anatomic structures of the urinary system.

2 Define and spell word parts related to the urinary system.

3 Define, pronounce, and spell disease and disorder terms related to the urinary system.

4 Define, pronounce, and spell surgical terms related to the urinary system.

5 Define, pronounce, and spell diagnostic terms related to the urinary system.

6 Define, pronounce, and spell complementary terms related to the urinary system.

7 Interpret the meaning of abbreviations related to the urinary system.

8 Apply medical language in clinical contexts.

ANATOMY

Organs of the urinary system are the kidneys, ureters, bladder, and urethra (Figs. 6.1, 6.2, and 6.3).

Function

The urinary system removes waste material from the body, regulates fluid volume, maintains electrolyte concentration in the body fluid, and assists in blood pressure regulation. The kidneys secrete urine formed from water and waste materials such as urea, potassium chloride, sodium chloride, phosphates, and other elements. Urea is the primary compound in human urine. The liver breaks down proteins in the blood to produce ammonia. Because ammonia is toxic, it is combined with other elements to form urea, which is transported in the bloodstream to the kidneys. The kidneys filter the blood and extract urea to form urine. Urine is collected in the renal pelvis of the kidney and is transported through the ureters into the bladder, where it is stored until it can be eliminated. Urine passes from the bladder through the urethra and urinary meatus to the outside of the body (Fig. 6.4).

Organs and Anatomic Structures of the Urinary System

TERM	DEFINITION
kidney (KID-nē)	one of two bean-shaped organs located on each side of the vertebral column on the posterior wall of the abdominal cavity covered anteriorly by the parietal peritoneum. Their function is to remove waste products from the blood and to aid in maintaining water and electrolyte balances.
nephron (NEF-ron)	urine-producing microscopic structure. Approximately 1 million nephrons are located in each kidney.
glomerulus (*pl.* glomeruli) (glō-MER-ū-lus) (glō-MER-ū-lī)	cluster of capillaries at the entrance of the nephron. The process of filtering the blood, thereby forming urine, begins here.
GLOMERULUS is derived from the Latin **glomus,** which means **ball of thread.** It was thought that the rounded cluster of capillary loops at the nephron's entrance resembled thread in a ball.	
renal pelvis (RĒ-nal) (PEL-vis)	funnel-shaped reservoir in the kidney that collects the urine and passes it to the ureter
hilum (HĪ-lum)	indentation on the medial side of the kidney where the renal artery, vein, and pelvis are located and the ureter leaves the kidney
ureters (Ū-re-ters)	two slender tubes, approximately 10 to 13 inches (26 to 33 cm) long, that receive the urine from the kidneys and carry it to the posterior portion of the bladder
urinary bladder (Ū-ri-nar-ē) (BLAD-er)	muscular, hollow organ that temporarily holds the urine. As it fills, the thick, muscular wall becomes thinner, and the organ increases in size.
BLADDER is a derivative of the Anglo-Saxon **blaeddre,** meaning a **blister** or **windbag.**	
urethra (ū-RĒ-thra)	lowest part of the urinary tract, through which the urine passes from the urinary bladder to the outside of the body. This narrow tube varies in length by sex. It is approximately 1.5 inches (3.8 cm) long in the female and approximately 8 inches (20 cm) in the male, in whom it is also part of the reproductive system. It carries seminal fluid (semen) at the time of ejaculation.
urinary meatus (Ū-ri-nar-ē) (mē-Ā-tus)	opening through which the urine passes to the outside
MEATUS is derived from the Latin **meare,** meaning **to pass** or **to go.** Other anatomic passages share the same name, such as the auditory meatus.	

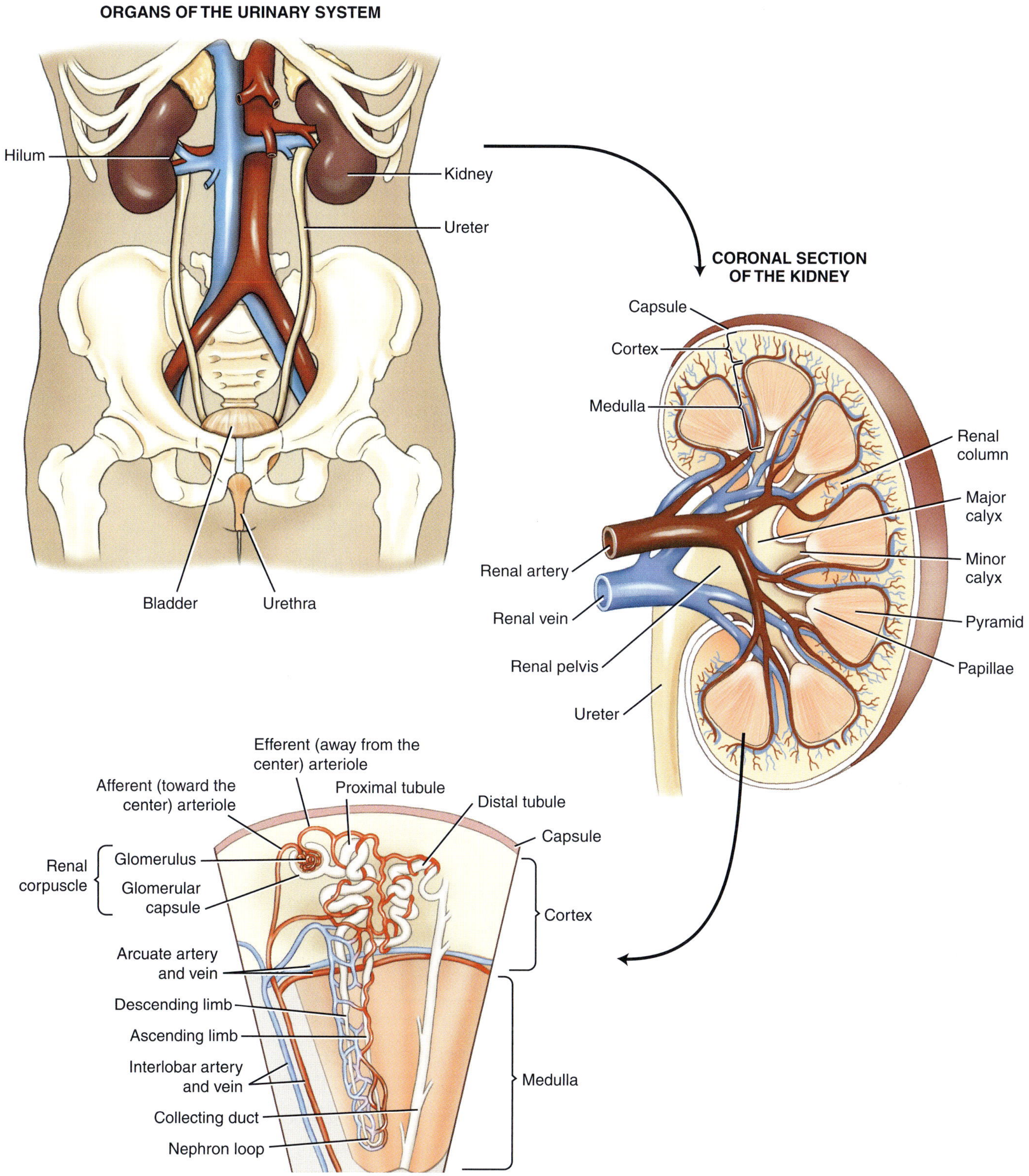

FIG. 6.1 The urinary system.

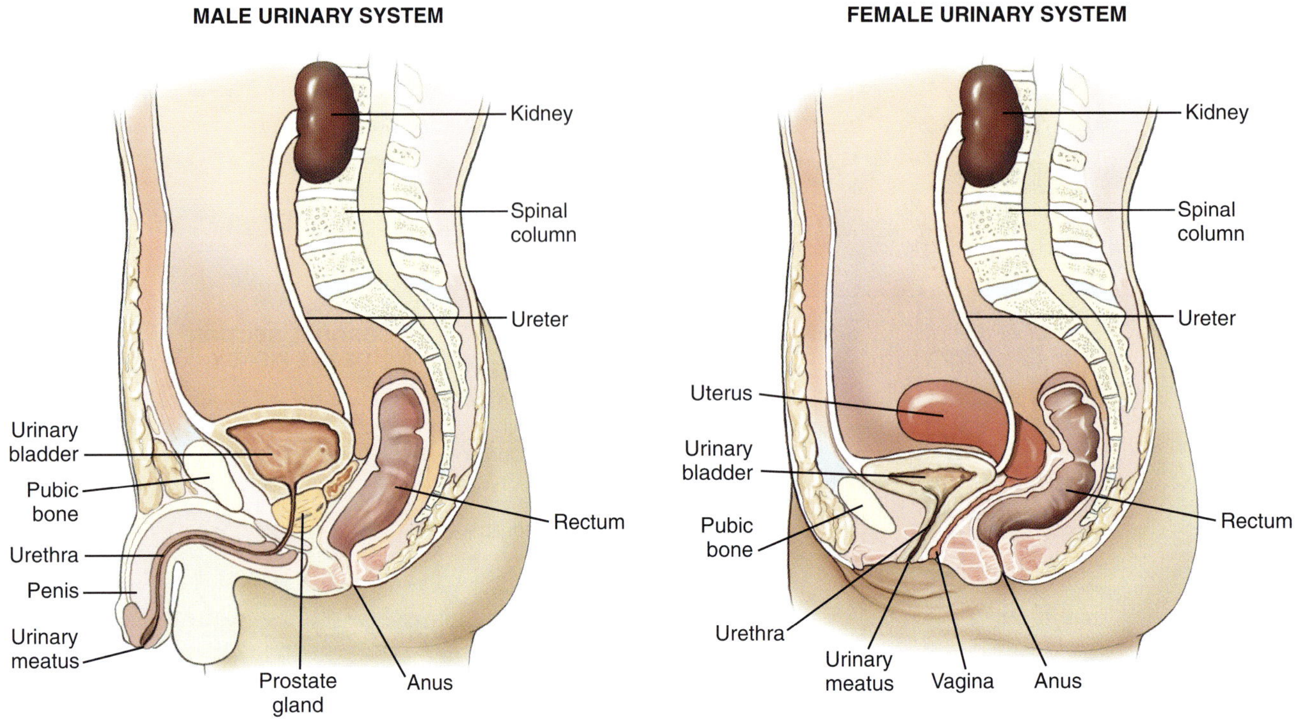

FIG. 6.2 Male and female urinary systems, sagittal view. The male urethra is approximately 8 inches (20 cm) in length compared with the female urethra, which is approximately 1.5 inches (3.8 cm) in length.

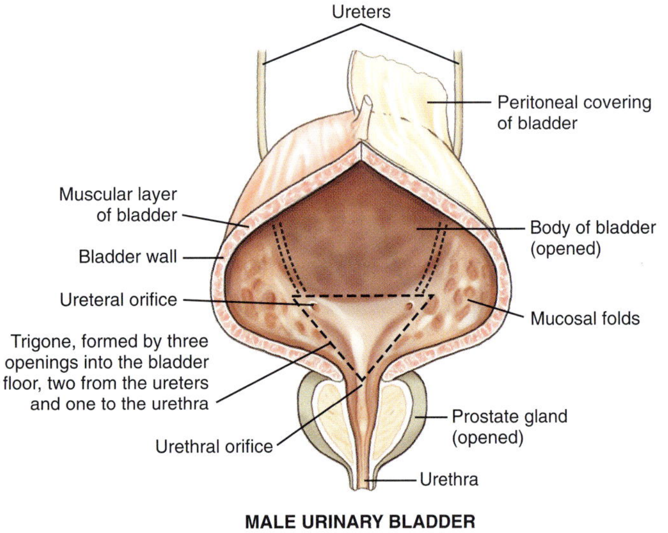

FIG. 6.3 Male urinary bladder.

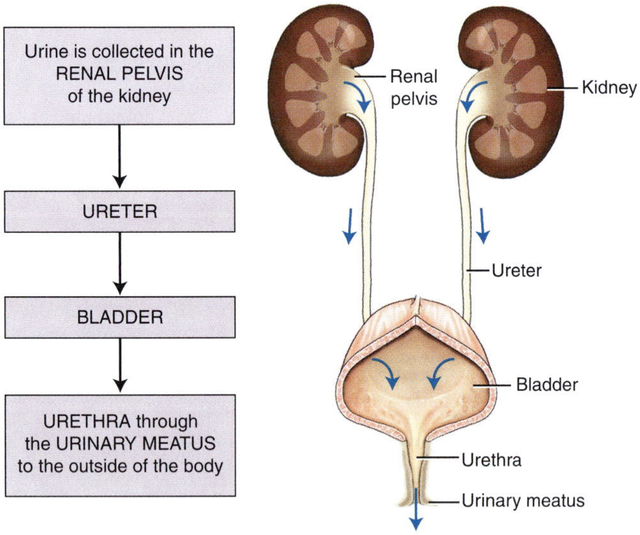

FIG. 6.4 Flow of urine.

PRONOUNCE ANATOMIC STRUCTURES

Practice saying aloud each of the organs and specific structures on the previous pages.

To hear the terms, go to Evolve Resources at www.evolve.elsevier.com and select:
Student Resources > Audio Glossary > Chapter 6 > **Anatomic Structures**

❑ Check the box when complete.

WORD PARTS

Use paper flashcards or electronic flashcards on Evolve to assist with memorization of word parts used to analyze, define, and build terms presented in this chapter. To reinforce learning, study one section of the Word Parts Table at a time, then complete the corresponding exercise on the following pages.

1 ■ Urinary System Combining Forms

COMBINING FORM	DEFINITION
cyst/o	bladder, sac (*Note:* refers to the urinary bladder unless otherwise identified.)
glomerul/o	glomerulus
meat/o	meatus (opening)
nephr/o	kidney
pyel/o	renal pelvis
ren/o	kidney
ureter/o	ureter
urethr/o	urethra
vesic/o	bladder, sac (*Note:* refers to the urinary bladder unless otherwise identified.)

PYELOS is the Greek word for **tub-shaped vessel,** which describes the renal pelvis shape.

2 ■ Combining Forms Used with Urinary System Terms

COMBINING FORM	DEFINITION
albumin/o	albumin
azot/o	urea, nitrogen
blast/o	developing cell, germ cell
glycos/o	sugar
hem/o	blood
hydr/o	water
lith/o	stone(s), calculus (*pl.* calculi)
noct/i	night *(Note: the combining vowel is i.)*
olig/o	scanty, few
son/o	sound
ur/o	urine, urinary tract
urin/o	urine, urinary tract

3 ■ Prefixes

PREFIX	DEFINITION
a-	absence of, without
dys-	painful, abnormal, difficult, labored
poly-	many, much
trans-	through, across, beyond

4 ■ Suffixes

SUFFIX	DEFINITION
-al	pertaining to
-ary	pertaining to
-cele	hernia, protrusion
-ectomy	excision, surgical removal
-emia	in the blood
-gram	the record, radiographic image
-graphy	process of recording, radiographic imaging
-ia	diseased or abnormal state, condition of
-iasis	condition
-itis	inflammation
-lith	stone(s), calculus (*pl.* calculi)
-logist	one who studies and treats (specialist, physician)
-logy	study of

4 ■ Suffixes—cont'd

SUFFIX	DEFINITION	SUFFIX	DEFINITION
-lysis	loosening, dissolution, separating	**-scope**	instrument used for visual examination
-megaly	enlargement	**-scopy**	visual examination
-oma	tumor, swelling	**-stenosis**	constriction or narrowing
-osis	abnormal condition	**-stomy**	creation of an artificial opening
-pexy	surgical fixation	**-tomy**	cut into, incision
-plasty	surgical repair	**-tripsy**	surgical crushing
-ptosis	drooping, sagging, prolapse	**-uria**	urine, urination

Refer to **Appendix B** and **Appendix C** for alphabetized lists of word parts and their meanings.

EXERCISE 1 ■ Urinary System Combining Forms

Refer to the first section of the word parts table.

A Label

Fill in the blanks with combining forms for this diagram of the urinary system. *To check your answers, go to Appendix A.*

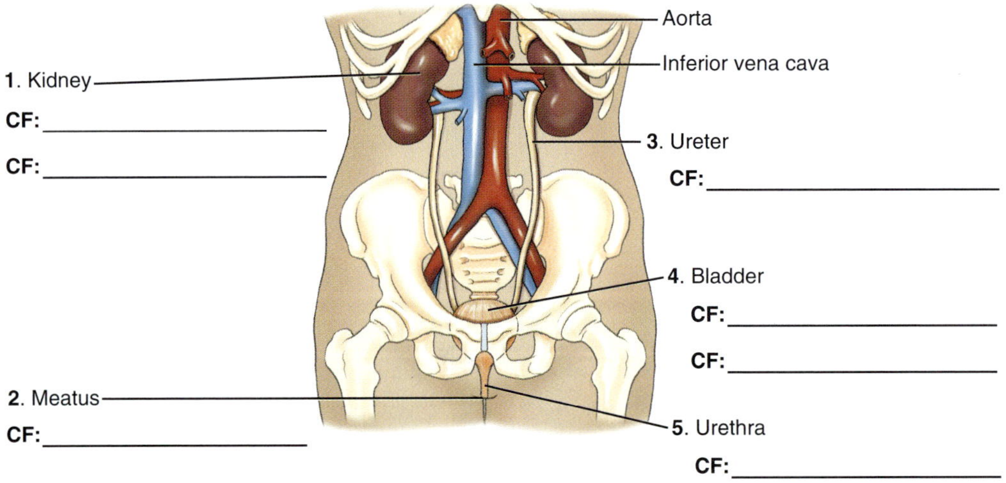

B Define and Match

Step 1: Write the definitions after the following combining forms.
Step 2: Match the descriptions on the right with the combining forms and definitions. Answers may be used more than once.

_____ 1. ren/o, ______________________
_____ 2. vesic/o, ______________________
_____ 3. nephr/o, ______________________
_____ 4. glomerul/o, ______________________
_____ 5. pyel/o, ______________________
_____ 6. ureter/o, ______________________
_____ 7. cyst/o, ______________________
_____ 8. meat/o, ______________________
_____ 9. urethr/o, ______________________

a. stores urine
b. outside opening through which the urine passes
c. carries urine from the kidney to the urinary bladder
d. cluster of capillaries in the kidney where the urine begins to form
e. carries urine from the bladder to the urinary meatus
f. reservoir within the kidney that collects the urine
g. organ that removes waste products from the blood

C Label

Fill in the blanks with combining forms to label these diagrams of the internal kidney structure.

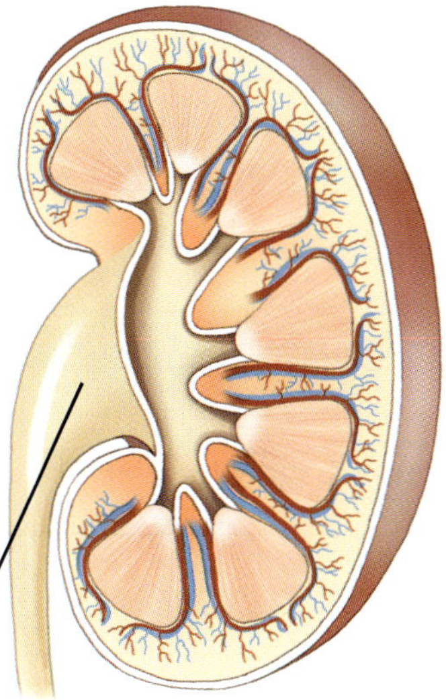

1. Renal pelvis
CF: ______________________

2. Glomerulus
CF: ______________________

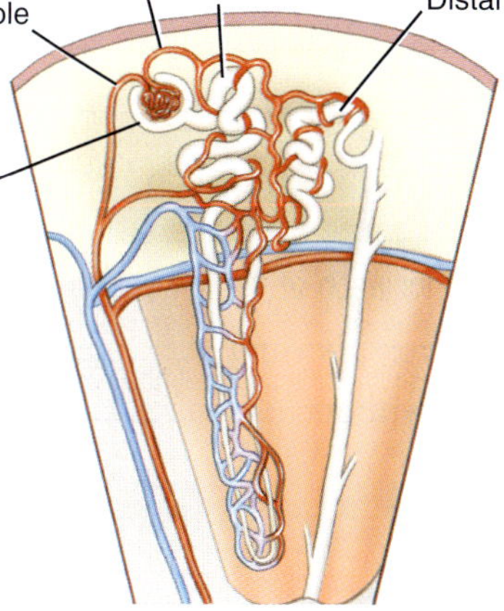

EXERCISE 2 ■ Combining Forms Used with Urinary System Terms

Refer to the second section of the word parts table.

A Define

Write the definitions of the following combining forms.

1. hydr/o ______________________
2. azot/o ______________________
3. noct/i ______________________
4. lith/o ______________________
5. albumin/o ______________________
6. urin/o ______________________
7. blast/o ______________________
8. olig/o ______________________
9. ur/o ______________________
10. glycos/o ______________________
11. son/o ______________________
12. hem/o ______________________

B Identify

Write the combining form for each of the following.

1. sugar ______________________
2. urine, urinary tract a. ______________________
   b. ______________________
3. water ______________________
4. developing cell, germ cell ______________________
5. albumin ______________________
6. night ______________________
7. urea, nitrogen ______________________
8. stone(s), calculus (*pl.* calculi) ______________________
9. scanty, few ______________________
10. blood ______________________
11. sound ______________________

EXERCISE 3 ■ Prefixes

Refer to the third section of the word parts table.

A Define

Write the definitions of the following prefixes.

1. dys- ____________________
2. trans- ____________________
3. a- ____________________
4. poly- ____________________

B Identify

Write the prefix for each of the following.

1. through, across, beyond ____________________
2. absence of, without ____________________
3. painful, abnormal, difficult, labored ____________________
4. many, much ____________________

EXERCISE 4 ■ Suffixes

Refer to the fourth section of the word parts table.

A Label

Write the suffixes pictured and defined.

1. ____________________
loosening, dissolution, separating

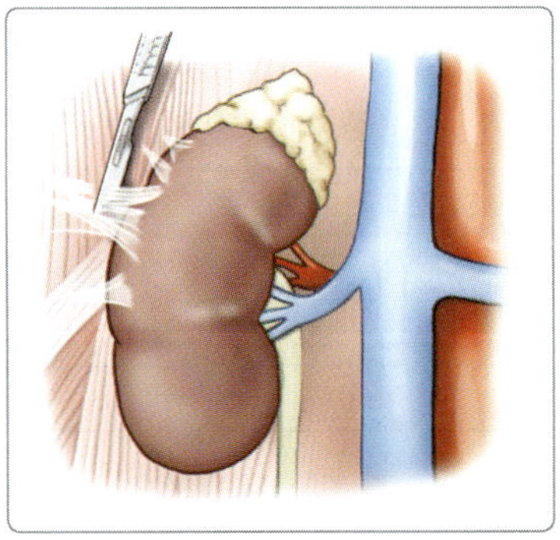

2. ____________________
drooping, sagging, prolapse

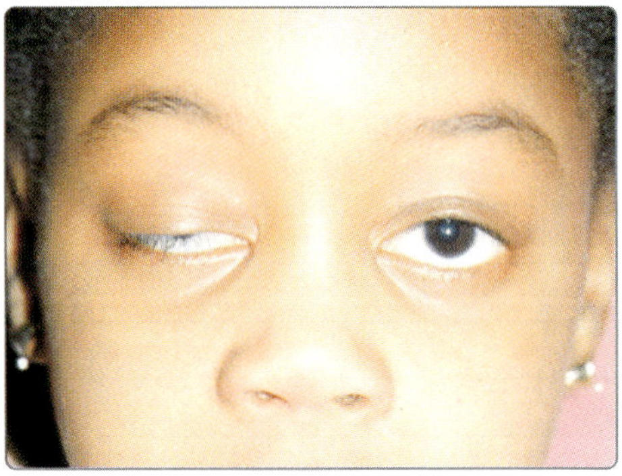

3. ____________________
surgical crushing

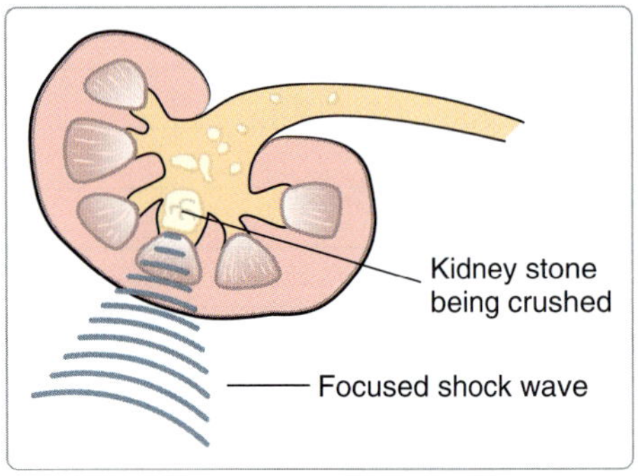

4. ____________________
stone(s), calculus (*pl.* calculi)

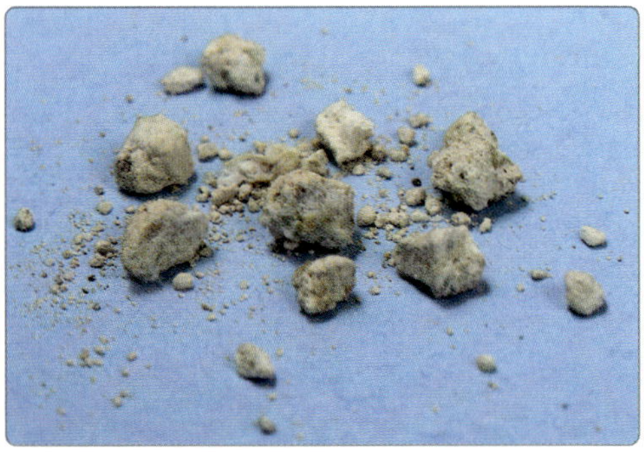

5. ______________________ surgical fixation	6. ______________________ urine, urination
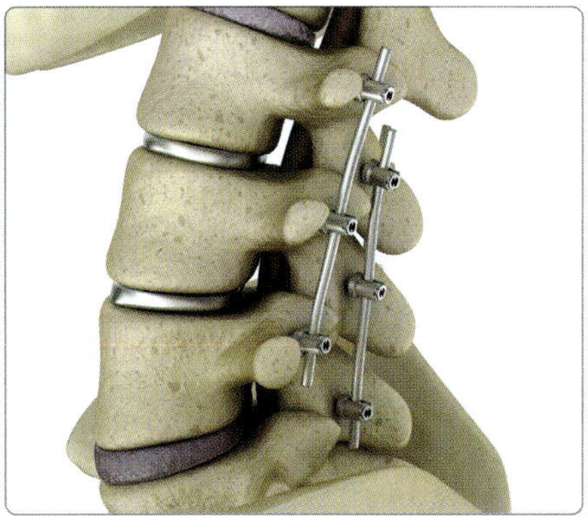	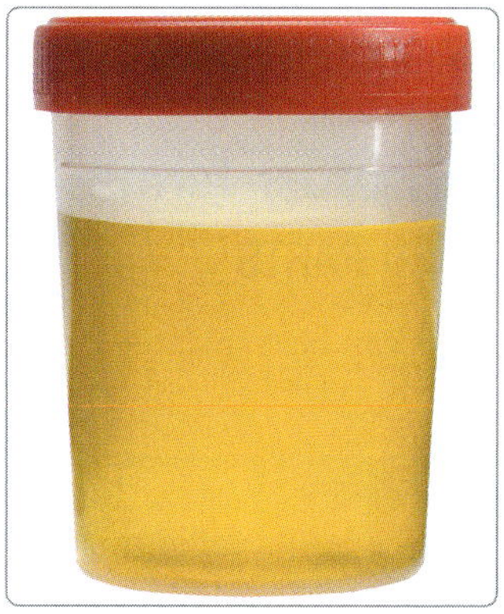

B Match

Match the suffixes in the first column with their correct definitions in the second column.

______	1. -logist	a. excision, surgical removal
______	2. -oma	b. hernia, protrusion
______	3. -graphy	c. instrument used for visual examination
______	4. -ectomy	d. enlargement
______	5. -al	e. pertaining to
______	6. -cele	f. one who studies and treats (specialist, physician)
______	7. -megaly	g. creation of an artificial opening
______	8. -stomy	h. process of recording, radiographic imaging
______	9. -plasty	i. tumor, swelling
______	10. -scope	j. surgical repair

C Define

Write the definitions of the following suffixes.

1. -stenosis ______________________
2. -itis ______________________
3. -iasis ______________________
4. -logy ______________________
5. -emia ______________________
6. -gram ______________________
7. -ary ______________________
8. -ia ______________________
9. -tomy ______________________
10. -osis ______________________
11. -scopy ______________________

MEDICAL TERMS

Medical terms relevant to this chapter have been grouped by topics, such as Disease and Disorder, and are listed in tables designated as Built from Word Parts or *NOT* Built from Word Parts. The exercises following each table assist with learning term definitions, pronunciations, and spellings.

Disease and Disorder Terms

BUILT FROM WORD PARTS

The following terms can be translated using definitions of word parts. Further explanation is provided within parentheses as needed.

TERM	DEFINITION
1. **cystitis** (sis-TĪ-tis)	inflammation of the bladder (Fig. 6.5)
2. **cystocele** (SIS-tō-sēl)	protrusion of the bladder
3. **cystolith** (SIS-tō-lith)	stone(s) in the bladder
4. **glomerulonephritis** (glō-*mer*-ū-lō-ne-FRĪ-tis)	inflammation of the glomeruli of the kidney
5. **hydronephrosis** (*hī*-drō-ne-FRŌ-sis)	abnormal condition of water in the kidney (swelling of the kidney due to a build up of urine; usually from a blockage in the ureter)
6. **nephritis** (ne-FRĪ-tis)	inflammation of a kidney
7. **nephroblastoma** (*nef*-rō-blas-TŌ-ma)	kidney tumor containing developing (germ) cells (malignant tumor) (also called **Wilms tumor**)
8. **nephrolithiasis** (*nef*-rō-lith-Ī-a-sis)	condition of stone(s) in the kidney
9. **nephroma** (nef-RŌ-ma)	tumor of the kidney

WILMS TUMOR also called nephroblastoma, is a rare malignancy of the kidney that primarily affects children. Named for German surgeon Dr. Max Wilms who described the disease in 1899, Wilms tumors are generally **unilateral** and can be successfully managed with appropriate surgical and oncology treatment.

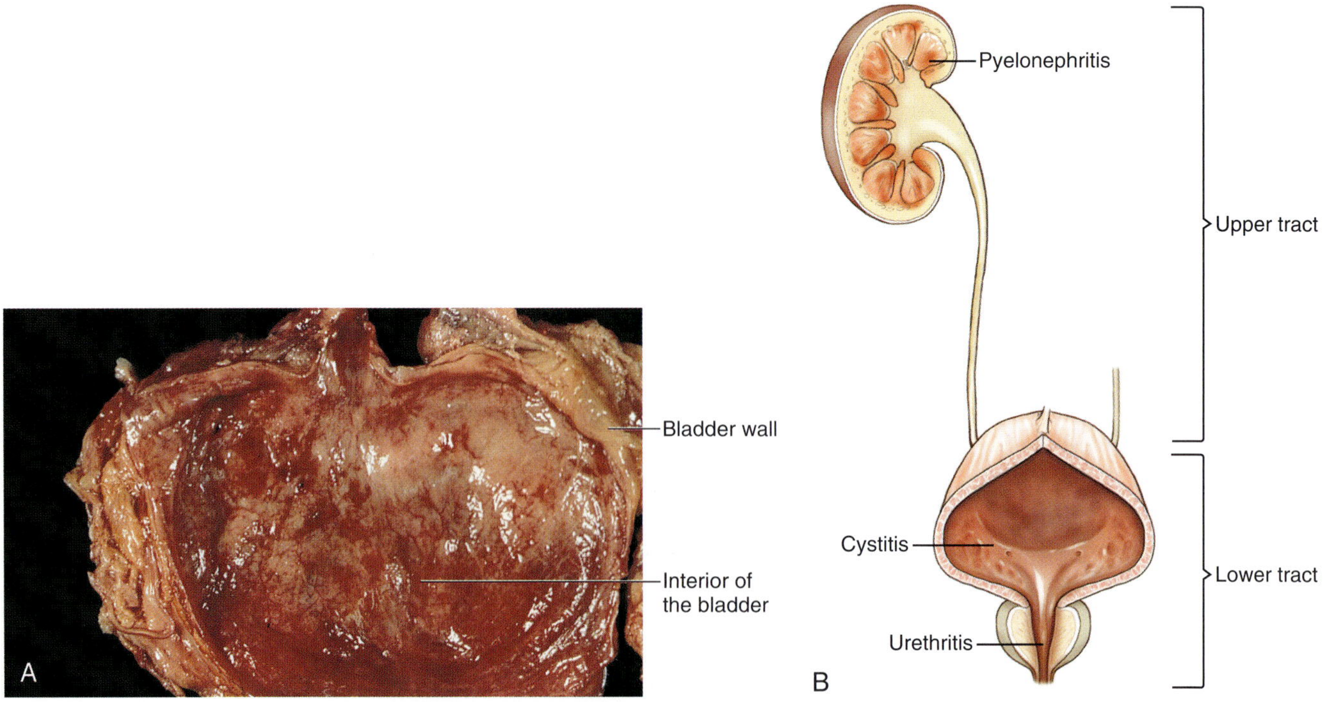

FIG. 6.5 Urinary tract infection. **A,** Acute cystitis. The swollen and red mucosa demonstrates inflammation. Cystitis is more common in women because the urethra is short, allowing easy access of bacteria to the urinary bladder. **B,** Upper and lower urinary tract infections. If cystitis is not treated promptly, the infection can spread to the kidneys, causing pyelonephritis.

TERM	DEFINITION
10. nephromegaly (*nef*-rō-MEG-a-lē)	enlargement of a kidney
11. nephroptosis (*nef*-rop-TŌ-sis)	drooping kidney (also called **floating kidney**)

NEPHROPTOSIS occurs when the kidney is no longer held in place and drops out of its normal position. The kidney is held in place by connective and adipose tissue, so it is susceptible to injury that may also cause the ureter to twist. Truck drivers and horseback riders are prone to this condition

TERM	DEFINITION
12. pyelitis (*pī*-e-LĪ-tis)	inflammation of the renal pelvis
13. pyelonephritis (*pī*-e-lō-ne-FRĪ-tis)	inflammation of the renal pelvis and the kidney (Fig. 6.5B, and Fig. 6.6)
14. uremia (ū-RĒ-mē-a)	urine (urea nitrogen) in the blood (refers the presence of azotemia and a wide range of signs and symptoms associated with chronic kidney disease, including polyuria [excessive urination], polydipsia [excessive thirst], vomiting, and weight loss; associated with renal failure) (also called **uremic syndrome**)

UREMIA was first used by Pierre Piorry, a French physician (1794-1879). He also created the medical terms **toxin, toxemia,** and **septicemia.**

TERM	DEFINITION
15. ureteritis (ū-*rē*-ter-Ī-tis)	inflammation of a ureter
16. ureterocele (ū-RĒ-ter-ō-*sēl*)	protrusion of a ureter (distally into the bladder)
17. ureterolithiasis (ū-*rē*-ter-ō-lith-Ī-a-sis)	condition of stone(s) in the ureter
18. urethritis (ū-rē-THRĪ-tis)	inflammation of the urethra
19. ureterostenosis (ū-*rē*-ter-ō-sten-Ō-sis)	narrowing of the ureter
20. urethrocystitis (ū-*rē*-thrō-sis-TĪ-tis)	inflammation of the urethra and the bladder
21. vesicoureteral reflux (VUR) (ves-i-kō-ū-RĒ-ter-al) (RĒ-fluks)	reflux pertaining to the bladder and ureter (condition in which urine flows backward towards the kidneys. May occur in up to 10% of children, and in some adults)

REFLUX is the flow of fluid through a vessel or valve in a direction opposite to normal.

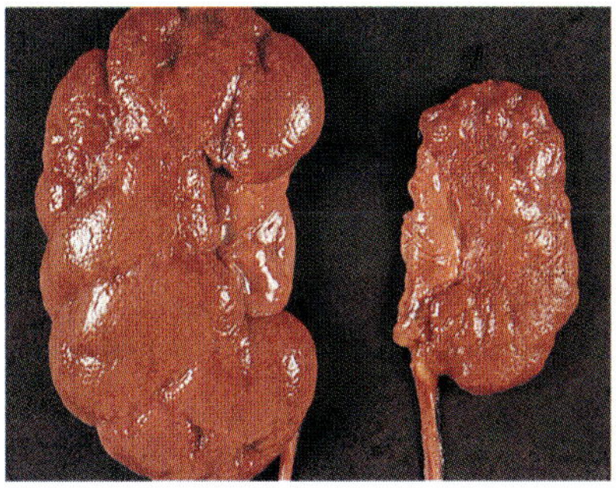

FIG. 6.6 *Kidney on left,* chronic pyelonephritis. *Kidney on right,* normal size with some scarring.

EXERCISE 5 ■ Pronounce and Spell

Practice pronunciation and spelling on paper and online.

1. Practice on Paper

a. **Pronounce:** Read the phonetic spelling and say aloud the terms listed in the previous table. Refer to the pronunciation key on p. 20 as necessary.
b. **Spell:** Have a study partner read the terms aloud. Write the spelling of the terms on a separate sheet of paper.

2. Practice Online

a. **Access** online learning resources. Go to evolve.elsevier.com > Evolve Resources > Student Resources.
b. **Pronounce:** Select Audio Glossary > Chapter 6 > Exercise 5. Select a term to hear its pronunciation and repeat aloud.
c. **Spell:** Select Activities > Chapter 6 > Spell Terms > Exercise 5. Select the audio icon and type the correct spelling of the term.

❑ Check the box when complete.

EXERCISE 6 ■ Analyze and Define

Analyze and define the following terms by drawing slashes between word parts, writing word part abbreviations above the term, underlining combining forms, and writing combining form abbreviations below the term.

EXAMPLE:

WR CV WR S
glomerul / o / nephr / itis
CF
inflammation of the glomeruli of the kidney

1. nephroblastoma
2. ureterostenosis
3. uremia
4. nephroptosis
5. cystocele
6. nephritis
7. pyelitis
8. ureterolithiasis
9. pyelonephritis
10. ureteritis

EXERCISE 7 ■ Build

A Fill In

Build disease and disorder terms for the following definitions by using the word parts you have learned.

EXAMPLE: inflammation of the ureter ureter / itis
WR / S

1. protrusion of a ureter _____ WR / CV / S
2. inflammation of the urethra and bladder _____ WR / CV / WR / S

3. reflux pertaining to the bladder and ureter (condition in which urine flows backwards toward the kidneys)

_____ / _____ / _____ / _____ reflux
WR / CV / WR / S

4. inflammation of the glomeruli of the kidney

_____ / _____ / _____ / _____
WR / CV / WR / S

5. tumor of the kidney

_____ / _____
WR / S

B Label

Build terms pictured by writing word parts above definitions.

1.

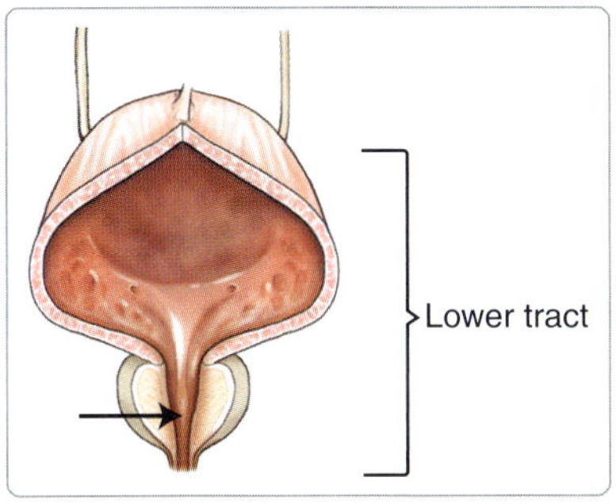

_____ / _____
urethra / inflammation

2.

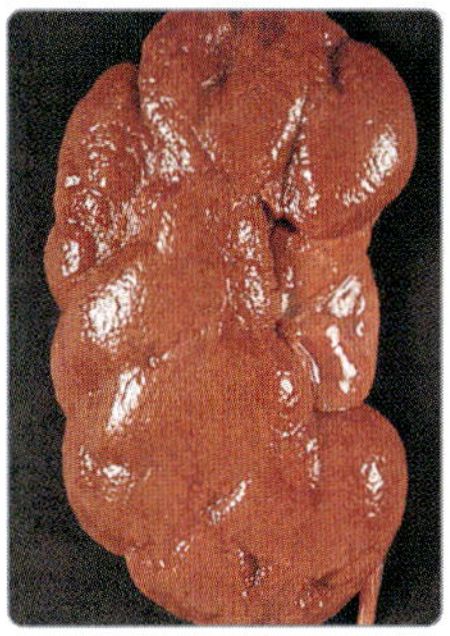

_____ / _____ / _____
kidney / CV / enlargement

3.

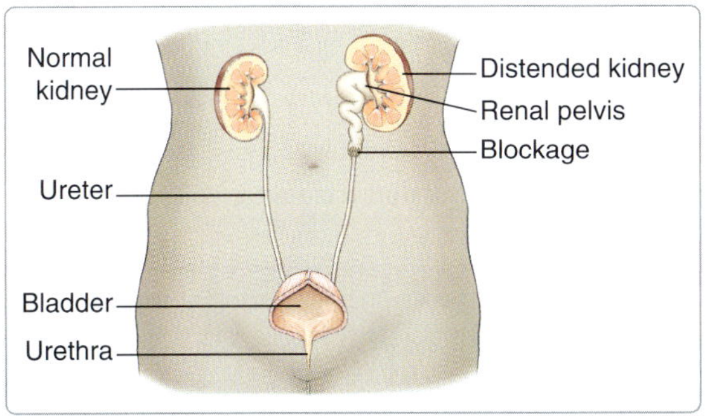

_____ / _____ / _____ / _____
water / CV / kidney / abnormal condition

4.

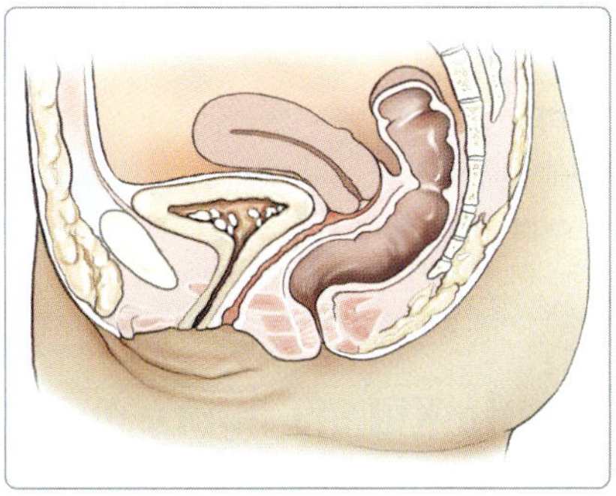

_____ / _____ / _____
bladder / CV / stone(s)

5.

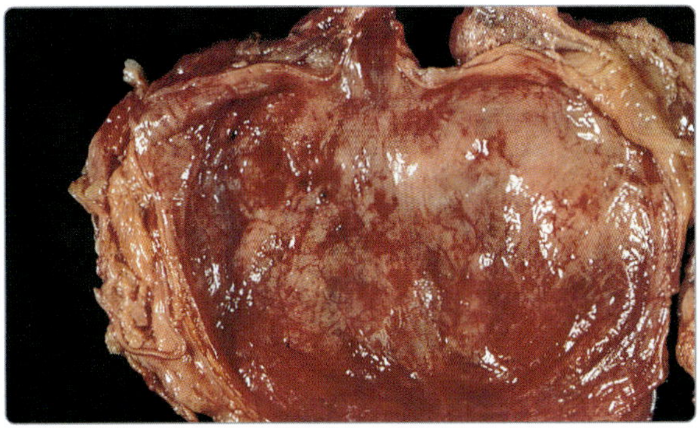

_____ / _____
bladder / inflammation

6.

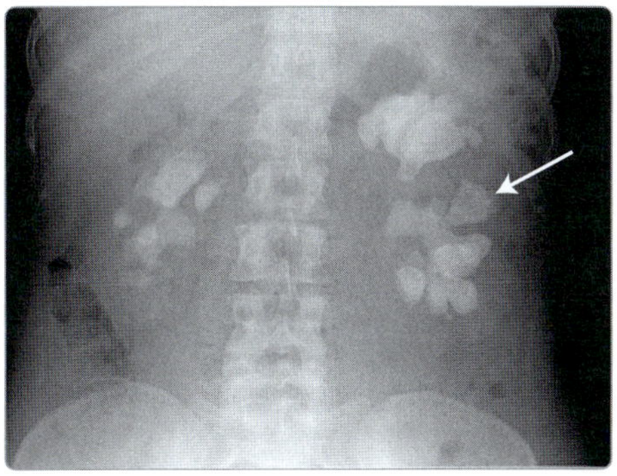

_____ / _____ / _____ / _____
kidney / CV / stone(s) / condition

Disease and Disorder Terms

NOT BUILT FROM WORD PARTS

Word parts may be present in the following terms; however, their full meanings cannot be translated using definitions of word parts alone.

TERM	DEFINITION
1. **acute kidney injury (AKI)** (a-KŪT) (KID-nē) (IN-ja-rē)	abrupt decline in kidney function that occurs over hours to days and is usually reversible (also called **acute renal failure [ARF]**) (Table 6.1)
2. **chronic kidney disease (CKD)** (KRON-ik) (KID-nē) (di-ZĒZ)	progressive, irreversible loss of kidney function (also called **chronic renal failure [CRF]**) (Table 6.1)
3. **end-stage renal disease (ESRD)** (end) (stāj) (RĒ-nal) (di-ZĒZ)	condition in which kidneys no longer function on their own. Dialysis or kidney transplantation is necessary for survival.
4. **epispadias** (*ep*-i-SPĀ-dē-as)	congenital defect in which the urinary meatus is located on the upper surface of the penis
5. **hypospadias** (*hī*-pō-SPĀ-dē-as)	congenital defect in which the urinary meatus is located on the underside of the penis. Females may also have a form of hypospadias where the urinary meatus is unusually located.
6. **polycystic kidney disease (PKD)** (*pol*-ē-SIS-tik) (KID-nē) (di-ZĒZ)	condition in which the kidney contains many cysts causing progressive interference with the ability to form urine
7. **renal calculus (*pl.* calculi)** (RĒ-nal) (KAL-kū-lus), (KAL-kū-lī)	stone in the kidney
8. **renal hypertension** (RĒ-nal) (*hī*-per-TEN-shun)	elevated blood pressure resulting from kidney disease
9. **urinary retention** (Ū-rin-*ār-ē*) (rē-TEN-shun)	abnormal accumulation of urine in the bladder because of an inability to urinate
10. **urinary suppression** (Ū-rin-*ār*-ē) (sū-PRESH-un)	sudden stoppage of urine formation
11. **urinary tract infection (UTI)** (Ū-rin-*ār*-ē) (trakt) (in-FEK-shun)	infection of one or more organs of the urinary tract (Fig. 6.5)

TABLE 6.1 Acute Kidney Injury vs. Chronic Kidney Disease

	Onset	Causes	Prognosis
Acute Kidney Injury (AKI)	Sudden	Trauma, obstruction, adverse drug reactions, or decreased blood flow from dehydration, burns, hemorrhage, and septic shock	Reversible with prompt treatment.
Chronic Kidney Disease (CKD)	Gradual	Hypertension, diabetes mellitus, and glomerulonephritis	Permanent. **End-stage renal disease (ESRD)** is the final outcome for patients with CKD, and reflects kidney function that is too poor to sustain life.

EXERCISE 8 ■ Pronounce and Spell

Practice pronunciation and spelling on paper and online.

1. Practice on Paper

a. **Pronounce:** Read the phonetic spelling and say aloud the terms listed in the previous table. Refer to the pronunciation key on p. 20 as necessary.

b. **Spell:** Have a study partner read the terms aloud. Write the spelling of the terms on a separate sheet of paper.

2. Practice Online

a. **Access** online learning resources. Go to evolve.elsevier.com > Evolve Resources > Student Resources.
b. **Pronounce:** Select Audio Glossary > Chapter 6 > Exercise 8. Select a term to hear its pronunciation and repeat aloud.
c. **Spell:** Select Activities > Chapter 6 > Spell Terms > Exercise 8. Select the audio icon and type the correct spelling of the term.

❑ Check the box when complete.

EXERCISE 9 ■ Fill In

A Label

Write the medical terms pictured and defined.

1. ____________________
congenital defect in which the urinary meatus is located on the underside of the penis

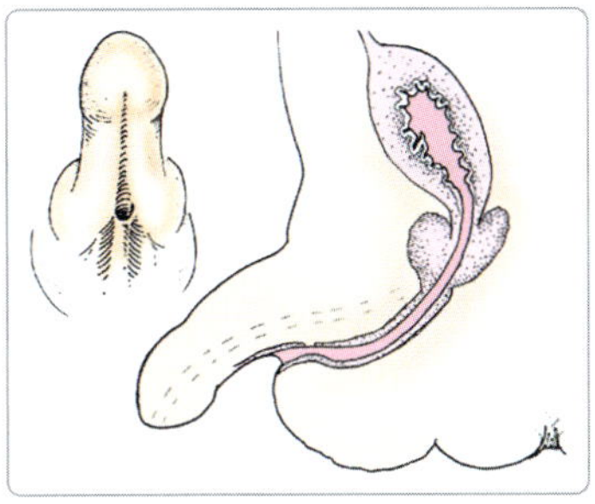

2. ____________________
condition in which the kidney contains many cysts causing progressive interference with the ability to form urine

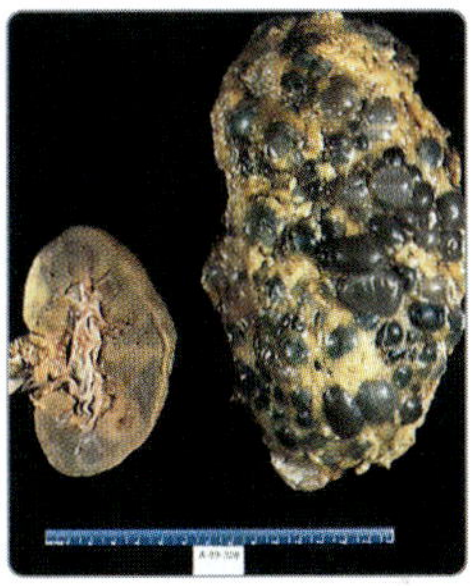

Kidney on left is a cross-section of normal kidney.

B Identify

Fill in the blanks with the correct terms.

1. Stone in the kidney is also called ____________________.
2. The inability to urinate, which results in an abnormal amount of urine in the bladder, is known as ____________________.
3. Elevated blood pressure resulting from kidney disease is ____________________.
4. Sudden stoppage of urine formation is referred to as ____________________.
5. ____________________ is a condition in which the urinary meatus is located on the upper surface of the penis.
6. Infection of one or more organs of the urinary system is called ____________________.
7. Progressive, irreversible loss of kidney function is called ____________________
8. ____________________ is a condition in which the kidneys can no longer function independently.
9. ____________________ is abrupt and usually reversible.

EXERCISE 10 ■ Match

Match the terms in the first column with their correct definitions in the second column.

______	1. end-stage renal disease	a. kidney with many cysts
______	2. hypospadias	b. sudden stoppage of urine formation
______	3. acute kidney injury	c. urinary meatus on the upper surface of the penis
______	4. renal hypertension	d. kidney stone
______	5. polycystic kidney disease	e. abnormal accumulation of urine in the bladder
______	6. urinary retention	f. urinary meatus on the underside of the penis
______	7. urinary suppression	g. infection of one or more organs of the urinary system
______	8. urinary tract infection	h. characterized by elevated blood pressure
______	9. chronic kidney disease	i. condition in which kidneys can no longer function on their own
______	10. renal calculus	j. abrupt decline in kidney function that is reversible
______	11. epispadias	k. progressive, irreversible loss of kidney function

EXERCISE 11 ■ Review of Disease and Disorder Terms

Can you define, pronounce, and spell the following terms?

acute kidney injury (AKI)
chronic kidney disease (CKD)
cystitis
cystocele
cystolith
end-stage renal disease (ESRD)
epispadias
glomerulonephritis
hydronephrosis
hypospadias
nephritis
nephroblastoma
nephrolithiasis
nephroma
nephromegaly
nephroptosis
polycystic kidney disease (PKD)
pyelitis
pyelonephritis
renal calculus (*pl.* calculi)
renal hypertension
uremia
ureteritis
ureterocele
ureterolithiasis
ureterostenosis
urethritis
urethrocystitis
urinary retention
urinary suppression
urinary tract infection (UTI)
vesicoureteral reflux (VUR)

Surgical Terms

BUILT FROM WORD PARTS AND *NOT* BUILT FROM WORD PARTS

The first portion of the table contains Urinary System Terms that can be translated using definitions of word parts. The second portion of the table contains Urinary System Terms that cannot be fully understood using the definitions of word parts.

■ Built from Word Parts

TERM	DEFINITION
1. cystectomy (sis-TEK-to-mē)	excision of the bladder
2. cystolithotomy (*sis*-tō-li-THOT-o-mē)	incision into the bladder to remove stone(s)
3. cystostomy (sis-TOS-to-mē)	creation of an artificial opening into the bladder (for urinary drainage) (also called **vesicostomy**)
4. lithotripsy (LITH-ō-trip-sē)	surgical crushing of stone(s) (using shock waves)
5. meatotomy (*mē*-a-TOT-o-mē)	incision into the meatus (to enlarge it)
6. nephrectomy (ne-FREK-to-mē)	excision of the kidney
7. nephrolithotomy (*nef*-rō-li-THOT-o-mē)	incision into the kidney to remove stone(s) (Fig. 6.7)
8. nephrolithotripsy (*nef*-rō-LITH-o-trip-sē)	surgical crushing of stone(s) in the kidney (using shock waves) (Fig. 6.7)

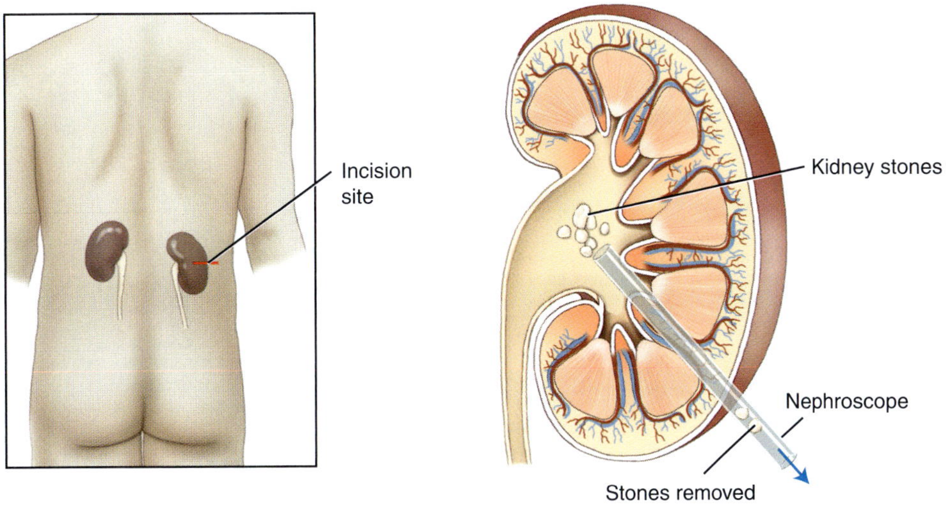

FIG. 6.7 Percutaneous nephrolithotomy or percutaneous lithotripsy uses a small incision in the back to remove medium or larger-size kidney stones. A nephroscope is passed into the kidney through the incision. In a **nephrolithotomy,** the surgeon removes the stone through the nephroscope. In a **nephrolithotripsy,** the stone is broken into fragments by a lithotripter and then removed through the nephroscope.

TERM	DEFINITION
9. **nephrolysis** (ne-FROL-i-sis)	separating the kidney (from other body structures)
10. **nephropexy** (NEF-rō-*peks*-ē)	surgical fixation of the kidney
11. **nephrostomy** (nef-ROS-to-mē)	creation of an artificial opening into the kidney
12. **pyelolithotomy** (*pī*-el-ō-lith-OT-o-mē)	incision into the renal pelvis to remove stone(s)
13. **pyeloplasty** (PĪ-el-ō-*plas*-tē)	surgical repair of the renal pelvis
14. **ureterectomy** (ū-*rē*-ter-EK-to-mē)	excision of the ureter
15. **ureterostomy** (ū-*rē*-ter-OS-to-mē)	creation of an artificial opening into the ureter (for drainage of urine)
16. **urethroplasty** (ū-RĒ-thrō-*plas*-tē)	surgical repair of the urethra
17. **urostomy** (ū-ROS-tō-mē)	creation of an artificial opening into the urinary system
18. **vesicourethral suspension** (*ves*-i-kō-ū-RĒ-thral) (*sus*-PEN-shun)	suspension pertaining to the bladder and urethra

VESICOURETHRAL SUSPENSION with a midurethral sling, called the Marshall-Marchetti Krantz technique, is performed to treat stress incontinence, the involuntary intermittent leakage of urine as a result of pressure from a cough or a sneeze on a weakened area around the urethra and bladder.

NOT Built from Word Parts

TERM	DEFINITION
1. **extracorporeal shock wave lithotripsy (ESWL)** (*eks*-tra-kor-POR-ē-al) (shok) (wāv) (LITH-ō-*trip*-sē)	noninvasive surgical procedure to crush stone(s) in the kidney or ureter by administration of repeated shock waves. Stone fragments are eliminated from the body in urine. (also called **shock wave lithotripsy [SWL]**).
EXTRACORPOREAL means occurring outside the body.	
2. **fulguration** (*ful*-gū-RĀ-shun)	destruction of living tissue with an electric spark (a method commonly used to destroy bladder growths) (Fig. 6.8)
3. **renal transplant** (RĒ-nal) (TRANS-plant)	surgical implantation of a donor kidney into a patient with inadequate renal function (Fig. 6.9)

RENAL FUNCTION REPLACEMENT THERAPIES
- Hemodialysis
- Peritoneal dialysis
- Renal transplant

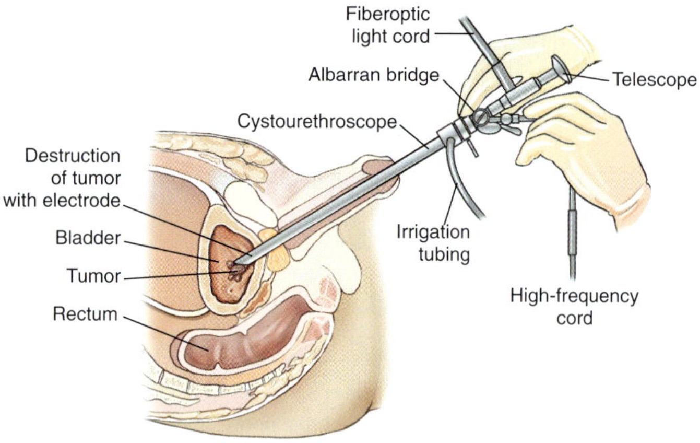

FIG. 6.8 Bladder fulguration.

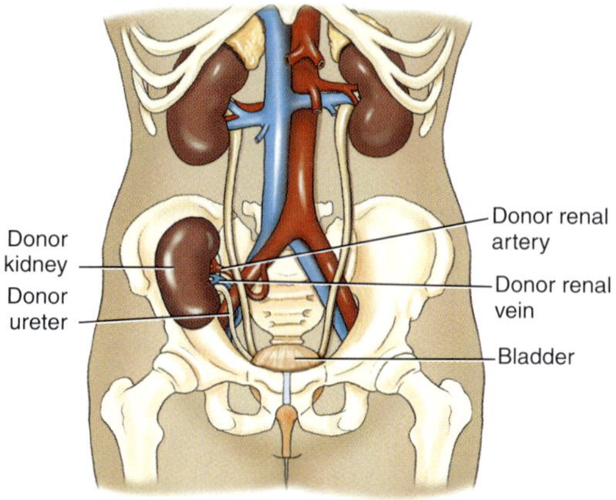

FIG. 6.9 Renal transplant showing donor kidney and blood vessels in place. Recipient's kidney is not always removed unless it is infected or is a cause of hypertension.

EXERCISE 12 ▪ Pronounce and Spell

Practice pronunciation and spelling on paper and online.

1. Practice on Paper

a. **Pronounce:** Read the phonetic spelling and say aloud the terms listed in the previous table. Refer to the pronunciation key on p. 20 as necessary.
b. **Spell:** Have a study partner read the terms aloud. Write the spelling of the terms on a separate sheet of paper.

2. Practice Online

a. **Access** online learning resources. Go to evolve.elsevier.com > Evolve Resources > Student Resources.
b. **Pronounce:** Select Audio Glossary > Chapter 6 > Exercise 12. Select a term to hear its pronunciation and repeat aloud.
c. **Spell:** Select Activities > Chapter 6 > Spell Terms > Exercise 12. Select the audio icon and type the correct spelling of the term.

❏ Check the box when complete.

EXERCISE 13 ▪ Surgical Terms Built from Word Parts

A Analyze and Define

Analyze and define the following terms by drawing slashes between word parts, writing word part abbreviations above the term, underlining combining forms, and writing combining form abbreviations below the term.

1. ureterostomy
____
____

2. nephrolithotomy
____
____

3. nephrostomy
____
____

4. nephrolysis
____
____

5. cystectomy
____
____

6. pyelolithotomy
____
____

7. nephropexy

____

____

8. cystolithotomy

____

____

9. nephrectomy

____

____

10. ureterectomy

____

____

11. cystostomy

____

____

12. pyeloplasty

____

____

13. urostomy

____

____

14. meatotomy

____

____

15. lithotripsy

____

____

16. urethroplasty

____

____

17. nephrolithotripsy

____

____

18. vesicourethral suspension

____

____

B Label

Build terms pictured by writing word parts above definitions.

1.

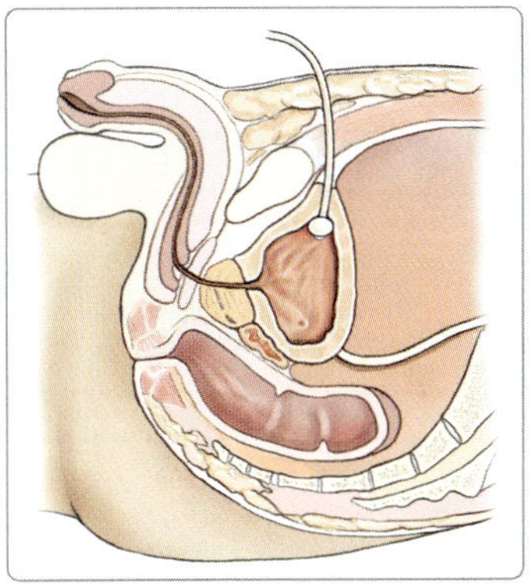

_______ / _______ / _______________
bladder / CV / creation of an artificial opening

2.

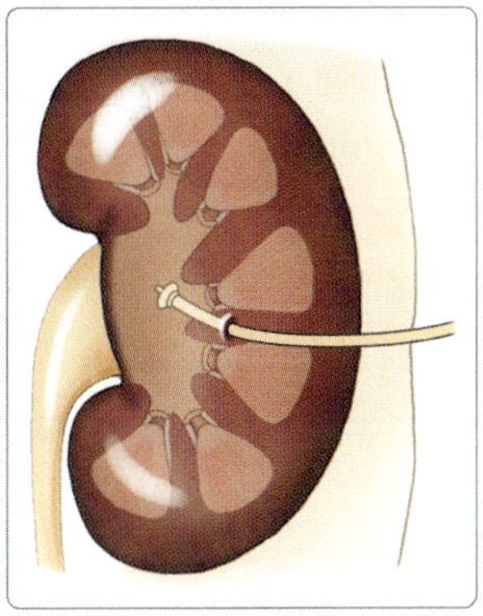

percutaneous _______ / _______ / _______________
kidney / CV / creation of an artificial opening

3.

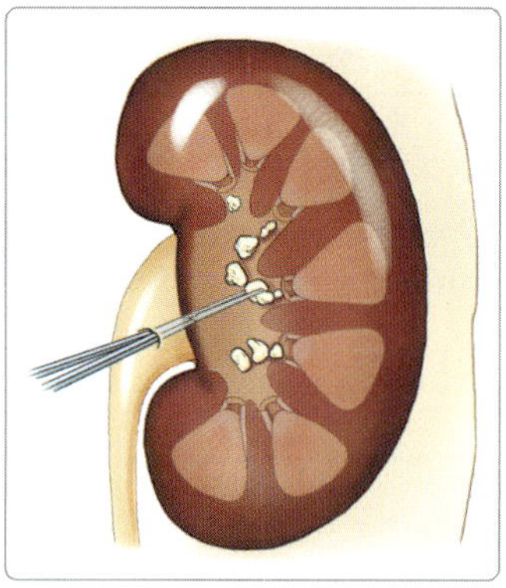

_______ / _______ / _______ / _______ / _______
renal pelvis | CV | stone | CV | incision

4.

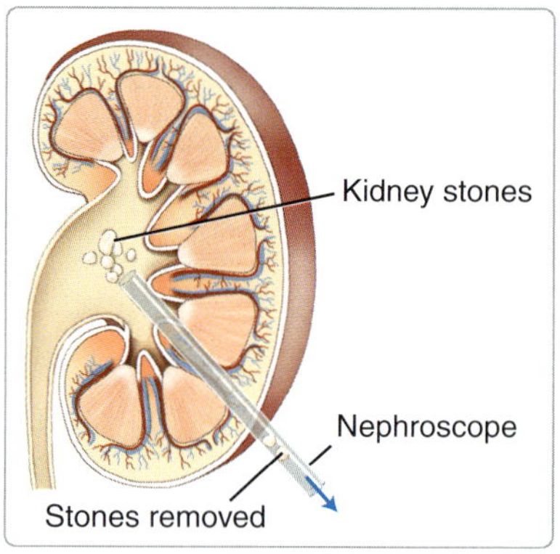

_______ / _______ / _______ / _______ / _______
kidney | CV | stone | CV | incision

5.

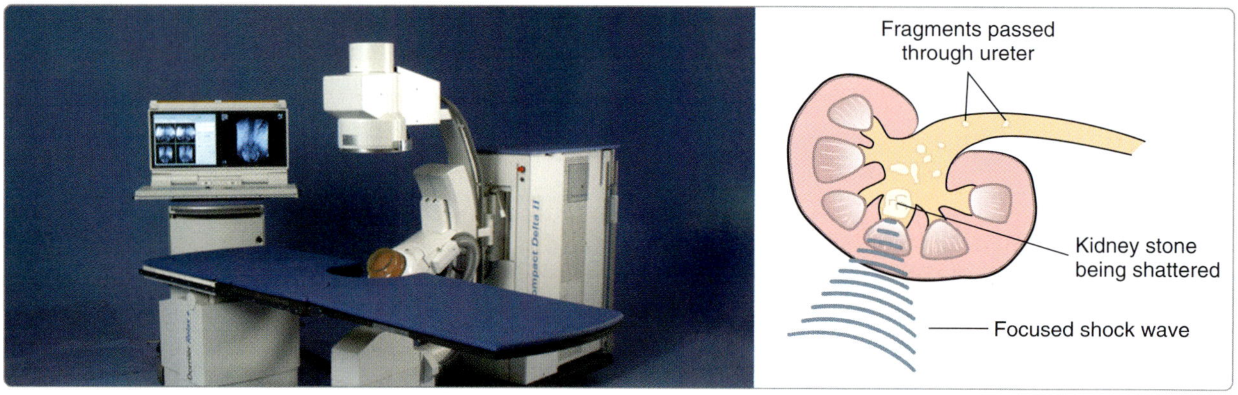

extracorporeal shock wave _______ / _______ / _______
stone | CV | surgical crushing

C Fill In

Build surgical terms for the following definitions by using the word parts you have learned.

1. creation of an artificial opening into the ureter
   _______ / _______ / _______
   WR / CV / S

2. excision of the kidney
   _______ / _______
   WR / S

3. surgical crushing of stone(s) in the kidney (using shock waves)
   _______ / _______ / _______ / _______ / _______
   WR / CV / WR / CV / S

4. creation of an artificial opening into the urinary system
   _______ / _______ / _______
   WR / CV / S

5. separating the kidney (from other structures)
   _______ / _______ / _______
   WR / CV / S

6. surgical repair of the renal pelvis
   _______ / _______ / _______
   WR / CV / S

7. surgical repair of the urethra ______ WR / CV / ______ S

8. excision of the bladder ______ WR / ______ S

9. incision into the meatus ______ WR / CV / ______ S

10. surgical fixation of the kidney ______ WR / CV / ______ S

11. excision of the ureter ______ WR / ______ S

12. incision into the bladder to remove stone(s) ______ WR / CV / ______ WR / CV / ______ S

13. suspension pertaining to the bladder and urethra ______ WR / CV / ______ WR / ______ S suspension

EXERCISE 14 ▪ Surgical Terms *NOT* Built from Word Parts

A Identify

Fill in the blanks with the correct terms.

1. The surgical implantation of a donor kidney into a patient with inadequate renal function is called ______ ______.
2. The destruction of living tissue with an electric spark is ______.
3. ______ ______ ______ ______ is a noninvasive surgical procedure for removal of kidney or ureteral stones.

B Match

Match the terms in the first column with their correct definitions in the second column.

______ 1. fulguration	a. implantation of a donor kidney
______ 2. renal transplant	b. used to destroy bladder growths
______ 3. ESWL	c. also called shock wave lithotripsy

EXERCISE 15 ▪ Review of Surgical Terms

Can you define, pronounce, and spell the following terms?

cystectomy	fulguration	nephrolysis	ureterectomy
cystolithotomy	lithotripsy	nephropexy	ureterostomy
cystostomy	meatotomy	nephrostomy	urethroplasty
extracorporeal shock wave lithotripsy (ESWL)	nephrectomy	pyelolithotomy	urostomy
	nephrolithotomy	pyeloplasty	vesicourethral suspension
	nephrolithotripsy	renal transplant	

Diagnostic Terms

BUILT FROM WORD PARTS AND *NOT* BUILT FROM WORD PARTS

The first portion of the table contains diagnostic terms that can be translated using definitions of word parts. The second portion of the table contains diagnostic terms that cannot be fully understood using the definitions of word parts.

Built from Word Parts

DIAGNOSTIC IMAGING

TERM	DEFINITION
1. **cystogram** (SIS-tō-gram)	radiographic image of the bladder
2. **cystography** (sis-TOG-ra-fē)	radiographic imaging of the bladder
3. **nephrosonography** (*nef*-rō-so-NOG-ra-fē)	process of recording the kidney using sound (ultrasonography)
4. **renogram** (RĒ-nō-gram)	radiographic record of the kidney (an imaging test, used to evaluate kidney function); (also called **nephrogram**) (Fig. 6.10B)
5. **retrograde urogram** (RET-rō-grād) (Ū-rō-gram)	radiographic image of the urinary tract (retrograde means to move in a direction opposite from normal; contrast medium is instilled into the bladder through a urethral catheter, and may extend to the ureters or kidneys in patients with vesicoureteral reflux)
6. **urogram** (Ū-rō-gram)	radiographic image of the urinary tract (Fig. 6.11)
7. **voiding cystourethrography (VCUG)** (VOID-ing) (*sis*-tō-*ū*-rē-THROG-ro-fē)	radiographic imaging of the bladder and the urethra (Fig. 6.12). (Radiographic images are taken of the bladder before and during urination using a contrast agent [fluoroscopy] or a radioactive material [nuclear medicine].)

ENDOSCOPY

TERM	DEFINITION
8. **cystoscope** (SIS-tō-skōp)	instrument used for visual examination of the bladder
9. **cystoscopy** (sis-TOS-ko-pē)	visual examination of the bladder
10. **nephroscopy** (ne-FROS-ko-pē)	visual examination of the kidney
11. **ureteroscopy** (ū-*rē*-ter-OS-ko-pē)	visual examination of the ureter

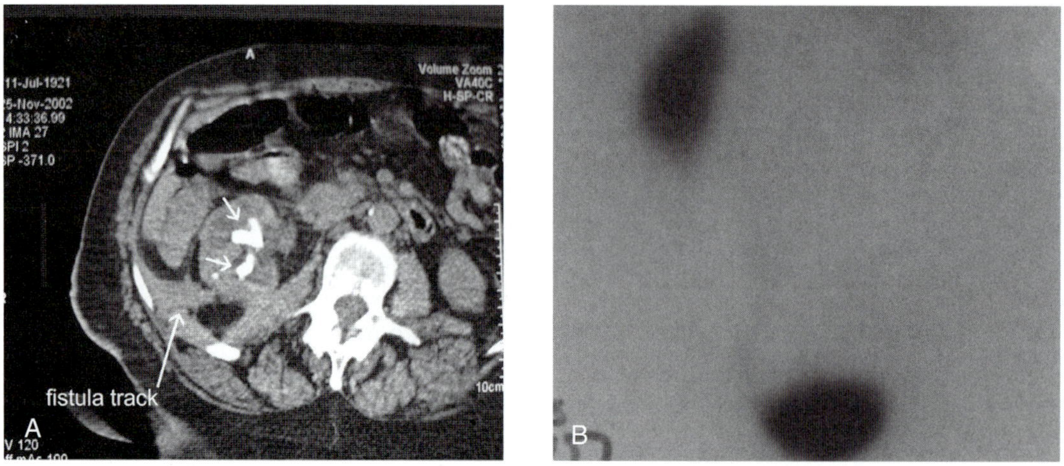

FIG. 6.10 **A,** CT scan of the kidney. Small arrows point to a large calculus within the renal pelvis (axial view). **B,** Renogram. Nuclear medicine image from the same patient, showing no function of the affected kidney (posterior view).

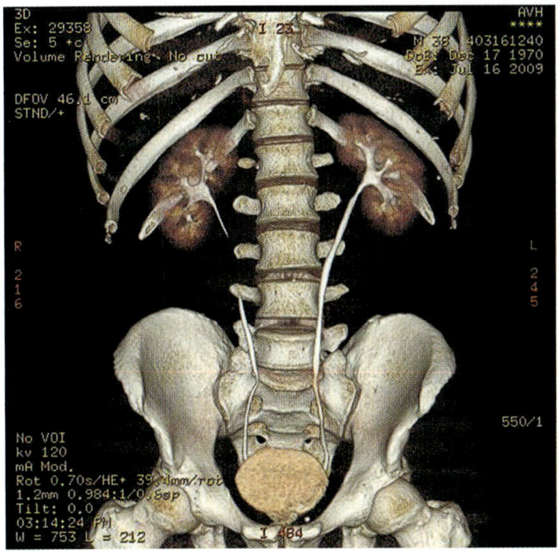

FIG. 6.11 CT urogram showing three-dimensional, reconstructed view of the kidneys, ureters, and bladder. CT urogram scans are now the primary diagnostic tool for detecting **urinary tract stones** and **perirenal infections. Intravenous urograms (IVU)** may still be used to evaluate an obstructing mass.

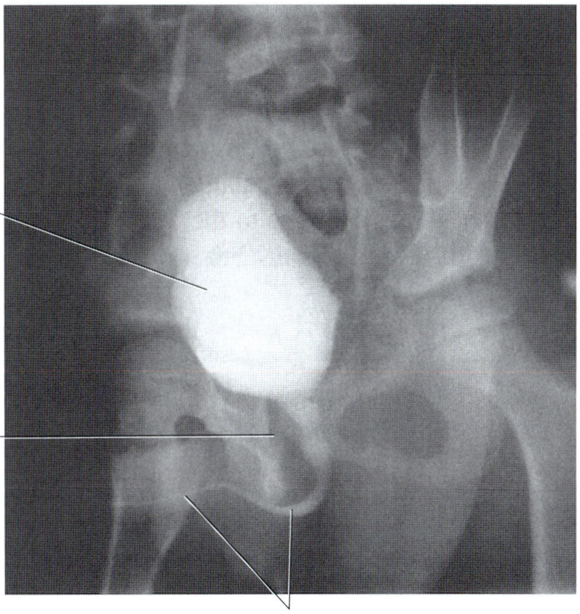

FIG. 6.12 Voiding cystourethrogram, male (lateral view).

NOT Built from Word Parts

DIAGNOSTIC IMAGING

TERM	DEFINITION
1. KUB (K-Ū-B) *each letter is said*	simple radiographic image of the abdomen. It is often used to view the **kidneys, ureters**, and **bladder** to determine their size, shape, and location, or to identify radiopaque calculi in these structures. A KUB may also be used to diagnose intestinal obstruction. (also called **flat plate of the abdomen**)

LABORATORY

TERM	DEFINITION
2. blood urea nitrogen (BUN) (blud) (ū-RĒ-a) (NĪ-trō-jen)	test that measures the amount of nitrogen in the blood that comes from urea. An increased BUN detects an abnormality in renal function.
BUN, the abbreviation for blood urea nitrogen, is almost exclusively used to refer to the test. It is pronounced letter by letter, B-Ū-N, not as a whole word.	
3. creatinine (crē-AT-i-nin)	blood test that measures the amount of a waste product in the blood that comes from the normal wear and tear of muscles. An elevated amount may indicate impaired kidney function.
4. specific gravity (SG) (spe-SIF-ik) (GRAV-i-tē)	test performed on a urine specimen to measure the concentrating or diluting ability of the kidneys
5. urinalysis (UA) (*ū*-rin-AL-is-is)	multiple routine tests performed on a urine specimen. Visual examination and chemical analysis of a urine specimen provides screening for blood, glucose, protein, and other substances in the urine and offers a picture of overall health.
6. urine culture and sensitivity (Ū-rin) (KUL-cher) (and) (*sen*-si-TIV-i-tē)	test performed on a urine specimen to determine the presence of bacteria and yeast; used to diagnose urinary tract infections
7. urodynamics (*ū*-rō-dī-NAM-iks)	pertaining to the force and flow of urine within the urinary tract. Urodynamic studies examine the process of voiding and tests bladder tone, capacity, and pressure along with urine flow and perineal muscle function. An enlarged prostate and urethral stricture will diminish urine flow rate.

EXERCISE 16 ■ Pronounce and Spell

Practice pronunciation and spelling on paper and online.

1. Practice on Paper

a. **Pronounce:** Read the phonetic spelling and say aloud the terms listed in the previous table. Refer to the pronunciation key on p. 20 as necessary.
b. **Spell:** Have a study partner read the terms aloud. Write the spelling of the terms on a separate sheet of paper.

2. Practice Online

a. **Access** online learning resources. Go to evolve.elsevier.com > Evolve Resources > Student Resources.
b. **Pronounce:** Select Audio Glossary > Chapter 6 > Exercise 16. Select a term to hear its pronunciation and repeat aloud.
c. **Spell:** Select Activities > Chapter 6 > Spell Terms > Exercise 16. Select the audio icon and type the correct spelling of the term.

❑ Check the box when complete.

EXERCISE 17 ■ Diagnostic Terms Built from Word Parts

A Analyze and Define

Analyze and define the following terms by drawing slashes between word parts, writing word part abbreviations above the term, underlining combining forms, and writing combining form abbreviations below the term.

1. (voiding) cystourethrography

____

____

2. cystography

____

____

3. nephrosonography

____

____

4. cystoscope

____

____

5. cystogram

____

____

6. cystoscopy

____

____

7. urogram

____

____

8. renogram

____

____

9. nephroscopy

____

____

10. ureteroscopy

____

____

B Label

Build terms pictured by writing word parts above definitions.

1.

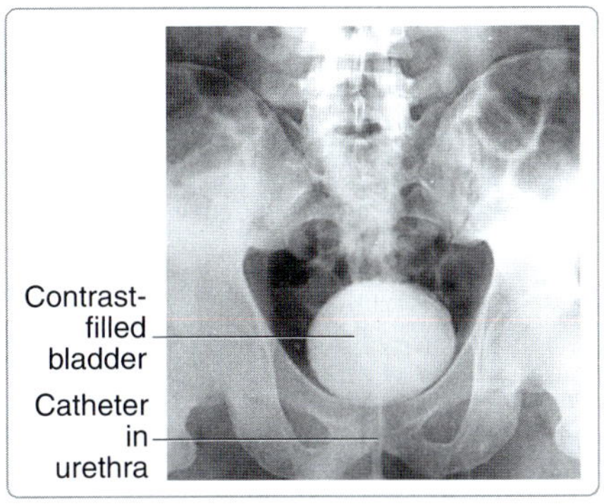

_______ / _______ / _______
bladder CV radiographic image

2.

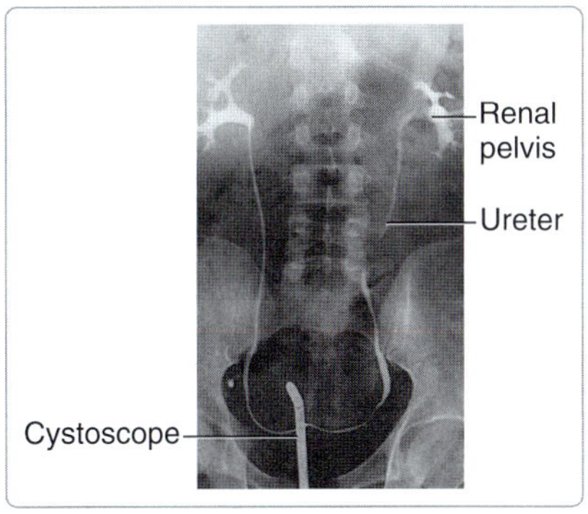

retrograde _______ / _______ / _______
urinary tract CV radiographic image

3.

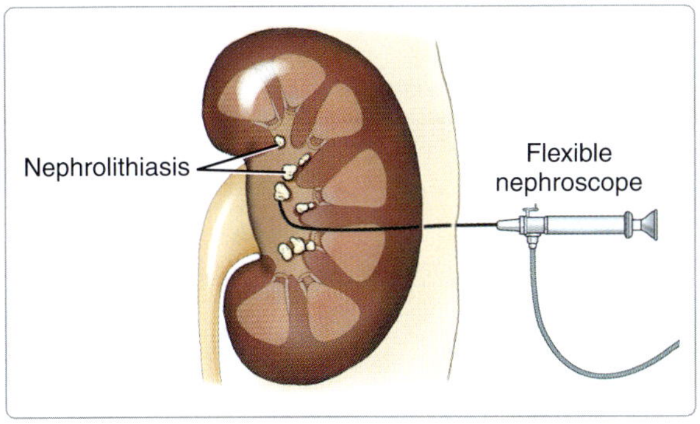

_______ / _______ / _______
kidney CV visual examination

4.

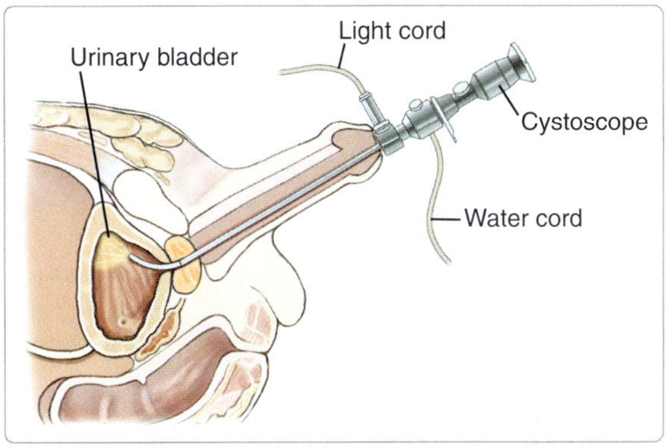

_______ / _______ / _______
bladder CV visual examination

C Fill In

Build diagnostic terms that correspond to the following definitions by using the word parts you have learned.

1. visual examination of the ureter _______ / _______ / _______
WR / CV / S

2. radiographic image of the urinary tract _______ / _______ / _______
WR / CV / S

3. process of radiographic recording the kidney using sound _______ / _______ / _______ / _______ / _______
WR / CV / WR / CV / S

4. instrument used for visual examination of the bladder _______ / _______ / _______
WR / CV / S

5. radiographic imaging of the bladder and the urethra

voiding _______ / _______ / _______ / _______ / _______
WR / CV / WR / CV / S

6. radiographic imaging of the bladder

_______ / _______ / _______
WR / CV / S

7. radiographic record of the kidney, used to evaluate kidney function

_______ / _______ / _______
WR / CV / S

EXERCISE 18 ■ Diagnostic Terms *NOT* Built from Word Parts

A Label

Write the medical terms pictured and defined.

1. _______________________________
test that measures the amount of nitrogen in the blood that comes from urea

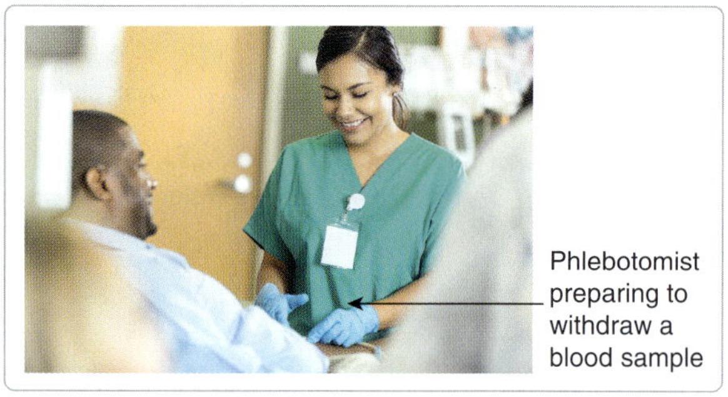

2. _______________________________
multiple tests performed on a urine specimen

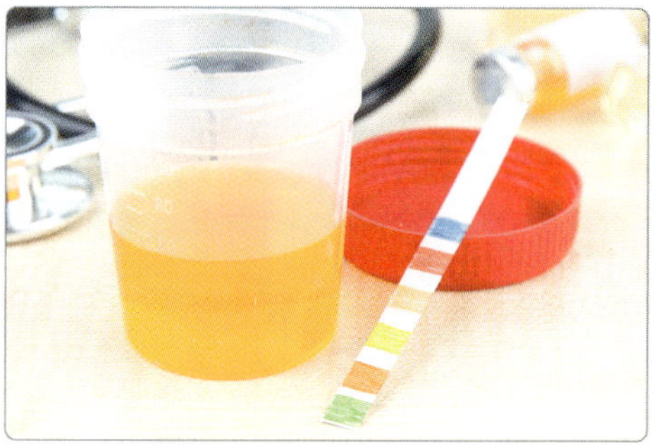

3. _______________________________
radiographic image of the abdomen to view kidneys, ureters, and bladder

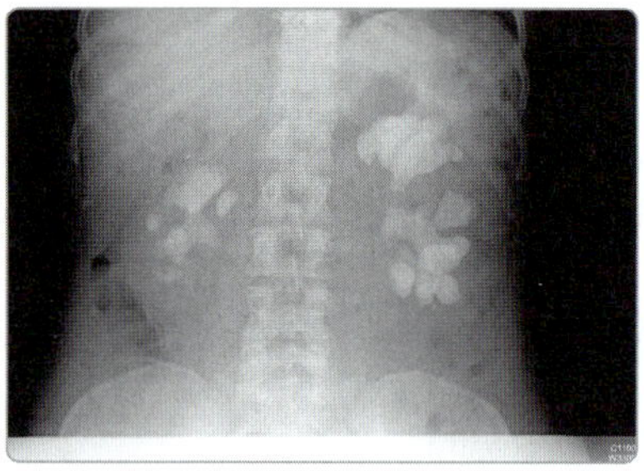

Note the bilateral calculi that fill the renal pelvis. Due to the distinctive shape, these are called **staghorn calculi** because of the resemblance to the antlers of a stag.

4. _______________________________
test on urine specimen to measure the concentrating and diluting abilities of the kidneys

Laboratory results

URINE
COLOR__________
APPEARANCE__________
PH__________
SG__________
ACETONE__________
GLUCOSE__________
BACTERIA__________
WBC__________
RBC__________
CASTS__________
OCCULT BLOOD__________
OTHER__________

B Match

Match the terms in the first column with their correct definitions in the second column.

______ 1. specific gravity	a. radiographic image of the kidneys, ureters, and bladder
______ 2. urodynamics	b. test that measures the amount of nitrogen in the blood that comes from urea
______ 3. urinalysis	c. urine test to measure concentrating or diluting abilities of the kidneys
______ 4. KUB	d. multiple routine tests performed on a urine sample
______ 5. creatinine	e. test that measures the amount of a waste product in the blood that comes from the normal wear and tear of muscles
______ 6. blood urea nitrogen	f. test performed on a urine specimen to determine the presence of bacteria and yeast
______ 7. urine culture and sensitivity	g. pertaining to the force and flow of urine within the urinary tract

EXERCISE 19 ■ Review of Diagnostic Terms

Can you define, pronounce, and spell the following terms?

blood urea nitrogen (BUN)
creatinine
cystogram
cystoscope
cystoscopy
KUB
nephrography
nephroscopy
nephrosonography
renogram
retrograde urogram
specific gravity (SG)
ureteroscopy
urinalysis (UA)
urine culture and sensitivity
urodynamics
urogram
voiding cystourethrography (VCUG)

Complementary Terms

BUILT FROM WORD PARTS

The following terms can be translated using definitions of word parts. Further explanation is provided within parentheses as needed.

SIGNS AND SYMPTOMS

TERM	DEFINITION
1. albuminuria (*al*-bū-min-Ū-rē-a)	albumin in the urine (albumin is an important protein in the blood, but when found in the urine, may indicate kidney disease; small amounts may be present in the absence of kidney disease)
2. anuria (an-Ū-rē-a)	absence of urine (failure of the kidney to produce urine)
3. azotemia (az-ō-TĒ-mē-a)	nitrogen in the blood (laboratory abnormality indicating an increase in nitrogen-containing compounds, including urea and creatinine. One of many signs and symptoms of uremia.)
4. dysuria (dis-Ū-rē-a)	difficult or painful urination
5. glycosuria (*glī*-kō-SŪ-rē-a)	sugar (glucose) in the urine
6. hematuria (*hēm*-a-TŪ-rē-a)	blood in the urine
7. nocturia (nok-TŪ-rē-a)	night urination
8. oliguria (*ol*-i-GŪ-rē-a)	scanty urine (amount)
9. polyuria (*pol*-ē-Ū-rē-a)	much (excessive) urine
10. pyuria (pī-Ū-rē-a)	pus in the urine

Complementary Terms—cont'd

BUILT FROM WORD PARTS

MEDICAL SPECIALTIES

TERM	DEFINITION
11. nephrologist (ne-FROL-o-jist)	physician who studies and treats diseases of the kidney
12. nephrology (ne-FROL-o-jē)	study of the kidney (a branch of medicine dealing with diseases of the kidney)
13. urologist (ū-ROL-o-jist)	physician who studies and treats diseases of the urinary tract
14. urology (ū-ROL-o-jē)	study of the urinary tract (a branch of medicine dealing with diseases of the male and female urinary systems and the male reproductive system)

UROLOGIST/NEPHROLOGIST A **urologist** treats diseases of the male and female urinary system and the male reproductive system both medically and surgically. A **nephrologist** treats kidney diseases and prescribes and manages dialysis therapy.

DESCRIPTIVE TERMS

TERM	DEFINITION
15. intravesical (*in*-tra-VES-i-kal)	pertaining to within the (urinary) bladder
16. meatal (mē-Ā-tal)	pertaining to the meatus
17. transurethral (*trans*-ū-RĒ-thral)	pertaining to through the urethra
18. urinary (Ū-rin-*ār*-ē)	pertaining to urine

EXERCISE 20 ■ Pronounce and Spell

Practice pronunciation and spelling on paper and online.

1. Practice on Paper

a. **Pronounce:** Read the phonetic spelling and say aloud the terms listed in the previous table. Refer to the pronunciation key on p. 20 as necessary.
b. **Spell:** Have a study partner read the terms aloud. Write the spelling of the terms on a separate sheet of paper.

2. Practice Online

a. **Access** online learning resources. Go to evolve.elsevier.com > Evolve Resources > Student Resources.
b. **Pronounce:** Select Audio Glossary > Chapter 6 > Exercise 20. Select a term to hear its pronunciation and repeat aloud.
c. **Spell:** Select Activities > Chapter 6 > Spell Terms > Exercise 20. Select the audio icon and type the correct spelling of the term.

❑ Check the box when complete.

EXERCISE 21 ■ Analyze and Define

Analyze and define the following terms by drawing slashes between word parts, writing word part abbreviations above the term, underlining combining forms, and writing combining form abbreviations below the term.

1. nocturia
____
____

2. urologist
____
____

3. oliguria
____
____

4. nephrologist
____
____

5. hematuria

____
____

6. urology

____
____

7. polyuria

____
____

8. albuminuria

____
____

9. anuria

____
____

10. azotemia

____
____

11. pyuria

____
____

12. urinary

____
____

13. glycosuria

____
____

14. dysuria

____
____

15. nephrology

____
____

16. intravesical

____
____

17. meatal

____
____

18. transurethral

____
____

EXERCISE 22 ■ Build

A Fill In

Build complementary terms for the following definitions by using the word parts you have learned.

1. night urination _______ / _______
   WR / S

2. scanty urine _______ / _______
   WR / S

3. pus in the urine _______ / _______
   WR / S

4. physician who studies and treats diseases of the urinary tract ______ / ___ / ______
WR / CV / S

5. much (excessive) urine ______ / ______
P / S(WR)

6. study of the kidney ______ / ___ / ______
WR / CV / S

7. pertaining to urine ______ / ______
WR / S

8. nitrogen in the blood ______ / ______
WR / S

9. study of the urinary tract ______ / ___ / ______
WR / CV / S

10. pertaining to through the urethra ______ / ______ / ______
P / WR / S

11. sugar (glucose) in the urine ______ / ______
WR / S

12. pertaining to within the (urinary) bladder ______ / ______ / ______
P / WR / S

13. absence of urine ______ / ______
P / S(WR)

14. albumin in the urine ______ / ______
WR / S

B Label

Build terms pictured by writing word parts above definitions.

1.

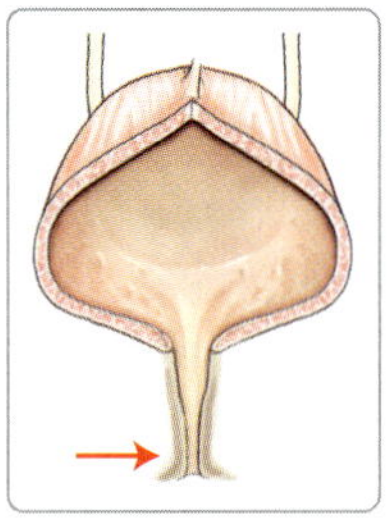

______ / ______
meatus / pertaining to

2.

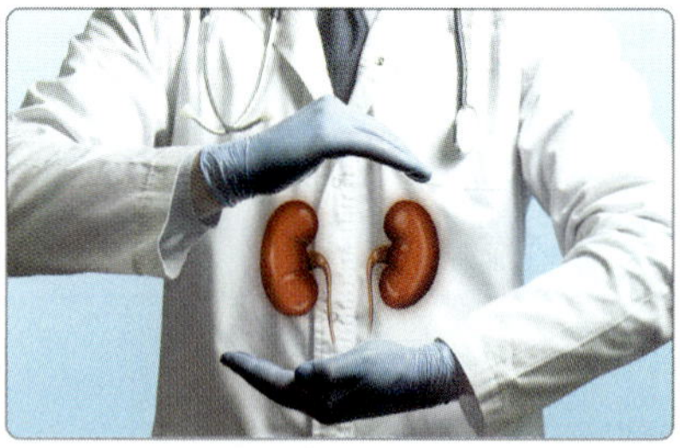

______ / ___ / ______
kidneys / CV / physician who studies and treats

3.

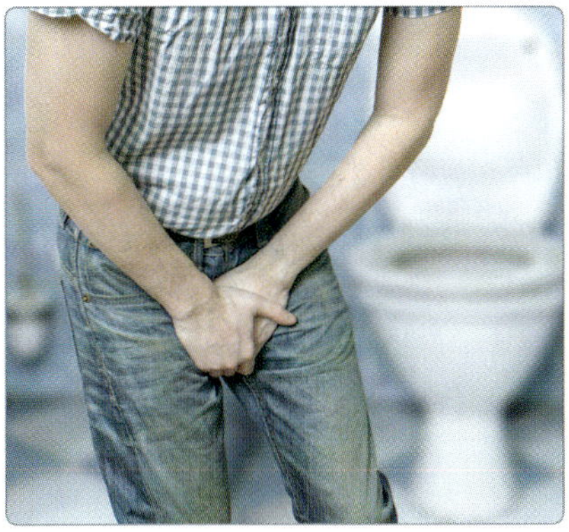

_____________ / _________________
difficult or painful — urination

4.

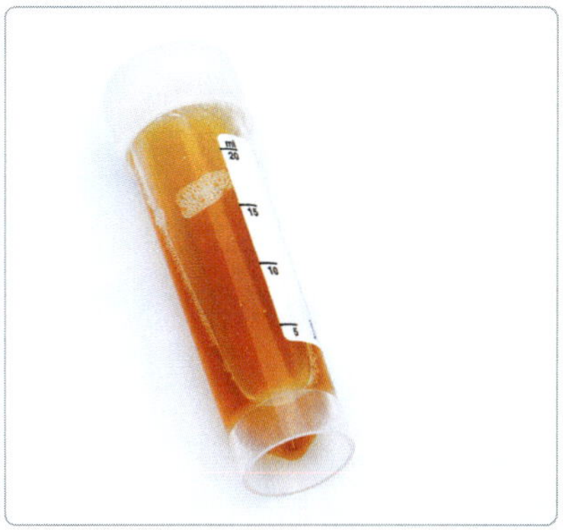

_____________ / _________________
blood — urine

Complementary Terms

NOT BUILT FROM WORD PARTS

Word parts may be present in the following terms; however, their full meanings cannot be translated using definitions of word parts alone.

SIGNS AND SYMPTOMS

TERM	DEFINITION
1. enuresis (*en*-ū-RĒ-sis)	involuntary urination. **Nocturnal enuresis**, or bed-wetting, has been described in early literature and continues to be a problem affecting 15% to 20% of school-aged children. There is no one cause for bed wetting. **Diurnal enuresis** is daytime wetting, which may be caused by a small bladder. Various treatments are used to treat diurnal enuresis. Children generally outgrow daytime wetting.
2. prolapse (prō-LAPS)	displacement of an organ or anatomic structure from its normal position (also called **ptosis**)
3. stricture (STRIK-chūr)	abnormal narrowing, such as a urethral stricture
4. urinary incontinence (Ū-rin-*ār*-ē) (in-KON-ti-nens)	inability to control the bladder causing leakage of urine

TREATMENTS

TERM	DEFINITION
5. diuretic (*dī*-ū-RET-ik)	agent that promotes the formation and excretion of urine
6. hemodialysis (HD) (*hē*-mō-dī-AL-i-sis)	procedure for removing impurities from the blood because of an inability of the kidneys to do so (Fig. 6.13)
7. peritoneal dialysis (*pār*-i-tō-NĒ-al) (dī-AL-i-sis)	procedure for removing toxic wastes when the kidney is unable to do so; the peritoneal cavity is used as the receptacle for the fluid used in the dialysis (Fig. 6.14)
8. urinary catheterization (Ū-rin-*ār*-ē) (*kath*-e-*ter*-i-ZĀ-shun)	passage of a catheter into the urinary bladder to withdraw urine

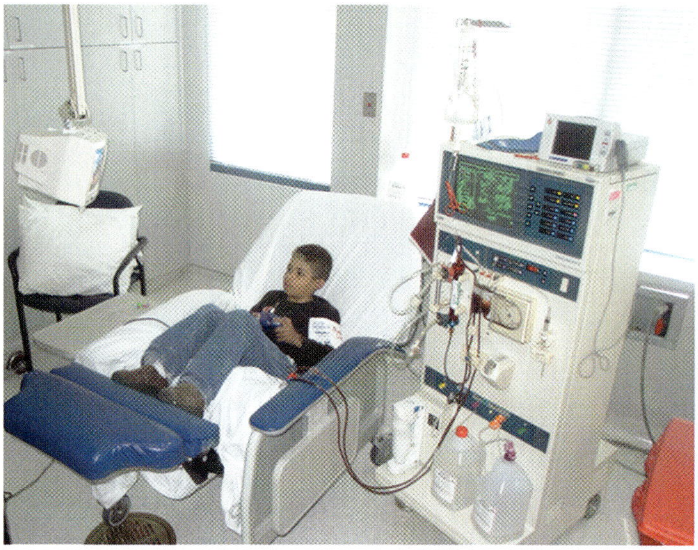

FIG. 6.13 Hemodialysis.

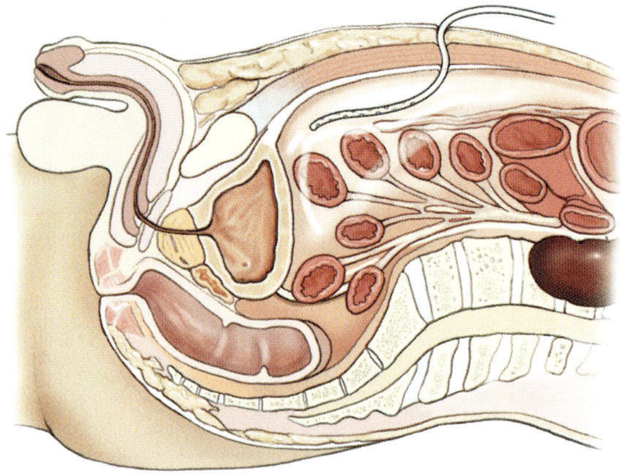

FIG. 6.14 Peritoneal dialysis. A sterile dialyzing fluid is instilled into the peritoneal cavity by gravity and dwells there for a period of time ordered by the physician. The fluid, containing the nitrogenous wastes and excess water that a healthy kidney normally removes, is drained from the cavity.

Complementary Terms—cont'd

NOT BUILT FROM WORD PARTS

EQUIPMENT

TERM	DEFINITION
9. catheter (cath) (KATH-e-ter)	flexible, tubelike device, such as a urinary catheter, for withdrawing or instilling fluids
CATHETER is derived from the Greek **katheter,** meaning a **thing let down.** A catheter lets down the urine from the bladder.	
10. urinal (Ū-rin-al)	receptacle for urine

OTHER

TERM	DEFINITION
11. distended (dis-TEN-ded)	stretched out (a bladder is distended when filled with urine)
12. electrolytes (ē-LEK-trō-lītz)	minerals in the body, such as sodium and potassium, that carry an electrolyte charge. Electrolyte balance is necessary for the body to function normally and is maintained by the kidneys.
13. void (voyd)	to empty or evacuate waste material, especially urine

Refer to Appendix E for pharmacology terms related to the urinary system.

EXERCISE 23 ■ Pronounce and Spell

Practice pronunciation and spelling on paper and online.

1. Practice on Paper

a. **Pronounce:** Read the phonetic spelling and say aloud the terms listed in the previous table. Refer to the pronunciation key on p. 20 as necessary.
b. **Spell:** Have a study partner read the terms aloud. Write the spelling of the terms on a separate sheet of paper.

2. Practice Online

a. **Access** online learning resources. Go to evolve.elsevier.com > Evolve Resources > Student Resources.
b. **Pronounce:** Select Audio Glossary > Chapter 6 > Exercise 23. Select a term to hear its pronunciation and repeat aloud.

c. **Spell:** Select Activities > Chapter 6 > Spell Terms > Exercise 23. Select the audio icon and type the correct spelling of the term.

❑ Check the box when complete.

EXERCISE 24 ■ Fill In

A Label

Write the medical terms pictured and defined.

1. ______________________
procedure for removing impurities from the blood because of an inability of the kidneys to do so

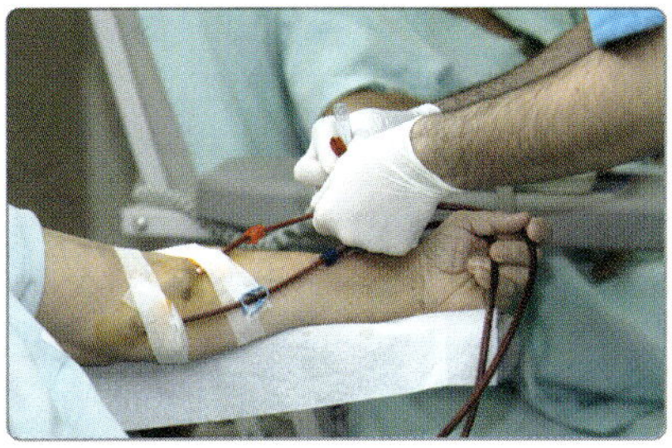

2. ______________________
flexible, tubelike device for withdrawing or instilling fluids

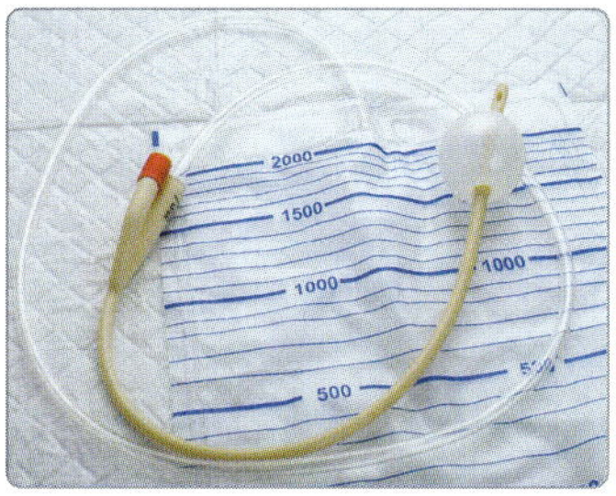

3. ______________________
stretched out

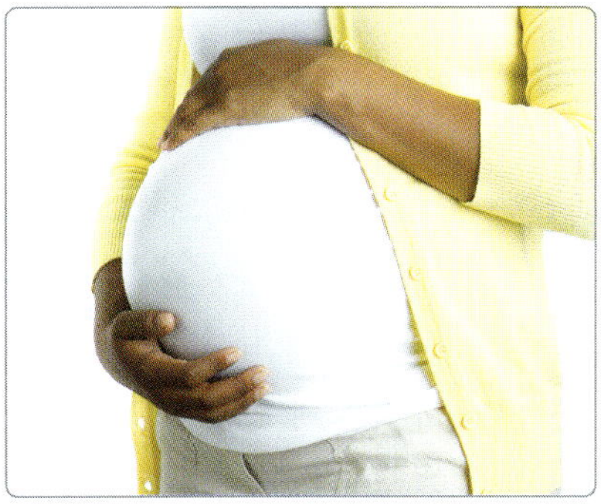

4. ______________________
involuntary urination

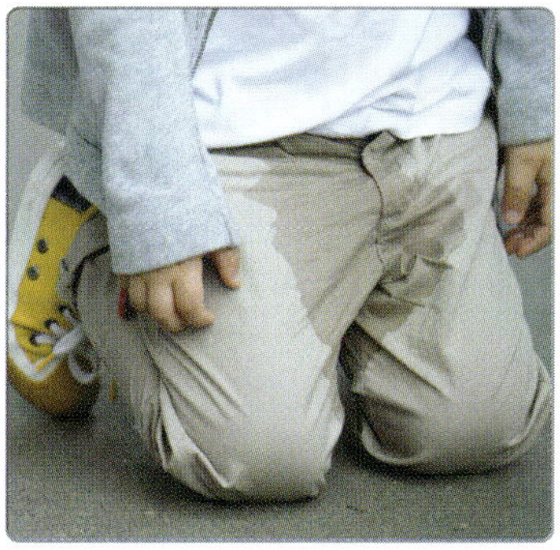

5. ______________________
receptacle for urine

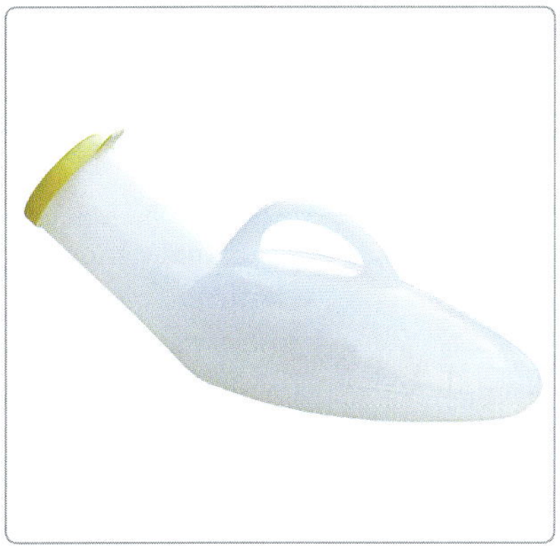

6. ______________________
procedure for removing toxic wastes when the kidney is unable to do so; uses the abdominal cavity as the fluid receptacle

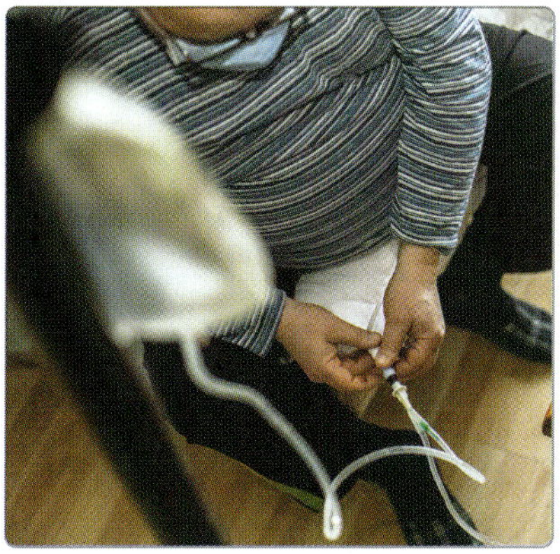

B Identify

Fill in the blanks with the correct terms.

1. Minerals in the body, such as sodium and potassium, are called ______________________________.
2. A(n) __________________________ agent promotes the formation and excretion of urine.
3. Ptosis is another name for _______________, which is displacement of an organ or anatomic structure from its normal position.
4. The inability to control the bladder, causing leaking of urine, is called ______________________________.
5. The passage of a tubelike device into the urinary bladder to withdraw urine is a(n) ___________________________.
6. To evacuate waste material, especially urine, is to _______________.
7. A(n) ____________________ is an abnormal narrowing.

EXERCISE 25 ▪ Match

A

Match the terms in the first column with their correct definitions in the second column.

______ 1. catheter	a. to evacuate or empty waste material, especially urine
______ 2. urinary catheterization	b. inability to control the bladder causing leakage of urine
______ 3. distended	c. process for removing impurities from the blood when the kidneys are unable to do so
______ 4. void	d. flexible, tubelike device for withdrawing or instilling fluids
______ 5. hemodialysis	e. stretched out
______ 6. urinary incontinence	f. passage of a tubelike device into the urinary bladder to remove urine

B

Match the terms in the first column with their correct definitions in the second column.

______ 1. prolapse	a. displacement of an organ or anatomic structure from its normal position
______ 2. peritoneal dialysis	b. receptacle for urine
______ 3. stricture	c. agent that promotes the formation and excretion of urine
______ 4. urinal	d. use of abdominal cavity to hold dialyzing fluid in the removal of toxic wastes
______ 5. enuresis	e. balance is necessary for the body to function normally
______ 6. diuretic	f. involuntary urination
______ 7. electrolytes	g. abnormal narrowing

EXERCISE 26 ▪ Review of Complementary Terms

Can you define, pronounce, and spell the following terms?

albuminuria	enuresis	nocturia	urinary
anuria	glycosuria	oliguria	urinary incontinence
azotemia	hematuria	peritoneal dialysis	urinary catheterization
catheter (cath)	hemodialysis (HD)	polyuria	urinal
distended	intravesical	prolapse	urologist
diuretic	meatal	pyuria	urology
dysuria	nephrologist	stricture	void
electrolytes	nephrology	transurethral	

Abbreviations

DISEASE AND DISORDERS

ABBREVIATION	TERM	ABBREVIATION	TERM
AKI	acute kidney injury	**OAB**	overactive bladder
ARF	acute renal failure	**PKD**	polycystic kidney disease
CKD	chronic kidney disease	**UTI**	urinary tract infection
CRF	chronic renal failure	**VUR**	vesicoureteral reflux
ESRD	end-stage renal disease		

DIAGNOSTIC

ABBREVIATION	TERM	ABBREVIATION	TERM
BUN	blood urea nitrogen	**UA**	urinalysis
KUB	kidneys ureters (and) bladder	**VCUG**	voiding cystourethrography
SG	specific gravity		

TREATMENT AND EQUIPMENT

ABBREVIATION	TERM	ABBREVIATION	TERM
cath	catheterization, catheter	**HD**	hemodialysis
ESWL	extracorporeal shock wave lithotripsy		

Refer to Appendix D for a complete list of abbreviations.

EXERCISE 27 ■ Fill In

Write the terms abbreviated.

1. When imaging is used to diagnose obstructive uropathy, a **KUB** ______________________ (and) ______________ is usually performed first. A urogram may be used for confirming or excluding obstruction and determining its level and cause. For further examination, **VCUG** ______________________ may be performed to evaluate the posterior urethra and check for **VUR** ______________________.
2. **SG** ______________________ is one of many tests performed on the urine specimen during a **UA** ______________. It measures the concentration of particles, including water and electrolytes in the urine.
3. **BUN** ______________________ is a laboratory test done on a blood sample to determine kidney function.
4. The number, size, and type of stones are important in determining if **ESWL** ______________________ is the best method for treating renal calculi.
5. Bladder **cath** ______________________ carries the risk of **UTI** ______________________.
6. Peritoneal dialysis, **HD** ______________________, and renal transplant are known as renal replacement therapies.
7. The more current term for **ARF** ______________________ is **AKI** ______________________. Onset is sudden and full recovery can occur with prompt treatment. **CKD** ______________________ is a more modern term for **CRF** ______________________. It is irreversible and progressive. **ESRD** ______________________ is when kidney function will not sustain life. A kidney transplant or dialysis may be used as treatment.
8. Urge incontinence is another name for **OAB** ______________________ and involves a sudden, strong need to urinate. As the bladder contracts, leakage of urine occurs.
9. Nephrosonography, or renal ultrasound, may be used to help diagnose **PKD**, ______________________, which is usually hereditary, and may be accompanied by renal hypertension, hematuria, or nephrolithiasis.

PRACTICAL APPLICATION

EXERCISE 28 ■ Case Study: Translate Between Everyday Language and Medical Language

CASE STUDY: Tyrone Parker

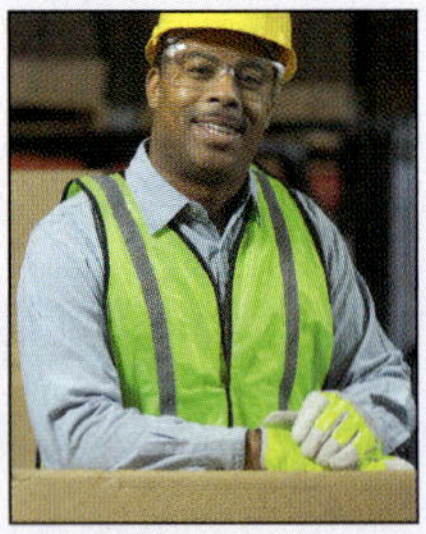

Tyrone Parker was feeling fine until about 3 days ago. He was at his job at a warehouse when he noticed pain in his back, but only on the left side. At first he thought maybe he pulled something when he was moving inventory. He took some over-the-counter pain medicine, but this didn't really seem to help. In the past when he had back pain, it got better after a night of sleep. When he woke up the next morning, the pain was worse and had spread into the lower part of his belly and his groin, still on the left side. He also noticed blood when he urinated. He was worried that he might have an infection of his bladder. He did not experience difficulty urinating but decided to make an appointment to see a physician who treats diseases of the urinary tract.

Now that you have worked through Chapter 6, on the urinary system, consider the medical terms that might be used to describe Tyrone's experience. See the Chapter at a Glance section at the end of the chapter for a list of terms that might apply.

A. *Underline phrases in the case study that could be substituted with medical terms.*

B. *Write the medical term and its definition for three of the phrases you underlined.*

MEDICAL TERM	DEFINITION
1. ____________________	______________________________
	______________________________
2. ____________________	______________________________
	______________________________
3. ____________________	______________________________
	______________________________

DOCUMENTATION: Excerpt from the Urgent Care Visit

Tyrone decided to go to Urgent Care because he could receive care right away. The following was noted in the Subjective section of the Electronic Health Record (EHR).

The patient is a 38-year-old man who was in his usual state of good health when he began to experience left-sided flank pain accompanied by gross hematuria 3 days ago. He denies chills or fever. He has no prior history of renal calculi but was treated for UTI 1 year ago. His father had end-stage renal disease requiring hemodialysis.

C. *Underline medical terms presented in Chapter 6 in the previous excerpt from Tyrone's medical record. See the Chapter at a Glance section at the end of the chapter for a complete list.*

D. *Select and define three of the medical terms you underlined. To check your answers, go to Appendix A.*

MEDICAL TERM	DEFINITION
1. ____________________	______________________________
	______________________________
2. ____________________	______________________________
	______________________________
3. ____________________	______________________________
	______________________________

EXERCISE 29 ■ Interact with Medical Documents

A

Read the report and complete it by writing medical terms on answer lines within the document. Definitions of terms to be written appear after the document.

83658 OLIVER, Bruno

File Patient Navigate Custom Fields Help

Chart Review | Encounters | Notes | Labs | Imaging | Procedures | Rx | Documents | Referrals | Scheduling | Billing

Name: **OLIVER, Bruno** MR#: **7463802** DOB: **07/30/19XX** Gender: M Age: 32 **Allergies: NKDA** **PCP:** Betsy Bathilde MD

Date of Admssion: 09/20/20XX
Date of Discharge: 09/23/20XX

Discharge Summary: Bruno Oliver is a 32-year-old male, appearing his stated age, who was admitted to the hospital after presenting to the emergency department on 09/20/20XX in acute distress. He complained of intermittent pain in the right posterior lumbar area, radiating to the right flank. He has a family history of 1. ____________________ and has been treated for this condition two other times in the past 10 years.

The white blood count, hemoglobin, and hematocrit were normal. The urinalysis showed microscopic 2. ____________________ .

This patient was admitted to the 3. ____________________ Unit and was administered intravenous morphine sulfate for pain control. VITAL SIGNS: Low-grade temperature of 99.4°F. Initial blood pressure was 146/92 mm Hg.

A 4. ______________revealed 5. ____________________ in the region of the right renal pelvis. A 6. ____________________with a right retrograde 7. __________________ confirmed the presence of the three stones in the right kidney. Significant ureteral obstruction was present.

A percutaneous 8. __________________________________ was completed with no complications. A ureteral stent was inserted as was an indwelling Foley 9. __________. Drainage from the right kidney was pale yellow in 48 hours. The Foley catheter was removed 3 days postoperatively.

At discharge, the patient is voiding without difficulty. The stones were sent to the laboratory for analysis. The report indicated that they were calcium oxalate.

The patient is to follow up with his urologist in a week to have his ureteral stent removed.

Electronically signed: Evan Landis, DO 09/23/20XX 09:18

Start | Log On/Off | Print | Edit

Definitions of Medical Terms to Complete the Document

Write the medical terms defined on corresponding answer lines in the document.

1. condition of stones in the kidney
2. blood in the urine
3. study of the urinary tract
4. radiographic image of the abdomen
5. stones
6. visual examination of the bladder
7. radiographic image of the urinary tract
8. incision into the kidney to remove a stone
9. flexible, tubelike device

EXERCISE 29 ■ Interact with Medical Documents—cont'd

B

Read the medical report and answer the questions below it.

2478 HEARNE, Allen

File Patient Navigate Custom Fields Help

Chart Review | Encounters | Notes | Labs | Imaging | Procedures | Rx | Documents | Referrals | Scheduling | Billing

Name: **HEARNE, Allen** MR#: 2478 DOB: 01/01/19XX Gender: M Age: 31 **Allergies:** None **PCP:** Frank Peterson MD

Operative Report

Preoperative diagnosis: Urinary tract obstruction
Postoperative diagnosis: Ureterolithiasis
Surgery Performed: Ureteroscopy with calculus extraction

The patient, a 31-year-old previously healthy male, presented with complaints of left flank pain, oliguria, nausea, and chills. The patient denied gross hematuria. CT urogram revealed presence of a left proximal ureteral stone.

Procedure: Anesthesia was induced and the patient was then placed in the dorsal lithotomy position. The area was draped and prepared in the standard manner, 30 mL of topical anesthesia (1% Lidocaine) was administered, and a penile clamp was applied to ensure retention. The ureteroscope was inserted, with access to the middle third of the ureter gained by passing a guidewire under fluoroscopic control. The guidewire was advanced beyond the stone, and the calculus was delivered through the ureter, engaged in a retrieval basket, and removed. The patient tolerated the procedure well and left the operating room in good condition.

Electronically signed: Martina Blancartt, MD 05/21/20XX 15:37

Start | Log On/Off | Print | Edit

Use the medical report above to answer the questions.

1. The patient presented with a complaint of
   a. difficult or painful urination.
   b. excessive urine.
   c. scanty urine.
   d. pus in the urine.
2. The presence of a ureteral stone was revealed by
   a. radiographic imaging.
   b. magnetic resonance imaging.
   c. ultrasound.
   d. computed tomography.
3. T F More than one stone was removed from the ureter.
4. Ureteroscope and ureteral are terms not included in the chapter. Using your knowledge of the meaning of word parts, define these terms.
   a. ureteral ______________________
   b. ureteroscope ______________________
   ____

EXERCISE 30 ■ Use Medical Language in Online Electronic Health Records

Select the correct medical terms to complete three medical records in one patient's electronic file.

Access online resources at evolve.elsevier.com > Evolve Resources > Student Resources > Activities > Chapter 6 > Electronic Health Records

Topic: Renal Calculus
Record 1: Office Visit
Record 2: Operative Report
Record 3: Post-Operative Office Visit

❑ Check the box when complete.

EXERCISE 31 ■ Pronounce Medical Terms in Use

Practice pronunciation of terms by reading aloud the following paragraph. Use the phonetic spellings to assist with pronunciation. The script also contains medical terms not presented in the chapter. If interested, research their meanings in a medical dictionary or a reliable online source.

A 76-year-old woman consulted with her primary care physician because of **hematuria** (*hēm*-a-TŪ-rē-a) and **dysuria** (dis-Ū-rē-a). She was referred to a **urologist** (ū-ROL-o-jist). **Urinalysis** (ū-rin-AL-is-is) disclosed 1+ albumin and mild **pyuria** (pī-Ū-rē-a) in addition to the hematuria. A spiral CT scan was obtained. Mild **nephrolithiasis** (*nef*-rō-lith-Ī-a-sis) was observed but no **hydronephrosis** (*hī*-drō-ne-FRŌ-sis). Finally a **cystoscopy** (sis-TOS-ko-pē) was performed, which showed mild **cystitis** (sis-TĪ-tis). A **urinary tract infection** (Ū-rin-*ār*-ē) (trakt) (in-FEK-shun) was diagnosed and the patient responded favorably to antibiotics. The urologist did not advise **lithotripsy** (LITH-ō-trip-sē) for the **renal calculi** (RĒ-nal) (KAL-kū-lī).

CHAPTER REVIEW

EXERCISE 32 ■ Chapter Content Quiz

Test your understanding of terms and abbreviations introduced in this chapter. Circle the letter for the medical term or abbreviation related to the words in italics.

1. The patient was diagnosed with a *drooping kidney*, or:
   a. nephromegaly
   b. nephroblastoma
   c. nephroptosis
2. The patient's radiographic image showed *condition of stones in the ureter*, or a condition known as:
   a. ureterocele
   b. ureterolithiasis
   c. ureterostenosis
3. The patient was scheduled for a right ureteral pelvic junction *ESWL*, a surgical procedure to:
   a. separate tissue
   b. create an artificial opening
   c. remove a stone
4. The physician first suspected diabetes when told of the *excessive amounts of urine* voided, or:
   a. oliguria
   b. polyuria
   c. dysuria
5. The urologist told the patient with the drooping kidney that it is necessary to *secure the kidney in place* by performing a:
   a. nephropexy
   b. nephrolysis
   c. nephrolithotripsy
6. The patient had a *sudden stoppage of urine formation*, or:
   a. urinary suppression
   b. urinary retention
   c. azotemia
7. The patient was scheduled for a *radiographic image of the urinary bladder*, or:
   a. cystoscopy
   b. cystogram
   c. cystography
8. The patient's mother informed the doctor of her son's *involuntary urination*, or:
   a. diuresis
   b. dysuria
   c. enuresis
9. The patient presented with a(n) *abnormal accumulation of urine in the bladder because of an inability to urinate*, or:
   a. polycystic kidney disease
   b. urinary retention
   c. urinary tract infection
10. The nurse practitioner ordered a *UA* on the patient or:
    a. urine
    b. urinary
    c. urinalysis

11. *Albuminuria* indicates a kidney problem because of albumin in the:
    a. blood
    b. urine
    c. urea
12. In the term nephrolithotripsy, *which word part indicates surgery?*
    a. first combining form
    b. second combining form
    c. suffix
13. When the bladder is *stretched out* because of urine, it is considered to be:
    a. distended
    b. contracted
    c. flexible
14. *Peritoneal dialysis* is the procedure for removing which of the following when the kidney cannot do so?
    a. urine
    b. toxic waste
    c. nitrogen
15. A ureteral *stricture* means the ureter is:
    a. ballooning
    b. narrowing
    c. blocked
16. The patient with *urine* (urea nitrogen) *in the blood* presented with polyuria, polydipsia, vomiting, and weight loss.
    a. azotemia
    b. hematuria
    c. uremia
17. A *creation of an artificial opening into the urinary system* was required for the patient who had a cystectomy due to carcinoma of the bladder.
    a. urostomy
    b. ureterostomy
    c. urethroplasty
18. Two types of *inability to control the bladder causing leakage of urine* are stress, caused by sneezing, coughing, or bearing down, and urge, which results when patients have to rush to get to the bathroom.
    a. urinary incontinence
    b. stricture
    c. prolapse
19. A(n) *pertaining to within the (urinary) bladder treatment* with mitomycin may be used to treat bladder cancer.
    a. meatal
    b. transurethral
    c. intravesical
20. Furosemide is a common *agent that promotes the formation and excretion of urine* that is used to treat edema and congestive heart failure.
    a. urinary catheterization
    b. diuretic
    c. peritoneal dialysis

CHAPTER AT A GLANCE Word Parts New to This Chapter

COMBINING FORMS

albumin/o
azot/o
blast/o
cyst/o
glomerul/o
glycos/o
hydr/o
lith/o
meat/o
nephr/o
noct/i
olig/o
pyel/o
ren/o
ur/o
ureter/o
urethr/o
urin/o
vesic/o

SUFFIXES

-iasis
-lith
-lysis
-pexy
-ptosis
-tripsy
-uria

CHAPTER AT A GLANCE Urinary System Terms Built from Word Parts

DISEASE AND DISORDER

cystitis
cystocele
cystolith
glomerulonephritis
hydronephrosis
nephritis
nephroblastoma
nephrolithiasis
nephroma
nephromegaly
nephroptosis
pyelitis
pyelonephritis
uremia
ureteritis
ureterocele
ureterolithiasis
urethritis
ureterostenosis
urethrocystitis
vesicoureteral reflux (VUR)

SURGICAL

cystectomy
cystolithotomy
cystostomy
lithotripsy
meatotomy
nephrectomy
nephrolithotomy
nephrolithotripsy
nephrolysis
nephropexy
nephrostomy
pyelolithotomy
pyeloplasty
ureterectomy
ureterostomy
urethroplasty
urostomy
vesicourethral suspension

DIAGNOSTIC

cystogram
cystography
cystoscope
cystoscopy
nephroscopy
nephrosonography
renogram
retrograde urogram
ureteroscopy
urogram
voiding cystourethrography (VCUG)

COMPLEMENTARY

albuminuria
anuria
azotemia
dysuria
glycosuria
hematuria
intravesical
meatal
nephrologist
nephrology
nocturia
oliguria
polyuria
pyuria
transurethral
urinary
urologist
urology

CHAPTER AT A GLANCE Urinary System Terms *NOT* Built from Word Parts

DISEASE AND DISORDER

acute kidney injury (AKI)
chronic kidney disease (CKD)
end-stage renal disease (ESRD)
epispadias
hypospadias
polycystic kidney disease (PKD)
renal calculus (*pl.* calculi)
renal hypertension
urinary retention
urinary suppression
urinary tract infection (UTI)

SURGICAL

extracorporeal shock wave lithotripsy (ESWL)
fulguration
renal transplant

DIAGNOSTIC

blood urea nitrogen (BUN)
creatinine
KUB
specific gravity (SG)
urinalysis (UA)
urine culture and sensitivity
urodynamics

COMPLEMENTARY

catheter (cath)
distended
diuretic
electrolytes
enuresis
hemodialysis (HD)
peritoneal dialysis
prolapse
stricture
urinal
urinary catheterization
urinary incontinence
void

Chapter 7

Male Reproductive System

Objectives

Upon completion of this chapter, you will be able to:

1. Pronounce organs and anatomic structures of the male reproductive system.
2. Define and spell word parts related to the male reproductive system.
3. Define, pronounce, and spell disease and disorder terms related to the male reproductive system.
4. Define, pronounce, and spell surgical terms related to the male reproductive system.
5. Define, pronounce, and spell diagnostic terms related to the male reproductive system.
6. Define, pronounce, and spell complementary terms related to the male reproductive system.
7. Interpret the meaning of abbreviations related to the male reproductive system.
8. Apply medical language in clinical contexts.

Outline

ANATOMY

The organs of the male reproductive system include external genitalia and internal structures (Fig. 7.1). The male external genitalia include the penis and scrotum, which contains the testes and an initial section of each vas deferens. Internal structures, located within the male pelvis, include a major portion of each vas deferens, the seminal vesicles, and the prostate gland. The penis and urethra are shared with the urinary system.

Function

The function of the male reproductive system is to produce, sustain, and transport sperm, the male reproductive germ cells, and to secrete the hormone testosterone (Fig. 7.2).

Organs and Anatomic Structures of the Male Reproductive System

TERM	DEFINITION
testis (*pl.* testes) (TES-tis), (TES-tēs)	primary male sex organ, paired, oval-shaped, and enclosed in a sac called the **scrotum**. The testes produce spermatozoa (sperm cells) and the hormone testosterone. (also called **testicle**)
seminiferous tubules (*sem*-i-NIF-er-es) (TOO-bū-elz)	approximately 900 coiled tubes within the testes in which spermatogenesis occurs
sperm (spurm)	the microscopic male germ cell, which, when united with the ovum, produces a zygote (fertilized egg) that with subsequent development becomes an embryo (also called **spermatozoon, *pl.* spermatozoa**) (Fig. 7.2)
testosterone (tes-TOS-te-rōn)	the principal male sex hormone. Its chief function is to stimulate the development of the male reproductive organs and secondary sex characteristics such as facial hair.
epididymis (*pl.* epididymides) (*ep*-i-DID-a-mis) (*ep*-i-DID-i-mē-dēz)	coiled tube attached to each testis that provides for storage, transit, and maturation of sperm; continuous with each vas deferens

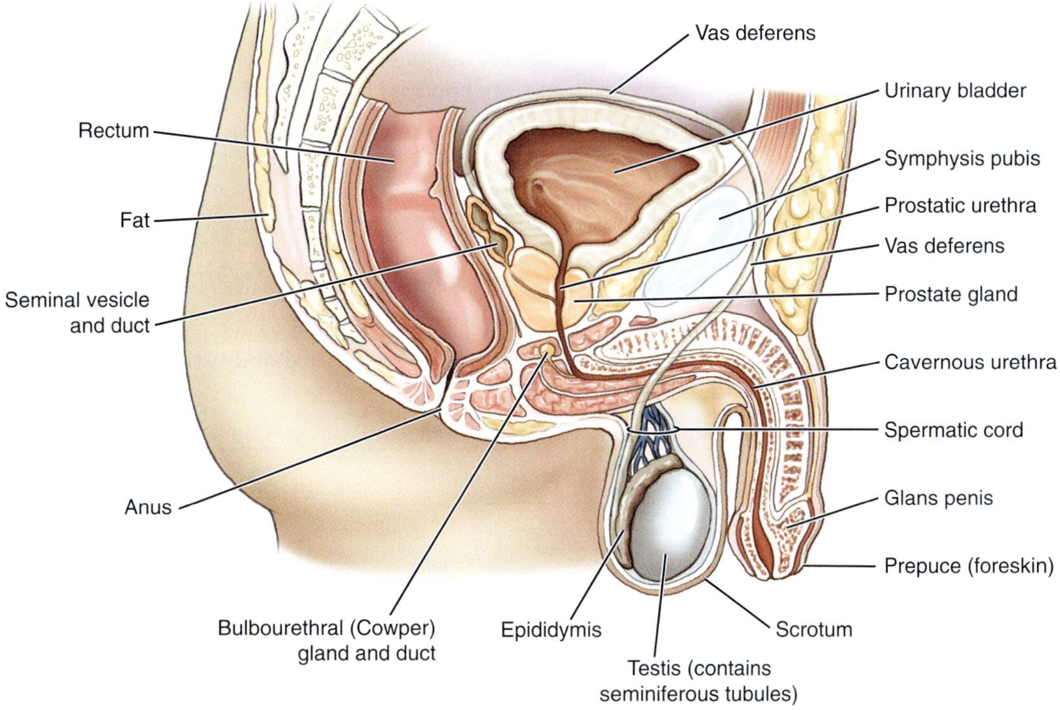

FIG. 7.1 Male reproductive organs and associated structures.

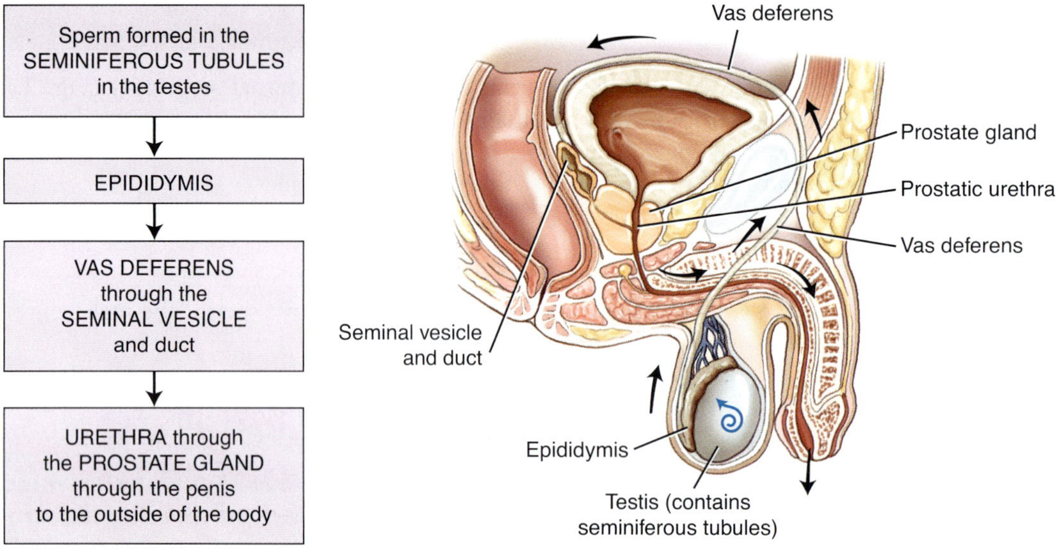

FIG. 7.2 Origination and transportation of sperm.

TERM	DEFINITION
vas deferens (vas) (DEF-ar-enz)	duct (tube) carrying the sperm from the epididymis to the urethra. The **spermatic cord** encloses each vas deferens with nerves, lymphatics, arteries, and veins. The urethra also connects with the urinary bladder and carries urine outside the body. A circular muscle constricts during intercourse to prevent urination. (also called **ductus deferens**)
seminal vesicles (SEM-e-nel) (VES-i-kelz)	two accessory glands located posterior to the base of the bladder that open into the vas deferens. The glands secrete a thick fluid that forms part of the semen.
prostate gland (PROS-tāt) (gland)	walnut-shaped gland that encircles the proximal section of the urethra. The prostate gland secretes a fluid that aids in the movement of the sperm and ejaculation.
PROSTATE is derived from the Greek **pro**, meaning **before**, and **statis**, meaning **standing** or **sitting**. Anatomically it is the gland standing before the bladder.	
semen (SĒ-men)	composed of sperm, seminal fluids, and other secretions
scrotum (SKRŌ-tem)	sac containing the testes and their corresponding epididymides, from which each vas deferens begins. The scrotum is suspended on both sides of and posterior to the penis.
penis (PĒ-nis)	male organ of urination and coitus (sexual intercourse)
glans penis (glanz) (PĒ-nis)	enlarged tip on the end of the penis
prepuce (PRE-pūs)	fold of skin covering the glans penis in uncircumcised males (foreskin of the penis)
genitalia (*jen*-i-TĀ-lē-a)	reproductive organs (male or female); includes internal and external reproductive organs (also called **genitals**)
gonads (GŌ-nadz)	primary reproductive organs; testes in males, ovaries in females

PRONOUNCE ANATOMIC STRUCTURES

Practice saying aloud each of the organs and specific structures on the previous pages.

To hear the terms, go to Evolve Resources at www.evolve.elsevier.com and select:
Student Resources > Audio Glossary > Chapter 7 > **Anatomic Structures**

❑ Check the box when complete.

WORD PARTS

Use paper flashcards or electronic flashcards on Evolve to memorize word parts used to analyze, define, and build medical terms in this chapter. To reinforce learning, study one section of the Word Parts Table at a time, then complete the corresponding exercise on the following pages.

1 ■ Male Reproductive System Combining Forms

COMBINING FORM	DEFINITION	COMBINING FORM	DEFINITION
andr/o	male	**prostat/o**	prostate gland
balan/o	glans penis	**sperm/o**	sperm, spermatozoon (*pl.* spermatozoa)
epididym/o	epididymis	**spermat/o**	sperm, spermatozoon (*pl.* spermatozoa)
orch/o	testis, testicle	**vas/o**	vessel, duct (vas deferens in terms describing the male reproductive system)
orchi/o	testis, testicle	**vesicul/o**	seminal vesicle(s)
orchid/o	testis, testicle		

2 ■ Combining Forms Used with Male Reproductive System Terms

COMBINING FORM	DEFINITION	COMBINING FORM	DEFINITION
cyst/o	bladder, sac	**lith/o**	stone(s), calculus (*pl.* calculi)
crypt/o	hidden	**olig/o**	scanty, few

3 ■ Prefixes

PREFIX	DEFINITION	PREFIX	DEFINITION
a-	absence of, without	**hyper-**	above, excessive
an-	absence of, without		

4 ■ Suffixes

SUFFIX	DEFINITION	SUFFIX	DEFINITION
-algia	pain	**-tomy**	cut into, incision
-ectomy	excision, surgical removal	**-pexy**	surgical fixation
-ia	diseased or abnormal state, condition of	**-pathy**	disease
-ic	pertaining to	**-plasia**	condition of formation, development, growth
-ism	state of	**-plasty**	surgical repair
-itis	inflammation	**-rrhea**	flow, discharge
-lith	stone(s), calculus (*pl.* calculi)	**-stomy**	creation of an artificial opening

Refer to **Appendix B** and **Appendix C** for alphabetized word parts and their meanings.

EXERCISE 1 ■ Male Reproductive System Combining Forms

Refer to the first section of the Word Parts Table.

A Label

Fill in the blanks with combining forms for this diagram of the male reproductive system. *To check your answers, go to Appendix A.*

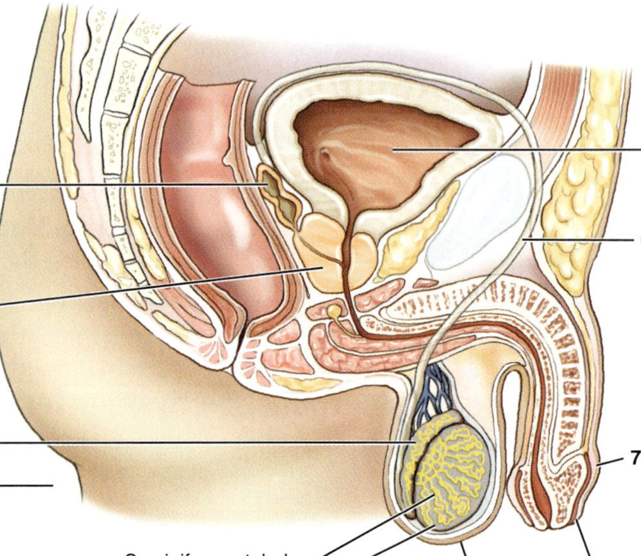

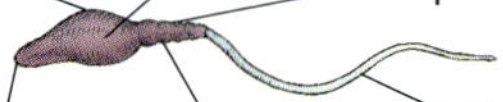

B Define and Match

Step 1: Write the definitions after the following combining forms.
Step 2: Match the descriptions on the right with the combining forms and definitions. Answers may be used more than once; no answer line appears for those not described in a lettered item.

_____ 1. sperm/o, ____________________

_____ 2. vas/o (vas deferens), ____________________

_____ 3. spermat/o, ____________________

_____ 4. balan/o, ____________________

_____ 5. prostat/o, ____________________

_____ 6. orch/o, ____________________

_____ 7. vesicul/o, ____________________

_____ 8. orchi/o, ____________________

_____ 9. epididym/o, ____________________

_____ 10. orchid/o, ____________________

11. andr/o, ____________________

a. duct (tube) carrying the sperm from the epididymis to the urethra
b. enlarged tip on the end of the penis
c. two accessory glands located posterior to the base of the bladder that open into the vas deferens
d. primary male sex organ, paired, oval-shaped, and enclosed in a sac
e. coiled tube attached to each testis that provides for storage, transit, and maturation of sperm
f. walnut-sized gland that encircles a proximal section of the urethra; secretes fluid that aids in the movement of the sperm and ejaculation
g. microscopic male germ cell, which, when united with the ovum, produces a zygote

EXERCISE 2 ■ Combining Forms Used with Male Reproductive System Terms

Refer to the second section of the Word Parts Table.

A Define

Write the definitions of the following combining forms.

1. olig/o ______________________
2. crypt/o ______________________
3. lith/o ______________________
4. cyst/o ______________________

B Identify

Write the combining forms for the following definitions.

1. stone(s), calculus (*pl.* calculi) ______________________
2. bladder, sac ______________________
3. hidden ______________________
4. scanty, few ______________________

EXERCISE 3 ■ Prefixes

Refer to the third section of the Word Parts Table.

A Identify

Write the prefixes for the following definitions.

1. absence of, without a. ______________________
   b. ______________________
2. above, excessive ______________________

B Define

Write the definitions of the following prefixes.

1. hyper- ______________________
2. an- ______________________
3. a- ______________________

EXERCISE 4 ■ Suffixes

Refer to the fourth section of the Word Parts Table.

A Match

Match the suffixes in the first column with the correct definitions in the second column. A definition may be used more than once.

______	1. -plasia	a. flow, discharge
______	2. -algia	b. cut into, incision
______	3. -ia	c. disease
______	4. -tomy	d. condition of formation, development, growth
______	5. -rrhea	e. pertaining to
______	6. -ic	f. diseased or abnormal state, condition of
______	7. -pathy	g. pain

B Match

Match the suffixes in the first column with the correct definitions in the second column. A definition may be used more than once.

______	1. -stomy	a. surgical repair
______	2. -ectomy	b. stone(s), calculus (*pl.* calculi)
______	3. -pexy	c. surgical fixation
______	4. -itis	d. state of
______	5. -plasty	e. inflammation
______	6. -ism	f. excision, surgical removal
______	7. -lith	g. creation of an artificial opening

MEDICAL TERMS

Medical terms relevant to this chapter have been grouped by topics, such as Disease and Disorder, and are listed in tables designated as Built from Word Parts or *NOT* Built from Word Parts. The exercises following each table assist with learning term definitions, pronunciations, and spellings.

Disease and Disorder Terms

BUILT FROM WORD PARTS

The following terms can be translated using definitions of word parts. Further explanation is provided within parentheses as needed.

TERM	DEFINITION
1. **andropathy** (an-DROP-a-thē)	disease of the male (specific to the male, such as orchitis)
2. **anorchism** (an-OR-kizm)	state of absence of testis (unilateral or bilateral)
3. **balanitis** (*bal*-a-NĪ-tis)	inflammation of the glans penis
4. **balanorrhea** (*bal*-a-nō-RĒ-a)	discharge from the glans penis
5. **benign prostatic hyperplasia (BPH)** (be-NĪN) (pros-TAT-ik) (*hī*-per-PLĀ-zha)	excessive development pertaining to the prostate gland (non-malignant enlargement of the prostate gland; causes narrowing of the urethra, which interferes with the passage of urine. Symptoms include frequency of urination, nocturia, urinary retention, and incomplete emptying of the bladder.) (also called **benign prostatic hypertrophy**) (Fig. 7.3)
6. **cryptorchidism** (krip-TOR-ki-*diz*-em)	state of hidden testis (during fetal development, testes are located in the abdominal area near the kidneys. Before birth they move down into the scrotal sac. Failure of one or both of the testes to descend from the abdominal cavity into the scrotum before birth results in cryptorchidism.) (also called **undescended testicle** and **undescended testicles**) (Fig. 7.4)
7. **epididymitis** (*ep*-i-*did*-i-MĪ-tis)	inflammation of the epididymis
8. **orchiepididymitis** (*or*-kē-*ep*-i-*did*-i-MĪ-tis)	inflammation of the testis and the epididymis
9. **orchitis** (or-KĪ-tis)	inflammation of the testis (also called **orchiditis**)
10. **prostatitis** (*pros*-ta-TĪ-tis)	inflammation of the prostate gland
11. **prostatocystitis** (*pros*-ta-tō-sis-TĪ-tis)	inflammation of the prostate gland and the (urinary) bladder
12. **prostatolith** (pros-TAT-ō-lith)	stone(s) in the prostate gland

PROSTATIC HYPERPLASIA refers to tissue changes resulting from an abnormal increase in the number of cells as may occur with age. While **benign prostatic hyperplasia** is the correct term for the pathologic process, **benign prostatic hypertrophy** is sometimes used to describe this condition.

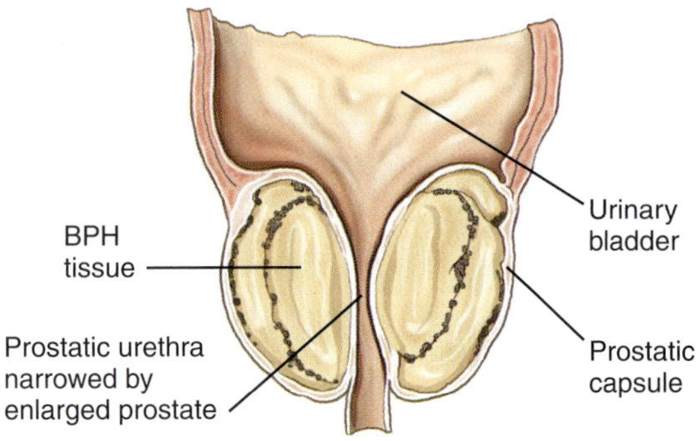

FIG. 7.3 Benign prostatic hyperplasia grows inward, causing narrowing of the urethra.

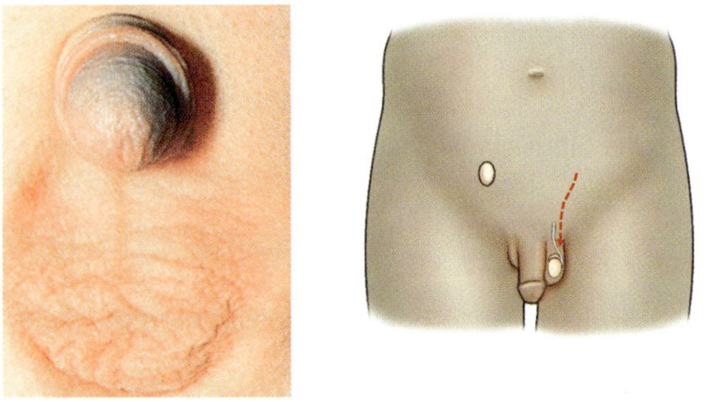

FIG. 7.4 A, Bilateral cryptorchidism. **B,** The arrow indicates the descent of the testis into the scrotal sac, which occurs before birth.

TERM	DEFINITION	TERM	DEFINITION
13. prostatorrhea (*pros*-ta-tō-RĒ-a)	discharge from the prostate gland	**14. prostatovesiculitis** (*pros*-ta-tō-ves-*ik*-ū-LĪ-tis)	inflammation of the prostate gland and the seminal vesicles

EXERCISE 5 ■ Pronounce and Spell

Practice pronunciation and spelling on paper and online.

1. Practice on Paper

a. **Pronounce:** Read the phonetic spelling and say aloud the terms listed in the previous table. Refer to the pronunciation key on p. 20 as necessary.
b. **Spell:** Have a study partner read the terms aloud. Write the spelling of the terms on a separate sheet of paper.

2. Practice Online

a. **Access** online learning resources. Go to evolve.elsevier.com > Evolve Resources > Student Resources.
b. **Pronounce:** Select Audio Glossary > Chapter 7 > Exercise 5. Select a term to hear its pronunciation and repeat aloud.
c. **Spell:** Select Activities > Chapter 7 > Spell Terms > Exercise 5. Select the audio icon and type the correct spelling of the term.

❑ Check the box when complete.

EXERCISE 6 ■ Analyze and Define

Analyze and define the following terms by drawing slashes between word parts, writing word part abbreviations above the term, underlining combining forms, and writing combining form abbreviations below the term.

1. prostatolith
____
____

2. balanitis
____
____

3. orchitis
____
____

4. prostatovesiculitis
____
____

5. prostatocystitis
____
____

6. orchiepididymitis
____
____

7. prostatorrhea
____
____

8. epididymitis
____
____

9. (benign) prostatic hyperplasia
____
____

10. cryptorchidism
____
____

11. balanorrhea

____

____

12. prostatitis

____

____

13. anorchism

____

____

14. andropathy

____

____

EXERCISE 7 ■ Build

A Label

Build terms pictured by writing word parts above definitions.

1.

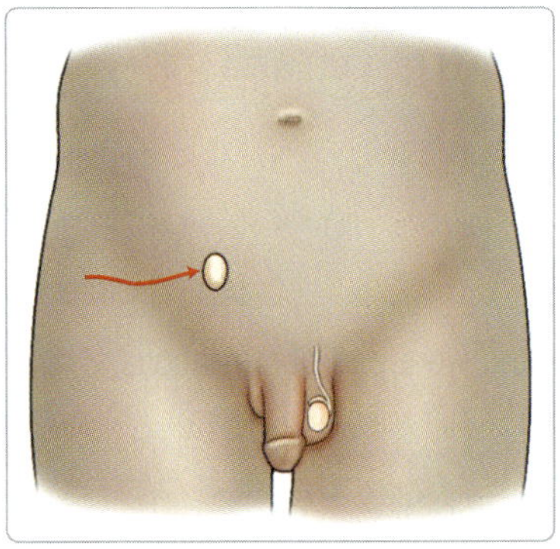

_______ / _______ / _______
hidden testis state of

2.

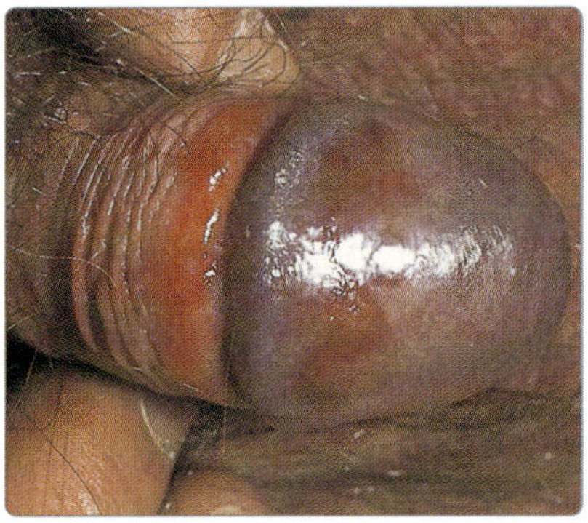

_______ / _______
glans penis inflammation

3.

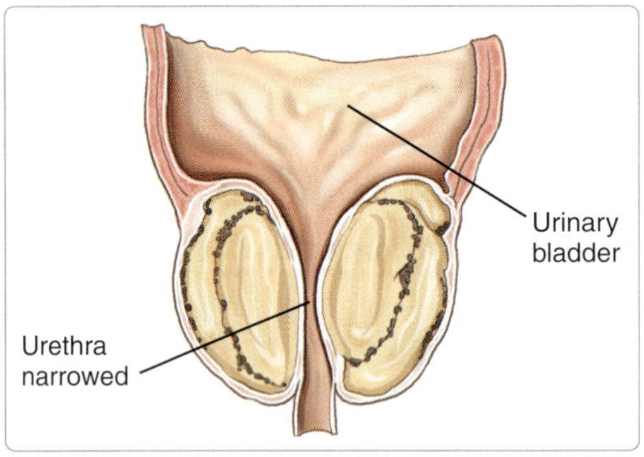

benign _______ / _______ _______ / _______
prostate pertaining to excessive development

B Fill In

Build disease and disorder terms for the following definitions with the word parts you have learned.

EXAMPLE: inflammation of the glans penis balan / itis (WR / S)

1. inflammation of the prostate gland and the (urinary) bladder ______ WR / CV / WR / S
2. stone(s) in the prostate gland ______ WR / CV / S
3. inflammation of the testis ______ WR / S
4. inflammation of the epididymis ______ WR / S
5. discharge from the prostate gland ______ WR / CV / S
6. inflammation of the prostate gland and the seminal vesicles ______ WR / CV / WR / S
7. state of absence of testis ______ P / WR / S
8. inflammation of the prostate gland ______ WR / S
9. inflammation of the testis and the epididymis ______ WR / WR / S
10. discharge from the glans penis ______ WR / CV / S
11. disease of the male ______ WR / CV / S

Disease and Disorder Terms

NOT BUILT FROM WORD PARTS

Word parts may be present in the following terms; however, their full meanings cannot be translated using definitions of word parts alone.

TERM	DEFINITION
1. erectile dysfunction (ED) (e-REK-tīl) (dis-FUNK-shun)	the inability of the male to attain or maintain an erection sufficient to perform sexual intercourse (formerly called **impotence**)

ERECTILE DYSFUNCTION (ED) Oral therapies, such as sildenafil, vardenafil, tadalafil, and avanafil are currently first-line treatment for erectile dysfunction and work by increasing the flow of blood in the genital area. Second-line treatment includes penile self-injectable drugs and vacuum devices. Surgical implantation of a penile prosthesis may be considered when other treatments are not effective.

Disease and Disorder Terms—cont'd

NOT BUILT FROM WORD PARTS

TERM	DEFINITION
2. **hydrocele** (HĪ-drō-sēl)	fluid-filled sac around the testicle; causes scrotal swelling
3. **infertility** (*in*-fer-TIL-i-tē)	reduced or absent ability to achieve pregnancy; generally defined after one year of frequent, unprotected sexual intercourse; may relate to male or female
4. **phimosis** (fī-MŌ-sis)	tightness of the prepuce (foreskin of the penis) that prevents its retraction over the glans penis; it may be congenital or a result of balanitis. Circumcision is the usual treatment.
5. **priapism** (PRĪ-a-*piz*-m)	persistent abnormal erection of the penis accompanied by pain and tenderness
6. **prostate cancer** (PROS-tāt) (KAN-cer)	cancer of the prostate gland, usually occurring in men middle-aged and older (Table 7.1)
7. **spermatocele** (SPER-ma-tō-sēl)	distention of the epididymis containing an abnormal cyst-like collection of fluid and sperm cells; may cause scrotal swelling
8. **testicular cancer** (tes-TIK-ū-ler) (KAN-cer)	cancer of the testicle, usually occurring in men 15 to 35 years of age

TABLE 7.1 Prostate Cancer

Prostate cancer is the most commonly diagnosed cancer in men and the second most common cause of cancer death among men in the United States. Approximately 95% of all cancers of the prostate are adenocarcinomas, arising from epithelial cells.

DIAGNOSTIC AND STAGING PROCEDURES

1. Digital rectal examination (DRE)
2. Prostate-specific antigen (PSA)
3. Transrectal ultrasound (TRUS)
4. Transrectal ultrasonically guided biopsy
5. MRI ultrasound fusion biopsy
6. MRI with endorectal surface coil (used for staging, not diagnosis)
7. Multiparametric MRI (used for staging, not diagnosis)

TREATMENT

Treatment depends on the stage of the prostate cancer, the age of the patient, and the choices of therapy by the patient and his physician. Options include the following:

1. Active Surveillance, with the intent to pursue active therapy if the disease progresses. Used in the earliest stages of cancer, or for men who are much older or have other serious health problems.
2. Radiation therapy, which may be performed with an external beam or with radioactive seeds (brachytherapy). It may be used in all stages of prostate cancer and is often combined with other therapies, especially in more advanced stages.
3. Radical Prostatectomy, which may be performed as an open surgery, laparoscopically, or with the use of robotic-assisted devices. Used in all stages of prostate cancer; in later stages, removal of the pelvic lymph nodes is also performed.
4. Hormonal therapy, to reduce the production of testosterone, which fuels the growth of prostate cancer. May be accomplished with medications or with surgical orchiectomy (castration). Used mainly in later stages.
5. Chemotherapy, treating cancer with drugs. Used mainly in later stages.
6. Treatments used for prostate cancer that returns (recurrence) or doesn't respond to other therapies include **cryotherapy**, the use of very cold temperatures to freeze and kill prostate cells, and **immunotherapy**, which helps boost the body's response to the cancer cells.

TABLE 7.1 Prostate Cancer—cont'd

PROGRESSION OF PROSTATE CANCER

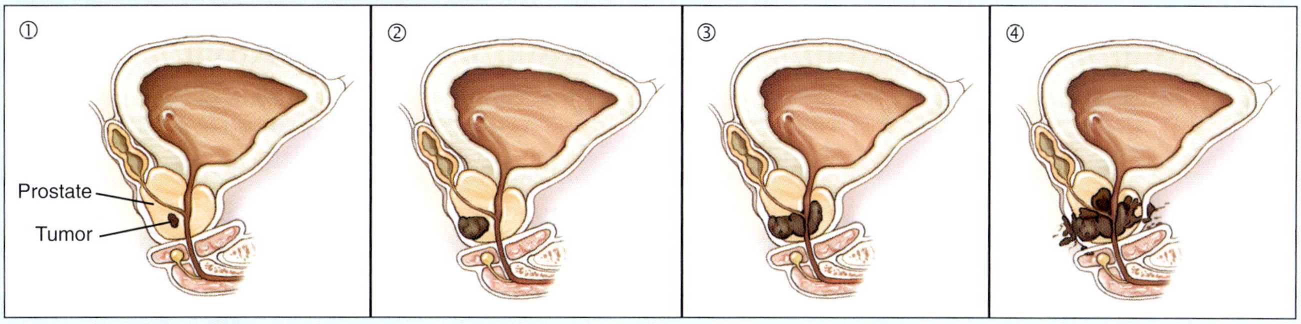

TERM	DEFINITION
9. testicular torsion (tes-TIK-ū-ler) (TOR-shun)	twisting of the spermatic cord causing decreased blood flow to the testis; occurs most often during puberty and often presents with a sudden onset of severe testicular or scrotal pain. Because of lack of blood flow to the testis, it is considered a surgical emergency.
10. varicocele (VAR-i-kō-*sēl*)	enlarged veins of the spermatic cord; may cause scrotal swelling

EXERCISE 8 ■ Pronounce and Spell

Practice pronunciation and spelling on paper and online.

1. Practice on Paper

a. **Pronounce:** Read the phonetic spelling and say aloud the terms listed in the previous table. Refer to the pronunciation key on p. 20 as necessary.
b. **Spell:** Have a study partner read the terms aloud. Write the spelling of the terms on a separate sheet of paper.

2. Practice Online

a. **Access** online learning resources. Go to evolve.elsevier.com > Evolve Resources > Student Resources.
b. **Pronounce:** Select Audio Glossary > Chapter 7 > Exercise 8. Select a term to hear its pronunciation and repeat aloud.
c. **Spell:** Select Activities > Chapter 7 > Spell Terms > Exercise 8. Select the audio icon and type the correct spelling of the term.

❑ Check the box when complete.

EXERCISE 9 ■ Fill In

A Identify

Fill in the blanks with the correct terms.

1. Another way of referring to cancer of the testicle is ____________________.
2. Inability to attain or maintain an erection is called ____________________.
3. Persistent abnormal erection is called ____________________.
4. ____________________ is the twisting of the spermatic cord causing decreased blood flow.
5. Distention of the epididymis containing an abnormal cyst-like collection of fluid and sperm cells is called a(n) ____________________.
6. ____________________ is the reduced or absent ability to achieve pregnancy, generally after one year of unprotected sexual intercourse.

B Label

Write the medical terms pictured and defined.

1. ______________________________
cancer of the prostate gland

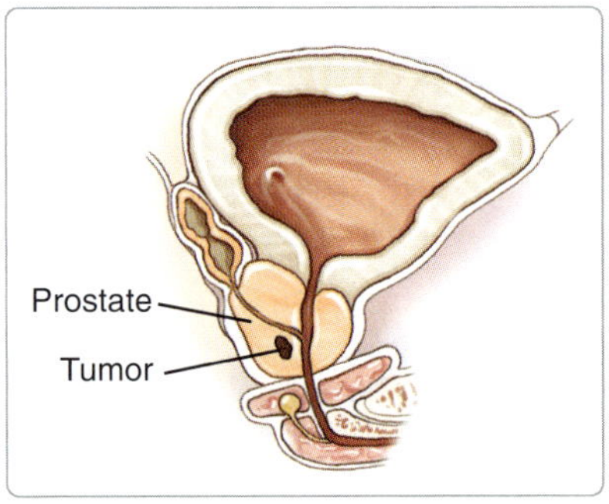

2. ______________________________
tightness of the prepuce (foreskin of the penis) that prevents its retraction over the glans penis

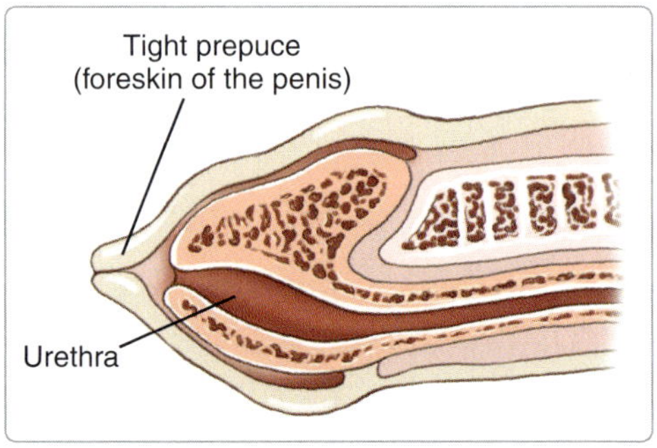

3. ______________________________
fluid-filled sac around the testicle; causes scrotal swelling

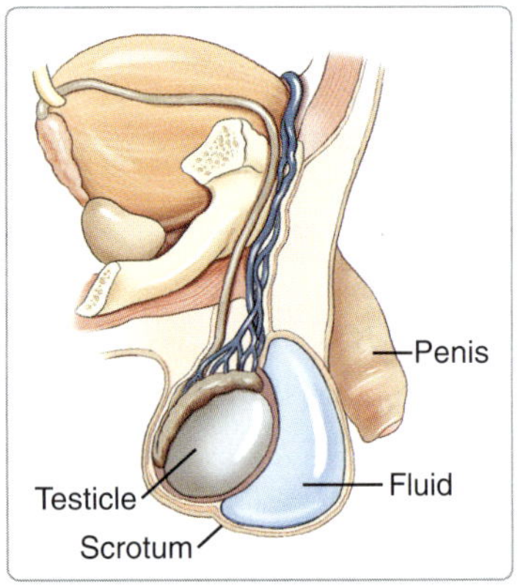

4. ______________________________
enlarged veins of the spermatic cord

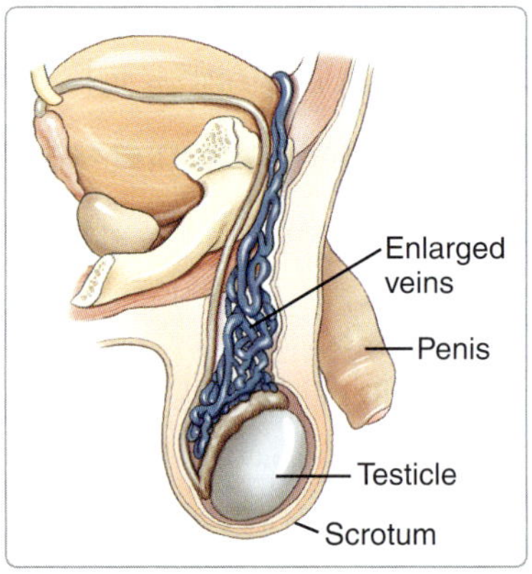

EXERCISE 10 ■ Match

Match the terms in the first column with the correct definitions in the second column.

_____ 1. varicocele	a. reduced or absent ability to achieve pregnancy
_____ 2. phimosis	b. inability to attain or maintain an erection
_____ 3. testicular cancer	c. tightness of the prepuce
_____ 4. erectile dysfunction	d. enlarged veins of the spermatic cord; may cause scrotal swelling
_____ 5. hydrocele	e. cancer of the testicle
_____ 6. prostate cancer	f. cancer of the prostate gland
_____ 7. testicular torsion	g. distention of the epididymis containing an abnormal cyst-like collection of fluid and sperm cells
_____ 8. priapism	h. persistent abnormal erection
_____ 9. spermatocele	i. twisting of the spermatic cord causing decreased blood flow
_____ 10. infertility	j. fluid-filled sac around the testicle; causes scrotal swelling

EXERCISE 11 ■ Review of Disease and Disorder Terms

Can you define, pronounce, and spell the following terms?

andropathy	epididymitis	phimosis	prostatovesiculitis
anorchism	erectile dysfunction (ED)	priapism	spermatocele
balanitis	hydrocele	prostate cancer	testicular cancer
balanorrhea	infertility	prostatitis	testicular torsion
benign prostatic hyperplasia (BPH)	orchiepididymitis	prostatocystitis	varicocele
cryptorchidism	orchitis	prostatolith	
		prostatorrhea	

Surgical Terms

BUILT FROM WORD PARTS

The following terms can be translated using definitions of word parts. Further explanation is provided within parentheses as needed.

TERM	DEFINITION
1. **balanoplasty** (BAL-a-nō-*plas*-tē)	surgical repair of the glans penis
2. **epididymectomy** (*ep*-i-*did*-i-MEK-to-mē)	excision of the epididymis
3. **orchiectomy** (*or*-kē-EK-to-mē)	excision of the testis (bilateral orchiectomy is called **castration**) (also called **orchidectomy**)
4. **orchiopexy** (OR-kē-ō-pek-sē)	surgical fixation of the testicle (performed to bring undescended testicle[s] into the scrotum) (also called **orchidopexy**)
5. **orchioplasty** (OR-kē-ō-*plas*-tē)	surgical repair of the testis
6. **orchiotomy** (*or*-kē-OT-o-mē)	incision into the testis (also called **orchidotomy**)
7. **prostatectomy** (*pros*-ta-TEK-to-mē)	excision of the prostate gland (Tables 7.1, 7.2, and 7.3)
8. **prostatocystotomy** (*pros*-tat-ō-sis-TOT-o-mē)	incision into the prostate gland and the (urinary) bladder
9. **prostatolithotomy** (*pros*-tat-ō-li-THOT-o-mē)	incision into the prostate gland to remove stone(s)

TABLE 7.2 Types of Prostatectomies

SIMPLE PROSTATECTOMY	RADICAL PROSTATECTOMY (RP)
The inside portion of the prostate gland is excised through an abdominal incision made above the pubic bone and through an incision in the bladder and prostate capsule. Laparoscopic and robotic simple prostatectomy are increasingly common techniques for this surgery.	The prostate gland with its capsule, seminal vesicles, vas deferens, and sometimes pelvic lymph nodes are excised. The procedure may be performed by various approaches, including retropubic, perineal, and laparoscopic. Retropubic and perineal approaches are performed using large, open incisions. Laparoscopic and robotic surgeries use smaller incisions.
Used to treat **benign prostatic hyperplasia (BPH)**, most often when the prostate is very large, or when the patient has not had success with BPH medication or minimally invasive procedures.	Used to treat **prostate cancer**.
Also called **open prostatectomy.**	Also called **radical retropubic prostatectomy, laparoscopic radical prostatectomy,** and **robotic-assisted laparoscopic radical prostatectomy (RALRP).**

Continued

TABLE 7.2 Types of Prostatectomies—cont'd

SIMPLE PROSTATECTOMY	RADICAL PROSTATECTOMY (RP)
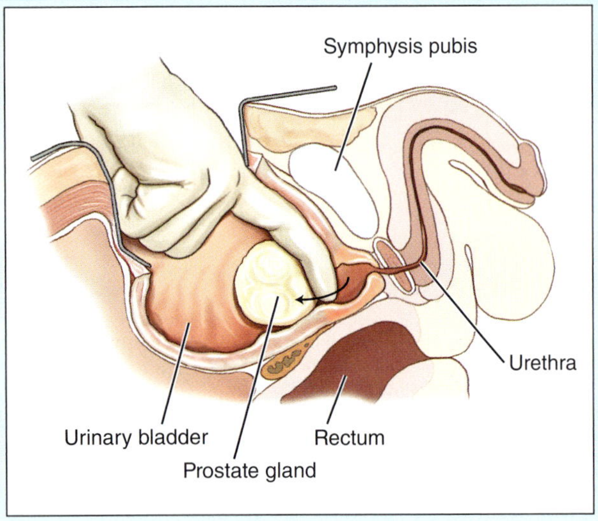	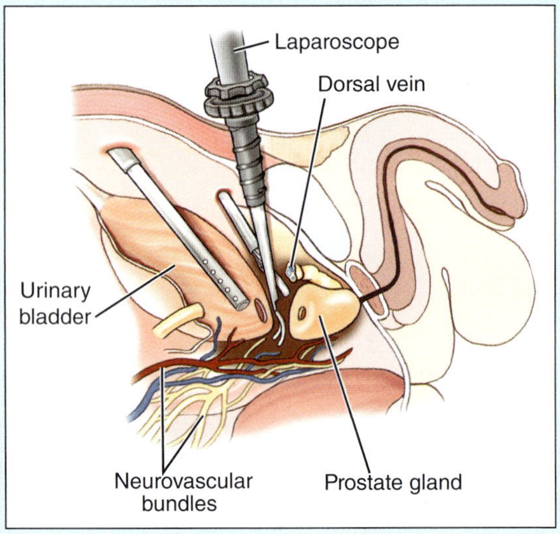
Simple prostatectomy with a suprapubic approach (large incision surgery). The surgeon approaches the prostate gland through an incision in the urinary bladder and uses a finger to remove the hyperplastic tissue.	**Radical prostatectomy** with a laparoscopic approach (small incision surgery). Laparoscopic radical prostatectomy and robotic-assisted laparoscopic radical prostatectomy (RALRP) are procedures used to treat early stages of prostate cancer.

Surgical Terms–cont'd

BUILT FROM WORD PARTS

TERM	DEFINITION	TERM	DEFINITION
10. prostatovesiculectomy (*pros*-tat-ō-ves-*ik*-ū-LEK-to-mē)	excision of the prostate gland and the seminal vesicles	**12. vasovasostomy** (*vas*-ō-vā-ZOS-to-mē)	creation of artificial openings between ducts (the severed ends of the vas deferens are reconnected in an attempt to restore fertility in men who have had a vasectomy)
11. vasectomy (va-SEK-to-mē)	excision of a duct (partial excision of the vas deferens bilaterally, resulting in male sterilization)	**13. vesiculectomy** (ve-*sik*-ū-LEK-to-mē)	excision of the seminal vesicle(s)

EXERCISE 12 ■ Pronounce and Spell

Practice pronunciation and spelling on paper and online.

1. Practice on Paper

a. **Pronounce:** Read the phonetic spelling and say aloud the terms listed in the previous table. Refer to the pronunciation key on p. 20 as necessary.
b. **Spell:** Have a study partner read the terms aloud. Write the spelling of the terms on a separate sheet of paper.

2. Practice Online

a. **Access** online learning resources. Go to evolve.elsevier.com > Evolve Resources > Student Resources.
b. **Pronounce:** Select Audio Glossary > Chapter 7 > Exercise 12. Select a term to hear its pronunciation and repeat aloud.
c. **Spell:** Select Activities > Chapter 7 > Spell Terms > Exercise 12. Select the audio icon and type the correct spelling of the term.

❑ Check the box when complete.

EXERCISE 13 ■ Analyze and Define

Analyze and define the following terms by drawing slashes between word parts, writing word part abbreviations above the term, underlining combining forms, and writing combining form abbreviations below the term.

EXAMPLE:

WR CV WR CV S
prostat / o / lith / o / tomy
CF CF
incision into the prostate gland to remove stone(s)

1. vasectomy
2. prostatocystotomy
3. orchiotomy
4. epididymectomy
5. orchiopexy
6. prostatovesiculectomy
7. orchioplasty
8. vesiculectomy
9. prostatectomy
10. balanoplasty
11. vasovasostomy
12. orchiectomy

EXERCISE 14 ■ Build

A Label

Build the surgical terms pictured by writing word parts above definitions.

1.

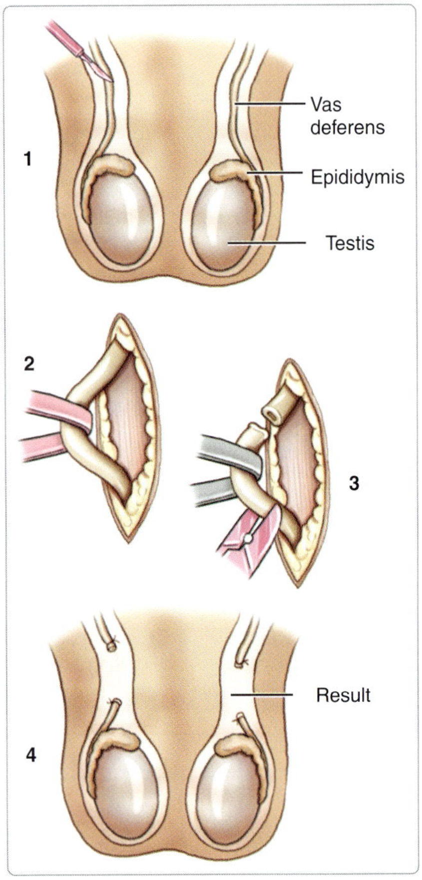

_____ / _____
duct excision

1. incision is made into the covering of the vas deferens
2. vas deferens is exposed and ligated (tied off)
3. segment of vas deferens is excised
4. vas deferens is repositioned and skin is sutured

2.

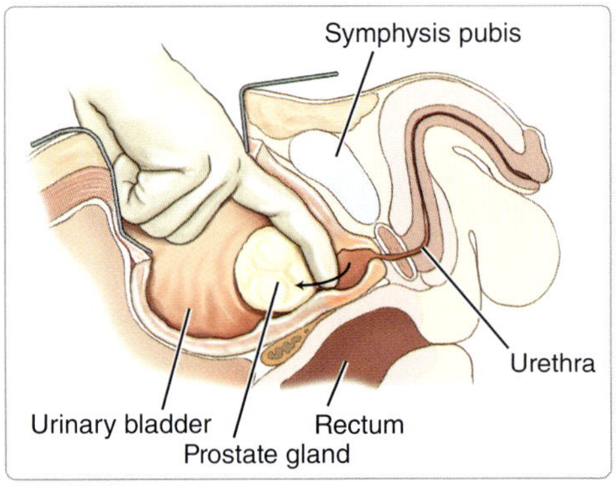

_____ / _____
prostate excision

3.

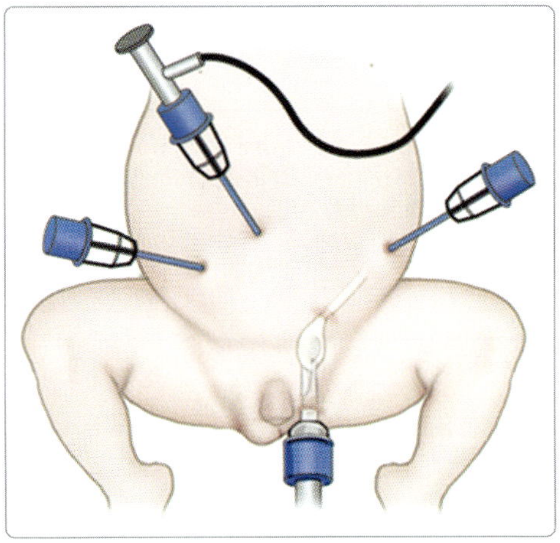

_____ / _____ / _____
testicle CV surgical fixation

4.

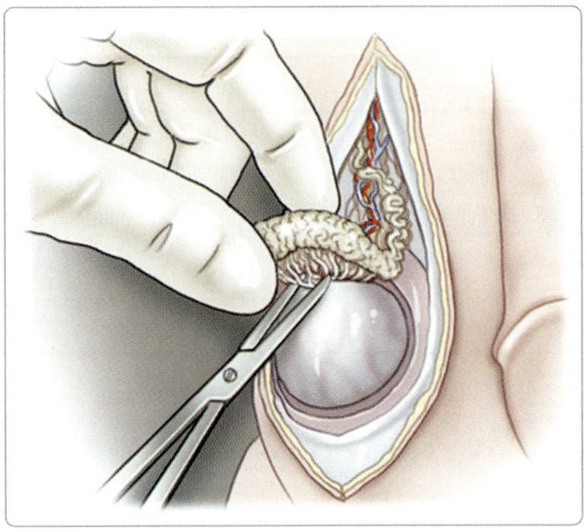

_____ / _____
epididymis excision

B Fill In

Build surgical terms for the following definitions by using the word parts you have learned.

EXAMPLE: excision of the prostate gland prostat / ectomy (WR / S)

1. excision of the testis ______ / ______ (WR / S)

2. surgical repair of the glans penis ______ / CV / ______ (WR / CV / S)

3. incision into the prostate gland and the (urinary) bladder ______ / CV / ______ / CV / ______ (WR / CV / WR / CV / S)

4. excision of the seminal vesicle(s) ______ / ______ (WR / S)

5. incision into the prostate gland to remove stone(s) ______ / CV / ______ / CV / ______ (WR / CV / WR / CV / S)

6. incision into the testis ______ / CV / ______ (WR / CV / S)

7. excision of the prostate gland and the seminal vesicles ______ / CV / ______ / ______ (WR / CV / WR / S)

8. surgical repair of the testis ______ / CV / ______ (WR / CV / S)

9. creation of artificial openings between ducts ______ / CV / ______ / CV / ______ (WR / CV / WR / CV / S)

Surgical Terms

NOT BUILT FROM WORD PARTS

Word parts may be present in the following terms; however, their full meanings cannot be translated using definitions of word parts alone.

TERM	DEFINITION
1. ablation (ab-LĀ-shun)	destruction of abnormal or excessive tissue by melting, vaporizing, or eroding
2. circumcision (*ser*-kum-SI-zhun)	surgical removal of the prepuce (foreskin); all or part of the foreskin may be removed
3. enucleation (ē-*nū*-klē-Ā-shun)	excision of a whole organ or mass without cutting into it
4. hydrocelectomy (*hī*-drō-sē-LEK-to-mē)	surgical removal of a fluid-filled sac around the testicle causing scrotal swelling (hydrocele)
5. laser surgery (LĀ–ser) (SUR-jer-ē)	use of a focused beam of light to excise or vaporize abnormal tissue and to control bleeding; uses a variety of non-invasive and minimally invasive procedures. Two common types of laser surgery used to treat BPH are **holmium laser enucleation of the prostate gland (HoLEP)** and **photoselective vaporization of the prostate gland (PVP)**. (Table 7.3, Fig 7.5)

Surgical Terms—cont'd

NOT BUILT FROM WORD PARTS

TERM	DEFINITION
6. morcellation (*mor*-se-LĀ-shun)	cutting or grinding solid tissue into smaller pieces for removal
7. robotic surgery (rō-BOT-ik) (SUR-jer-ē)	use of small surgical instruments attached to a computer and operated by the surgeon from a console several feet from the operating table (Table 7.2, Fig. 7.6)
8. sterilization (*stār*-i-li-ZĀ-shun)	surgical procedure that prevents pregnancy, either the ability of the female to conceive or of the male to induce conception
9. transurethral incision of the prostate gland (TUIP) (*trans*-ū-RĒ-thral) (in-SIZH-en) (of) (the) (PROS-tāt) (gland)	surgical procedure that widens the urethra by making a few small incisions in the bladder neck and the prostate gland. No prostate tissue is removed. TUIP may be used instead of TURP when the prostate gland is less enlarged. (Table 7.3)
10. transurethral microwave thermotherapy (TUMT) (*trans*-ū-RĒ-thral) (MĪ-krō-wāv) (*ther*-mō-THER-a-pē)	treatment that eliminates excess tissue present in benign prostatic hyperplasia by using heat generated by microwave (Table 7.3)
11. transurethral resection of the prostate gland (TURP) (*trans*-ū-RĒ-thral) (rē-SEK-shun) (of) (the) (PROS-tāt) (gland)	surgical removal of pieces of the prostate gland tissue by using an instrument inserted through the urethra. The capsule is left intact; usually performed when the enlarged prostate gland interferes with urination. (Table 7.3)

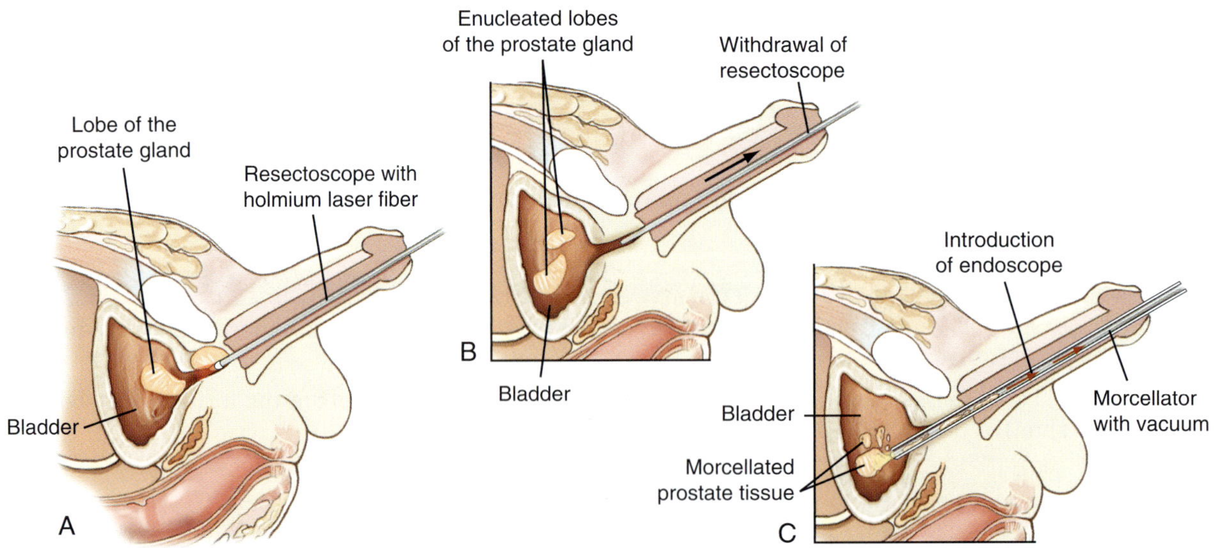

FIG. 7.5 Holmium laser enucleation of the prostate (HoLEP) is a minimally invasive laser surgery performed endoscopically to treat benign prostatic hyperplasia. **A,** The lobes of the prostate gland are removed intact from surrounding structures using a holmium laser. **B,** The enucleated lobes are temporarily placed in the urinary bladder. **C,** The lobes of the prostate are morcellated within the urinary bladder and removed through the endoscope using suction.

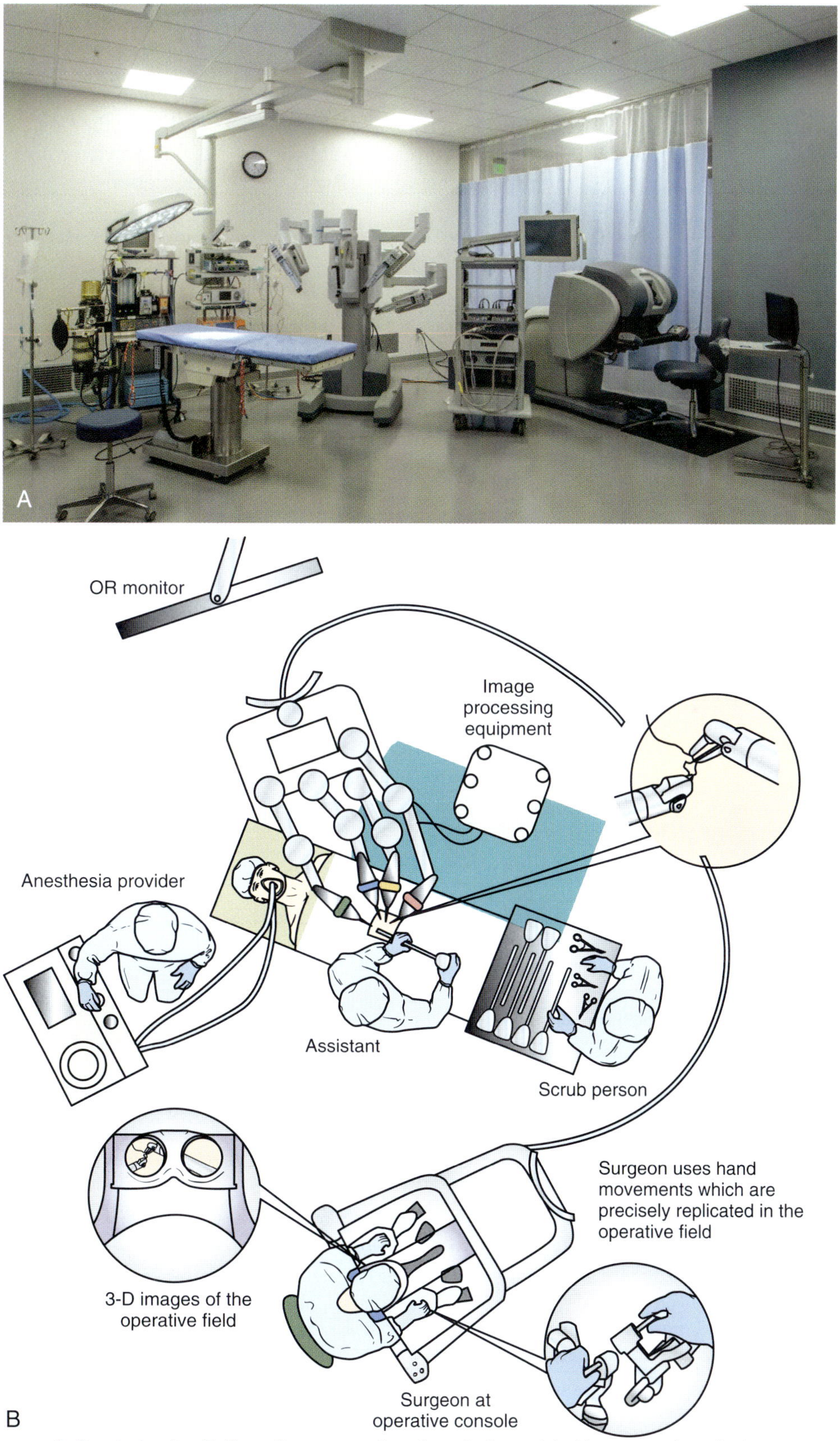

FIG. 7.6 Robotic surgery. **A,** Surgical suite. **B,** Operating room set-up for robotic-assisted laparoscopic radical prostatectomy (RALRP) with a robotic system. Note the surgeon performs the procedure at an operative console rather than hands-on surgery.

TABLE 7.3 Surgical Treatments for Benign Prostatic Hyperplasia

INCISIONAL SURGERIES	LASER SURGERIES	OTHER SURGICAL PROCEDURES
1. Simple prostatectomy 2. Transurethral incision of the prostate gland (TUIP) 3. Transurethral resection of the prostate gland (TURP)	1. Holmium laser enucleation of the prostate gland (HoLEP) 2. Photoselective vaporization of the prostate gland (PVP)	1. Transurethral microwave thermotherapy (TUMT) 2. Water vapor energy (WAVE) ablation

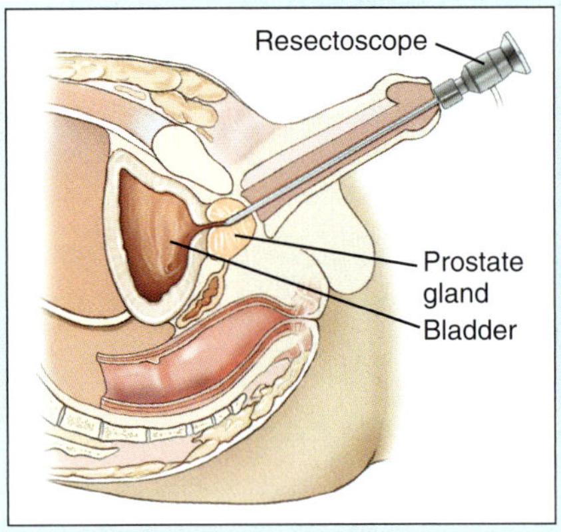

Transurethral resection of the prostate gland (TURP) uses a resectoscope inserted through the urethra to the prostate gland. The end of the instrument is equipped to remove pieces of the enlarged prostate gland to relieve bladder outlet obstruction (BOO).

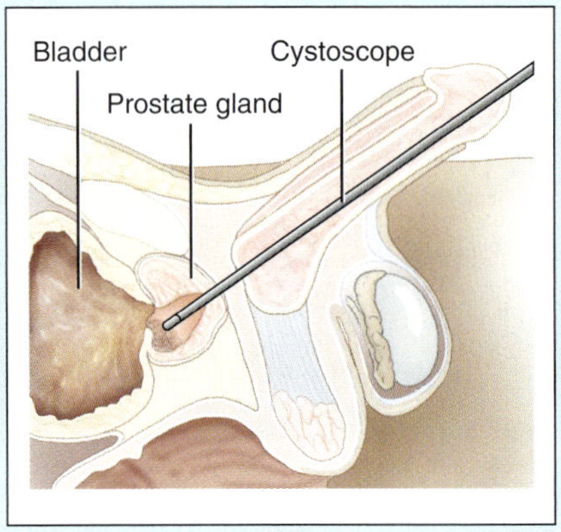

Photoselective vaporization of the prostate gland (PVP) uses a laser system operated through a cystoscope inserted through the urethra to the prostate gland. Overgrown prostate tissue is vaporized using heat generated by the laser.

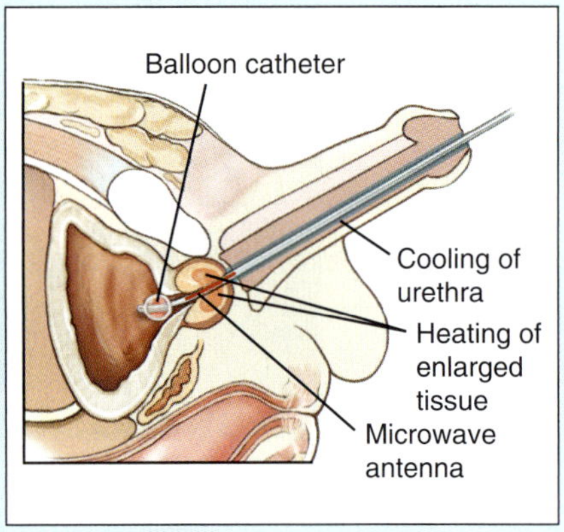

Transurethral microwave thermotherapy (TUMT) destroys prostate tissue with heat from microwaves emitted by an antenna guided by a catheter, which has been inserted through the urethra. A cooling mechanism protects surrounding tissue.

EXERCISE 15 ■ Pronounce and Spell

Practice pronunciation and spelling on paper and online.

1. Practice on Paper

a. **Pronounce:** Read the phonetic spelling and say aloud the terms listed in the term table. Refer to the pronunciation key on p. 20 as necessary.
b. **Spell:** Have a study partner read the terms aloud. Write the spelling of the terms on a separate sheet of paper.

2. Practice Online

a. **Access** online learning resources. Go to evolve.elsevier.com > Evolve Resources > Student Resources.
b. **Pronounce:** Select Audio Glossary > Chapter 7 > Exercise 15. Select a term to hear its pronunciation and repeat aloud.
c. **Spell:** Select Activities > Chapter 7 > Spell Terms > Exercise 15. Select the audio icon and type the correct spelling of the term.

❑ Check the box when complete.

EXERCISE 16 ■ Fill In

A Label

Write the surgical terms pictured and defined.

1. ______________________________
use of small surgical instruments attached to a computer and operated by the surgeon from a console several feet from the operating table

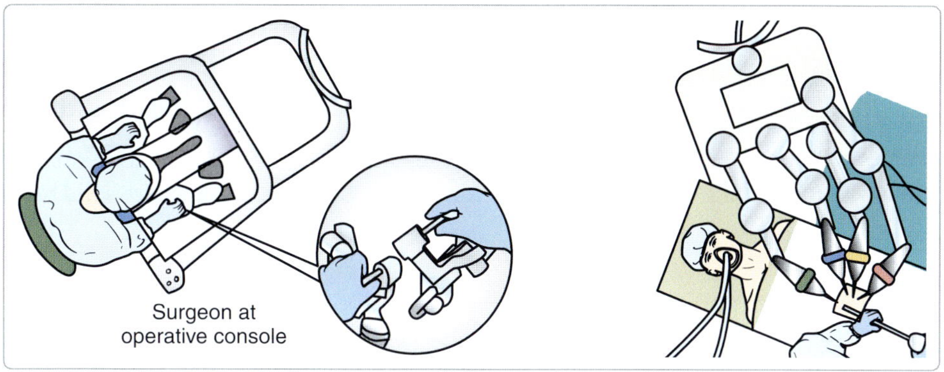

2. ______________________________
____
surgical removal of pieces of the prostate gland tissue by using an instrument inserted through the urethra.

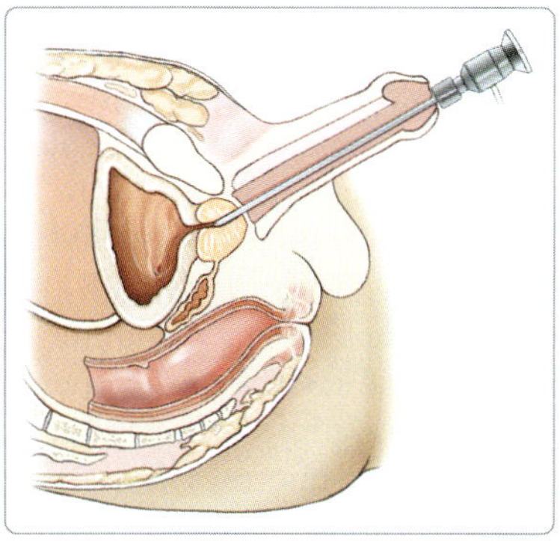

3. ______________________________
____
treatment that eliminates excess tissue present in benign prostatic hyperplasia by using heat generated by microwave

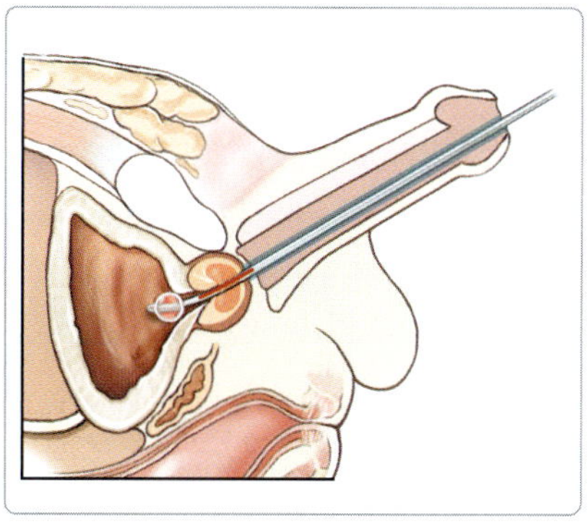

4. ______________________________
surgical removal of the prepuce (foreskin)

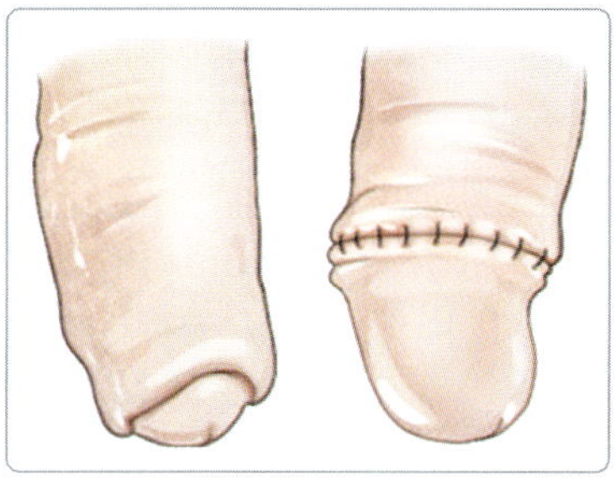

5. ______________________________
excision of a whole organ or mass without cutting into it

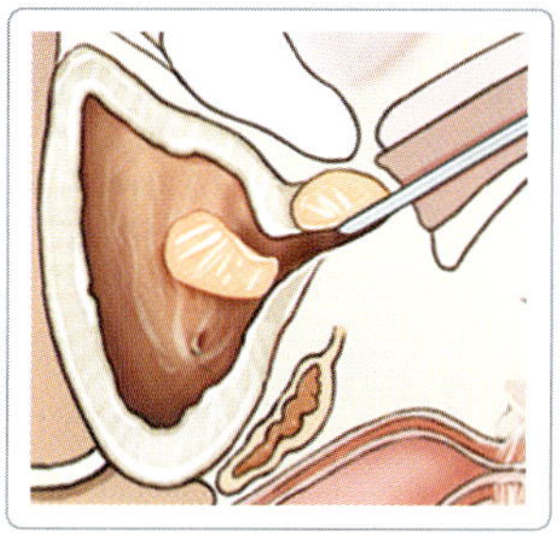

B Identify

Fill in the blanks with the correct term.

1. A surgical procedure that prevents pregnancy, either the ability of the female to conceive or of the male to induce conception is called ______.
2. Photoselective vaporization of the prostate (PVP) is one form of ______, the destruction of abnormal or excessive tissue by melting, vaporizing, or eroding.
3. Surgical removal of a fluid-filled sac around the testicle causing scrotal swelling is ______.
4. A surgical procedure for benign prostatic hyperplasia that widens the urethra by making small incisions is called ______.
5. One type of ______, where a focused beam of light is used to excise or vaporize abnormal tissue and to control bleeding, is holmium laser enucleation of the prostate gland (HoLEP).
6. Endoscopic surgeries often involve ______, where solid tissue is cut or ground into smaller pieces for removal.

EXERCISE 17 ■ Match

Match the terms in the first column with the correct definitions in the second column.

_____ 1. hydrocelectomy	a. destruction of abnormal or excessive tissue by melting, vaporizing, or eroding
_____ 2. transurethral resection of the prostate gland (TURP)	b. surgical procedure that widens the urethra by making a few small incisions in the bladder neck and the prostate gland
_____ 3. robotic surgery	c. use of a focused beam of light to excise or vaporize abnormal tissue and to control bleeding
_____ 4. morcellation	d. surgical removal of the prepuce (foreskin)
_____ 5. transurethral microwave thermotherapy (TUMT)	e. excision of a whole organ or mass without cutting into it
_____ 6. sterilization	f. surgical procedure that prevents pregnancy, either the ability of the female to conceive or of the male to induce conception
_____ 7. transurethral incision of the prostate gland (TUIP)	g. surgical removal of a fluid-filled sac around the testicle causing scrotal swelling
_____ 8. ablation	h. use of small surgical instruments attached to a computer and operated by the surgeon from a console several feet from the operating table
_____ 9. circumcision	i. treatment that eliminates excess tissue present in benign prostatic hyperplasia by using heat generated by microwave
_____ 10. laser surgery	j. cutting or grinding solid tissue into smaller pieces for removal
_____ 11. enucleation	k. surgical removal of pieces of the prostate gland tissue by using an instrument inserted through the urethra

EXERCISE 18 ■ Review of Surgical Terms

Can you define, pronounce, and spell the following terms?

ablation
balanoplasty
circumcision
enucleation
epididymectomy
hydrocelectomy
laser surgery
morcellation
orchiectomy
orchiopexy
orchioplasty
orchiotomy
prostatectomy
prostatocystotomy
prostatolithotomy
prostatovesiculectomy
robotic surgery
sterilization
transurethral incision of the prostate gland (TUIP)
transurethral microwave thermotherapy (TUMT)
transurethral resection of the prostate gland (TURP)
vasectomy
vasovasostomy
vesiculectomy

Diagnostic Terms

NOT BUILT FROM WORD PARTS

Word parts may be present in the following terms; however, their full meanings cannot be translated using definitions of word parts alone.

DIAGNOSTIC IMAGING

TERM	DEFINITION
1. MRI ultrasound fusion biopsy (M-R-I) (UL-tra-sound) (FŪ-shun) (BĪ-op-sē)	combination of magnetic resonance imaging with transrectal ultrasound (TRUS) to obtain a tissue from a prostate lesion. Software merges an existing MR image with live ultrasound images. The combined, or fused, MRI-TRUS image is used to direct the biopsy needle into the area of the prostate that looks suspicious on MRI. (also called **MRI-TRUS fusion**, **MR-ultrasound fusion**, and **fusion guided biopsy**) (Table 7.1)
2. multiparametric MRI (MUL-ti-par-a-*met*-rik) (M-R-I)	magnetic resonance imaging procedure providing information of anatomic structure and physiology for the staging of prostate cancer. It uses a combination of different MRI modalities to better understand the size and extent of prostate tumors. (Table 7.1)
3. transrectal ultrasound (TRUS) (trans-REK-tal) (UL-tra-sound)	ultrasound procedure used to diagnose prostate cancer. Sound waves are sent and received by a transducer probe that is placed into the rectum. (Table 7.1)

LABORATORY

TERM	DEFINITION
4. prostate-specific antigen (PSA) (PROS-tāt) (spe-SIF-ik) (AN-ti-jen)	blood test that measures the level of prostate-specific antigen in the blood. Elevated test results may indicate the presence of prostate cancer, urinary or prostatic infection, or excess prostate tissue, as found in benign prostatic hyperplasia or prostatitis. (Table 7.1)
5. semen analysis (SĒ-men) (a-NAL-i-sis)	microscopic observation of ejaculated semen, revealing the size, structure, and movement of sperm; used to evaluate male infertility and to determine the effectiveness of a vasectomy (also called **sperm count** and **sperm test**)
6. total testosterone (TŌ-tal) (tes-TOS-ta-rōn)	blood test to measure the level of the hormone responsible for male physical characteristics (testosterone); used to detect multiple conditions in men and women, including infertility

OTHER

TERM	DEFINITION
7. digital rectal examination (DRE) (DIJ-i-tal) (REK-tal) (eg-*zam*-i-NĀ-shun)	physical examination in which the healthcare provider inserts a gloved finger into the rectum and palpates the prostate through the rectal wall to determine the size, shape, and consistency of the gland; used to screen for BPH and prostate cancer. BPH usually presents as a uniform, nontender enlargement, whereas cancer usually presents as a stony hard nodule. (Table 7.1)

EXERCISE 19 ■ Pronounce and Spell

Practice pronunciation and spelling on paper and online.

1. Practice on Paper

a. **Pronounce:** Read the phonetic spelling and say aloud the terms listed in the previous table. Refer to the pronunciation key on p. 20 as necessary.

b. **Spell:** Have a study partner read the terms aloud. Write the spelling of the terms on a separate sheet of paper.

2. Practice Online

a. **Access** online learning resources. Go to evolve.elsevier.com > Evolve Resources > Student Resources.
b. **Pronounce:** Select Audio Glossary > Chapter 7 > Exercise 19. Select a term to hear its pronunciation and repeat aloud.
c. **Spell:** Select Activities > Chapter 7 > Spell Terms > Exercise 19. Select the audio icon and type the correct spelling of the term.

❑ Check the box when complete.

EXERCISE 20 ■ Fill In

Fill in the blanks with the correct terms.

1. A physical examination in which the healthcare provider palpates the prostate through the rectal wall to determine the size, shape, and consistency of the gland is called ______________________.
2. A blood test that, when elevated, may indicate the presence of prostate cancer is called ______________________.
3. A diagnostic ultrasound procedure used to obtain images of the prostate gland is called ______________________.
4. A laboratory test for microscopic observation of ejaculated semen to evaluate male infertility is called ______________________.
5. A magnetic resonance imaging procedure that provides structural and physiological information for the staging of prostate cancer is called ______________________.
6. ______________________ is a blood test to measure the level of the hormone responsible for male physical characteristics and may be used to detect infertility.
7. A diagnostic imaging test that uses a combination of magnetic resonance imaging with transrectal ultrasound (TRUS) to obtain a tissue from a prostate lesion is called ______________________.

EXERCISE 21 ■ Match

Match the terms in the first column with the correct definitions in the second column.

_____ 1. semen analysis
_____ 2. prostate-specific antigen (PSA)
_____ 3. transrectal ultrasound (TRUS)
_____ 4. total testosterone
_____ 5. MRI ultrasound fusion biopsy
_____ 6. digital rectal examination (DRE)
_____ 7. multiparametric MRI

a. test that uses a combination of different MRI modalities to better understand the size and extent of prostate tumors
b. a gloved finger palpates the prostate through the rectal wall to determine the size, shape, and consistency of the gland
c. blood test to measure the level of the hormone responsible for male physical characteristics
d. elevated results of this blood test may indicate the presence of prostate cancer, urinary or prostatic infection, or excess prostate tissue
e. microscopic observation of ejaculated semen, used to evaluate male infertility and to determine the effectiveness of a vasectomy
f. ultrasound procedure used to diagnose prostate cancer
g. combination of magnetic resonance imaging with transrectal ultrasound to obtain a tissue from a prostate lesion

EXERCISE 22 ■ Review of Diagnostic Terms

Can you define, pronounce, and spell the following terms?

digital rectal examination (DRE)	prostate-specific antigen (PSA)	total testosterone
MRI ultrasound fusion biopsy	semen analysis	transrectal ultrasound (TRUS)
multiparametric MRI		

Complementary Terms

Included in this section of the chapter are a few terms, including sexually transmitted infections, that apply to all genders. These infections can cause damage to reproductive organs and other potentially serious health consequences if left untreated. Any sexual behavior involving contact with the body fluids of another person puts an individual at risk for infection.

BUILT FROM WORD PARTS AND *NOT* BUILT FROM WORD PARTS

The first portion of the table contains Male Reproductive System Terms that can be translated using definitions of word parts. The second portion of the table contains terms that cannot be fully understood using the definitions of word parts.

Built from Word Parts

SIGNS AND SYMPTOMS

TERM	DEFINITION	TERM	DEFINITION
1. **aspermia** (a-SPER-mē-a)	condition of without sperm (characterized by absence of semen or ejaculation)	2. **oligospermia** (*ol*-i-gō-SPER-mē-a)	condition of scanty sperm (in the semen; may contribute to infertility)
ASPERMIA may indicate the lack of production of spermatozoa, the lack of production of semen, or the lack of ejaculation of semen.		3. **orchialgia** (*ōr*-kē-AL-ja)	pain in the testis (also called **testalgia**)

NOT Built from Word Parts

INFECTIONS

TERM	DEFINITION
1. **chlamydia** (kla-MID-ē-a)	sexually transmitted infection, caused by the bacterium *C. trachomatis*; sometimes referred to as a **silent STI** because many people are not aware they have the disease. Symptoms that occur when the disease becomes serious are painful urination and discharge from the penis in men and genital itching, vaginal discharge, and bleeding between menstrual periods in women.
2. **genital herpes** (JEN-i-tal) (HER-pēz)	sexually transmitted infection caused by herpes simplex virus type 2
3. **gonorrhea** (gon-ō-RĒ-a)	sexually transmitted infection caused by a bacterial organism that inflames the mucous membranes of the genitourinary tract
4. **human immunodeficiency virus (HIV)** (HŪ-man) (*im*-ū-nō-de-FISH-en-sē) (VĪ-rus)	sexually transmitted infection caused by a retrovirus that infects T-helper cells of the immune system; may also be acquired in utero or transmitted through infected blood via needle sharing. Advanced HIV infection progresses to AIDS (acquired immunodeficiency syndrome).
5. **human papillomavirus (HPV)** (HŪ-man) (*pap*-i-LŌ-ma-*vī*-rus)	sexually transmitted infection caused by viral infection; there are more than 40 types of HPV that cause benign or cancerous growths in male and female genitals (also called **genital warts**)
HUMAN PAPILLOMAVIRUS is the cause of most cervical cancers. Some penile, vulvar, vaginal, throat, and anal cancers are also linked to HPV infection. HPV is the most prevalent sexually transmitted disease and vaccines are available to protect men and women from HPV infection.	
6. **sexually transmitted infection (STI)** (SEK-shū-al-ē) (TRANS-mi-ted)(in-FEK-shun)	infection spread through sexual contact; STIs affect both males and females, causing damage to reproductive organs and potentially serious health consequences if left untreated (also called **sexually transmitted disease [STD]**)
SEXUALLY TRANSMITTED INFECTION (STI) VS. SEXUALLY TRANSMITTED DISEASE (STD): WHAT'S THE DIFFERENCE? Usually, a "disease" refers to a clear medical problem, often with signs or symptoms. But patients with an infection may have no signs or symptoms and still have the problem. While **STI** is medically more accurate, you will also frequently hear the term **STD**.	
7. **syphilis** (SIF-i-lis)	infection caused by the bacterium *Treponema pallidum*. Rapidly spreads throughout the body, and if untreated becomes systemic and can progress through three stages separated by latent periods. Usually sexually transmitted, but may be acquired in utero and by direct contact with infected skin. (Fig. 7.7)

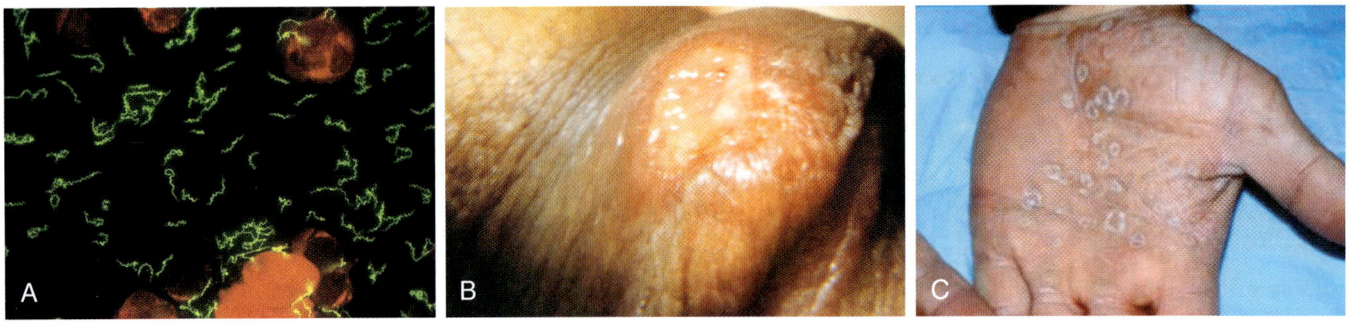

FIG. 7.7 Syphilis. **A,** *Treponema pallidum*, organism responsible for syphilis viewed microscopically. **B,** Primary syphilis, depicting a syphilitic chancre. **C,** Secondary syphilis, depicting rash on palms of hands.

Complementary Terms—cont'd

NOT Built from Word Parts

INFECTIONS

TERM	DEFINITION
8. trichomoniasis (*trik*-ō-mō-NĪ-a-sis)	sexually transmitted infection caused by a one-cell organism *Trichomonas.* It infects the genitourinary tract. Men may be asymptomatic or may develop urethritis, an enlarged prostate gland, or epididymitis. Women may have vaginal itching, dysuria, and vaginal or urethral discharge.

TREATMENTS

TERM	DEFINITION
9. artificial insemination (ar-ti-FISH-al) (in-*sem*-i-NĀ-shun)	introduction of washed and concentrated sperm into the female reproductive tract; used as a treatment for infertility
10. condom (KON-dum)	cover for the penis worn to prevent conception and the spread of sexually transmitted infections
11. spermicide (SPUR-mi-sīd)	an agent that destroys spermatozoa; used to prevent conception

Refer to **Appendix E** for pharmacology terms.

OTHER

TERM	DEFINITION
12. azoospermia (ā-*zō*-a-SPUR-mē-a)	lack of live sperm in the semen (characterized by absence of semen or ejaculation)

AZOOSPERMIA may be:
- obstructive, caused by blocked vessels or ducts
- nonobstructive, caused by infection, lack of production of spermatozoa, or retrograde ejaculation where semen travels into the urinary bladder rather than exiting through the urethra

TERM	DEFINITION
13. ejaculation (ē-*jak*-ū-LĀ-shun)	ejection of semen from the male urethra
14. orgasm (ŌR-gazm)	climax of sexual stimulation
15. puberty (PŪ-ber-tē)	period when secondary sex characteristics (such as pubic and armpit hair, deepening of voice in men, breast development in women, etc.) develop and the ability to reproduce sexually begins

EXERCISE 23 ■ Pronounce and Spell

Practice pronunciation and spelling on paper and online.

1. Practice on Paper

a. **Pronounce:** Read the phonetic spelling and say aloud the terms listed in the previous table. Refer to the pronunciation key on p. 20 as necessary.
b. **Spell:** Have a study partner read the terms aloud. Write the spelling of the terms on a separate sheet of paper.

2. Practice Online

a. **Access** online learning resources. Go to evolve.elsevier.com > Evolve Resources > Student Resources.
b. **Pronounce:** Select Audio Glossary > Chapter 7 > Exercise 23. Select a term to hear its pronunciation and repeat aloud.
c. **Spell:** Select Activities > Chapter 7 > Spell Terms > Exercise 23. Select the audio icon and type the correct spelling of the term.

❑ Check the box when complete.

EXERCISE 24 ■ Complementary Terms Built from Word Parts

A Analyze and Define

Analyze and define the following terms by drawing slashes between word parts, writing word part abbreviations above the term, underlining combining forms, and writing combining form abbreviations below the term.

1. o r c h i a l g i a

____

____

2. o l i g o s p e r m i a

____

____

3. a s p e r m i a

____

____

B Build

Build the complementary terms for the following definitions by using the word parts you have learned.

1. condition of without sperm (or semen or ejaculation) ______ / ______ / ______
P / WR / S

2. condition of scanty sperm (in the semen) ______ / ______ / ______ / ______
WR / CV / WR / S

3. pain in the testis ______ / ______
WR / S

EXERCISE 25 ■ Complementary Terms *NOT* Built from Word Parts

A Match

Match the terms in the first column with their correct definitions in the second column.

_____ 1. ejaculation
_____ 2. human papillomavirus
_____ 3. genital herpes
_____ 4. gonorrhea
_____ 5. orgasm
_____ 6. condom
_____ 7. azoospermia

a. climax of sexual stimulation
b. STI caused by herpes simplex virus type 2
c. ejection of semen
d. lack of live sperm in the semen
e. cover for the penis worn to prevent conception and the spread of sexually transmitted infections
f. also called genital warts
g. STI caused by a bacterium that inflames mucous membranes

B Match

Match the terms in the first column with their correct definitions in the second column.

_____ 1. sexually transmitted infection
_____ 2. spermicide
_____ 3. syphilis
_____ 4. puberty
_____ 5. human immunodeficiency virus
_____ 6. trichomoniasis
_____ 7. artificial insemination
_____ 8. chlamydia

a. infection spread through sexual contact
b. period when secondary sex characteristics develop and the ability to reproduce sexually begins
c. retrovirus that progresses to AIDS
d. infection caused by *Treponema pallidum*; if untreated, progresses through three stages
e. introduction of washed and concentrated sperm into the female reproductive tract
f. STI caused by a bacterium, *C. trachomatis* (silent STD)
g. an agent that destroys spermatozoa; used to prevent conception
h. STI caused by a one-cell organism, *Trichomonas*

EXERCISE 26 ■ Review of Complementary Terms

Can you define, pronounce, and spell the following terms?

artificial insemination
aspermia
azoospermia
chlamydia
condom
ejaculation
genital herpes
gonorrhea
human immunodeficiency virus (HIV)
human papillomavirus (HPV)
oligospermia
orchialgia
orgasm
puberty
sexually transmitted infection (STI)
spermicide
syphilis
trichomoniasis

Abbreviations

SIGNS AND SYMPTOMS

ABBREVIATION	TERM	ABBREVIATION	TERM
BOO	bladder outlet obstruction	**LUTS**	lower urinary tract symptoms

DISEASE AND DISORDERS

ABBREVIATION	TERM	ABBREVIATION	TERM
BPH	benign prostatic hyperplasia	**HPV**	human papillomavirus
ED	erectile dysfunction	**STD**	sexually transmitted disease
HIV	human immunodeficiency virus	**STI**	sexually transmitted infection

DIAGNOSTIC

ABBREVIATION	TERM	ABBREVIATION	TERM
DRE	digital rectal examination	**TRUS**	transrectal ultrasound
PSA	prostate-specific antigen		

TREATMENT

ABBREVIATION	TERM	ABBREVIATION	TERM
HoLEP	holmium laser enucleation of the prostate gland	**TUIP**	transurethral incision of the prostate gland
PVP	photoselective vaporization of the prostate gland	**TUMT**	transurethral microwave thermotherapy
RP	radical prostatectomy	**TURP**	transurethral resection of the prostate gland

Refer to **Appendix D** for a complete list of abbreviations.

EXERCISE 27 ■ Fill In

Write the terms abbreviated.

1. The patient experienced **LUTS** ______________________ caused by **BOO** ______________________.
2. The physician performed a **DRE** ______________________ on the patient to assist in diagnosing **BPH** ______________________.
3. Surgical treatments for BPH include:
   TUIP ______________________ of the prostate gland
   TURP ______________________ of the prostate gland
   TUMT ______________________
   PVP ______________________ of the prostate gland
   HoLEP ______________________ of the prostate gland
4. **HIV** ______________________ is a type of retrovirus that infects T-helper cells of the immune system.
5. **HPV** ______________________ causes female and male genital warts and most cervical cancers.
6. **STI** ______________________ is the preferred term for **STD** ______________________.
7. **PSA** ______________________ is a laboratory test used to diagnose cancer of the prostate.
8. **RP** ______________________ is a surgical procedure to treat prostate cancer.
9. **ED** ______________________ was formerly referred to as impotence.
10. **TRUS** ______________________, used in the diagnosis of prostate cancer, provides imaging of the prostate gland and is used as a guide for biopsy of the prostate.

PRACTICAL APPLICATION

EXERCISE 28 ■ Case Study: Translate Between Everyday Language and Medical Language

CASE STUDY: Jimmie Zeller

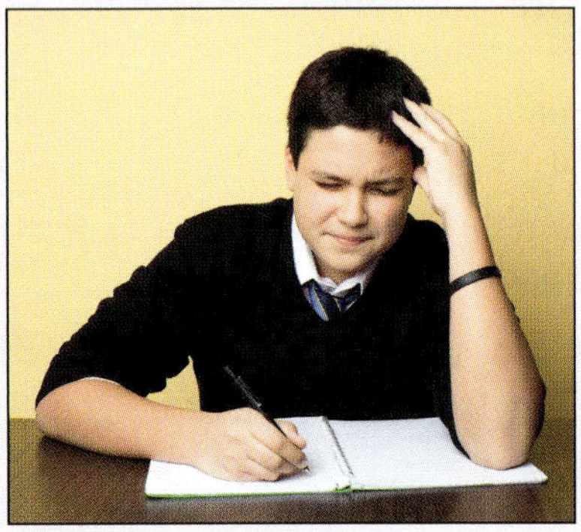

Jimmie, a 15-year-old male, is in the emergency department (ED) because of pain in his testicle that started about 6 hours ago. The pain started suddenly, he felt nauseated, and vomited twice. The ED physician examined him and found that his scrotum was swollen, and the painful testicle was higher than the other. A Doppler ultrasound was performed and the findings suggested twisting of the spermatic cord with decreased blood flow to the testis. A surgeon was called immediately to examine Jimmie, since this condition requires immediate surgical fixation of the testis or even surgical removal of the testis. The surgeon examined him quickly and took him immediately to the operating room, since she knew that the risk of reduced or absent ability to achieve pregnancy increases when this condition is left untreated.

Now that you have worked through Chapter 7, on the male reproductive system, consider the medical terms that might be used to describe Jimmie's experience. See the Chapter at a Glance section at the end of the chapter for a list of terms that might apply.

A. *Underline phrases in the case study that could be substituted with medical terms.*

B. *Write the medical term and its definition for three of the phrases you underlined.*

MEDICAL TERM	DEFINITION
1. ______________	______________
2. ______________	______________
3. ______________	______________

DOCUMENTATION: Excerpt From Operative Note

This 15-year-old male presented to the emergency department with orchialgia and a swollen scrotum of approximately 6 hours duration. A Doppler ultrasound was suspicious for testicular torsion and my examination was also highly suggestive of this. He was brought to the operating room for surgical exploration. The patient and his mother received informed consent in which the possibilities of orchiectomy and future infertility were addressed. After appropriate anesthesia and sterile preparation of the surgical field were performed, a transscrotal approach was used to bring the affected testicle into the operative field. Testicular torsion was confirmed and the spermatic cord was detorsed until no twists were visible. Orchiopexy was then performed on both testes using permanent sutures.

C. *Underline medical terms presented in Chapter 7 used in the previous excerpt from Jimmie's medical record. See the Chapter at a Glance section at the end of the chapter for a complete list.*

D. *Select and define three of the medical terms you underlined. To check your answers, go to Appendix A.*

MEDICAL TERM	DEFINITION
1. ______________	______________
2. ______________	______________
3. ______________	______________

EXERCISE 29 ■ Interact with Medical Documents

A

Read the report and complete it by writing medical terms on answer lines within the document. Definitions of terms to be written appear after the document.

19504 NGUYEN, Andrew

File Patient Navigate Custom Fields Help

Chart Review | Encounters | Notes | Labs | Imaging | Procedures | Rx | Documents | Referrals | Scheduling | Billing

Name: **NGUYEN, Andrew** MR#: 19504 DOB: 07/27/19XX Gender: M Age: 75 **Allergies: Erythromycin, Penicillin** **PCP:** Joe Larson, MD

Emergency Department Report

Chief complaint: Severe lower abdominal pain and the inability to void for the past 12 hours.

Present illness: Andrew Nguyen is a 75-year-old male who presented to the emergency department at 0300 stating that he was in great pain and could not urinate. He had not been seen by a physician for several years but claimed to be in good health except for "a little high blood pressure." The patient reports previous urinary frequency, 1.________________x 2, hesitancy, intermittency, and diminished force and caliber of the urinary stream. He also has had postvoid dribbling and the sensation of not having completely emptied the bladder for some weeks or even several months. Earlier today, he had 2. ________________________ at the end of urination.

Current medications: Benadryl 25 mg at bedtime.

Physical exam: Temperature, 98.6°F. Blood pressure, 140/90 mm Hg. Pulse, 98. Respirations, 24. Palpation of the abdomen reveals a suprapubic mass approximately three fingerbreadths below the umbilicus, dull to percussion and slightly tender. DRE reveals an enlarged prostate gland without hard nodules.

Impression: Urinary bladder outlet obstruction (abbreviated as 3.____________) with 4.______________bladder distention. 5.____________________ __________________ ___________________is the probable diagnosis.

Plan: Indwelling Foley catheter for relief of urinary obstruction.
6.____________________ consult.

Electronically signed: Eleanor Adams MD 08/23/20XX 03:57

Start | Log On/Off | Print | Edit

Definitions of Medical Terms to Complete the Document

Write the medical terms defined on corresponding answer lines in the document.

1. night urination
2. blood in the urine
3. abbreviation for bladder outlet obstruction
4. pertaining to urine
5. nonmalignant excessive development pertaining to the prostate gland (enlargement of the prostate gland)
6. study of the urinary tract

EXERCISE 29 ■ Interact with Medical Documents—cont'd

B

Read the medical report and answer the questions below it.

Michigan Oncology Group **44976 East Lincoln** **Detroit, MI 97654**

January 23, 20XX

Kathryn S. Marcus, MD
Internal Medicine Services
2301 North Brinkley
Detroit, MI 97654

Re: Brindley, Javier
DOB: 08/24/19XX

Dear Dr. Marcus:

It is now 3 years since this patient had brachytherapy using radioactive seeds for his T2a, Gleason 5 prostate cancer. He continues to experience nocturia and some erectile dysfunction with a prostate obstruction score of 3.

His weight is stable at 209 pounds and blood pressure is 122/82 mm Hg. He has no adenopathy. DRE reveals a smooth prostate with no nodules. There is a slight asymmetry with greater prominence on the right side. The PSA remains 0.1 as of August 20, 20XX.

He is doing well and is likely cured of his cancer. I would like to continue seeing him on a yearly basis with a repeat PSA. He will continue seeing you as needed.

Joseph P. Potter, MD
JPP/bko

Use the medical report above to answer the questions.

1. In addition to erectile dysfunction, the patient's symptoms include:
   a. pus in the urine
   b. excessive urine
   c. night urination
   d. blood in the urine
2. Brachytherapy using radioactive seeds was used to treat:
   a. benign prostatic hyperplasia
   b. prostate cancer
   c. erectile dysfunction
3. Which diagnostic test revealed "a smooth prostate"?
   a. transrectal ultrasound
   b. prostate-specific antigen
   c. digital rectal examination
4. Three years after treatment, the patient:
   a. appears to be cancer free
   b. shows disease progression
   c. has been recommended for a radical prostatectomy

EXERCISE 30 ■ Use Medical Language in Online Electronic Health Records

Select the correct medical terms to complete three medical records in one patient's electronic file.

Access online resources at evolve.elsevier.com > Evolve Resources > Student Resources > Activities > Chapter 7 > Electronic Health Records

Topic: Prostate Cancer
Record 1: Office Visit
Record 2: Pathology Report
Record 3: Progress Note

❏ Check the box when complete.

EXERCISE 31 ■ Pronounce Medical Terms in Use

Practice pronunciation of terms by reading aloud the following paragraph. Use the phonetic spellings to assist with pronunciation. The script also contains medical terms not presented in the chapter. If interested, research their meanings in a medical dictionary or a reliable online source.

A 62-year-old male was found to have an elevated **prostate-specific antigen** (PROS-tāt) (spe-SIF-ik) (AN-ti-jen) test during a routine physical examination. At the age of 42 years he underwent a **vasectomy** (va-SEK-to-mē). The patient denies having nocturia or any significant change in his urinary stream. **Digital rectal examination** (DIJ-i-tal) (REK-tal) (eg-*zam*-i-NĀ-shun) revealed a mildly enlarged prostate gland with a 1.0 cm stony hard nodule of the right lobe. The urologist performed a **transrectal ultrasound** (trans-REK-tal) (UL-tra-sound) and biopsy. A diagnosis of adenocarcinoma of the prostate was made. The patient elected to undergo a robot-assisted radical **prostatectomy** (*pros*-ta-TEK-to-mē). Urinary incontinence complicated his postoperative course but this lasted for only 3 months. No **erectile dysfunction** (e-REK-tīl) (dis-FUNK-shun) was reported. His prognosis for full recovery should be excellent.

CHAPTER REVIEW

EXERCISE 32 ■ Chapter Content Quiz

Test your understanding of terms and abbreviations introduced in this chapter. Circle the letter for the medical term or abbreviation related to the words in italics.

1. *Inflammation of the testis* is often caused by a bacterial or viral infection.
   a. orchitis
   b. epididymitis
   c. prostatitis

2. The medical term for *discharge from the glans penis* is:
   a. balanitis
   b. balanorrhea
   c. balanorrhaphy

3. Radical *excision of the prostate gland* is used to treat prostate cancer.
   a. prostatectomy
   b. orchiectomy
   c. epididymectomy

4. HoLEP and PVP are surgical procedures used to treat *nonmalignant enlargement of the prostate gland.*
   a. anorchism
   b. testicular cancer
   c. benign prostatic hyperplasia

5. *State of hidden testicles* is an associated risk factor for the development of *cancer of the testicle.*
   a. cryptorchidism, testicular cancer
   b. anorchism, testicular torsion
   c. prostatitis, prostate cancer

6. *Inflammation of the testis and the epididymis* may be caused by an STI.
   a. prostatocystitis
   b. prostatovesiculitis
   c. orchiepididymitis

7. *A fluid-filled sac around the testicle causing scrotal swelling* is common in newborns.
   a. spermatocele
   b. hydrocele
   c. varicocele

8. *Surgical repair of the glans penis* is performed to correct anterior hypospadias.
   a. balanoplasty
   b. orchioplasty
   c. prostatocystotomy

9. The surgical procedure circumcision is the removal of all or part of the *foreskin.*
   a. glans penis
   b. testes
   c. prepuce

10. A surgical procedure that *destroys abnormal or excessive tissue by melting, vaporizing, or eroding* utilizes:
    a. morcellation
    b. enucleation
    c. ablation

11. The abbreviation for the *ultrasound procedure used to diagnose prostate cancer* with use of a transducer probe placed in the rectum is:
    a. TUMT
    b. TRUS
    c. PSA
12. Sudden onset of *pain in the testis* can be a symptom of *twisting of the spermatic cord.*
    a. orchialgia, testicular torsion
    b. aspermia, anorchism
    c. prostatolith, prostatolithotomy
13. A *microscopic observation of ejaculated semen* was ordered after the patient's *excision of a duct (vas deferens)* to evaluate the success of the procedure.
    a. prostate-specific antigen, prostatovesiculectomy
    b. digital rectal examination, vasovasostomy
    c. semen analysis, vasectomy
14. Upon diagnosis of an intratesticular mass, a radical inguinal *excision of the testis* was recommended as a diagnostic and therapeutic procedure.
    a. orchiectomy
    b. prostatectomy
    c. vasectomy
15. The term meaning *reduced or absent ability to achieve pregnancy* does not mean complete inability to create offspring.
    a. erectile dysfunction
    b. sterilization
    c. infertility
16. *Condition of scanty sperm* and *lack of live sperm in semen* are terms frequently used in discussions of male infertility.
    a. oligospermia, azoospermia
    b. puberty, ejaculation
    c. chlamydia, syphilis
17. A *procedure in which sound waves are sent and received by a transducer probe that is placed into the rectum* is used to assess the prostate and the surrounding tissues.
    a. multiparametric MRI
    b. transrectal ultrasound
    c. prostate-specific antigen (PSA)
18. A *blood test to measure the level of the hormone responsible for male physical characteristics* level may be sufficient for screening, but additional tests may be necessary for those with mild symptoms of deficiency.
    a. total testosterone
    b. prostate-specific antigen (PSA)
    c. semen analysis
19. A vaccine for *sexually transmitted infection caused by viral infection that causes benign or cancerous growths in male and female genitals* can help prevent the majority of infections that cause cervical cancer.
    a. chlamydia
    b. human immunodeficiency virus
    c. human papillomavirus
20. *A tightness of the prepuce (foreskin of the penis) that prevents its retraction over the glans penis* is normal in babies and toddlers, but may be caused by infection in older boys and adults.
    a. priapism
    b. phimosis
    c. balanitis

CHAPTER AT A GLANCE Word Parts New to This Chapter

COMBINING FORMS

andr/o
balan/o
epididym/o
orch/o
orchi/o
orchid/o
prostat/o
sperm/o
spermat/o
vas/o
vesicul/o

SUFFIXES

-algia
-ism

CHAPTER AT A GLANCE Male Reproductive System Terms Built from Word Parts

DISEASE AND DISORDER
andropathy
anorchism
balanitis
balanorrhea
benign prostatic hyperplasia (BPH)
cryptorchidism
epididymitis
orchiepididymitis
orchitis
prostatitis
prostatocystitis
prostatolith
prostatorrhea
prostatovesiculitis

SURGICAL
balanoplasty
epididymectomy
orchiectomy
orchiopexy
orchioplasty
orchiotomy
prostatectomy
prostatocystotomy
prostatolithotomy
prostatovesiculectomy
vasectomy
vasovasostomy
vesiculectomy

COMPLEMENTARY
aspermia
oligospermia
orchialgia

CHAPTER AT A GLANCE Male Reproductive System Terms *NOT* Built from Word Parts

DISEASE AND DISORDER
erectile dysfunction (ED)
hydrocele
infertility
phimosis
priapism
prostate cancer
spermatocele
testicular cancer
testicular torsion
varicocele

SURGICAL
ablation
circumcision
enucleation
hydrocelectomy
laser surgery
morcellation
robotic surgery
sterilization
transurethral incision of the prostate gland (TUIP)
transurethral microwave thermotherapy (TUMT)
transurethral resection of the prostate gland (TURP)

DIAGNOSTIC
digital rectal examination (DRE)
MRI ultrasound fusion biopsy
multiparametric MRI
prostate-specific antigen (PSA)
semen analysis
total testosterone
transrectal ultrasound (TRUS)

COMPLEMENTARY
artificial insemination
azoospermia
chlamydia
condom
ejaculation
genital herpes
gonorrhea
human immunodeficiency virus (HIV)
human papillomavirus (HPV)
orgasm
puberty
sexually transmitted infection (STI)
spermicide
syphilis
trichomoniasis

Chapter 8

Female Reproductive System

Objectives

Upon completion of this chapter, you will be able to:

1 Pronounce organs and anatomic structures of the female reproductive system.

2 Define and spell word parts related to the female reproductive system.

3 Define, pronounce, and spell disease and disorder terms related to the female reproductive system.

4 Define, pronounce, and spell surgical terms related to the female reproductive system.

5 Define, pronounce, and spell diagnostic terms related to the female reproductive system.

6 Define, pronounce, and spell complementary terms related to the female reproductive system.

7 Interpret the meaning of abbreviations related to the female reproductive system.

8 Apply medical language in clinical contexts.

Outline

Answers to Chapter Exercises, Appendix A

ANATOMY

Externally, the female reproductive system consists of the vulva, clitoris, and mammary glands. Internally, this system consists of the vagina, uterus, fallopian tubes, and ovaries (Fig. 8.1).

Function

The female reproductive system comprises external and internal organs, glands, and structures and is responsible for supporting conception and pregnancy. As the female matures throughout her lifespan, this system develops and changes based on the influence of hormones produced by the ovaries. Estrogen and progesterone are female hormones essential for sexual maturation and the overall health of the female. These hormones affect the structure and function of the integumentary, urinary, cardiac, musculoskeletal, and neurologic systems.

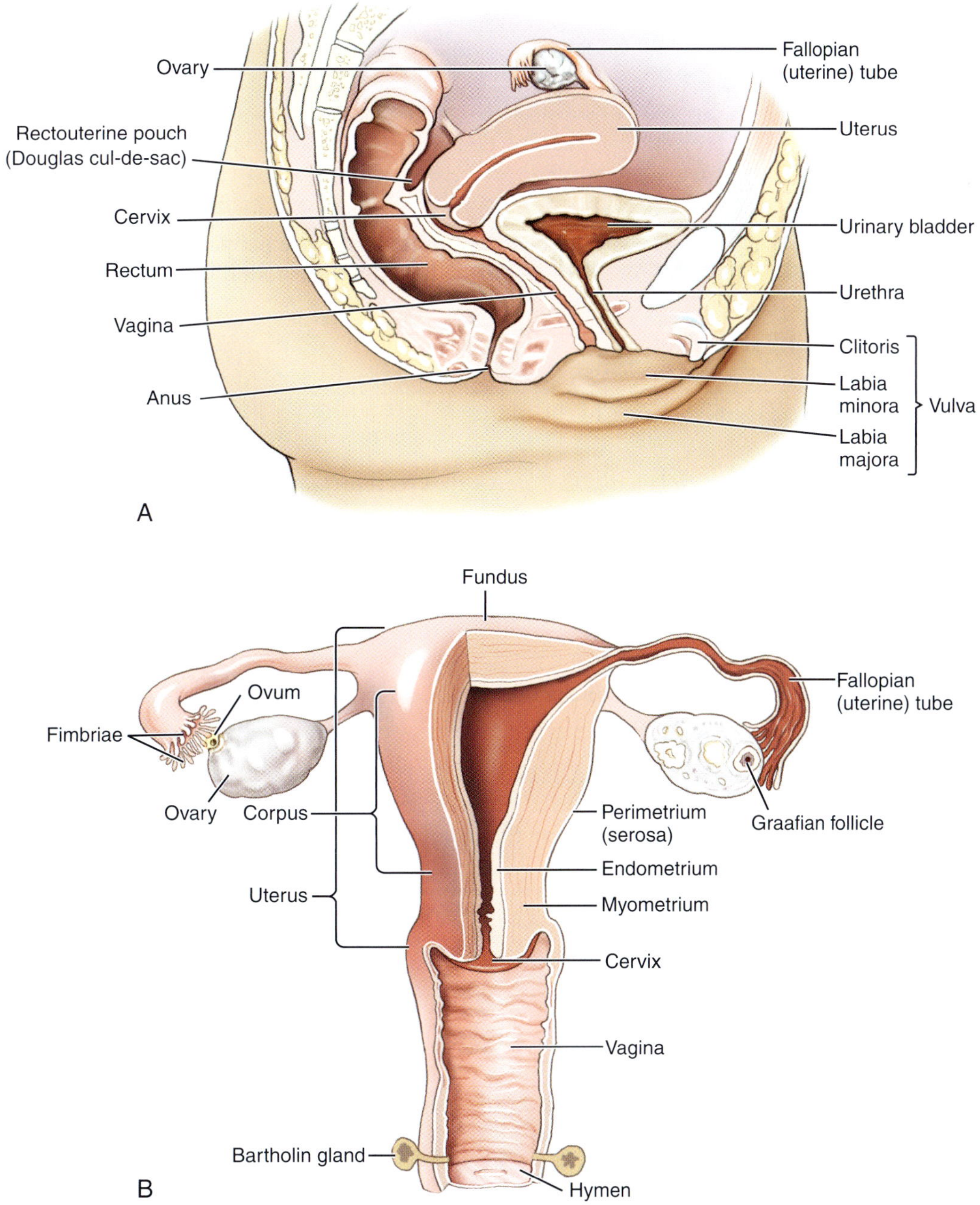

FIG. 8.1 Female reproductive organs. A, Sagittal view. **B,** Frontal view.

Internal Organs and Anatomic Structures of the Female Reproductive System

TERM	DEFINITION
ovaries (Ō-var-ēs)	almond-shaped organs located in the pelvic cavity; form and store egg cells (ova) and produce the hormones estrogen and progesterone. **Ovulation** is the release of an egg from the ovaries, which can then travel through the fallopian tubes to the uterus.
ovum *(pl.* ova) (Ō-vum) (Ō-va)	female egg cell
graafian follicles (GRA-fē-en) (FOL-i-kels)	100,000 microscopic sacs that make up a large portion of the ovaries. Each follicle contains an immature ovum. Normally one graafian follicle develops to maturity monthly between puberty and menopause. It moves to the surface of the ovary and releases the ovum, which passes into the fallopian tube.
THE GRAAFIAN FOLLICLE is named for Dutch anatomist Reinier de Graaf, who discovered the sac in 1672.	
fallopian tubes (fa-LŌ-pē-an) (toobz)	pair of tubes attached to the uterus that provide a passageway for the ovum to move from the ovary to the uterus (also called **uterine tubes**)
THE FALLOPIAN TUBE was named in honor of Gabriele Falloppio, 1523-1562, one of the most important anatomists and physicians of the sixteenth century. Falloppio also gave the **vagina** and the **placenta** their names. Fallopian, an eponym, has become so common in medical terminlogy that it is often not capitalized.	
fimbria *(pl.* fimbriae) (FIM-brē-a) (FIM-brē-ā)	finger-like projection at the free end of the fallopian tube
uterus (Ū-ter-us)	pear-sized and shaped muscular organ that lies in the pelvic cavity, except during pregnancy when it enlarges and extends up into the abdominal cavity. Its functions are menstruation, pregnancy, and labor.
endometrium (*en*-dō-MĒ-trē-um)	inner lining of the uterus
myometrium (*mī*-ō-MĒ-trē-um)	muscular middle layer of the uterus
perimetrium (*per*-i-MĒ-trē-um)	outer protective layer of the uterus that secretes watery serous fluid to reduce friction (also called **uterine serosa**)
corpus (KŌR-pus)	large central portion of the uterus (also called **uterine body**)
fundus (FUN-dus)	rounded upper portion of the uterus
cervix (Cx) (SER-vicks)	narrow lower portion of the uterus
vagina (va-JĪ-nah)	passageway between the uterus and the outside of the body
hymen (HĪ-men)	fold of membrane found near the opening of the vagina

External Female Reproductive Structures

TERM	DEFINITION
vulva (VUL-va)	external genitals of the female, including the mons pubis, labia majora, labia minora, clitoris, urinary meatus, and vaginal opening
perineum (*per*-i-NĒ-um)	pelvic floor in both the male and female. In females it refers to the area between the vaginal opening and the anus.

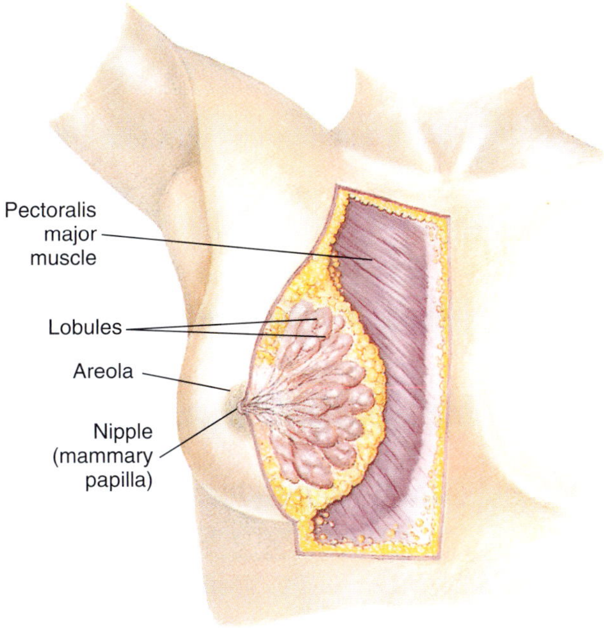

FIG. 8.2 Female breast.

Glands of the Female Reproductive System

TERM	DEFINITION
Bartholin glands (BAR-tō-lin) (glans)	pair of mucus-producing glands located on each side of the vagina, just above the vaginal opening (also called **greater vestibular glands**)
BARTHOLIN GLANDS were described by Caspar Bartholin, a Danish anatomist, in 1675.	
breasts (brests)	milk-producing glands. Each breast consists of 15 to 20 divisions or lobules. (also called **mammary glands**) (Fig. 8.2)
mammary papilla (MAM-a-rē) (pa-PIL-a)	breast nipple
areola (a-RĒ-ō-la)	pigmented area around the breast nipple

PRONOUNCE ANATOMIC STRUCTURES

Practice saying aloud each of the organs and specific structures on the previous pages.

To hear the terms, go to Evolve Resources at www.evolve.elsevier.com and select: Student Resources > Audio Glossary > Chapter 8 > **Anatomic Structures.**

❑ Check the box when complete.

WORD PARTS

Use paper flashcards or electronic flashcards on Evolve to memorize word parts used to analyze, define, and build medical terms in this chapter. To reinforce learning, study one section of the Word Parts Table at a time, then complete the corresponding exercise on the following pages.

1 ■ Female Reproductive System Combining Forms

COMBINING FORM	DEFINITION	COMBINING FORM	DEFINITION
cervic/o	cervix	**endometri/o**	endometrium
colp/o	vagina	**episi/o**	vulva

1 ■ Female Reproductive System Combining Forms—cont'd

COMBINING FORM	DEFINITION	COMBINING FORM	DEFINITION
gynec/o	woman, female reproductive organs	**oophor/o**	ovary
hymen/o	hymen	**pelv/i**	pelvis, pelvic cavity (*Note: the combining vowel is an **i***)
hyster/o	uterus	**perine/o**	perineum
mamm/o	breast	**salping/o**	fallopian tube (uterine tube) (Fig. 8.3)
mast/o	breast	**trachel/o**	cervix
men/o	menstruation	**vagin/o**	vagina
metr/o	uterus	**vulv/o**	vulva

2 ■ Combining Forms Used with Female Reproductive System Terms

COMBINING FORM	DEFINITION	COMBINING FORM	DEFINITION
hemat/o	blood	**my/o**	muscle
hydr/o	water	**olig/o**	scanty, few
leuk/o	white	**py/o**	pus

3 ■ Prefixes

PREFIX	DEFINITION	PREFIX	DEFINITION
a-	absence of, without	**endo-**	within
dys-	painful, abnormal, difficult, labored	**peri-**	surrounding (outer)

4 ■ Suffixes

SUFFIX	DEFINITION	SUFFIX	DEFINITION
-al	pertaining to	**-osis**	abnormal condition
-algia	pain	**-pexy**	surgical fixation
-cele	hernia, protrusion	**-plasty**	surgical repair
-cleisis	surgical closure	**-rrhagia**	excessive bleeding
-ectomy	excision, surgical removal	**-rrhaphy**	suturing, repairing
-gram	the record, radiographic image	**-rrhea**	flow, discharge
-graphy	process of recording, radiographic imaging	**-salpinx**	fallopian tube (uterine tube)
-ic	pertaining to	**-scope**	instrument used for visual examination
-itis	inflammation	**-scopic**	pertaining to visual examination
-logist	one who studies and treats (specialist, physician)	**-scopy**	visual examination
-logy	study of	**-tomy**	cut into, incision

Refer to **Appendix B** and **Appendix C** for alphabetized word parts and their meanings.

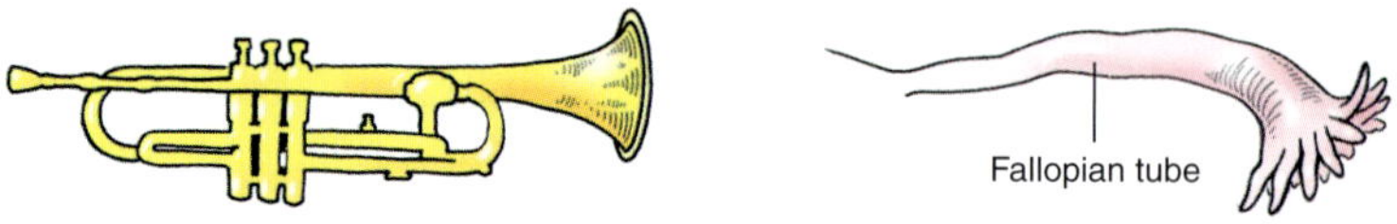

FIG. 8.3 Salpinx is derived from the Greek term for trumpet. The term was used for the fallopian tubes because of their trumpet-like shape.

EXERCISE 1 ■ Female Reproductive System Combining Forms

Refer to the first section of the word parts table.

A Label

Fill in the blanks with combining forms in this diagram of internal female reproductive organs and anatomic structures. *To check your answers, go to Appendix A at the back of the textbook.*

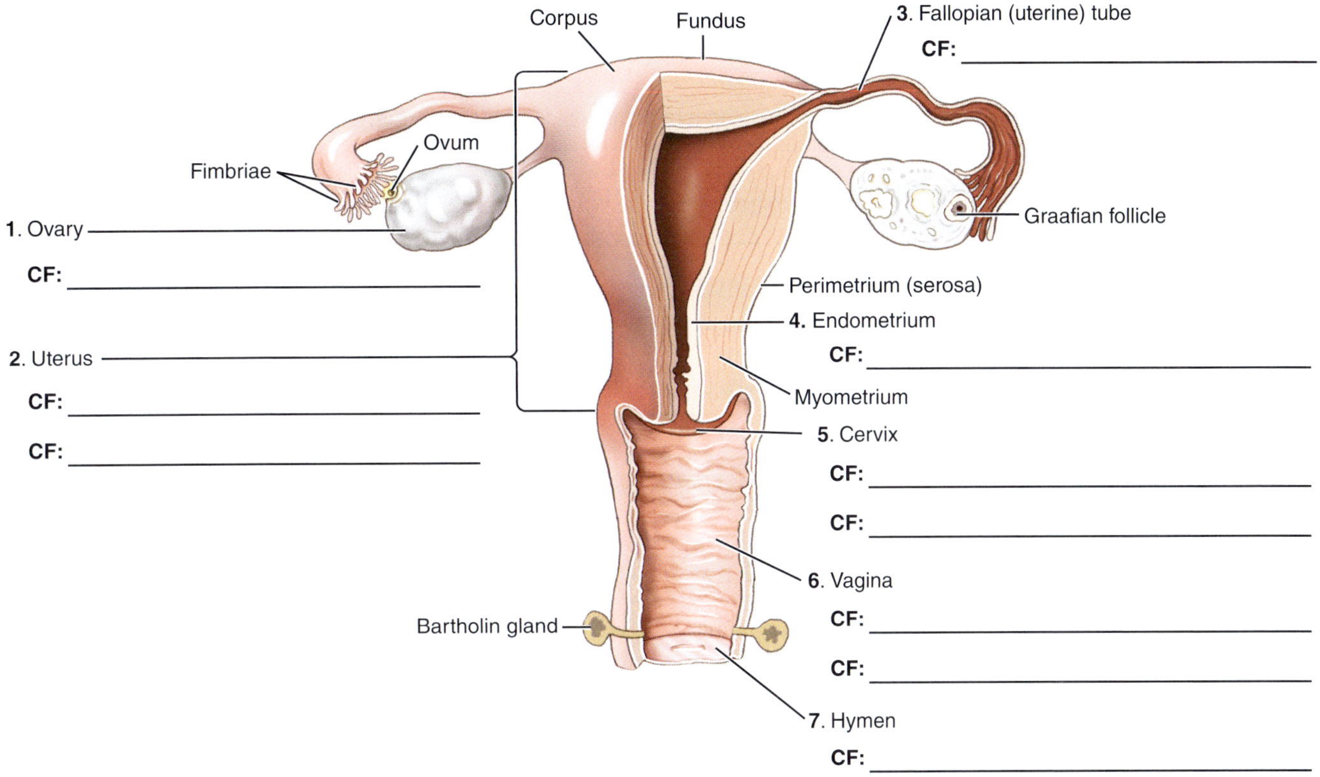

B Label

Fill in the blanks with combining forms in this diagram of external female reproductive organs and anatomic structures.

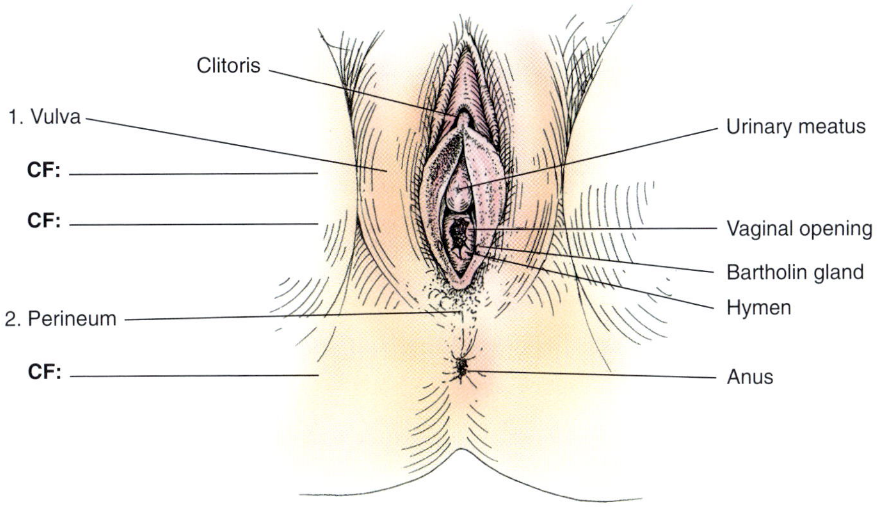

C Identify

Write the combining form for each of the following.

1. menstruation ____________________
2. woman, female reproductive organs ____________________
3. breast a. ____________________, b. ____________________
4. pelvis, pelvic cavity ____________________

D Define and Match

Step 1: Write the definitions after the following combining forms.
Step 2: Match the descriptions on the right with the combining forms and definitions. Answers may be used more than once; no answer line appears for those not described in a lettered item.

_____ 1. salping/o, ____________________
_____ 2. metr/o, ____________________
_____ 3. perine/o, ____________________
_____ 4. cervic /o, ____________________
_____ 5. colp/o, ____________________
_____ 6. trachel/o, ____________________
_____ 7. mamm/o, ____________________
8. pelv/i, ____________________

a. pelvic floor in male and female anatomy
b. passageway between the uterus and the outside of the body
c. narrow lower portion of the uterus
d. milk-producing glands
e. pear-sized and shaped muscular organ
f. passageway for ovum to move from the ovary to the uterus

E Define and Match

Step 1: Write the definitions after the following combining forms.
Step 2: Match the descriptions on the right with the combining forms and definitions. Answers may be used more than once; no answer line appears for those not described in a lettered item.

_____ 1. vagin/o, ____________________
_____ 2. hymen/o, ____________________
_____ 3. episi/o, ____________________
_____ 4. hyster/o, ____________________
_____ 5. mast/o, ____________________
_____ 6. oophor/o, ____________________
_____ 7. vulv/o, ____________________
_____ 8. endometri/o, ____________________
9. men/o, ____________________
10. gynec/o, ____________________

a. fold of membrane near the opening of the vagina
b. passageway between the uterus and the outside of the body
c. inner lining of the uterus
d. external genitals of the female
e. milk-producing glands
f. pear-sized and shaped muscular organ
g. almond-shaped organs located in the pelvic cavity that produce and store female reproductive cells

EXERCISE 2 ■ Combining Forms Used with Female Reproductive System Terms

Refer to the second section of the word parts table.

A Define

Write the definitions of the following combining forms.

1. olig/o ____________________
2. hemat/o ____________________
3. my/o ____________________
4. leuk/o ____________________
5. py/o ____________________
6. hydr/o ____________________

B Identify

Write the combining form for each of the following.

1. pus ______
2. water ______
3. blood ______
4. muscle ______
5. scanty, few ______
6. white ______

EXERCISE 3 ■ Prefixes

Refer to the third section of the word parts table.

A Define

Write the definitions of the following prefixes.

1. endo- ______
2. a- ______
3. peri- ______
4. dys- ______

B Identify

Write the prefix for each of the following definitions.

1. painful, abnormal, difficult, labored ______
2. within ______
3. absence of, without ______
4. surrounding (outer) ______

EXERCISE 4 ■ Suffixes

Refer to the fourth section of the word parts table.

A Match

Match the suffixes in the first column with their correct definitions in the second column.

______	1. -graphy	a. pertaining to visual examination
______	2. -pexy	b. pertaining to
______	3. -cele	c. process of recording, radiographic imaging
______	4. -scopic	d. inflammation
______	5. -logy	e. study of
______	6. -itis	f. hernia, protrusion
______	7. -al	g. suturing, repairing
______	8. -rrhaphy	h. surgical fixation

B Define

Write the definitions of the following suffixes.

1. -gram ______
2. -osis ______
3. -algia ______
4. -rrhea ______
5. -scopy ______
6. -ic ______
7. -ectomy ______
8. -plasty ______
9. -rrhagia ______
10. -scope ______
11. -tomy ______
12. -logist ______

C Label

Write the suffixes pictured and defined.

1. ______________________
fallopian tube (uterine tube)

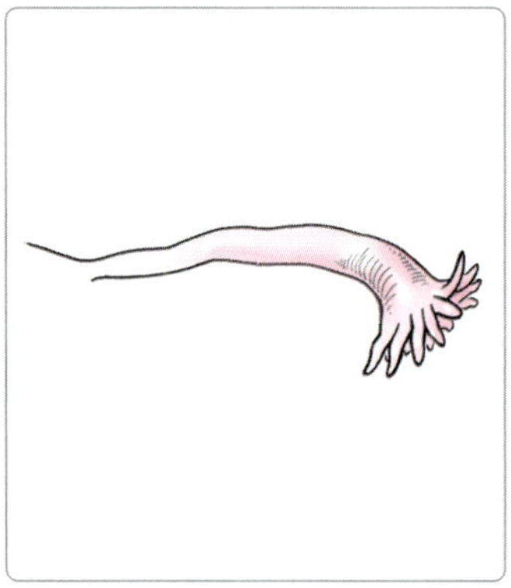

2. ______________________
surgical closure

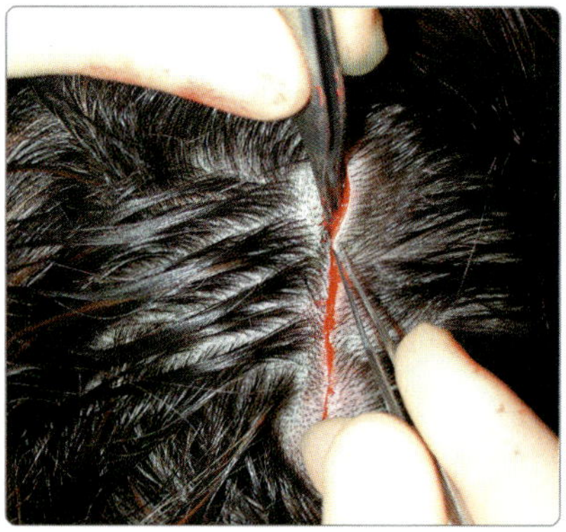

MEDICAL TERMS

Medical terms relevant to this chapter have been grouped by topics, such as Disease and Disorder, and are listed in tables designated as Built from Word Parts or *NOT* Built from Word Parts. The exercises following each table assist with learning term definitions, pronunciations, and spellings.

Disease and Disorder Terms

BUILT FROM WORD PARTS

The following terms can be translated using definitions of word parts. Further explanation is provided within parentheses as needed.

TERM	DEFINITION
1. **amenorrhea** (a-*men*-ō-RĒ-a)	absence of menstrual flow
2. **cervicitis** (*ser*-vi-SĪ-tis)	inflammation of the cervix (Fig. 8.7)
3. **dysmenorrhea** (dis-*men*-ō-RĒ-a)	painful menstrual flow
4. **endometriosis** (*en*-dō-*mē*-trē-Ō-sis)	abnormal condition of the endometrium (endometrial tissue grows outside of the uterus in various areas in the pelvic cavity, including ovaries, fallopian tubes, intestines, and uterus) (Fig. 8.4)
5. **endometritis** (*en*-dō-mē-TRĪ-tis)	inflammation of the endometrium (Fig. 8.7)
6. **hematosalpinx** (*hem*-a-tō-SAL-pinks)	blood in the fallopian tube
7. **hydrosalpinx** (*hī*-drō-SAL-pinks)	water in the fallopian tube (a clear, watery fluid collects in the tube, and can cause blockage)
8. **mastitis** (*mas*-TĪ-tis)	inflammation of the breast
9. **menometrorrhagia** (*men*-ō-*met*-rō-RĀ-jea)	excessive bleeding from the uterus at menstruation (and between menstrual cycles; heavy and irregular bleeding)
10. **menorrhagia** (*men*-ō-RĀ-jea)	excessive bleeding at menstruation (heavy bleeding in regular, cyclical pattern)
11. **metrorrhagia** (*mē*-trō-RĀ-jea)	excessive bleeding from the uterus (irregular, out-of-cycle bleeding ranging from heavy to light, including spotting)

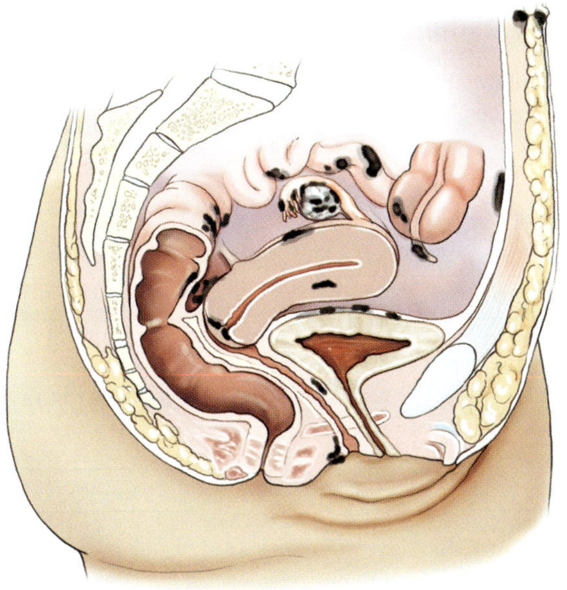

FIG. 8.4 Endometriosis. Spots indicate common sites of endometrial deposits.

TERM	DEFINITION	TERM	DEFINITION
12. myometritis (*mī*-o-me-TRĪ-tis)	inflammation of the uterine muscle (myometrium)	**17. salpingitis** (*sal*-pin-JĪ-tis)	inflammation of the fallopian tube (Fig. 8.7)
13. oligomenorrhea (*ol*-i-gō-*men*-ō-RĒ-a)	scanty menstrual flow (infrequent menstrual flow)	**18. salpingocele** (sal-PING-gō-sēl)	hernia of the fallopian tube
14. oophoritis (*ō*-of-o-RĪ-tis)	inflammation of the ovary	**19. vaginitis** (*vaj*-i-NĪ-tis)	inflammation of the vagina (Fig. 8.7)
15. perimetritis (*per*-i-me-TRĪ-tis)	inflammation surrounding the uterus (perimetrium)	**20. vaginosis** (*vaj*-i-NŌ-sis)	abnormal condition of the vagina (caused by a bacterial imbalance) (also called **bacterial vaginosis**)
16. pyosalpinx (*pī*-ō-SAL-pinks)	pus in the fallopian tube	**21. vulvovaginitis** (*vul*-vō-*vaj*-i-NĪ-tis)	inflammation of the vulva and vagina

EXERCISE 5 ■ Pronounce and Spell

Practice pronunciation and spelling on paper and online.

1. Practice on Paper

a. **Pronounce:** Read the phonetic spelling and say aloud the terms listed in the previous table. Refer to the pronunciation key on p. 20 as necessary.
b. **Spell:** Have a study partner read the terms aloud. Write the spelling of the terms on a separate sheet of paper.

2. Practice Online

a. **Access** online learning resources. Go to evolve.elsevier.com > Evolve Resources > Student Resources.
b. **Pronounce:** Select Audio Glossary > Chapter 8 > Exercise 5. Select a term to hear its pronunciation and repeat aloud.
c. **Spell:** Select Activities > Chapter 8 > Spell Terms > Exercise 5. Select the audio icon and type the correct spelling of the term.

❑ Check the box when complete.

EXERCISE 6 ■ Analyze and Define

Analyze and define the following terms by drawing slashes between word parts, writing word part abbreviations above the term, underlining combining forms, and writing the combining form abbreviations below the term.

1. oligomenorrhea

____

____

2. cervicitis

____

____

3. vaginosis

____

____

4. hematosalpinx

____

____

5. metrorrhagia

____

____

6. oophoritis

____

____

7. perimetritis

____

____

8. vulvovaginitis

____

____

9. salpingocele

____

____

10. menometrorrhagia

____

____

EXERCISE 7 ■ Build

A Label

Build terms pictured by writing word parts above definitions.

1.

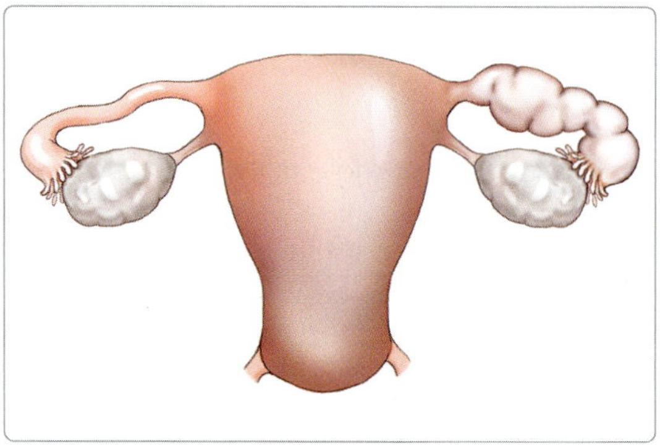

_______ / _______ / _______
water CV fallopian tube

2.

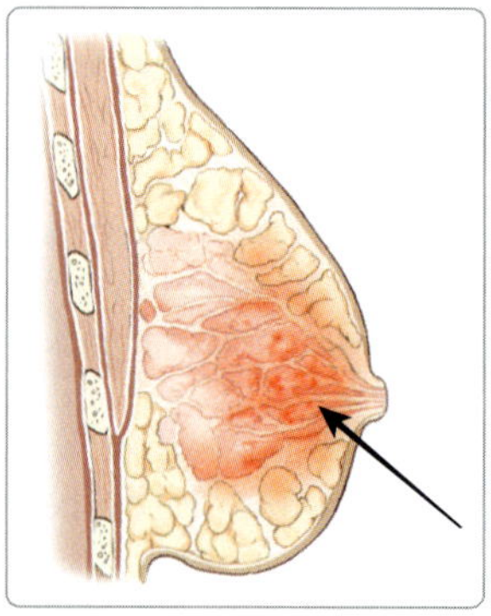

_______ / _______
inflammation breast

3.

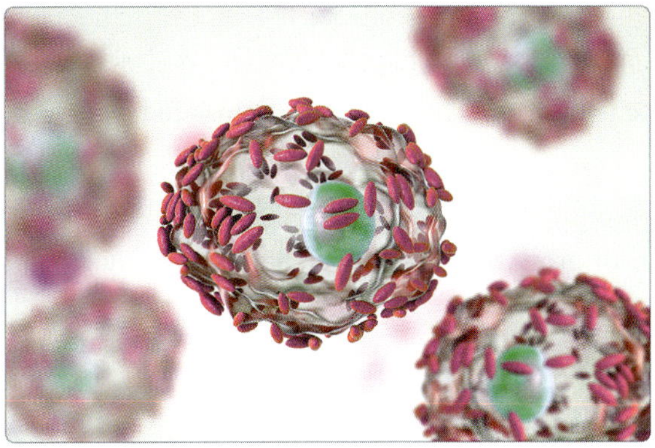

_______________ / _______________
vagina abnormal condition
(caused by a bacterial imbalance)

4.

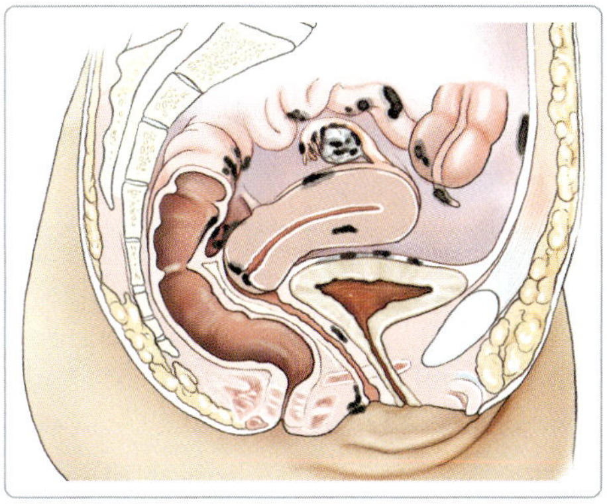

_______________ / _______________
endometrium abnormal condition

5.

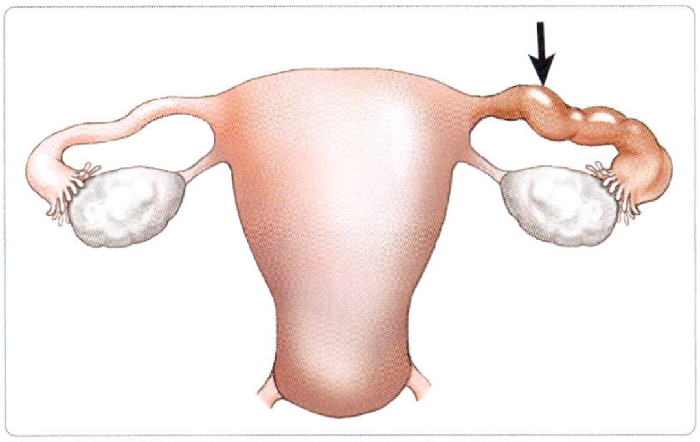

_______________ / _______________
fallopian tube inflammation

6.

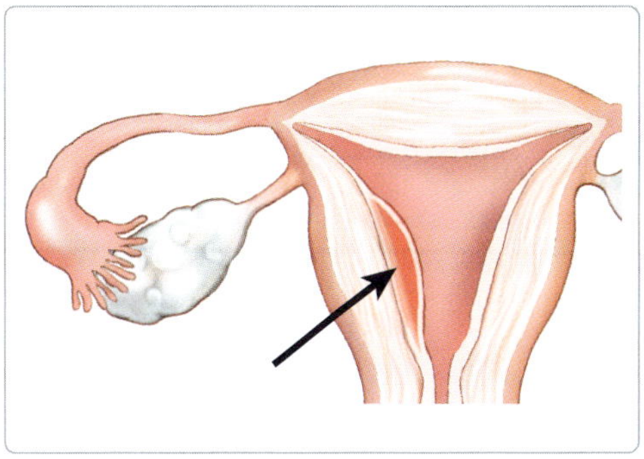

_______________ / _______________
endometrium inflammation

B Fill In

Build disease and disorder terms for the following definitions by using the word parts you have learned.

1. inflammation of the uterine muscle
   ______ / ______ / ______ / ______
   WR / CV / WR / S

2. excessive bleeding at menstruation (heavy bleeding in regular, cyclical pattern)
   ______ / ______ / ______
   WR / CV / S

3. pus in the fallopian tube
   ______ / ______ / ______
   WR / CV / S

4. absence of menstrual flow
   ______ / ______ / ______ / ______
   P / WR / CV / S

5. painful menstrual flow
   ______ / ______ / ______ / ______
   P / WR / CV / S

Disease and Disorder Terms

NOT BUILT FROM WORD PARTS

Word parts may be present in the following terms; however, their full meanings cannot be translated using definitions of word parts alone.

TERM	DEFINITION
1. **abnormal uterine bleeding (AUB)** (ab-NOR-mul) (Ū-ter-in) (BLĒD-ing)	irregular bleeding in the absence of pregnancy; menometrorrhagia, menorrhagia, and metrorrhagia are some types of AUB
2. **adenomyosis** (*ad*-e-nō-mī-Ō-sis)	growth of endometrium into the muscular portion of the uterus
3. **Bartholin cyst** (BAR-tō-lin) (sist)	blockage of one of the glands on either side of the vagina; usually causes a tender, swollen lump on the affected side, which may become infected, resulting in a Bartholin abscess
4. **breast cancer** (brest) (KAN-cer)	malignant tumor of the breast (Fig. 8.5)
5. **cervical cancer** (SER-vi-kal) (KAN-cer)	malignant tumor of the cervix, which progresses from cervical dysplasia to carcinoma. Its cause is linked to human papillomavirus (HPV) infection.

HPV VACCINE The Food and Drug Administration (FDA) approved a vaccine for human papillomavirus (HPV) in 2006, directly impacting the prevention of **cervical cancer**. The vaccine is highly effective in protecting against several forms of HPV as long as it is administered before a male or female becomes sexually active. Because vaccination does not combat all strains of HPV and is not 100% effective, periodic cervical cancer screening is strongly recommended.

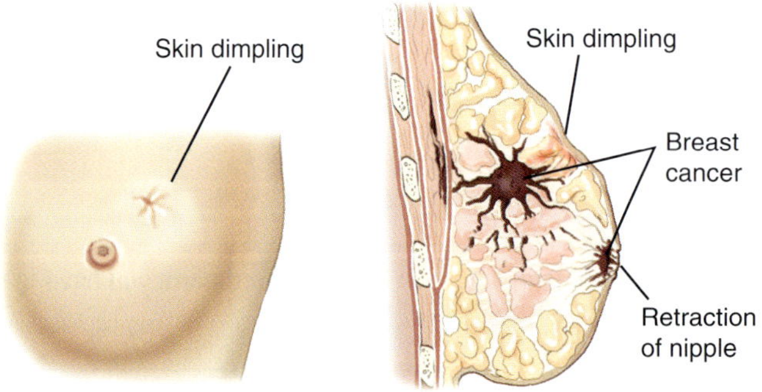

FIG. 8.5 Clinical signs of breast cancer.

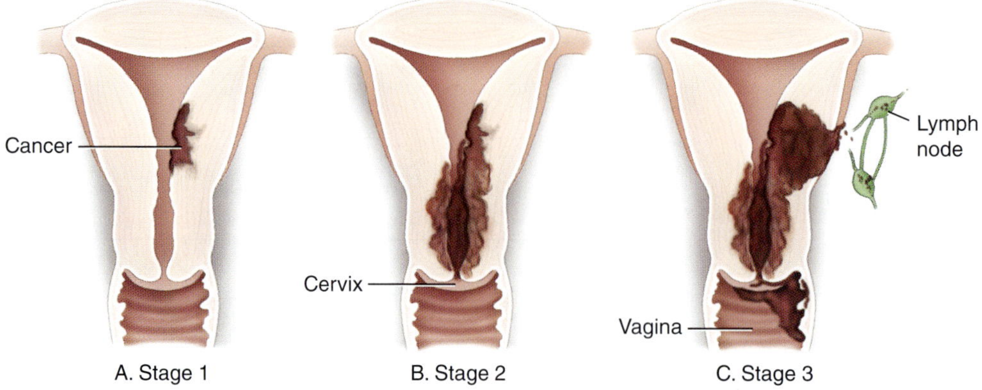

FIG. 8.6 Endometrial cancer. A, Stage 1: Confined to the endometrium. **B,** Stage 2: Spread into support structures of the cervix from the body of the uterus. **C,** Stage 3: Spreads to other organs such as the vagina.

TERM	DEFINITION
6. endometrial cancer (*en*-dō-MĒ-trē-al) (KAN-cer)	malignant tumor of the endometrium (also called **uterine cancer**) (Fig. 8.6)
7. fibrocystic breast changes (FCC) (*fī*-brō-SIS-tik) (brest) (CHĀN-jiz)	thickening of tissue (fibrosis), benign cysts, and pain or tenderness in one or both breasts; thought to be caused by monthly hormonal changes (also called **fibrocystic breasts**; formerly called **fibrocystic breast disease**)
8. ovarian cancer (ō-VAR-ē-an) (KAN-cer)	malignant tumor of the ovary
9. pelvic inflammatory disease (PID) (PEL-vik) (in-FLAM-a-*tor*-ē) (di-ZĒZ)	inflammation of some or all of the female pelvic organs; can be caused by many different pathogens. If untreated, the infection may spread upward from the vagina, involving the uterus, fallopian tubes, ovaries, and other pelvic organs. An ascending infection may result in infertility and, in acute cases, fatal septicemia (Fig. 8.7).
10. polycystic ovary syndrome (PCOS) (*pol*-ē-SIS-tik) (Ō-vah-rē) (SIN-drōm)	condition typically characterized by hormonal imbalances, ovulatory dysfunction, and multiple ovarian cysts; symptoms can include irregular menstruation, acne, excess facial and body hair, and infertility. People with this condition have increased risks of cardiovascular disease, obesity, and glucose intolerance.
11. premenstrual syndrome (PMS) (prē-MEN-stroo-al) (SIN-drōm)	syndrome involving physical and emotional symptoms occurring up to 10 days before menstruation. Symptoms include nervous tension, irritability, mastalgia, edema, and headache.
12. toxic shock syndrome (TSS) (TOK-sik) (shok) (SIN-drōm)	severe illness characterized by high fever, rash, vomiting, diarrhea, and myalgia, followed by hypotension and, in severe cases, shock and death; usually affects menstruating women using tampons; caused by *Staphylococcus aureus* and *Streptococcus pyogenes*
13. uterine fibroid (Ū-ter-in) (FĪ-broyd)	benign tumor of the uterine muscle (also called **myoma of the uterus** or **leiomyoma**)
14. uterovaginal prolapse (*ū*-ter-ō-VAJ-i-nal) (prō-LAPS)	dropping of the uterus (and sometimes vagina) due to weakened pelvic muscles; the uterus moves downward into and is sometimes visible outside the vagina
15. vaginal fistula (VAJ-i-nal) (FIS-tū-la)	abnormal connection between the vagina and another organ, such as the urinary bladder, colon, or rectum (Table 8.1)

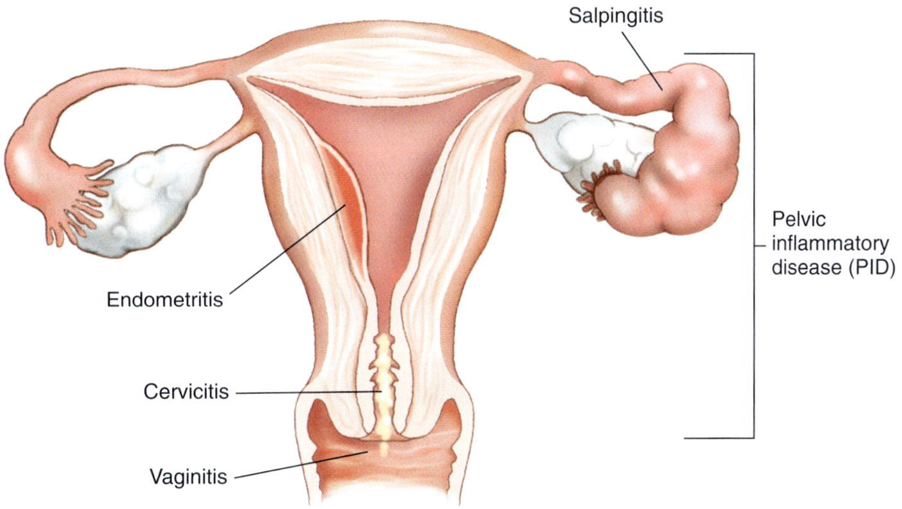

FIG. 8.7 Ascending infection of the female reproductive system as seen in pelvic inflammatory disease.

TABLE 8.1 Types, Symptoms, and Causes of Vaginal Fistulas

TYPES OF VAGINAL FISTULAS	SYMPTOMS	CAUSES OF VAGINAL FISTULAS
• **Vesicovaginal fistula,** abnormal connection between the urinary bladder and the vagina • **Colovaginal fistula,** abnormal connection between the colon (large intestine) and the vagina • **Rectovaginal fistula,** abnormal connection between the rectum and the vagina	• **Vesicovaginal fistula,** urine may leak or flow out of the vagina, causing incontinence, bad smells, sores or discomfort • **Colovaginal and rectovaginal fistulas,** foul smelling discharge (feces) or gas may come out of the vagina, which may be painful or cause infections	• **Gynecologic surgery,** including hysterectomy and caesarean section, and injuries during childbirth (occurs more frequently in developing countries where access to medical care may be limited) • **Gastrointestinal diseases** including inflammatory bowel disease (Crohn disease and ulcerative colitis) and diverticulitis • **Malignancies** in the pelvic region and radiation therapy for pelvic cancers

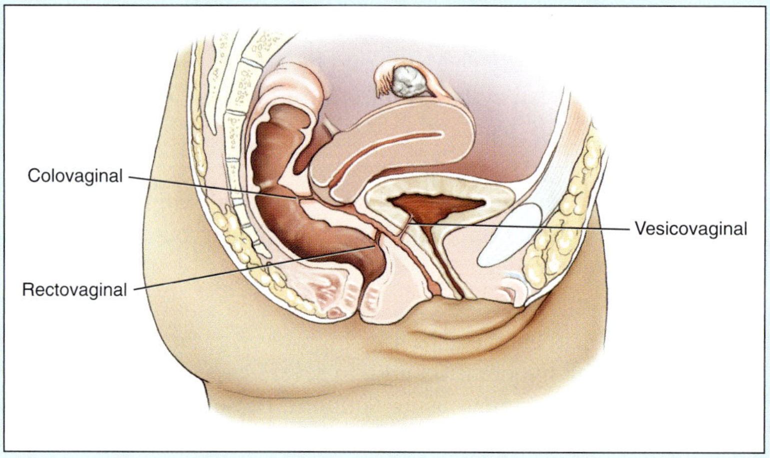

Vaginal fistulas: vesicovaginal, colovaginal, and rectovaginal.

EXERCISE 8 ■ Pronounce and Spell

Practice pronunciation and spelling on paper and online.

1. Practice on Paper

a. **Pronounce:** Read the phonetic spelling and say aloud the terms listed in the term table. Refer to the pronunciation key on p. 20 as necessary.
b. **Spell:** Have a study partner read the terms aloud. Write the spelling of the terms on a separate sheet of paper.

2. Practice Online

a. **Access** online learning resources. Go to evolve.elsevier.com > Evolve Resources > Student Resources.
b. **Pronounce:** Select Audio Glossary > Chapter 8 > Exercise 8. Select a term to hear its pronunciation and repeat aloud.
c. **Spell:** Select Activities > Chapter 8 > Spell Terms > Exercise 8. Select the audio icon and type the correct spelling of the term.

❑ Check the box when complete.

EXERCISE 9 ■ Match

Match the terms in the first column with their correct definitions in the second column.

_____ 1. vaginal fistula
_____ 2. uterovaginal prolapse
_____ 3. uterine fibroid
_____ 4. fibrocystic breast changes
_____ 5. endometrial cancer
_____ 6. breast cancer
_____ 7. adenomyosis

a. abnormal connection between the vagina and another organ
b. also called myoma of the uterus or leiomyoma
c. also called uterine cancer
d. dropping of the uterus (and sometimes vagina) due to weakened pelvic muscles
e. growth of endometrium into the muscular portion of the uterus
f. malignant tumor of the breast
g. thickening of tissue (fibrosis), benign cysts, and pain or tenderness in one or both breasts

EXERCISE 10 ■ Match

Match the terms in the first column with their correct definitions in the second column.

_____ 1. toxic shock syndrome
_____ 2. premenstrual syndrome
_____ 3. polycystic ovary syndrome
_____ 4. pelvic inflammatory disease
_____ 5. ovarian cancer
_____ 6. cervical cancer
_____ 7. Bartholin cyst
_____ 8. abnormal uterine bleeding

a. blockage of one of the glands on either side of the vagina
b. hormonal imbalances, ovulatory dysfunction, and multiple ovarian cysts
c. inflammation of some or all of the female pelvic organs
d. irregular bleeding in the absence of pregnancy
e. malignant tumor of the ovary
f. physical and emotional symptoms occurring up to 10 days before menstruation
g. progresses from cervical dysplasia to carcinoma
h. severe illness characterized by high fever, rash, vomiting, diarrhea, and myalgia, followed by hypotension and, in severe cases, shock and death

EXERCISE 11 ■ Fill In

A Identify

Fill in the blanks with the correct terms.

1. A malignant tumor of the ovary is referred to as __________ __________.
2. __________ is growth of endometrium into the muscular portion of the uterus.
3. A severe illness characterized by high fever, rash, vomiting, diarrhea, and myalgia, followed by hypotension, which is associated with the use of tampons. is known as __________ __________ __________.
4. __________ __________ is a malignant tumor, which progresses from cervical dysplasia to carcinoma, and is linked to human papillomavirus (HPV) infection.
5. A syndrome involving physical and emotional symptoms occurring up to 10 days before menstruation is called __________ __________.
6. Irregular bleeding in the absence of pregnancy is __________ __________ __________; menometrorrhagia, menorrhagia, and metrorrhagia are examples.
7. __________ __________ __________ refers to thickening of tissue (fibrosis), benign cysts, and pain or tenderness in one or both breasts.

B Label

Write the medical terms pictured and defined.

1. ______________________
dropping of the uterus (and sometimes vagina) due to weakened pelvic muscles

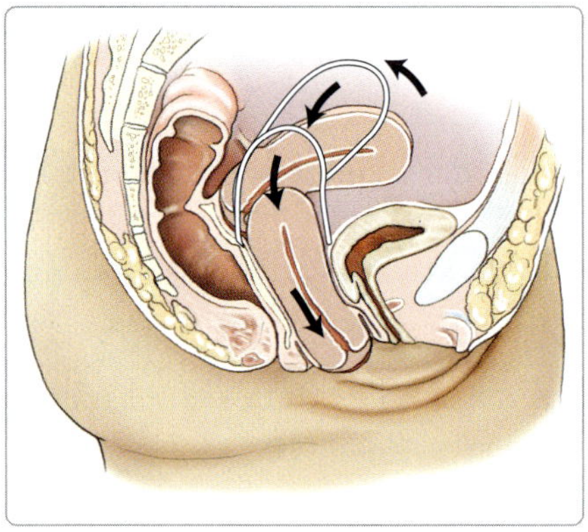

2. ______________________
benign tumor of the uterine muscle

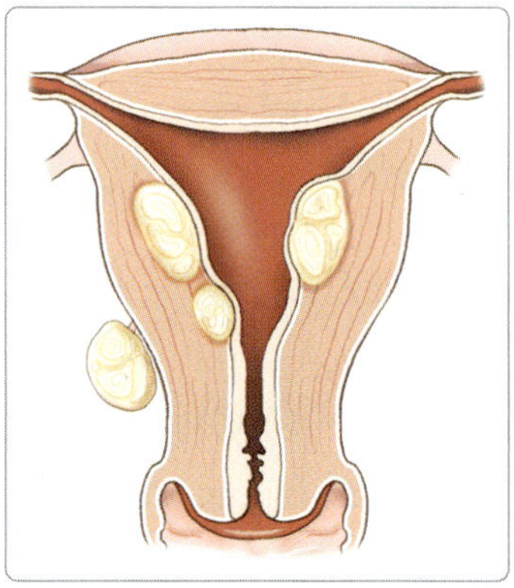

3. ______________________
malignant tumor of the endometrium

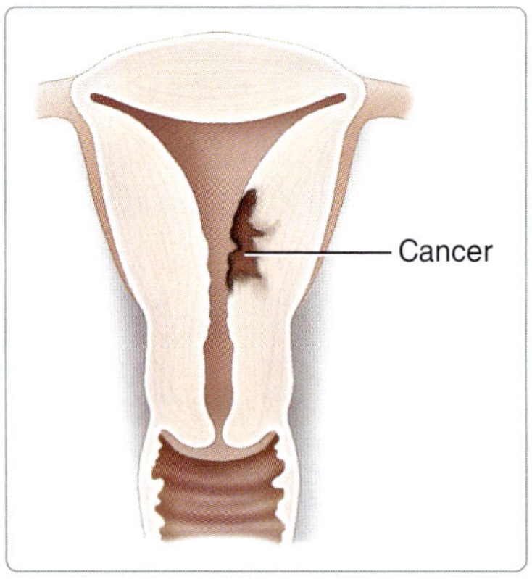

4. ______________________
malignant tumor of the breast

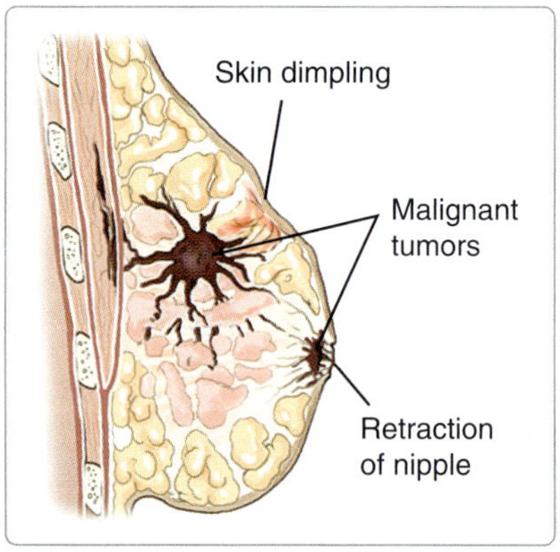

5. ______________________
inflammation of some or all of the female pelvic organs

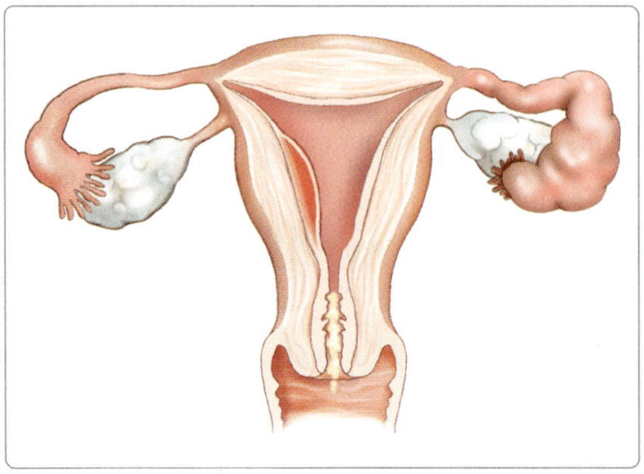

6. ______________________
abnormal connection between the vagina and another organ, such as the urinary bladder, colon, or rectum

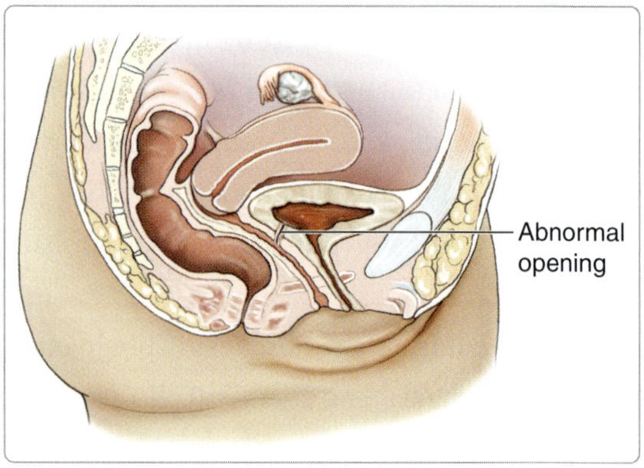

7. ______________________________
condition typically characterized by hormonal imbalances, ovulatory dysfunction, and multiple ovarian cysts

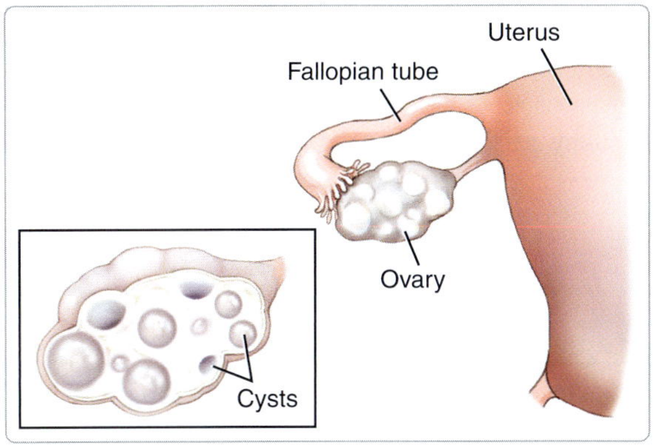

8. ______________________________
blockage of one of the glands on either side of the vagina; usually causes a tender, swollen lump on the affected side

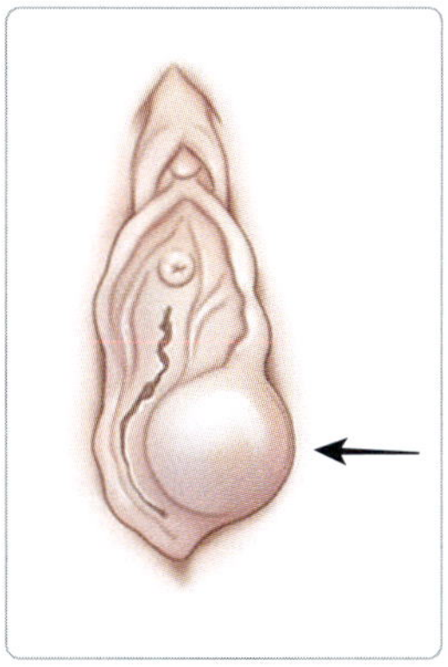

EXERCISE 12 ■ Review of Disease and Disorder Terms

Can you define, pronounce, and spell the following terms?

abnormal uterine bleeding (AUB)
adenomyosis
amenorrhea
Bartholin cyst
breast cancer
cervical cancer
cervicitis
dysmenorrhea
endometrial cancer
endometriosis
endometritis
fibrocystic breast changes (FCC)
hematosalpinx
hydrosalpinx
mastitis
menometrorrhagia
menorrhagia
metrorrhagia
myometritis
oligomenorrhea
oophoritis
ovarian cancer
pelvic inflammatory disease (PID)
perimetritis
polycystic ovary syndrome (PCOS)
premenstrual syndrome (PMS)
pyosalpinx
salpingitis
salpingocele
toxic shock syndrome (TSS)
uterine fibroid
uterovaginal prolapse
vaginal fistula
vaginitis
vaginosis
vulvovaginitis

Surgical Terms

BUILT FROM WORD PARTS

The following terms can be translated using definitions of word parts. Further explanation is provided within parentheses as needed.

TERM	DEFINITION
1. colpocleisis (*kol*-pō-KLĪ-sis)	surgical closure of the vagina
2. colpoperineorrhaphy (kol-pō-*per*-i-nē-OR-a-fē)	suturing of the vagina and the perineum (performed to mend perineal vaginal tears)
3. colpoplasty (KOL-pō-*plas*-tē)	surgical repair of the vagina
4. colporrhaphy (kol-POR-a-fē)	suturing of the vagina (wall of the vagina)
5. episiorrhaphy (e-*piz*-ē-OR-a-fē)	suturing of (a tear in) the vulva
6. hymenotomy (*hī*-men-OT-o-mē)	incision into the hymen
7. hysterectomy (*his*-te-REK-to-mē)	excision of the uterus (Table 8.2, Fig. 8.8)
8. hysteropexy (HIS-ter-ō-*pek*-sē)	surgical fixation of the uterus
9. mammoplasty (MAM-ō-*plas*-tē)	surgical repair of the breast (performed to enlarge or reduce in size, and to reconstruct after removal of a tumor) (Fig. 8.9)

TYPES OF MAMMOPLASTY include **implants**, which use a silicone or saline insert to create a breast, and **flap reconstruction**, which transfers the patient's muscle or fat and surrounding tissue from another area to the chest to create a breast mound.

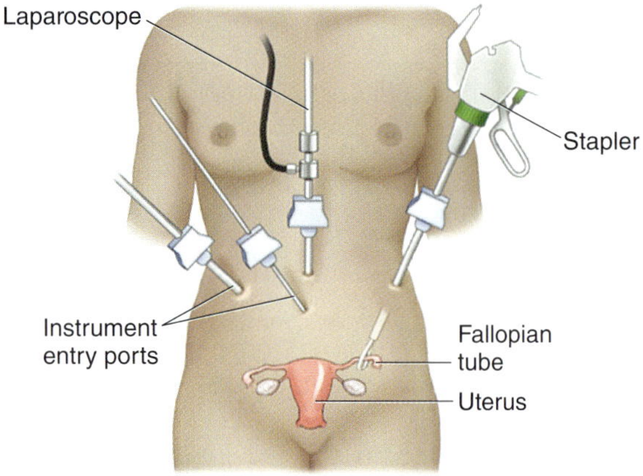

FIG. 8.8 Laparoscopically assisted vaginal hysterectomy (LAVH). The laparoscope, a type of endoscope, is inserted into the abdominopelvic cavity through a tiny incision near the umbilicus, allowing direct observation of the pelvic organs and structures. Three or four additional tiny incisions may be made to accommodate other instruments and devices. Numerous gynecological surgeries can be performed laparoscopically, including **hysterectomy, hysteropexy, myomectomy, oophorectomy, salpingectomy, salpingostomy,** and **tubal ligation.**

TABLE 8.2 Types of Hysterectomies

Total hysterectomy	Excision of the entire uterus, including the cervix; can be performed abdominally, vaginally, or laparoscopically
Subtotal hysterectomy	Excision of the upper part of the uterus leaving the cervix in place; can be performed abdominally or laparoscopically (also called **supracervical hysterectomy**)
Radical hysterectomy	Excision of the entire uterus, upper portion of the vagina, and surrounding tissues; performed abdominally

Surgical Terms—cont'd

BUILT FROM WORD PARTS

TERM	DEFINITION
10. mastectomy (mas-TEK-to-mē)	excision of the breast (Table 8.3, Fig. 8.9)
11. mastopexy (MAS-tō-pek-sē)	surgical fixation of the breast (performed to lift sagging breast tissue or to create symmetry) (Fig. 8.9)
12. oophorectomy (*ō*-of-o-REK-to-mē)	excision of the ovary
13. perineorrhaphy (*per*-i-nē-OR-a-fē)	suturing of (a tear in) the perineum
14. salpingectomy (*sal*-pin-JEK-to-mē)	excision of the fallopian tube
15. salpingo-oophorectomy (sal-*ping*-gō-ō-*of*-o-REK-to-mē)	excision of the fallopian tube and the ovary
16. salpingostomy (*sal*-ping-GOS-to-mē)	creation of an artificial opening in the fallopian tube (performed to restore patency)
17. trachelectomy (*trā*-ke-LEK-to-mē)	excision of the cervix (also called **cervicectomy**)
18. vulvectomy (vul-VEK-to-mē)	excision of the vulva

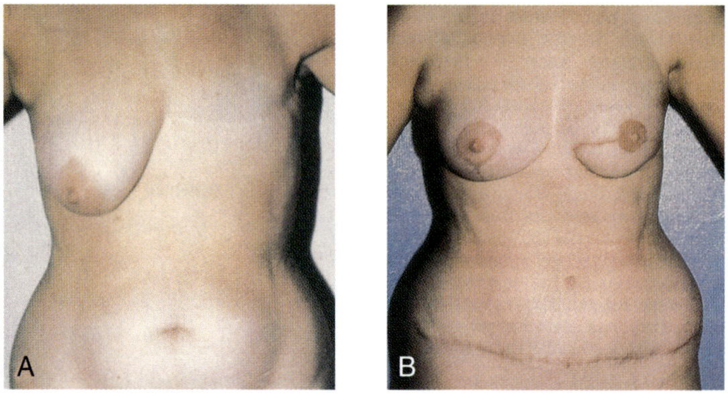

FIG. 8.9 Breast surgery and reconstruction. A, Left breast shows modified radical mastectomy scar. **B,** Left breast shows mammoplasty by TRAM (transverse rectus abdominis muscle) reconstruction (note the extensive lower abdominal scar, repositioned navel, and reconstructed nipple) and right mastopexy.

TABLE 8.3 Types of Surgeries Performed to Treat Malignant Breast Tumors

TRADITIONAL SURGERIES	
Radical mastectomy	Removal of breast tissue, nipple, lymph nodes, and underlying chest wall muscle (rarely performed)
Modified radical mastectomy	Removal of breast tissue, nipple, and lymph nodes
Simple mastectomy	Removal of breast tissue, nipple, and skin (also called **total mastectomy**)
BREAST CONSERVING SURGERIES	Less invasive procedures that preserve more of the breast are now an option for many people with breast cancer
Lumpectomy	Removal of the cancerous lesion along with a margin of surrounding healthy breast tissue. Radiation therapy may be needed as well.
Segmental mastectomy	Removal of a quadrant, or wedge, of breast tissue (also called **quadrantectomy**)
Skin-sparing mastectomy	Removal of the breast tissue, nipple, and areola, leaving most of the skin over the breast intact. Used only for smaller tumors that are not close to the skin.
Nipple-sparing mastectomy	Removal of breast tissue only, preserving the overlying skin, nipple and areola (also called **subcutaneous mastectomy**). Used mainly for small, early stage cancers that are near the outer part of the breast.
BREAST RECONSTRUCTION	Type of surgery that can restore the original appearance of the breasts. It may be performed at the time of mastectomy or during a second surgery, 6-12 months later. Some people choose not to have reconstructive surgery.

EXERCISE 13 ■ Pronounce and Spell

Practice pronunciation and spelling on paper and online.

1. Practice on Paper

a. **Pronounce:** Read the phonetic spelling and say aloud the terms listed in the term table. Refer to the pronunciation key on p. 20 as necessary.
b. **Spell:** Have a study partner read the terms aloud. Write the spelling of the terms on a separate sheet of paper.

2. Practice Online

a. **Access** online learning resources. Go to evolve.elsevier.com > Evolve Resources > Student Resources.
b. **Pronounce:** Select Audio Glossary > Chapter 8 > Exercise 13. Select a term to hear its pronunciation and repeat aloud.
c. **Spell:** Select Activities > Chapter 8 > Spell Terms > Exercise 13. Select the audio icon and type the correct spelling of the term.

❑ Check the box when complete.

EXERCISE 14 ■ Analyze and Define

Analyze and define the following terms by drawing slashes between word parts, writing word part abbreviations above the term, underlining combining forms, and writing the combining form abbreviations below the term.

1. colpoplasty
____
____

2. hymenotomy
____
____

3. vulvectomy

____

____

4. perineorrhaphy

____

____

5. salpingostomy

____

____

6. oophorectomy

____

____

7. mastopexy

____

____

8. colpoperineorrhaphy

____

____

EXERCISE 15 ■ Build

A Label

Build surgical terms pictured by writing word parts above definitions.

1.

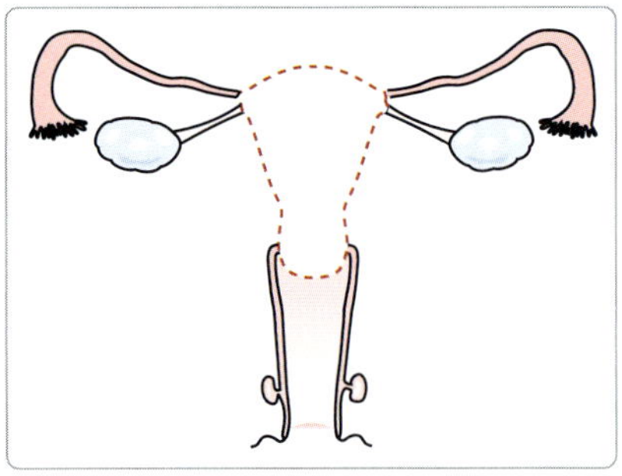

_______________ / _______________
uterus excision

2.

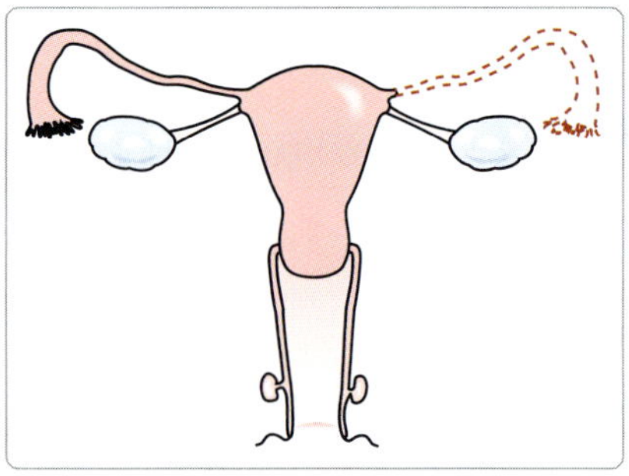

_______________ / _______________
fallopian tube excision

3.

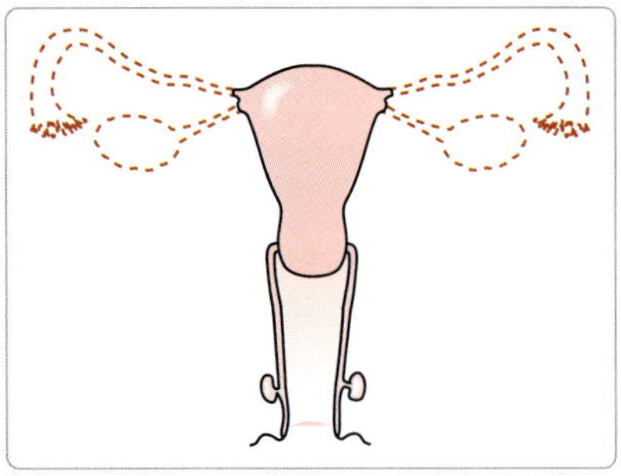

bilateral _______________ / ____ /- _______ / ________
fallopian tube CV ovary excision

4.

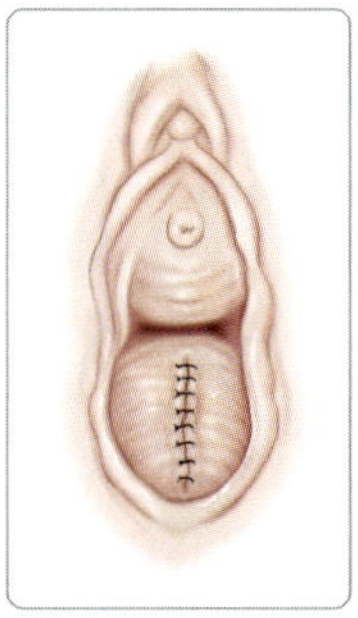

________ / _____ / ___________________
vulva CV suturing (of a tear)

5.

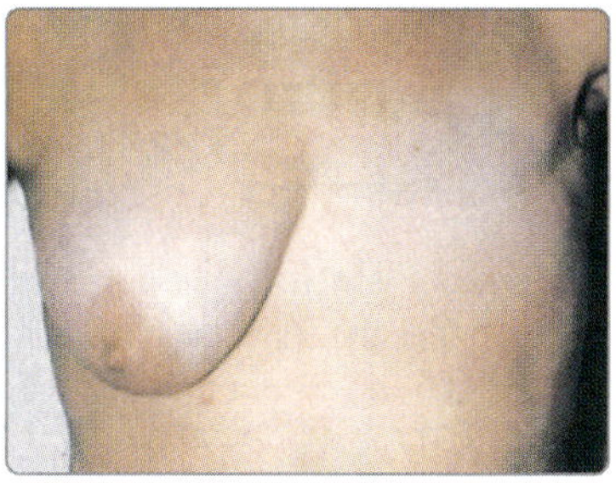

_______________/_______________
breast excision

6.

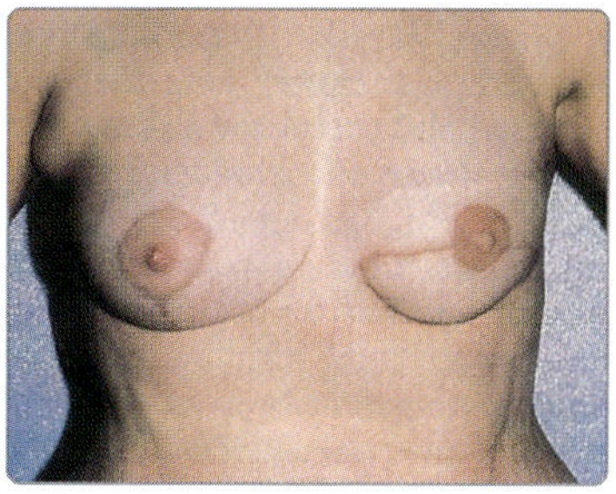

_______/_______/_______________
breast CV surgical repair

B Fill In

Build surgical terms for the following definitions by using the word parts you have learned.

1. suturing of the vagina ________ / ____ / ________ (WR / CV / S)
2. excision of the cervix ________ / ________ (WR / S)
3. surgical closure of the vagina ________ / ____ / ________ (WR / CV / S)
4. surgical fixation of the uterus ________ / ____ / ________ (WR / CV / S)

Surgical Terms

NOT BUILT FROM WORD PARTS

Word parts may be present in the following terms; however, their full meanings cannot be translated using definitions of word parts alone.

TERM	DEFINITION
1. anterior and posterior colporrhaphy (A&P repair) (an-TĒR-ē-or) (pos-TĒR-ē-or) (kol-POR-a-fē)	surgical repair of a weakened vaginal wall to correct a cystocele (protrusion of the bladder against the anterior wall of the vagina) and a rectocele (protrusion of the rectum against the posterior wall of the vagina)
2. conization (*kon*-i-ZĀ-shun)	surgical removal of a cone-shaped area of the cervix; used in the treatment for noninvasive cervical cancer. Types of conization include loop electrosurgical excision procedure (LEEP), cryosurgery (cold knife conization), and laser ablation. (also called **cone biopsy**)
3. dilation and curettage (D&C) (dī-LĀ-shun) (kū-re-TAHZH)	surgical procedure to widen the cervix and remove contents from the uterus using a curette, an instrument for scraping or suctioning; the procedure can be diagnostic or therapeutic (Fig. 8.10)
4. endometrial ablation (*en*-dō-MĒ-trē-al) (ab-LĀ-shun)	procedure to destroy or remove the endometrium by use of laser, electrical, or thermal energy; used to treat abnormal uterine bleeding (Fig. 8.11)

ABLATION is from the Latin **ablatum**, meaning **to carry away**. In surgery, **ablation** means **excision or eradication**, especially by cutting with laser or electrical energy.

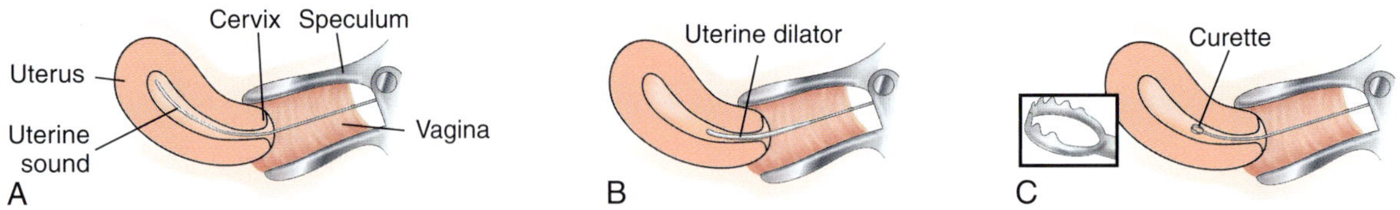

FIG. 8.10 Dilation and curettage (D&C). A, Uterine sound is a device used to measure the size of the uterus, to help determine how far to insert the instruments. **B,** Uterine dilator helps to open the cervix to allow easier access. **C,** Curette scrapes the endometrium and removes contents.

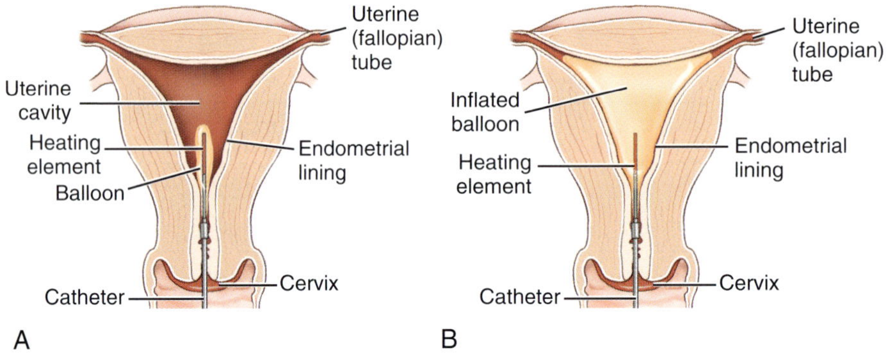

FIG. 8.11 Endometrial ablation using thermal energy. A, The balloon catheter (deflated) is inserted through the cervix into the uterine cavity. **B,** The balloon is inflated with a solution of 5% dextrose and water and heated to 87°C for 8 minutes, ablating the endometrial lining.

Surgical Terms—cont'd

NOT BUILT FROM WORD PARTS

TERM	DEFINITION
5. myomectomy (*mī*-ō-MEK-to-mē)	excision of a uterine fibroid (myoma)
6. tubal ligation (TOO-bul) (lī-GĀ-shun)	surgical closure of the fallopian tubes for sterilization; tubes may be cut and tied (ligated), cut and cauterized, or closed off with a clip, clamp, ring, or band (also called **tubal sterilization** and **female surgical sterilization**) (Fig. 8.12)
7. uterine artery embolization (UAE) (Ū-ter-in) (AR-ter-ē) (*em*-be-li-ZĀ-shun)	placement of metal coils or small gelatin beads into uterine arteries to stop blood flow supplying uterine fibroids or to stop severe hemorrhage after childbirth; performed by an interventional radiologist (also called **uterine fibroid embolization** when used to treat uterine fibroids)

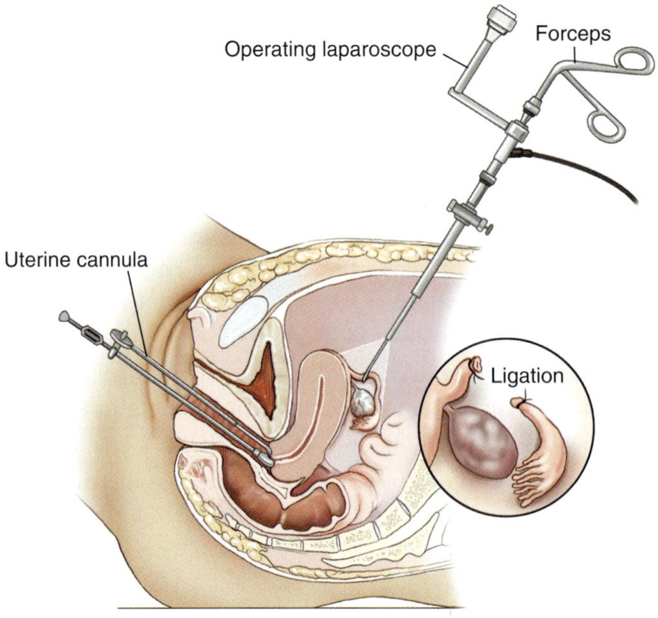

FIG. 8.12 Laparoscopic tubal ligation.

EXERCISE 16 ■ Pronounce and Spell

Practice pronunciation and spelling on paper and online.

1. Practice on Paper

a. **Pronounce:** Read the phonetic spelling and say aloud the terms listed in the term table. Refer to the pronunciation key on p. 20 as necessary.
b. **Spell:** Have a study partner read the terms aloud. Write the spelling of the terms on a separate sheet of paper.

2. Practice Online

a. **Access** online learning resources. Go to evolve.elsevier.com > Evolve Resources > Student Resources.
b. **Pronounce:** Select Audio Glossary > Chapter 8 > Exercise 16. Select a term to hear its pronunciation and repeat aloud.
c. **Spell:** Select Activities > Chapter 8 > Spell Terms > Exercise 16. Select the audio icon and type the correct spelling of the term.

❑ Check the box when complete.

EXERCISE 17 ■ Fill In

A Label

Write the surgical terms pictured and defined.

1. ______________________
surgical closure of the fallopian tubes for sterilization

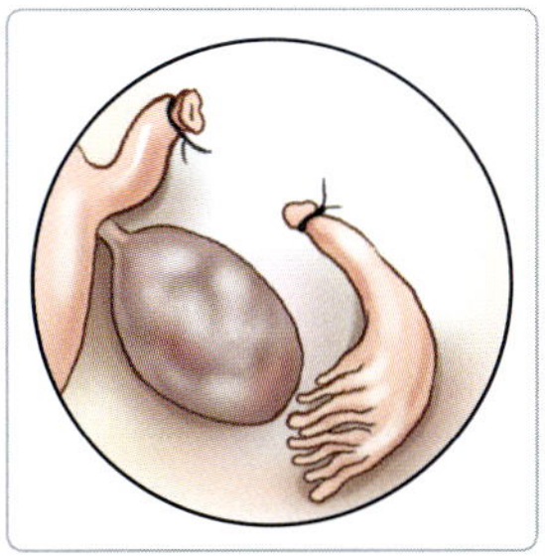

2. ______________________
surgical procedure to widen the cervix and remove contents from the uterus using an instrument for scraping or suctioning

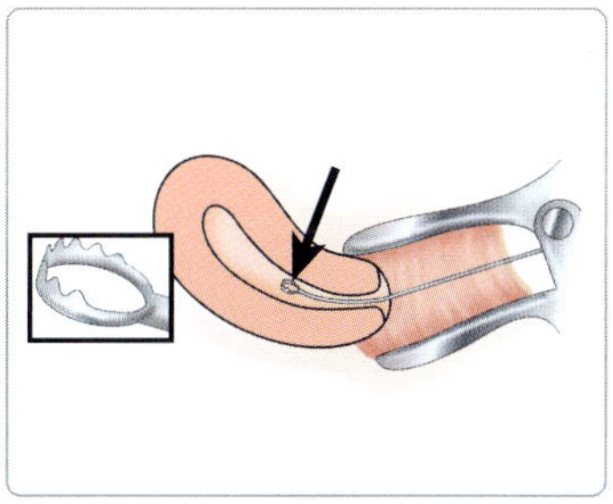

3. ______________________
procedure to destroy or remove the endometrium by use of laser, electrical, or thermal energy

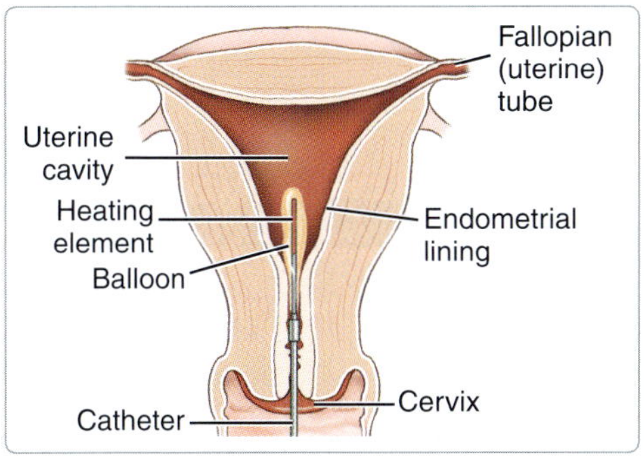

4. ______________________
excision of a uterine fibroid

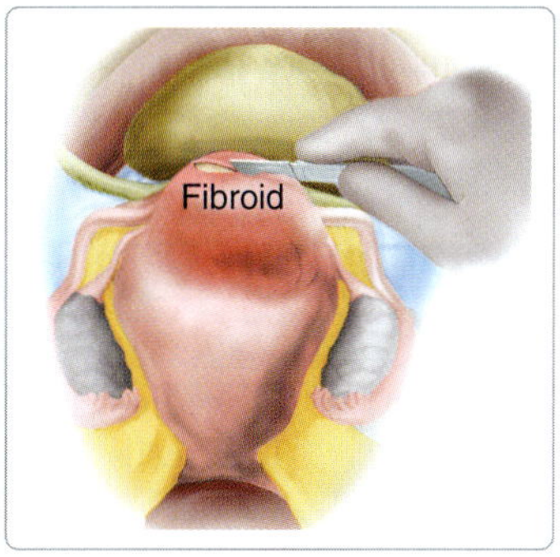

B Identify

Fill in the blanks with the correct terms.

1. The surgery used to repair a cystocele and rectocele is a(n) ______________________ and ______________ ______________.
2. A procedure used to treat uterine fibroids by blocking the blood supply is called ______________ ______________ ______________.
3. Surgical removal of a cone-shaped area of the cervix is called ______________________.

C Match

Match the surgical procedures in the first column with their corresponding organs in the second column. You may use the answers in the second column more than once.

_____ 1. dilation and curettage	a. fallopian tubes
_____ 2. tubal ligation	b. vagina
_____ 3. anterior and posterior colporrhaphy	c. uterus
_____ 4. myomectomy	d. ovaries
_____ 5. conization	e. vulva
_____ 6. endometrial ablation	f. lymph nodes
_____ 7. uterine artery embolization	g. cervix

EXERCISE 18 ■ Review of Surgical Terms

Can you define, pronounce, and spell the following terms?

anterior and posterior colporrhaphy (A&P repair)
colpocleisis
colpoperineorrhaphy
colpoplasty
colporrhaphy
conization
dilation and curettage (D&C)
endometrial ablation
episiorrhaphy
hymenotomy
hysterectomy
hysteropexy
mammoplasty
mastectomy
mastopexy
myomectomy
oophorectomy
perineorrhaphy
salpingectomy
salpingo-oophorectomy
salpingostomy
trachelectomy
tubal ligation
uterine artery embolization (UAE)
vulvectomy

Diagnostic Terms

BUILT FROM WORD PARTS AND *NOT* BUILT FROM WORD PARTS

The first portion of the table contains Female Reproductive System Terms that can be translated using definitions of word parts. The second portion of the table contains Female Reproductive System Terms that cannot be fully understood using the definitions of word parts.

■ Built from Word Parts

DIAGNOSTIC IMAGING

TERM	DEFINITION	TERM	DEFINITION
1. hysterosalpingogram (HSG) (*his*-ter-ō-*sal*-PING-gō-gram)	radiographic image of the uterus and fallopian tubes (after an injection of a contrast agent)	**2. mammogram** (MAM-ō-gram)	radiographic image of the breast

TERM	DEFINITION	TERM	DEFINITION
3. mammography (ma-MOG-ra-fē)	radiographic imaging of the breast (also called **digital mammography** when images are obtained electronically and viewed on a computer)	**4. sonohysterography (SHG)** (*son*-ō-*his*-ter-OG-ra-fē)	process of recording the uterus by use of sound (Saline solution is injected into the uterine cavity during transvaginal sonography. Used to diagnose abnormalities inside the uterus, including polyps, fibroids, adhesions.) (also called **hysterosonography**)

ENDOSCOPY

TERM	DEFINITION	TERM	DEFINITION
5. colposcope (KOL-pō-skōp)	instrument used for visual examination of the vagina (and cervix)	**9. pelviscopic** (pel-vi-SKOP-ik)	pertaining to visual examination of the pelvic cavity (female reproductive organs)
6. colposcopy (kol-POS-ko-pē)	visual examination (with a magnified view) of the vagina (and cervix)	**10. pelviscopy** (pel-VIS-ku-pē)	visual examination of the pelvic cavity (female reproductive organs) (also called **gynecologic laparoscopy**)
7. hysteroscope (HIS-ter-ō-skōp)	instrument used for visual examination of the uterus (uterine cavity)		
8. hysteroscopy (*his*-ter-OS-ko-pē)	visual examination of the uterus (uterine cavity)		

NOT Built from Word Parts

DIAGNOSTIC IMAGING

TERM	DEFINITION
1. sentinel lymph node biopsy (SEN-tin-el) (limf) (nōd) (BĪ-op-sē)	injection of blue dye and/or radioactive isotope used to identify the sentinel lymph node(s), the first in the axillary chain and most likely to contain metastasis of breast cancer. The nodes are removed and microscopically examined. If the nodes closest to the cancer (called "sentinel nodes") are negative, additional nodes are not removed. (Fig. 8.13)
2. stereotactic breast biopsy (*ster*-ē-ō-TAK-tik) (brest) (BĪ-op-sē)	technique that combines mammography and computer-assisted biopsy to obtain tissue from a breast lesion (Fig. 8.14)

TYPES OF BREAST BIOPSY

- **Image-guided breast biopsy** uses mammography, sonography, or magnetic resonance (MR) images to guide a biopsy needle.
- **Surgical breast biopsy** involves making an incision to remove a palpable breast lesion (also called **open** or **incisional biopsy**).
- **Wire localization biopsy** uses image guidance to place a thin, flexible wire directly into a breast lesion. The lesion is removed surgically with the wire intact.

TERM	DEFINITION
3. transvaginal sonography (TVS) (trans-VAJ-i-nal) (so-NOG-ra-fē)	ultrasound procedure that uses a transducer placed in the vagina to obtain images of the ovaries, uterus, cervix, fallopian tubes, and surrounding structures; used to diagnose masses such as ovarian cysts or tumors, to monitor pregnancy, and to evaluate ovulation for the treatment of infertility (Fig. 8.15)

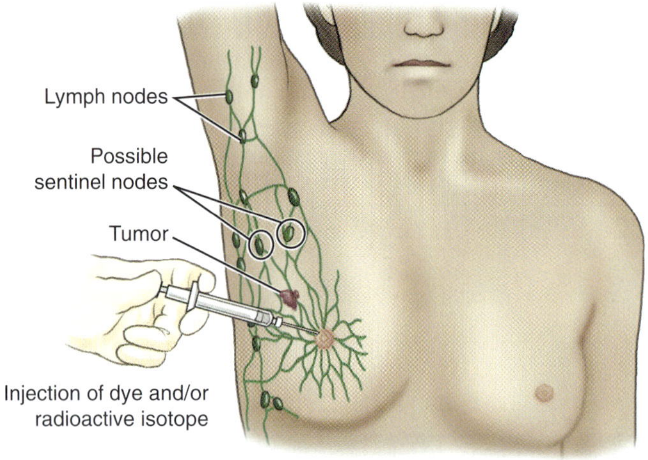

FIG. 8.13 Preparation for sentinel lymph node biopsy. The process of identifying the sentinel node(s) is performed in the nuclear medicine department of radiology. The biopsy is performed in surgery. The sentinel lymph node biopsy procedure was first developed for patients with melanoma. It is now also used to determine metastasis of breast cancer to the lymph nodes. Previously, surgeons would remove 10 to 20 lymph nodes to determine the spread of cancer, which often caused lymphedema and painful swelling of the affected arm.

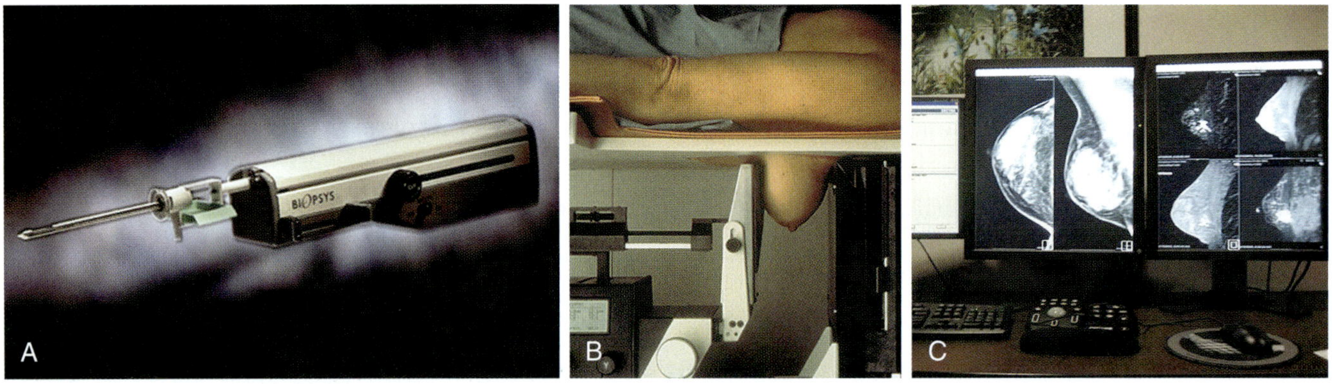

FIG. 8.14 Stereotactic breast biopsy, which is used for nonpalpable lesions that are visible on mammography. The patient is placed prone on a special table with the breast suspended through an opening. The breast is placed in a mammography machine under the table, which produces a digital mammography image that identifies the exact location of the lesion. The biopsy instrument is guided by a radiologist or surgeon. **A,** The stereotactic needle is used to obtain the specimen for biopsy. **B,** The patient is positioned for stereotactic breast biopsy. **C,** The mammogram appears digitally and is used to determine the placement of the biopsy needle.

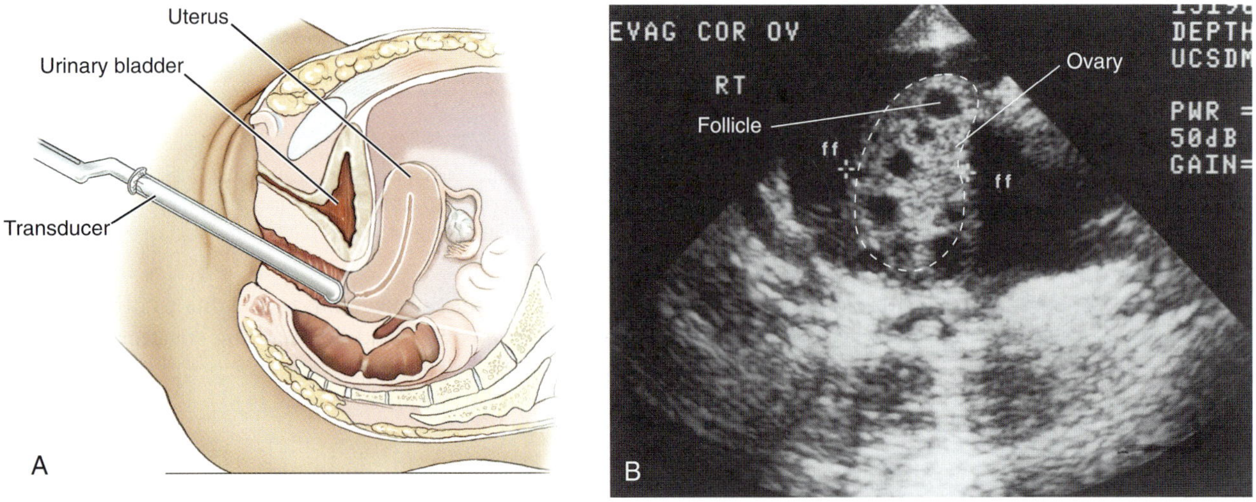

FIG. 8.15 Transvaginal sonography. A, Transducer placed in the vagina. **B,** Transvaginal coronal image of the right ovary with multiple follicles, showing free fluid surrounding the ovary.

Diagnostic Terms—cont'd

BUILT FROM WORD PARTS AND *NOT* BUILT FROM WORD PARTS

NOT Built from Word Parts

LABORATORY

TERM	DEFINITION
4. CA-125 test (C-A-1-25) (test)	blood test primarily used to monitor treatment for ovarian cancer and to detect recurrence once treatment is complete. CA-125 (cancer antigen 125) is a protein found on the surface of most ovarian cancer cells and is released into the bloodstream. Elevated amounts of CA-125 in the blood may indicate the presence of ovarian cancer. (also called **CA-125** and **CA 125 tumor marker**)
5. HPV test (H-P-V) (test)	cytological study of cervical and vaginal secretions to detect high-risk forms of the human papillomavirus (HPV) that can cause abnormal cervical cells and cervical cancer; used for cervical cancer screening (Table 8.4)
6. Pap test (pap) (test)	cytological study of cervical and vaginal secretions to detect abnormal and cancerous cells; primarily used for cervical cancer screening (also called **Papanicolaou** [*pap*-a-NIK-kō-lā-oo] **test**; formerly called **Pap smear**) (Table 8.4)

PAP TEST is named after Dr. George N. Papanicolaou (1883-1962), a Greek physician practicing in the United States, who developed the cell smear method for the diagnosis of cancer in 1943. Though the smear method could be used to sample cells from any organ, it has been commonly used on cervical and vaginal secretions to detect cervical cancer. In 1966 the FDA approved a liquid-based screening system, which improved the detection of squamous intraepithelial lesions. With use of the liquid-based method surpassing use of the smear method, the procedure is more commonly called a Pap test, rather than a Pap smear.

EXERCISE 19 ■ Pronounce and Spell

Practice pronunciation and spelling on paper and online.

1. Practice on Paper

a. **Pronounce:** Read the phonetic spelling and say aloud the terms listed in the term table. Refer to the pronunciation key on p. 20 as necessary.
b. **Spell:** Have a study partner read the terms aloud. Write the spelling of the terms on a separate sheet of paper.

2. Practice Online

a. **Access** online learning resources. Go to evolve.elsevier.com > Evolve Resources > Student Resources.
b. **Pronounce:** Select Audio Glossary > Chapter 8 > Exercise 19. Select a term to hear its pronunciation and repeat aloud.
c. **Spell:** Select Activities > Chapter 8 > Spell Terms > Exercise 19. Select the audio icon and type the correct spelling of the term.

❑ Check the box when complete.

EXERCISE 20 ■ Diagnostic Terms Built from Word Parts

A Analyze and Define

Analyze and define the following diagnostic terms by drawing slashes between word parts, writing word part abbreviations above the term, underlining combining forms, and writing combining form abbreviations below the term.

1. colposcopy

____

____

2. mammogram

____

____

3. colposcope

____

____

4. hysteroscopy

____

____

5. hysterosalpingogram

____

____

6. pelviscopic

____

____

TABLE 8.4 Comparison of the Pap Test and the HPV Test

	PAP TEST	HPV TEST
Purpose of the test	Checks the cervix for any abnormal cells that could lead to cervical cancer	Looks for DNA from humanpapilloma virus in cells from the cervix
Who should have the test	Women between the ages of 21 and 65, every 3 to 5 years	Women age 30 to 65, every 5 years with or without a Pap test at the same time; performing the tests at the same time is called **co-testing**
How the tests are performed	The healthcare provider inserts a speculum (an instrument used to see the cervix) into the vagina and uses a flat stick and a soft brush to collect cells from the cervix (A). This sample of cells is then placed in a bottle with a liquid preservative (B) and sent to the lab for interpretation. 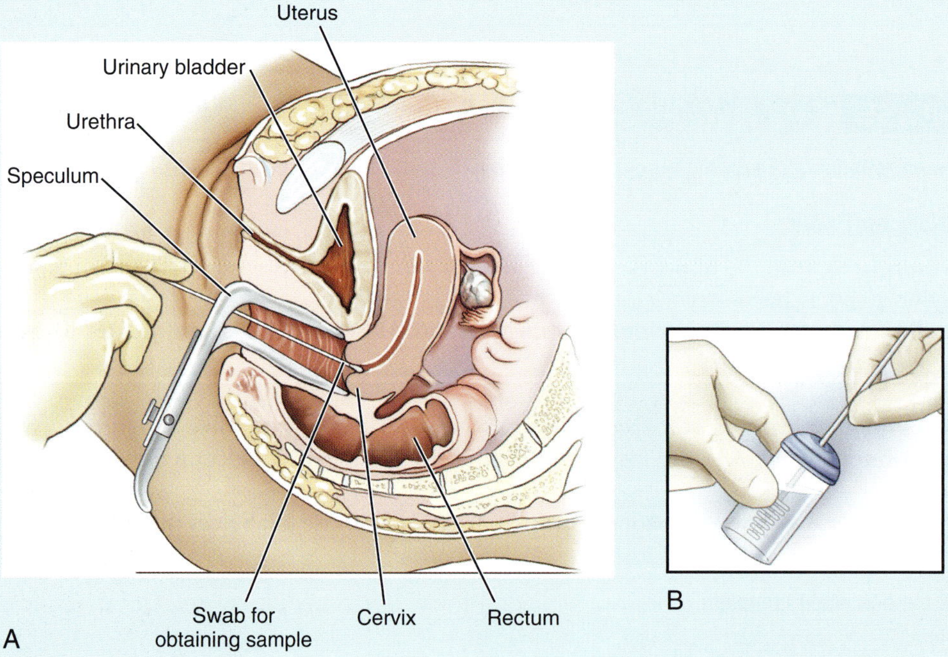 	
Interpreting the results	• **Normal** • **ASC-US** (unclear, could be abnormal) • **Abnormal** (low grade or high grade)	• **Positive** (an HPV type is present that is associated with cervical cancer) • **Negative** (no HPV type associated with cervical cancer is present)
Next steps	• **Normal:** return to usual screening recommendations • **ASC-US:** perform HPV testing if not yet done, more frequent testing or colposcopy • **Abnormal:** more frequent testing, colposcopy and biopsy, or immediate treatment (depending on level of abnormality, age, and HPV test results)	• **Negative:** return to usual screening recommendations • **Positive:** Further testing may be done to determine the virus subtype (HPV 16 and 18 have to strongest association to cervical cancer). Options also include watchful waiting (many HPV infections will resolve on their own), colposcopy, biopsy, and possible treatment depending on results.

7. pelviscopy

____

____

8. mammography

____

____

9. hysteroscope

____

____

10. sonohysterography

____

____

B Build

Build diagnostic terms pictured by writing word parts above definitions.

1.

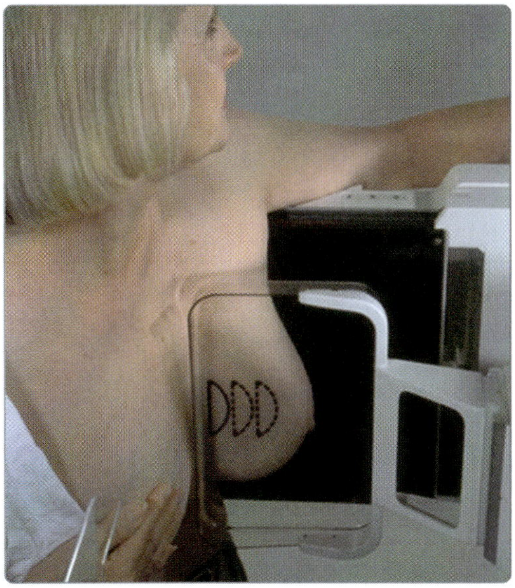

_____ / _____ / _____
breast CV radiographic imaging

2.

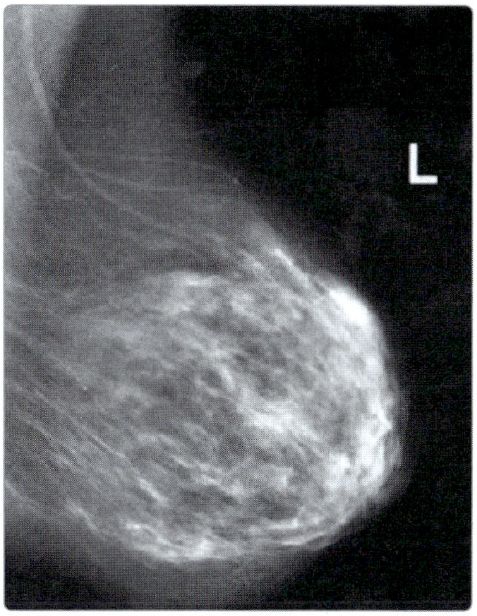

_____ / _____ / _____
breast CV radiographic image

3.

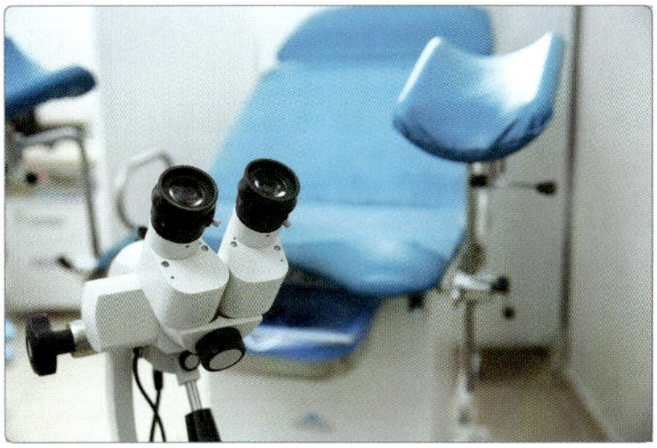

_____ / _____ / _____
vagina CV instrument used for visual examination

4.

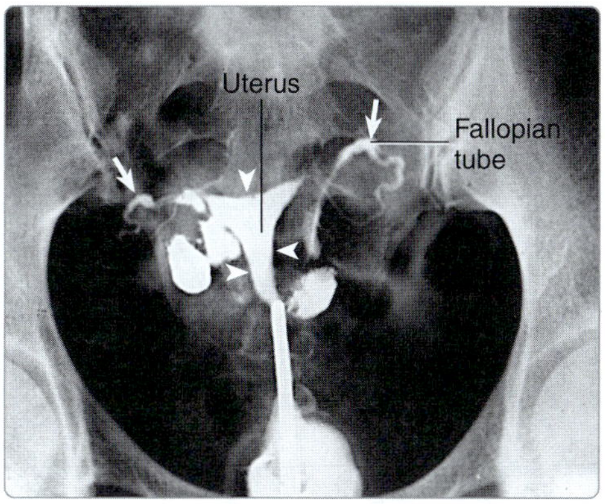

_____ / _____ / _____ / _____ / _____
uterus CV fallopian tubes CV radiographic image

C Build

Build diagnostic terms for the following definitions by using the word parts you have learned.

1. visual examination of the vagina (and cervix) ______ WR / CV / ______ S
2. visual examination of the uterus ______ WR / CV / ______ S
3. pertaining to visual examination of the pelvic cavity (female reproductive organs) ______ WR / CV / ______ S
4. visual examination of the pelvic cavity (female reproductive organs) ______ WR / CV / ______ S
5. instrument used for visual examination of the uterus ______ WR / CV / ______ S
6. process of recording the uterus with sound ______ WR / CV / ______ WR / CV / ______ S

EXERCISE 21 ▪ Diagnostic Terms *NOT* Built from Word Parts

A Label

Write the diagnostic terms pictured and defined.

1. ______________________
procedure that uses a transducer placed in the vagina to obtain images of the ovaries, uterus, cervix, fallopian tubes, and surrounding structures

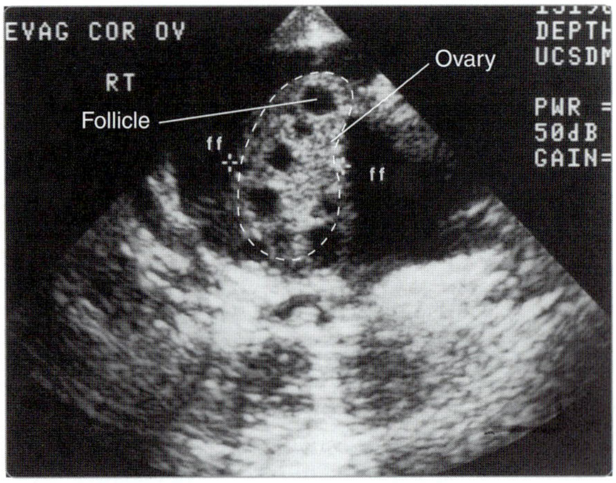

2. ______________________
cytological study of cervical and vaginal secretions; primarily used for cervical cancer screening

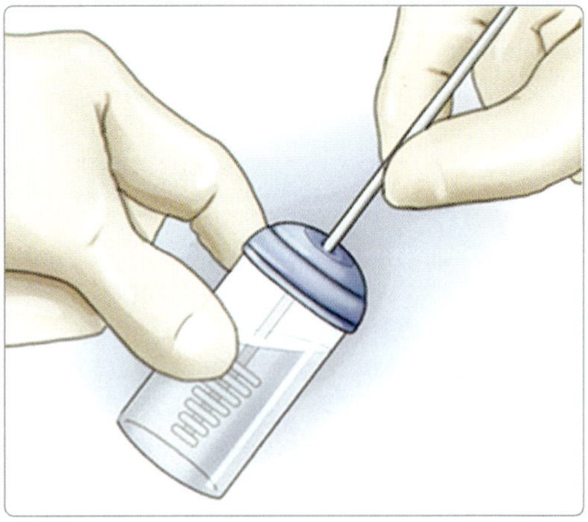

B Match

Match the terms in the first column with their correct definitions in the second column

______ 1. Pap test	a. blood test used to monitor treatment for ovarian cancer and to detect recurrence
______ 2. transvaginal sonography	b. combines mammography and computer-assisted biopsy to obtain tissue from a breast lesion
______ 3. sentinel lymph node biopsy	c. cytological study of cervical and vaginal secretions to detect abnormal and cancerous cells
______ 4. HPV test	d. ultrasound procedure that uses a transducer placed in the vagina to obtain images of internal female reproductive structures
______ 5. CA-125 test	e. Identification of the first lymph nodes in the axillary chain using blue dye and/or radioactive isotope
______ 6. stereotactic breast biopsy	f. cytological study of cervical and vaginal secretions to detect high-risk forms of the human papillomavirus

C Identify

Fill in the blanks with the correct terms.

1. ____________ ____________ ____________ ____________ uses a blue dye to identify lymph nodes most likely to contain metastasis of breast cancer.
2. A technique that combines mammography and computer-assisted biopsy of the breast is known as ____________ ____________ ____________.
3. ____________ ____________ is a blood test used to monitor treatment and detect recurrence of ovarian cancer.
4. A cytological study of cervical and vaginal secretions used to test for the virus that can cause cervical cancer is called ____________ ____________.

EXERCISE 22 ■ Review of Diagnostic Terms

Can you define, pronounce, and spell the following terms?

CA-125 test
colposcope
colposcopy
HPV test
hysterosalpingogram (HSG)
hysteroscope
hysteroscopy
mammogram
mammography
Pap test
pelviscopic
pelviscopy
sentinel lymph node biopsy
sonohysterography (SHG)
stereotactic breast biopsy
transvaginal sonography (TVS)

Complementary Terms

BUILT FROM WORD PARTS AND *NOT* BUILT FROM WORD PARTS

The first portion of the table contains Female Reproductive System Terms that can be translated using definitions of word parts. The second portion of the table contains terms that cannot be fully understood using the definitions of word parts.

■ Built from Word Parts

SIGNS AND SYMPTOMS

TERM	DEFINITION	TERM	DEFINITION
1. leukorrhea (*lū*-kō-RĒ-a)	white discharge (from the vagina)	**2. mastalgia** (mas-TAL-ja)	pain in the breast

Complementary Terms—cont'd

BUILT FROM WORD PARTS AND *NOT* BUILT FROM WORD PARTS

Built from Word Parts

MEDICAL SPECIALTIES

TERM	DEFINITION	TERM	DEFINITION
3. **gynecologist** (*gīn*-ek-OL-o-jist)	physician who studies and treats diseases of women (female reproductive system)	4. **gynecology (GYN)** (*gīn*-ek-OL-o-jē)	study of women (branch of medicine dealing with health and diseases of the female reproductive system)

DESCRIPTIVE TERMS

TERM	DEFINITION	TERM	DEFINITION
5. **endocervical** (*en*-dō-SER-vi-kal)	pertaining to within the cervix	8. **vesicovaginal** (*ves*-i-kō-VAJ-i-nal)	pertaining to the (urinary) bladder and the vagina
6. **pelvic** (PEL-vik)	pertaining to the pelvis	9. **vulvovaginal** (*vul*-vō-VAJ-i-nal)	pertaining to the vulva and vagina
7. **vaginal** (VAJ-i-nal)	pertaining to the vagina		

NOT Built from Word Parts

SIGNS AND SYMPTOMS

TERM	DEFINITION
1. **anovulation** (*an*-ov-ū-LĀ-shun)	failure of the ovary to release an egg
2. **dyspareunia** (*dis*-pa-RŪ-nē-a)	difficult or painful intercourse
3. **fistula** (FIS-tū-la)	abnormal passageway between two organs or between an internal organ and the body surface
4. **oligoovulation** (*ol*-i-gō-ov-ū-LĀ-shun)	infrequent release of an egg

TREATMENTS

TERM	DEFINITION
5. **contraception** (*kon*-tra-SEP-shen)	intentional prevention of conception (pregnancy) (also called **birth control [BC]**) (Fig. 8.16)
METHODS OF CONTRACEPTION include barrier (condoms), chemical (spermicides), oral pharmaceutical (birth control pills), and long-acting reversible contraception (LARC) such as an intrauterine device (IUD), intrauterine system (IUS), implant, and injection.	
6. **hormone replacement therapy (HRT)** (HŌR-mōn) (rē-PLĀS-ment) (THER-a-pē)	replacement of hormones, estrogen and progesterone, to treat symptoms associated with menopause

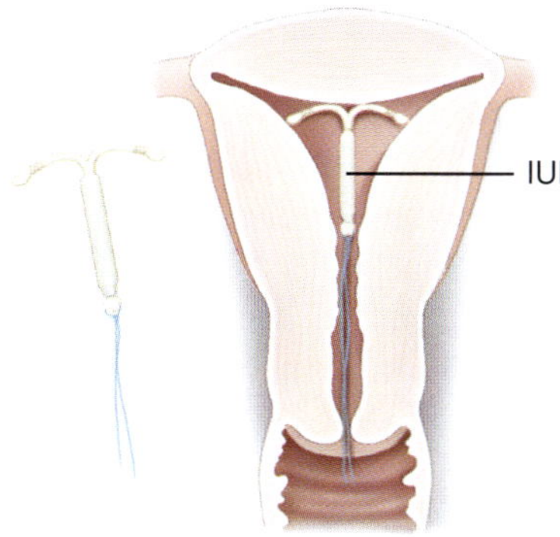

FIG. 8.16 Intrauterine device (IUD). Inserted through the cervix, this T-shaped device provides long-term contraception by changing the intrauterine environment.

EQUIPMENT

TERM	DEFINITION
7. speculum (SPEK-ū-lum)	instrument for opening a body cavity to allow visual inspection

OTHERS

TERM	DEFINITION
8. menarche (me-NAR-kē)	beginning of menstruation (specifically, onset of the first menstrual period)
9. menopause (MEN-o-pawz)	cessation of menstruation, usually around the ages of 48 to 53 years; may be induced at an earlier age surgically (bilateral oophorectomy) or medically (side effect of chemotherapy treatment)

Refer to **Appendix E** for pharmacology terms related to the female reproductive system.

EXERCISE 23 ■ Pronounce and Spell

Practice pronunciation and spelling on paper and online.

1. Practice on Paper

a. **Pronounce:** Read the phonetic spelling and say aloud the terms listed in the previous table. Refer to the pronunciation key on p. 20 as necessary.
b. **Spell:** Have a study partner read the terms aloud. Write the spelling of the terms on a separate sheet of paper.

2. Practice Online

a. **Access** online learning resources. Go to evolve.elsevier.com > Evolve Resources > Student Resources.
b. **Pronounce:** Select Audio Glossary > Chapter 8 > Exercise 23. Select a term to hear its pronunciation and repeat aloud.
c. **Spell:** Select Activities > Chapter 8 > Spell Terms > Exercise 23. Select the audio icon and type the correct spelling of the term.

❑ Check the box when complete.

EXERCISE 24 ■ Complementary Terms Built from Word Parts

A Analyze and Define

Analyze and define the following complementary terms by drawing slashes between word parts, writing word part abbreviations above the term, underlining combining forms, and writing combining form abbreviations below the term.

1. gynecologist

____

____

2. gynecology

____

____

3. vulvovaginal

____

____

4. mastalgia

____

____

5. pelvic

____

____

6. leukorrhea

____

____

7. vesicovaginal

____

____

8. vaginal

____

____

9. endocervical

____

____

B Build

Build complementary terms for the following definitions by using the word parts you have learned.

1. white discharge (from the vagina) _____ / _____ / _____
WR / CV / S

2. pertaining to the pelvis _____ / _____
WR / S

3. pain in the breast _____ / _____
WR / S

4. pertaining to the vulva and vagina _____ / _____ / _____ / _____
WR / CV / WR / S

5. physician who studies and treats diseases of women

______ / ______ / ______
WR / CV / S

6. study of women (branch of medicine dealing with health and diseases of the female reproductive system)

______ / ______ / ______
WR / CV / S

7. pertaining to the (urinary) bladder and the vagina

______ / ______ / ______ / ______
WR / CV / WR / S

8. pertaining to the vagina

______ / ______
WR / S

9. pertaining to within the cervix

______ / ______ / ______
P / WR / S

EXERCISE 25 ■ Complementary Terms *NOT* Built from Word Parts

A Match

Match the terms in the first column with their correct definitions in the second column.

______ 1. dyspareunia
______ 2. contraception
______ 3. hormone replacement therapy
______ 4. speculum
______ 5. anovulation
______ 6. menarche
______ 7. fistula
______ 8. menopause
______ 9. oligoovulation

a. abnormal passageway between two organs
b. instrument for opening a body cavity to allow visual inspection
c. failure of the ovary to release an egg
d. also called birth control
e. onset of the first menstrual period
f. infrequent release of an egg
g. difficult or painful intercourse
h. cessation of menstruation
i. replacement of hormones to treat symptoms associated with menopause

B Label

Write the medical terms pictured and defined.

1. ______________________________
instrument for opening a body cavity to allow visual inspection

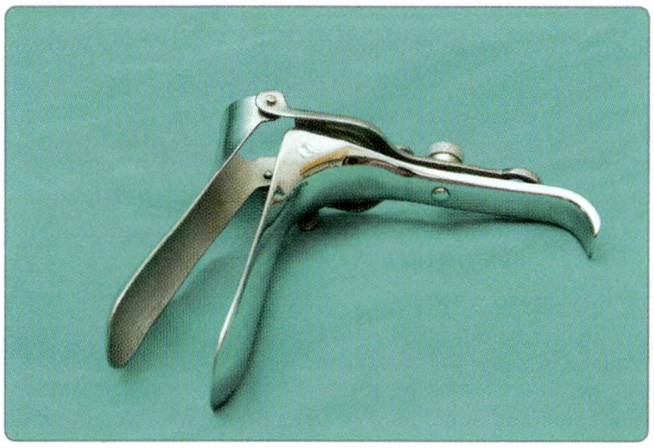

2. ______________________________
intentional prevention of conception (pregnancy)

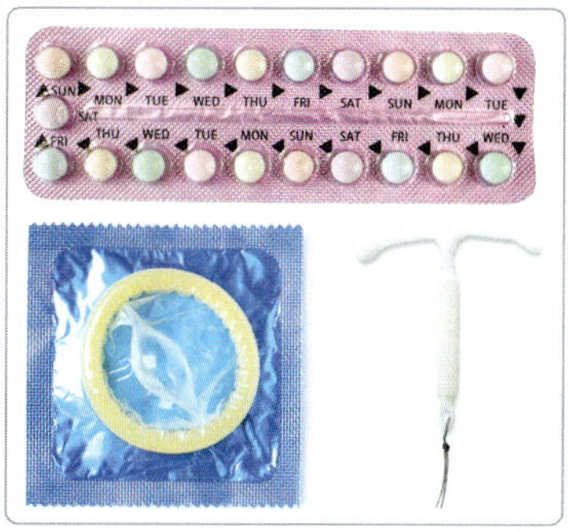

C Identify

Write the term for each of the following.

1. abnormal passageway ______
2. beginning of menstruation (specifically, onset of the first menstrual period) ______
3. painful intercourse ______
4. cessation of menstruation ______
5. replacement of hormones to treat symptoms associated with menopause ______
6. failure of the ovary to release an egg ______
7. infrequent release of an egg ______

EXERCISE 26 ■ Review of Complementary Terms

Can you define, pronounce, and spell the following terms?

anovulation
contraception
dyspareunia
endocervical
fistula
gynecologist
gynecology (GYN)
hormone replacement therapy (HRT)
leukorrhea
mastalgia
menarche
menopause
oligoovulation
pelvic
speculum
vaginal
vesicovaginal
vulvovaginal

Abbreviations

DISEASES AND DISORDERS

ABBREVIATION	TERM	ABBREVIATION	TERM
AUB	abnormal uterine bleeding	**PID**	pelvic inflammatory disease
FCC	fibrocystic breast changes	**PMS**	premenstrual syndrome
PCOS	polycystic ovary syndrome	**TSS**	toxic shock syndrome

DIAGNOSTIC

ABBREVIATION	TERM	ABBREVIATION	TERM
HSG	hysterosalpingogram	**TVS**	transvaginal sonography
SHG	sonohysterography		

TREATMENT

ABBREVIATION	TERM	ABBREVIATION	TERM
A&P repair	anterior and posterior colporrhaphy	**LAVH**	laparoscopically assisted vaginal hysterectomy
BC	birth control	**TAH/BSO**	total abdominal hysterectomy/bilateral salpingo-oophorectomy
D&C	dilation and curettage	**TLH**	total laparoscopic hysterectomy
HRT	hormone replacement therapy	**UAE**	uterine artery embolization
IUD	intrauterine device	**VH**	vaginal hysterectomy
IUS	intrauterine system		

MEDICAL SPECIALTIES

ABBREVIATION	TERM
GYN	gynecology

OTHER	
ABBREVIATION	TERM
Cx	cervix

Refer to **Appendix D** for a complete list of abbreviations.

EXERCISE 27 ■ Fill In

Write the terms abbreviated.

1. To repair a cystocele and rectocele the patient is scheduled in surgery for an **A&P repair** ______________ and ______________ ______________.
2. Following a **TAH/BSO** ______________ ______________ ______________ and ______________ ______________-______________ the gynecologist prescribed **HRT** ______________ ______________ ______________ for the patient to take for 3 months after surgery.
3. **SHG** ______________ and **TVS** ______________ ______________ are diagnostic ultrasound procedures used to assist in diagnosing diseases and disorders of the female reproductive organs.
4. When performing a **VH** ______________ ______________ the surgeon removes the uterus through the vagina without a surgical incision into the abdomen. During a(n) **LAVH** ______________-______________ ______________ ______________ the surgeon uses a fiberoptic laparoscope inserted through a tiny incision near the umbilicus to visualize the uterus and guide removal through the vagina. In a **TLH** ______________ ______________ ______________, morcellation is used to remove the uterus through the laparoscope.
5. **D&C** ______________ and ______________ is the dilation of the **Cx** ______________ and scraping of the endometrium.
6. **FCC** ______________ ______________ ______________ is the most common breast problem of women in their 20s.
7. A female patient with probable **PID** ______________ ______________ ______________ was referred to the **GYN** ______________ clinic for evaluation and care.
8. The medical management of **PMS** ______________ ______________ emphasizes the relief of symptoms.
9. **UAE** ______________ ______________ ______________ offers a minimally invasive treatment option for some women with symptomatic uterine fibroids.
10. For long-acting reversible contraception, the female patient considered an **IUD** ______________ ______________ and **IUS** ______________ ______________ either of which would be inserted by a gynecologist. While these methods of **BC** ______________ ______________ are effective in preventing pregnancy, they do not protect against sexually transmitted infections.
11. A diagnosis of **PCOS** ______________ ______________ ______________ may be made if two of the following criteria are met: 1) chronic anovulation, 2) hyperandrogenism (excessive secretion of androgens with clinical or biological manifestations), and 3) polycystic ovaries.
12. When investigating the cause of **AUB** ______________ ______________ ______________ in women over 50, endometrial cancer must be considered and ruled out.

PRACTICAL APPLICATION

EXERCISE 28 ■ Case Study: Translate Between Everyday Language and Medical Language

CASE STUDY: Cindy Collier and Rajive Modi

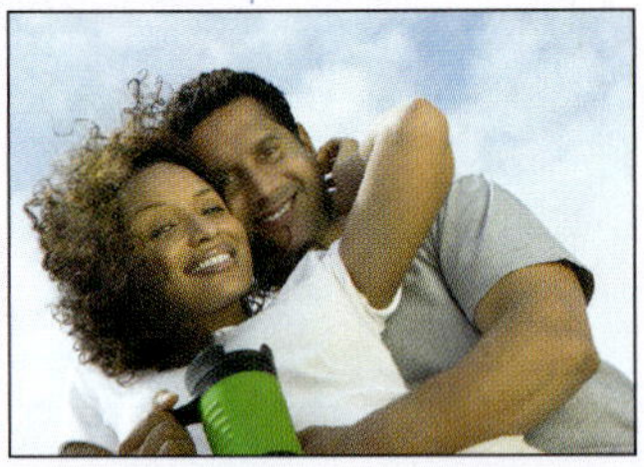

Cindy and Rajive want to have a baby. They have been trying for over a year to get pregnant, but it hasn't happened. Cindy worries something is wrong. Even though she has her period every month, menstruating is very painful, and she bleeds a lot. She often has pain low in her belly. She had sexual partners before Rajive, and she is worried that one may have given her a disease. Rajive is also concerned, and wonders if something might be wrong with him that is keeping Cindy from getting pregnant. When he was born only one of his testicles was down, and they had to do surgery to fix the other one. He hasn't had any problems since then. He had partners before Cindy, and he is worried that he may have passed something on to her.

Now that you have worked through Chapters 7 and 8 on the reproductive systems, consider the medical terms that might be used to describe Cindy and Rajive's experience. See the Chapter at a Glance sections at the end of Chapters 7 and 8 for a list of terms that might apply.

A. *Underline phrases in the case study that could be substituted with medical terms.*

B. *Write the medical term and its definition for three of the phrases you underlined.*

MEDICAL TERM	DEFINITION
1. ______________________	______________________________________
2. ______________________	______________________________________
3. ______________________	______________________________________

DOCUMENTATION: Excerpt from Infertility Clinic Consultation

Cindy, a 31-year-old female, and her husband Rajive, a 32-year-old male, present for workup and treatment for infertility. They have been trying to conceive for 14 months. Rajive: past medical history is significant for cryptorchidism at birth, which was repaired by orchidopexy at age 2. Cindy: menarche at 14, symptoms of dysmenorrhea and menorrhagia, both of which have worsened since discontinuing birth control pills. She had a normal Pap test approximately 1 year ago.

Diagnostic Studies: A complete blood count (CBC) was ordered as well as serum tests for thyroid-stimulating hormone (TSH), follicle-stimulating hormone (FSH), and prolactin level (PRL). A urine pregnancy test was negative.

Impression: Primary infertility; cause undetermined. Possible cervicitis caused by chlamydia and possible pelvic inflammatory disease.

Recommendation: We will await culture results and treat both partners with antibiotics if necessary. If labs are normal, we will proceed with a semen analysis for Rajive. We should consider a hysterosalpingogram (HSG) for Cindy based on her history and physical exam findings.

C. *Underline medical terms presented in Chapters 7 and 8 used in the previous excerpt from the infertility consultation. See the Chapter at a Glance sections at the end of the chapter for a complete list.*

D. *Select and define three of the medical terms you underlined. To check your answers, go to Appendix A.*

MEDICAL TERM	DEFINITION
1. ______________________	______________________________________
2. ______________________	______________________________________
3. ______________________	______________________________________

EXERCISE 29 ■ Interact with Medical Documents

A

Read the report and complete it by writing medical terms on answer lines within the document. Definitions of terms to be written appear after the document.

234-5678BR GARCIA, Evelina

File Patient Navigate Custom Fields Help

Chart Review | Encounters | Notes | Labs | Imaging | Procedures | Rx | Documents | Referrals | Scheduling | Billing

Name: **GARCIA, Evelina** MR#: 234-5678BR DOB: 10/08/19XX Gender: F Age: 48 **Allergies:** Peanuts **PCP:** Emily Fowler MD

Surgical Progress Note: Evelina Garcia is a 48-year-old woman here for follow-up after a suspicious lesion in the left breast was discovered during routine 1.________________.
Her husband and sister are present for this visit.

Family history is positive for breast 2.__________________ in two maternal aunts, both under age 50 at diagnosis.

Past medical history includes 3.____________________ for 4.________________ and 5.__________________. She has been on 6.____________________ since age 46 years.

The patient consented to a 7.____________________________________.

The pathology report is as follows:
Gross description: Received in formalin are four, pink-tan, cylindrical fragments of fibroadipose tissue, which range from 0.8 to 1.3 cm in length, each with a 0.1-cm diameter. The specimen is entirely submitted in one cassette.

Final diagnosis: Mammary parenchyma, left breast guided needle biopsy: Infiltrating, moderately differentiated ductal carcinoma with focal ductal carcinoma in situ, Grade 2, involving all four specimens. Lymphovascular invasion is identified.

Upon examination, the biopsy site reveals a 1-cm, healing surgical scar on the 8.__________________________ aspect of the left breast. The patient reports mild tenderness, alleviated with ibuprofen, but denies any signs or symptoms of infection.

Extensive education provided to patient and family regarding diagnosis and surgical treatment options. Patient states that she is interested in 9.____________________ with immediate reconstruction. Due to presence of lymphovascular invasion, 10.________ ___________________________ will be scheduled at the time of definitive surgery.

Consultation appointments arranged through Breast Center with medical oncology and plastic surgery clinics within 1 week. Follow-up appointment scheduled for next week.

Electronically signed: Meredith Woolridge, MD 11/17/20XX 09:17

Start | Log On/Off | Print | Edit

Definitions of Medical Terms to Complete the Document

Write the medical terms defined on corresponding answer lines in the document.

1. radiographic imaging of the breast
2. cancerous tumor
3. excision of the uterus
4. growth of endometrium into the muscular portion of the uterus
5. abnormal condition in which endometrial tissue occurs in various areas of the pelvic cavity
6. abbreviation for replacement of hormones to treat menopause
7. combines mammography and computer-assisted biopsy to obtain tissue from a breast lesion
8. pertaining to the middle and to (one) side
9. surgical removal of a breast
10. an injection of blue dye and/or radioactive isotope used to identify the first in the axillary chain and most likely to contain metastasis of breast cancer

EXERCISE 29 ■ Interact with Medical Documents—cont'd

B

Read the medical report and answer the questions below it.

47820 CARLSON, AKELAH

File Patient Navigate Custom Fields Help

Patient Chart | Lab | Rad | Notes | Documents | Rx | Scheduling | Images | Billing

Name: **CARLSON, Akelah** MR#: **47820** DOB: **2/15/19XX** Gender: **F** Age: **37** Allergies: **Neomycin, Bacitracin** PCP: **Robert Stone, MD**

CHART NOTE

ENCOUNTER DATE: 11/13/20XX

HISTORY: This 37-year-old gravida 2 para 2 woman was referred by her primary care provider. She complains of fullness in the pelvic region and menometrorrhagia. She admits to frequency and urgency of urination. Also, she complains of fatigue. The patient's last menstrual period was 2 weeks ago. Her mother was treated for ovarian cancer.

PHYSICAL EXAMINATION: Upon bimanual pelvic examination, an ill-defined mass was palpable on left lateral portion of the uterus.

DIAGNOSTIC STUDIES: Pap test results showed normal cytology. CA-125 test results were normal. Transvaginal sonography confirmed the presence of a pedunculated fallopian fibroid. The fallopian tubes and ovaries were normal.

IMPRESSION: Uterine fibroids.

RECOMMENDATION: We discussed the benefits of having a vaginal hysterectomy with bilateral salpingo-oophorectomy in view of her mother's history of ovarian cancer. The patient declined this approach because of the desire to have another child. A laparoscopic myomectomy is therefore recommended.

Electronically signed by: Elizabeth Fuller, MD 11/14/20XX 15:34

Use the medical report above to answer the questions.

1. The patient's symptoms include:
   a. absence of menstrual flow
   b. scanty menstrual flow
   c. increased amount of menstrual flow during menses and bleeding between periods
   d. painful menstruation
2. The CA-125 diagnostic study was used to detect the presence of:
   a. ovarian cancer
   b. cervical cancer
   c. endometrial cancer
   d. endometriosis
3. The recommended procedure, a myomectomy, will entail the surgical excision of:
   a. the breast
   b. the uterus
   c. ovarian cancer
   d. uterine fibroids

EXERCISE 30 ■ Use Medical Language in Online Electronic Health Records

Select the correct medical terms to complete three medical records in one patient's electronic file.

Access online resources at evolve.elsevier.com > Evolve Resources > Student Resources > Activities > Chapter 8 > Electronic Health Records

Topic: Invasive Ductal Carcinoma
Record 1: Gynecology Clinic Visit
Record 2: Radiology Final Report
Record 3: Pathology Final Diagnosis

❑ Check the box when complete.

EXERCISE 31 ■ Pronounce Medical Terms in Use

Practice pronunciation of terms by reading aloud the following paragraphs. Use the phonetic spellings to assist with pronunciation. The script also contains medical terms not presented in the chapter. If interested, research their meanings in a medical dictionary or a reliable online source.

CANCERS OF THE FEMALE REPRODUCTIVE SYSTEM

Breast Cancer

The breast is the most common site of cancer in women. More than 80% of **breast cancer** (brest) (KAN-cer) is infiltrating ductal cancer (IDC), which originates in the mammary ducts. The rate of growth depends on hormonal influences. As long as the cancer remains in the duct, it is considered noninvasive and is called *ductal carcinoma in situ (DCIS).*

Mammography (ma-MOG-ra-fē) is the most common method used for diagnosing cancer of the breast. Confirmation is done with a biopsy obtained by conventional surgery or guided breast biopsy, such as **stereotactic breast biopsy** (ster-ē-ō-TAK-tik) (brest) (BĪ-op-sē).Treatment may include lumpectomy, **mastectomy** (mas-TEK-to-mē),chemotherapy, radiation therapy, and hormonal therapy.

Cervical Cancer

In many regions of the world **cervical cancer** (SER-vi-kal) (KAN-cer) is the leading cause of death in women. Cervical cancer frequently results from a sexually transmitted infection, a feature that distinguishes it from other cancers. Abnormal **vaginal** (VAJ-i-nal) bleeding is the most common symptom. **Pap tests** (pap) (tests) and **HPV tests** (H-P-V) (tests), followed by **colposcopy** (kol-POS-ko-pē) with biopsy is used to diagnose this disease. Surgical treatment options include **conization** (*kon*-i-ZĀ-shun), such as LEEP, and **hysterectomy** (*his*-te-REK-to-mē). Chemotherapy and radiation therapy may also be used. A vaccine for human papillomavirus is now available for both boys and girls and can be used for the prevention of cervical cancer.

Endometrial Cancer

Currently 75% of women diagnosed with **endometrial cancer** (en-dō-MĒ-trē-al) (KAN-cer) are postmenopausal. Inappropriate bleeding is a warning sign; hence early diagnosis is common. **Pelvic** (PEL-vik) examination, Pap test, and endometrial sampling are used to diagnose this disease. Treatment is **hysterosalpingo-oophorectomy** (*his*-ter-ō-sal-*ping*-gō-ō-*of*-o-REK-to-mē), which may be followed by chemotherapy and radiation therapy. Laparoscopically assisted vaginal hysterectomy may also be used.

Ovarian Cancer

Ovarian cancer (ō-VAR-ē-an) (KAN-cer) is the ninth most common form of cancer in women, yet it is the most challenging to diagnose and causes more deaths than any other cancer of the female reproductive system. Early symptoms are often absent or associated with other problems; thus early diagnosis is uncommon. Early symptoms include abdominal discomfort and bloating; later stages include abdominal or pelvic pain and urinary or menstrual irregularities. **CA-125 test** (C-A-1-25) (test) and **transvaginal sonography** (trans-VAJ-i-nal) (so-NOG-ra-fē) are used in diagnosing this disease. Treatment is total abdominal hysterectomy and bilateral **salpingo-oophorectomy** (sal-ping-gō-ō-*of*-o-REK-to-mē) and removal of as much additional involved tissue as possible, including lymph nodes in the pelvic area. Chemotherapy is usually prescribed following surgery.

CHAPTER REVIEW

EXERCISE 32 ■ Chapter Content Quiz

Test your understanding of terms and abbreviations introduced in this chapter. Circle the letter for the medical term or abbreviation related to the words in italics.

1. *A severe illness that may affect menstruating women after using tampons* is abbreviated as:
   a. TSS
   b. TVS
   c. TLH

2. *Blockage of one of the glands on either side of the vagina* can lead to infection, which may result in an abscess.
   a. cervicitis
   b. vulvovaginitis
   c. Bartholin cyst

3. *Inflammation of the breast*, is an infection characterized by *pain in the breast*, edema, warmth, and erythema and most commonly occurs with breast-feeding.
   a. mastitis, mastalgia
   b. myometritis, mastopexy
   c. perimetritis, mammoplasty

4. Bilateral *water in the fallopian tube* indicates both tubes are blocked by watery liquid and can be a cause of female infertility.
   a. salpingocele
   b. hematosalpinx
   c. hydrosalpinx

5. Symptoms of *growth of the endometrium into the muscular portion of the uterus* include dysmenorrhea, menorrhagia, and *difficult or painful intercourse*.
   a. endometriosis, mastalgia
   b. adenomyosis, dyspareunia
   c. myometritis, amenorrhea

6. Monthly hormonal changes may cause *thickening of tissue (fibrosis), benign cysts, and pain or tenderness in one or both breasts*.
   a. FCC
   b. PMS
   c. PID

7. Cryosurgery, laser ablation, and LEEP are various surgical techniques performed to *remove a cone-shaped area of the cervix*.
   a. colporrhaphy
   b. conization
   c. myomectomy

8. The *surgical procedure to widen the cervix and remove contents from the uterus* can be used for both diagnosis and treatment.
   a. CX
   b. D&C
   c. SHG

9. A *surgical repair of the breast* to reduce size is called reduction:
   a. mammoplasty
   b. mammogram
   c. mastectomy

10. Partial *surgical closure of the vagina* may be used to treat vaginal prolapse for patients who are not candidates for more complex reconstructive surgeries and who are no longer sexually active.
    a. colpocleisis
    b. episiorrhaphy
    c. trachelectomy

11. In *total excision of the uterus performed laparoscopically*, the uterus, including the cervix, is morcellated and withdrawn through the laparoscope.
    a. TAH/BSO
    b. TLH
    c. TSS

12. The *instrument used for visual examination of the uterus* is a thin, lighted device inserted through the vagina that transmits images of the inside of the uterus to a computer screen.
    a. hysteroscope
    b. colposcope
    c. pelviscopy

13. The *cytological study of cervical and vaginal secretions to detect high-risk forms of the human papillomavirus* is a lab test conducted to screen for cervical cancer.
    a. CA-125 test
    b. Pap test
    c. HPV test

14. *Infrequent release of an ovum from a mature graafian follicle* generally refers to having 8 or fewer menstrual cycles in 1 year.
    a. oligomenorrhea
    b. oligoovulation
    c. anovulation

15. A *vesicovaginal* fistula is an abnormal passage way between the vagina and the:
    a. rectum
    b. urinary bladder
    c. vulva

16. The *instrument used to open* the vagina to conduct a pelvic exam is called:
    a. speculum
    b. hysteroscope
    c. colposcope

17. *The beginning of menstruation*, when the first menstrual period occurs, is called
    a. menopause
    b. anovulation
    c. menarche
18. Symptoms of *dropping of the uterus (and sometimes vagina) due to weakened pelvic muscles* may include urine leaks, discomfort in the *pertaining to the pelvis* area, and lower back pain.
    a. vaginal fistula, endocervical
    b. uterovaginal prolapse, pelvic
    c. abnormal uterine bleeding, vulvovaginal
19. *Syndrome involving physical and emotional symptoms occurring up to 10 days before menstruation* may range from mild to severe, and affect up to 90% of women of reproductive age.
    a. Premenstrual syndrome
    b. Toxic shock syndrome
    c. Polycystic ovary syndrome
20. A *technique that combines mammography and computer-assisted biopsy to obtain tissue from a breast lesion* may be performed if the lesion can be seen on imaging but cannot be felt by the patient or medical care provider.
    a. transvaginal sonography
    b. sentinel lymph node biopsy
    c. stereotactic breast biopsy

CHAPTER AT A GLANCE Word Parts New to This Chapter

COMBINING FORMS

cervic/o
colp/o
endometri/o
episi/o
gynec/o
hymen/o
hyster/o
mamm/o
mast/o
men/o
metr/o
oophor/o
pelv/i
perine/o
salping/o
trachel/o
vagin/o
vulv/o

PREFIXES

peri-

SUFFIXES

-cleisis
-rrhaphy
-salpinx

CHAPTER AT A GLANCE Female Reproductive System Terms Built from Word Parts

DISEASE AND DISORDER

amenorrhea
cervicitis
dysmenorrhea
endometriosis
endometritis
hematosalpinx
hydrosalpinx
mastitis
menometrorrhagia
menorrhagia
metrorrhagia
myometritis
oligomenorrhea
oophoritis
perimetritis
pyosalpinx
salpingitis
salpingocele
vaginitis
vaginosis
vulvovaginitis

SURGICAL

colpocleisis
colpoperineorrhaphy
colpoplasty
colporrhaphy
episiorrhaphy
hymenotomy
hysterectomy
hysteropexy
mammoplasty
mastectomy
mastopexy
oophorectomy
perineorrhaphy
salpingectomy
salpingo-oophorectomy
salpingostomy
trachelectomy
vulvectomy

DIAGNOSTIC

colposcope
colposcopy
hysterosalpingogram (HSG)
hysteroscope
hysteroscopy
mammogram
mammography
pelviscopic
pelviscopy
sonohysterography (SHG)

COMPLEMENTARY

endocervical
gynecologist
leukorrhea
mastalgia
pelvic
vaginal
vesicovaginal
vulvovaginal

CHAPTER AT A GLANCE Female Reproductive System Terms *NOT* Built from Word Parts

DISEASE AND DISORDER

abnormal uterine bleeding (AUB)
adenomyosis
Bartholin cyst
breast cancer
cervical cancer
endometrial cancer
fibrocystic breast changes (FCC)
ovarian cancer
pelvic inflammatory disease (PID)
polycystic ovary syndrome (PCOS)
premenstrual syndrome (PMS)
toxic shock syndrome (TSS)
uterine fibroid
uterovaginal prolapse
vaginal fistula

SURGICAL

anterior and posterior colporrhaphy (A&P repair)
conization
dilation and curettage (D&C)
endometrial ablation
myomectomy
tubal ligation
uterine artery embolization (UAE)

DIAGNOSTIC

CA-125 test
HPV test
Pap test
sentinel lymph node biopsy
stereotactic breast biopsy
transvaginal sonography (TVS)

COMPLEMENTARY

anovulation
contraception
dyspareunia
fistula
hormone replacement therapy (HRT)
menarche
menopause
oligoovulation
speculum

Chapter 9

Obstetrics and Neonatology

Outline

Objectives

Upon completion of this chapter, you will be able to:

1. Pronounce organs and anatomic structures relating to pregnancy.
2. Define and spell word parts related to obstetrics and neonatology.
3. Define, pronounce, and spell disease and disorder terms related to obstetrics and neonatology.
4. Define, pronounce, and spell surgical and diagnostic terms related to obstetrics and neonatology.
5. Define, pronounce, and spell complementary terms related to obstetrics and neonatology.
6. Interpret the meaning of abbreviations related to obstetrics and neonatology.
7. Apply medical language in clinical contexts.

ANATOMY

Obstetrics is the branch of medicine that deals with childbirth and the care of the mother before, during, and after birth. **Neonatology** is the branch of medicine that deals with the diagnosis and treatment of disorders of the newborn.

Terms Relating to Pregnancy

TERM	DEFINITION
gamete (GAM-ēt)	mature germ cell, either sperm (male) or ovum (female)
conception (kon-SEP-shun)	beginning of pregnancy, when the sperm enters the ovum. Conception normally occurs in the fallopian tubes. (also called **fertilization**) (Fig. 9.1A)
zygote (ZĪ-gōt)	cell formed by the union of the sperm and the ovum
embryo (EM-brē-ō)	unborn offspring in the stage of development from implantation of the zygote to the end of the eighth week of pregnancy. This period is characterized by rapid growth of the embryo.
fetus (FĒ-tus)	unborn offspring from the beginning of the ninth week of pregnancy until birth (Fig. 9.1B)
gestation (jes-TĀ-shun)	development of a new individual from conception to birth (also called **pregnancy**)
gestation period (jes-TĀ-shun) (PĒR-ē-ed)	duration of pregnancy; normally 38 to 42 weeks, which can be divided into three equal periods, called *trimesters*
implantation (*im*-plan-TĀ-shun)	embedding of the zygote in the uterine lining. The process normally begins about 7 days after fertilization and continues for several days. (Fig. 9.1A)
placenta (pla-SEN-ta)	structure that grows on the wall of the uterus during pregnancy and allows for nourishment of the fetus (commonly referred to as **afterbirth**) (Fig. 9.1B)
amniotic sac (*am*-nē-OT-ic) (sak)	membranous bag that surrounds the fetus before delivery (also called **amnionic sac** and commonly referred to as **bag of waters**) (Fig. 9.1B)
chorion (KOR-ē-on)	outermost layer of the fetal membrane

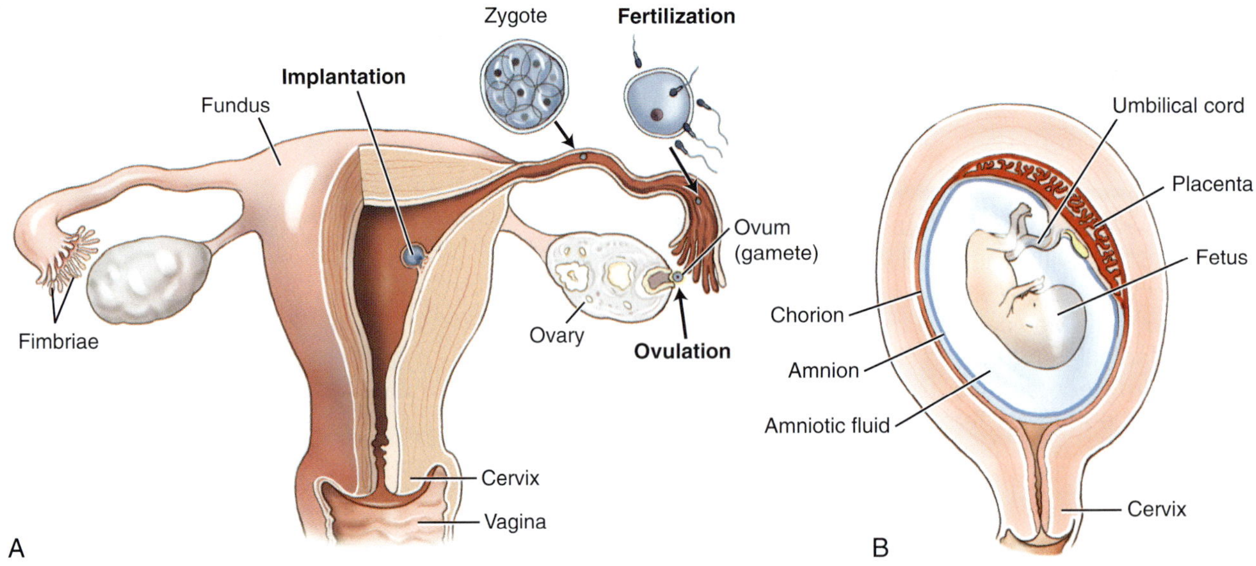

FIG. 9.1 **A,** Ovulation, fertilization, and implantation. **B,** Development of the fetus.

TERM	DEFINITION
amnion (*am*-nē-ON)	innermost layer of the fetal membrane
amniotic fluid (*am*-nē-OT-ic) (flu-id)	fluid within the amniotic sac, which surrounds the fetus (also called **amnionic fluid**)
umbilicus (um-BIL-i-cus)	navel (belly button); marks the site of attachment of the umbilical cord to the fetus

SKIN CHANGES THAT OCCUR THROUGHOUT PREGNANCY

- **striae gravidarum**: "stretch marks" occurring on the abdomen, breast, buttocks, and thighs from weakening of elastic tissues
- **linea nigra**: dark medial line extending from the pubis upward
- **chloasma**: hyperpigmentation of blotchy brown macules usually evenly distributed over the cheeks and forehead

PRONOUNCE ANATOMIC STRUCTURES

Practice saying aloud each of the organs and specific structures on the previous pages.

To hear the terms, go to Evolve Resources at www.evolve.elsevier.com and select:
Student Resources > Audio Glossary > Chapter 9 > **Anatomic Structures.**

❏ Check the box when complete.

WORD PARTS

Use paper flashcards or electronic flashcards on Evolve to memorize word parts used to analyze, define, and build medical terms in this chapter. To reinforce learning, study one section of the Word Parts Table at a time, then complete the corresponding exercise on the following pages.

1 ■ Obstetric and Neonatology Combining Forms

COMBINING FORM	DEFINITION
amni/o	amnion, amniotic fluid
amnion/o	amnion, amniotic fluid
chori/o	chorion
fet/i, fet/o	fetus, unborn offspring *(Note: both i and o may be used as combining vowels with fet/.)*
gravid/o	pregnancy
lact/o	milk
nat/o	birth
omphal/o	umbilicus, navel
par/o	bear, give birth to, labor, childbirth
part/o	bear, give birth to, labor, childbirth
puerper/o	childbirth

PUERPER is made up of two Latin word roots: **puer,** meaning **child,** and **per**, meaning **through.**

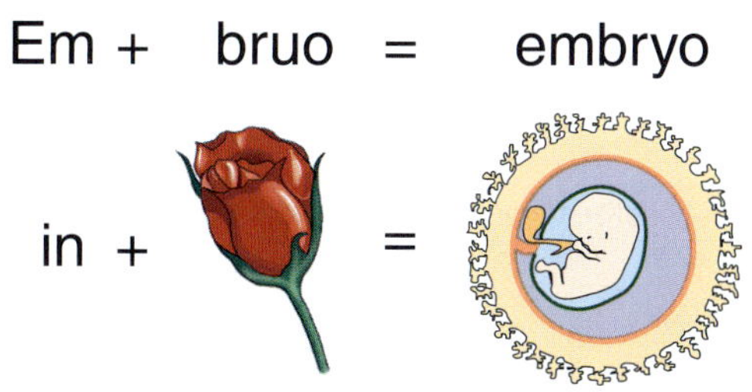

FIG. 9.2 ***Embryo*** comes from the Greek ***em,*** meaning "in," plus ***bruo,*** meaning "to bud" or "to shoot."

2 ■ Combining Forms Used with Obstetric and Neonatology Terms

COMBINING FORM	DEFINITION
carcin/o	cancer
cephal/o	head
episi/o	vulva
esophag/o	esophagus (tube leading from the throat to the stomach) (see Fig. 11.1)
hydr/o	water
hyster/o	uterus
olig/o	scanty, few
pelv/i	pelvis, pelvic cavity
prim/i	first *(Note: the combining vowel is* i.*)*
pseud/o	false
pylor/o	pylorus, pyloric sphincter (see Fig. 11.4)

PYLORUS refers to portion of the stomach that connects to the small intestine, and the **pyloric sphincter** is ring of muscle between the two.

COMBINING FORM	DEFINITION
son/o	sound
terat/o	malformations

TERAT/O is translated literally as **monster**; however, in terms containing terat/o relating to obstetrics, terat/o refers to malformations or abnormal development.

COMBINING FORM	DEFINITION
trache/o	trachea

3 ■ Prefixes

PREFIX	DEFINITION
ante-	before
dys-	painful, abnormal, difficult, labored
intra-	within
micro-	small
multi-	many
neo-	new
nulli-	none
poly-	many, much
post-	after
pre-	before

4 ■ Suffixes

SUFFIX	DEFINITION
-a	noun suffix, no meaning
-al	pertaining to
-amnios	amnion, amniotic fluid
-cele	hernia, protrusion
-centesis	surgical puncture to aspirate fluid (with a sterile needle)
-cyesis	pregnancy
-e	noun suffix, no meaning
-gen	substance or agent that produces or causes
-genic	producing, originating, causing
-graphy	process of recording, radiographic imaging
-ic	pertaining to
-is	noun suffix, no meaning
-itis	inflammation
-logist	one who studies and treats (specialist, physician)
-logy	study of
-oma	tumor, swelling
-rrhea	flow, discharge
-rrhexis	rupture
-stenosis	constriction or narrowing
-tocia	birth, labor
-tomy	cut into, incision
-um	noun suffix, no meaning
-us	noun suffix, no meaning

Refer to **Appendix B** and **Appendix C** for alphabetized word parts and their meanings.

EXERCISE 1 ■ Obstetric and Neonatology Combining Forms

Refer to the first section of the word parts table.

A Label

Fill in the blanks with combining forms to label this diagram of fetal development. *To check your answers, go to Appendix A* at the back of the textbook.

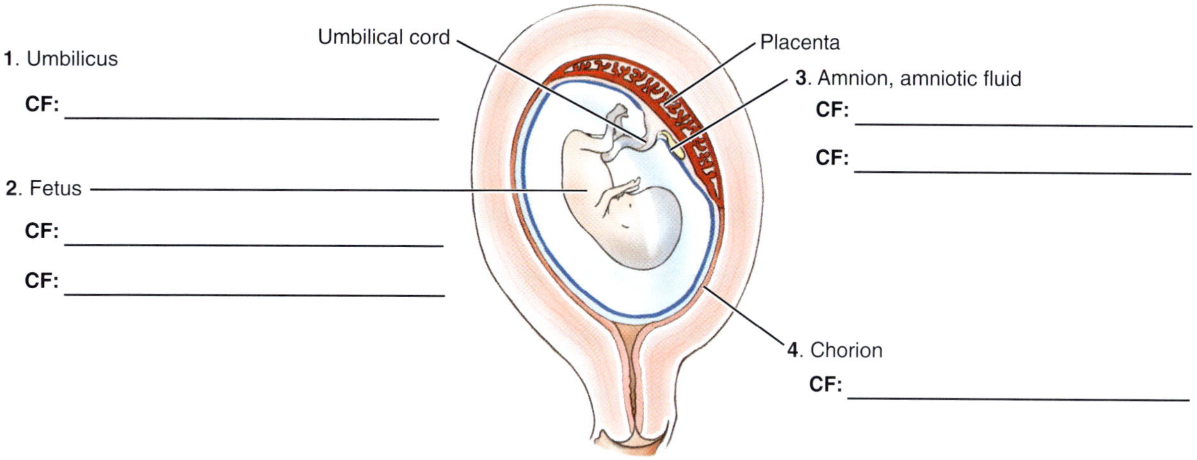

B Identify

Write the combining form for each of the following definitions.

1. childbirth ____
2. bear, give birth to, labor, childbirth a. ____ b. ____
3. pregnancy ____
4. milk ____
5. birth ____

C Define and Match

Step 1: Write the definitions after the following combining forms.
Step 2: Match the descriptions on the right with the combining forms and definitions. Answers may be used more than once.

____ 1. amni/o, ____
____ 2. omphal/o, ____
____ 3. amnion/o, ____
____ 4. fet/o, fet/i, ____
____ 5. chori/o, ____

a. outermost layer of the fetal membrane
b. 9 weeks of pregnancy to birth
c. innermost layer of fetal membrane; fluid surrounding the fetus
d. site of the umbilical cord attachment to the fetus

D Define

Write the definitions of the following combining forms.

1. lact/o ____
2. par/o, part/o ____
3. puerper/o ____
4. gravid/o ____
5. nat/o ____

EXERCISE 2 ■ Combining Forms Used with Obstetric and Neonatology Terms

Refer to the second section of the word parts table.

A Define

Write the definitions of the following combining forms.

1. prim/i ______
2. olig/o ______
3. pylor/o ______
4. hydr/o ______
5. cephal/o ______
6. episi/o ______
7. hyster/o ______
8. esophag/o ______
9. carcin/o ______
10. pseud/o ______
11. terat/o ______
12. trache/o ______
13. son/o ______
14. pelv/i ______

B Identify

Write the combining form for each of the following definitions.

1. head ______
2. scanty, few ______
3. first ______
4. uterus ______
5. pylorus, pyloric sphincter ______
6. pelvis, pelvic cavity ______
7. false ______
8. vulva ______
9. malformations ______
10. esophagus ______
11. cancer ______
12. trachea ______
13. water ______
14. sound ______

EXERCISE 3 ■ Prefixes

Refer to the third section of the word parts table.

A Define

Write the definitions of the following prefixes.

1. pre- ______
2. micro- ______
3. neo- ______
4. multi- ______
5. post- ______
6. dys- ______
7. ante- ______
8. poly- ______
9. intra- ______
10. nulli- ______

B Identify

Write the prefix for each of the following definitions.

1. none ______
2. after ______
3. small ______
4. within ______
5. before a. ______
   b. ______
6. many, much ______
7. many ______
8. new ______
9. painful, abnormal, difficult, labored ______

EXERCISE 4 ■ Suffixes

Refer to the fourth section of the word parts table.

A Define

Write the definitions of the following suffixes.

1. -logy ______________________
2. -gen ______________________
3. -oma ______________________
4. -ic ______________________
5. -tomy ______________________
6. -logist ______________________
7. -cele ______________________
8. -genic ______________________
9. -stenosis ______________________
10. -itis ______________________
11. -rrhea ______________________
12. -graphy ______________________

B Label

Write the suffixes pictured and defined.

1. ______________________
birth, labor

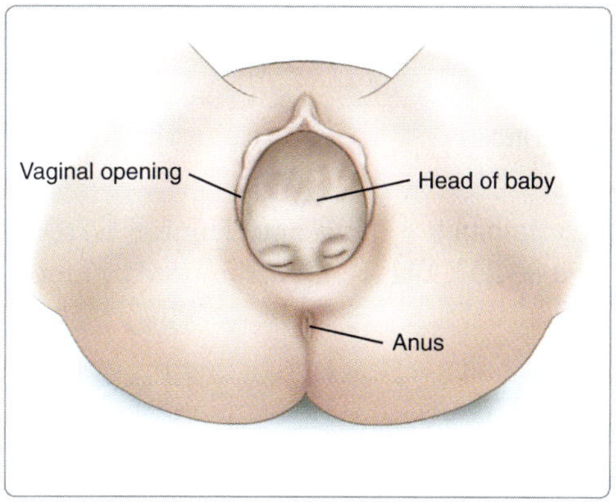

2. ______________________
rupture

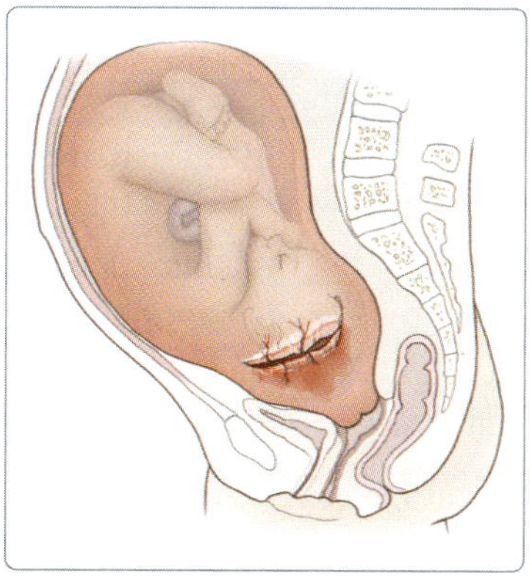

3. ______________________
pregnancy

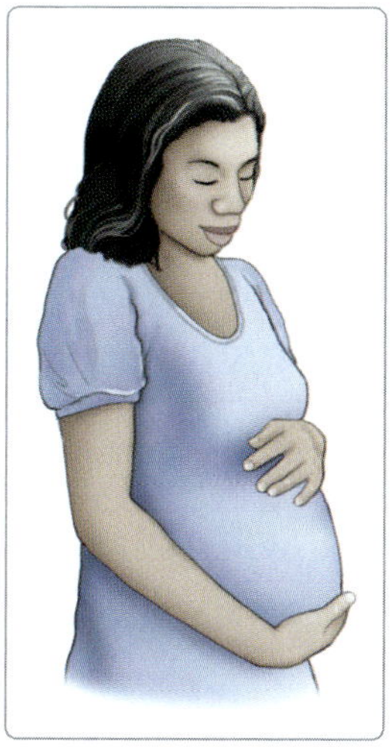

4. ______________________
amnion, amniotic fluid

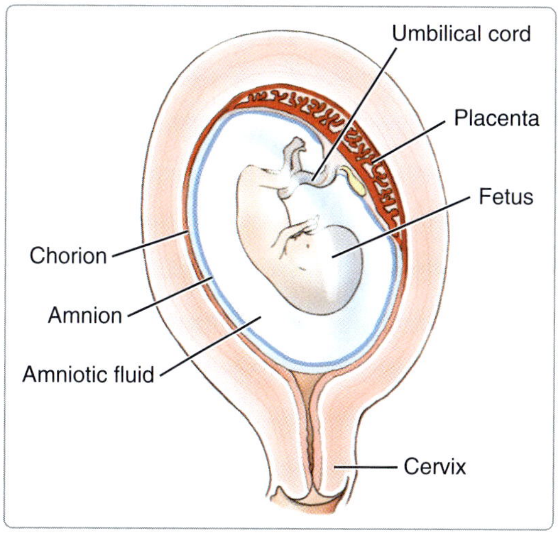

C Identify

Write the suffixes in this chapter that have no meaning. Place in alphabetical order.

1. ______________________
2. ______________________
3. ______________________
4. ______________________
5. ______________________

MEDICAL TERMS

Medical terms relevant to this chapter have been grouped by topics, such as Disease and Disorder, and are listed in tables designated as Built from Word Parts or *NOT* Built from Word Parts. The exercises following each table assist with learning term definitions, pronunciations, and spellings.

Obstetric Disease and Disorder Terms

BUILT FROM WORD PARTS AND *NOT* BUILT FROM WORD PARTS

The first portion of the table contains Obstetric Disease and Disorder Terms that can be translated using definitions of word parts. The second portion of the table contains Obstetric Disease and Disorder Terms that cannot be fully understood using the definitions of word parts.

Built from Word Parts

TERM	DEFINITION
1. amnionitis (*am*-nē-ō-NĪ-tis)	inflammation of the amnion
2. chorioamnionitis (*kor*-ē-ō-*am*-nē-ō-NĪ-tis)	inflammation of the chorion and amnion
3. choriocarcinoma (*kor*-ē-ō-*kar*-si-NŌ-ma)	cancerous tumor of the chorion
4. dystocia (dis-TŌ-sha)	difficult labor (obstructed or prolonged; causes may be from maternal factors, such as ineffective uterine contractions and abnormal pelvic shape, or from fetal causes, such as large size and abnormal birth presentation)
5. hysterorrhexis (*his*-ter-ō-REK-sis)	rupture of the uterus
6. oligohydramnios (*ol*-i-gō-hī-DRAM-nē-os)	scanty amnion water (less than the normal amount of amniotic fluid; 500 mL or less)
7. polyhydramnios (*pol*-ē-hī-DRAM-nē-os)	much amnion water (more than the normal amount of amniotic fluid; 2000 mL or more) (also called **hydramnios**)
8. pseudocyesis (sū-dō-sī-Ē-sis)	false pregnancy (a woman who believes she is pregnant—this may be a psychological condition or related to underlying pathology, such as a uterine tumor)

NOT Built from Word Parts

TERM	DEFINITION
1. abortion (AB) (a-BŌR-shun)	termination of pregnancy by the expulsion from the uterus of an embryo or fetus before viability, usually before 20 weeks of gestation. Spontaneous abortion is the termination of pregnancy that occurs naturally and is commonly referred to as *miscarriage*. Induced abortion is the intentional termination of pregnancy by surgical or medical intervention.
2. abruptio placentae (ab-RUP-shē-ō) (pla-SEN-tē)	premature separation of the placenta from the uterine wall (Fig. 9.4A)

TERM	DEFINITION
3. eclampsia (e-KLAMP-sē-a)	severe complication and progression of preeclampsia characterized by convulsion (see *preeclampsia* later). Eclampsia is a potentially life-threatening disorder.
4. ectopic pregnancy (ek-TOP-ik) (PREG-nan-sē)	pregnancy occurring outside the uterus, commonly in the fallopian tubes (Fig. 9.3)
5. placenta previa (pla-SEN-ta) (PRĒ-vē-a)	abnormally low implantation of the placenta on the uterine wall completely or partially covering the cervix. Dilation of the cervix can cause separation of the placenta from the uterine wall, resulting in bleeding. With severe hemorrhage, a cesarean section is necessary to save the mother and baby's life. (Fig. 9.4B)
6. preeclampsia (prē-ē-KLAMP-sē-a)	abnormal condition encountered during pregnancy or shortly after delivery characterized by high blood pressure and proteinuria, but with no convulsions. The cause is unknown; if not successfully treated, the condition can progress to eclampsia.

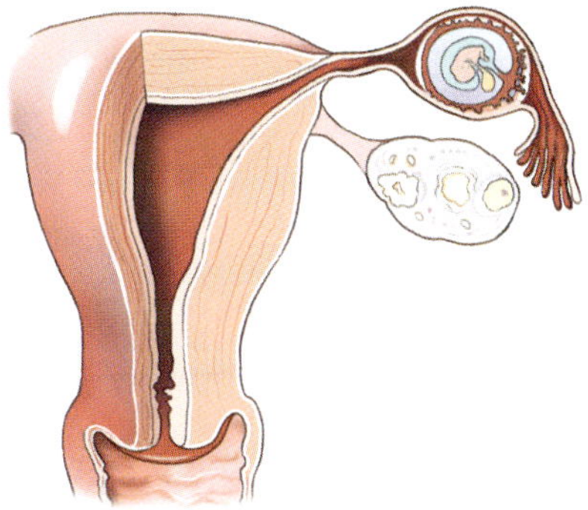

FIG. 9.3 Ectopic pregnancy.

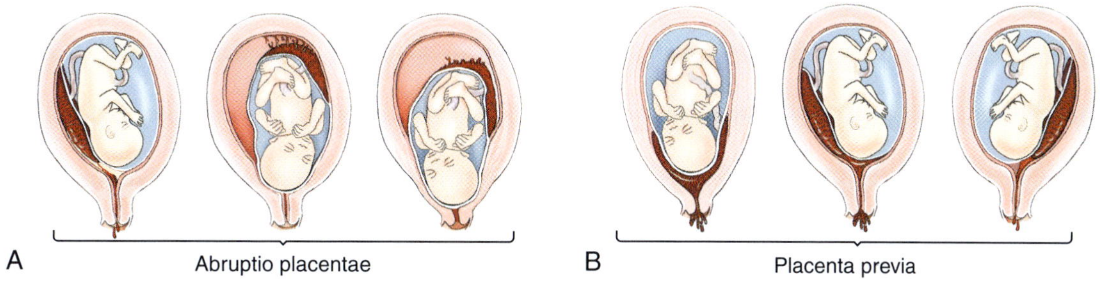

FIG. 9.4 Various presentations of abruptio placentae **(A)** and placenta previa **(B)**.

EXERCISE 5 ■ Pronounce and Spell

Practice pronunciation and spelling on paper and online.

1. Practice on Paper

a. **Pronounce:** Read the phonetic spelling and say aloud the terms listed in the previous table. Refer to the pronunciation key on p. 20 as necessary.
b. **Spell:** Have a study partner read the terms aloud. Write the spelling of the terms on a separate sheet of paper.

2. Practice Online

a. **Access** online learning resources. Go to evolve.elsevier.com > Evolve Resources > Student Resources.
b. **Pronounce:** Select Audio Glossary > Chapter 9 > Exercise 5. Select a term to hear its pronunciation and repeat aloud.
c. **Spell:** Select Activities > Chapter 9 > Spell Terms > Exercise 5. Select the audio icon and type the correct spelling of the term.

❑ Check the box when complete.

EXERCISE 6 ■ Obstetric Disease and Disorder Terms Built from Word Parts

A Analyze and Define

Analyze and define the following disease and disorder terms.

1. chorioamnionitis
____
____

2. choriocarcinoma
____
____

3. pseudocyesis
____
____

4. amnionitis
____
____

5. hysterorrhexis
____
____

6. oligohydramnios
____
____

7. polyhydramnios
____
____

8. dystocia
____
____

B Label

Build terms pictured by writing word parts above definitions.

1.

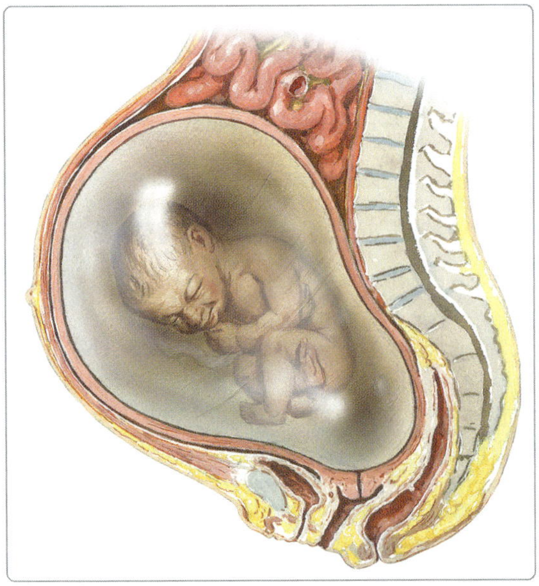

_______ / _______ / _______
much water amnion

2.

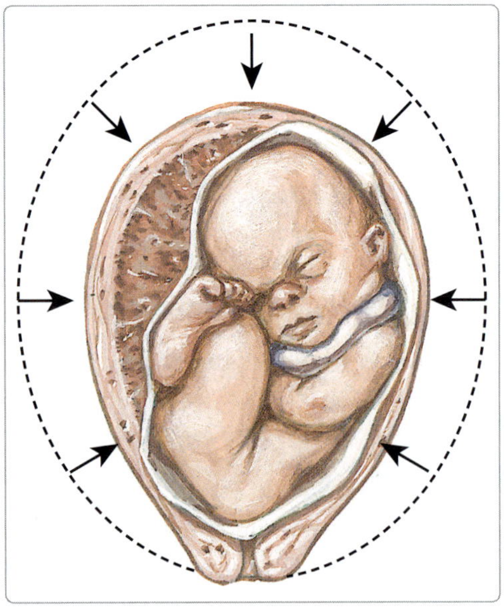

_______ / ___ / _______ / _______
scanty CV water amnion

3.

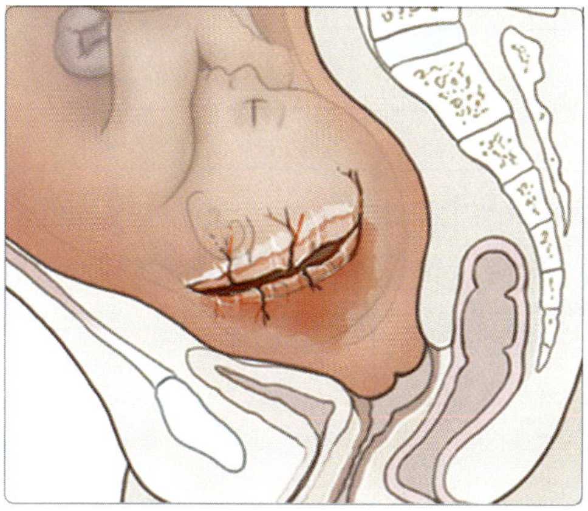

_________ / _____ / _____________
uterus CV rupture

4.

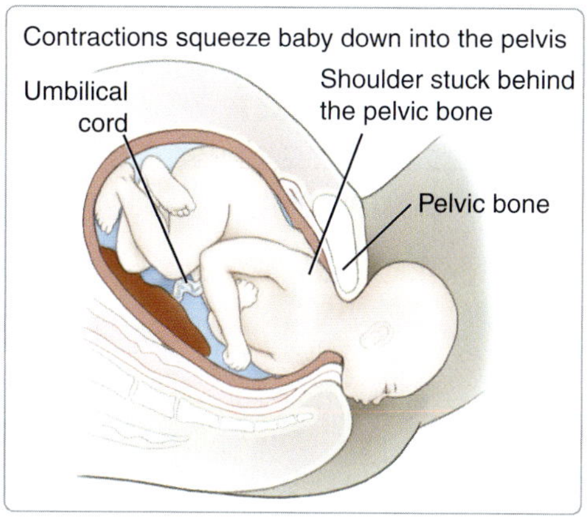

_____________ / _____________
difficult labor

C Fill In

Build disease and disorder terms for the following definitions by using the word parts you have learned.

1. cancerous tumor of the chorion
_______ / ___ / _______ / _______
WR CV WR S

2. inflammation of the amnion
_______ / _______
WR S

3. inflammation of the chorion and amnion
_______ / ___ / _______ / _______
WR CV WR S

4. false pregnancy
_______ / ___ / _______
WR CV S

EXERCISE 7 ▪ Obstetric Disease and Disorder Terms *NOT* Built from Word Parts

A Match

Match the terms in the first column with their correct definitions in the second column.

_____ 1. abruptio placentae
_____ 2. preeclampsia
_____ 3. ectopic pregnancy
_____ 4. placenta previa
_____ 5. eclampsia
_____ 6. abortion

a. severe complication and progression of preeclampsia characterized by convulsion
b. abnormally low implantation of the placenta on the uterine wall
c. termination of pregnancy by the expulsion from the uterus of an embryo or fetus before viability
d. premature separation of the placenta from the uterine wall
e. pregnancy occurring outside the uterus
f. abnormal condition characterized by high blood pressure and proteinuria, but with no convulsions

B Label

Write the medical terms pictured and defined.

1. ______________________________
pregnancy occurring outside the uterus, commonly in the fallopian tubes

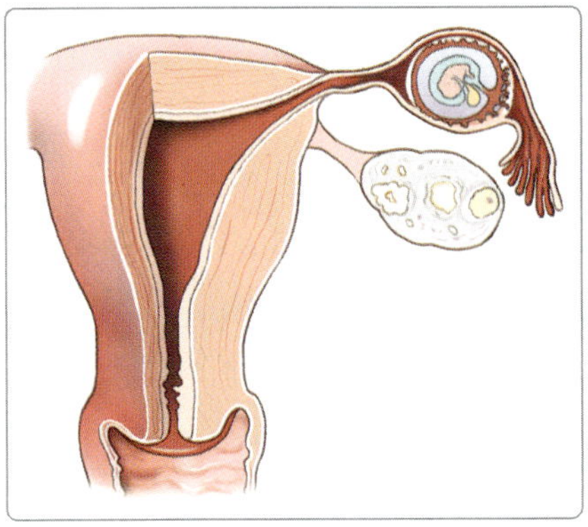

2. ______________________________
premature separation of the placenta from the uterine wall

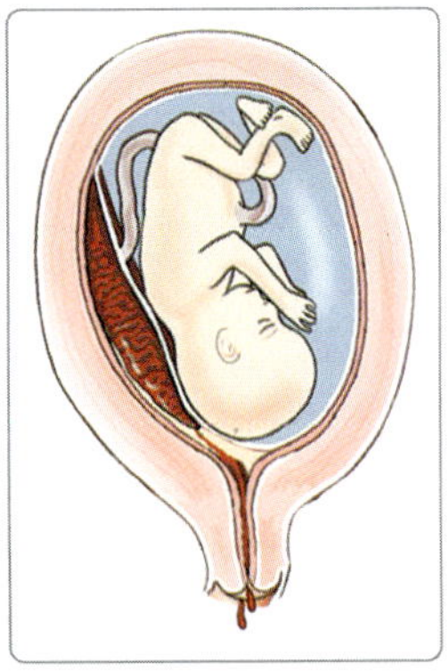

3. ______________________________
abnormally low implantation of the placenta on the uterine wall

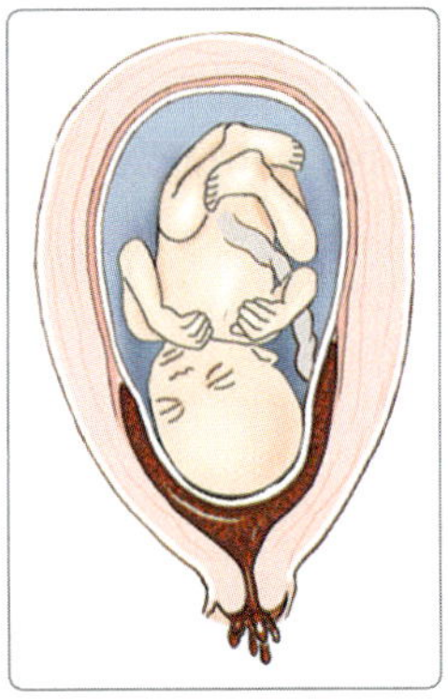

C Identify

Fill in the blanks with the correct terms.

1. severe complication and progression of preeclampsia ______________________________
2. termination of pregnancy by the expulsion from the uterus of an embryo or fetus ______________________________
3. characterized by high blood pressure and proteinuria, but with no convulsions ______________________________

EXERCISE 8 ■ Review of Obstetric Disease and Disorder Terms

Can you define, pronounce, and spell the following terms?

abortion (AB)
abruptio placentae
amnionitis
chorioamnionitis
choriocarcinoma
dystocia
eclampsia
ectopic pregnancy
hysterorrhexis
oligohydramnios
placenta previa
polyhydramnios
preeclampsia
pseudocyesis

Neonatology Disease and Disorder Terms

BUILT FROM WORD PARTS AND *NOT* BUILT FROM WORD PARTS

The first portion of the table contains Neonatology Disease and Disorder Terms that can be translated using definitions of word parts. The second portion of the table contains Neonatology Disease and Disorder Terms that cannot be fully understood using the definitions of word parts.

Built from Word Parts

TERM	DEFINITION
1. **microcephalus** (*mī*-krō-SEF-a-lus)	(fetus with a very) small head
2. **omphalitis** (*om*-fa-LĪ-tis)	inflammation of the umbilicus
3. **omphalocele** (OM-fal-ō-*sēl*)	hernia at the umbilicus (a part of the intestine protrudes through the abdominal wall at birth)
4. **pyloric stenosis** (pī-LOR-ik) (ste-NŌ-sis)	narrowing pertaining to the pyloric sphincter (Congenital pyloric stenosis occurs in 1 of every 200 newborns.)
5. **tracheoesophageal fistula** (*trā*-kē-ō-ē-*sof*-a-JĒ-al) (FIS-tū-la)	abnormal passageway pertaining to the trachea and esophagus (between the trachea and esophagus)

STENOSIS comes from the Greek word of the same spelling meaning to *narrow*. In medical language, it may appear as a suffix, -stenosis, or a standalone word as in pyloric stenosis.

NOT Built from Word Parts

TERM	DEFINITION
1. **cleft lip or palate** (kleft) (lip) (or) (PAL-at)	congenital split of the lip or roof of the mouth, one or both deformities may be present (*cleft* indicates a fissure) (Fig. 9.5)
2. **coarctation of the aorta** (kō-ark-TĀ-shun) (of) (the) (ā-OR-ta)	congenital stenosis (narrowing) that occurs in the arch of the aorta
3. **congenital cytomegalovirus (CMV) infection** (kon-JEN-i-tal) (*sī*-to-MEG-a-lō-*vī*-rus) (in-FEK-shun)	herpes-type virus that crosses the placenta. Symptoms in newborns may include jaundice, microcephaly, developmental delay and hearing loss; some infants may have no symptoms.
4. **congenital heart disease** (kon-JEN-i-tal) (hart) (di-ZĒZ)	heart abnormality present at birth
5. **Down syndrome** (down) (SIN-drōm)	genetic condition caused by a chromosomal abnormality characterized by varying degrees of intellectual, developmental, and physical disorders or defects (there is an extra 21st chromosome; hence, it is also called **trisomy 21**) (Fig. 9.6)
6. **erythroblastosis fetalis** (e-*rith*-rō-blas-TŌ-sis) (fē-TAL-is)	condition of the newborn characterized by hemolysis of the erythrocytes. The condition is usually caused by incompatibility of the infant's and mother's blood, occurring when the mother's blood is Rh negative and the infant's blood is Rh positive.
7. **esophageal atresia** (e-*sof*-a-JĒ-al) (a-TRĒ-zha)	congenital absence of part of the esophagus. Food cannot pass from the baby's mouth to the stomach.
8. **fetal alcohol syndrome (FAS)** (FĒ-tal) (AL-kō-hol) (SIN-drōm)	condition caused by excessive alcohol consumption by the mother during pregnancy. Various birth defects may be present, including central nervous system dysfunction and malformations of the skull and face.
9. **gastroschisis** (gas-TROS-ki-sis)	congenital fissure of the abdominal wall that is not at the umbilicus. Enterocele, protrusion of the intestine, is usually present.

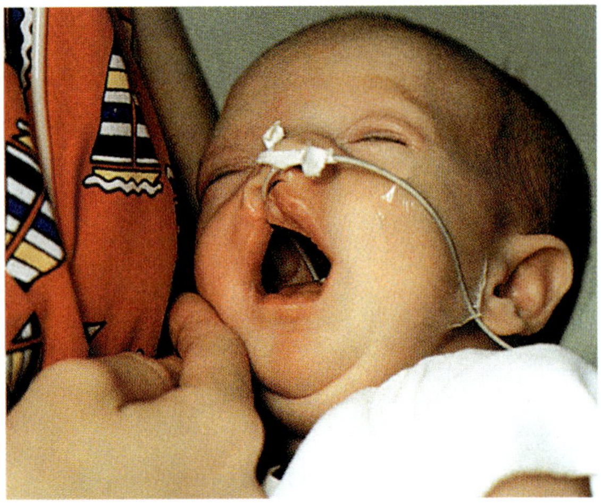

FIG. 9.5 Unilateral cleft lip. Note the nasogastric feeding tube in place. Neonates born with a cleft lip, palate, or both may require assistive feeding due to an impaired ability to suck.

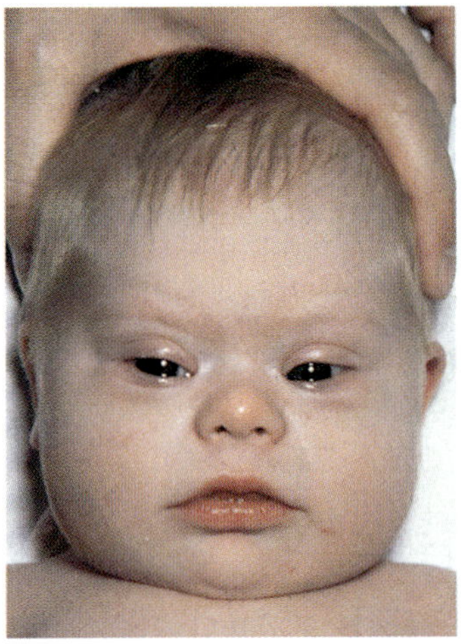

FIG. 9.6 Neonate with Down syndrome.

Neonatal Disease and Disorder Terms—cont'd

BUILT FROM WORD PARTS AND *NOT* BUILT FROM WORD PARTS

NOT Built from Word Parts

TERM	DEFINITION
10. respiratory distress syndrome (RDS) (RES-pi-ra-*tōr*-ē) (di-STRESS) (SIN-drōm)	respiratory complication in the newborn, especially in premature infants. In premature infants RDS is caused by normal immaturity of the respiratory system resulting in compromised respiration. (formerly called **hyaline membrane disease**)
11. spina bifida (SPĪ-na) (BIF-i-da)	congenital defect in the vertebral column caused by the failure of the vertebral arch to close. If the meninges protrude through the opening the condition is called meningocele. Protrusion of both the meninges and spinal cord is called meningomyelocele. (Fig. 9.7)

BIRTHMARKS are benign discolorations in the neonate's skin. Common birthmarks include: **congenital dermal melanocytosis**, which are bluish-black areas of hyperpigmentation often found on the lower back or buttocks of darker-skinned neonates, and **hemangiomas**, which are various benign vascular tumors or stains that cause reddish discoloration and/or malformations of the skin surface. **Nevus flammeus**, also called port-wine stain, is common, often temporary, and is caused by the dilation of certain blood vessels.

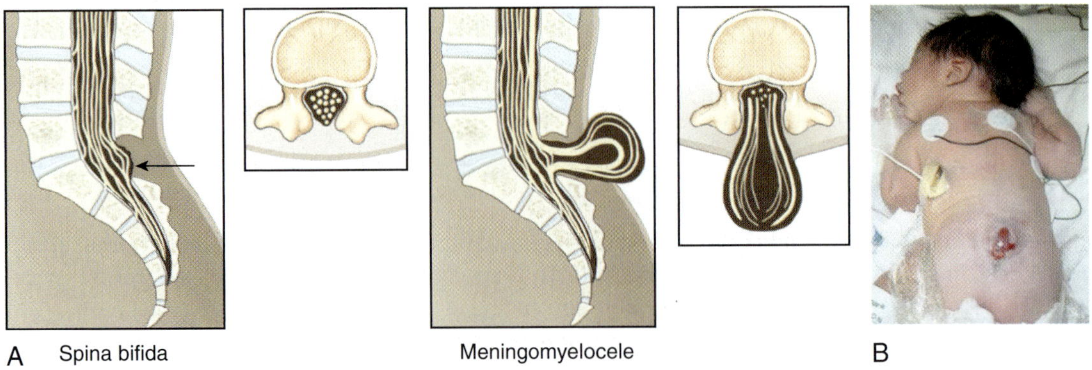

FIG. 9.7 **A,** Drawings of spina bifida and meningomyelocele. **B,** Photograph of meningomyelocele.

EXERCISE 9 ■ Pronounce and Spell

Practice pronunciation and spelling on paper and online.

1. Practice on Paper

a. **Pronounce:** Read the phonetic spelling and say aloud the terms listed in the previous table. Refer to the pronunciation key on p. 20 as necessary.
b. **Spell:** Have a study partner read the terms aloud. Write the spelling of the terms on a separate sheet of paper.

2. Practice Online

a. **Access** online learning resources. Go to evolve.elsevier.com > Evolve Resources > Student Resources.
b. **Pronounce:** Select Audio Glossary > Chapter 9 > Exercise 9. Select a term to hear its pronunciation and repeat aloud.
c. **Spell:** Select Activities > Chapter 9 > Spell Terms > Exercise 9. Select the audio icon and type the correct spelling of the term.

❑ Check the box when complete.

EXERCISE 10 ■ Neonatology Disease and Disorder Terms Built from Word Parts

A Analyze and Define

Analyze and define the following disease and disorder terms.

1. pyloric (stenosis)

____
____

2. omphalocele

____
____

3. omphalitis

____
____

4. microcephalus

____
____

5. tracheoesophageal (fistula)

____
____

B Label

Build terms pictured by writing word parts above definitions.

1.

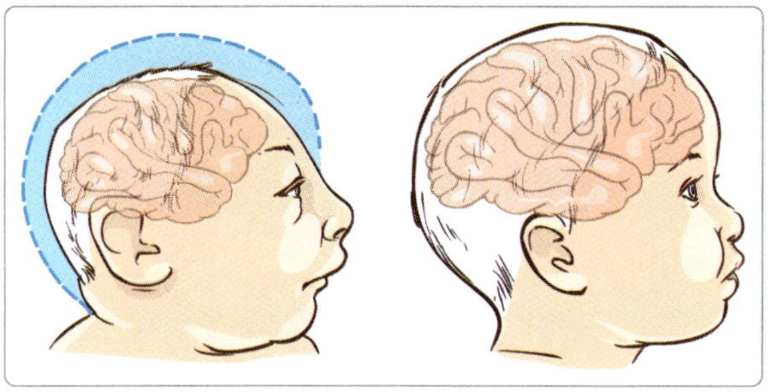

A. _______ / _______ / us
small head

B. normal-sized head

2.

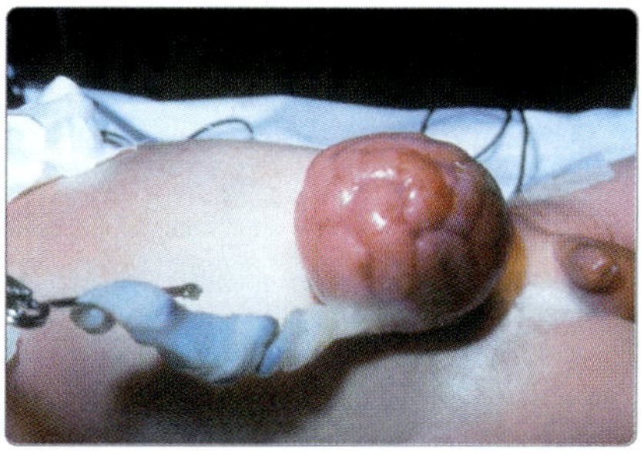

_______ / ___ / _______
umbilicus CV hernia

C Fill In

Build disease and disorder terms for the following definitions by using the word parts you have learned.

1. (narrowing) pertaining to the pyloric sphincter ______ WR / ______ S stenosis

2. abnormal passageway pertaining to the trachea and the esophagus (between the trachea and esophagus) ______ WR / CV / ______ WR / ______ S fistula

3. inflammation of the umbilicus ______ WR / ______ S

EXERCISE 11 ■ Neonatology Disease and Disorder Terms *NOT* Built from Word Parts

A Match

Match the terms in the first column with their correct definitions in the second column.

______ 1. Down syndrome
______ 2. cleft lip or palate
______ 3. spina bifida
______ 4. coarctation of the aorta
______ 5. congenital cytomegalovirus infection
______ 6. respiratory distress syndrome
______ 7. esophageal atresia
______ 8. gastroschisis
______ 9. fetal alchohol syndrome
______ 10. congenital heart disease
______ 11. erythroblastosis fetalis

a. heart abnormality present at birth
b. respiratory complication of neonates
c. split of the lip or roof of the mouth
d. caused by incompatibility of the infant's and the mother's blood
e. congenital fissure of the abdominal wall
f. congenital stenosis of the aorta
g. congenital absence of part of the esophagus
h. causes various birth defects, including central nervous system dysfunction
i. genetic condition caused by chromosomal abnormality
j. defect of the vertebral column
k. herpes-type virus that crosses the placenta

B Label

Write the medical terms pictured and defined.

1. ______________________
congenital absence of part of the esophagus

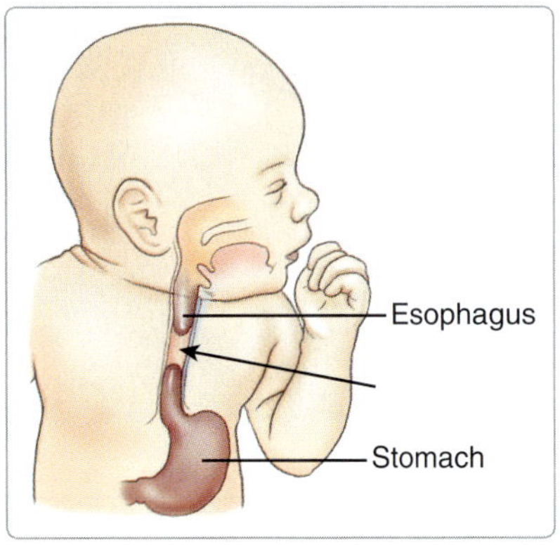

2. ______________________
congenital stenosis (narrowing) that occurs in the arch of the aorta

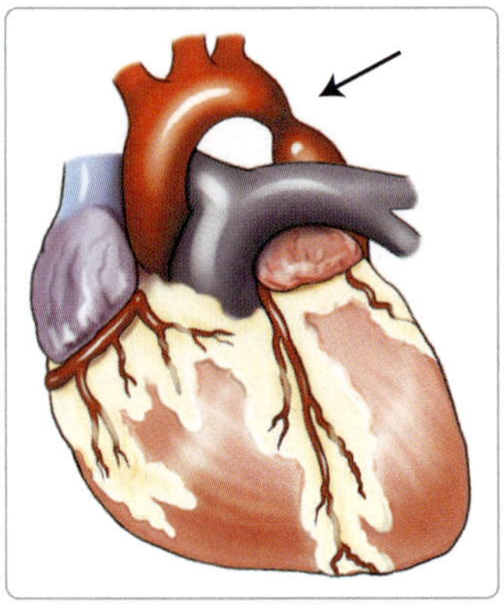

3. ______________________ congenital defect in the vertebral column caused by the failure of the vertebral arch to close. 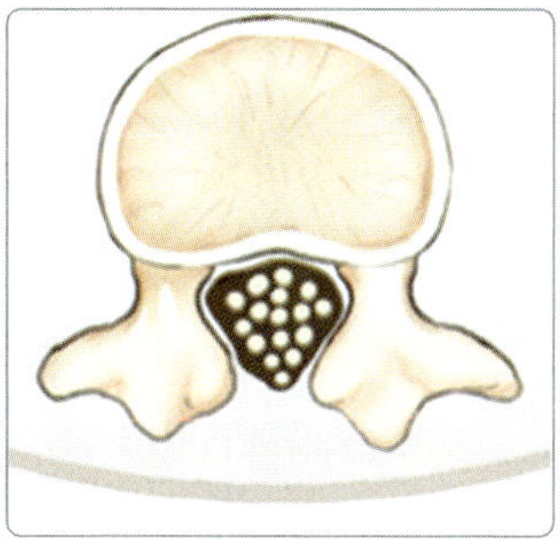	4. ______________________ congenital fissure of the abdominal wall that is not at the umbilicus. 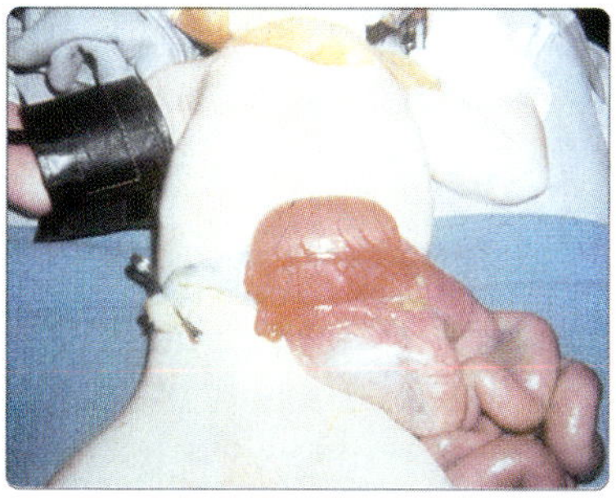

C Identify

Fill in the blanks with the correct terms.

1. ______________ ______________ is a condition of the newborn caused by hemolysis of the erythrocytes, and may occur when a mother has an Rh negative blood type and the infant is Rh positive.
2. Ventricular septal defect is an example of ______________ ______________ ______________, a heart abnormality present at birth.
3. A respiratory complication that occurs more commonly in premature infants is ______________ ______________ ______________.
4. While some infants have no symptoms, ______________ ______________ ______________, a herpes-type virus, may cause jaundice, microcephaly, developmental delay, and hearing loss.
5. ______________ ______________ ______________ is a condition caused by excessive alcohol consumption by the mother during pregnancy.
6. A congenital split of the lip or roof of the mouth is called ______________ ______________ or ______________.
7. ______________ ______________, a genetic condition caused by a chromosomal abnormality, is also called trisomy 21.

EXERCISE 12 ■ Review of Neonatology Disease and Disorder Terms

Can you define, pronounce, and spell the following terms?

cleft lip or palate
coarctation of the aorta
congenital cytomegalovirus (CMV) infection
congenital heart disease
Down syndrome
erythroblastosis fetalis
esophageal atresia
fetal alcohol syndrome (FAS)
gastroschisis
microcephalus
omphalitis
omphalocele
pyloric stenosis
respiratory distress syndrome (RDS)
spina bifida
tracheoesophageal fistula

Obstetric Surgical Terms

BUILT FROM WORD PARTS AND *NOT* BUILT FROM WORD PARTS

The first portion of the table contains Obstetric Surgical Terms that can be translated using definitions of word parts. The second portion of the table contains Obstetric Surgical Terms that cannot be fully understood using the definitions of word parts.

Built from Word Parts

TERM	DEFINITION	TERM	DEFINITION
1. **amniotomy** (*am*-nē-OT-o-mē)	incision into the amnion (rupture of the fetal membrane to induce labor; a special hook is generally used to make the incision) (Fig. 9.8)	2. **episiotomy** (e-*piz*-ē-OT-o-mē)	incision into the vulva (perineum) (sometimes performed during delivery to prevent a traumatic tear of the vulva) (also called **perineotomy**) (Fig. 9.9)

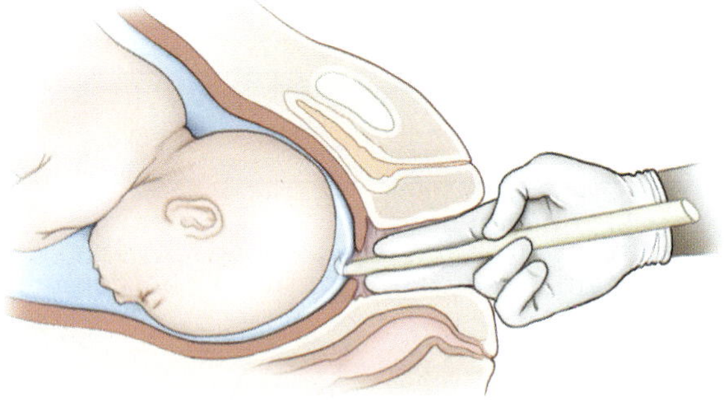

FIG. 9.8 Amniotomy.

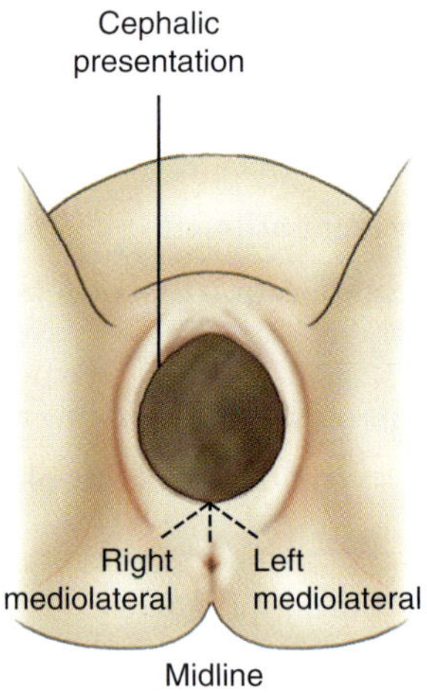

FIG. 9.9 Episiotomies.

NOT Built from Word Parts

TERM	DEFINITION
1. **cervical cerclage** (SER-vi-kal) (ser-KLAHZH)	suturing the cervix closed to prevent dilation and premature delivery
2. **cesarean section (CS, C-section)** (se-ZĀR-ē-an) (SEK-shun)	birth of a fetus through an incision in the mother's abdomen and uterus (may also be spelled **caesarean**)
CESAREAN SECTION (C-SECTION) The origin of this term has no relation to the birth of Julius Caesar, as is commonly believed. One suggested etymology is that, from 715 to 672 BC, it was Roman law that the operation be performed on dying women in the last few months of pregnancy in the hope of saving the child. At that time the operation was called a **caeso matris utero**, which means **the cutting of the mother's uterus**.	
3. **in vitro fertilization (IVF)** (in) (VĒ-trō) (*fer*-ti-li-ZĀ-shun)	method of fertilizing human ova outside the body and placing the zygote into the uterus; used when infertility is present. Infertility management techniques that artificially combine both the ova and the sperm are called **assisted reproductive technology (ART)**. (Fig. 9.10)

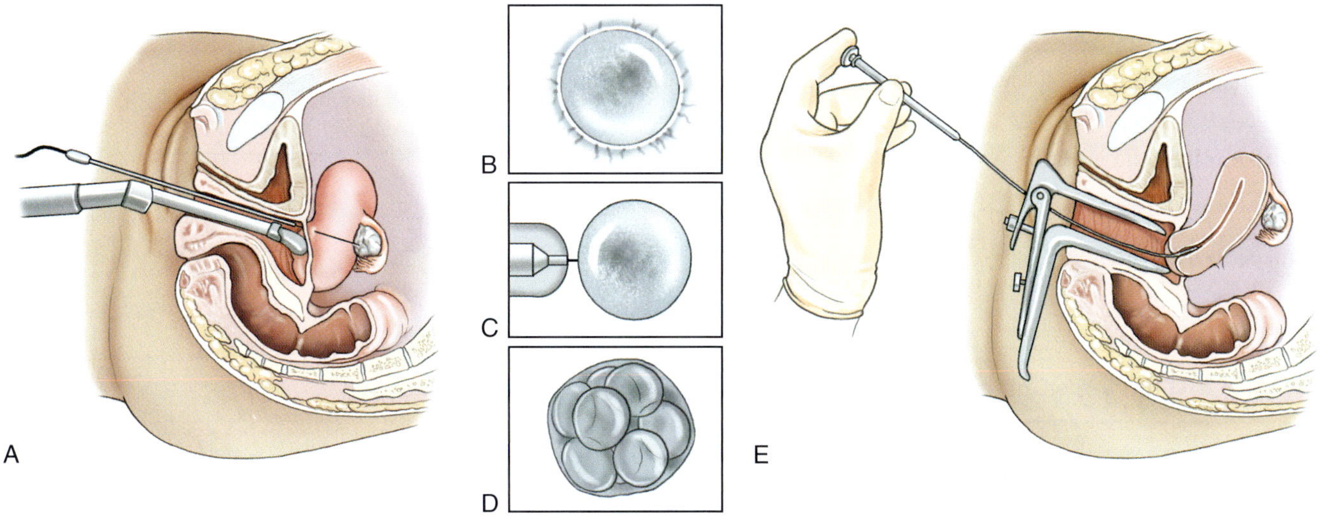

FIG. 9.10 In vitro fertilization (IVF). After ovarian stimulation, ova are retrieved from the ovary by ultrasound-guided transvaginal needle aspiration **(A).** The ova are fertilized outside the body in a dish with spermatozoa obtained from semen **(B).** A technique using a single sperm called intracytoplasmic sperm injection may also be used **(C).** After 48 hours the fertilized ova (zygotes) **(D)** are injected into the uterus for implantation **(E).** The first pregnancy after in vitro fertilization was reported more than 3 decades ago. Since then **assisted reproductive technology (ART)** has achieved millions of pregnancies worldwide.

EXERCISE 13 ■ Pronounce and Spell

Practice pronunciation and spelling on paper and online.

1. Practice on Paper

a. **Pronounce:** Read the phonetic spelling and say aloud the terms listed in the previous table. Refer to the pronunciation key on p. 20 as necessary.
b. **Spell:** Have a study partner read the terms aloud. Write the spelling of the terms on a separate sheet of paper.

2. Practice Online

a. **Access** online learning resources. Go to evolve.elsevier.com > Evolve Resources > Student Resources.
b. **Pronounce:** Select Audio Glossary > Chapter 9 > Exercise 13. Select a term to hear its pronunciation and repeat aloud.
c. **Spell:** Select Activities > Chapter 9 > Spell Terms > Exercise 13. Select the audio icon and type the correct spelling of the term.

❑ Check the box when complete.

EXERCISE 14 ■ Obstetric Surgical Terms Built from Word Parts

A Analyze and Define

Analyze and define the following surgical terms.

1. episiotomy

____

____

2. amniotomy

____

____

B Build

Build surgical terms for the following definitions by using the word parts you have learned.

1. incision into the amnion ______ WR / CV / S

2. incision into the vulva ______ WR / CV / S

EXERCISE 15 ■ Obstetric Surgical Terms *NOT* Built from Word Parts

A Label

Write the surgical terms pictured and defined.

1. ______
suturing the cervix closed to prevent premature delivery

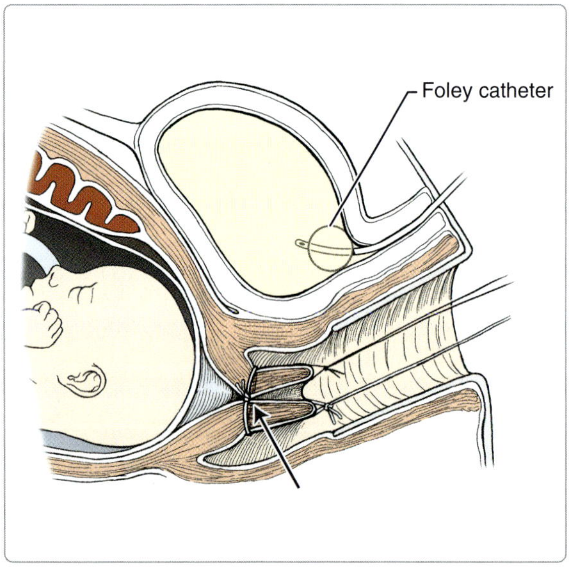

2. ______
method of fertilizing human ova outside the body and placing the zygote into the uterus

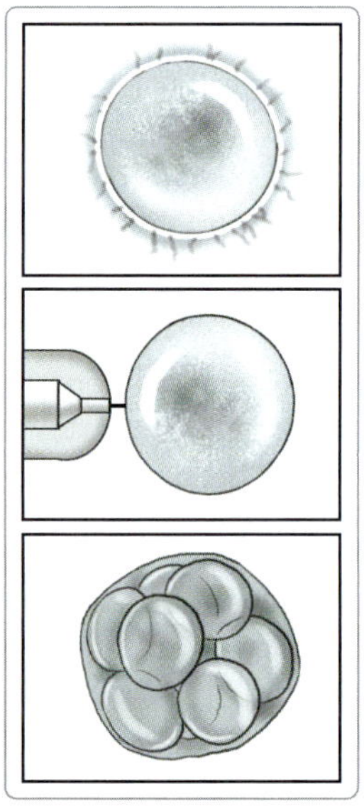

3. ______
birth of a fetus through an incision in the mother's abdomen and uterus

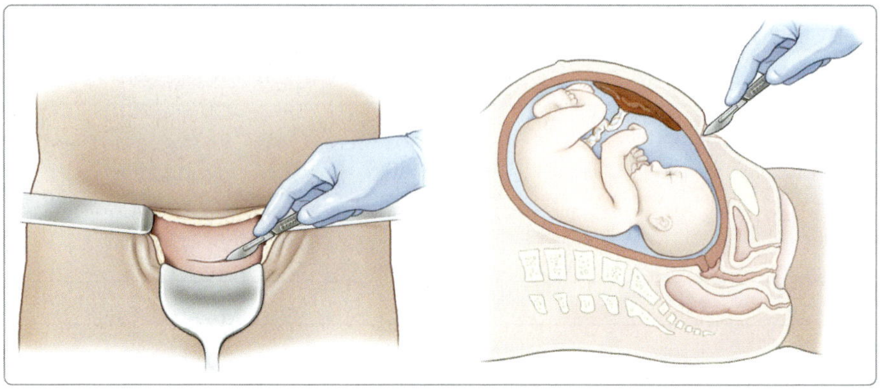

B Match

Match the terms in the first column with their correct definitions in the second column.

_____ 1. cesarean section	a. method of fertilizing human ova outside the body
_____ 2. cervical cerclage	b. birth of a fetus through an incision in the mother's abdomen
_____ 3. in vitro fertilization	c. suturing the cervix closed

EXERCISE 16 ■ Review of Obstetric Surgical Terms

Can you define, pronounce, and spell the following terms?

amniotomy cervical cerclage	cesarean section (CS, C-section)	episiotomy	in vitro fertilization (IVF)

Obstetric and Neonatology Diagnostic Terms

BUILT FROM WORD PARTS AND *NOT* BUILT FROM WORD PARTS

The first portion of the table contains Obstetric and Neonatology Diagnostic Terms that can be translated using definitions of word parts. The second portion of the table contains Obstetric and Neonatology Diagnostic Terms that cannot be fully understood using the definitions of word parts.

■ Built from Word Parts

DIAGNOSTIC IMAGING

TERM	DEFINITION	TERM	DEFINITION
1. **amniocentesis** (*am*-nē-ō-sen-TĒ-sis)	surgical puncture to aspirate amniotic fluid (The needle is inserted through the abdominal and uterine walls, using ultrasound to guide the needle. It is a prenatal test in which the fluid is used for the assessment of fetal health and maturity to aid in diagnosing fetal abnormalities.) (Fig. 9.11)	2. **pelvic sonography** (PEL-vik) (so-NOG-ra-fē)	pertaining to the pelvis, process of recording sound (pelvic ultrasound is used extensively to evaluate the fetus and pregnancy) (also called **pelvic ultrasonography, pelvic ultrasound,** and **obstetric ultrasonography**) (Fig. 9.12)

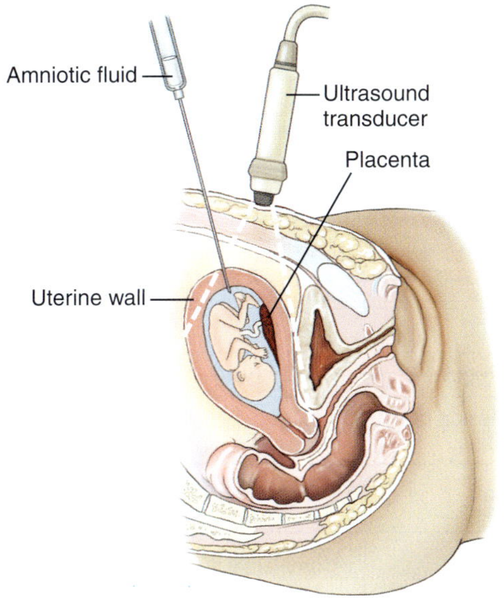

FIG. 9.11 Amniocentesis. Ultrasound is used to guide the needle through the abdominal and uterine walls.

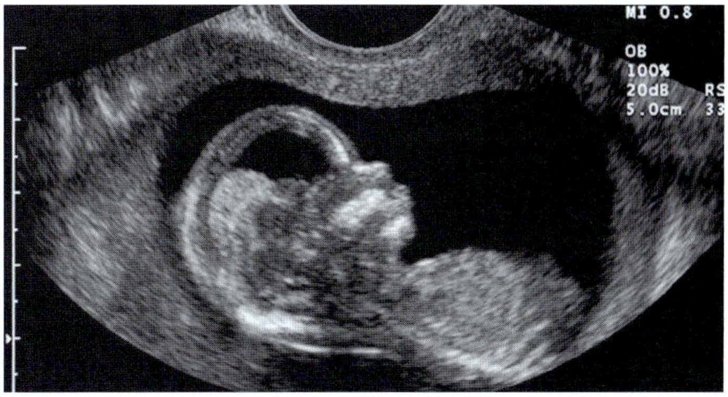

FIG. 9.12 Pelvic sonography image showing a fetal profile. Some specific uses are to: (1) diagnose early abnormal pregnancy, (2) determine the age of the fetus, (3) measure fetal growth, and (4) determine fetal position.

Obstetric and Neonatology Diagnostic Terms—cont'd

BUILT FROM WORD PARTS AND *NOT* BUILT FROM WORD PARTS

NOT Built from Word Parts

DIAGNOSTIC IMAGING

TERM	DEFINITION
1. **nuchal translucency screening** (NŪ-kal) (trans-LŪ-sen-sē) (SKRĒN-ing)	ultrasound test to check the back of the fetal neck for extra fluid or thickening. It is usually performed between 11 and 13 weeks of pregancy and, when combined with first trimester screening blood tests, may reveal an increased risk for Down syndrome or other congenital disorders.

LABORATORY

TERM	DEFINITION
2. **quad screen** (kwod) (skrēn)	blood test performed during the second trimester measuring four hormone levels that can reveal an increased risk of certain disorders in the developing fetus. It measures the levels of alpha-fetoprotein, human chorionic gonadotropin, unconjugated estriol and inhibin and can indicate the possibility of Down syndrome (trisomy 21), trisomy 18, and neural tube defects such as spina bifida. An abnormal quad screen requires a confirming diagnostic test such as ultrasound or amniocentesis, and genetic counselling is an important part of the work-up.

OTHER

TERM	DEFINITION
3. **Apgar score** (AP-gar) (skor)	system for rapid neonatal assessment at 1 and 5 minutes after birth. Five vital criteria, including heart rate, respiration, muscle tone, response to stimulation, and color, are assessed and scored on a 0-2 scale, with 7-10 considered normal. (Fig. 9.13)

APGAR SCORE Developed in 1952 by Virginia Apgar, MD, the Apgar score provides a basic framework for rapid neonatal assessment by health care providers at 1 minute and 5 minutes after birth. Five vital criteria (**heart rate**, **respiration**, **muscle tone**, **response to stimulation**, and **color**) are assessed and scored on a 0-2 scale. The score is totaled, with a 5-minute Apgar score of 7 to 10 considered normal. The Apgar score is used only for quickly reporting a neonate's status and does not predict future health outcomes.

TERM	DEFINITION
4. **chorionic villus sampling (CVS)** (kor-ē-A-nik) (VIL-us) (SAM-pling)	prenatal test that takes a sample of the the area of blood supply in the placenta either through the abdominal wall or the vagina. It is usually performed between 10 and 13 weeks of pregnancy and tests for chromosome and other genetic problems. It has a small risk of miscarriage and is thus usually performed only in high-risk pregnancies or when a screening test is positive for an abnormality. (Fig. 9.14)

SIGN	SCORE		
	0	1	2
Heart rate	Absent	Below 100	Over 100
Respiratory effort	Absent	Slow, irregular	Good, crying
Muscle tone	Limp	Some flexion of extremities	Active motion
Response to catheter in nostril (tested after oropharynx is clear)	No response	Grimace	Cough or sneeze
Color	Blue, pale	Body pink, extremities blue	Completely pink

FIG. 9.13 Apgar Score

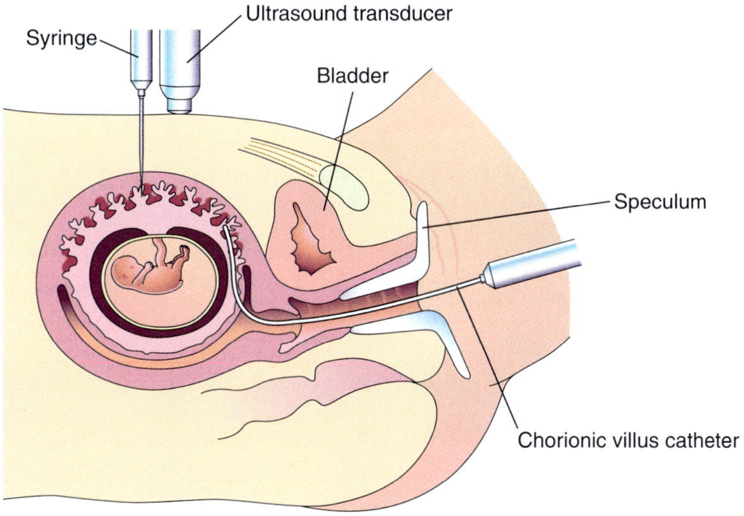

FIG. 9.14 Chorionic villus sampling.

EXERCISE 17 ■ Pronounce and Spell

Practice pronunciation and spelling on paper and online.

1. Practice on Paper

a. **Pronounce:** Read the phonetic spelling and say aloud the terms listed in the previous table. Refer to the pronunciation key on p. 20 as necessary.
b. **Spell:** Have a study partner read the terms aloud. Write the spelling of the terms on a separate sheet of paper.

2. Practice Online

a. **Access** online learning resources. Go to evolve.elsevier.com > Evolve Resources > Student Resources.
b. **Pronounce:** Select Audio Glossary > Chapter 9 > Exercise 17. Select a term to hear its pronunciation and repeat aloud.
c. **Spell:** Select Activities > Chapter 9 > Spell Terms > Exercise 17. Select the audio icon and type the correct spelling of the term.

❑ Check the box when complete.

EXERCISE 18 ■ Obstetric and Neonatology Diagnostic Terms Built from Word Parts

A Analyze and Define

Analyze and define the following obstetric and neonatology diagnostic terms.

1. amniocentesis

____

____

2. pelvic sonography

____

____

B Label

Build diagnostic terms pictured by writing word parts above definitions.

1.

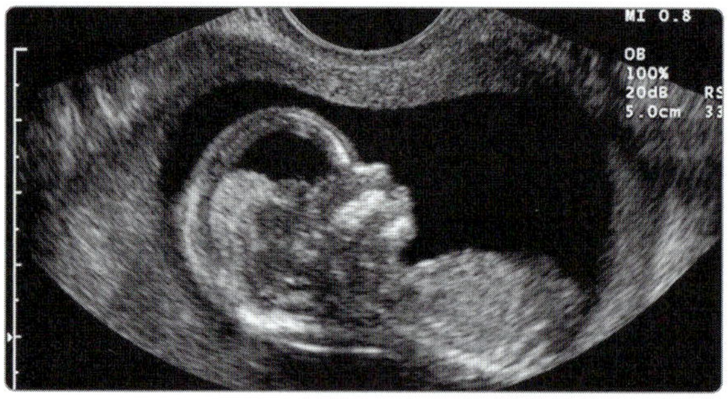

_____________ / _______________
pelvis   pertaining to

________ / ____ / _______________
sound   CV   process of recording

2.

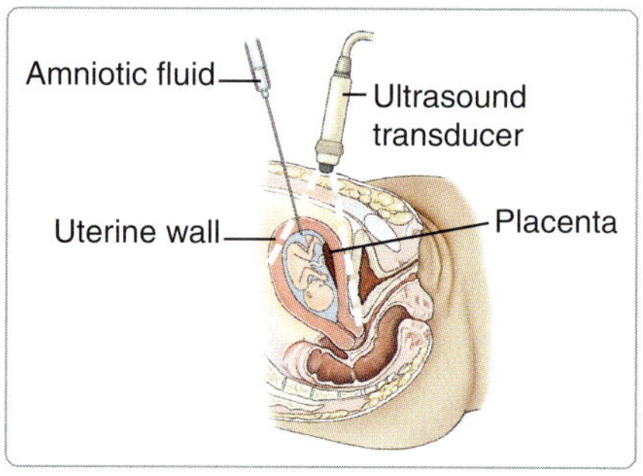

________ / ____ / _______________
amnion   CV   surgical puncture to aspirate fluid

EXERCISE 19 ■ Diagnostic Terms *NOT* Built from Word Parts

A Match

Match the terms in the first column with their correct definitions in the second column.

_____ 1. quad screen
_____ 2. Apgar score
_____ 3. nuchal translucency screening
_____ 4. chorionic villus sampling

a. system for rapid neonatal assessment at 1 and 5 minutes after birth
b. takes a sample of the the area of blood supply in the placenta
c. test that measures four hormone levels, can reveal increased risk
d. ultrasound test to check the back of the fetal neck for extra fluid or thickening

B Identify

Fill in the blanks with the correct terms.

1. A system for rapid neonatal assessment judging five vital criteria is called ______________ ______________.
2. ______________ ______________ ______________ is usually performed between 10 and 13 weeks of pregnancy and tests for chromosome and other genetic problems.
3. A blood test that measures levels of alpha-fetoproten, human chorionic gonadotropin, unconjugated estriol and inhibin is called a ______________ ______________.
4. ______________ ______________ ______________ uses ultrasound to look for extra fluid or thickening, and when combined with first trimester screening blood tests, may reveal an increased risk for Down syndrome or other congenital disorders.

EXERCISE 20 ■ Review of Obstetric and Neonatology Diagnostic Terms

Can you define, pronounce, and spell the following terms?

amniocentesis	chorionic villus sampling (CVS)	nuchal translucency screening	pelvic sonography
Apgar score			quad screen

Obstetric Complementary Terms

BUILT FROM WORD PARTS AND *NOT* BUILT FROM WORD PARTS

The first portion of the table contains Obstetric Complementary Terms that can be translated using definitions of word parts. The second portion of the table contains Obstetric Complementary Terms that cannot be fully understood using the definitions of word parts.

Built from Word Parts

SIGNS AND SYMPTOMS

TERM	DEFINITION	TERM	DEFINITION
1. amniorrhea (*am*-nē-ō-RĒ-a)	discharge (escape) of amniotic fluid	**3. lactorrhea** (*lak*-tō-RĒ-a)	(spontaneous) discharge of milk
2. amniorrhexis (*am*-nē-ō-REK-sis)	rupture of the amnion		

DESCRIPTIVE TERMS

TERM	DEFINITION	TERM	DEFINITION
4. antepartum (*an*-tē-PAR-tum)	before childbirth (reference to the mother)	**11. nulligravida** (*nul*-li-GRAV-i-da)	no pregnancies (a woman who has never been pregnant)
5. gravida (GRAV-i-da)	pregnant (a woman who is or has been pregnant, regardless of pregnancy outcome)	**12. nullipara** (nu-LIP-a-ra)	no births (a woman who has not given birth to a viable offspring)
6. gravidopuerperal (*grav*-i-dō-pū-ER-per-al)	pertaining to pregnancy and childbirth (from delivery until reproductive organs return to normal)	**13. para** (PAR-a)	birth (a woman who has given birth to an offspring after the point of viability—20 weeks, whether the fetus is alive or stillborn)
7. intrapartum (*in*-tra-PAR-tum)	within (during) labor and childbirth	**14. postpartum** (pōst-PAR-tum)	after childbirth (reference to the mother)
8. lactogenic (*lak*-tō-JEN-ik)	producing milk (by stimulation)	**15. primigravida** (prī-mi-GRAV-i-da)	first pregnancy (a woman in her first pregnancy)
9. multigravida (*mul*-ti-GRAV-i-da)	many pregnancies (a woman who has been pregnant two or more times)	**16. primipara (primip)** (*prī*-MIP-a-ra)	first birth (a woman who has given birth to an offspring after the point of viability—20 weeks)
10. multipara (multip) (mul-TIP-a-ra)	many births (a woman who has given birth to two or more viable offspring)	**17. puerperal** (pū-ER-per-al)	pertaining to (immediately after) childbirth

OTHER

TERM	DEFINITION
18. puerpera (pū-ER-per-a)	childbirth (a woman who has just given birth)

TABLE 9.1 Comparing Terms: Gravid/o and Par/o

GRAVID/O (PREGNANCY)	PAR/O (BIRTH)
nulli/gravid/a – no pregnancies	nulli/par/a – no births
primi/gravid/a – first pregnancy	primi/par/a – first birth
multi/gravid/a – many pregnancies	multi/par/a – many births

AN EXAMPLE OF USING GRAVIDA AND PARA IN MEDICAL SHORTHAND IN A CLINICAL SETTING

A 27 y/o **G4P2113** is a woman who has had **four** pregnancies, **two** term births, **one** preterm birth, **one** abortion, and has **three** living children.

Obstetric Complementary Terms—cont'd

BUILT FROM WORD PARTS AND *NOT* BUILT FROM WORD PARTS

NOT Built from Word Parts

SIGNS AND SYMPTOMS

TERM	DEFINITION
1. colostrum (ke-LOS-trem)	thin, milky fluid secreted by the breast during pregnancy and during the first days after birth before lactation begins
2. lochia (LŌ-kē-a)	vaginal discharge after childbirth
3. quickening (KWIK-en-ing)	first feeling of movement of the fetus in utero by the pregnant woman. It usually occurs between 16 and 20 weeks of gestation.

MEDICAL SPECIALTIES

TERM	DEFINITION
4. midwife (MID-wīf)	individual who practices midwifery
5. midwifery (MID-wif-rē)	practice of assisting in childbirth

COMPARE MIDWIFE AND DOULA **Midwives** practice midwifery and supervise pregnancy, labor, delivery, and puerperium. They assist with delivery independently, care for the newborn, and obtain medical assistance as necessary. A **midwife** may or may not be a registered nurse. Education, certification, and licensure vary by state and country. A **doula** (DOO-la) is a trained birth attendant who provides continual physical and emotional support to the laboring woman. **Doulas** provide a complementary role to the obstetric healthcare team.

TERM	DEFINITION
6. obstetrician (*ob*-ste-TRISH-an)	physician who specializes in obstetrics
7. obstetrics (OB) (ob-STET-riks)	medical specialty dealing with pregnancy, childbirth, and puerperium

DESCRIPTIVE TERMS

TERM	DEFINITION
8. breech presentation (brēch) (prē-zen-TĀ-shun)	birth position in which the buttocks, feet, or knees emerge first
9. cephalic presentation (se-FAL-ik) (prē-zen-TĀ-shun)	birth position in which any part of the head emerges first. It is the most common presentation.
10. in vitro (in) (VĒ-trō)	outside the body or in a lab setting
11. in vivo (in) (VĒ-vō)	within the living body

OTHER

TERM	DEFINITION
12. lactation (lak-TĀ-shun)	secretion of milk
13. parturition (*par*-tū-RISH-un)	act of giving birth
14. puerperium (*pū*-er-PĒ-rē-um)	period from delivery until the reproductive organs return to normal (approximately 6 weeks)

Refer to **Appendix E** for pharmacology terms related to obstetrics and neonatology.

EXERCISE 21 ■ Pronouce and Spell

Practice pronunciation and spelling on paper and online.

1. Practice on Paper

a. **Pronounce:** Read the phonetic spelling and say aloud the terms listed in the previous table. Refer to the pronunciation key on p. 20 as necessary.
b. **Spell:** Have a study partner read the terms aloud. Write the spelling of the terms on a separate sheet of paper.

2. Practice Online

a. **Access** online learning resources. Go to evolve.elsevier.com > Evolve Resources > Student Resources.
b. **Pronounce:** Select Audio Glossary > Chapter 9 > Exercise 21. Select a term to hear its pronunciation and repeat aloud.
c. **Spell:** Select Activities > Chapter 9 > Spell Terms > Exercise 21. Select the audio icon and type the correct spelling of the term.

❑ Check the box when complete.

EXERCISE 22 ■ Obstetric Complementary Terms Built from Word Parts

A Analyze and Define

Analyze and define the following obstetric complementary terms.

1. multigravida
____
____

2. lactorrhea
____
____

3. puerperal
____
____

4. amniorrhea
____
____

5. nullipara
____
____

6. amniorrhexis
____
____

7. postpartum
____
____

8. primipara
____
____

9. gravida
____
____

10. puerpera
____
____

B Label

Build terms pictured by writing word parts above definitions.

1.

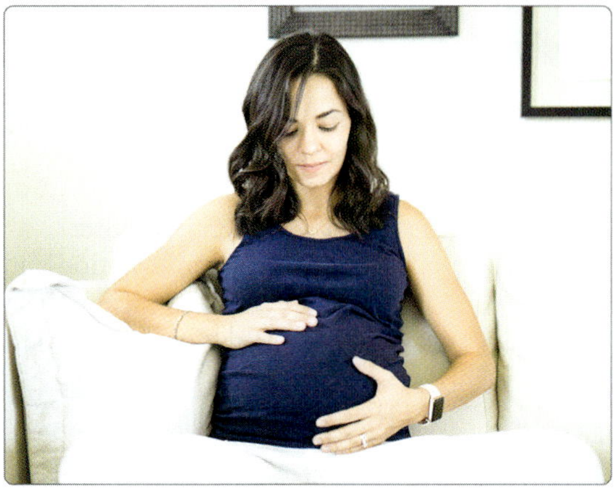

_______________ / _______________ / um
before childbirth
(reference to the mother)

2.

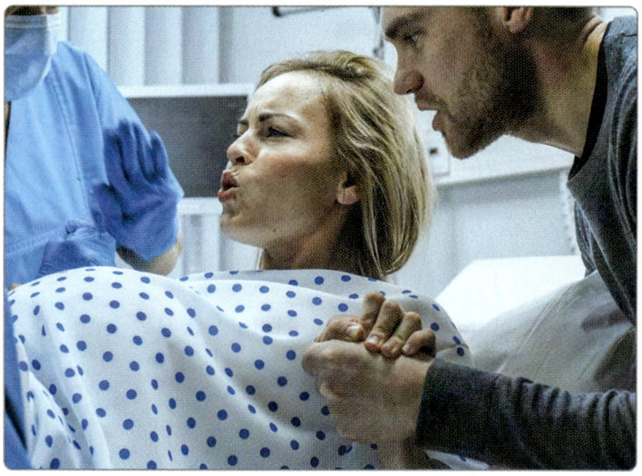

_______________ / _______________ / um
within (during) labor and childbirth

3.

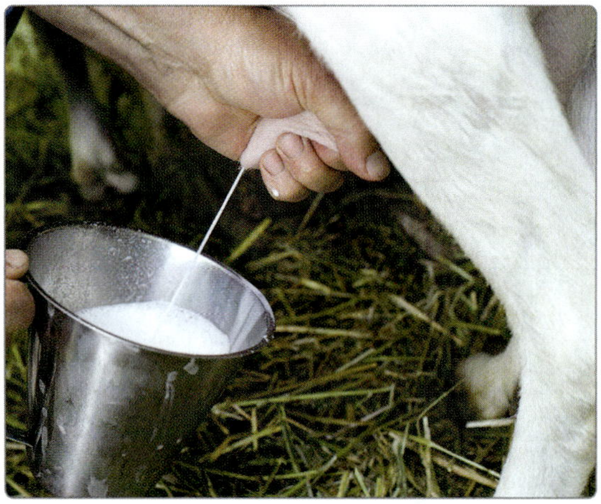

__________ / _____ / _______________
milk CV producing

4.

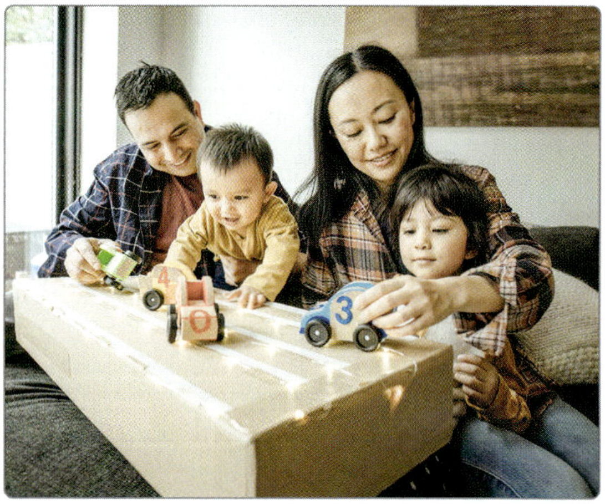

_______ / _______ / a
many births

C Fill In

Build obstetric complementary terms for the following definitions by using the word parts you have learned.

1. pertaining to pregnancy and childbirth ______ / ___ / ______ / ______ (WR / CV / WR / S)

2. first pregnancy ______ / ___ / ______ / ______ (WR / CV / WR / S)

3. birth (a woman who has given birth to an offspring after the point of viability) ______ / ______ (WR / S)

4. no pregnancies (a woman who has never been pregnant) ______ / ______ / ______ (P / WR / S)

EXERCISE 23 ■ Obstetric Complementary Terms *NOT* Built from Word Parts

A Identify

Fill in the blanks with the correct terms.

1. The act of giving birth is called ______________________.
2. ______________________ is the practice of assisting in childbirth.
3. The period from delivery until the reproductive system returns to normal, or ______________________, lasts about 6 weeks.
4. ______________________ is the first feeling of fetal movement by the pregnant woman and usually occurs between 16 and 20 weeks of gestation.
5. The medical specialty dealing with pregnancy, childbirth, and puerperium is called ______________________.
6. ______________________ ______________________ means within the living body.
7. The thin, milky fluid secreted by the breast during pregnancy, and shortly after birth is called ______________________.
8. ______________________ is vaginal discharge after childbirth.

B Label

Write the medical terms pictured and defined.

1. ______________________
birth position in which any part of the head emerges first.

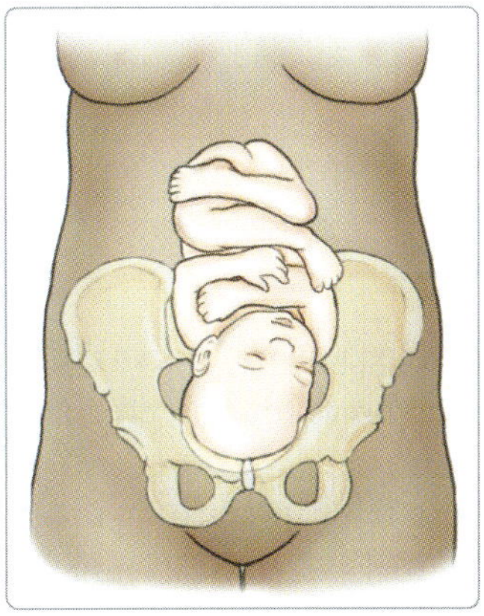

2. ______________________
birth position in which the buttocks, feet, or knees emerge first

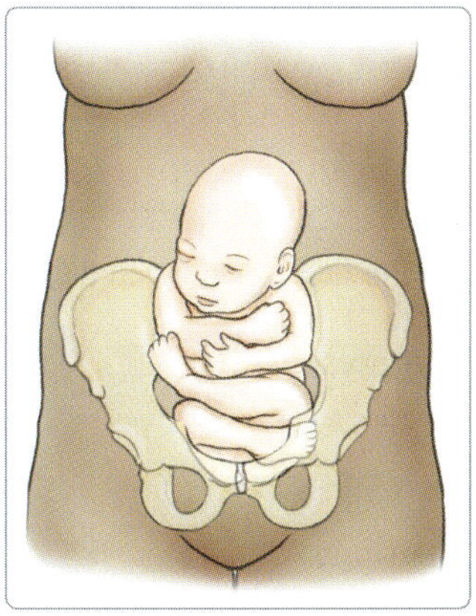

3. ______________________
secretion of milk

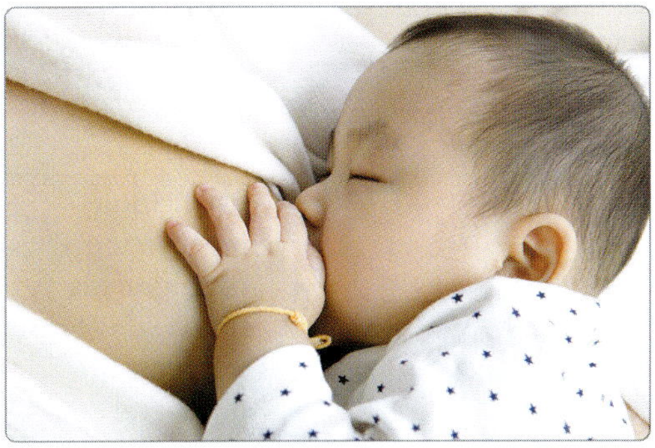

4. ______________________
outside the body or in a lab setting

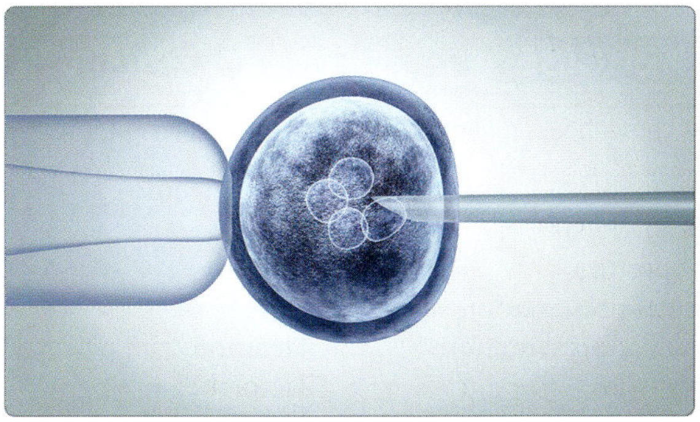

5. ______________________________
individual who practices the assistance of childbirth

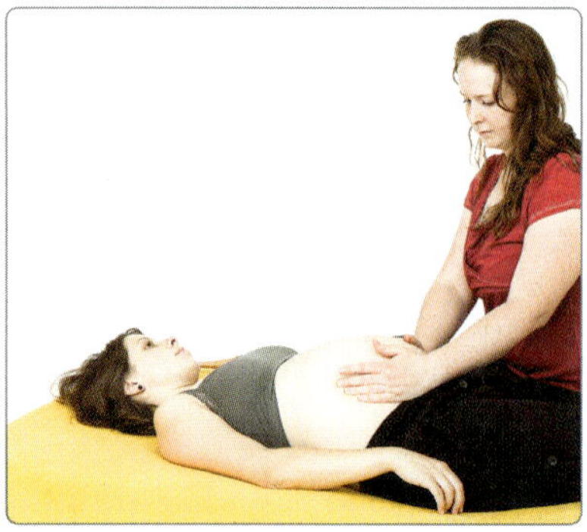

6. ______________________________
physician who specializes in pregnancy, childbirth, and the puerperium

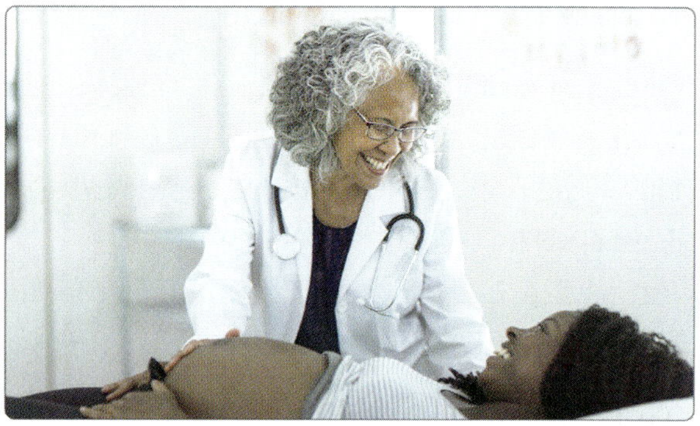

C Match

Match the terms in the first column with their correct definitions in the second column.

_____ 1. parturition	a. within the living body
_____ 2. lochia	b. secretion of milk
_____ 3. in vivo	c. practice of assisting in childbirth
_____ 4. lactation	d. physician who specializes in pregnancy, childbirth, and the puerperium
_____ 5. midwifery	e. act of giving birth
_____ 6. obstetrician	f. birth position in which any part of the head emerges first
_____ 7. cephalic presentation	g. vaginal discharge after childbirth

D Match

Match the terms in the first column with their correct definitions in the second column.

_____ 1. breech presentation	a. period from delivery until the reproductive organs return to normal
_____ 2. midwife	b. thin, milky fluid secreted by the breast during pregnancy and in the first few days after
_____ 3. quickening	c. first feeling of movement of the fetus in utero by the pregnant woman
_____ 4. puerperium	d. birth position in which the buttocks, feet, or knees emerge first
_____ 5. colostrum	e. outside the body or in a lab setting
_____ 6. obstetrics	f. individual who practices assisting in childbirth
_____ 7. in vitro	g. medical specialty dealing with pregnancy, childbirth, and the puerperium

EXERCISE 24 ■ Review of Obstetric Complementary Terms

Can you define, pronounce, and spell the following terms?

amniorrhea	intrapartum	midwifery	parturition
amniorrhexis	in vitro	multigravida	postpartum
antepartum	in vivo	multipara (multip)	primigravida
breech presentation	lactogenic	nulligravida	primipara (primip)
cephalic presentation	lactation	nullipara	puerpera
colostrum	lactorrhea	obstetrician	puerperal
gravida	lochia	obstetrics (OB)	puerperium
gravidopuerperal	midwife	para	quickening

Neonatalogy Complementary Terms

The first portion of the table contains Neonatalogy Complementary Terms that can be translated using definitions of word parts. The second portion of the table contains Neonatal Complementary Terms that cannot be fully understood using the definitions of word parts.

BUILT FROM WORD PARTS AND *NOT* BUILT FROM WORD PARTS

Built from Word Parts

MEDICAL SPECIALTIES

TERM	DEFINITION
1. **neonatologist** (*nē*-ō-nā-TOL-o-jist)	physician who studies and treats disorders of the newborn
2. **neonatology** (*nē*-ō-nā-TOL-o-jē)	study of the newborn (branch of medicine that deals with diagnosis and treatment of disorders in newborns)
3. **teratology** (*ter*-a-TOL-o-jē)	study of malformations (usually in regard to malformations caused by teratogens on the developing embryo)

DESCRIPTIVE TERMS

TERM	DEFINITION
4. **fetal** (FĒ-tal)	pertaining to the fetus
5. **natal** (NĀ-tal)	pertaining to birth
6. **neonate** (NĒ-ō-nāt)	new birth (an infant from birth to 4 weeks of age) (synonymous with **newborn [NB]**)
7. **postnatal** (pōst-NĀ-tal)	pertaining to after birth (reference to the newborn)
8. **prenatal** (prē-NĀ-tal)	pertaining to before birth (reference to the newborn)
9. **teratogen** (ter-A-tō-jen)	(any agent) producing malformations (in the developing embryo)
10. **teratogenic** (*ter*-a-tō-JEN-ik)	producing malformations (in the developing embryo)

TERATOGENS include chemical agents such as drugs, alcohol, viruses, x-rays, and environmental factors.

NOT Built from Word Parts

SIGNS AND SYMPTOMS

TERM	DEFINITION
1. **congenital anomaly** (kon-JEN-i-tal) (a-NOM-a-lē)	abnormality present at birth; often discovered before birth by sonography or amniocentesis
2. **meconium** (me-KŌ-nē-um)	first stool of the newborn (greenish-black)

TREATMENTS

TERM	DEFINITION
3. **gavage** (ga-VOZH)	process of feeding through a tube; used for critically ill newborns and others who are unconscious, unable to swallow, or too weak to eat (also called **gastric gavage**)

DESCRIPTIVE TERMS

TERM	DEFINITION
4. **premature infant** (PRĒ-ma-tur) (IN-fent)	infant born before completing 37 weeks of gestation (also called **preterm infant**)
5. **stillborn** (STIL-born)	born dead (death of fetus after 20 weeks of pregnancy)

TABLE 9.2 Terms Relating to Mother and Newborn

	BEFORE BIRTH	AFTER BIRTH
Mother	antepartum	postpartum
Newborn	prenatal	postnatal

EXERCISE 25 ■ Pronouce and Spell

Practice pronunciation and spelling on paper and online.

1. Practice on Paper

a. **Pronounce:** Read the phonetic spelling and say aloud the terms listed in the previous table. Refer to the pronunciation key on p. 20 as necessary.
b. **Spell:** Have a study partner read the terms aloud. Write the spelling of the terms on a separate sheet of paper.

2. Practice Online

a. **Access** online learning resources. Go to evolve.elsevier.com > Evolve Resources > Student Resources.
b. **Pronounce:** Select Audio Glossary > Chapter 9 > Exercise 25. Select a term to hear its pronunciation and repeat aloud.
c. **Spell:** Select Activities > Chapter 9 > Spell Terms > Exercise 25. Select the audio icon and type the correct spelling of the term.

❑ Check the box when complete.

EXERCISE 26 ■ Neonatalogy Complementary Terms Built from Word Parts

A Analyze and Define

Analyze and define the following neonatology complementary terms.

1. teratogenic
____
____

2. neonatology
____
____

3. neonate
____
____

4. fetal
____
____

5. prenatal
____
____

6. teratology
____
____

7. natal
____
____

8. neonatologist
____
____

9. teratogen

____

____

10. postnatal

____

____

B Label

Build terms pictured by writing word parts above definitions.

1.

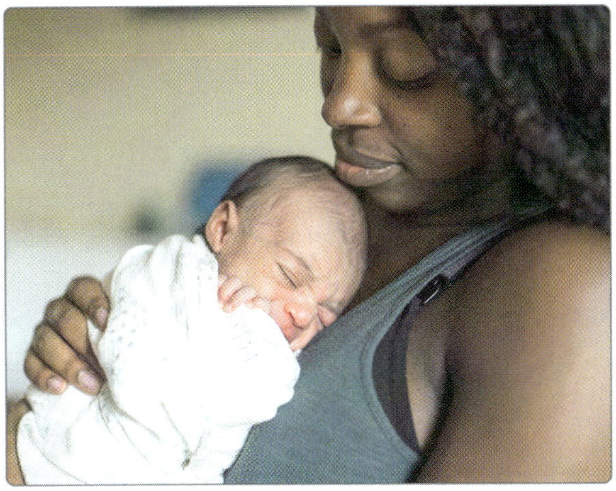

_____ / _____ / _____
new / birth / noun suffix (no meaning)

2.

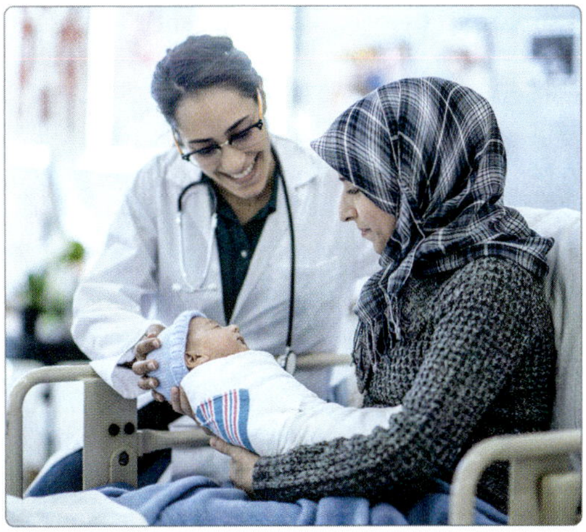

_____ / _____ / _____ / _____
new / birth / CV / physician who studies and treats

3.

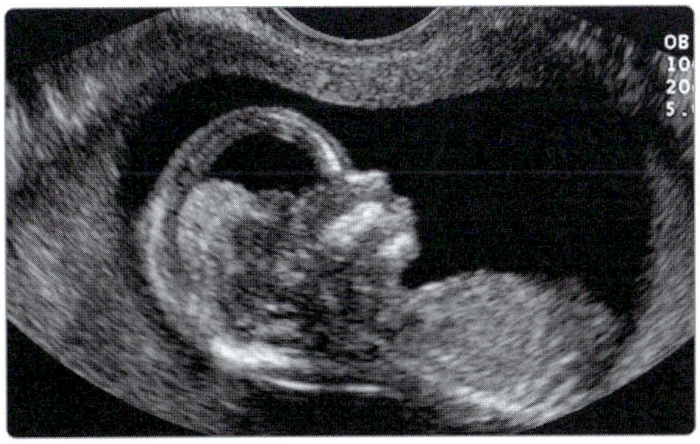

_____ / _____
fetus / pertaining to

4.

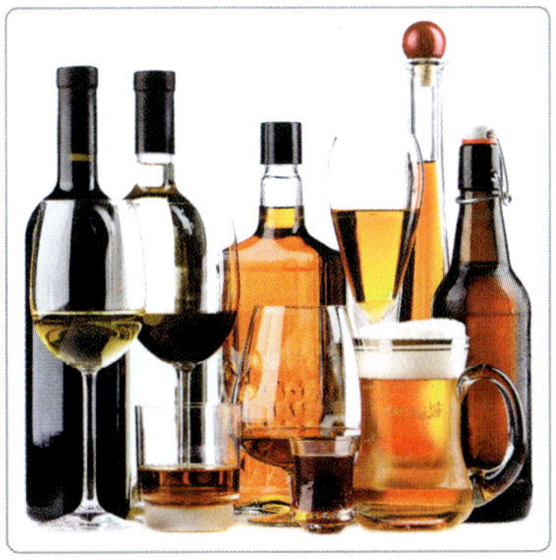

_____ / _____ / _____
malformations / CV / agent that produces

C Fill In

Build neonatology complementary terms for the following definitions by using the word parts you have learned.

1. pertaining to after birth (reference to the newborn)

_____ / _____ / _____
P / WR / S

2. study of malformations

_____ / _____ / _____
WR / CV / S

3. study of the newborn ______ P / ______ WR / ______ CV / ______ S

4. producing malformations ______ WR / ______ CV / ______ S

5. pertaining to birth ______ WR / ______ S

6. pertaining to before birth (reference to the newborn) ______ P / ______ WR / ______ S

EXERCISE 27 ■ Neonatology Complementary Terms *NOT* Built from Word Parts

A Identify

Fill in the blanks with the correct terms.

1. An abnormality present at birth, ______________ ______________, may be discovered before birth by sonography or amniocentesis.
2. ______________ is the term for the death of a fetus after 20 weeks of pregnancy.
3. The first stool of the newborn is called ______________.

B Label

Write the medical terms pictured and defined.

1. ______________________________
process of feeding through a tube

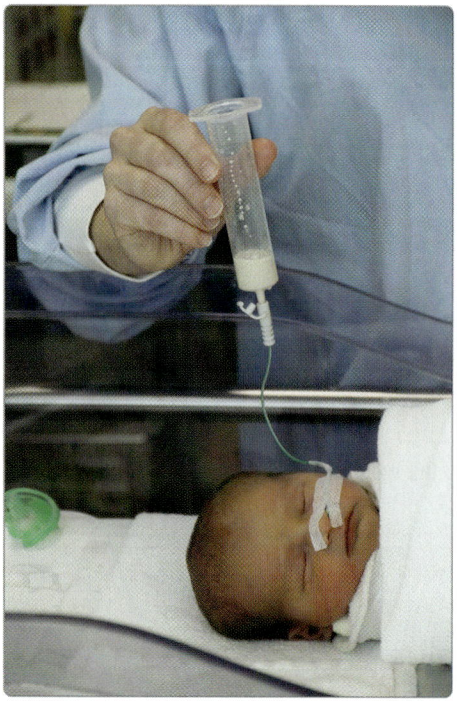

2. ______________________________
infant born before completing 37 weeks of gestation

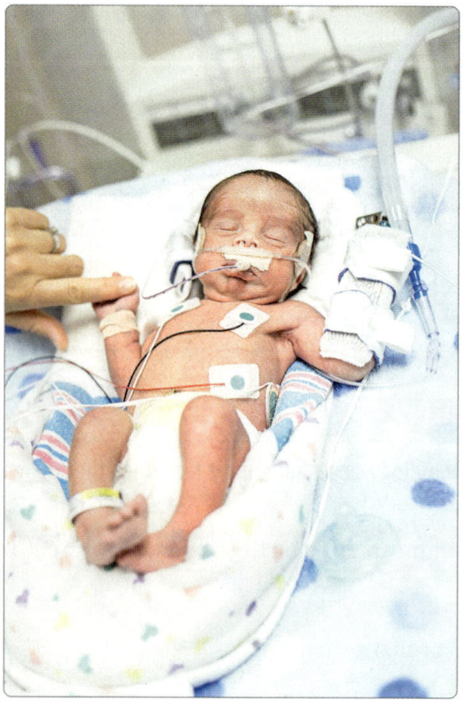

C Match

Match the terms in the first column with their correct definitions in the second column.

_____ 1. meconium	a. infant born before completing 37 weeks of gestation
_____ 2. stillborn	b. abnormality present at birth
_____ 3. gavage	c. process of feeding through a tube
_____ 4. premature infant	d. first stool of the newborn
_____ 5. congenital anomaly	e. born dead (death of fetus after 20 weeks of pregnancy)

EXERCISE 28 ■ Review of Neonatalogy Complementary Terms

Can you define, pronounce, and spell the following terms?

congenital anomaly	natal	postnatal	teratogen
fetal	neonate	premature infant	teratogenic
gavage	neonatologist	prenatal	teratology
meconium	neonatology	stillborn	

Abbreviations

DISEASES AND DISORDERS

ABBREVIATION	TERM	ABBREVIATION	TERM
CMV	cytomegalovirus	**RDS**	respiratory distress syndrome
FAS	fetal alcohol syndrome		

DIAGNOSTIC

ABBREVIATION	TERM
CVS	chorionic villus sampling

TREATMENT

ABBREVIATION	TERM	ABBREVIATION	TERM
AB	abortion	**IVF**	in vitro fertilization
CS, C-section	cesarean section	**VBAC**	vaginal birth after cesarean (section)

MEDICAL SPECIALTIES

ABBREVIATION	TERM
OB	obstetrics

DESCRIPTIVE

ABBREVIATION	TERM	ABBREVIATION	TERM
multip	multipara	**primip**	primipara
NB	newborn		

OTHER

ABBREVIATION	TERM	ABBREVIATION	TERM
DOB	date of birth	**LMP**	last menstrual period
EDD	expected (estimated) date of delivery		

Refer to **Appendix D** for a complete list of abbreviations.

EXERCISE 29 ■ Fill In

Write the terms abbreviated.

1. The **EDD** ________________ ________________ ________________ for a pregnant woman is based on the date of the first day of her **LMP** ________________ ________________ ________________; a first trimester ultrasound may help if this date is unclear. An infant's **DOB** ________________ ________________ ________________ may occur before or after this date.
2. **OB** ________________ pertains to the care of the mother during pregnancy, delivery, and the puerperium, while neonatology deals with care of the **NB** ________________.
3. A **primip** ________________ has given birth to only one offspring, but a **multip** ________________ has given birth to two or more.
4. **CVS** ________________ ________________ ________________ can be used earlier in pregnancy than amniocentesis to diagnose genetic disorders such as Down Syndrome; however, it has a greater risk of spontaneous **AB** ________________, and thus is usually only used when quad screens or other tests are abnormal, or in very high-risk pregnancies.
5. **FAS** ________________ ________________ ________________ is caused by a known teratogen, and no amount of alcohol is considered safe during pregnancy.
6. Congenital **CMV** ________________ infection can be acquired from the mother at any time during pregnancy, but most occurs often in the third trimester (the last 13 weeks of pregnancy).
7. For women who are at risk of premature delivery, corticosteroids can be given to help reduce the symptoms of **RDS** ________________ ________________ ________________.
8. **CS** ________________ ________________, also abbreviated as **c-section**, may be performed for a number of reasons, including nonreassuring fetal status, failure to progress during labor, or breech presentation.
9. On a later pregnancy, women who have had a previous c-section may choose to repeat this procedure, or they may consider **VBAC** ________________ ________________ ________________ ________________ (section), provided their risk for hysterorrhexis is low.
10. Since the first birth due to **IVF** ________________ ________________ ________________ in 1978, more than 7 million pregnancies have been achieved by this and other assisted reproductive technologies.

PRACTICAL APPLICATION

EXERCISE 30 ■ Case Study: Translate Between Everyday Language and Medical Language

CASE STUDY: Charlene Birch

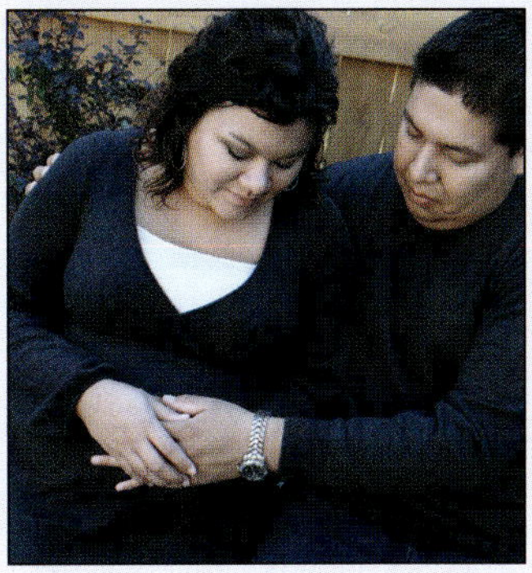

Charlene Birch is pregnant for the third time. She gave birth to one healthy baby about 4 years ago. The other baby was born dead when she was about 7 months into her pregnancy. Now she is about 3 months pregnant. She had an ultrasound test done when she first found out she was pregnant. This week she had some blood tests done and the doctor told her that the results suggest that her developing baby may have a genetic condition that causes physical and mental problems. He is suggesting a test where they use a needle to take fluid out of her womb and look at it under a microscope. She and her husband are very concerned and are not sure what to do.

Now that you have worked through Chapter 9 on obstetrics and neonatology, consider the medical terms that might be used to describe Charlene's experience. See the Chapter at a Glance section at the end of the chapter for a list of terms that might apply.

A. *Underline phrases in the case study that could be substituted with medical terms presented in Chapter 9 and previous chapters.*

B. *Write the medical term and its definition for three of the phrases you underlined.*

MEDICAL TERM	DEFINITION
1. ______________________	______________________________________
	______________________________________
2. ______________________	______________________________________
	______________________________________
3. ______________________	______________________________________
	______________________________________

DOCUMENTATION: Excerpt from the Obstetrics Clinic Visit

Charlene is a 37-year-old gravida 3 para 2 female with an EDD of January 15, 20xx. Her prenatal history has been unremarkable up to this point. Recently, however, her prenatal screening tests came back suspicious for Down syndrome. I have recommended an amniocentesis to confirm this diagnosis. She is aware of the risks of the procedure, including the small possibility of spontaneous abortion. I have recommended that she have a very close follow-up. We will attempt to detect any conditions including cardiac congenital anomalies or gastrointestinal malformation such as tracheoesophageal fistula. We will plan to have a neonatologist present at the time of birth.

C. *Underline medical terms presented in Chapter 9 used in the previous excerpt from Charlene's medical record. See the Chapter at a Glance section at the end of the chapter for a complete list.*

D. *Select and define three of the medical terms you underlined. To check your answers, go to Appendix A.*

MEDICAL TERM	DEFINITION
1. ______________________	______________________________________
	______________________________________
2. ______________________	______________________________________
	______________________________________
______________________	______________________________________
	______________________________________

EXERCISE 31 ■ Interact with Medical Documents

A

Read the report and complete it by writing medical terms on answer lines within the document. Definitions of terms to be written appear after the document.

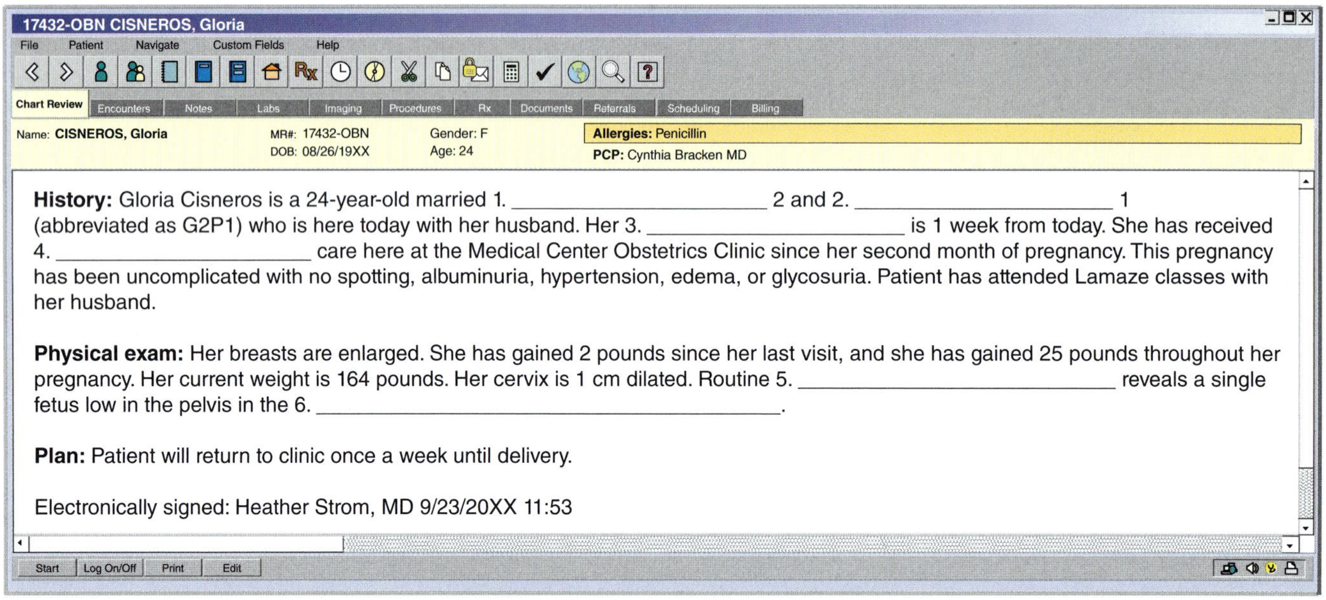

17432-OBN CISNEROS, Gloria

File Patient Navigate Custom Fields Help

Chart Review | Encounters | Notes | Labs | Imaging | Procedures | Rx | Documents | Referrals | Scheduling | Billing

Name: **CISNEROS, Gloria** MR#: 17432-OBN DOB: 08/26/19XX Gender: F Age: 24 **Allergies:** Penicillin **PCP:** Cynthia Bracken MD

History: Gloria Cisneros is a 24-year-old married 1. ______________________ 2 and 2. ______________________ 1 (abbreviated as G2P1) who is here today with her husband. Her 3. ______________________ is 1 week from today. She has received 4. ______________________ care here at the Medical Center Obstetrics Clinic since her second month of pregnancy. This pregnancy has been uncomplicated with no spotting, albuminuria, hypertension, edema, or glycosuria. Patient has attended Lamaze classes with her husband.

Physical exam: Her breasts are enlarged. She has gained 2 pounds since her last visit, and she has gained 25 pounds throughout her pregnancy. Her current weight is 164 pounds. Her cervix is 1 cm dilated. Routine 5. ______________________ reveals a single fetus low in the pelvis in the 6. ______________________.

Plan: Patient will return to clinic once a week until delivery.

Electronically signed: Heather Strom, MD 9/23/20XX 11:53

Start | Log On/Off | Print | Edit

LAMAZE is a method of psychophysical preparation for childbirth started in the 1950s by a French obstetrician, Fernand Lamaze. The method requires classes and practice before and coaching during labor and delivery.

Definitions of Medical Terms to Complete the Document

Write the medical terms defined on corresponding answer lines in the document.

1. pregnant (woman)
2. birth
3. abbreviation for expected delivery date
4. pertaining to before birth (reference to the newborn)
5. pertaining to the pelvis, process of recording sound
6. birth position in which any part of the head emerges first

B

Read the medical report and answer the questions below it.

053447 SMITH, EMMALINE

File Patient Navigate Custom Fields Help

Patient Chart | Lab | Rad | Notes | Documents | Rx | Scheduling | Images | Billing

Name: **SMITH, EMMALINE** MR#: **053447** Gender: **F** Allergies: **ASA, Phenergan**

DOB: **3/17/XX** Age: **32** PCP: **Joseph Plains, MD**

RADIOLOGY REPORT

DATE: 04/17/20XX

INDICATION: Lower abdominal pain

EXAMINATION: Pelvic sonography

HISTORY: Thirty-two-year-old primip with menstrual irregularity and abdominal pain. History of pelvic inflammatory disease and spontaneous abortion x1.

FINDINGS: Sagittal and transverse images reveal an extrauterine sac containing a fetus in the left fallopian tube. Cystic mass (hematoma) is evident in the rectouterine pouch. No fetal heart activity is noted.

OPINION: Ectopic pregnancy, left fallopian tube.

Electronically signed by: A.W. Tyat, MD 4/17/20XX 21:07

Start | Log On/Off | Print | Edit

Use the medical report above to answer the questions.

1. The patient has:
   a. never been pregnant
   b. given birth to two or more viable offspring
   c. borne one viable offspring
2. **True** or **False** The patient has experienced one abortion.
3. **True** or **False** Radiographic images were used to determine the findings.

EXERCISE 32 ▪ Use Medical Language in Online Electronic Health Records

Select the correct medical terms to complete three medical records in one patient's electronic file.

Access online resources at evolve.elsevier.com > Evolve Resources > Student Resources > Activities > Chapter 9 > Electronic Health Records

Topic: Cesarean Section
Record 1: Operative Report
Record 2: Ultrasound Report
Record 3: Obstetrics Delivery Note

❏ Check the box when complete.

EXERCISE 33 ■ Pronounce Medical Terms in Use

Practice pronunciation of terms by reading aloud the following paragraph. Use the phonetic spellings to assist with pronunciation. The script also contains medical terms not presented in the chapter. If interested, research their meanings in a medical dictionary or a reliable online source.

> Josephine Alcotts is a 34-year-old **gravida** (GRAV-i-da) 2 **para** (PAR-a) 1 woman. Her LMP was April 20, 20XX. The EDD is January 25, 20XX. The **obstetrician** (*ob*-ste-TRISH-an) prescribed folic acid to prevent **spina bifida** (SPĪ-na) (BIF-i-da). The patient's first pregnancy was complicated by **preeclampsia** (prē-ē-KLAMP-sē-a) and a **breech presentation** (brēch) (prē-zen-TĀ-shun), which required a **cesarean section** (se-ZĀR-ē-an) (SEK-shun). **Pelvic sonography** (PEL-vik) (so-NOG-ra-fē) showed a single female fetus with normal development. She went on to deliver a healthy baby by VBAC 3 days before her expected delivery date.

CHAPTER REVIEW

EXERCISE 34 ■ Chapter Content Quiz

Test your understanding of terms and abbreviations introduced in this chapter. Circle the letter for the medical term, definition, or abbreviation related to the words in italics.

1. During the second trimester, the patient had a pelvic sonogram, which revealed *less than the normal amount of amniotic fluid*. Etiology may be related to disorders of fetal urinary system.
   a. chorioamnionitis
   b. oligohydramnios
   c. polyhydramnios

2. Because of inadequate uterine contractions, the patient was experiencing *difficult labor*.
   a. dysphasia
   b. dystocia
   c. dysuria

3. Down syndrome can be diagnosed by two prenatal tests: chorionic villus sampling done at 10 to 13 weeks of pregnancy, or a *surgical puncture to aspirate amniotic fluid* after 15 weeks of pregnancy.
   a. amniocentesis
   b. CVS
   c. amniorrhea

4. Infection of the Zika virus during pregnancy is linked to an increase in premature births, blindness, neurological disorders, and *small heads* in newborns.
   a. microcephalus
   b. omphalocele
   c. gastroschisis

5. *Antepartum* hemorrhage is considered an emergency.
   a. during labor
   b. after childbirth
   c. before childbirth

6. In the EHR, the medical assistant recorded that the patient *has never been pregnant*.
   a. nullipara
   b. nulligravida
   c. prenatal

7. At 20 weeks of gestation, the patient was diagnosed with preeclampsia. The *disease progressed and she began having convulsions*. She was then diagnosed as having:
   a. eclampsia
   b. abruptio placentae
   c. placenta previa

8. The premature newborn was diagnosed with *RDS*.
   a. respiratory distress symptom
   b. right dominate syndrome
   c. respiratory distress syndrome

9. The mother was experiencing *vaginal discharge* throughout her postpartum period.
   a. lactation
   b. lochia
   c. meconium

10. The drug thalidomide taken by the mother was a *producing malformation* risk for the fetus.
    a. lactogenic
    b. teratogenic
    c. embryogenic
11. After a complete infertility evaluation, the physician recommended *IVF* for the couple.
    a. in vivo fertilization
    b. in vitro fertilization
    c. in vitro fetus
12. The patient was *pregnant with her third child.* She was referred to as:
    a. multigravida
    b. multipara
    c. nullipara
13. The patient required a *cesarean section* when her labor failed to progress, and a low fetal heart rate was detected.
    a. CMV
    b. CVS
    c. CS
14. The premature infant was unable to nurse on her own, thus *process of feeding through a tube* was recommended.
    a. cesarean section
    b. gavage
    c. amniocentesis
15. *Congenital stenosis which occurs in the arch of the aorta* was discovered on the fetal ultrasound.
    a. coarctation of the aorta
    b. congenital cytomegalovirus infection
    c. Down syndrome
16. A woman with a previous history of premature labor and delivery underwent *suturing the cervix closed to prevent dilation and premature delivery* during her second trimester.
    a. cervicitis
    b. cervical cerclage
    c. cervicectomy
17. *Congenital fissure of the abdominal wall that is not at the umbilicus* is most commonly diagnosed by ultrasound around 18 to 20 weeks of pregnancy.
    a. omphalitis
    b. omphalocele
    c. gastroschisis
18. The physician ordered an amniocentesis after the patient had an abnormal *blood test performed during the second trimester measuring four hormone levels that can reveal an increased risk of certain disorders in the developing fetus.*
    a. quad screen
    b. Apgar score
    c. pelvic sonography
19. The obstetrician ordered a(n) *ultrasound test to check the back of the fetal neck for extra fluid or thickening*, along with blood tests, at the patient's first prenatal visit.
    a. chorionic villus sampling
    b. pelvic sonography
    c. nuchal translucency screening
20. Gamete intrafallopian transfer is another form of reproductive technology that is performed *outside the body or in a lab setting.*
    a. in vivo
    b. in vitro
    c. en vivo

CHAPTER AT A GLANCE Word Parts New to This Chapter

COMBINING FORMS			PREFIXES	SUFFIXES	
amni/o	fet/o	part/o	ante-	-amnios	-rrhexis
amnion/o	gravid/o	prim/i	multi-	-cyesis	-tocia
cephal/o	lact/o	pseud/o	nulli-	-e	-um
chori/o	nat/o	puerper/o	post-	-is	-us
esophag/o	omphal/o	pylor/o	pre-		
fet/i	par/o	terat/o			

CHAPTER AT A GLANCE Obstetric and Neonatology Terms Built from Word Parts

OBSTETRIC DISEASE AND DISORDER
amnionitis
chorioamnionitis
choriocarcinoma
dystocia
hysterorrhexis
oligohydramnios
polyhydramnios
pseudocyesis

NEONATAL DISEASE AND DISORDER
microcephalus
omphalitis
omphalocele
pyloric stenosis
tracheoesophageal fistula

OBSTETRIC SURGICAL
amniotomy
episiotomy

DIAGNOSTIC
amniocentesis
pelvic sonography

OBSTETRIC COMPLEMENTARY
amniorrhea
amniorrhexis
antepartum
gravida
gravidopuerperal
intrapartum
lactogenic
lactorrhea
multigravida
multipara (multip)
nulligravida
nullipara
para
postpartum
primigravida
primipara (primip)
puerpera
puerperal

NEONATAL COMPLEMENTARY
fetal
natal
neonate
neonatologist
neonatology
postnatal
prenatal
teratogen
teratogenic
teratology

CHAPTER AT A GLANCE Obstetric and Neonatal Terms *NOT* Built from Word Parts

OBSTETRIC DISEASE AND DISORDER
abortion (AB)
abruptio placentae
eclampsia
ectopic pregnancy
placenta previa
preeclampsia

NEONATAL DISEASE AND DISORDER
cleft lip or palate
coarctation of the aorta
congenital cytomegalovirus infection (CMV)
congenital heart disease
Down syndrome
erythroblastosis fetalis
esophageal atresia
fetal alcohol syndrome (FAS)
gastroschisis
respiratory distress syndrome (RDS)
spina bifida

OBSTETRIC SURGICAL
cervical cerclage
cesarean section (CS, C-section)
in vitro fertilization (IVF)

DIAGNOSTIC
Apgar score
chorionic villus sampling (CVS)
nuchal translucency screening
quad screen

OBSTETRIC COMPLEMENTARY
breech presentation
cephalic presentation
colostrum
in vitro
in vivo
lactation
lochia
midwife
midwifery
obstetrician
obstetrics (OB)
parturition
puerperium
quickening

NEONATAL COMPLEMENTARY
congenital anomaly
gavage
meconium
premature infant
stillborn

Chapter 10

Cardiovascular, Immune, Lymphatic Systems and Blood

Outline

Objectives

Upon completion of this chapter, you will be able to:

1. Pronounce organs and anatomic structures.
2. Define and spell word parts.
3. Define, pronounce, and spell cardiovascular system terms.
4. Define, pronounce, and spell blood terms.
5. Define, pronounce, and spell lymphatic system terms.
6. Define, pronounce, and spell immune system terms.
7. Interpret the meaning of abbreviations presented in the chapter.
8. Apply medical language in clinical contexts.

ANATOMY

At first glance this may seem like an overabundance of material in one chapter. It is a lot to cover, but as you will see **the systems have interactive functions**. The lymphatic and immune systems support each other by providing an immune response to invading microorganisms and foreign substances. The lymphatic system and blood share macrophages and lymphocytes. Lymph is drained into large veins of the cardiovascular system, and the cardiovascular system is responsible for circulating blood throughout the body.

Cardiovascular System

The cardiovascular system consists of the heart and a closed network of blood vessels composed of arteries, capillaries, and veins (Fig. 10.1).

FUNCTION

The heart functions as two pumps operating simultaneously. The right side of the heart pumps blood to the lungs while the left side pumps blood to the rest of the body. The exchange of gases, nutrients, and waste between the blood and body tissue takes place in the capillaries. The blood with carbon dioxide and waste is carried from the tissues through veins to organs of excretion. The cardiovascular system also serves a critical role in the body's ability to regulate temperature.

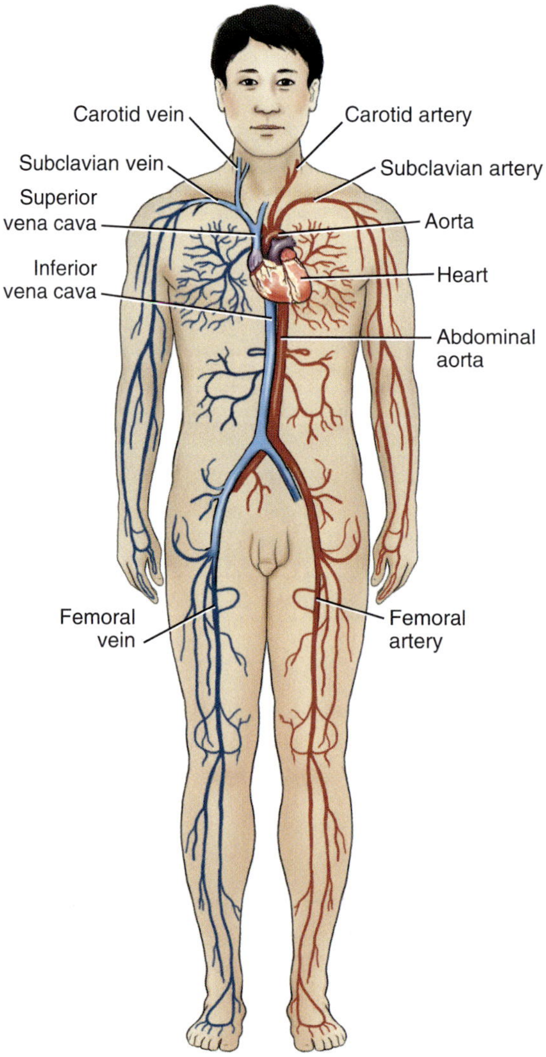

FIG. 10.1 Cardiovascular system.

Organs and Anatomic Structures of the Cardiovascular System

TERM	DEFINITION
heart (hart)	muscular cone-shaped organ the size of a fist, located behind the sternum (breast bone) and between the lungs. The pumping action of the heart circulates blood throughout the body. The heart consists of two smaller upper chambers, the **right atrium** and the **left atrium** (*pl.* **atria**), and two larger lower chambers, the **right ventricle** and the **left ventricle** (*pl.* **ventricles**). The right atrium receives blood returning from the body through the veins and contracts to fill the right ventricle, which then pumps blood to the lungs. The left atrium receives blood from the lungs and contracts to fill the left ventricle, which then contracts to pump blood from the heart through the arteries to body tissues. The **atrial septum** separates the atria and the **ventricular septum** separates the ventricles. (Fig. 10.2)
atrioventricular valves (*ā*-trē-ō-ven-TRIK-ū-ler) (valvz)	consist of the **tricuspid** and **mitral** valves, which lie between the right atrium and the right ventricle and the left atrium and left ventricle, respectively. Valves of the heart keep blood flowing in one direction.
semilunar valves (*sem*-ē-LOO-ner) (valvz)	**pulmonary** and **aortic** valves located between the right ventricle and the pulmonary artery and between the left ventricle and the aorta, respectively.
pericardium (*per*-i-KAR-dē-um)	two-layer sac surrounding the heart, consisting of an external fibrous and an internal serous layer. The internal serous layer is then divided into two parts: the outer layer, called the parietal pericardium, and the inner layer, called the epicardium. Between these is the pericardial space, which contains fluid produced by the serous layer that facilitates movement of the heart.
epicardium (*ep*-i-KAR-dē-um)	outer lining covering the heart; also part of the pericardium (see above)
myocardium (*my*-ō-KAR-dē-um)	middle, thick, muscular layer of the heart
endocardium (*en*-dō-KAR-dē-um)	inner lining of the heart
blood vessels (blud) (VES-els)	tubelike structures that carry blood throughout the body (Fig. 10.3)
arteries (AR-ter-ēz)	blood vessels that carry blood away from the heart. All arteries, with the exception of the pulmonary artery, carry oxygen and other nutrients from the heart to the body cells. The **pulmonary artery**, in contrast, carries carbon dioxide and other waste products from the heart to the lungs.
arterioles (ar-TĒR-ē-ōlz)	smallest arteries
aorta (ā-OR-ta)	largest artery in the body, which originates at the left ventricle, briefly ascends as the arch of the aorta, then descends through the thorax and abdomen
veins (vānz)	blood vessels that carry blood back to the heart. All veins, with the exception of the pulmonary veins, carry blood containing carbon dioxide and other waste products. The **pulmonary veins** carry oxygenated blood from the lungs to the heart.
venules (VEN-ūlz)	smallest veins
venae cavae (VĒ-nā) (KĀ-vā)	largest veins in the body. The **inferior vena cava** carries blood to the heart from body parts below the diaphragm, and the **superior vena cava** returns the blood to the heart from the upper part of the body.
capillaries (KAP-i-*lār*-ēz)	microscopic blood vessels that connect arterioles with venules. Materials are passed between the blood and tissue through the capillary walls.

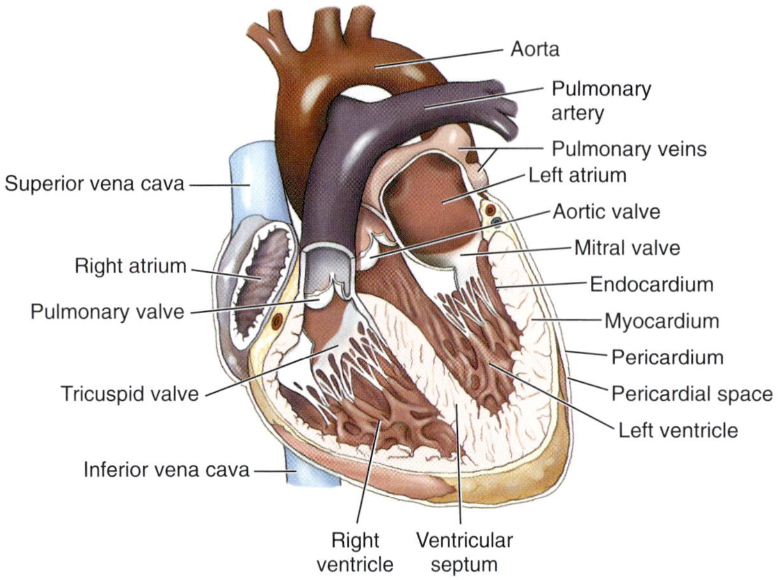

FIG. 10.2 Interior of the heart.

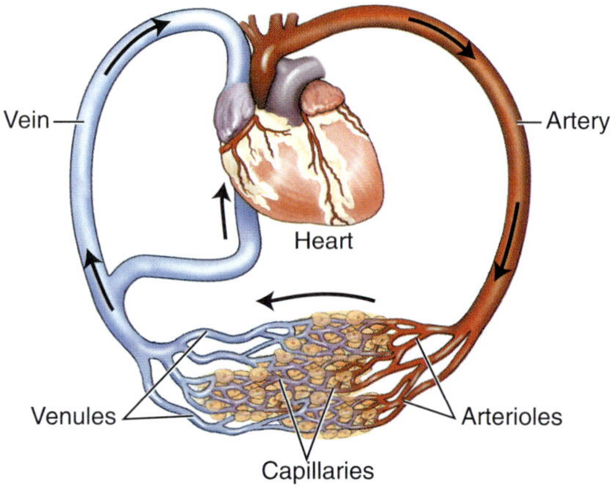

FIG. 10.3 Types of blood vessels.

Blood

The adult body contains about 5 liters of blood. Blood cells, also known as formed elements, make up 45% of blood, while plasma accounts for 55% (Fig. 10.4). All blood cells originate from bone marrow, which is the soft inner tissue found in flat bones, such as the hip and shoulder blade, and also at the ends of long bones, such as the femur and humerus. Stem cells in the bone marrow develop into different types of blood cells in a process known as a **hematopoiesis**. These blood cells increase in number and mature, giving rise to specialized blood cells such as erythrocytes, leukocytes and thrombocytes (platelets).

FUNCTION

Activities of the blood include transportation of nutrients, waste, oxygen, carbon dioxide, and hormones; protection of the body against microorganisms; and regulation by controlling body temperature and maintaining fluid and electrolyte balance.

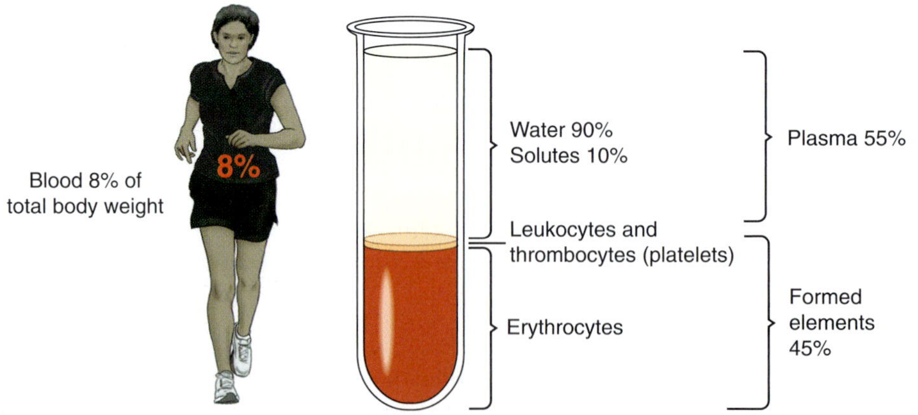

FIG. 10.4 Composition of blood.

Composition of Blood

TERM	DEFINITION
blood (blud)	fluid circulated through the heart, arteries, capillaries, and veins; composed of **plasma** and **formed elements**, such as erythrocytes, leukocytes, and thrombocytes (platelets)
plasma (PLAZ-ma)	clear, straw-colored, liquid portion of blood in which cells are suspended. Plasma is approximately 90% water. The other 10% is composed of solutes (dissolved substances), which include proteins, electrolytes, and vitamins. Plasma comprises approximately 55% of the total blood volume.
serum (SĒR-um)	clear, watery fluid portion of the blood that remains after a clot has formed
cells (formed elements)	production of new blood cells takes place in bone marrow, the spongy tissue inside some bones
erythrocytes (e-RITH-rō-sītes)	red blood cells that carry oxygen
leukocytes (LOO-kō-sītes)	white blood cells that combat infection and respond to inflammation. There are five types of white blood cells. (Fig. 10.5)
thrombocytes (THROM-bō-sītes)	one of the formed elements in the blood that is responsible for aiding in the clotting process (also called **platelets**)

STEM CELLS

Hematopoietic stem cells are immature cells found in the bone marrow and peripheral blood. They have the potential to develop into all types of blood cells. Hematopoietic stem cells for transplantation may be obtained from the patient (**autologous**), from an identical twin (**synergetic**), or from a sibling or other individual (**allogenic**).

Embryonic stem cells are derived from the earliest stage of development of the embryo and have the potential to develop into mature body cells.

Stem cell transplantation is used to treat **leukemia** (cancer involving the white blood cells), **aplastic anemia** (disease in which there is inadequate production of blood cells), **multiple myeloma** (cancer that forms tumors in the bone marrow), **lymphoma** (cancer involving lymphoid cells), and **immune deficiency disorders**.

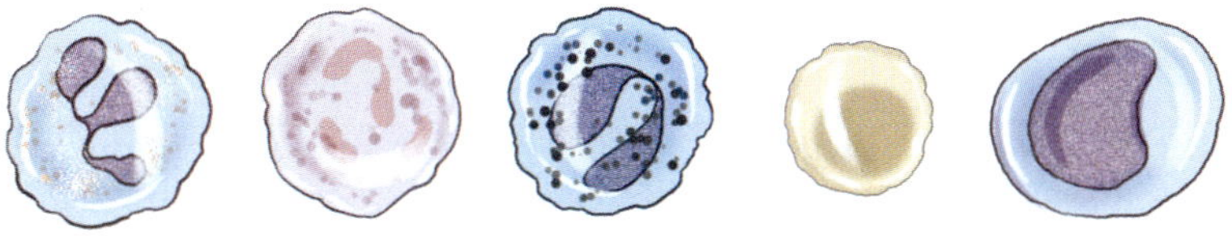

FIG. 10.5 Types of leukocytes. Each leukocyte plays a different role in providing immune responses to pathogens, foreign agents, allergies, and abnormal body cells.

Lymphatic System

The lymphatic system consists of lymph transported through lymphatic vessels, lymph nodes, the spleen, and thymus gland (Fig. 10.6).

FUNCTION

Three functions of the lymphatic system are to return excessive tissue fluid to the blood, absorb fats and fat-soluble vitamins from the small intestine and transport them to the blood, and provide defense against infections and other diseases. Collected extracellular fluid called lymph travels away from body tissue toward the heart and is drained into the cardiovascular system through ducts in the upper chest. Breathing and muscle action help propel lymph through the vessels.

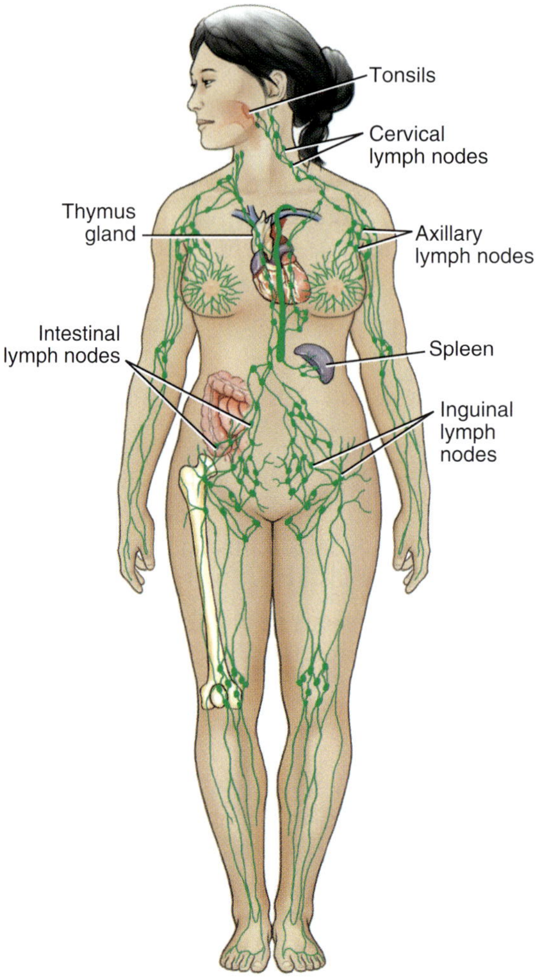

FIG. 10.6 Lymphatic system.

Organs and Anatomic Structures of the Lymphatic System

TERM	DEFINITION
lymph (limf)	transparent, colorless, tissue fluid; contains **lymphocytes** and **monocytes** and flows in a one-way direction toward the heart
lymphatic vessels (lim-FAT-ik) (VES-els)	transport lymph from body tissues into the right and left subclavian veins, which then empty into the superior vena cava. The lymphatic vessels begin as capillaries spread throughout the body then merge into larger tubes that eventually become ducts in the chest. They provide a one-way flow for lymph, which enters through veins into the circulatory system.
lymph nodes (limf) (nōdz)	small, spherical bodies composed of lymphoid tissue. They may be singular or grouped together along the path of the lymph vessels. The nodes filter lymph to keep substances such as bacteria and other foreign agents from entering the blood. They also contain lymphocytes.
spleen (splēn)	located in the left side of the abdominal cavity between the stomach and the diaphragm. In adulthood, the spleen is the largest lymphatic organ in the body. Blood, rather than lymph, flows through the spleen. Blood is cleansed of microorganisms in the spleen. The spleen stores blood and destroys worn out red blood cells.
thymus gland (THĪ-mus) (gland)	one of the primary lymphatic organs, it is located anterior to the ascending aorta and posterior to the sternum between the lungs. It plays an important role in the development of the body's immune system, particularly from infancy to puberty. Around puberty the thymus gland shrinks so that most of the gland is connective tissue.

Immune System

The immune system does not have its own organs and structures. Its function depends on organs and structures of other body systems, including the spleen, liver, intestinal tract, lymph nodes, and bone marrow.

FUNCTION

The immune system protects the body against pathogens (disease-causing organisms such as bacteria, fungi, and viruses), foreign agents that cause allergic reactions (e.g., peanuts), toxins (e.g., insect bites), and abnormal body cells (e.g., cancer). Immune function depends on three layers of protection, often referred to as lines of defense. (Fig. 10.7)

The first line of defense is the prevention of foreign substances from entering the body. Unbroken skin and mucous membranes act as mechanical barriers. Ear wax and saliva act as chemical barriers. If the first line of defense is penetrated by pathogens, a second line of defense continues to battle disease. Second-line defenses include inflammation and fever plus phagocytosis, a process in which some of the white blood cells destroy the invading microorganisms. Also activated are protective proteins such as interferons, which fight viruses, and natural killer (NK) cells, which are effective against microorganisms and cancer cells. Specific immunity, the third line of defense, provides protection against specific pathogens, such as the polio virus, by forming specific antibodies to fight against the infectious agent.

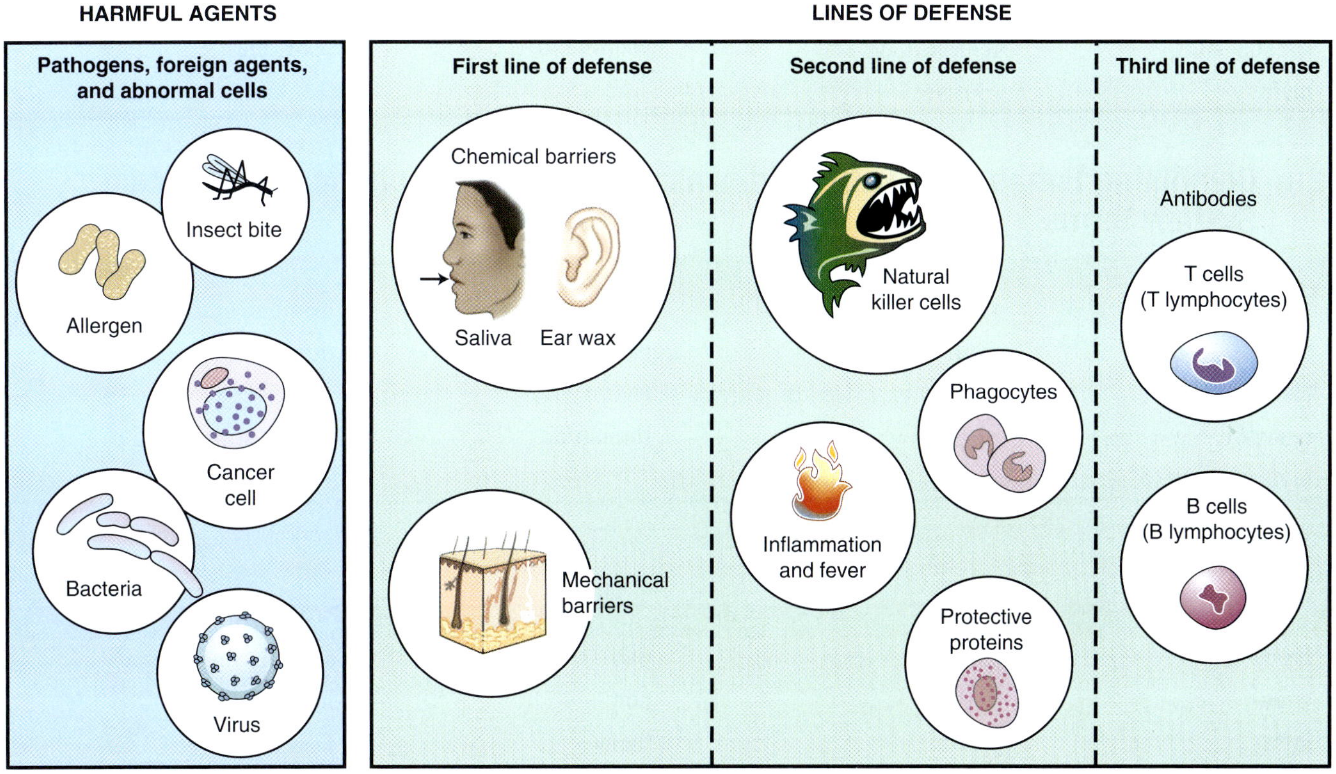

FIG. 10.7 Three lines of defense provided by the immune system to protect the body against pathogens, foreign agents, and cancer.

PRONOUNCE ANATOMIC STRUCTURES

Practice saying aloud each of the organs and specific structures on the previous pages.

To hear the terms, go to Evolve Resources at www.evolve.elsevier.com and select:
Student Resources > Audio Glossary > Chapter 10 > **Anatomic Structures**

❑ Check the box when complete.

WORD PARTS

Use paper flashcards or electronic flashcards on Evolve to assist with memorization of word parts used to analyze, define, and build terms presented in this chapter. To reinforce learning, study one section of the Word Parts Table at a time, then complete the corresponding exercise on the following pages.

1 ■ Anatomic Structures Combining Forms

COMBINING FORM	DEFINITION	COMBINING FORM	DEFINITION
angi/o	vessel(s); blood vessel(s)	**myel/o**	bone marrow
aort/o	aorta	**MYEL/O** also means spinal cord; see Chapter 15.	
arteri/o	artery *(s.)*, arteries *(pl.)*	**phleb/o**	vein(s)
atri/o	atrium	**plasm/o**	plasma
cardi/o	heart	**splen/o**	spleen
cyt/o	cell	**SPLEN/O** has only one "e" while its definition, spleen, has two.	
hem/o	blood	**thym/o**	thymus gland
hemat/o	blood	**valvul/o**	valve
lymph/o	lymph, lymph tissue	**ven/o**	vein(s)
lymphaden/o	lymph node	**ventricul/o**	ventricle
my/o	muscle		

2 ■ Combining Forms Used with Cardiovascular, Blood, Lymphatic, and Immune System Terms

COMBINING FORM	DEFINITION	COMBINING FORM	DEFINITION
ather/o	yellowish, fatty plaque	**immun/o**	immune system
ech/o	sound	**isch/o**	deficiency, blockage
electr/o	electricity, electrical activity	**leuk/o**	white
embol/o	plug	**thromb/o**	blood clot
erythr/o	red		

3 ■ Prefixes

PREFIX	DEFINITION	PREFIX	DEFINITION
brady-	slow	**peri-**	surrounding (outer)
endo-	within	**poly-**	many, much
intra-	within	**tachy-**	fast, rapid
pan-	all, total		

4 ■ Suffixes

SUFFIX	DEFINITION	SUFFIX	DEFINITION
-apheresis	removal	**-centesis**	surgical puncture to aspirate fluid (with a sterile needle)
-ar	pertaining to	**-ectomy**	excision, surgical removal

SUFFIX	DEFINITION	SUFFIX	DEFINITION
-emia	in the blood	**-osis**	abnormal condition (means increase when used with blood cell word roots)
-genic	producing, originating, causing	**-ous**	pertaining to
-gram	the record, radiographic image	**-pathy**	disease
-graphy	process of recording, radiographic imaging	**-penia**	abnormal reduction in number
-ia	diseased or abnormal state, condition of	**-plasty**	surgical repair
-ic	pertaining to	**-rrhage**	excessive flow
-ism	state of	**-rrhaphy**	suturing, repairing
-itis	inflammation	**-sclerosis**	hardening
-logist	one who studies and treats (specialist, physician)	**-scopy**	visual examination
-logy	study of	**-stasis**	control, stop, standing
-lysis	loosening, dissolution, separating	**-stenosis**	constriction or narrowing
-megaly	enlargement	**-us**	noun suffix, no meaning
-oma	tumor, swelling		

-RRH SUFFIXES, of which there are five, have all now been introduced, including **-rrhage** and **-rrhaphy**. The other three are **-rrhea**, meaning flow or discharge; **-rrhagia**, meaning excessive bleeding; and **-rrhexis**, meaning rupture.

Refer to **Appendix B** and **Appendix C** for alphabetical lists of word parts and their meanings.

EXERCISE 1 ■ Anatomic Structures Combining Forms

Refer to the first section of the word parts table.

A Label

Fill in the blanks with combining forms to label this diagram of a cutaway section of the heart. *To check your answers, go to Appendix A.*

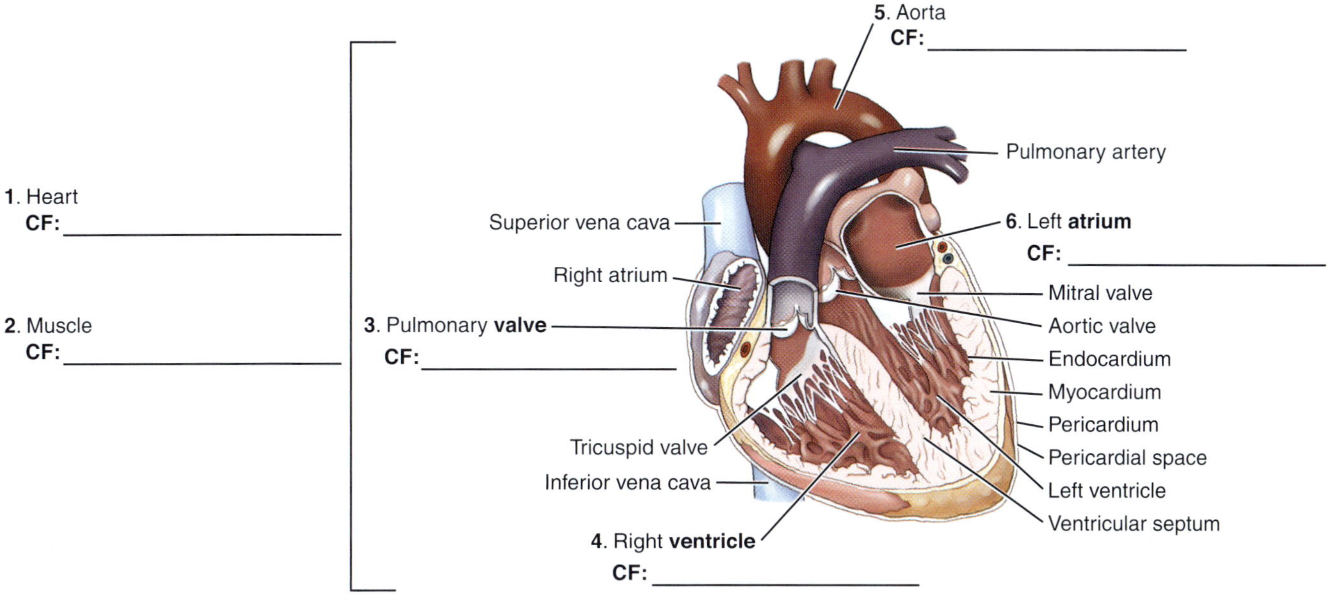

B Define and Match

Step 1: Write the definitions after the following combining forms.
Step 2: Match the descriptions on the right with the combining forms and definitions.

______ 1. cardi/o, ______________________

______ 2. atri/o, ______________________

______ 3. valvul/o, ______________________

______ 4. ventricul/o, ______________________

______ 5. aort/o, ______________________

______ 6. my/o, ______________________

a. structures that keep blood flowing in one direction

b. larger lower chamber in the heart

c. largest artery in the body

d. pumping action circulates blood throughout the body

e. small upper chamber in the heart

f. tissue that produces movement

C Label

Fill in the blanks to label the illustrations of blood vessels and blood.

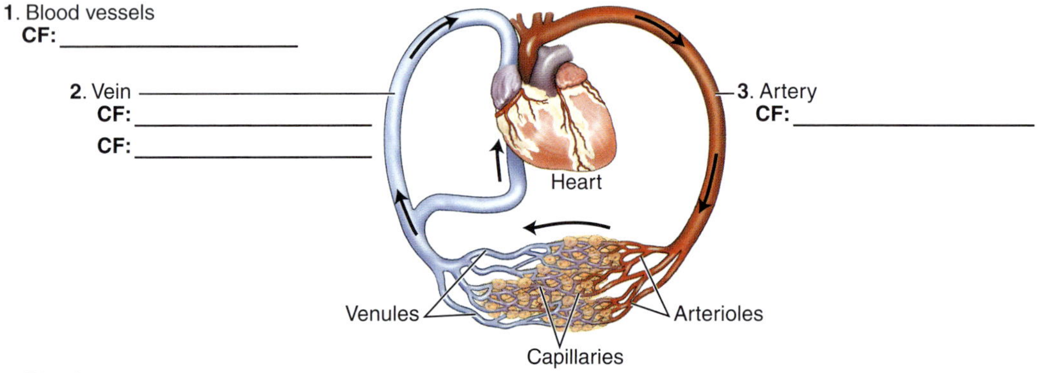

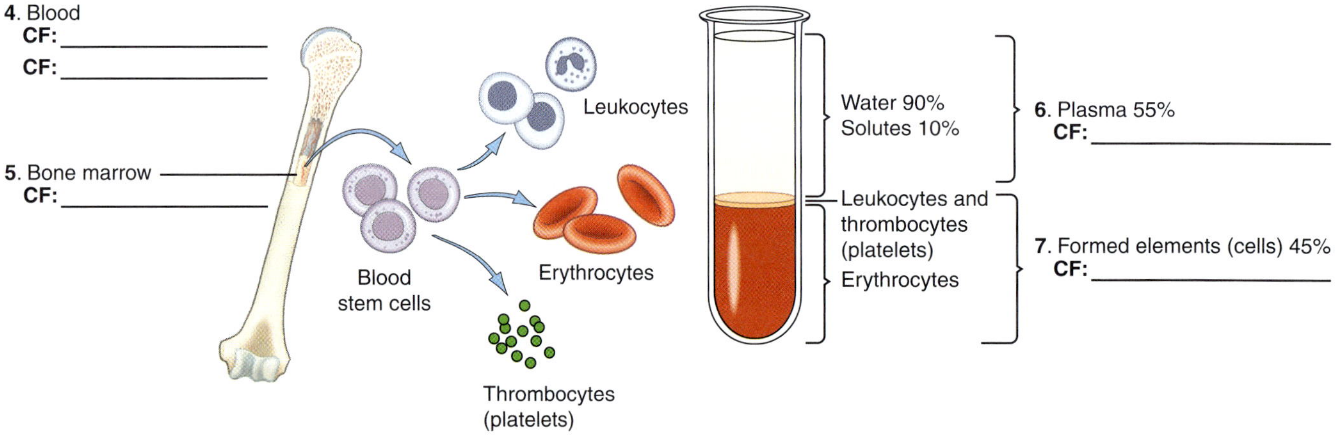

D Define and Match

Step 1: Write the definitions after the following combining forms.
Step 2: Match the descriptions on the right with the combining forms and definitions. Answers may be used more than once.

______ 1. arteri/o, ______________________

______ 2. myel/o, ______________________

______ 3. hemat/o, ______________________

______ 4. phleb/o, ______________________

______ 5. angi/o, ______________________

______ 6. ven/o, ______________________

______ 7. plasm/o, ______________________

______ 8. hem/o, ______________________

a. fluid circulated through the heart, arteries, capillaries, and veins

b. clear, straw-colored, liquid portion of blood

c. blood vessels that carry blood away from the heart

d. soft inner tissue of bones where blood cells are formed

e. blood vessels that carry blood back to the heart

f. tubelike structures that carry blood or other fluids

E Label

Fill in the blanks with combining forms to label the illustration of the lymphatic system.

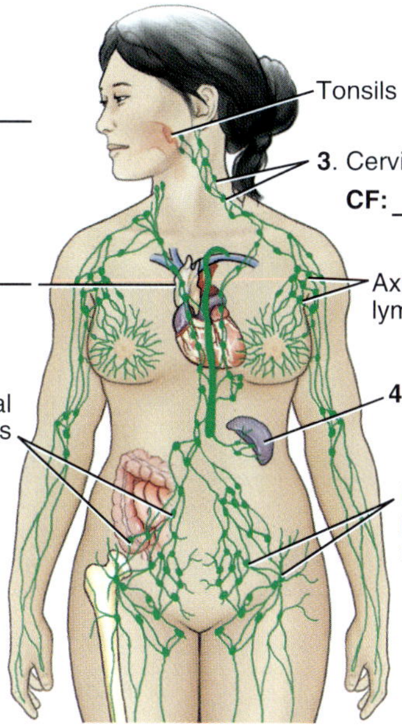

When used in reference to the lymphatic system, the combining form **lymphaden/o** refers to a collection of lymphatic tissue and is called a lymph **node** rather than the literal translation of lymph gland.

F Define and Match

Step 1: Write the definitions after the following combining forms.
Step 2: Match the descriptions on the right with the combining forms and definitions.

______ 1. splen/o, ______	a. small, spherical bodies of tissue that filter lymph
______ 2. lymph/o, ______	b. lymphatic organ important in the development of immunity
______ 3. thym/o, ______	c. largest lymphatic organ in adulthood that filters blood
______ 4. lymphaden/o, ______	d. transparent, colorless, tissue fluid

EXERCISE 2 ■ Combining Forms Used with Cardiovascular, Blood, Lymphatic, and Immune System Terms

Refer to the second section of the word parts table.

A Define

Write the definitions of the following combining forms.

1. ech/o ______
2. thromb/o ______
3. isch/o ______
4. erythr/o ______
5. ather/o ______
6. electr/o ______
7. leuk/o ______
8. immun/o ______
9. embol/o ______

B Identify

Write the combining form for each of the following.

1. blood clot ______
2. sound ______
3. deficiency, blockage ______
4. yellowish, fatty plaque ______
5. immune system ______
6. electricity, electrical activity ______
7. plug ______
8. white ______
9. red ______

EXERCISE 3 ■ Prefixes

Refer to the third section of the word parts table.

A Define

Write the definitions of the following prefixes.

1. brady- ______
2. pan- ______
3. poly- ______
4. tachy- ______
5. intra- ______
6. peri- ______
7. endo- ______

B Identify

Write the prefix for each of the following.

1. fast ______
2. slow ______
3. many, much ______
4. surrounding (outer) ______
5. all, total ______
6. within ______; ______

EXERCISE 4 ■ Suffixes

Refer to the fourth section of the word parts table.

A Identify

Write the suffix for each of the following.

1. excessive flow ______
2. producing, originating, causing ______
3. hardening ______
4. loosening, dissolution, separating ______
5. abnormal reduction in number ______
6. control, stop, standing ______
7. removal ______
8. study of ______
9. one who studies and treats (specialist, physician) ______
10. noun suffix, no meaning ______
11. pertaining to ______; ______; ______

B Match

Match the suffixes indicating disease or disorder in the first column with their correct definitions in the second column.

______	1. -stenosis	a. in the blood
______	2. -ia	b. inflammation
______	3. -rrhage	c. disease
______	4. -penia	d. state of
______	5. -pathy	e. hardening
______	6. -osis	f. constriction or narrowing
______	7. -oma	g. excessive flow
______	8. -itis	h. enlargement
______	9. -ism	i. abnormal reduction in number
______	10. -emia	j. tumor
______	11. -megaly	k. abnormal condition (means increase when used with blood cell word roots)
______	12. -sclerosis	l. diseased or abnormal state, condition of

C Match

Match the suffixes indicating diagnostic or surgical procedures in the first column with their correct definitions in the second column.

______	1. -centesis	a. suturing, repairing
______	2. -ectomy	b. the record, radiographic image
______	3. -plasty	c. visual examination
______	4. -rrhaphy	d. surgical puncture to aspirate fluid (with a sterile needle)
______	5. -scopy	e. process of recording, radiographic imaging
______	6. -gram	f. excision, surgical removal
______	7. -graphy	g. surgical repair

MEDICAL TERMS

Medical terms relevant to this chapter have been grouped by topics, such as Cardiovascular System Terms, and are listed in tables designated as Built from Word Parts or *NOT* Built from Word Parts. The exercises following each table assist with learning term definitions, pronunciations, and spellings.

Cardiovascular System Terms

BUILT FROM WORD PARTS

The following terms can be translated using definitions of word parts. Further explanation is provided within parentheses as needed.

DISEASE AND DISORDERS

TERM	DEFINITION	TERM	DEFINITION
1. angioma (an-jē-Ō-ma)	tumor composed of blood vessels	**4. arteriosclerosis** (ar-*tēr*-ē-ō-skle-RŌ-sis)	hardening of the arteries
2. angiostenosis (*an*-jē-ō-ste-NŌ-sis)	narrowing of a blood vessel	**5. atherosclerosis** (*ath*-er-ō-skle-RŌ-sis)	hardening of fatty plaque (deposited on the arterial wall)
3. aortic stenosis (ā-OR-tik) (ste-NŌ-sis)	narrowing, pertaining to aorta (narrowing of the aortic valve) (Fig. 10.8)		

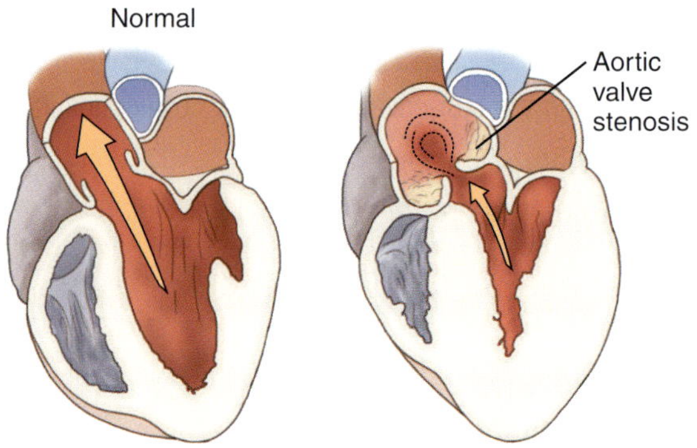

FIG. 10.8 Aortic stenosis.

Cardiovascular System Terms—cont'd

BUILT FROM WORD PARTS

TERM	DEFINITION
6. bradycardia (*brad*-ē-KAR-dē-a)	condition of a slow heart (rate less than 60 beats per minute) *(Note: The i in cardi/o has been dropped)*
7. cardiomegaly (*kar*-dē-ō-MEG-a-lē)	enlargement of the heart
8. cardiomyopathy (kar-dē-ō-mī-OP-a-thē)	disease of the heart muscle
9. endocarditis (*en*-dō-kar-DĪ-tis)	inflammation of the inner (lining) of the heart (particularly heart valves)
10. ischemia (is-KĒ-mē-a)	deficiency in blood (flow); (caused by constriction or obstruction of a blood vessel)

MYOCARDIAL ISCHEMIA is the deficient flow of blood to the heart muscle caused by vessel constriction commonly due to atherosclerosis and potentially leading to **myocardial infarction**.

TERM	DEFINITION
11. myocarditis (*mī*-ō-kar-DĪ-tis)	inflammation of the muscle of the heart
12. pericarditis (*per*-i-kar-DĪ-tis)	inflammation of the sac surrounding the heart (Fig. 10.9)
13. phlebitis (fle-BĪ-tis)	inflammation of a vein
14. polyarteritis (*pol*-ē-*ar*-te-RĪ-tis)	inflammation of many (sites in the) arteries *(Note: The i in arteri/o has been dropped)*
15. tachycardia (*tak*-i-KAR-dē-a)	condition of a rapid heart (rate of more than 100 beats per min) *(Note: The i in cardi/o has been dropped)*
16. thrombophlebitis (throm-bō-fle-BĪ-tis)	inflammation of a vein associated with a blood clot
17. valvulitis (*val*-vū-LĪ-tis)	inflammation of a valve (of the heart)

SURGICAL TERMS

TERM	DEFINITION
18. angioplasty (AN-jē-ō-*plas*-tē)	surgical repair of a blood vessel
19. atherectomy (ath-er-EK-to-mē)	excision of fatty plaque (from a blocked artery using a specialized catheter and a rotary cutter)
20. embolectomy (*em*-bo-LEK-to-mē)	excision of a plug (embolus or clot, usually with a balloon catheter, inflating the balloon beyond the clot, then pulling the balloon back to the incision and bringing the plug with it)
21. endarterectomy (*end*-ar-ter-EK-to-mē)	excision within the artery (excision of plaque from the arterial wall). *(Note: the o from endo- is dropped for easier pronunciation)*

ENDARTERECTOMY procedures are usually named for the artery to be cleaned out, such as **carotid endarterectomy**, which means removal of plaque from the wall of the carotid artery.

TERM	DEFINITION
22. pericardiocentesis (*per*-i-kar-dē-ō-sen-TĒ-sis)	surgical puncture to aspirate fluid from the sac surrounding the heart (usually to relieve cardiac tamponade and/or for diagnostic investigation) (Fig. 10.9)

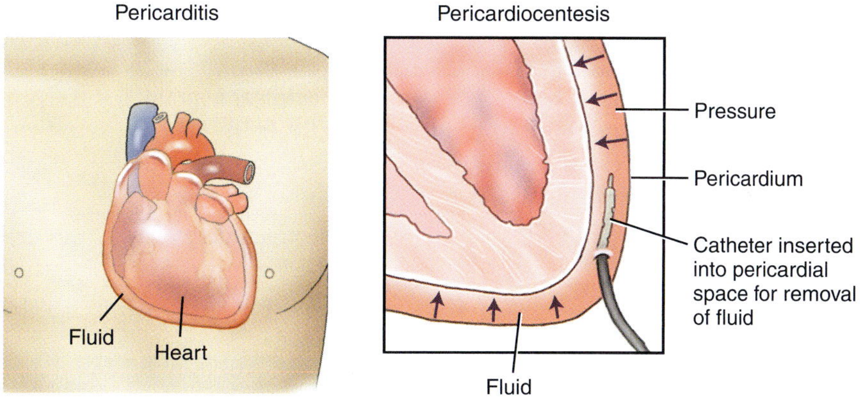

FIG. 10.9 Pericarditis may produce excess fluid in the pericardium. If the fluid seriously affects the heart's ability to pump blood, pericardiocentesis may be performed to remove the fluid.

TERM	DEFINITION	TERM	DEFINITION
23. phlebectomy (fle-BEK-to-mē)	excision of a vein	**24. valvuloplasty** (VAL-vū-lō-*plas*-tē)	surgical repair of a valve (cardiac or venous)

DIAGNOSTIC IMAGING TERMS

TERM	DEFINITION	TERM	DEFINITION
25. angiography (*an*-jē-OG-ra-fē)	radiographic imaging of blood vessels (the procedure is named for the vessel to be studied, e.g., **femoral angiography** or **coronary angiography**) (Table 10.1)	**27. aortogram** (ā-ŌR-to-gram)	radiographic image of the aorta (after an injection of contrast media)
26. angioscopy (*an*-jē-OS-ko-pē)	visual examination (of the inside) of a blood vessel	**28. arteriogram** (ar-TĒR-ē-ō-gram)	radiographic image of an artery (after an injection of contrast media)
		29. venogram (VĒ-nō-gram)	radiographic image of a vein (after an injection of contrast media)

TABLE 10.1 Types of Angiography

CORONARY ARTERY VISUALIZATION

Coronary angiography is an **invasive procedure** in which a catheter is inserted into an artery in the groin, arm or neck, then advanced into the coronary vessels. Next, contrast media are injected, and images are recorded. It is considered the best technique for determining the percentage of blockage in the coronary arteries.

OTHER VASCULAR VISUALIZATION

Magnetic resonance angiography (MRA) is a **noninvasive procedure** that does not require catheterization and uses specialized MR imaging to study vascular structures of the body. MRA may be chosen over computed tomography angiography because there is no exposure to ionizing radiation.

Computed tomography angiography (CTA) is a **noninvasive procedure** that uses a high-resolution CT system to study vascular structures of the body after the injection of intravenous contrast media.

Digital subtraction angiography (DSA) is an **invasive procedure** in which an image is taken and stored in the computer, then contrast medium is injected. A second image is taken and stored in the computer. The computer compares the two images and subtracts the first image from the second, removing structures not being studied. DSA enables better visualization of the arteries than regular angiography.

DIAGNOSTIC PROCEDURES

TERM	DEFINITION
30. echocardiogram (ECHO) (*ek*-ō-KAR-dē-ō-gram)	record of the heart (structure and motion) using sound (waves); (used to detect valvular disease and evaluate heart function)
31. electrocardiogram (ECG, EKG) (ē-*lek*-trō-KAR-dē-ō-gram)	record of the electrical activity of the heart
32. electrocardiography (ē-*lek*-trō-*kar*-dē-OG-ra-fē)	process of recording the electrical activity of the heart

MEDICAL SPECIALTIES

TERM	DEFINITION
33. cardiologist (*kar*-dē-OL-o-jist)	physician who studies and treats diseases of the heart
34. cardiology (*kar*-dē-OL-o-jē)	study of the heart (a branch of medicine that deals with diseases of the heart)

ELECTROPHYSIOLOGIST is a **cardiologist** who specializes in the diagnosis and treatment of patients with arrhythmias.

DESCRIPTIVE TERMS

TERM	DEFINITION
35. atrioventricular (AV) (ā-trē-ō-ven-TRIK-ū-ler)	pertaining to the atrium and ventricle
36. cardiogenic (kar-dē-ō-JEN-ik)	originating in the heart
37. intravenous (IV) (in-tra-VĒ-nus)	pertaining to within the vein

INTRAVENOUS (IV) THERAPY is **the infusion of a substance directly into a vein** for therapeutic purposes. **IV therapy** is a very common and essential component of medical care, serving as a direct, efficient route for the administration of fluids, medications, and blood products.

EXERCISE 5 ■ Pronounce and Spell

Practice pronunciation and spelling on paper and online.

1. Practice on Paper

a. **Pronounce:** Read the phonetic spelling and say aloud the terms listed in the previous table. Refer to the pronunciation key on p. 20 as necessary.
b. **Spell:** Have a study partner read the terms aloud. Write the spelling of the terms on a separate sheet of paper.

2. Practice Online

a. **Access** online learning resources. Go to evolve.elsevier.com > Evolve Resources > Student Resources.
b. **Pronounce:** Select Audio Glossary > Chapter 10 > Exercise 5. Select a term to hear its pronunciation and repeat aloud.
c. **Spell:** Select Activities > Chapter 10 > Spell Terms > Exercise 5. Select the audio icon and type the correct spelling of the term.

❑ Check the box when complete.

EXERCISE 6 ■ Analyze and Define

Analyze and define the following terms.

1. atrioventricular
2. electrocardiography
3. cardiologist
4. aortogram
5. valvulitis
6. phlebectomy
7. tachycardia
8. angioscopy
9. angiography
10. cardiogenic
11. ischemia
12. thrombophlebitis
13. atherectomy
14. valvuloplasty
15. angioma
16. cardiomyopathy

EXERCISE 7 ■ Build

A Label

Build terms pictured by writing word parts above definitions.

1.

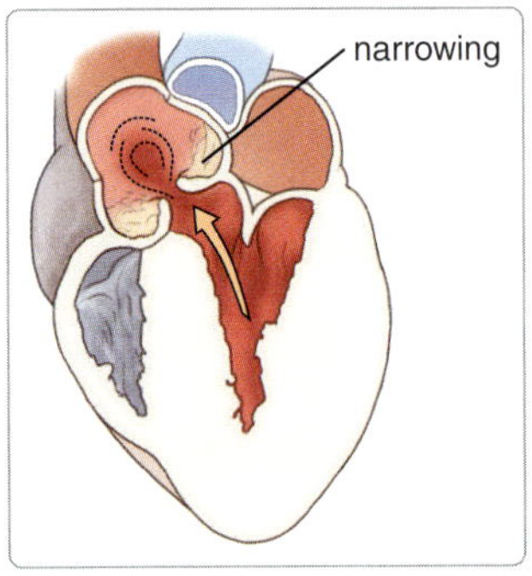

_______ /_________ _________
aorta pertaining to narrowing

2.

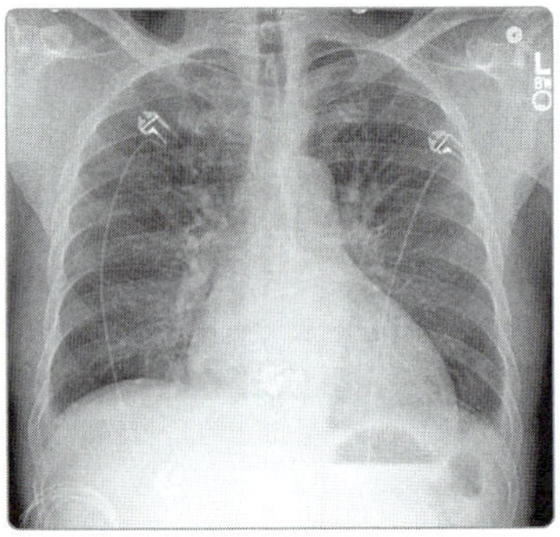

Chest radiography showing

_________ /_____ /__________
heart CV enlargement

3.

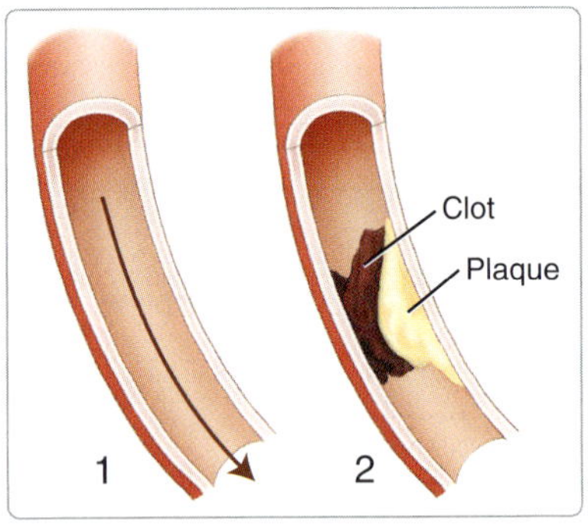

1. Healthy artery with smooth blood flow
2. Blocked artery due to blood clot and

_________ /______ /__________
fatty plaque CV hardening

4.

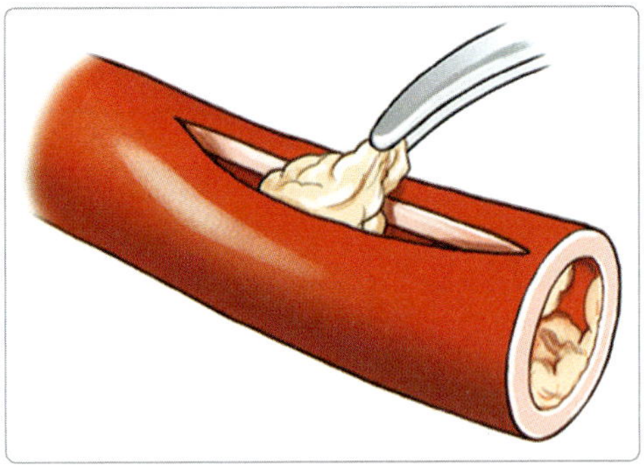

_________ /_______ /__________
within artery excision

5.

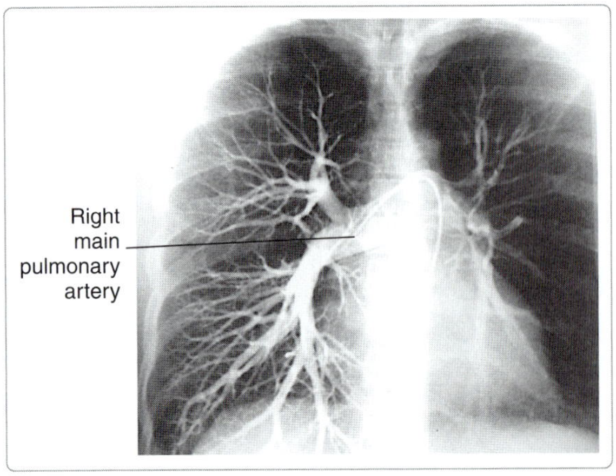

_________ /______ /______________,
artery CV radiographic image
performed after injection of contrast media

6.

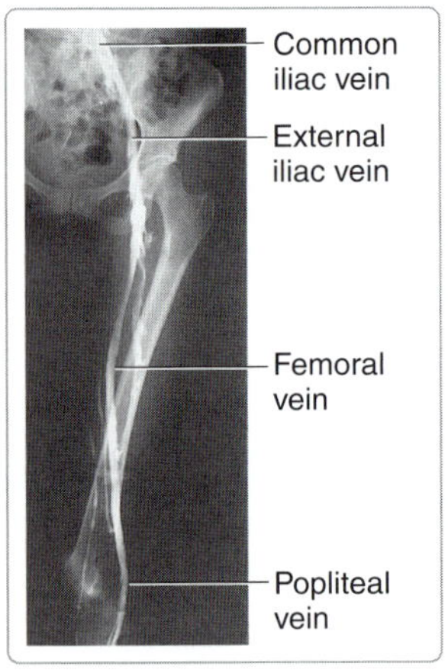

Normal _______ /_____ /__________, left lower limb
vein CV radiographic image

7.

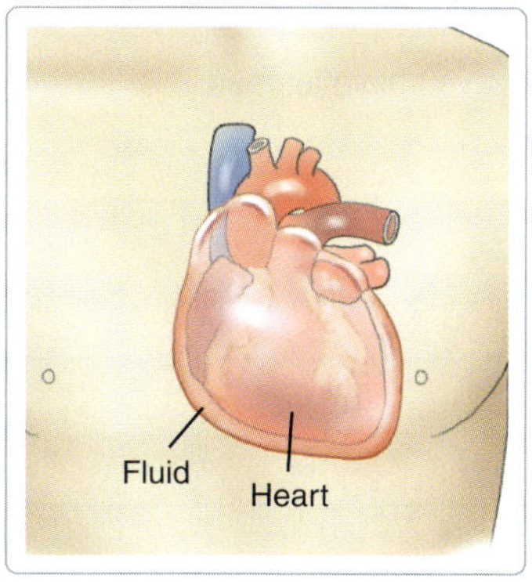

_______ / _______ / _______
surrounding heart inflammation

8.

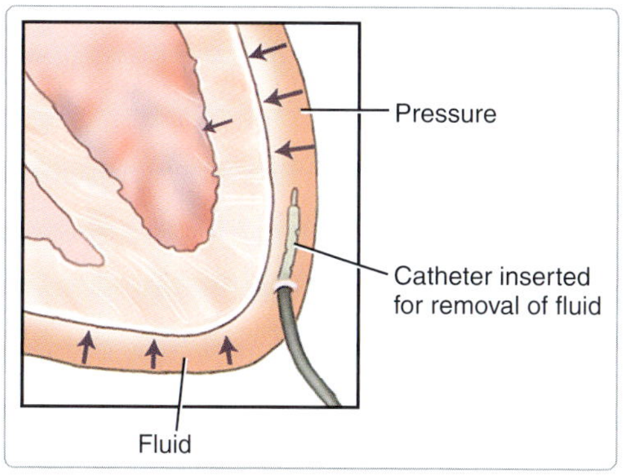

_______ / _______ / _______ / _______
surrounding heart CV surgical puncture

9.

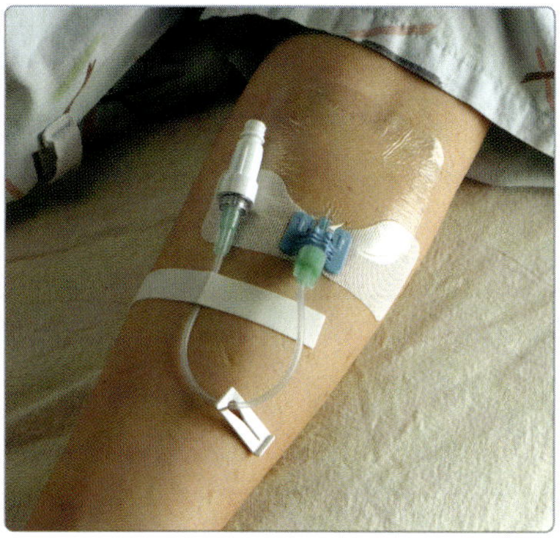

Patient's arm with an

_______ / _______ / _______ (IV) catheter
within vein pertaining to

10.

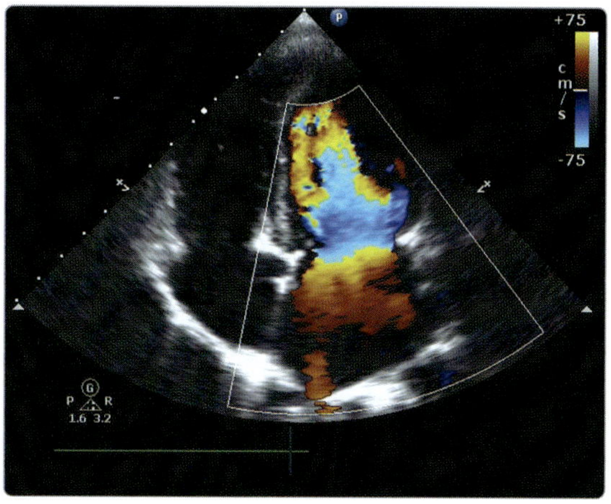

Transthoracic, two-dimensional color Doppler

_______ / _______ / _______ / _______ / _______
sound CV heart CV record

11.

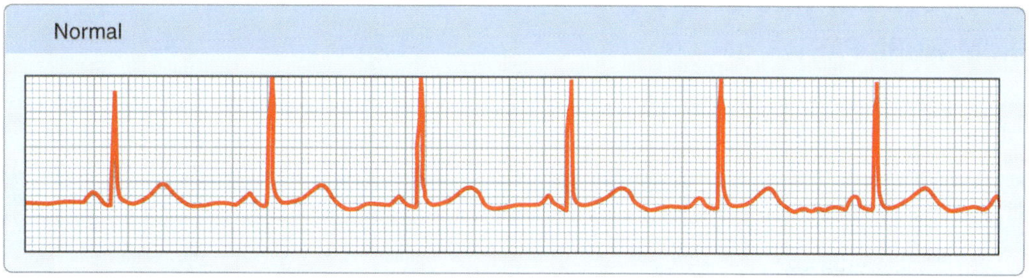

_______ / _______ / _______ / _______ / _______ showing a normal sinus rhythm
electrical activity CV heart CV record

B Fill In

Build cardiovascular system terms for the following definitions by using the word parts you have learned.

1. inflammation of a vein ____ / ____ (WR / S)
2. surgical repair of a blood vessel ____ / ____ / ____ (WR / CV / S)
3. inflammation of the inner (layer) of the heart ____ / ____ / ____ (P / WR / S)
4. condition of slow heart rate ____ / ____ / ____ (P / WR / S)
5. hardening of the arteries ____ / ____ / ____ (WR / CV / S)
6. excision of a plug ____ / ____ (WR / S)
7. inflammation of the muscle of the heart ____ / ____ / ____ / ____ / ____ (WR / CV / WR / CV / S)
8. narrowing of a blood vessel ____ / ____ / ____ (WR / CV / S)
9. inflammation of many (sites in the) arteries ____ / ____ / ____ (P / WR / S)
10. study of the heart ____ / ____ / ____ (WR / CV / S)

Cardiovascular System Terms

NOT BUILT FROM WORD PARTS

Word parts may be present in the following terms; however, their full meanings cannot be translated using definitions of word parts alone.

DISEASE AND DISORDERS	
TERM	**DEFINITION**
1. acute coronary syndrome (ACS) (a-KŪT) (KOR-o-nar-ē) (SIN-drōm)	sudden symptoms of insufficient blood supply to the heart indicating unstable angina or acute myocardial infarction. Rapid assessment is necessary to determine the diagnosis and treatment and to minimize heart damage.
2. aneurysm (AN-ū-riz-em)	ballooning of a weakened portion of an arterial wall (Fig. 10.10)
3. angina pectoris (an-JĪ-na) (PEK-to-ris)	chest pain, which may radiate to the left arm and jaw, that occurs when there is an insufficient supply of blood to the heart muscle

ANGINA PECTORIS was believed by the ancients to be a disorder of the breast. The Latin **angere**, meaning to throttle, was used to represent the sudden pain and was added to pectus, meaning breast.

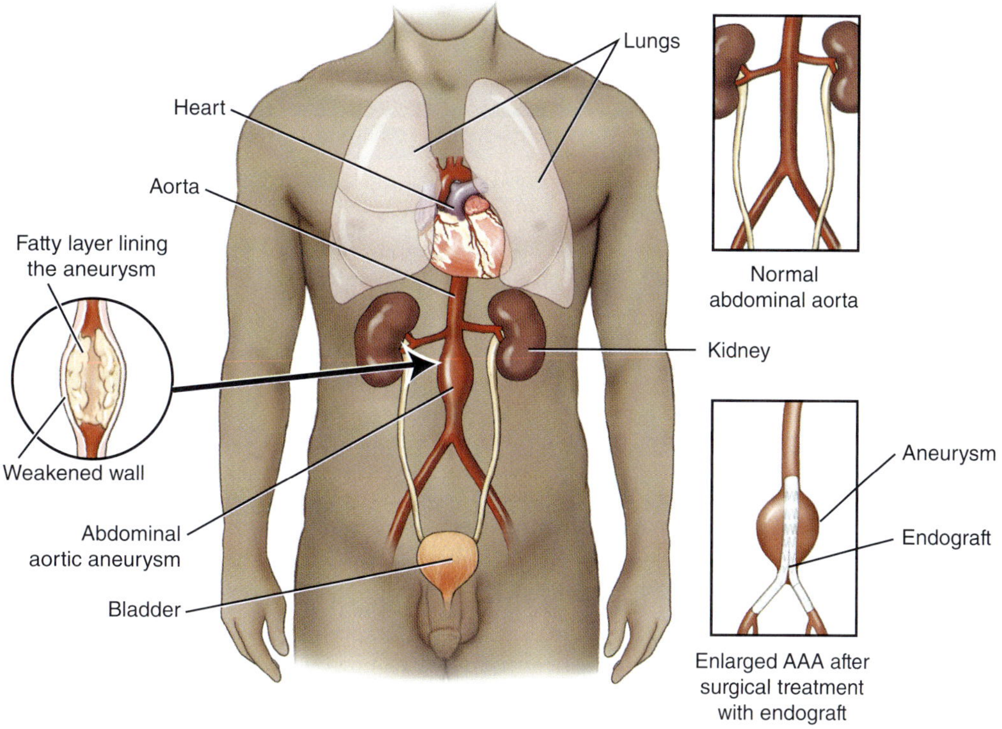

FIG. 10.10 Abdominal aortic aneurysm. An abdominal aortic aneurysm (AAA) is located in the abdominal area of the aorta, the main blood vessel that transports blood away from the heart. Because the success rate of surgery is much lower once an aneurysm has ruptured, more emphasis is being placed on diagnosis. AAAs can be detected by physical examination but are more frequently detected by abdominal ultrasound or computerized tomography (CT). Smaller AAAs have a very low risk of rupture and are usually followed closely to make sure they don't enlarge. Larger AAAs are usually repaired surgically. The preferred surgical intervention, called **endovascular stenting,** is performed through a puncture in the femoral artery, using a radiographic procedure called fluoroscopy. With this technique, an **endograft** can be placed within an aneurysm.

TERM	DEFINITION
4. arrhythmia (ā-RITH-mē-a)	any disturbance or abnormality in the heart's normal rhythmic pattern
5. cardiac arrest (KAR-dē-ak) (a-REST)	sudden cessation of cardiac output and effective circulation, which requires cardiopulmonary resuscitation **(CPR)**
6. cardiac tamponade (KAR-dē-ak) (tam-po-NĀD)	acute compression of the heart caused by fluid accumulation in the pericardial cavity
7. coronary artery disease (CAD) (KOR-o-nar-ē) (AR-te-rē) (di-ZĒZ)	condition that reduces the flow of blood through the coronary arteries to the myocardium that may progress to depriving the heart tissue of sufficient oxygen and nutrients to function normally; most often caused by coronary atherosclerosis. CAD is a common cause of heart failure and myocardial infarction.
CORONARY is derived from the Latin coronalis, meaning crown or wreath. It describes the arteries encircling the heart.	
8. cor pulmonale (kor) (pul-mō-NAL-ē)	enlargement of the heart's right ventricle due to pulmonary disease
9. deep vein thrombosis (DVT) (dēp) (vān) (throm-BŌ-sis)	condition of thrombus (blood clot) in a deep vein of the body. Most often occurs in the lower extremities. A clot, or part of a clot, can break off and travel to the lungs, causing a pulmonary embolism.

Cardiovascular System Terms—cont'd

NOT BUILT FROM WORD PARTS

DISEASE AND DISORDERS—cont'd

TERM	DEFINITION
10. fibrillation (fi-bri-LĀ-shun)	rapid, quivering, uncoordinated contractions of the atria or ventricles causing cardiac arrhythmia

TYPES OF FIBRILLATION In **atrial fibrillation (AFib)**, the atria quiver instead of contracting, causing an irregular ventricular response. Not all of the blood is ejected with each contraction, and the remaining blood flow becomes turbulent. This increases the risk of clot formation. Two types of AFib are **paroxysmal atrial fibrillation (PAF)**, which is intermittent, and **chronic atrial fibrillation**, which is sustained (Fig. 10.11). In **ventricular fibrillation (VF)**, the heart does not contract and blood flow stops, causing a medical emergency that may result in sudden death.

TERM	DEFINITION
11. heart failure (HF) (hart) (fāl-ŪR)	condition in which there is an inability of the heart to pump enough blood through the body to supply the tissues and organs with nutrients and oxygen (also called **congestive heart failure [CHF]**)
12. hypertensive heart disease (HHD) (hī-per-TEN-siv) (hart) (di-ZĒZ)	disorder of the heart caused by persistent high blood pressure; it may be associated with hypertrophy (abnormal thickening of the heart muscle) or dilation of the chambers of the heart (due to thinning and stretching of the heart muscle)
13. intermittent claudication (in-ter-MIT-ent) (klaw-di-KĀ-shun)	condition of pain, tension and weakness in a limb that starts when walking is begun, increases until walking is no longer possible, and then completely resolves when the patient is at rest. It is caused by reversible muscle ischemia that occurs with peripheral artery disease.
14. mitral valve stenosis (MĪ-tral) (ste-NŌ-sis)	narrowing of the mitral valve from scarring, usually caused by episodes of rheumatic fever
15. myocardial infarction (MI) (mī-ō-KAR-dē-al) (in-FARK-shun)	death (necrosis) of a portion of the myocardium caused by lack of oxygen resulting from an interrupted blood supply (also called **heart attack**)

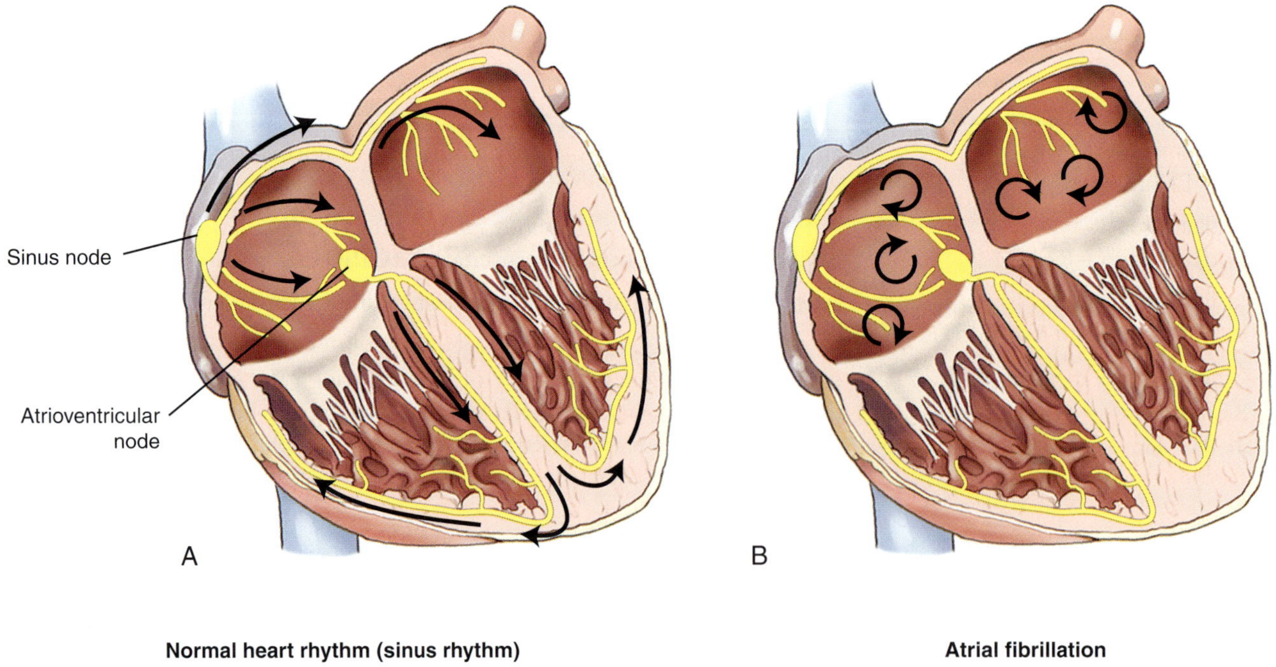

FIG. 10.11 Atrial fibrillation (AFib). **A,** Normal heart rhythm. *Arrows* indicate the normal travel of electrical impulses though the heart, stimulating coordinated contraction of chambers. **B,** Atrial fibrillation showing chaotic, rapid electrical impulses.

TERM	DEFINITION
16. peripheral artery disease (PAD) (pe-RIF-er-al) (AR-ter-ē) (di-ZĒZ)	disease of the arteries in the arms and legs, resulting in narrowing or complete obstruction of the artery. This is caused most commonly by atherosclerosis, but occasionally by inflammatory diseases, emboli, or thrombus formation. The most common symptom of peripheral artery disease is intermittent claudication. (also called **peripheral vascular disease [PVD]**)

RAYNAUD (RĀ-NŌ) PHENOMENON is classified as a **peripheral artery disease (PAD)**. The condition was first described by Maurice Raynaud, a French physician, in 1862. Symptoms include intermittent, symmetric attacks of cyanosis and pallor of the distal ends of the fingers and toes often caused by exposure to cold temperature.

TERM	DEFINITION
17. rheumatic heart disease (rū-MAT-ik) (hart) (di-ZĒZ)	damage to the heart muscle or heart valves caused by one or more episodes of rheumatic fever

RHEUMATIC FEVER is an inflammatory disease, usually occurring in children and young adults after an upper respiratory tract streptococcal infection. One of the most serious symptoms is valvulitis (inflammation of a cardiac valve). While antibiotics have greatly decreased the incidence of this disease in developed nations, it is still a significant threat in developing nations.

TERM	DEFINITION
18. varicose veins (VAR-i-kōs) (vānz)	distended or tortuous veins usually found in the lower extremities (Fig. 10.12)

VARICOSE VEINS AND TREATMENT Varicose veins usually occur in the superficial veins of the legs. One-way valves in the veins help move the blood upward. When these valves fail, or the veins lose their elasticity, the blood flows backward, pools, and forms varicose veins. Causes are heredity, obesity, pregnancy, illness, or injury. Treatments include laser ablation, ambulatory phlebectomy, and sclerotherapy.

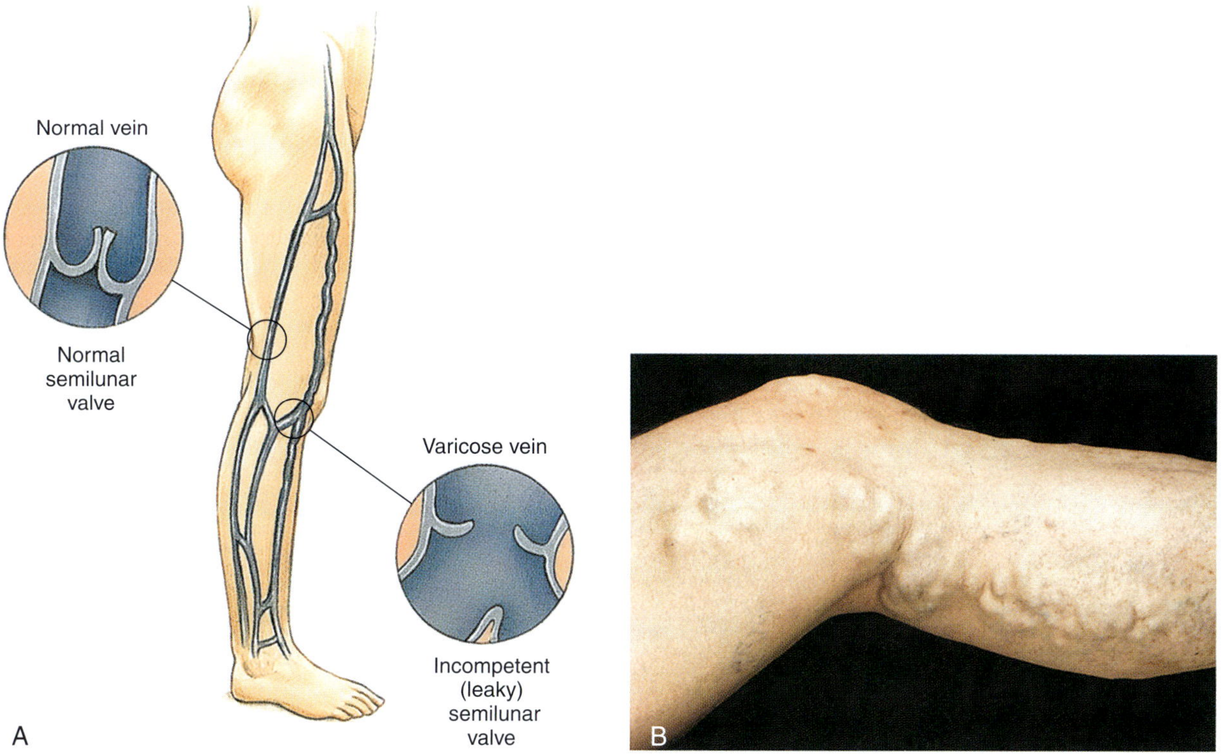

FIG. 10.12 A, Normal and varicose veins. **B,** Appearance of varicose veins.

Cardiovascular System Terms—cont'd

NOT BUILT FROM WORD PARTS

SURGICAL TERMS	
TERM	**DEFINITION**
19. artificial cardiac pacemaker (ar-ti-FISH-el) (KAR-dē-ak) (PĀS-mā-kr)	battery-powered apparatus implanted under the skin with leads placed on the heart or in the chamber of the heart used to treat an abnormal heart rhythm, usually one that is too slow, secondary to an abnormal sinus node
SINUS NODE of the heart is the body's natural pacemaker. Also called the sinoatrial or SA node, it consists of specialized fibers that are responsible for initiating nerve impulses that tell the heart muscles when to contract. When the SA node is working properly, the pumping motion of the heart chambers is coordinated and well-timed. If the SA node (or other parts of the heart's conduction system) doesn't work properly, arrhythmias may occur.	
20. automatic implantable cardiac defibrillator (AICD) (aw-to-MAT-ik) (im-PLANT-a-bl) (KAR-dē-ak) (dē-FIB-ri-lā-tor)	device implanted in the body that continuously monitors the heart rhythm. If life-threatening arrhythmias occur, the device delivers an electric shock to convert the arrhythmia back to a normal rhythm.
21. catheter ablation (KATH-e-ter) (ab-LĀ-shun)	procedure in which abnormal cells that trigger abnormal heart rhythms (arrhythmias) are destroyed by using a device that heats or freezes the cells (Fig. 10.13)
22. coronary artery bypass graft (CABG) (KOR-o-*nar*-ē) (AR-te-rē) (BĪ-pas) (graft)	surgical technique to bring a new blood supply to heart muscle by detouring around blocked arteries
23. coronary stent (KOR-o-*nar*-ē) (stent)	supportive scaffold device placed in the coronary artery; used to prevent closure of the artery after angioplasty or atherectomy; used to treat an artery occluded by plaque
24. femoropopliteal bypass (*fem*-o-rō-pop-LIT-ē-al) (BĪ-pass)	surgery to establish an alternate route from femoral artery to popliteal artery to bypass an obstruction
25. percutaneous transluminal coronary angioplasty (PTCA) (*per*-kū-TĀ-nē-us) (trans-LŪ-min-al) (KOR-o-*nar*-ē) (AN-jē-ō-*plas*-tē)	procedure in which a balloon is advanced into a coronary artery to the area where plaque has formed. When the balloon is inflated, the vessel wall expands, allowing blood to flow more freely. (also called **balloon angioplasty**)
26. thrombolytic therapy (*throm*-bō-LIT-ik) (THER-a-pē)	injection of a medication either intravenously or intra-arterially to dissolve blood clots. It is often used in emergency departments for acute myocardial infarction.

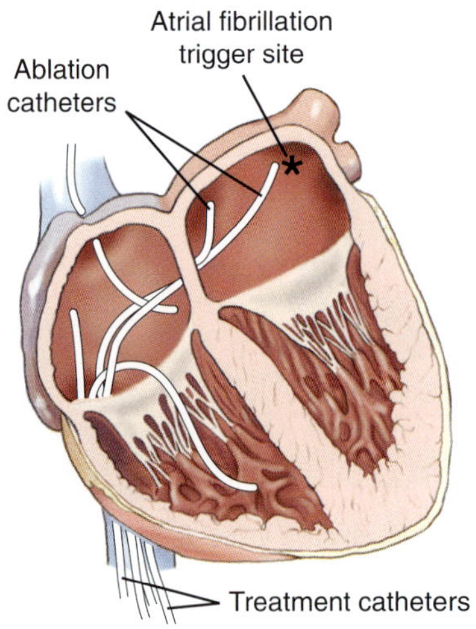

FIG. 10.13 Catheter ablation is used to treat atrial fibrillation if drug therapy is not effective.

DIAGNOSTIC IMAGING TERMS

TERM	DEFINITION
27. digital subtraction angiography (DSA) (DIJ-i-tal) (sub-TRAK-shun) (*an*-jē-OG-ra-fē)	process of digital radiographic imaging of the blood vessels that "subtracts" or removes structures not being studied (see Table 10.1)
28. Doppler ultrasound (DOP-ler) (UL-tra-sound)	study that uses high-frequency sound waves for detection of blood flow within the vessels; used to assess intermittent claudication, deep vein thrombosis, and other blood flow abnormalities
29. sestamibi test (*ses*-ta-MIB-ē) (test)	nuclear medicine test used to diagnose coronary artery disease and assess revascularization after coronary artery bypass surgery. Sestamibi, a radioactive isotope, is taken up by normal myocardial cells, but not in ischemia or infarction. These areas are identified as "cold" spots on the images produced.
30. single-photon emission computed tomography (SPECT) (SING-el) (FŌ-ton) (ē-MISH-on) (com-PŪ-ted) (tō-MOG-ra-fē)	nuclear medicine test that collects a series of images (projections) as a Gamma camera rotates around the patient. These projections are then used by a computer to generate three dimensional pictures; it also helps show the function of organs, such as coronary artery flow or active and inactive areas of the brain.
31. transesophageal echocardiogram (TEE) (*trans*-e-*sof*-a-JĒ-al) (*ek*-ō-KAR-dē-ō-*gram*)	ultrasound test that examines cardiac function and structure by using an ultrasound probe placed in the esophagus, which provides more direct views of the heart structures

DIAGNOSTIC PROCEDURES

TERM	DEFINITION
32. cardiac catheterization (KAR-dē-ak) (*kath*-e-ter-i-ZĀ-shun)	diagnostic procedure performed by passing a catheter into the heart from a blood vessel in the groin or arm to examine the condition of the heart and surrounding blood vessels; used to diagnose and treat cardiovascular conditions such as coronary artery disease
33. exercise stress test (EK-ser-sīz) (stres) (test)	study that evaluates cardiac function during physical stress by riding a bike or walking on a treadmill. **Electrocardiography** is the most common method, but **echocardiography** and **nuclear medicine scanning** (diagnostic imaging tests) can also be used to measure cardiac function while exercising.

CHEMICAL STRESS TESTING is the **use of drugs to simulate the stress of physical exercise** on the body. It is used to study cardiac function in patients who are unable to exercise.

OTHER DIAGNOSTIC MEASUREMENT TERMS

TERM	DEFINITION
34. blood pressure (BP) (blud) (PRES-ūr)	pressure exerted by the blood against the blood vessel walls. A blood pressure measurement written as **systolic** pressure (120) and **diastolic** pressure (80) is commonly recorded as 120/80 (blood pressure is measured in millimeters of mercury [mm Hg]).

SYSTOLE (SIS-tō-lē) is the cardiac-cycle phase in which the ventricles contract and eject blood. **Diastole** (dī-AS-tō-lē) is the phase in which the ventricles relax and fill with blood between contractions.

TERM	DEFINITION
35. pulse (puls)	contraction of the heart, which can be felt with a fingertip. The pulse is most commonly felt over the radial artery (in the wrist); however, the pulsations can be felt over a number of sites, including the femoral (groin) and carotid (neck) arteries.
36. sphygmomanometer (*sfig*-mō-ma-NOM-e-ter)	device used for measuring blood pressure

Cardiovascular System Terms—cont'd

NOT BUILT FROM WORD PARTS

LABORATORY TERMS

TERM	DEFINITION
37. C-reactive protein (CRP) (C)-(rē-AK-tiv) (PRŌ-tēn)	blood test to measure the amount of C-reactive protein in the blood, which when elevated, indicates inflammation in the body. It is sometimes used in assessing the risk of cardiovascular disease.
38. creatine phosphokinase (CPK) (KRĒ-a-tin) (*fos*-fō-KĪ-nās)	blood test used to measure the level of creatine phosphokinase, an enzyme of heart and skeletal muscle released into the blood after muscle injury or necrosis. The test is useful in evaluating patients with acute myocardial infarction.
39. lipid profile (LIP-id) (PRŌ-fīl)	blood test used to measure the amount and type of lipids (fat-like substances) in a sample of blood. This test is used to evaluate one of the risks of cardiovascular disease, and to monitor therapy for patients taking lipid-lowering medications. (Table 10.2)
40. troponin (TRŌ-pō-nin)	blood test that measures troponin, a heart muscle enzyme. Troponins are released into the blood approximately 3 hours after necrosis of the heart muscle and may remain elevated from 7 to 10 days. The test is useful in the diagnosis of a myocardial infarction.

BIOMARKER is a naturally occurring substance of certain body cells that can be measured in the blood and used to aid in the diagnosis of various disorders. **Troponin, creatine phosphokinase**, and **C-reactive protein** are biomarkers, and elevated levels are used in diagnosing various disorders occurring in the body.

SIGNS AND SYMPTOMS

TERM	DEFINITION
41. bruit (broo-Ē)	sound heard over an artery during auscultation resulting from vibration in the vessel wall caused by turbulent blood flow. Bruits are frequently caused by abnormal narrowing of an artery.

TABLE 10.2 Understanding a Lipid Profile

Cholesterol—a compound important in the production of sex hormones, steroids, cell membranes, and bile acids. Cholesterol is produced by the body and is also contained in foods such as animal fats. Cholesterol is transported by lipoproteins.
High-density lipoprotein (HDL)—a type of lipoprotein that removes cholesterol from the tissues and transports it to the liver to be excreted in the bile. Elevated levels of HDL are considered protective against development of atherosclerosis, which may lead to coronary artery disease. HDL is often referred to as the "good" cholesterol.
Low-density lipoprotein (LDL)—a type of lipoprotein that transports cholesterol to the tissue and deposits it on the walls of the arteries. High levels of LDL are associated with the presence of atherosclerosis, which may lead to coronary artery disease. LDL is often referred to as the "bad" cholesterol.
Total cholesterol—a measurement of the cholesterol components LDL, HDL, and VLDL (triglyceride carriers) in the blood.
Triglycerides (TGs)—a form of fat in the blood. Triglycerides are synthesized in the liver and used to store energy. Test results are used to assess the risk of coronary artery disease.
Very-low-density lipoprotein (VLDL)—a type of lipoprotein that transports most of the triglycerides in the blood. Elevated levels of VLDL, to a lesser degree than LDL, indicate a risk for developing coronary artery disease.

TERM	DEFINITION
42. hypercholesterolemia (*hī*-per-k-*les*-ter-ol-Ē-mē-a)	excessive amount of cholesterol in the blood; associated with an increased risk of cardiovascular disease
43. hyperlipidemia (*hī*-per-*lip*-i-DĒ-mē-a)	excessive amount of any type of fats (lipoproteins, triglycerides, and cholesterol) in the blood; associated with an increased risk of cardiovascular disease
44. hypertension (HTN) (*hī*-per-TEN-shun)	blood pressure that is above normal (greater than 130/80 mm Hg in adults under the age of 60)
45. hypertriglyceridemia (*hī*-per-trī-*glis*-er-rī-DĒ-mē-a)	excessive amount of triglycerides in the blood; associated with an increased risk of cardiovascular disease
46. hypotension (*hī*-pō-TEN-shun)	blood pressure that is below normal (less than 90/60 mm Hg in adults under the age of 60)
47. murmur (MER-mer)	unusual sound heard during auscultation of the heart caused by turbulent blood flow. It may be "innocent" (not indicating disease), or it may reflect disease or malformation, such as an abnormal heart valve.
48. occlusion (a-KLOO-shun)	closing or blockage of a blood vessel or hollow organ

TREATMENTS

TERM	DEFINITION
49. cardiopulmonary resuscitation (CPR) (*kar*-dē-ō-PUL-mo-nar-ē) (rē-*sus*-i-TĀ-shun)	emergency procedure consisting of external cardiac compressions; may be accompanied by artificial ventilation
50. defibrillation (dē-*fib*-ri-LĀ-shun)	application of an electric shock to the myocardium through the chest wall to restore normal cardiac rhythm (Fig. 10.14)
51. vasoconstrictor (*vās*-ō-kon-STRIK-tor)	agent that narrows the diameter of the blood vessels
52. vasodilator (*vās*-ō-DĪ-lā-tor)	agent that expands the diameter of the blood vessels

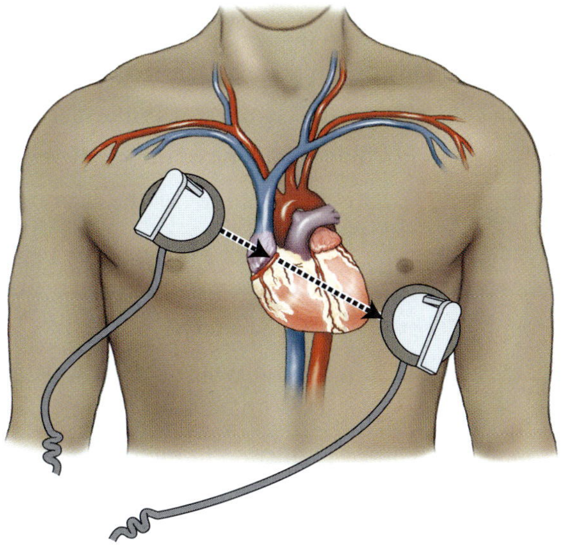

FIG. 10.14 Placement of defibrillator paddles on the chest.

EXERCISE 8 ■ Pronounce and Spell

Practice pronunciation and spelling on paper and online.

1. Practice on Paper

a. **Pronounce:** Read the phonetic spelling and say aloud the terms listed in the previous table. Refer to the pronunciation key on p. 20 as necessary.
b. **Spell:** Have a study partner read the terms aloud. Write the spelling of the terms on a separate sheet of paper.

2. Practice Online

a. **Access** online learning resources. Go to evolve.elsevier.com > Evolve Resources > Student Resources.
b. **Pronounce:** Select Audio Glossary > Chapter10 > Exercise 8. Select a term to hear its pronunciation and repeat aloud.
c. **Spell:** Select Activities > Chapter 10 > Spell Terms > Exercise 8. Select the audio icon and type the correct spelling of the term.

❑ Check the box when complete.

EXERCISE 9 ■ Fill In

A Disease and Disorder Terms

Fill in the blanks with the correct terms.

1. Sudden cessation of cardiac output and effective circulation is referred to as a(n) ____________________ ____________________.
2. Veins that are distended or tortuous are called ____________________ ____________________.
3. ____________________ is the name given to the ballooning of a weakened portion of an artery wall.
4. ____________________ ____________________ ____________________ is a condition most often caused by coronary atherosclerosis, which deprives the heart tissue of sufficient oxygen and nutrients to function normally.
5. ____________________ ____________________ is a cardiac condition characterized by chest pain caused by an insufficient blood supply to the cardiac muscle.
6. Death of a portion of myocardial muscle caused by lack of oxygen resulting from an interrupted blood supply is called a(n) ____________________ ____________________.
7. Rapid, quivering, uncoordinated contractions of the atria or ventricles called ____________________ creates a(n) ____________________ or disturbance or abnormality in the heart's normal rhythmic pattern.
8. A disorder of the heart caused by a persistently high blood pressure is called ____________________ heart disease.
9. ____________________ ____________________ is the inability of the heart to pump enough blood through the body to supply tissues and organs.
10. ____________________ ____________________ ____________________ is a disease of the arteries in the arms and legs resulting in narrowing or complete obstruction of an artery.
11. ____________________ ____________________ is a condition in which a patient has pain and discomfort in calf muscles while walking.
12. Acute compression of the heart caused by fluid accumulation in the pericardial cavity is known as ____________________ ____________________.

13. Episodes of rheumatic fever can cause ________________ ________________ ________________ and ________________ ________________ ________________.

14. ________________ ________________ ________________ is the condition of a thrombus, most often occurring in the lower extremities.

15. ________________ ________________ ________________ is a sudden insufficient blood supply to the heart, indicating unstable angina or myocardial infarction.

16. Enlargement of the heart's right ventricle due to pulmonary disease is called ________ ____________.

B Surgical Terms

Write the surgical terms pictured and defined.

1. ____

____

battery-powered apparatus implanted under the skin with leads placed on the heart or in the chamber of the heart used to treat an abnormal heart rhythm

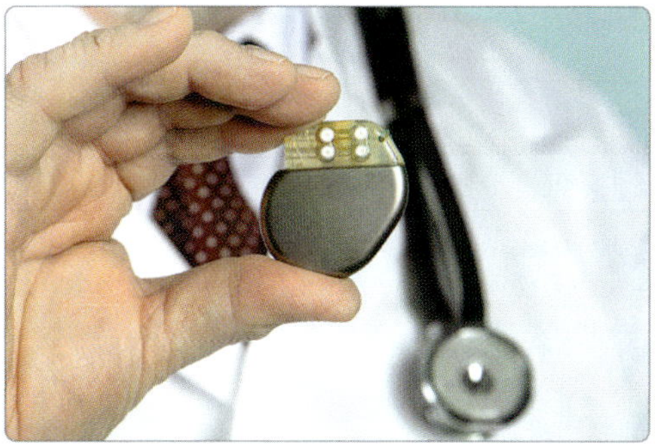

2. ____

____

injection of a medication either intravenously or intra-arterially to dissolve blood clots

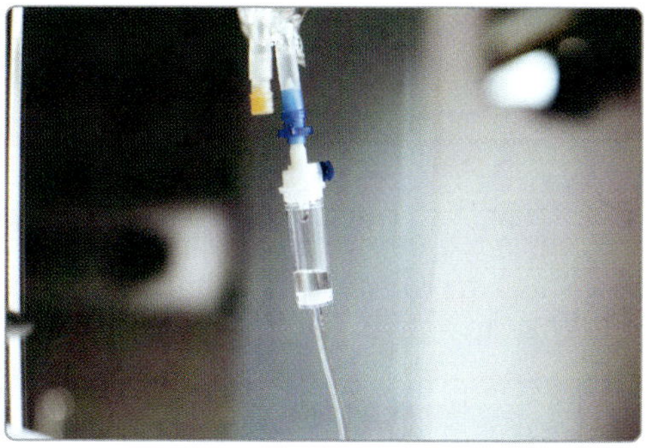

3. ____

____

surgical technique to bring a new blood supply to heart muscle by detouring around blocked arteries

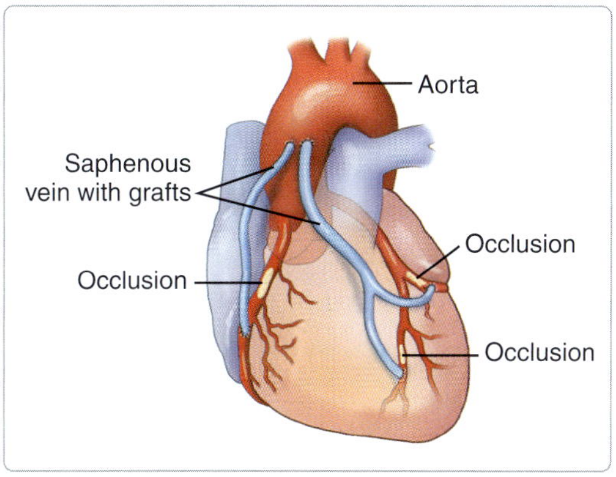

4. ____

____

procedure in which abnormal cells that trigger abnormal heart rhythms (arrhythmias) are destroyed by using a device that heats or freezes the cells

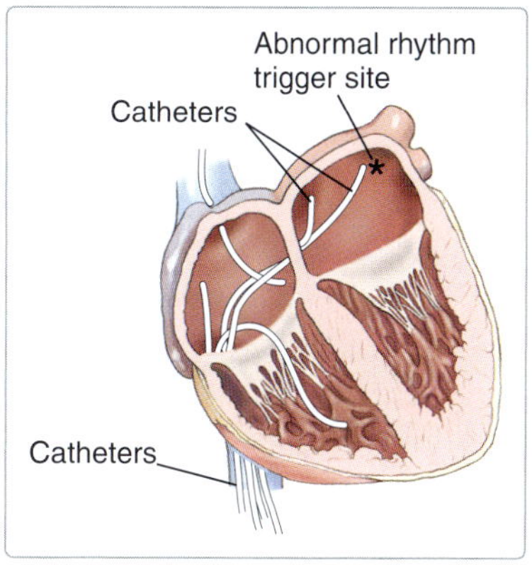

5. ______________________________

____

supportive scaffold device placed in the coronary artery; used to prevent closure of the artery after angioplasty or atherectomy

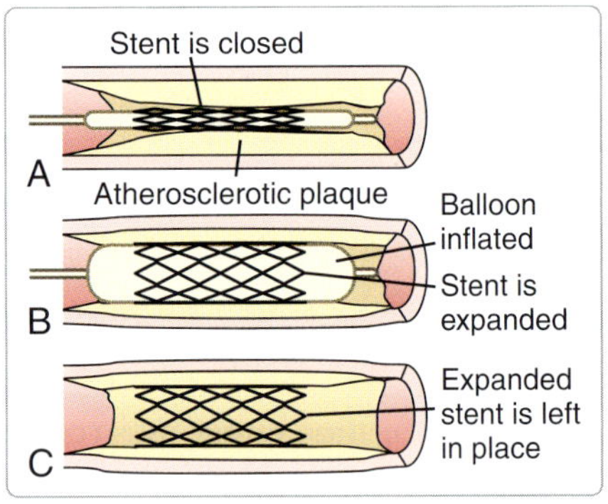

6. ______________________________

____

procedure in which a balloon is advanced into the coronary artery, to where plaque has formed. The balloon is inflated, the vessel wall expands, allowing blood to flow more freely

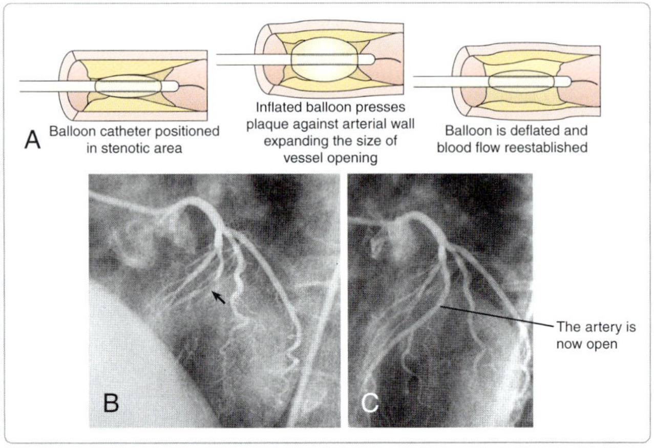

7. ______________________________

____

device implanted in the body that can deliver an electric shock to convert arrhythmia back to a normal rhythm

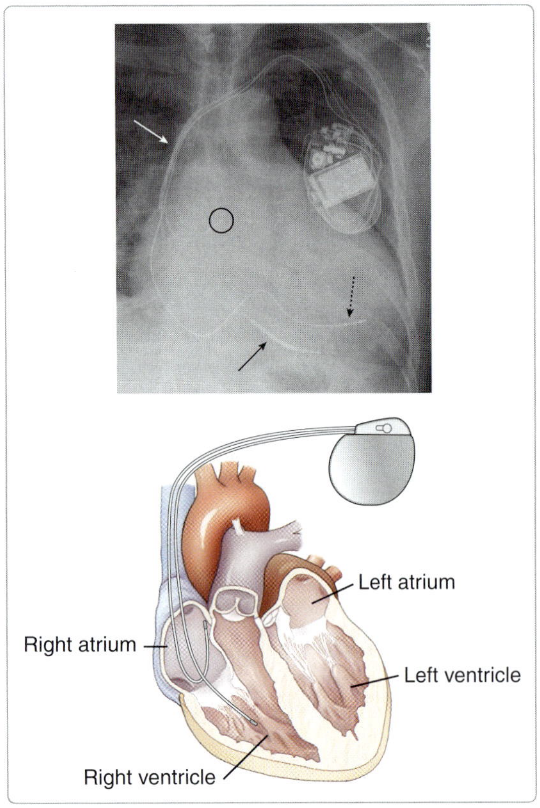

8. ______________________________

____

surgery to establish an alternate route from the femoral artery to the popliteal artery to bypass an obstruction

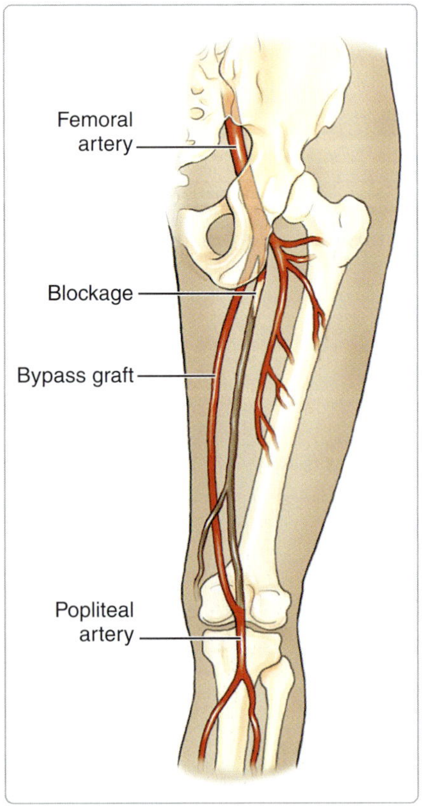

EXERCISE 10 ■ Diagnostic Terms

A Label

Write the diagnostic terms pictured and defined.

1. ______________________________
study that uses high-frequency sound waves for detection of blood flow within the vessels

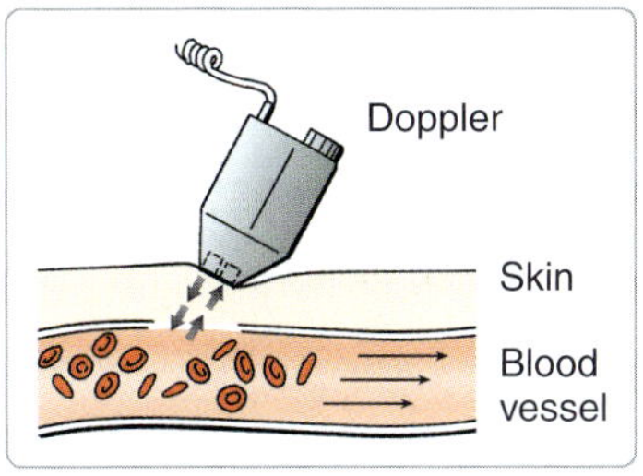

2. ______________________________
blood test used to measure the amount and type of fat-like substances in a sample of blood

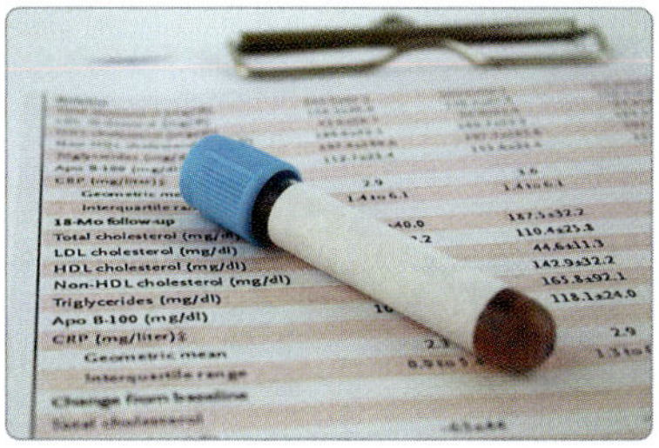

3. ______________________________
study that elevates cardiac function during physical stress by riding a bike or walking on a treadmill

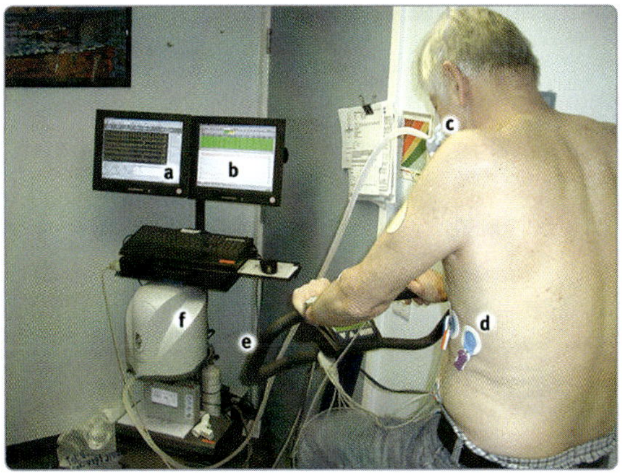

4. ______________________________
nuclear medicine test used to diagnose coronary artery disease and assess revascularization after CABG surgery

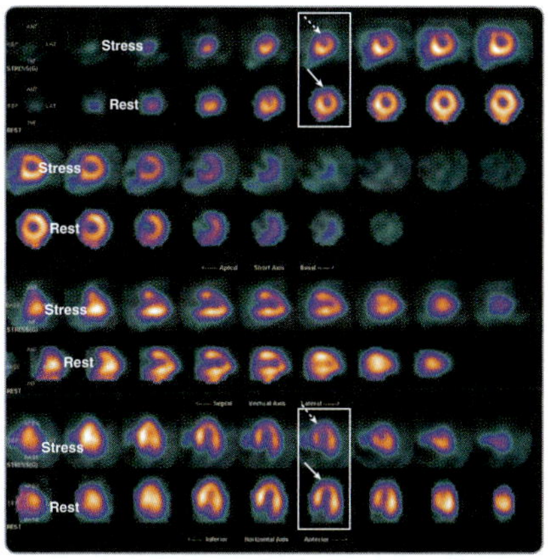

5. ______________________________
____
process of digital radiographic imaging of the blood vessels that "subtracts" or removes structures not being studied

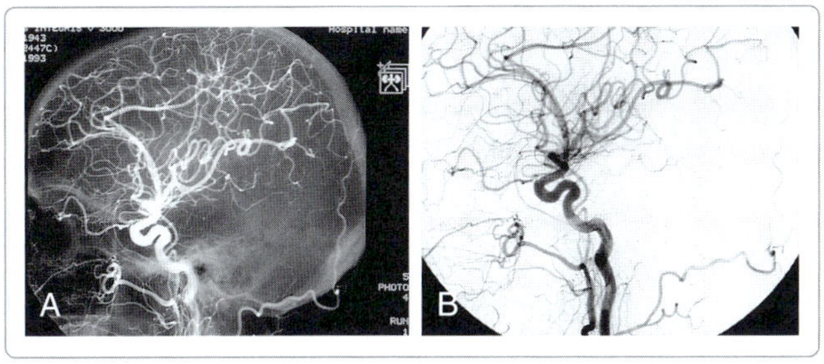

6. ______________________________
device used to measure blood pressure

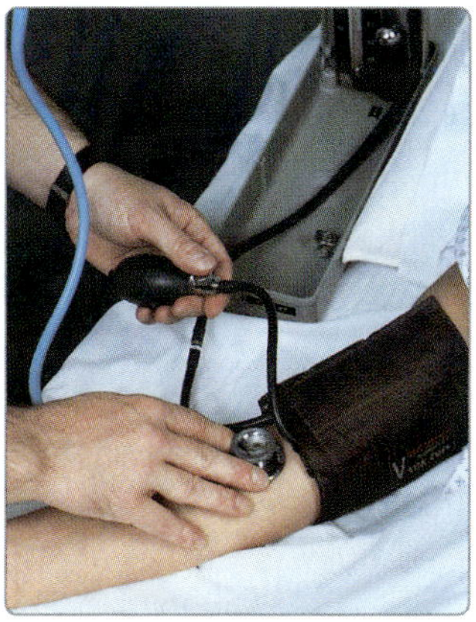

7. ______________________________
diagnostic procedure performed by passing a catheter into the heart from a vessel in the groin or arm to examine the condition of the heart and surrounding blood vessels

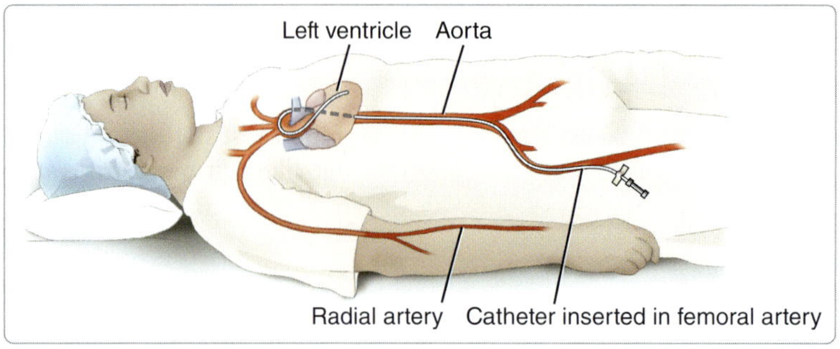

B Fill In

Fill in the blanks with the correct diagnostic terms.

1. ______________ ______________ is a test in which an ultrasound probe provides views of the heart structures from the esophagus.
2. A nuclear medicine test that visualizes the heart from several different angles, producing three dimensional images, is called a(n) ______________-______________ ______________ ______________ ______________.
3. A blood test to measure an enzyme of the heart released into the bloodstream after muscle injury is called ______________ ______________.
4. An elevated ______________ ______________ indicates inflammation in the body.
5. ______________ is the rhythmic expansion of an artery created by contraction of the heart that can be felt with a fingertip.
6. ______________ is a heart muscle enzyme released into the bloodstream approximately 3 hours after heart muscle necrosis.
7. The vital sign measured with the use of a sphygmomanometer and stethoscope that is recorded in millimeters of mercury is ______________ ______________.

EXERCISE 11 ■ Signs and Symptoms and Treatment Terms

A Match

Match the terms for signs and symptoms and treatments in the first column with the correct definitions in the second column.

_____ 1. vasodilator
_____ 2. vasoconstrictor
_____ 3. bruit
_____ 4. hypercholesterolemia
_____ 5. occlusion
_____ 6. murmur
_____ 7. hypotension
_____ 8. hypertriglyceridemia
_____ 9. hypertension
_____ 10. hyperlipidemia

a. blood pressure that is below normal (less than 90/60 mm Hg in adults under the age of 60)
b. excessive amount of cholesterol in the blood
c. blood pressure that is above normal (greater than 130/80 mm Hg in adults under the age of 60)
d. closing or blockage of a blood vessel or hollow organ
e. excessive amount of triglycerides in the blood
f. excessive amount of any type of fats (lipoproteins, triglycerides, and cholesterol) in the blood
g. agent or nerve that narrows the diameter of the blood vessels
h. sound heard over an artery during auscultation resulting from vibration in the vessel wall caused by turbulent blood flow
i. unusual sound heard during auscultation of the heart caused by turbulent blood flow
j. agent or nerve that expands the diameter of the blood vessels

B Label

Write the treatment terms pictured and defined.

1. ______________________________
application of an electric shock to the myocardium through the chest wall to restore normal cardiac rhythm

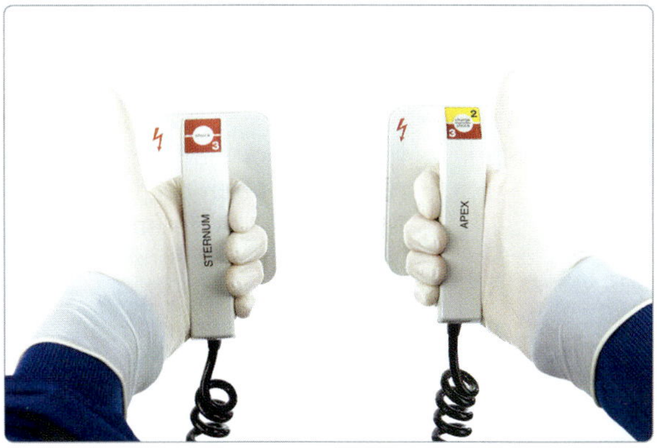

2. ______________________________
emergency procedure consisting of external cardiac compressions; may be accompanied by artificial ventilation

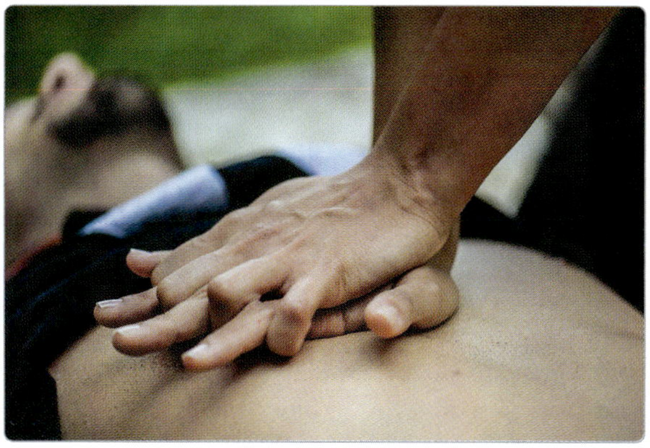

EXERCISE 12 ■ Review of Cardiovascular Terms

Can you define, pronounce, and spell the following cardiovascular system terms?

acute coronary syndrome (ACS)
aneurysm
angina pectoris
angiography
angioma
angioplasty
angioscopy
angiostenosis
aortic stenosis
aortogram
arrhythmia
arteriogram
arteriosclerosis
artificial cardiac pacemaker
atherectomy
atherosclerosis
atrioventricular (AV)
automatic implantable cardiac defibrillator (AICD)
blood pressure (BP)
bradycardia
bruit
cardiac arrest
cardiac catheterization
cardiac tamponade
cardiogenic
cardiologist
cardiology
cardiomegaly
cardiomyopathy
cardiopulmonary resuscitation (CPR)
catheter ablation
cor pulmonale
coronary artery bypass graft (CABG)
coronary artery disease (CAD)
coronary stent
C-reactive protein (CRP)
creatine phosphokinase (CPK)
deep vein thrombosis (DVT)
defibrillation
digital subtraction angiography (DSA)
Doppler ultrasound
echocardiogram (ECHO)
electrocardiogram (ECG, EKG)
electrocardiography
embolectomy
endarterectomy
endocarditis
exercise stress test
femoropopliteal bypass
fibrillation
heart failure (HF)
hypercholesterolemia
hyperlipidemia
hypertension (HTN)
hypertensive heart disease (HHD)
hypertriglyceridemia
hypotension
intermittent claudication
intravenous (IV)
ischemia
lipid profile
mitral valve stenosis
murmur
myocardial infarction (MI)
myocarditis
occlusion
percutaneous transluminal coronary angioplasty (PTCA)
pericardiocentesis
pericarditis
peripheral artery disease (PAD)
phlebectomy
phlebitis
polyarteritis
pulse
rheumatic heart disease
sestamibi test
single-photon emission computed tomography (SPECT)
sphygmomanometer
tachycardia
thrombolytic therapy
thrombophlebitis
transesophageal echocardiogram (TEE)
troponin
valvulitis
valvuloplasty
varicose veins
vasoconstrictor
vasodilator
venogram

Blood Terms

BUILT FROM WORD PARTS

The following terms can be translated using definitions of word parts. Further explanation is provided within parentheses as needed.

DISEASE AND DISORDERS

TERM	DEFINITION
1. **embolism** (EM-bō-lizm)	state of a plug (blood clot or foreign material, such as air or fat, lodged inside a blood vessel)
2. **embolus (*pl.* emboli)** (EM-bō-lus) (EM-bo-lī)	plug (blood clot or foreign material, such as air or fat, that enters the bloodstream and moves until it lodges at another point in the circulation)
3. **erythrocytopenia** (e-rith-rō-sī-tō-PĒ-nē-a)	abnormal reduction of red (blood) cells (also called **anemia**)
4. **hematoma** (*hē*-ma-TŌ-ma)	tumor of blood (collection of blood that has leaked out of a broken vessel into the surrounding tissue)
5. **hemorrhage** (HEM-o-rij)	excessive flow of blood (bleeding internally or externally)
6. **leukocytopenia** (lū-kō-sī-tō-PĒ-nē-a)	abnormal reduction of white (blood) cells (also called **leukopenia**)
7. **multiple myeloma** (MUL-te-pl) (*mī*-e-LŌ-ma)	tumors of the bone marrow (a blood malignancy that most often occurs after age 65. Signs and symptoms may include bone pain, infections, weight loss, anemia, and fatigue.)
8. **pancytopenia** (*pan*-sī-tō-PĒ-nē-a)	abnormal reduction of all (blood) cells
9. **thrombocytopenia** (throm-bō-sī-tō-PĒ-nē-a)	abnormal reduction of blood clotting cells (platelets)
10. **thrombosis** (throm-BŌ-sis)	abnormal condition of a blood clot
11. **thrombus** (THROM-bus)	blood clot (attached to the interior wall of an artery or vein)

EMBOLUS/THROMBUS An embolus circulates in the bloodstream until it becomes lodged in a vessel, whereas a thrombus is attached to the interior wall of a vessel. When any part of a thrombus breaks away and circulates in the bloodstream, it becomes known as an embolus.

SIGNS AND SYMPTOMS

TERM	DEFINITION
12. **hemolysis** (*hē*-MOL-i-sis)	dissolution of (red) blood (cells)
13. **lymphocytosis** (*lim*-fō-sī-TŌ-sis)	increase in the number of lymphocytes

HEMOLYSIS refers to the breakdown of red blood cells at the end of their life cycles. Diseases, genetic defects, and medications can increase the rate of hemolysis causing red blood cells to be destroyed too soon. The resulting shortage of healthy red blood cells leads to a form of anemia called **hemolytic anemia**.

OTHER TERMS

TERM	DEFINITION
14. **hematologist** (*hē*-ma-TOL-o-jist)	physician who studies and treats diseases of the blood
15. **hemostasis** (*hē*-mō-STĀ-sis)	stoppage of bleeding
16. **plasmapheresis** (*plaz*-ma-fe-RĒ-sis)	removal of plasma (from withdrawn blood; the cells, called formed elements, are then reinfused into the donor or into another patient who needs blood cells rather than whole blood)
17. **phlebotomy** (fle-BOT-o-mē)	incision into a vein (with a needle to remove blood for testing)
18. **thrombolysis** (throm-BOL-i-sis)	dissolution of a blood clot

EXERCISE 13 ■ Pronounce and Spell

Practice pronunciation and spelling on paper and online.

1. Practice on Paper

a. **Pronounce:** Read the phonetic spelling and say aloud the terms listed in the previous table. Refer to the pronunciation key on p. 20 as necessary.
b. **Spell:** Have a study partner read the terms aloud. Write the spelling of the terms on a separate sheet of paper.

2. Practice Online

a. **Access** online learning resources. Go to evolve.elsevier.com > Evolve Resources > Student Resources.
b. **Pronounce:** Select Audio Glossary > Chapter10 > Exercise 13. Select a term to hear its pronunciation and repeat aloud.
c. **Spell:** Select Activities > Chapter 10 > Spell Terms > Exercise 13. Select the audio icon and type the correct spelling of the term.

❑ Check the box when complete.

EXERCISE 14 ■ Analyze and Define

Analyze and define the following blood terms.

1. hemostasis

____
____

2. hematologist

____
____

3. hemolysis

____
____

4. lymphocytosis

____
____

5. pancytopenia

____
____

6. erythrocytopenia

____
____

7. embolism

____
____

8. thrombus

____
____

EXERCISE 15 ■ Build

A Fill In

Build blood terms for the following definitions by using the word parts you have learned.

1. abnormal reduction of white (blood) cells ______ / ______ / ______ / ______ / ______
WR / CV / WR / CV / S

2. excessive flow of blood ________ / CV / ________
WR / CV / S

3. dissolution of a blood clot ________ / CV / ________
WR / CV / S

4. abnormal reduction of blood clotting cells (platelets) ________ / CV / ________ / CV / ________
WR / CV / WR / CV / S

5. plug ________ / ________
WR / S

6. tumors of the bone marrow multiple ________ / ________
WR / S

B Label

Build terms pictured by writing word parts above definitions.

1.
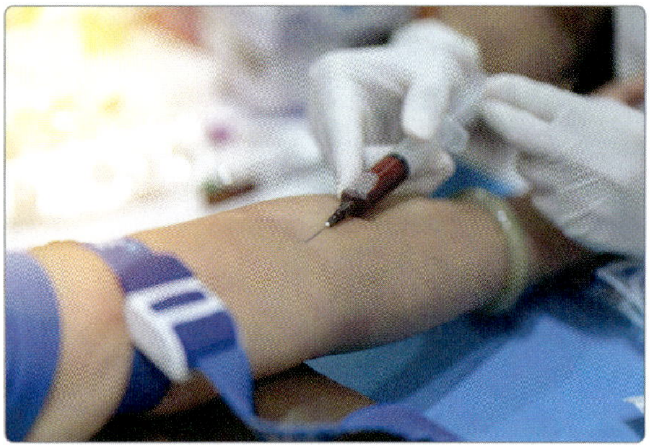

________ / ________ / ________
vein / CV / incision

2.
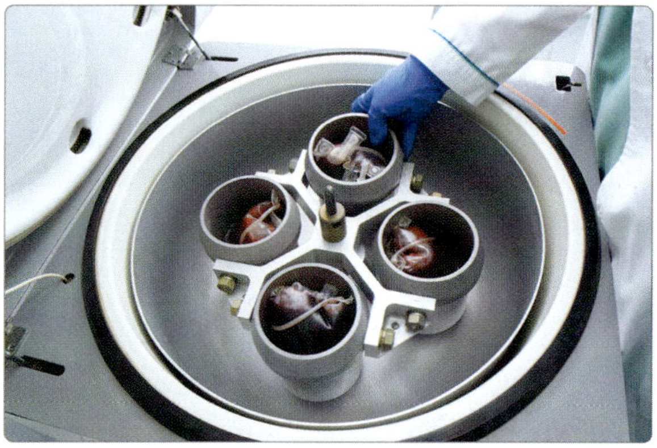

________ / ________
plasma / removal

3.
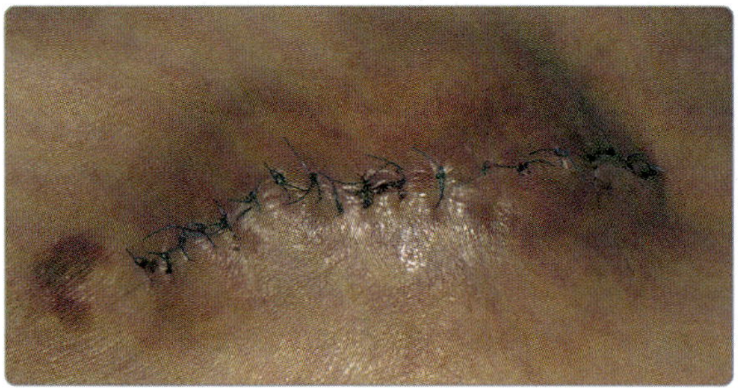

Post-surgical site displaying swelling and formation of a ________ / ________
blood / tumor

4.
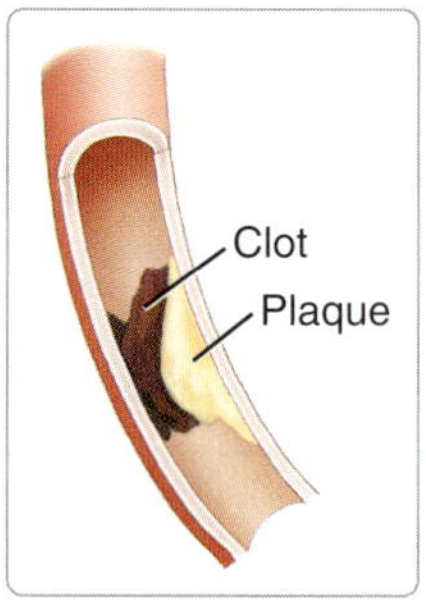

Blocked artery due to atherosclerosis and ________ / ________
blood clot / abnormal condition

Blood Terms

NOT BUILT FROM WORD PARTS

Word parts may be present in the following terms; however, their full meanings cannot be translated using definitions of word parts alone.

DISEASE AND DISORDERS

TERM	DEFINITION
1. anemia (a-NĒ-mē-a)	condition in which there is a reduction in the number of erythrocytes (RBCs). Anemia may be caused by blood loss, by decreased production of RBCs, or by increased destruction of RBCs. (Table 10.3)
2. bleeding disorder (BLĒD-ing) (dis-OR-der)	disease in which there is an inability to form proper blood clots; examples include hemophilia, von Willebrand disease, and bleeding factor deficiencies
3. hemophilia (hē-mō-FIL-ē-a)	inherited bleeding disorder most commonly caused by a deficiency of the coagulation factor VIII
4. leukemia (lū-KĒ-mē-a)	malignant disease characterized by excessive increase in abnormal leukocytes (white blood cells) formed in the bone marrow (Table 10.4)

TABLE 10.3 Common Types of Anemia

TYPE	DESCRIPTION
Anemia due to blood loss	• acute blood loss anemia as a result of hemorrhage
Anemia due to decreased production of red blood cells	• iron deficiency anemia: not enough iron in the body to produce hemoglobin • pernicious anemia: ineffective production of red blood cells due to vitamin B_{12} deficiency • aplastic anemia: resulting from bone marrow failure
Anemia due to increased destruction of red blood cells	• hemolytic anemia: reduced life of blood cells (such as in sickle cell disease)

TABLE 10.4 Leukemia

Leukemia is differentiated by the type of leukocyte that is affected and how quickly the disease develops and progresses.

Acute leukemia develops quickly with rapid progression of the disease. Both adults and children may develop acute leukemia. Acute leukemia is the most common form of cancer in children and adolescents.

Chronic leukemia develops slowly with gradual disease progression and most often occurs in adults.

Lymphocytic leukemia affects the lymphoid cells (lymphocytes), which form lymph tissue (part of the immune system).

Myelogenous leukemia affects the myeloid cells, which form red blood cells, white blood cells, and platelets.

MAJOR TYPES OF LEUKEMIA

- **acute lymphocytic leukemia (ALL):** the most common type in young children, can affect adults (also called acute lymphoblastic leukemia)
- **acute myelogenous leukemia (AML):** most common acute leukemia in adults, can also affect children
- **chronic lymphocytic leukemia (CLL):** most common chronic adult leukemia; patient may feel well for years without needing treatment
- **chronic myelogenous leukemia (CML):** occurs mostly in older adults

Rare types of leukemia include hairy cell leukemia **(HCL)**, myelodysplastic syndromes, and myeloproliferative disorders

Blood Terms—cont'd

NOT BUILT FROM WORD PARTS

DISEASE AND DISORDERS—CONT'D

TERM	DEFINITION
5. **sepsis** (SEP-sis)	systemic inflammatory response caused by pathogenic microorganisms, usually bacteria, entering the bloodstream and multiplying; life-threatening condition, which may lead to tissue damage, organ failure, and death. The overwhelming presence of pathogens in the blood is called septicemia.
6. **sickle cell disease** (SI-kl) (sel) (di-ZĒZ)	group of inherited red blood cell disorders (anemias) where hemoglobin is abnormally shaped and has a shorter life cycle
7. **thalassemia** (*thal*-a-SĒ-mē-ah)	inherited bleeding disorder causing reduced production of healthy blood cells and hemoglobin

DIAGNOSTIC PROCEDURES

TERM	DEFINITION
8. **bone marrow aspiration** (bōn) (MAR-ō) (*as*-pi-RĀ-shun)	procedure to obtain a sample of the **liquid** portion of the bone marrow, usually from the ilium (upper hip bone) for study; used to diagnose leukemia, infections, some types of anemia, and other blood disorders
9. **bone marrow biopsy** (bōn) (MAR-ō) (BĪ-op-sē)	procedure to obtain a sample of the **solid** portion of bone marrow, usually from the ilium, for study; used to diagnose leukemia, infections, some types of anemia, and other blood disorders. May be performed at the same time as bone marrow aspiration.

BONE MARROW is contained within spongy bone, which is located primarily at the ends of long bones and in the center of other bones. Stem cells within the bone marrow turn into thrombocytes (platelets), red blood cells, and white blood cells.

LABORATORY

TERM	DEFINITION
10. **activated partial thromboplastin time (aPTT)** (AK-ti-*vāt*-ed) (PAR-shel) (*throm*-bō-PLAS-tin) (tīm)	blood test that measures the ability of the blood to clot by assessing intrinsic blood factors. Used to evaluate bleeding disorders such as hemophilia A and B and monitor some types of anticoagulation therapy such as heparin. Frequently ordered in conjunction with prothrombin time (PT/INR).
11. **bleeding profile** (BLĒD-ing) (PRŌ-fīl)	series of tests that measure the ability of various factors in the blood to form a clot. Usually includes PT/INR, aPTT, thrombin time, and tests for platelets and fibrinogen.

COAGULATION ABNORMALITIES **Blood coagulation** is the process that causes blood to clot and helps prevent excessive blood loss through a cut, puncture, or other trauma to blood vessels. The coagulation cascade involves a series of components called **blood clotting factors**, which act together in a step-wise manner to stop the flow of blood. These factors may be **intrinsic** (originating in the blood) or **extrinsic** (originating from tissues outside the blood). An abnormality in any of these factors, or in the ways in which they come together to form a clot, may result in either an inability to form a clot, such as **hemophilia**, or a tendency for the blood to form clots too easily, such as **deep vein thrombosis**. There are a number laboratory tests to determine whether coagulation is functioning appropriately, and to find the source of the abnormality if a patient is bleeding too much, or clotting too easily.

TERM	DEFINITION
12. **complete blood count with differential (CBC with diff)** (com-PLĒT) (blud) (kownt) (with) (*dif*-er-EN-shal)	laboratory test for basic blood screening that measures various aspects of erythrocytes, leukocytes, and thrombocytes (platelets); this automated test quickly provides a tremendous amount of information about the blood
13. **hematocrit (Hct)** (hē-MAT-o-crit)	percentage of a blood sample that is composed of erythrocytes. It is used in the diagnosis and evaluation of anemic patients.

TERM	DEFINITION
14. hemoglobin (Hgb) (HĒ-mō-*glō*-bin)	blood test that measures the amount of hemoglobin (the protein in red blood cells that carries oxygen) in the blood
15. prothrombin time (PT/INR) (prō-THROM-bin) (tīm)	blood test that measures the ability of the blood to clot by assessing extrinsic blood factors. Used to evaluate bleeding disorders such as those caused by liver disease or vitamin K deficiency, or to monitor anticoagulation therapy such as warfarin. Frequently ordered in conjunction with activated partial thromboplastin time (aPTT).

PT/INR stands for **prothrombin time/international normalized ratio**. Most institutions, on the recommendation of the World Health Organization, report both absolute numbers and INR numbers, which provide uniform PT results to physicians worldwide.

TREATMENTS

TERM	DEFINITION
16. bone marrow transplant (BMT) (bōn) (MAR-ō) (TRANS-plant)	infusion of healthy bone marrow cells from a matched donor into a patient with severely diseased or damaged bone marrow; the donor cells may establish a colony of new, healthy tissue in the recipient's bone marrow
17. peripheral blood stem cell transplant (PBSCT) (pe-RIF-er-al)(blud) (stem) (sel) (TRANS-plant)	infusion of blood-forming cells (stem cells) to replace blood cells damaged by disease or treatments, such as chemotherapy; stem cells are collected by apheresis, a process in which blood is removed from the patient or a matched donor and spun through a machine to harvest stem cells

INFUSION is the introduction of fluid into the bloodstream through a vein.

MEDICAL SPECIALTIES

TERM	DEFINITION
18. perfusionist (per-FŪ-shun-ist)	person who operates the heart-lung machine during surgeries where the patient's blood must be oxygenated outside of the body; perfusionists monitor and are responsible for the circulatory and respiratory function of the patient during cardiothoracic surgery
19. phlebotomist (fle-BOT-ō-mist)	person who performs venipuncture for the purpose of drawing blood or injecting IV fluids

OTHER TERMS

TERM	DEFINITION
20. anticoagulant (*an*-tī-kō-AG-ū-lant)	agent that slows the blood clotting process
21. blood dyscrasia (blud) (dis-KRĀ-zha)	any abnormal or pathologic condition of the blood

DYSCRASIA is made up of the Greek word parts **dys-**, meaning difficult, painful or abnormal, and **-crasia**, meaning mixture. Blood disease in ancient Greek times was thought to be an abnormal mixture of the four humors: blood, black bile, yellow bile, and phlegm. Today the term remains, but its full meaning can no longer be directly translated from its word parts.

TERM	DEFINITION
22. extravasation (ek-*strav*-a-SĀ-shun)	escape of blood or other fluid from a vessel into the tissue
23. venipuncture (VEN-i-*punk*-chur)	procedure used to puncture a vein with a needle to remove blood, instill a medication, or start an intravenous infusion (also called **phlebotomy**)

EXERCISE 16 ■ Pronounce and Spell

Practice pronunciation and spelling on paper and online.

1. Practice on Paper

a. **Pronounce:** Read the phonetic spelling and say aloud the terms listed in the previous table. Refer to the pronunciation key on p. 20 as necessary.
b. **Spell:** Have a study partner read the terms aloud. Write the spelling of the terms on a separate sheet of paper.

2. Practice Online

a. **Access** online learning resources. Go to evolve.elsevier.com > Evolve Resources > Student Resources.
b. **Pronounce:** Select Audio Glossary > Chapter10 > Exercise 16. Select a term to hear its pronunciation and repeat aloud.
c. **Spell:** Select Activities > Chapter 10 > Spell Terms > Exercise 16. Select the audio icon and type the correct spelling of the term.

❑ Check the box when complete.

EXERCISE 17 ■ Match

Match the disease and disorder terms in the first column with their correct definitions in the second column.

_____ 1. anemia
_____ 2. thalassemia
_____ 3. leukemia
_____ 4. sepsis
_____ 5. sickle cell disease
_____ 6. hemophilia
_____ 7. bleeding disorder

a. disease in which there is an inability to form proper blood clots (general term)
b. systemic inflammatory response caused by pathogenic microorganisms, usually bacteria, entering the bloodstream and multiplying
c. inherited bleeding disorder most commonly caused by a deficiency of the coagulation factor VIII
d. group of inheritied red blood disorders where hemoglobin is abnormally shaped and has a shorter life cycle
e. condition in which there is a reduction in the number of erythrocytes
f. malignant disease characterized by excessive increase in abnormal leukocytes
g. inherited blood disorder causing reduced production of healthy blood cells and hemoglobin

EXERCISE 18 ■ Label

Write the medical term pictured and defined.

1. ______________________________

____

procedure to obtain a sample of the **liquid** portion of the bone marrow

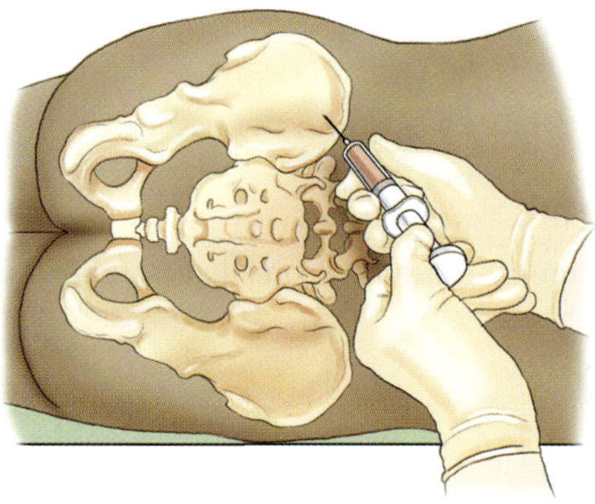

2. ______________________________

____

procedure to obtain a sample of the **solid** portion of bone marrow

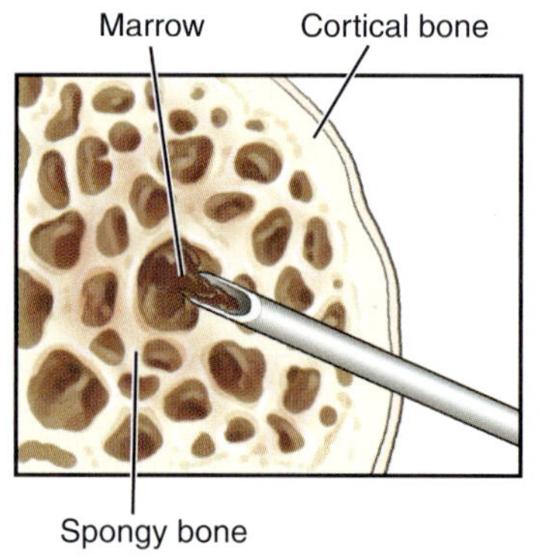

3. ______________________
person who performs venipuncture for the purpose of drawing blood or injecting IV fluids

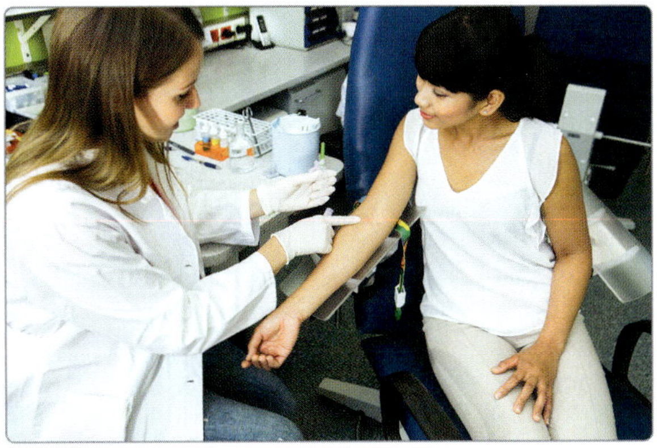

4. ______________________
person who operates the heart-lung machine during surgeries where the patient's blood must be oxygenated outside of the body

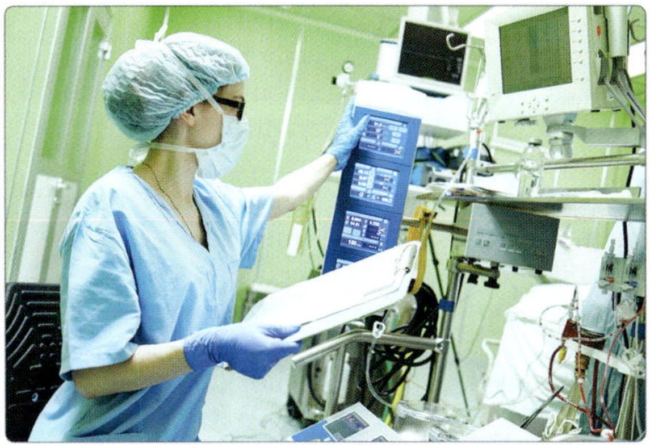

EXERCISE 19 ■ Fill In

Fill in the blanks with the correct terms.

1. Sickle cell disease, thalassemia, and leukemia are examples of ______________________ (plural form of the term), any abnormal or pathologic conditions of the blood.
2. A(n) ______________________, or agent that slows the blood clotting process, would be prescribed to prevent clots forming in blood vessels in patients diagnosed with atrial fibrillation, mechanical heart valves, and following certain surgeries.
3. A phlebotomist performs ______________________, the procedure used to puncture a vein with a needle to remove blood, instill a medication, or start an intravenous infusion. The escape of blood or fluid from a vessel or ______________________ may occur at a venipuncture site. Tissue damage may occur if infused medicine leaks into surrounding tissue.
4. The infusion of healthy bone marrow cells called ______________________ and the infusion of blood-forming cells called ______________________ are used to treat multiple myeloma and some forms of leukemia, anemia, and lymphoma. Both treatments introduce stem cells into the blood stream, where they can migrate to bone marrow and begin to make new blood cells.
5. This automated laboratory test for blood screening, or ______________________, measures various aspects of erythrocytes, leukocytes, and thrombocytes (platelets) and quickly gives a tremendous amount of information about the blood.
6. Two laboratory tests used in the diagnosis of anemia are ______________________, which reports the percentage of erythrocytes in a blood sample, and ______________________, which measures the amount of oxygen-carrying protein in erythrocytes.
7. A ______________________ measures the ability of various factors in the blood to form a clot using a series of tests, including ______________________, that assesses extrinsic blood factors, and ______________________, that assesses intrinsic blood factors.

EXERCISE 20 ■ Review of Blood Terms

Can you define, pronounce, and spell the following blood terms?

activated partial thromboplastin time (aPTT)
anemia
anticoagulant
bleeding disorder
bleeding profile
blood dyscrasia
bone marrow aspiration
bone marrow biopsy
bone marrow transplant (BMT)
complete blood count (CBC) and differential (Diff)
embolism
embolus (*pl.* emboli)
erythrocytopenia
extravasation
hematocrit (Hct)
hematologist
hematoma
hemoglobin (Hgb)
hemolysis
hemophilia
hemorrhage
hemostasis
leukemia
leukocytopenia
lymphocytosis
multiple myeloma
pancytopenia
perfusionist
peripheral blood stem cell transplant (PBSCT)
phlebotomist
phlebotomy
plasmapheresis
prothrombin time (PT/INR)
sepsis
sickle cell disease
thalassemia
thrombocytopenia
thrombolysis
thrombosis
thrombus
venipuncture

Lymphatic System Terms

BUILT FROM WORD PARTS AND *NOT* BUILT FROM WORD PARTS

The first portion of the table contains Lymphatic System Terms that can be translated using definitions of word parts. The second portion of the table contains Lymphatic System Terms that cannot be fully understood through translation of word parts.

■ Built from Word Parts

DISEASE AND DISORDERS

TERM	DEFINITION
1. **lymphadenitis** (*lim*-fad-e-NĪ-tis)	inflammation of lymph nodes
2. **lymphadenopathy** (lim-*fad*-e-NOP-a-thē)	disease of lymph nodes (characterized by abnormal enlargement of the lymph nodes associated with an infection or malignancy)
3. **lymphangitis** (lim-fan-JĪ-tis)	inflammation of lymph vessels
4. **lymphoma** (lim-FŌ-ma)	tumor of lymphatic tissue (malignant)

LYMPHOMAS are grouped into two general categories called **Hodgkin lymphoma** and **non-Hodgkin lymphoma**. While both forms are malignant and may involve painless swelling of lymph nodes, the diseases vary in pathology and progress differently.

TERM	DEFINITION
5. **splenomegaly** (*sple*-nō-MEG-a-lē)	enlargement of the spleen
6. **thymoma** (thī-MŌ-ma)	tumor of the thymus gland

SURGICAL TERMS

TERM	DEFINITION
7. **splenectomy** (sple-NEK-to-mē)	excision of the spleen
8. **splenorrhaphy** (sple-NOR-a-fē)	suturing, repairing of the spleen
9. **thymectomy** (thī-MEK-to-mē)	excision of the thymus gland

DIAGNOSTIC IMAGING

TERM	DEFINITION
10. **lymphangiography** (*lim*-fan-jē-OG-ra-fē)	radiographic imaging of lymph vessels

NOT Built from Word Parts

DISEASE AND DISORDERS

TERM	DEFINITION
1. infectious mononucleosis (in-FEK-shus) (*mon*-ō-*nū*-klē-Ō-sis)	acute infection caused by the Epstein-Barr virus characterized by swollen lymph nodes, sore throat, fatigue, and fever. The disease affects mostly young people and is often transmitted by saliva.
2. lymphedema (*lim*-fi-DĒ-ma)	swelling of tissue, usually of one arm or leg, caused by faulty lymphatic drainage

EXERCISE 21 ■ Pronounce and Spell

Practice pronunciation and spelling on paper and online.

1. Practice on Paper

a. **Pronounce:** Read the phonetic spelling and say aloud the terms listed in the previous table. Refer to the pronunciation key on p. 20 as necessary.
b. **Spell:** Have a study partner read the terms aloud. Write the spelling of the terms on a separate sheet of paper.

2. Practice Online

a. **Access** online learning resources. Go to evolve.elsevier.com > Evolve Resources > Student Resources.
b. **Pronounce:** Select Audio Glossary > Chapter10 > Exercise 21. Select a term to hear its pronunciation and repeat aloud.
c. **Spell:** Select Activities > Chapter 10 > Spell Terms > Exercise 21. Select the audio icon and type the correct spelling of the term.

❑ Check the box when complete.

EXERCISE 22 ■ Lymphatic System Terms Built from Word Parts

A Analyze and Define

Analyze and define the following lymphatic system terms.

1. lymphangiography
____
____

2. thymectomy
____
____

3. splenorrhaphy
____
____

4. splenomegaly
____
____

5. lymphoma
____
____

6. lymphadenitis
____
____

B Build

Build lymphatic system terms for the following definitions by using the word parts you have learned.

1. inflammation of lymph vessels ______ / ______ / ______ (WR / WR / S)

2. disease of lymph nodes ______ / ______ / ______ (WR / CV / S)

3. tumor of the thymus gland ______ / ______ (WR / S)

4. excision of the spleen ______ / ______ (WR / S)

EXERCISE 23 ■ Lymphatic System Terms *NOT* Built from Word Parts

A Label

Write the medical terms pictured and defined.

1. ______________________
acute infection caused by the Epstein-Barr virus characterized by swollen lymph nodes, sore throat, fatigue, and fever

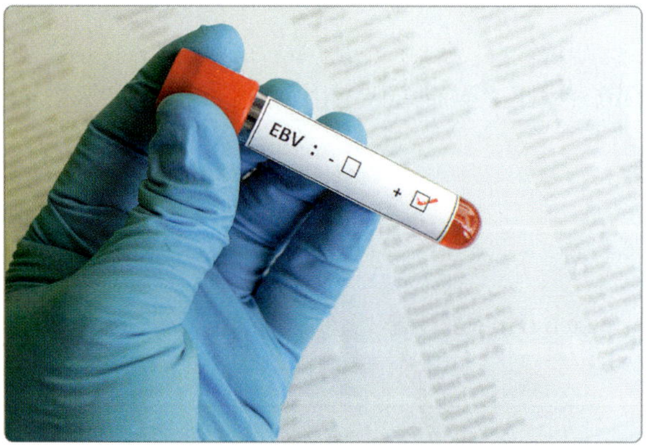

2. ______________________
swelling of tissue, usually of one arm or leg, caused faulty lymphatic drainage

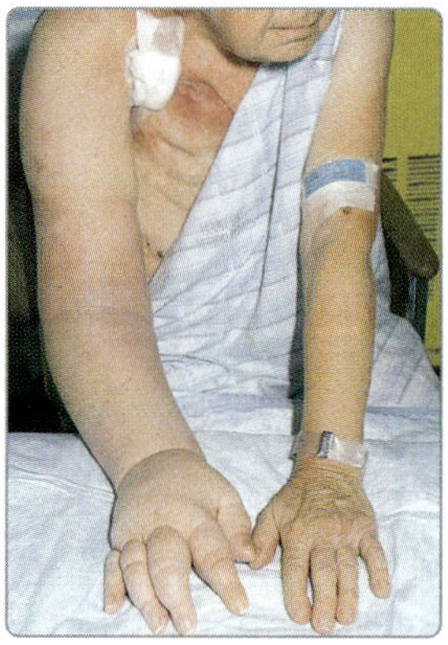

B Fill In

Fill in the blanks with the correct terms.

1. Hematologists and oncologists are medical specialists who treat ______________________, or tumor of lymphatic tissue. Treatment depends on the specific type, Hodgkin or non-Hodgkin, and sub-type of the disease.
2. Radiographic imaging of lymph vessels or ______________________ is a fluoroscopic procedure performed by an interventional radiologist; it can be used to assess the spread of cancer, determine the cause of lymphedema, and guide treatment.

3. Tumor of the thymus gland or ______________________ is associated with myasthenia gravis and other autoimmune diseases. Excision of the thymus gland or ______________________ is used as treatment for this type of tumor, which may be benign or malignant.
4. Excision of the spleen or ______________________ may be performed to ease symptoms of pain or feelings of fullness caused by an enlarged spleen or ______________________.
5. While a splenectomy would be used to treat a ruptured spleen, suturing of the spleen or ______________ would be used to repair a traumatic splenic injury.
6. Disease of the lymph nodes ______________________ is a palpable enlargement of lymph nodes commonly caused by upper respiratory infections.
7. Inflammation of lymph nodes or ______________________ is the term used when lymphadenopathy is present along with redness and tenderness; it usually results from an infection.
8. Inflammation of lymph vessels ______________________ is an infection of the lymphatic channels, often resulting from an acute streptococcal infection, and can appear as red streaks on the skin. If untreated, it can lead to cellulitis.

EXERCISE 24 ■ Review of Lymphatic System Terms

Can you define, pronounce, and spell the following lymphatic system terms?

infectious mononucleosis	lymphangiography	lymphoma	splenorrhaphy
lymphadenitis	lymphangitis	splenectomy	thymectomy
lymphadenopathy	lymphedema	splenomegaly	thymoma

Immune System Terms

BUILT FROM WORD PARTS AND *NOT* BUILT FROM WORD PARTS

The first portion of the table contains Immune System Terms that can be translated using definitions of word parts. The second portion of the table contains Immune System Terms that cannot be fully understood through translation of word parts.

■ Built from Word Parts

MEDICAL SPECIALTIES

TERM	DEFINITION	TERM	DEFINITION
1. immunologist (*im*-ū-NOL-o-jist)	physician who studies and treats immune system disorders	**2. immunology** (*im*-ū-NOL-o-jē)	study of the immune system (branch of medicine dealing with immune system disorders)

OTHER TERMS

TERM	DEFINITION
3. lymphocyte (*lim*-fa-SĪT)	lymph cell (type of leukocyte found in lymph tissue that is a part of the immune system and fights infection)

Immune System Terms—cont'd

BUILT FROM WORD PARTS AND *NOT* BUILT FROM WORD PARTS

NOT Built from Word Parts

DISEASE AND DISORDERS

TERM	DEFINITION
1. **acquired immunodeficiency syndrome (AIDS)** (a-KWĪRD) (*im*-ū-nō-de-FISH-en-sē) (SIN-drōm)	advanced, chronic immune system suppression caused by human immunodeficiency virus (HIV) infection; manifested by opportunistic infections (such as candidiasis and tuberculosis), neurologic disease (peripheral neuropathy and cognitive motor impairment), and secondary neoplasms (Kaposi sarcoma)
2. **allergy** (AL-er-jē)	hypersensitivity to a substance, resulting in an inflammatory immune response
3. **anaphylaxis** (*an*-a-fe-LAK-sis)	exaggerated reaction to a previously encountered antigen such as bee venom, peanuts, or latex. While symptoms may initially be mild, such as hives or sneezing, anaphylaxis can quickly become severe. When it leads to a drop in blood pressure and blockage of the airway (which can lead to death within minutes), it is called **anaphylactic shock**.
4. **autoimmune disease** (*aw*-tō-i-MŪN) (di-ZĒZ)	disease caused by the body's inability to distinguish its own cells from foreign bodies, thus producing antibodies that attack its own tissue. **Rheumatoid arthritis** and **systemic lupus erythematosus** are examples of autoimmune diseases.
5. **immunodeficiency** (*im*-ū-nō-de-FISH-en-sē)	disorder caused by an inability to produce an adequate immune response due to a lack of functioning antibodies, lymphocytes, or both. May be inherited, acquired by an infection, or caused by treatments, such as chemotherapy. (also called **immunocompromised**)
6. **opportunistic infections** (*op*-ar-too-NIS-tik) (in-FEK-shuns)	illnesses caused by microorganisms that are not usually pathogenic but result in disease because of a weakened immune system
7. **sarcoidosis** (*sar*-koi-DŌ-sis)	disease in which clumps of inflammatory cells form in one or more organs of the body, frequently the lungs and lymph nodes. Thought to be caused by an overreaction of the immune system to an unknown substance.

DIAGNOSTIC LABORATORY

TERM	DEFINITION
8. **erythrocyte sedimentation rate (ESR)** (e-RITH-rō-sīt) (*sed*-a-men-TĀ-shun) (rāt)	blood test that determines the amount of time it takes for red blood cells to settle at the bottom of a tube of blood. A faster than normal rate may indicate inflammation, part of the immune response. Because the test cannot identify a specific disease, it is usually combined with other, more specific tests. (also called **sed rate**)

MEDICAL SPECIALTY

TERM	DEFINITION
9. **allergist** (AL-er-jist)	physician who studies and treats allergic conditions

OTHER TERMS

TERM	DEFINITION
10. allergen (AL-er-jen)	environmental substance capable of producing a hypersensitivity reaction (allergy) in the body. Common allergens are house dust, pollen, animal dander, and various foods.
HYPERSENSITIVITY refers to a condition in which the body "overreacts" to something which it perceives to be a foreign substance, such as an allergen.	
11. antibody (AN-ti-*bod*-ē)	protective protein produced by the immune system in response to the presence of a foreign substance (antigen)
12. antigen (AN-ti-jen)	substance that triggers an immune response when introduced into the body. Examples of antigens are transplant tissue, toxins, and infectious organisms.
13. immunity (i-MŪ-ni-tē)	being resistant to specific invading pathogens
TYPES OF IMMUNITY **Inherited immunity** develops before birth and is also called inborn immunity. **Acquired immunity** develops after birth *naturally*, when antigen exposure is not deliberate, or *artificially*, when antigen exposure is deliberate.	
14. immunosuppression (*im*-ū-nō-su-PRESH-un)	state in which in the body's ability to fight infections or disease is reduced; may be caused by a disease process, be a treatment side effect, or induced with pharmaceuticals to prevent transplant rejection and to treat autoimmune diseases
15. vaccine (vak-SĒN)	suspension of weakened or killed microorganisms administered by injection, mouth, or nasal spray, which induces immunity to prevent an infectious disease

EXERCISE 25 ■ Pronounce and Spell

Practice pronunciation and spelling on paper and online.

1. Practice on Paper

a. **Pronounce:** Read the phonetic spelling and say aloud the terms listed in the previous table. Refer to the pronunciation key on p. 20 as necessary.
b. **Spell:** Have a study partner read the terms aloud. Write the spelling of the terms on a separate sheet of paper.

2. Practice Online

a. **Access** online learning resources. Go to evolve.elsevier.com > Evolve Resources > Student Resources.
b. **Pronounce:** Select Audio Glossary > Chapter10 > Exercise 25. Select a term to hear its pronunciation and repeat aloud.
c. **Spell:** Select Activities > Chapter 10 > Spell Terms > Exercise 25. Select the audio icon and type the correct spelling of the term.

❑ Check the box when complete.

EXERCISE 26 ■ Immune System Terms Built from Word Parts

Analyze and define the following immune system terms.

1. lymphocyte

____

____

2. immunology

____

____

3. i m m u n o l o g i s t

____

____

EXERCISE 27 ■ Immune System Terms *NOT* Built from Word Parts

Match the immune system terms in the first column with their definitions in the second column.

_____ 1. allergen
_____ 2. autoimmune disease
_____ 3. opportunistic infections
_____ 4. antigen
_____ 5. immunity
_____ 6. allergist
_____ 7. antibodies
_____ 8. immunodeficiency
_____ 9. sarcoidosis
_____ 10. vaccine
_____ 11. allergy
_____ 12. acquired immunodeficiency syndrome
_____ 13. anaphylaxis
_____ 14. erythrocyte sedimentation rate
_____ 15. immunosuppression

a. disorder caused by an inability to produce an adequate immune response due to a lack of functioning antibodies, lymphocytes, or both
b. advanced, chronic immune system suppression caused by HIV infection
c. administered by injection, nasal spray, or orally to prevent an infectious disease
d. protective protein produced by the immune system in response to the presence of a foreign substance
e. house dust, pollen, and animal dander are examples
f. transplant tissue, toxins, and infectious organisms are examples
g. physician who treats allergic conditions
h. disease in which clumps of inflammatory cells form in one or more organs of the body, frequently the lungs and lymph nodes
i. hypersensitivity to a substance
j. rheumatoid arthritis is an example
k. exaggerated reaction to a previously encountered antigen
l. resistant to specific invading pathogens
m. illnesses caused by microorganisms that are not usually pathogenic but result in disease becuase of a weakened immune system
n. the body's ability to fight infections or disease is reduced
o. blood test that determines the amount of time it takes for red blood cells to settle at the bottom of a tube of blood

EXERCISE 28 ■ Fill In

Fill in the blanks with the correct terms.

1. A(n) ______________________, an environmental substance capable of producing a hypersensitivity reaction, is a specific type of ______________________ or substance that triggers an immune response when introduced into the body. A(n) ______________________ is a protective protein produced by the immune system in response to the presence of an antigen.
2. An exaggerated reaction to a previously encountered antigen such as bee venom, peanuts, or latex is called ______________________. While symptoms may initially be mild, such as hives or sneezing, it can quickly become severe. When it leads to a drop in blood pressure and blockage of the airway (which can lead to death within minutes), it is called anaphylactic shock.
3. ______________________ is a disease in which clumps of inflammatory cells form in one or more organs of the body, frequently the lungs and lymph nodes. It is thought to be caused by an overreaction of the immune system to an unknown substance.
4. A blood test that determines the amount of time it takes for red blood cells to settle at the bottom of a tube of blood that may indicate inflammation is called ______________________ and is abbreviated as ________.

5. A lymph cell or ________________________ is a type of leukocyte found in lymph tissue that is a part of the immune system and fights infection.
6. The suspension of weakened or killed microorganisms administered by injection, mouth, or nasal spray, or a(n) ____________________, aims to prevent infectious disease by causing ____________________, or being resistant to specific invading pathogens.
7. Patients with ________________________________, abbreviated as ________, or advanced, chronic immune system suppression caused by human immunodeficiency virus are particularly at risk for ____________________ or illnesses caused by microorganisms that are not usually pathogenic but result in disease because of a weakened immune system.
8. A state in which in the body's ability to fight infections or disease is reduced or ____________________ may be caused by a disease process, be a treatment side effect, or induced with pharmaceuticals to prevent transplant rejection and to treat autoimmune diseases.
9. Study of the immune system or ____________________ is the branch of medicine concerned with how the body protects itself from pathogens and considers its underperformance, such as ____________________ or an inability to produce an adequate immune response, and overperformance, such as ____________________ or hypersensitivity to a substance, resulting in an inflammatory immune response
10. A clinical ____________________, or physician who studies and treats immune system disorders, treats patients with ____________________, or disease caused by the body's inability to distinguish its own cells from foreign bodies; they may also be involved in the care of those receiving transplants or immunotherapy. A(n) ____________________, or physician who studies and treats allergic conditions is a board-certified physician sometimes referred to as an allergist/immunologist, which indicates the ability to diagnose and treat allergies, asthma, and immune deficiency disorders.

EXERCISE 29 ■ Review of Immune System Terms

Can you define, pronounce, and spell the following immune system terms?

acquired immunodeficiency syndrome (AIDS)
allergen
allergist
allergy
anaphylaxis
antibody
antigen
autoimmune disease
erythrocyte sedimentation rate (ESR)
immunity
immunodeficiency
immunologist
immunology
immunosuppression
lymphocyte
opportunistic infections
sarcoidosis
vaccine

Abbreviations

DISEASE AND DISORDERS

ABBREVIATION	TERM	ABBREVIATION	TERM
ACS	acute coronary syndrome	**HF**	heart failure
AFib	atrial fibrillation	**HHD**	hypertensive heart disease
CAD	coronary artery disease	**MI**	myocardial infarction
DVT	deep vein thrombosis	**PAD**	peripheral artery disease

SIGNS AND SYMPTOMS

ABBREVIATION	TERM
HTN	hypertension

Abbreviations—cont'd

DIAGNOSTIC

ABBREVIATION	TERM	ABBREVIATION	TERM
aPTT	activated partial thromboplastin time	**ECHO**	echocardiogram
BP	blood pressure	**ESR**	erythrocyte sedimentation rate
CBC with diff	complete blood count with differential	**Hct**	hematocrit
CPK	creatine phosphokinase	**Hgb**	hemoglobin
CRP	C-reactive protein	**PT**	prothrombin time
DSA	digital subtraction angiography	**SPECT**	single-photon emission computed tomography
ECG, EKG	electrocardiogram	**TEE**	transesophageal echocardiogram

TREATMENTS

ABBREVIATION	TERM	ABBREVIATION	TERM
AICD	automatic implantable cardiac defibrillator	**CPR**	cardiopulmonary resuscitation
BMT	bone marrow transplant	**PBSCT**	peripheral blood stem cell transplant
CABG	coronary artery bypass graft	**PTCA**	percutaneous transluminal coronary angioplasty

DESCRIPTIVE

ABBREVIATION	TERM	ABBREVIATION	TERM
AV	atrioventricular	**IV**	intravenous

OTHER

ABBREVIATION	TERM	ABBREVIATION	TERM
CCU	coronary care unit	**WBC**	white blood cell (leukocyte)
RBC	red blood cell (erythrocyte)		

Refer to **Appendix D** for a complete list of abbreviations.

EXERCISE 30 ■ Abbreviations

Write the terms abbreviated.

1. **CAD** ______________ ______________ ______________ has received growing interest over the past several years. Diagnostic procedures for new patients usually begin with an exercise **ECG** ______________________________. Patients whose stress tests are borderline usually proceed to noninvasive imaging such as **SPECT** ______________-______________ ______________ ______________ ______________ and stress **ECHO** ______________________________.
2. **DVT** ______________ ______________ ______________ is common in hospitalized patients. Early detection is important because DVT can result in death from a pulmonary embolism. Doppler ultrasound is a noninvasive diagnostic procedure used to diagnose DVT. MRI and venography may be used as well.
3. The **CBC** ______________ ______________ ______________ **with diff** ______________ is a series of automated laboratory tests of the peripheral blood that provide a great deal of information about the blood and

other body organs. Tests performed as part of the CBC are **RBC** ________ ________ ________ count, **WBC** ________ ________ ________ count and differential, **Hgb** ________, and **Hct** ________.

4. Standard surgical treatment for CAD includes **CABG** ________ ________ ________ ________. There is a growth in the use of minimally invasive techniques to treat CAD, which include transmyocardial laser revascularization and **PTCA** ________ ________ ________ ________, atherectomy, and coronary stent placement.
5. Hospitalized patients diagnosed with **MI** ________ ________ are cared for in the **CCU** ________ ________ ________.
6. A sphygmomanometer is used to measure **BP** ________ ________.
7. Diagnosis used to indicate that a patient's heart is unable to pump enough blood through the body to supply tissues is **HF** ________ ________.
8. If the patient's heart and/or lungs have ceased to function, the medical team must begin **CPR** ________ ________.
9. A patient with persistently elevated blood pressure is likely to be diagnosed with **HHD** ________ ________ ________.
10. When scheduling blood tests for a patient on oral anticoagulant medication, the doctor is likely to include a **PT** ________ ________.
11. Any interruption of the conduction of electrical impulses from the atria to the ventricles is called **AV** ________ block.
12. The treatment of **ACS** ________ ________ ________ is aimed at preventing thrombus formation and restoring blood flow to the occluded coronary artery.
13. Stopping smoking, exercising, and proper diet are important in the medical management of **PAD** ________ ________ ________.
14. **DSA** ________ ________ ________ is especially valuable in cardiac diagnostic applications.
15. The physician ordered a **TEE** ________ ________ to examine the patient's heart structure and function.
16. Two blood tests used in assessing and evaluating cardiovascular diseases are **CRP** ________ ________ and **CPK** ________ ________.
17. A patient experiencing **AFib** ________ ________ may be referred to an electrophysiologist, a cardiology subspecialist.
18. An **AICD** ________ ________ ________ ________ delivers an electric shock to convert an arrhythmia back to normal rhythm.
19. The patient with dehydration was ordered **IV** ________ fluids by her physician.
20. **HTN** ________ is usually diagnosed when a patient has elevated blood pressure on two separate occasions.
21. The primary difference between **PBSCT** ________ ________ ________ ________ ________ and **BMT** ________ ________ ________ is whether stem cells are collected from blood or bone marrow.
22. **ESR** ________ ________ ________ or sed rate indirectly measures the degree of inflammation in the body and is used to help detect inflammation associated with infections, cancers, and autoimmune diseases.

PRACTICAL APPLICATION

EXERCISE 31 ■ Case Study: Translate Between Everyday Language and Medical Language

CASE STUDY: Natalia Krouse

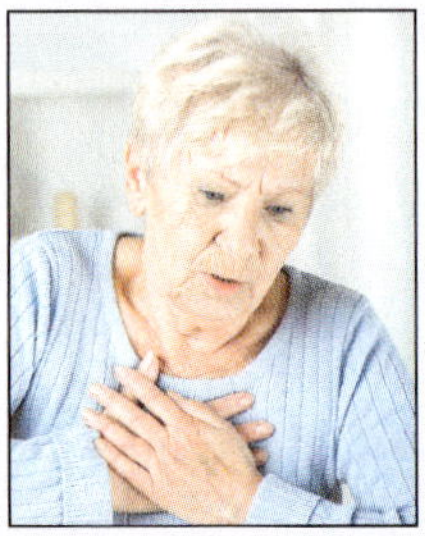

Natalia has not been feeling well lately. She seems to feel "wiped out" most of the time. She wonders if maybe her medicine for high blood pressure isn't working as well as it used to. Tonight she went for her usual walk after dinner with her dogs. She had barely made it down the driveway when she started feeling pain in her chest. It felt like something pushing down on her and squeezing her. She noticed pain in her left arm and even in her jaw. She noticed her heart was racing, and she was breathing faster than usual. She was also feeling dizzy at the same time and was afraid she might pass out. She stopped to sit down and after about 5 minutes she started feeling a little better. Her neighbor saw her and called 911. An ambulance came and took her to the emergency department.

Now that you have worked through Chapter 10 on the cardiovascular system, consider the medical terms that might be used to describe Natalia's experience. See the Chapter at a Glance section at the end of the chapter for a list of terms that might apply.

A. *Underline phrases in the case study that could be substituted with medical terms.*

B. *Write the medical term and its definition for three of the phrases you underlined.*

MEDICAL TERM	DEFINITION
1. ____________________	______________________________
2. ____________________	______________________________
3. ____________________	______________________________

DOCUMENTATION: Excerpt from Hospital Admission Report

Natalia was brought to the emergency department and was admitted to the cardiology floor of the hospital. A portion of her history from the electronic medical record is noted below.

The patient has an extensive history of chronic cardiovascular issues. Coronary artery disease risk factors include hypertension and hypercholesterolemia. She also has extensive varicose veins of the lower extremities bilaterally. Her family physician referred her to a cardiologist in 2003 for medical management of these complications. She smokes one pack of cigarettes a day and has previously declined participation in a smoking cessation program. She is not diabetic. Family history reveals a brother who had coronary artery bypass grafts and a mother deceased from abdominal aortic aneurysm rupture.

C. *Underline medical terms presented in Chapter 10 in the previous excerpt from Natalia's medical record. See the Chapter at a Glance section at the end of the chapter for a complete list.*

D. *Select and define three of the medical terms you underlined. To check your answers, go to Appendix A.*

MEDICAL TERM	DEFINITION
1. ____________________	______________________________
2. ____________________	______________________________
3. ____________________	______________________________

EXERCISE 32 ■ Interact With Medical Documents

A

Read the report and complete it by writing medical terms on answer lines within the document. Definitions of terms to be written appear after the document.

9011401 CALDWELL, Jack

File Patient Navigate Custom Fields Help

Chart Review | Encounters | Notes | Labs | Imaging | Procedures | Rx | Documents | Referrals | Scheduling | Billing

Name: **Jack Caldwell** MR#: 9011401 DOB: 02/13/19xx Gender: M Age: 22 **Allergies:** None known **PCP:** Alberto Salazar, DO

Family Practice Clinic Office Visit Note

CC: Swollen glands in neck

S: 22-year-old male with a 3-month history of swollen glands, fever and chills, fatigue and night sweats. Also notes decreased appetite and a 10-pound weight loss over last 2 months. Past medical history is significant for 1.______________ ______________ at age 15, with severe 2.____________________. A 3.____________________ was performed at that time. His PMH is otherwise unremarkable. He does not smoke and drinks alcohol approximately 2x weekly. He denies use of other drugs. Family history is significant for an uncle with 4.____________________________. He is up to date on all of his 5.__________________.

O. Vital signs: temp = 99.7° F, P = 98 bpm, BP = 102/68 mm Hg, R = 16. General: A thin white male in no acute distress. HEENT exam is significant for bilateral non-tender 6.__________________ in the anterior and posterior cervical neck, as well as in the supraclavicular and submental areas. Lungs are clear to auscultation and cardiovascular exam reveals a regular rate with no 7.____________, with normal pulses for all extremities. Abdominal exam is unremarkable. There is no evidence of enlarged lymph nodes in the groin or armpits.

A/P: This presentation is very suspicious for Hodgkin 8.___________________. We will order a complete blood count and differential to look for 9.__________________ and other blood diseases. We will schedule him for a lymph node biopsy and a CT scan of the chest, abdomen, and pelvis. A 10.__________ __________ ____________ may be necessary for staging if lymphoma is confirmed. We will also refer him to a 11._______________/oncologist.

Start | Log On/Off | Print | Edit

Definitions of Medical Terms to Complete the Document

Write the medical terms defined on corresponding answer lines in the document.

1. acute infection caused by the Epstein-Barr virus characterized by swollen lymph nodes, sore throat, fatigue, and fever
2. enlargement of the spleen
3. excision of the spleen
4. tumor of lymphatic tissue (malignant)
5. suspension of weakened or killed microorganisms administered by injection, mouth, or nasal spray (plural form of the term)
6. disease of lymph nodes
7. any disturbance or abnormality in the heart's normal rhythmic pattern
8. tumor of lymphatic tissue (malignant)
9. malignant disease characterized by excessive increase in abnormal leukocytes formed in the bone marrow
10. procedure to obtain a sample of the solid portion of bone marrow, usually from the ilium, for study
11. physician who studies and treats diseases of the blood

EXERCISE 32 ■ Interact With Medical Documents—cont'd

B

Read the medical report and answer the questions below it.

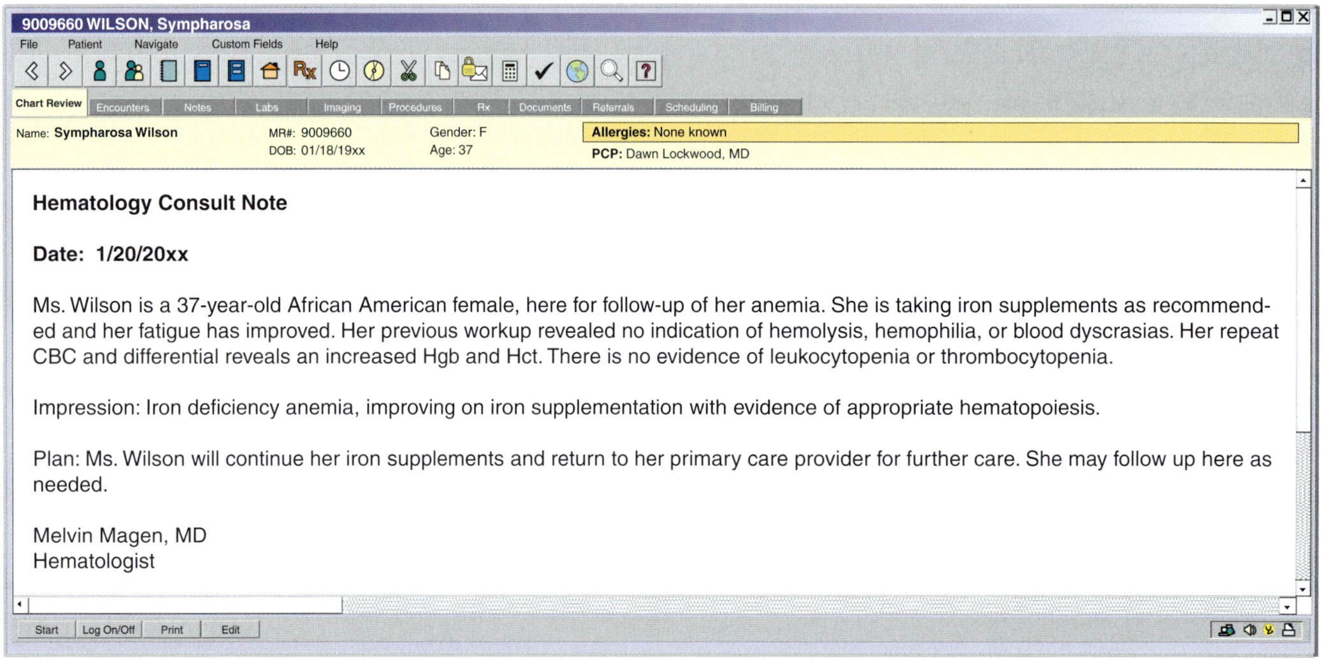

9009660 WILSON, Sympharosa

File Patient Navigate Custom Fields Help

Chart Review | Encounters | Notes | Labs | Imaging | Procedures | Rx | Documents | Referrals | Scheduling | Billing

Name: **Sympharosa Wilson** MR#: 9009660 DOB: 01/18/19xx Gender: F Age: 37 **Allergies:** None known **PCP:** Dawn Lockwood, MD

Hematology Consult Note

Date: 1/20/20xx

Ms. Wilson is a 37-year-old African American female, here for follow-up of her anemia. She is taking iron supplements as recommended and her fatigue has improved. Her previous workup revealed no indication of hemolysis, hemophilia, or blood dyscrasias. Her repeat CBC and differential reveals an increased Hgb and Hct. There is no evidence of leukocytopenia or thrombocytopenia.

Impression: Iron deficiency anemia, improving on iron supplementation with evidence of appropriate hematopoiesis.

Plan: Ms. Wilson will continue her iron supplements and return to her primary care provider for further care. She may follow up here as needed.

Melvin Magen, MD
Hematologist

Start | Log On/Off | Print | Edit

Use the medical report above to answer the questions.

1. Ms. Wilson was seen in the hematology clinic for:
   a. a low platelet count
   b. a low erythrocyte count
   c. a low white blood cell count
2. Her repeat CBC and differential revealed an improved:
   a. hemoglobin and C-reactive protein
   b. hematocrit and troponin
   c. hemoglobin and hematocrit
3. The consulting doctor was a physician who studies and treats:
   a. immune system disorders
   b. diseases of the blood
   c. diseases of the heart
4. **True** or **False**: the patient had evidence of dissolution of red blood cells.
5. **True** or **False**: the reason for the hematology consult was erythrocytopenia.

EXERCISE 33 ■ Use Medical Language in Online Electronic Health Records

Select the correct medical terms to complete three medical records in one patient's electronic file.

Access online resources at evolve.elsevier.com > Evolve Resources > Student Resources > Activities > Chapter 10 > Electronic Health Records

Topic: CAD
Record 1: Echocardiogram Report
Record 2: Cardiovascular Operative Report
Record 3: Discharge Summary

❑ Check the box when complete.

EXERCISE 34 ■ Pronounce Medical Terms in Use

Practice pronunciation of terms by reading aloud the following paragraph. Use the phonetic spellings to assist with pronunciation. The script also contains medical terms not presented in the chapter. If interested, research their meanings in a medical dictionary or a reliable online source.

A 55-year-old man presented to his doctor with pain in the calf and swelling in the left foot and ankle. Three days prior, the patient had completed trans-Pacific airline travel, spending several hours in a sitting position. He has a history of **varicose veins** (VAR-i-kōs) (vānz). No previous history of **hypertension** (*hī*-per-TEN-shun) or **thrombophlebitis** (*throm*-bō-fle-BĪ-tis) existed. Physical examination revealed an edematous left lower extremity and a tender calf. The pedal **pulse** (puls) was intact. A **Doppler ultrasound** (DOP-ler) (UL-tra-sound) was obtained, which revealed **deep vein thrombosis** (dēp) (vān) (throm-BŌ-sis). He was treated as an outpatient with apixaban and will continue this therapy for at least 3 months. Unlike warfarin, this oral **anticoagulant** (an-tī-kō-AG-ū-lant) therapy does not require routine monitoring of the **prothrombin time** (prō-THROM-bin) (tīm).

CHAPTER REVIEW

EXERCISE 35 ■ Chapter Content Quiz

Test your understanding of terms and abbreviations introduced in this chapter. Circle the letter for the medical term or abbreviation related to the words in italics.

1. Ms. Tompkins was diagnosed with sickle cell disease and was sent to a *physician who studies and treats diseases of the blood* for further evaluation.
   a. cardiologist
   b. immunologist
   c. hematologist
2. Following a trans-Pacific flight, Kenji Makoto developed *inflammation of the vein associated with a blood clot*, which was probably due to sitting for a long period of time.
   a. thrombophlebitis
   b. lymphadenitis
   c. atherosclerosis
3. Ted Lauer had a *record of the electrical activity of the heart* to follow up on his atrial fibrillation.
   a. CPR
   b. ECG
   c. ECHO
4. Mr. Schonfeld was diagnosed with a 6-cm abdominal aortic *ballooning of a weakened portion of a vessel wall*, which required surgical repair with an endograft.
   a. embolism
   b. thrombosis
   c. aneurysm
5. On physical examination of the neck, Samantha Winslow was noted to have *disease of lymph nodes (abnormal enlargement of the lymph nodes)*.
   a. lymphoma
   b. lymphadenopathy
   c. lymphadenitis
6. After finishing a course of immunosuppressive medication for cancer treatment, a CBC revealed that the patient had *abnormal reduction of white blood cells*.
   a. leukocytopenia
   b. anemia
   c. thrombocytopenia
7. Mr. Matthews has an allergy to peanuts; he carries an EpiPen to prevent *episodes of exaggerated reaction to a previously encountered antigen, which can lead to death within minutes*.
   a. immunodeficiency
   b. anaphylaxis
   c. autoimmune disease
8. Mrs. Patel was experiencing *episodes of chest pain that occurs when there is an insufficient amount of blood to the heart muscle* and was scheduled for an exercise stress test.
   a. acute coronary syndrome
   b. atrial fibrillation
   c. angina pectoris
9. Because Mr. Jiang is taking warfarin, he needs to have his *blood test used to determine certain coagulation activity defects and to monitor anticoagulation therapy* tested regularly.
   a. prothrombin time
   b. hematocrit
   c. hemoglobin
10. Mr. MacDougal was brought to the emergency department after suffering chest trauma in a motor vehicle accident. His symptoms and chest x-ray were suspicious for aortic rupture, so a(n) *radiographic image of the aorta* was obtained.
    a. arteriogram
    b. aortogram
    c. venogram
11. After her myocardial infarction, Mrs. Alvarez was found to have 95% blockage in three sections of her coronary arteries. Thus, a *surgical technique to bring a new blood supply to heart muscle by detouring around blocked arteries* was performed.
    a. coronary stent
    b. angiography
    c. coronary artery bypass graft
12. Mr. Williams suffered from pancytopenia after his chemotherapy, so the hematologist ordered a(n) *infusion of healthy bone marrow cells from a matched donor into a patient with severely diseased or damaged bone marrow*.
    a. bone marrow aspiration
    b. bone marrow biopsy
    c. bone marrow transplant
13. Kelly Anastopoulis was recently diagnosed with rheumatoid arthritis, a(n) *disease caused by the body's inability to distinguish its own cells from foreign bodies*, when she had symptoms of joint pain and swelling in her hands.
    a. immunodeficiency
    b. blood dyscrasia
    c. autoimmune disease

14. Mrs. Rosenberg was admitted to the hospital to rule out a myocardial infarction. A phlebotomist performed a venipuncture to obtain labs, including a *blood test to measure the level of an enzyme of heart and skeletal muscle released into the blood after muscle injury or necrosis*.
    a. CPK
    b. CRP
    c. CBC
15. Ryan Lee developed *inflammation of the sac surrounding the heart* after a viral upper respiratory infection.
    a. myocarditis
    b. pericarditis
    c. endocarditis
16. Mr. O'Leary presented with symptoms of a stroke. *Process of digital radiographic imaging of the blood vessels that "subtracts" or removes structures not being studied* was performed to see if thrombolytic therapy was appropriate.
    a. digital subtraction angiography
    b. transesophageal echocardiogram
    c. single-photon emission computed tomography
17. During his high school sports physical, Habib El-Amin was found to have a(n) *unusual sound heard during auscultation of the heart caused by turbulent blood flow*.
    a. extravasation
    b. murmur
    c. bruit
18. The surgeon performed an emergency *suturing, repairing of the spleen* after Theresa Pangilinan ruptured it playing lacrosse.
    a. splenectomy
    b. thymectomy
    c. splenorrhaphy
19. The cardiologist recommended a *battery-powered apparatus implanted under the skin to treat an abnormal heart rhythm* for Mr. Jones, who had episodes of severe bradycardia.
    a. artificial cardiac pacemaker
    b. automatic implantable cardiac defibrillator
    c. percutaneous transluminal coronary angioplasty
20. Because she was over the age of 65, the physician recommended a pneumonia *suspension of weakened or killed microorganisms administered by injection, mouth, or nasal spray* for Mrs. Kurtz.
    a. venipuncture
    b. vaccine
    c. vasoconstrictor

CHAPTER AT A GLANCE Word Parts New to This Chapter

COMBINING FORMS

angi/o
aort/o
arteri/o
ather/o
atri/o
cardi/o
ech/o
electr/o
embol/o
immun/o
isch/o
lymph/o
lymphaden/o
myel/o
phleb/o
plasm/o
splen/o
thromb/o
thym/o
valvul/o
ven/o
ventricul/o

PREFIXES

-brady
-pan

SUFFIXES

-apheresis
-penia
-rrhage
-sclerosis

CHAPTER AT A GLANCE Terms Built from Word Parts

CARDIOVASCULAR

angiography
angioma
angioplasty
angioscopy
angiostenosis
aortic stenosis
aortogram
arteriogram
arteriosclerosis
atherectomy
atherosclerosis
atrioventricular (AV)
bradycardia
cardiogenic
cardiologist
cardiology
cardiomegaly
cardiomyopathy
echocardiogram (ECHO)
electrocardiogram (ECG, EKG)
electrocardiography
embolectomy
endarterectomy
endocarditis
intravenous (IV)
ischemia
myocarditis
pericardiocentesis
pericarditis
phlebectomy
phlebitis
polyarteritis
tachycardia
thrombophlebitis
valvulitis
valvuloplasty
venogram

BLOOD

embolism
embolus (*pl.* emboli)
erythrocytopenia
hematologist
hematoma
hemolysis
hemorrhage
hemostasis
leukocytopenia
lymphocytosis
multiple myeloma
pancytopenia
phlebotomy
plasmapheresis
thrombocytopenia
thrombolysis
thrombosis
thrombus

LYMPHATIC

lymphadenitis
lymphadenopathy
lymphangiography
lymphangitis
lymphoma
splenectomy
splenomegaly
splenorrhaphy
thymectomy
thymoma

IMMUNE

immunologist
immunology
lymphocyte

CHAPTER AT A GLANCE Terms *NOT* Built from Word Parts

CARDIOVASCULAR

acute coronary syndrome (ACS)
aneurysm
angina pectoris
arrhythmia
artificial cardiac pacemaker
automatic implantable cardiac defibrillator (AICD)
blood pressure (BP)
bruit
cardiac arrest
cardiac catheterization
cardiac tamponade
cardiopulmonary resuscitation (CPR)
catheter ablation
cor pulmonale
coronary artery bypass graft (CABG)
coronary artery disease (CAD)
coronary stent
C-reactive protein (CRP)
creatine phosphokinase (CPK)
deep vein thrombosis (DVT)
defibrillation
digital subtraction angiography (DSA)
Doppler ultrasound
exercise stress test
femoropopliteal bypass
fibrillation
heart failure (HF)
hypercholesterolemia
hyperlipidemia
hypertension (HTN)
hypertensive heart disease (HHD)
hypertriglyceridemia
hypotension
intermittent claudication
lipid profile
mitral valve stenosis
murmur
myocardial infarction (MI)
occlusion
percutaneous transluminal coronary angioplasty (PTCA)
peripheral artery disease (PAD)
pulse
rheumatic heart disease
sestamibi test
single-photon emission computed tomography (SPECT)
sphygmomanometer
thrombolytic therapy
transesophageal echocardiogram (TEE)
troponin
varicose veins
vasoconstrictor
vasodilator

BLOOD

activated partial thromboplastin time (aPTT)
anemia
anticoagulant
bleeding disorder
bleeding profile
blood dyscrasia
bone marrow aspiration
bone marrow biopsy
bone marrow transplant (BMT)
complete blood count (CBC) and differential (Diff)
extravasation
hematocrit (Hct)
hemoglobin (Hgb)
hemophilia
leukemia
perfusionist
peripheral blood stem cell transplant (PBSCT)
phlebotomist
prothrombin time (PT/INR)
sepsis
sickle cell disease
thalassemia
venipuncture

LYMPHATIC

infectious mononucleosis
lymphedema

IMMUNE

acquired immunodeficiency syndrome (AIDS)
allergen
allergist
allergy
anaphylaxis
antibody
antigen
autoimmune disease
erythrocyte
immunodeficiency
opportunistic infections
sarcoidosis
sedimentation rate (ESR)
vaccine

Chapter 11

Digestive System

Outline

Objectives

Upon completion of this chapter, you will be able to:

1. Pronounce organs and anatomic structures of the digestive system.
2. Define and spell word parts related to the digestive system.
3. Define, pronounce, and spell disease and disorder terms related to the digestive system.
4. Define, pronounce, and spell surgical terms related to the digestive system.
5. Define, pronounce, and spell diagnostic terms related to the digestive system.
6. Define, pronounce, and spell complementary terms related to the digestive system.
7. Interpret the meaning of abbreviations related to the digestive system.
8. Apply medical language in clinical contexts.

ANATOMY

The digestive system, also known as the alimentary canal or the gastrointestinal tract and abbreviated as GI tract, is a long continuous tube comprising the mouth, pharynx, esophagus, stomach, small intestine, large intestine, rectum, and anus. Accessory organs of the digestive system are the salivary glands, liver, bile ducts, gallbladder, and pancreas. (Figs. 11.1 through 11.5)

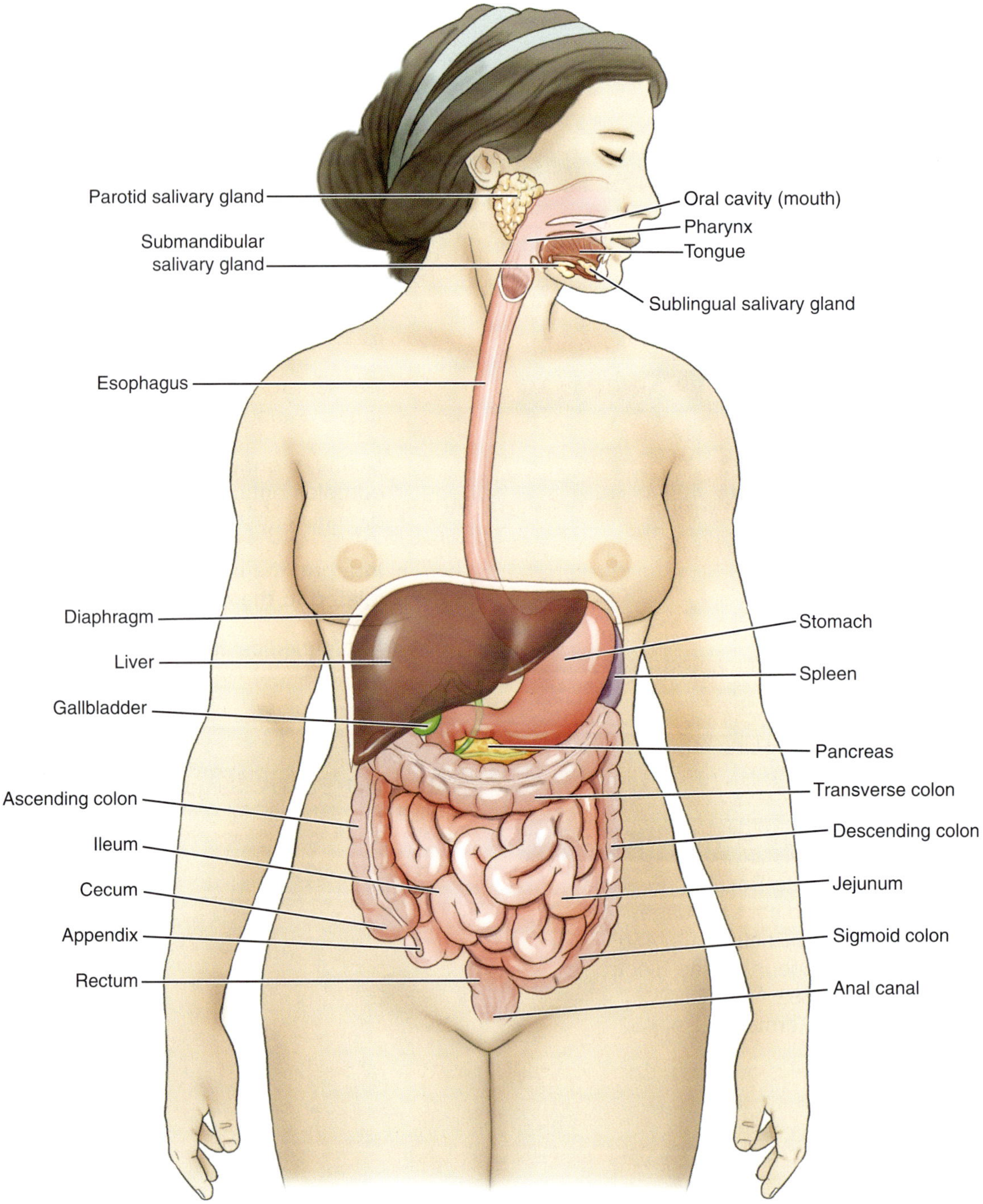

FIG. 11.1 Organs of the digestive system.

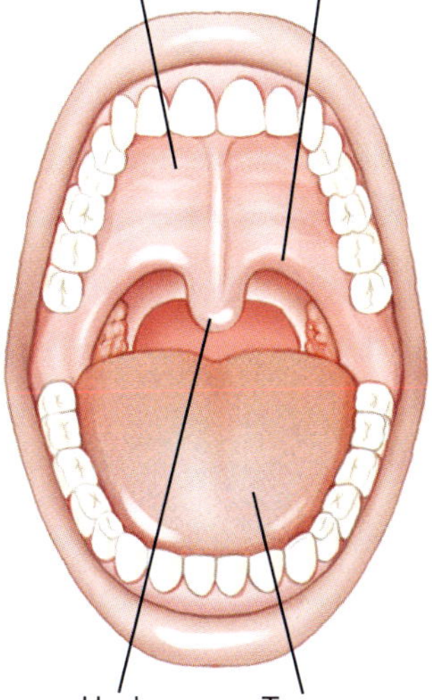

FIG. 11.2 The oral cavity.

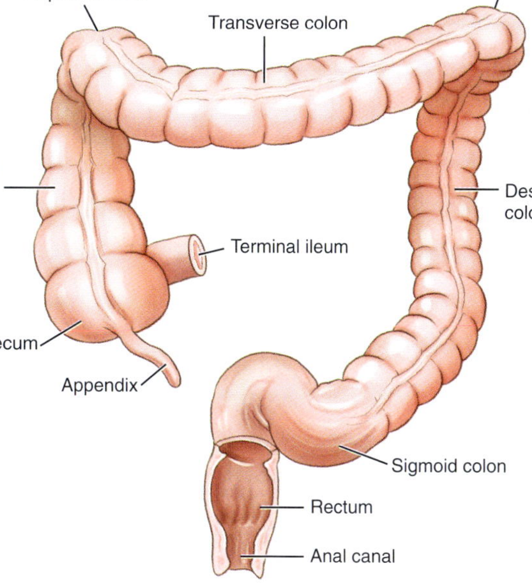

FIG. 11.3 Anatomy of the large intestine.

Function

Functions of the digestive system are **ingestion**, the taking in of nutrients through the mouth; **digestion**, the mechanical and chemical breakdown of food for use by body cells; **absorption**, the transfer of digested food from the small intestine to the blood stream; and **elimination**, the removal of solid waste from the body.

Organs and Anatomic Structures of the Digestive System

TERM	DEFINITION
mouth (mouth)	opening through which food passes into the body; breaks food into small particles by mastication (chewing) and mixing with saliva (Fig. 11.2)
tongue (tung)	consists mostly of skeletal muscle; attached in the posterior region of the mouth. It provides movement of food for mastication, directs food to the pharynx for swallowing, and is a major organ for taste and speech.
palate (PAL-et)	separates the nasal cavity from the oral cavity
soft palate (sawft) (PAL-et)	posterior portion, not supported by bone
hard palate (hawrd) (PAL-et)	anterior portion, supported by bone
uvula (Ū-vū-la)	soft V-shaped structure that extends from the soft palate; directs food into the throat
pharynx (FAR-inks)	performs the swallowing action that passes food from the mouth into the esophagus (also called **throat**)

Organs and Anatomic Structures of the Digestive System—cont'd

TERM	DEFINITION
esophagus (e-SOF-a-gus)	10-inch (25-cm) tube that is a passageway for food extending from the pharynx to the stomach. **Peristalsis**, involuntary wavelike movements that propel food along the gastrointestinal tract, begins in the esophagus.
stomach (STUM-ek)	J-shaped sac that mixes and stores food. It secretes chemicals for digestion and hormones that act locally to control digestive system functions.
cardia (KAR-dē-a)	area around the opening of the esophagus
fundus (FUN-dus)	proximal domed portion of the stomach
body (BOD-ē)	central portion of the stomach, distal to the fundus
antrum (AN-trum)	distal portion of the stomach
pylorus (pī-LOR-us)	portion of the stomach that connects to the small intestine
pyloric sphincter (pī-LOR-ik) (SFINK-ter)	ring of muscle that guards the opening between the stomach and the duodenum
small intestine (smal) (in-TES-tin)	20-foot (6-m) tube extending from the pyloric sphincter to the large intestine. **Digestion** is completed in the small intestine. **Absorption**, the passage of the nutrients (end products of digestion) from the small intestine to the bloodstream, takes place through the **villi**, tiny fingerlike projections that line the walls of the small intestine.
duodenum (dū-OD-e-num)	first 10 to 12 inches (25 cm) of the small intestine
DUODENUM is derived from the Latin **duodeni**, meaning **12 each**, a reference to its length. It was named in 240 BC by a Greek physician. **Jejunum** is derived from the Latin **jejunus**, meaning **empty**; it was so named because the early anatomists always found it empty. **Ileum** is derived from the Greek **eilein**, meaning to **roll**, a reference to the peristaltic waves that move food along the gastrointestinal tract. This term was first used in the early part of the 17th century.	
jejunum (je-JŪ-num)	second portion of the small intestine, approximately 8 feet (2.4 m) long
ileum (IL-ē-um)	third portion of the small intestine, approximately 11 feet (3.3 m) long, which connects with the large intestine
large intestine (larj) (in-TES-tin)	approximately 5 feet (1.5 m) long tube that extends from the ileum to the anus (Fig. 11.3). **Absorption** of water and transit of the solid waste products of digestion take place in the large intestine.
cecum (SĒ-kum)	U-shaped pouch that is the first portion of the large intestine
colon (KŌ-lun)	main portion of the large intestine. The colon is divided into four parts: ascending colon, transverse colon, descending colon, and sigmoid colon.
rectum (REK-tum)	distal portion of the large intestine, approximately 8 to 10 inches (20 cm) long, extending from the sigmoid colon to the anus
anus (Ā-nus)	sphincter muscle (ringlike band of muscle fiber that keeps an opening tight) at the end of the gastrointestinal tract. Provides for **elimination** of solid waste products of digestion.

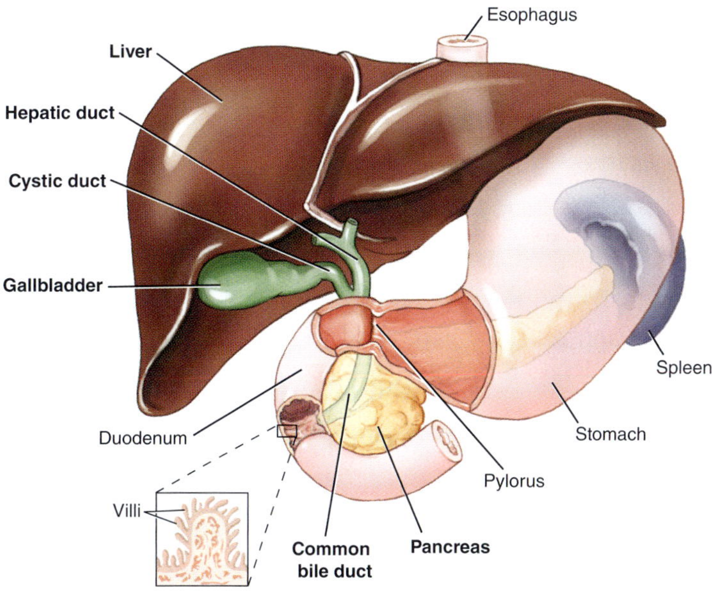

FIG. 11.4 Accessory organs: liver, hepatic duct, cystic duct, gallbladder, common bile duct, and pancreas. Salivary glands, also accessory organs, are shown in Fig. 11.1.

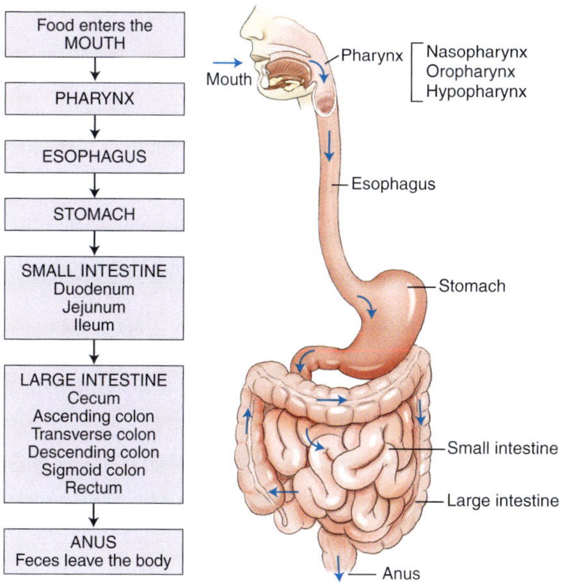

FIG. 11.5 Pathway of food.

TERM	DEFINITION
ACCESSORY ORGANS (Fig. 11.4)	
salivary glands (SAL-i-*ver*-ē) (glans)	produce saliva, which flows into the mouth (Fig. 11.1)
liver (LIV-er)	produces bile, which is necessary for the digestion of fats. The liver performs many other functions concerned with digestion and metabolism.
biliary tract (BIL-ē-ar-ē) (trakt)	organs and ducts (passageways) that transport, store, and release bile (also called **biliary system**)
bile ducts (bīl) (dukts)	passageways that carry bile. The **hepatic duct** collects bile formed in the liver. The **cystic duct** transports bile to and from the gallbladder for storage.
common bile duct (ka-mon)(bīl) (dukt)	small, tubelike structure where the hepatic duct and cystic duct join; conveys bile to the duodenum to aid in the breakdown of fats
gallbladder (GAWL-blad-er)	small, saclike structure that stores bile produced by the liver
pancreas (PAN-krē-us)	produces pancreatic juice, which helps digest all types of food; secretes insulin for carbohydrate metabolism
PANCREAS is derived from the Greek **pan**, meaning **all**, and **krea**, meaning **flesh**. The pancreas was first described in 300 BC. It was so named because of its fleshy appearance.	
OTHER STRUCTURES	
peritoneum (*per*-i-tō-NĒ-um)	serous saclike lining of the abdominal and pelvic cavities
appendix (a-PEN-diks)	small pouch, which has no known function in digestion; attached to the cecum (also called **vermiform appendix**)
abdomen (AB-duh-men)	portion of the body between the thorax and the pelvis

PRONOUNCE ANATOMIC STRUCTURES

Practice saying aloud each of the organs and specific structures on the previous pages.

To hear the terms, go to Evolve Resources at www.evolve.elsevier.com and select:
Student Resources > Audio Glossary > Chapter 11 > Anatomic Structures

❑ Check the box when complete.

WORD PARTS

Use paper flashcards or electronic flashcards on Evolve to memorize word parts used to analyze, define, and build medical terms in this chapter. To reinforce learning, study one section of the Word Parts Table at a time, then complete the corresponding exercise on the following pages.

1 ■ Digestive System Combining Forms

COMBINING FORM	DEFINITION
an/o	anus
antr/o	antrum
cec/o	cecum
col/o	colon (large intestine)
colon/o	colon (large intestine)
duoden/o	duodenum
enter/o	intestines (usually the small intestine)
esophag/o	esophagus
gastr/o	stomach
ile/o	ileum
jejun/o	jejunum
or/o	mouth
proct/o	rectum
rect/o	rectum
sigmoid/o	sigmoid colon
stomat/o	mouth

2 ■ Accessory Organs and Combining Forms Used with Digestive System Terms

COMBINING FORM	DEFINITION
abdomin/o	abdomen, abdominal cavity
append/o	appendix
appendic/o	appendix
celi/o	abdomen, abdominal cavity
cheil/o	lip(s)
cholangi/o	bile duct(s)
chol/e	gall, bile *(Note: the combining vowel is* e.*)*
choledoch/o	common bile duct
cyst/o	bladder, sac
diverticul/o	diverticulum, *pl.* diverticula (pouch extending from a hollow organ) (Fig. 11.6)
gingiv/o	gum(s)
gloss/o	tongue
hepat/o	liver
herni/o	hernia (protrusion of an organ through a membrane or cavity wall)
lapar/o	abdomen, abdominal cavity
lith/o	stone(s), calculus (*pl.* calculi)
lingu/o	tongue
nas/o	nose
palat/o	palate
pancreat/o	pancreas
peritone/o	peritoneum
pharyng/o	pharynx
polyp/o	polyp, small growth
pylor/o	pylorus, pyloric sphincter
sial/o	saliva, salivary gland
steat/o	fat
uvul/o	uvula

HERNIA Types in the digestive system include abdominal, hiatal or diaphragmatic, inguinal, and umbilical hernia. (Fig. 11.7)

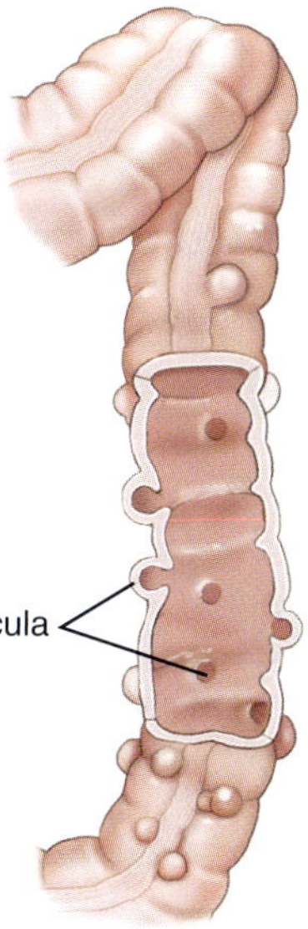

FIG. 11.6 Diverticula of the large intestine.

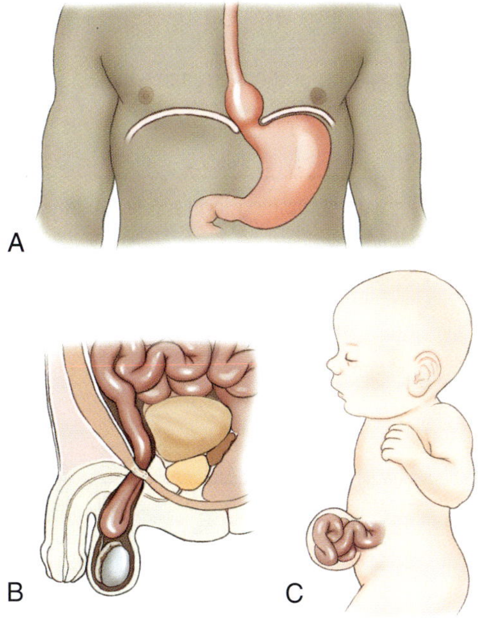

FIG. 11.7 Digestive hernias. **A**, Hiatal. **B**, Inguinal. **C**, Umbilical.

3 ■ Prefixes

PREFIX	DEFINITION	PREFIX	DEFINITION
a-	absence of, without	**hemi-**	half
dys-	painful, abnormal, difficult, labored		

4 ■ Suffixes

SUFFIX	DEFINITION	SUFFIX	DEFINITION
-ac	pertaining to	**-logy**	study of
-al	pertaining to	**-megaly**	enlargement
-cele	hernia, protrusion	**-oma**	tumor, swelling
-centesis	surgical puncture to aspirate fluid (with a sterile needle)	**-osis**	abnormal condition (means increase when used with blood cell word roots)
-eal	pertaining to	**-pathy**	disease
-ectomy	excision, surgical removal	**-pepsia**	digestion
-gram	the record, radiographic image	**-plasty**	surgical repair
-graphy	process of recording, radiographic imaging	**-rrhaphy**	suturing, repairing
		-rrhea	flow, discharge
-iasis	condition	**-scope**	instrument used for visual examination
-ia	diseased or abnormal state, condition of	**-scopy**	visual examination
-ic	pertaining to	**-stomy**	creation of an artificial opening
-itis	inflammation	**-tomy**	cut into, incision
-lith	stone(s), calculus (*pl.* calculi)	**-y**	noun suffix, no meaning
-logist	one who studies and treats (specialist, physician)		

Refer to **Appendix B** and **Appendix C** for a complete listing of word parts.

EXERCISE 1 ■ Digestive System Combining Forms

Refer to the first section of the word parts table.

A Label

Fill in the blanks with combining forms to label this diagram of the digestive system. *To check your answers, go to Appendix A at the back of the textbook.*

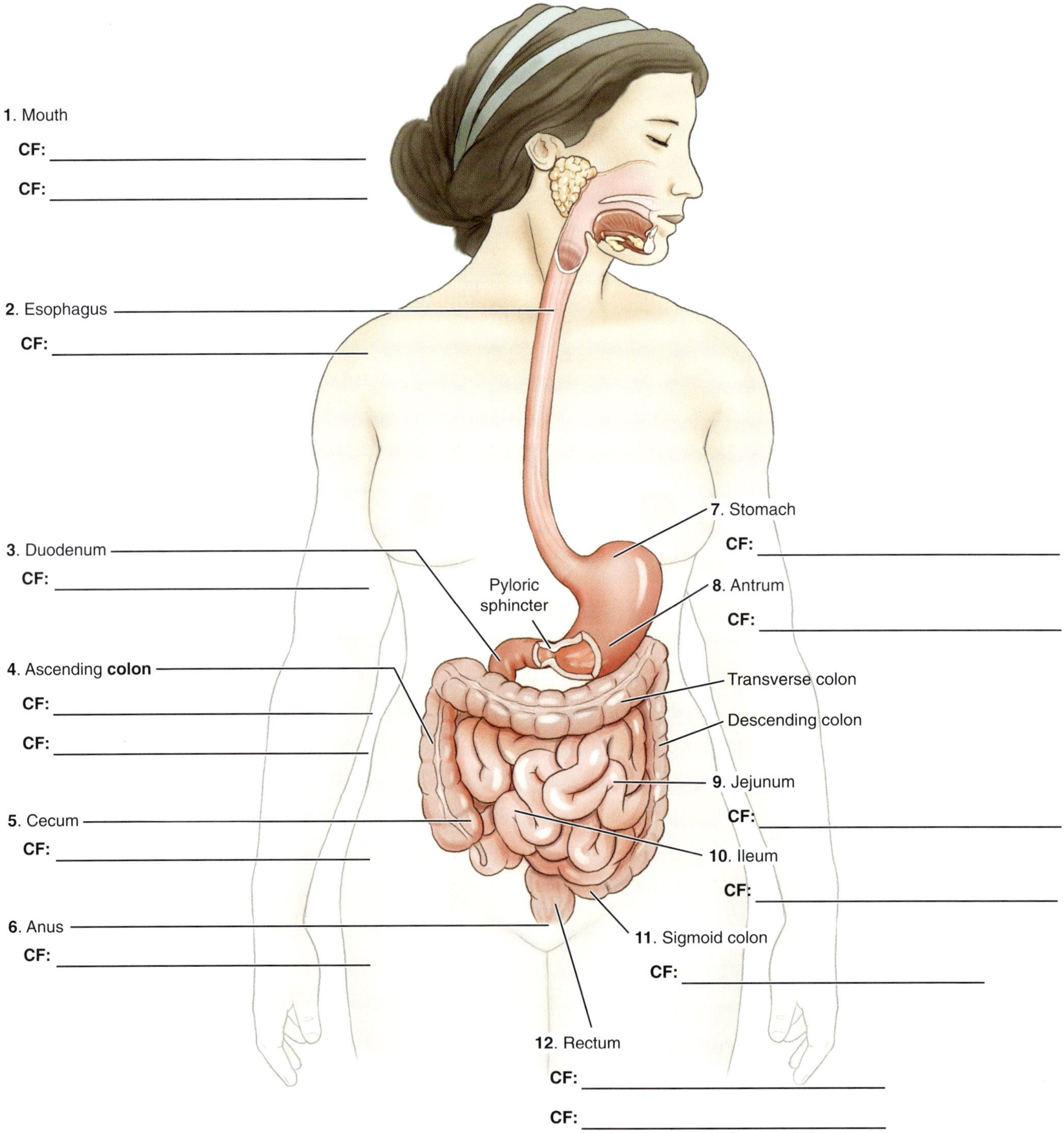

B Define and Match

Step 1: Write the definitions after the following combining forms.
Step 2: Match the descriptions on the right with the combining forms and definitions.

_____ 1. jejun/o, ______________________
_____ 2. an/o, ______________________
_____ 3. gastr/o, ______________________
_____ 4. rect/o, ______________________
_____ 5. or/o, ______________________
_____ 6. col/o, ______________________
_____ 7. sigmoid/o, ______________________
_____ 8. enter/o, ______________________

a. opening through which food passes into the body
b. distal portion of the large intestine
c. main portion of the large intestine
d. 20-foot (6-m) tube extending from the pyloric sphincter to the large intestine
e. second portion of the small intestine
f. portion of large intestine between descending colon and rectum
g. sphincter muscle at the end of the gastrointestinal tract
h. J-shaped sac that mixes and stores food

C Define and Match

Step 1: Write the definitions after the following combining forms.
Step 2: Match the descriptions on the right with the combining forms and definitions.

_____ 1. ile/o, ______________________
_____ 2. stomat/o, ______________________
_____ 3. proct/o, ______________________
_____ 4. esophag/o, ______________________
_____ 5. antr/o, ______________________
_____ 6. colon/o, ______________________
_____ 7. duoden/o, ______________________
_____ 8. cec/o, ______________________

a. distal portion of the stomach
b. first 10 to 12 inches (25 cm) of the small intestine
c. U-shaped pouch that is the first portion of the large intestine
d. third portion of the small intestine, approximately 11 feet (3.3 m) long
e. 10-inch (25-cm) tube that is a passageway for food extending from the pharynx to the stomach
f. main portion of the large intestine
g. opening through which food passes into the body
h. distal portion of the large intestine

EXERCISE 2 ■ Accessory Organs and Combining Forms Used with Digestive System Terms

Refer to the second section of the word parts table.

A Identify

Write the combining form for each of the following.

1. peritoneum ______________________
2. gall, bile ______________________
3. hernia ______________________
4. diverticulum ______________________
5. polyp, small growth ______________________
6. fat ______________________

B Define

Write the definitions of the following combining forms.

1. herni/o ______________________
2. abdomin/o ______________________
3. sial/o ______________________
4. chol/e ______________________
5. diverticul/o ______________________
6. gingiv/o ______________________
7. appendic/o ______________________
8. gloss/o ______________________

9. hepat/o ______________________
10. cheil/o ______________________
11. peritone/o ______________________
12. palat/o ______________________
13. pancreat/o ______________________
14. lapar/o ______________________
15. lingu/o ______________________
16. choledoch/o ______________________
17. pylor/o ______________________
18. uvul/o ______________________
19. cholangi/o ______________________
20. polyp/o ______________________
21. celi/o ______________________
22. steat/o ______________________
23. append/o ______________________
24. pharyng/o ______________________
25. cyst/o ______________________

C Label

Fill in the blanks with combining forms to label this diagram of the digestive system and associated structures.

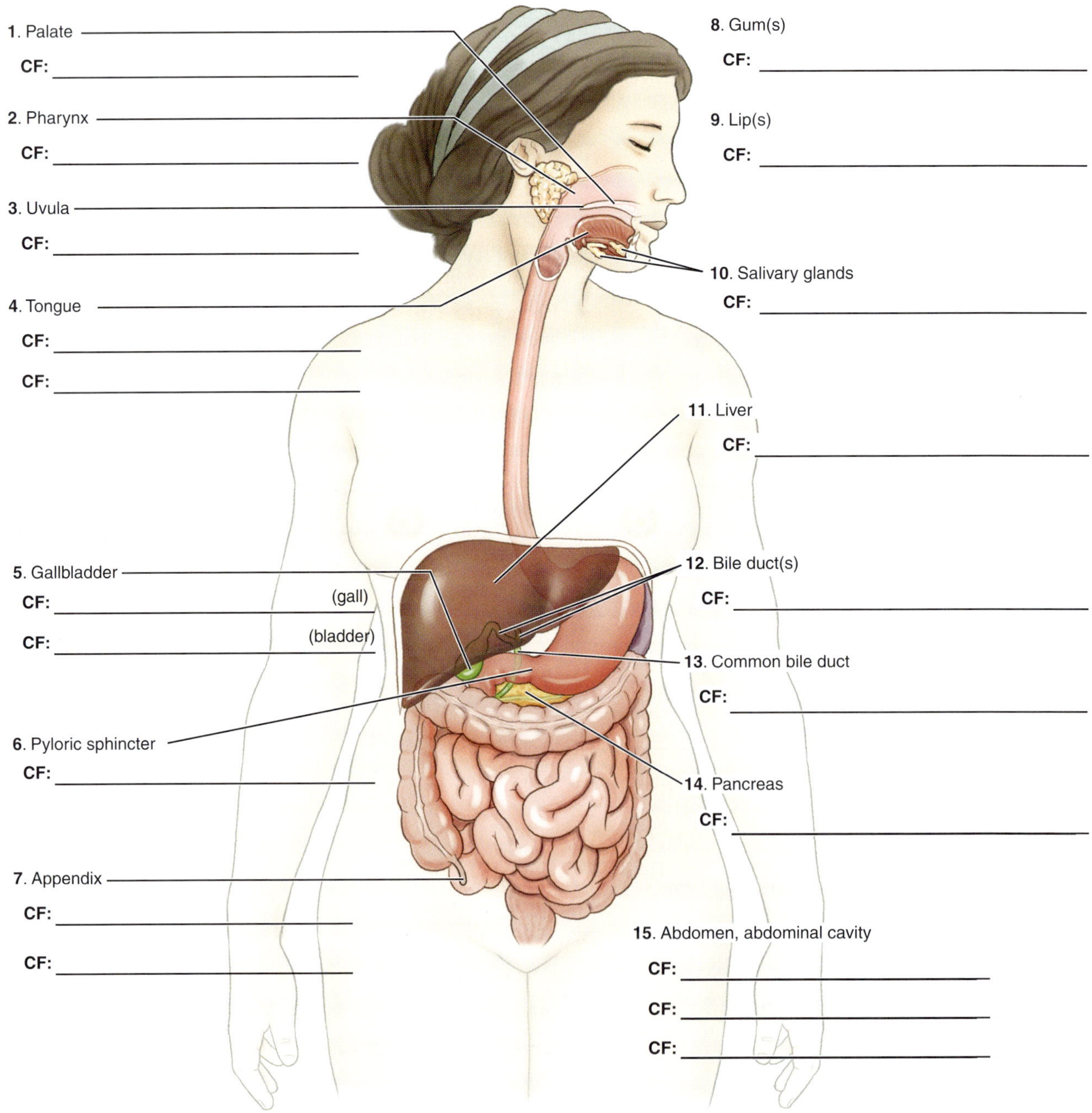

EXERCISE 3 ■ Prefixes

Refer to the third section of the word parts table.

A Define

Write the definitions of the following prefixes.

1. dys- ______________________
2. hemi- ______________________
3. a- ______________________

B Identify

Write the prefixes for the following definitions.

1. absence of, without ______________________
2. half ______________________
3. painful, abnormal, difficult, labored ______________________

EXERCISE 4 ■ Suffixes

Refer to the fourth section of the word parts table.

A Define

Write the definitions of the following suffixes.

1. -pepsia ______________________
2. -ac, -al, -ic ______________________
3. -y ______________________
4. -osis ______________________
5. -iasis ______________________
6. -ia ______________________

B Identify

Write the suffixes for the following definitions.

1. instrument used for visual examination ______________________
2. process of recording, radiographic imaging ______________________
3. one who studies and treats (specialist, physician) ______________________
4. study of ______________________
5. the record, radiographic image ______________________
6. visual examination ______________________

C Match

Match the suffixes in the first column with their correct definitions in the second column.

______ 1. -rrhea	a. disease
______ 2. -pathy	b. enlargement
______ 3. -oma	c. flow, discharge
______ 4. -megaly	d. hernia, protrusion
______ 5. -lith	e. inflammation
______ 6. -itis	f. tumor, swelling
______ 7. -cele	g. stone(s), calculus (*pl.* calculi)

D Match

Match the suffixes in the first column with their correct definitions in the second column.

_____ 1. -centesis	a. creation of an artificial opening
_____ 2. -ectomy	b. cut into, incision
_____ 3. -plasty	c. excision, surgical removal
_____ 4. -rrhaphy	d. surgical puncture to aspirate fluid (with a sterile needle)
_____ 5. -stomy	e. pertaining to
_____ 6. -tomy	f. suturing, repairing
_____ 7. -eal	g. surgical repair

MEDICAL TERMS

Medical terms relevant to this chapter have been grouped by topics, such as Disease and Disorder, and are listed in tables designated as Built from Word Parts or *NOT* Built from Word Parts. The exercises following each table assist with learning term definitions, pronunciations, and spellings.

Disease and Disorder Terms

BUILT FROM WORD PARTS

The following terms can be translated using definitions of word parts. Further explanation is provided within parentheses as needed.

TERM	DEFINITION
1. appendicitis (a-*pen*-di-SĪ-tis)	inflammation of the appendix
2. cheilitis (kī-LĪ-tis)	inflammation of the lips
3. cholangioma (kō-*lan*-jē-Ō-ma)	tumor of the bile duct
4. cholecystitis (*kō*-lē-sis-TĪ-tis)	inflammation of the gallbladder
5. choledocholithiasis (kō-*led*-o-kō-li-THĪ-a-sis)	condition of stones in the common bile duct
6. cholelithiasis (*kō*-le-li-THĪ-a-sis)	condition of gallstones
7. colitis (ko-LĪ-tis)	inflammation of the colon

ANTIBIOTIC-ASSOCIATED COLITIS is caused by a bacterium called ***Clostridium difficile*** (***C. difficile***). Though usually occurring in hospitalized patients, it is also now occurring more frequently in the general community. Symptoms include diarrhea and abdominal pain. Treatments include stopping the antibiotic and frequent hand washing to limit the spread of disease between patients. Oral vancomycin and other antibiotics work directly in the colon to kill *C. difficile* bacteria.

TERM	DEFINITION
8. diverticulitis (*dī*-ver-*tik*-ū-LĪ-tis)	inflammation of a diverticulum
9. diverticulosis (*dī*-ver-*tik*-ū-LŌ-sis)	abnormal condition of having diverticula (Figs. 11.6 and 11.15B)
10. dysentery (DIS-en-ter-ē)	painful intestines (disorder that involves inflammation of the intestines, usually the large intestine, associated with abdominal pain and diarrhea that is often bloody)
11. enteritis (*en*-ter-Ī-tis)	inflammation of the intestines
12. enteropathy (en-ter-OP-a-thē)	disease of the intestines
13. esophagitis (e-*sof*-a-JĪ-tis)	inflammation of the esophagus
14. gastritis (gas-TRĪ-tis)	inflammation of the stomach
15. gastroenteritis (*gas*-trō-*en*-te-RĪ-tis)	inflammation of the stomach and intestines
16. gingivitis (*jin*-ji-VĪ-tis)	inflammation of the gums
17. glossitis (glos-Ī-tis)	inflammation of the tongue
18. hepatitis (*hep*-a-TĪ-tis)	inflammation of the liver
19. hepatoma (*hep*-a-TŌ-ma)	tumor of the liver

TERM	DEFINITION
20. pancreatitis (*pan*-krē-a-TĪ-tis)	inflammation of the pancreas
21. peritonitis (*per*-i-tō-NĪ-tis)	inflammation of the peritoneum
In the term **peritonitis**, the final **e** is dropped from the combining form **peritone/o**.	
22. polyposis (*pol*-i-PŌ-sis)	abnormal condition of (multiple) polyps (in the mucous membrane of the intestine, especially the colon.)
FAMILIAL POLYPOSIS is a syndrome with a high potential for malignancy if polyps are not removed when they are small.	
23. proctitis (prok-TĪ-tis)	inflammation of the rectum
24. rectocele (REK-tō-sēl)	hernia of the rectum
25. sialolith (sī-AL-ō-lith)	stone in the salivary gland
26. steatohepatitis (*stē*-a-tō-*hep*-a-TĪ-tis)	inflammation of the liver associated with (excess) fat; (often caused by alcohol abuse and obesity; over time may lead to cirrhosis)
NASH SYNDROME or **nonalcoholic steatohepatitis** may occur in nonalcoholic patients who are obese and/or suffer from type 2 diabetes mellitus.	
27. stomatitis (stō-ma-TĪ-tis)	inflammation of the mouth (mucous membrane)
28. uvulitis (*ū*-vū-LĪ-tis)	inflammation of the uvula

EXERCISE 5 ■ Pronounce and Spell

Practice pronunciation and spelling on paper and online.

1. Practice on Paper

a. **Pronounce:** Read the phonetic spelling and say aloud the terms listed in the previous table. Refer to the pronunciation key on p. 20 as necessary.
b. **Spell:** Have a study partner read the terms aloud. Write the spelling of the terms on a separate sheet of paper.

2. Practice Online

a. **Access** online learning resources. Go to evolve.elsevier.com > Evolve Resources > Student Resources.
b. **Pronounce:** Select Audio Glossary > Chapter 11 > Exercise 5. Select a term to hear its pronunciation and repeat aloud.
c. **Spell:** Select Activities > Chapter 11 > Spell Terms > Exercise 5. Select the audio icon and type the correct spelling of the term.

❑ Check the box when complete.

EXERCISE 6 ■ Analyze and Define

Analyze and define the following terms.

1. steatohepatitis

____

____

2. diverticulosis

____

____

3. cholangioma

____

____

4. hepatoma

____

____

5. uvulitis

____

____

6. pancreatitis

____

____

7. proctitis

____

____

8. cheilitis

____

____

9. gastritis

____

____

10. rectocele

____

____

11. enteropathy

____

____

12. peritonitis

____

____

13. enteritis

____

____

14. glossitis

____

____

EXERCISE 7 ■ Build

A Label

Build terms pictured by writing word parts above definitions.

1.

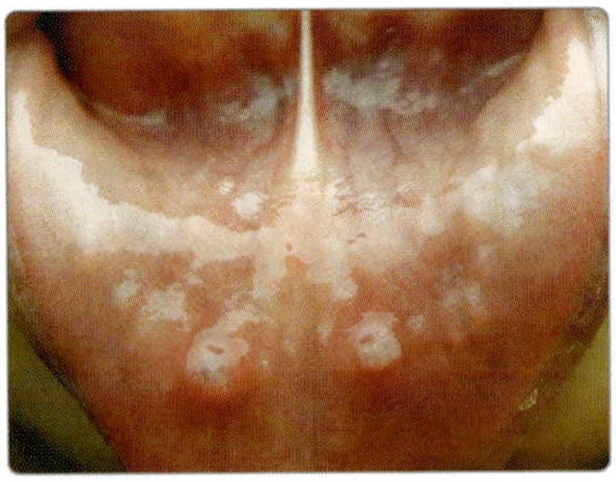

________ / ________
mouth inflammation

2.

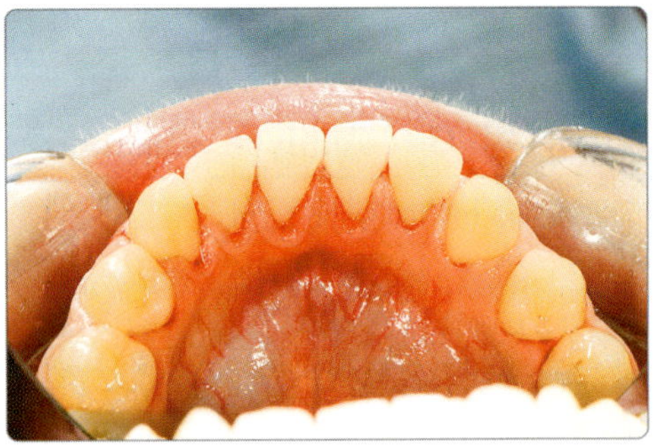

________ / ________
gums inflammation

3.

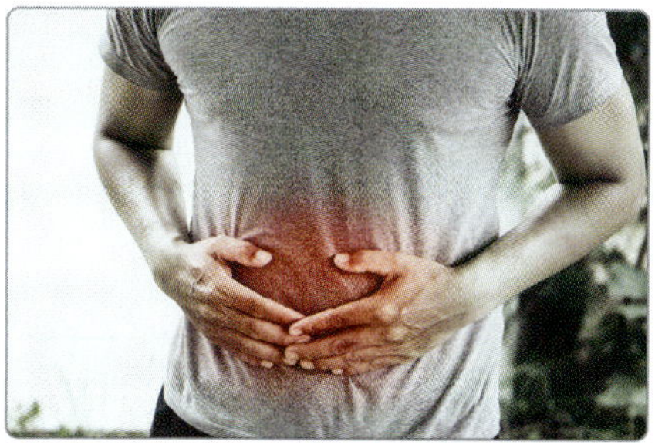

_______ / _______ / y
painful / intestines

4.

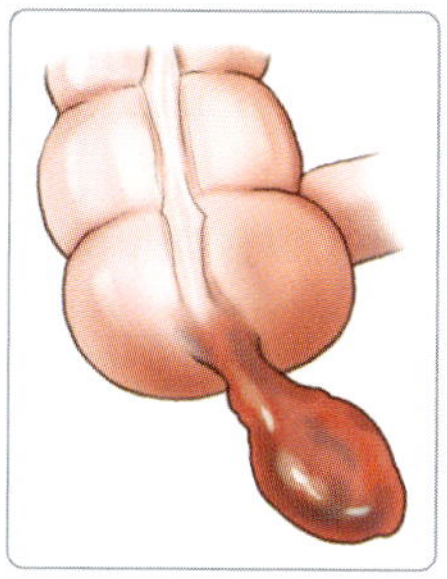

_______ / _______
appendix / inflammation

5.

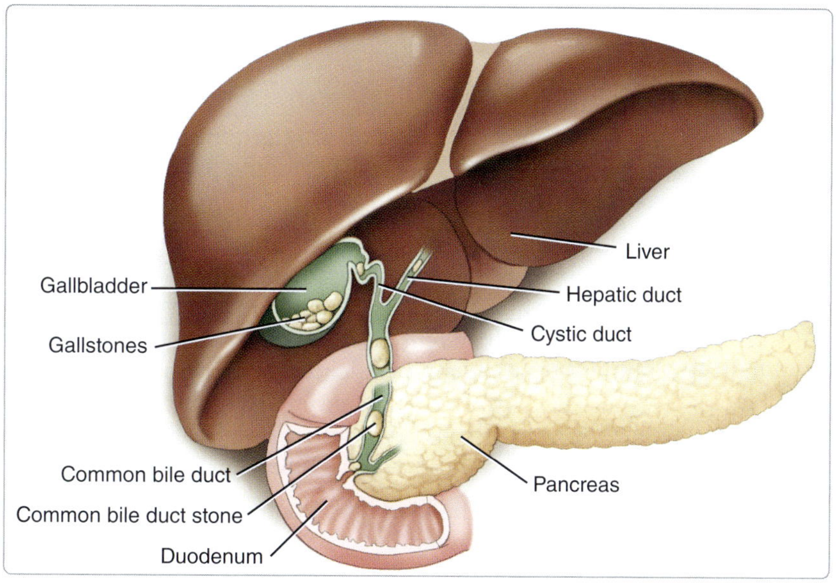

Common sites of

_______ / _______ / _______ / _______ and _______ / _______ / _______ / _______
gall / CV / stone / condition of — common bile duct / CV / stone / condition of

B Fill In

Build disease and disorder terms for the following definitions by using the word parts you have learned.

1. inflammation of the liver _______ / _______ (WR / S)
2. inflammation of the colon _______ / _______ (WR / S)
3. stone in the salivary gland _______ / CV / _______ (WR / CV / S)
4. inflammation of the esophagus _______ / _______ (WR / S)
5. inflammation of a diverticulum _______ / _______ (WR / S)

6. inflammation of the gallbladder ______ WR / CV / WR / S

7. abnormal condition of (multiple) polyps ______ WR / S

8. inflammation of the stomach and intestines ______ WR / CV / WR / S

Disease and Disorder Terms

NOT BUILT FROM WORD PARTS

Word parts may be present in the following terms; however, their full meanings cannot be translated using definitions of word parts alone.

TERM	DEFINITION
1. adhesion (ad-HĒ-zhun)	abnormal growing together of two peritoneal surfaces that normally are separated. This may occur after abdominal surgery. Surgical treatment is called **adhesiolysis** or **adhesiotomy.**
2. celiac disease (SĒ-lē-ak) (di-ZĒZ)	malabsorption syndrome caused by an immune reaction to gluten (a protein in wheat, rye, and barley), which may damage the lining of the small intestine that is responsible for absorption of food into the bloodstream. Celiac disease is considered a multisystem disorder with varying signs and symptoms, including abdominal bloating and pain, chronic diarrhea or constipation, steatorrhea (excessive fat in the stool), vomiting, weight loss, fatigue, and iron deficiency anemia. A pruritic skin rash known as dermatitis herpetiformis may be associated with celiac disease. (also called **gluten enteropathy**)
3. cirrhosis (sir-RŌ-sis)	chronic disease of the liver with gradual destruction of cells and formation of scar tissue; commonly caused by alcoholism and certain types of viral hepatitis
4. Crohn disease (krōn) (di-ZĒZ)	chronic inflammation of the intestinal tract usually affecting the ileum and colon; characterized by cobblestone ulcerations and the formation of scar tissue that may lead to intestinal obstruction (also called **regional ileitis** or **regional enteritis**)
5. gastroesophageal reflux disease (GERD) (gas-trō-e-sof-a-JĒ-al) (RĒ-fluks) (di-ZĒZ)	abnormal backward flow of the gastrointestinal contents into the esophagus, causing heartburn and the gradual breakdown of the mucous barrier of the esophagus

GASTROESOPHAGEAL REFLUX DISEASE (GERD) is a common gastrointestinal disorder. The acidity of the regurgitated stomach contents causes inflammation of the esophagus (reflux esophagitis). In addition to heartburn, GERD may also cause chronic cough and excessive throat clearing. **Chronic GERD** may cause cellular changes in the lower esophagus called **Barrett esophagus**, which increases the risk of cancer.

TERM	DEFINITION
6. hemochromatosis (hē-mō-krō-ma-TŌ-sis)	iron metabolism disorder that occurs when too much iron is absorbed from food, resulting in excessive deposits of iron in the tissue; can cause heart failure, diabetes, cirrhosis, or cancer of the liver
7. hemorrhoids (HEM-o-roydz)	swollen or distended veins in the rectum or anus, which are called internal or external, respectively, and can be a source of rectal bleeding and pain
8. ileus (IL-ē-us)	nonmechanical obstruction of the intestine, caused by a lack of effective peristalsis (involuntary wavelike movements that propel food along the gastrointestinal tract)
9. intussusception (*in*-tu-sus-SEP-shun)	prolapse of one part of the intestine inside the part next to it. It is most common in infants; symptoms may include intestinal blockage, abdominal pain with cramping, or a lump that can be felt from the outside.

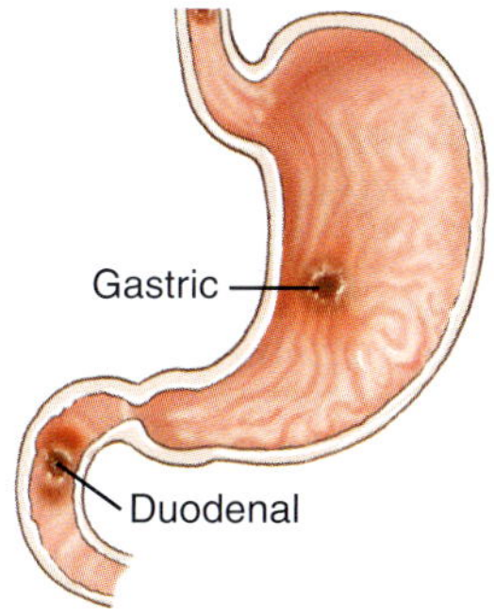

FIG. 11.8 Sites of peptic ulcers.

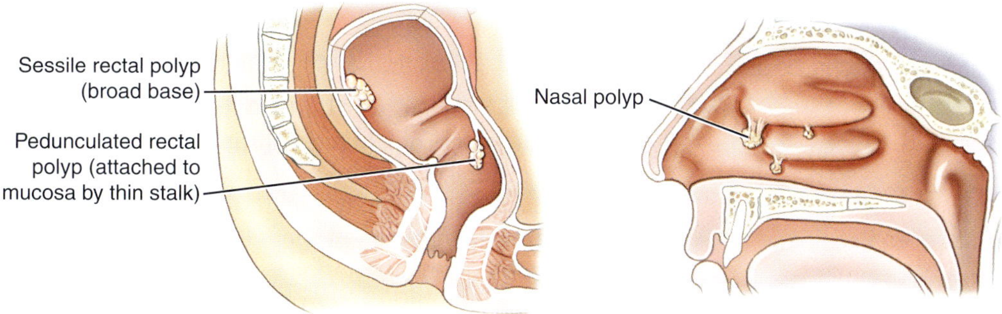

FIG. 11.9 Polyp is a general term used to describe a protruding growth from a mucous membrane. Polyps are commonly found in the nose, throat, intestines, uterus, and urinary bladder.

TERM	DEFINITION
10. irritable bowel syndrome (IBS) (IR-i-ta-bl) (BOW-el) (SIN-drōm)	periodic disturbances of bowel function, such as diarrhea and/or constipation, usually associated with abdominal pain
11. obesity (ō-BĒS-i-tē)	excess of body fat, which increases body weight; a condition in which body mass index (BMI) is greater than 30 kg/m^2. **Overweight** is defined as BMI between 25 and 29.9 kg/m^2. **Morbid obesity** is defined as a BMI over 40 kg/m^2.
12. peptic ulcer (PEP-tik) (UL-ser)	erosion of the mucous membrane of the stomach or duodenum associated with increased secretion of acid from the stomach, bacterial infection (*H. pylori*), or medications such as nonsteroidal anti-inflammatory drugs (often referred to as **gastric** or **duodenal ulcer**, depending on its location) (Fig. 11.8)
13. polyp (POL-ip)	tumorlike growth extending outward from a mucous membrane; usually benign; common sites are in the nose, throat, and intestines (Figs. 11.9 and 11.11)
14. ulcerative colitis (UC) (UL-ser-a-tiv) (kō-LĪ-tis)	disease characterized by inflammation of the colon with the formation of ulcers, which can cause bloody diarrhea. A proctocolectomy with permanent ileostomy may become necessary if the patient doesn't respond to medical therapy.
15. volvulus (VOL-vū-lus)	twisting or kinking of the intestine, causing intestinal obstruction

EXERCISE 8 ■ Pronounce and Spell

Practice pronunciation and spelling on paper and online.

1. Practice on Paper

a. **Pronounce:** Read the phonetic spelling and say aloud the terms listed in the previous table. Refer to the pronunciation key on p. 20 as necessary.
b. **Spell:** Have a study partner read the terms aloud. Write the spelling of the terms on a separate sheet of paper.

2. Practice Online

a. **Access** online learning resources. Go to evolve.elsevier.com > Evolve Resources > Student Resources.
b. **Pronounce:** Select Audio Glossary > Chapter 11 > Exercise 8. Select a term to hear its pronunciation and repeat aloud.
c. **Spell:** Select Activities > Chapter 11 > Spell Terms > Exercise 8. Select the audio icon and type the correct spelling of the term.

❑ Check the box when complete.

EXERCISE 9 ■ Match

Match the terms in the first column with their definitions in the second column.

_____ 1. hemochromatosis
_____ 2. cirrhosis
_____ 3. ulcerative colitis
_____ 4. ileus
_____ 5. celiac disease
_____ 6. irritable bowel syndrome
_____ 7. Crohn disease
_____ 8. obesity

a. excess of body fat, which increases body weight
b. nonmechanical obstruction of the intestine
c. disease characterized by inflammation of the colon with the formation of ulcers, which can cause bloody diarrhea
d. chronic inflammation of the intestinal tract usually affecting the ileum and colon with cobblestone ulcerations
e. iron metabolism disorder resulting in excessive deposits of iron in the tissue; can cause cirrhosis or liver cancer
f. malabsorption syndrome caused by an immune reaction to gluten
g. chronic disease of the liver with gradual destruction of cells and formation of scar tissue
h. periodic disturbances of bowel function, such as diarrhea and/or constipation, usually associated with abdominal pain

EXERCISE 10 ■ Label

Write the medical terms pictured and defined.

1. ______________________
erosion of the mucous membrane of the stomach or duodenum associated with increased secretion of acid from the stomach

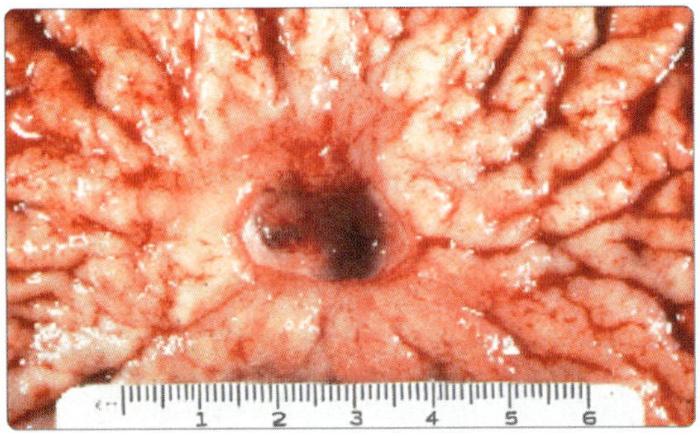

2. ______________________
twisting or kinking of the intestine, causing intestinal obstruction

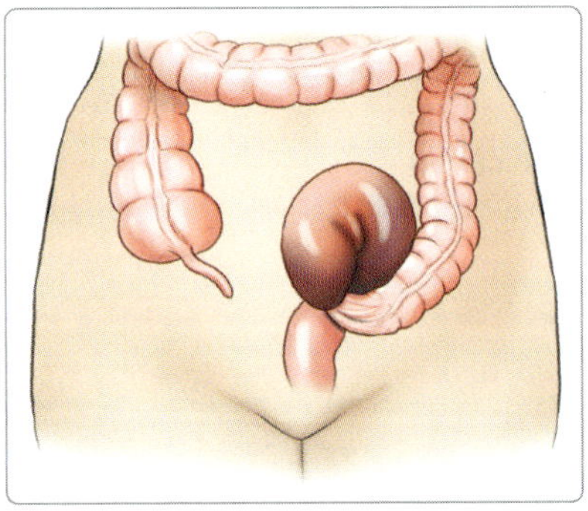

3. ______________________
tumor like growth extending outward from a mucous membrane; usually benign

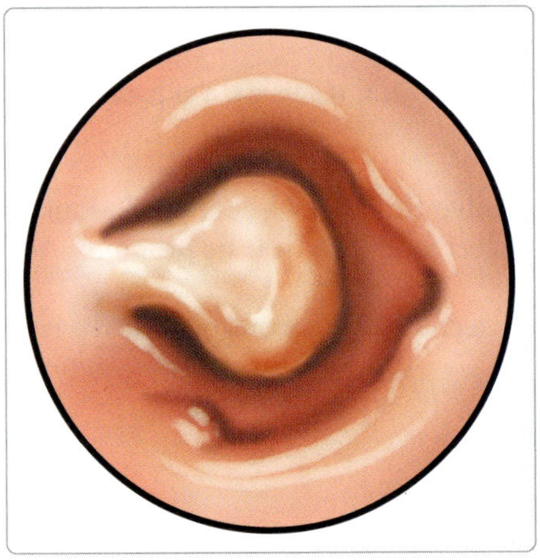

4. ______________________
abnormal backward flow of the gastrointestinal contents into the esophagus

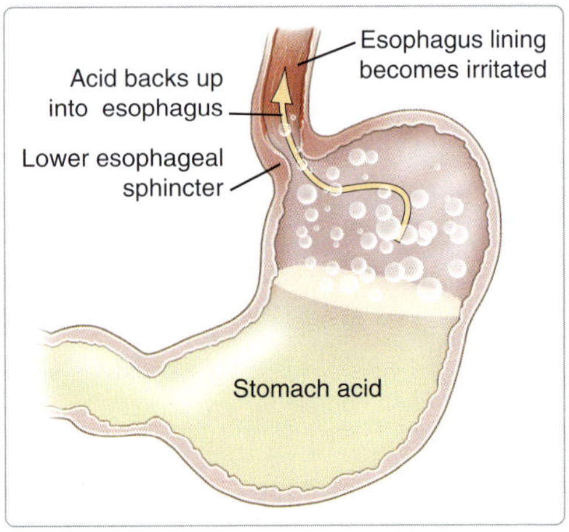

5. ___________________________________

abnormal growing together of two peritoneal surfaces that normally are separated

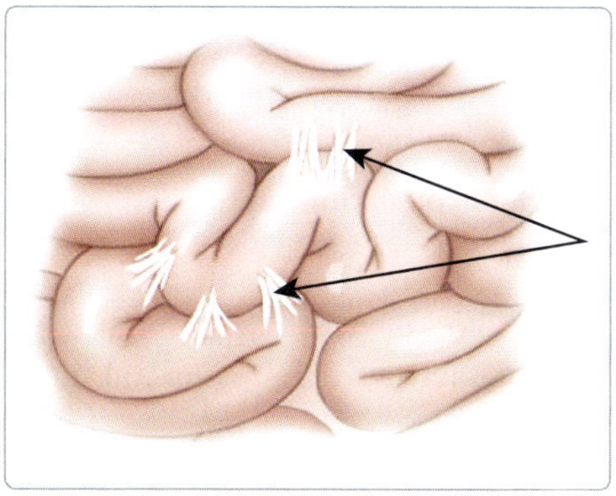

6. ___________________________________

prolapse of one part of the intestine inside the part next to it

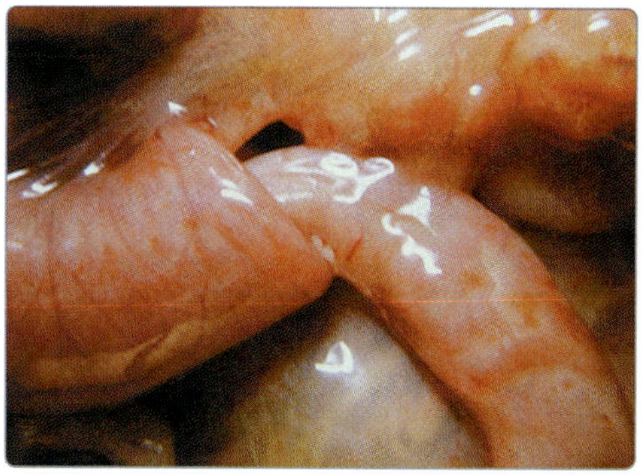

7. ___________________________________

swollen or distended veins in the rectum or anus, which can be a source of rectal bleeding and pain

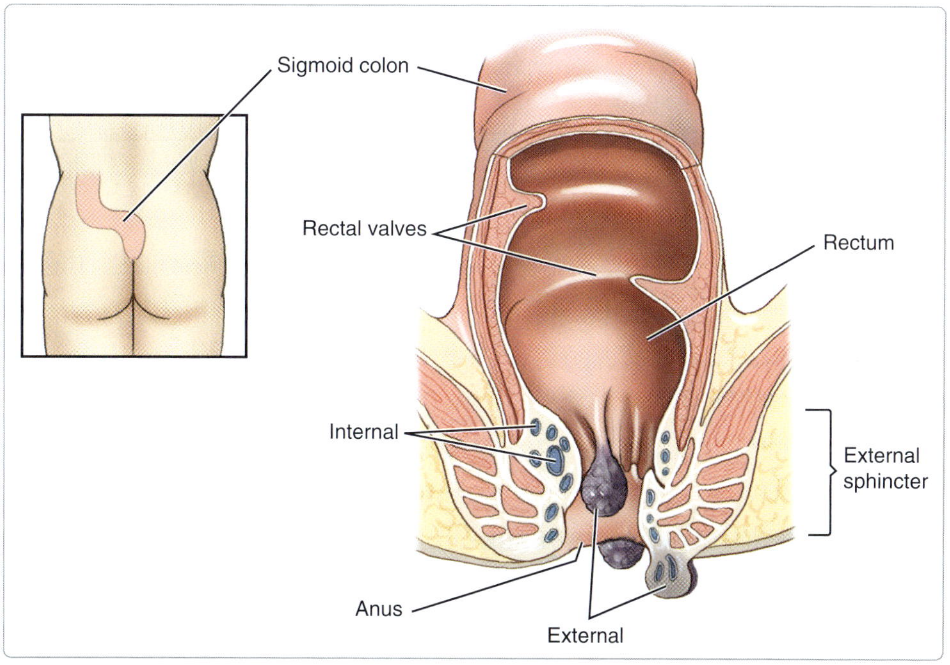

EXERCISE 11 ■ Review of Disease and Disorder Terms

Can you define, pronounce, and spell the following terms?

adhesion
appendicitis
celiac disease
cheilitis
cholangioma
cholecystitis
choledocholithiasis
cholelithiasis
cirrhosis
colitis
Crohn disease
diverticulitis
diverticulosis
dysentery
enteritis
enteropathy
esophagitis
gastritis
gastroenteritis
gastroesophageal reflux disease (GERD)
gingivitis
glossitis
hemochromatosis
hemorrhoids
hepatitis
hepatoma
ileus
intussusception
irritable bowel syndrome (IBS)
obesity

pancreatitis
peptic ulcer
peritonitis
polyp
polyposis
proctitis
rectocele
sialolith
steatohepatitis
stomatitis
ulcerative colitis (UC)
uvulitis
volvulus

Surgical Terms

BUILT FROM WORD PARTS

The following terms can be translated using definitions of word parts. Further explanation is provided within parentheses as needed.

TERM	DEFINITION
1. **abdominocentesis** (ab-*dom*-i-nō-sen-TĒ-sis)	surgical puncture to aspirate fluid from the abdominal cavity (also called **paracentesis**)
2. **abdominoplasty** (ab-DOM-i-nō-*plas*-tē)	surgical repair of the abdomen
3. **anoplasty** (Ā-nō-*plas*-tē)	surgical repair of the anus
4. **antrectomy** (an-TREK-to-mē)	excision of the antrum (of the stomach)
5. **appendectomy** (*ap*-en-DEK-to-mē)	excision of the appendix
6. **cheiloplasty** (KĪ-lō-*plas*-tē)	surgical repair of the lip
7. **cholecystectomy** (*kō*-le-sis-TEK-to-mē)	excision of the gallbladder (Fig. 11.10)

CHOLECYSTECTOMY was first performed in 1882 by a German surgeon. **Laparoscopic cholecystectomy** was first performed in 1985.

TERM	DEFINITION
8. **choledocholithotomy** (kō-*led*-o-kō-li-THOT-o-mē)	incision into the common bile duct to remove a stone
9. **colectomy** (kō-LEK-to-mē)	excision of the colon
10. **colostomy** (ko-LOS-to-mē)	creation of an artificial opening into the colon (through the abdominal wall; used for the passage of stool)

COLOSTOMY is a surgical procedure that creates a mouthlike opening called a **stoma** and may be permanent or temporary. It is performed as a treatment for bowel obstruction, cancer, or diverticulitis.

TERM	DEFINITION
11. **diverticulectomy** (*dī*-ver-*tik*-ū-LEK-to-mē)	excision of a diverticulum
12. **enterorrhaphy** (*en*-ter-OR-a-fē)	suturing of the (small) intestine

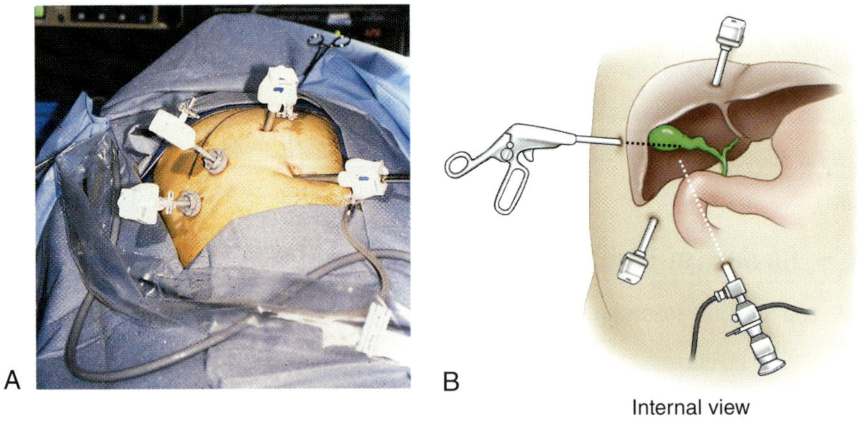

FIG. 11.10 In **laparoscopic cholecystectomy**, a type of endoscopic surgery, carbon dioxide (CO_2) is introduced into the abdominal cavity for better visualization. A tiny camera and surgical instruments, including a laparoscope, are passed through small incisions. **A,** External view. **B,** Internal view.

TERM	DEFINITION
13. esophagogastroplasty (e-*sof*-a-gō-GAS-trō-*plas*-tē)	surgical repair of the esophagus and the stomach
14. gastrectomy (gas-TREK-to-mē)	excision of the stomach (or part of the stomach)
15. gastrojejunostomy (*gas*-trō-je-jū-NOS-to-mē)	creation of an artificial opening between the stomach and jejunum
16. gastroplasty (GAS-trō-*plas*-tē)	surgical repair of the stomach
17. gastrostomy (gas-TROS-to-mē)	creation of an artificial opening into the stomach (through the abdominal wall)

GASTROSTOMY is a surgical procedure used to insert a tube, often referred to as a "G-tube," through the abdomen and into the stomach. This provides a route for long-term tube feeding if swallowing is impossible and to vent the stomach for air or drainage

TERM	DEFINITION
18. gingivectomy (*jin*-ji-VEK-to-mē)	surgical removal of gum (tissue)
19. glossorrhaphy (glo-SOR-a-fē)	suturing of the tongue
20. hemicolectomy (*hem*-ē-kō-LEK-to-mē)	excision of half of the colon
21. herniorrhaphy (*her*-nē-OR-a-fē)	suturing of a hernia (for repair)
22. ileostomy (*il*-ē-OS-to-mē)	creation of an artificial opening into the ileum (through the abdominal wall; used for passage of stool)

ILEOSTOMY is a surgical procedure that creates a mouthlike opening called a **stoma**. It is performed following total proctocolectomy for ulcerative colitis, Crohn disease, or cancer.

TERM	DEFINITION
23. laparotomy (*lap*-a-ROT-o-mē)	incision into the abdominal cavity (also called **celiotomy**)
24. palatoplasty (PAL-a-tō-*plas*-tē)	surgical repair of the palate
25. pancreatectomy (pan-crē-a-TEK-ta-mē)	excision of the pancreas
26. polypectomy (*pol*-i-PEK-to-mē)	excision of a polyp (Fig. 11.11)
27. pyloroplasty (pī-LOR-ō-*plas*-tē)	surgical repair of the pylorus
28. uvulectomy (*ū*-vū-LEK-to-mē)	excision of the uvula
29. uvulopalatopharyngoplasty (UPPP) (*ū*-vū-lō-*pal*-a-*tō*-fa-RING-gō-*plas*-tē)	surgical repair of the uvula, palate, and pharynx (performed to correct obstructive sleep apnea) (see Fig. 5.6)

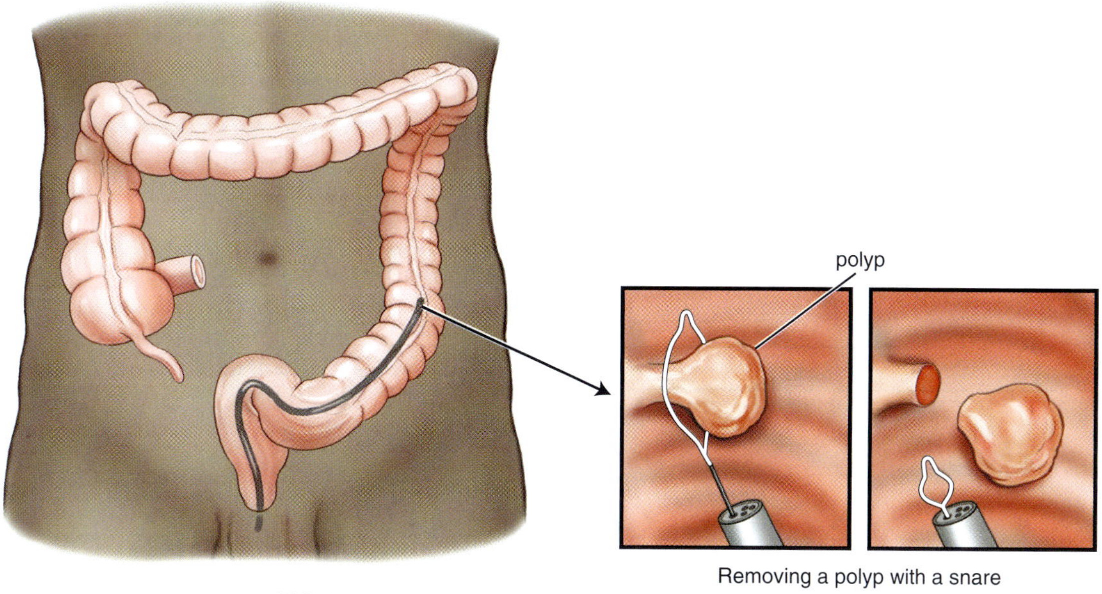

FIG. 11.11 Polypectomy performed using a colonoscope.

EXERCISE 12 ■ Pronounce and Spell

Practice pronunciation and spelling on paper and online.

1. Practice on Paper

a. **Pronounce:** Read the phonetic spelling and say aloud the terms listed in the previous table. Refer to the pronunciation key on p. 20 as necessary.
b. **Spell:** Have a study partner read the terms aloud. Write the spelling of the terms on a separate sheet of paper.

2. Practice Online

a. **Access** online learning resources. Go to evolve.elsevier.com > Evolve Resources > Student Resources.
b. **Pronounce:** Select Audio Glossary > Chapter 11 > Exercise 12. Select a term to hear its pronunciation and repeat aloud.
c. **Spell:** Select Activities > Chapter 11 > Spell Terms > Exercise 12. Select the audio icon and type the correct spelling of the term.

❑ Check the box when complete.

EXERCISE 13 ■ Analyze and Define

Analyze and define the following terms.

1. herniorrhaphy
____
____

2. gastroplasty
____
____

3. hemicolectomy
____
____

4. antrectomy
____
____

5. enterorrhaphy
____
____

6. uvulectomy
____
____

7. gastrojejunostomy
____
____

8. cholecystectomy
____
____

9. abdominoplasty
____
____

10. pancreatectomy
____
____

11. pyloroplasty

____

____

12. choledocholithotomy

____

____

13. uvulopalatopharyngoplasty

____

____

14. abdominocentesis

____

____

EXERCISE 14 ■ Build

A Label

Build terms pictured by writing word parts above definitions.

1.

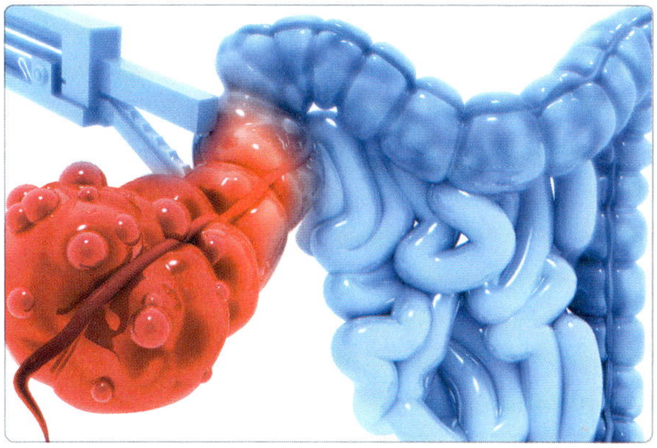

_______________ / _______________
appendix excision

2.

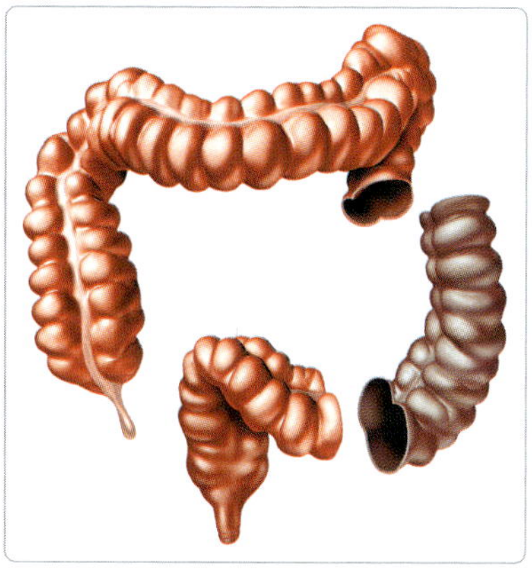

_______________ / _______________
colon excision

3.

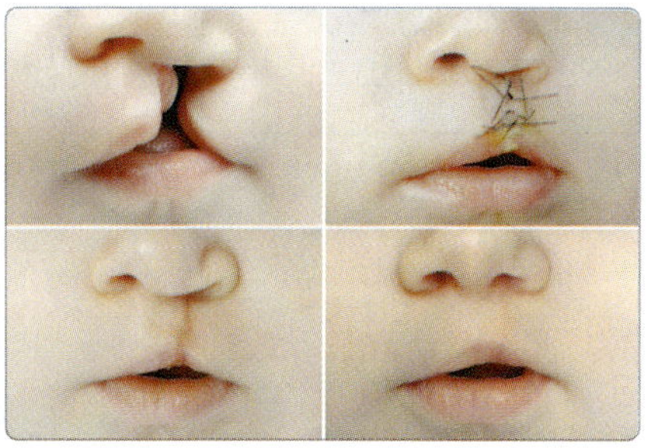

_______________ / ______ / _______________
palate CV surgical repair

4.

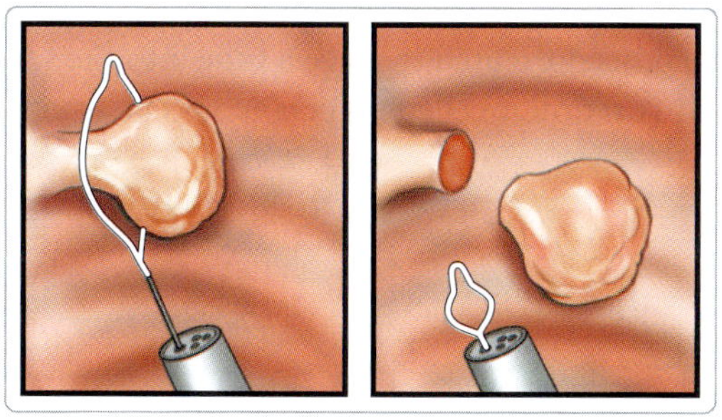

_______________ / _______________
polyp excision

5.

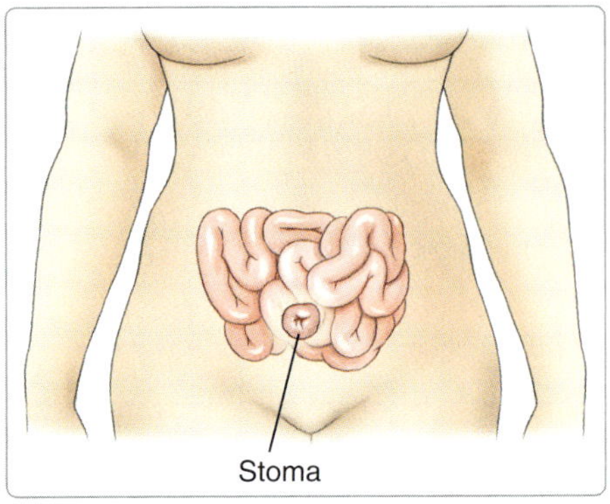

_________ /_____ /_________________
ileum CV creation of an artificial opening

after a total colectomy.

6.

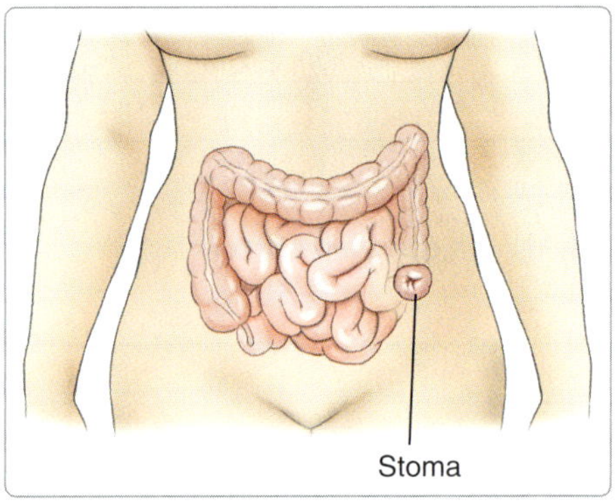

_________ /_____ /_________________
colon CV creation of an artificial opening

after an abdominoperineal resection.

7.

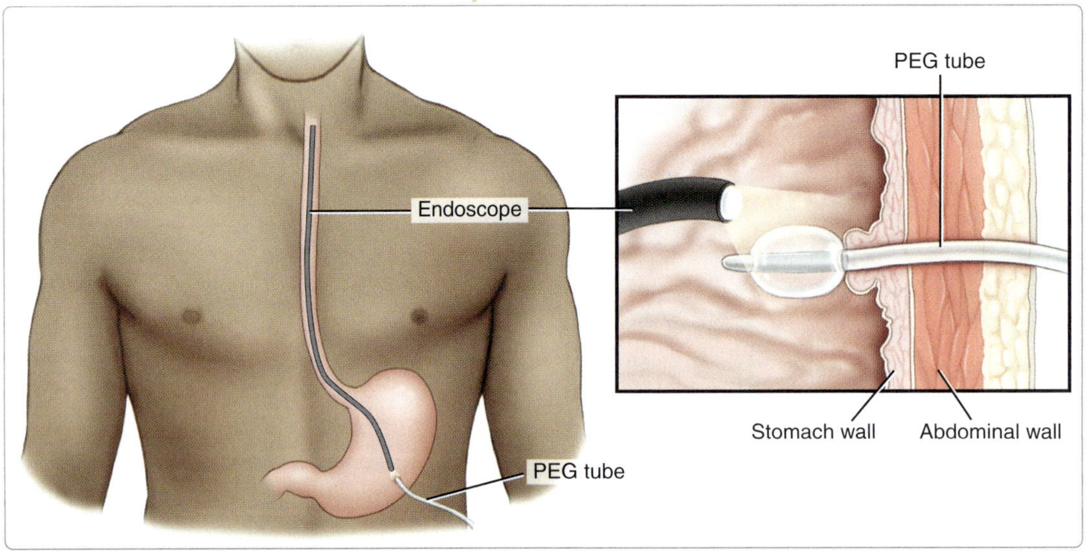

The procedure used to place a tube into the stomach through the abdominal wall to administer liquids for nutrition and hydration is called percutaneous endoscopic ___________ /______ /______________________.
stomach CV creation of an artificial opening

8.

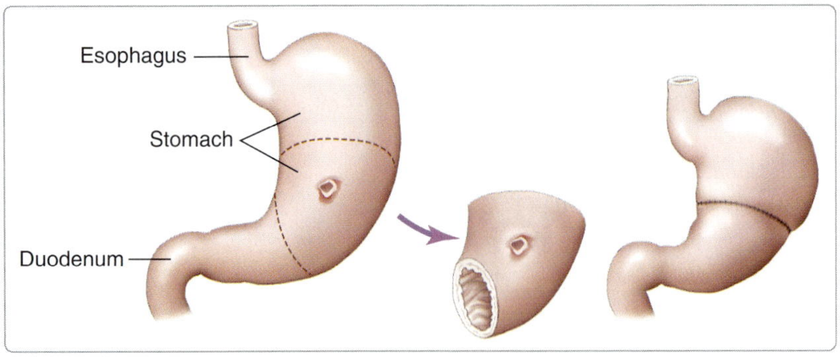

Partial ________ /__________________ may be performed to treat chronic gastric ulcers.
stomach surgical removal

B Fill In

Build surgical terms for the following definitions by using the word parts you have learned.

1. suturing of the tongue ______ WR / CV / ______ S
2. surgical repair of the esophagus and stomach ______ WR / CV / ______ WR / CV / ______ S
3. excision of a diverticulum ______ WR / ______ S
4. surgical removal of gum (tissue) ______ WR / ______ S
5. incision into the abdominal cavity ______ WR / CV / ______ S
6. surgical repair of the anus ______ WR / CV / ______ S
7. excision of the gallbladder ______ WR / CV / ______ WR / ______ S

Surgical Terms

NOT BUILT FROM WORD PARTS

Word parts may be present in the following terms; however, their full meanings cannot be translated using definitions of word parts alone.

TERM	DEFINITION
1. abdominoperineal resection (APR) (ab-*dom*-i-nō-per-i-NĒ-el) (rē-SEK-shun)	removal of the distal colon, rectum, and anal sphincter through both abdominal and perineal approaches; performed to treat some colorectal cancers and inflammatory diseases of the lower large intestine. The patient will have a colostomy.
2. anastomosis (*pl.* anastomoses) (a-*nas*-to-MŌ-sis) (a-*nas*-to-MŌ-sēz)	connection created by surgically joining two structures, such as blood vessels or bowel segments (Fig. 11.12)
3. bariatric surgery (*bar*-ē-AT-rik) (SUR-jer-ē)	surgical reduction of gastric capacity to treat morbid obesity, a condition that can cause serious illness (Table 11.1)
BARIATRIC contains the word roots **bar**, meaning **weight**, and **iatr**, meaning **treatment**.	
4. hemorrhoidectomy (*hem*-o-royd-EK-to-mē)	excision of hemorrhoids, the swollen or distended veins in the lower rectum and anus
5. vagotomy (vā-GOT-o-mē)	cutting of certain branches of the vagus nerve, performed with gastric surgery to reduce the amount of gastric acid produced and thus reduce the recurrence of ulcers

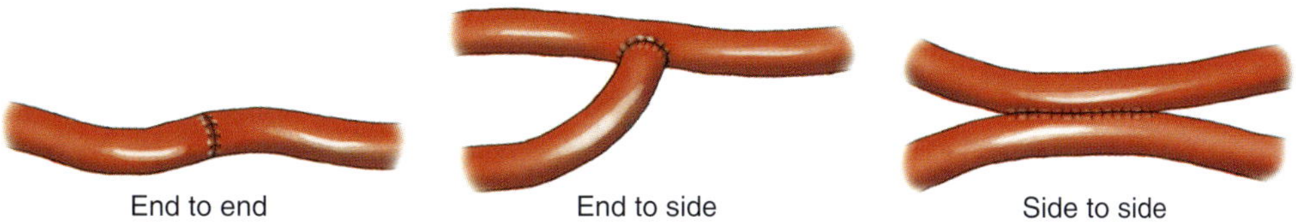

FIG. 11.12 Types of anastomoses.

TABLE 11.1 Bariatric Surgery

Bariatric surgery may be used to treat morbid obesity for patients with a BMI greater than 40 or those with a BMI greater than 35 associated with a serious medical condition. During surgery, a small stomach pouch is created for the purpose of restricting the amount of food an individual can eat. The following are three types of surgeries performed.

ROUX-EN-Y GASTRIC BYPASS (RYGB)

Creation of a small gastric pouch with drainage of food to the rest of the gastrointestinal tract through a restricted stoma; the duodenum and part of the jejunum are bypassed. RYGB, the most common form of bariatric surgery performed in the United States, restricts food intake and calorie absorption rate.

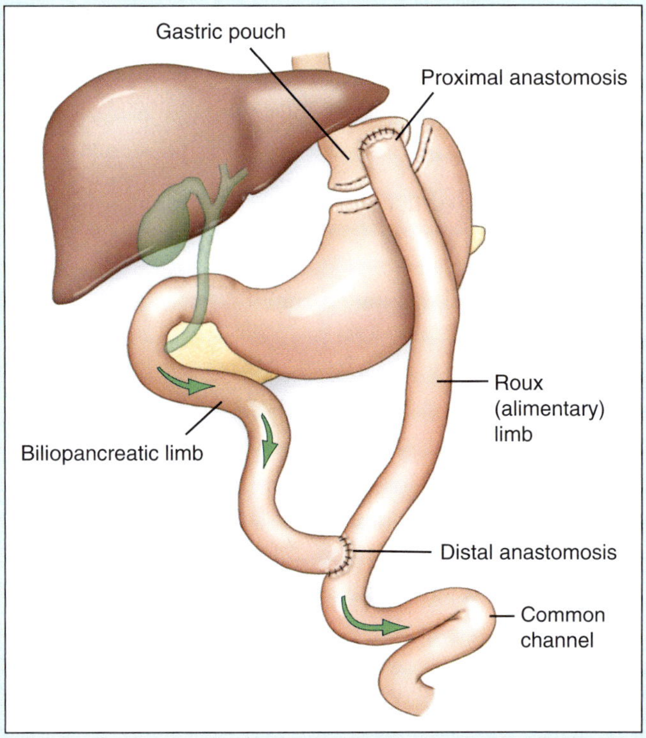

SLEEVE GASTRECOMY

The majority of the stomach is removed and a smaller tubular stomach is created. The capacity of the stomach is therefore significantly reduced.

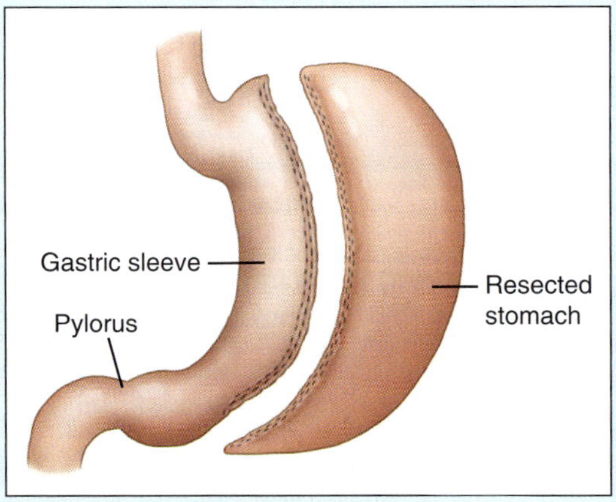

LAPAROSCOPIC ADJUSTABLE GASTRIC BANDING (LAGB)

Creation of a small gastric pouch by the placement of a band around the upper portion of the stomach; the band can be adjusted to change the size of the stomach through a subcutaneous port.

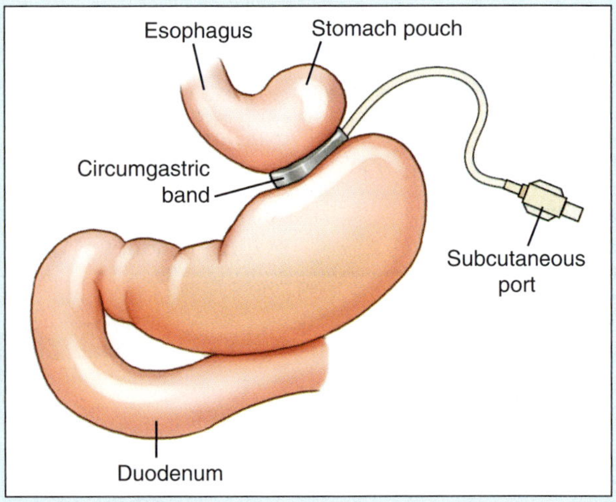

EXERCISE 15 ■ Pronounce and Spell

Practice pronunciation and spelling on paper and online.

1. Practice on Paper

a. **Pronounce:** Read the phonetic spelling and say aloud the terms listed in the previous table. Refer to the pronunciation key on p. 20 as necessary.
b. **Spell:** Have a study partner read the terms aloud. Write the spelling of the terms on a separate sheet of paper.

2. Practice Online

a. **Access** online learning resources. Go to evolve.elsevier.com > Evolve Resources > Student Resources.
b. **Pronounce:** Select Audio Glossary > Chapter 11 > Exercise 15. Select a term to hear its pronunciation and repeat aloud.
c. **Spell:** Select Activities > Chapter 11 > Spell Terms > Exercise 15. Select the audio icon and type the correct spelling of the term.

❑ Check the box when complete.

EXERCISE 16 ■ Identify

Write the term for each of the following definitions.

1. cutting certain branches of the vagus nerve ____________________
2. connection created by surgically joining two structures ____________________
3. removal of the distal colon, rectum, and anal sphincter ____________________
____
4. surgical reduction of gastric capacity to treat morbid obesity ____________________
5. excision of swollen or distended veins in the lower rectum and anus ____________________
____

EXERCISE 17 ■ Review of Surgical Terms

Can you define, pronounce, and spell the following terms?

abdominocentesis
abdominoperineal resection (APR)
abdominoplasty
anastomosis (*pl.* anastomoses)
anoplasty
antrectomy
appendectomy
bariatric surgery
cheiloplasty
cholecystectomy
choledocholithotomy
colectomy
colostomy
diverticulectomy
enterorrhaphy
esophagogastroplasty
gastrectomy
gastrojejunostomy
gastroplasty
gastrostomy
gingivectomy
glossorrhaphy
hemicolectomy
hemorrhoidectomy
herniorrhaphy
ileostomy
laparotomy
palatoplasty
pancreatectomy
polypectomy
pyloroplasty
uvulectomy
uvulopalatopharyngoplasty (UPPP)
vagotomy

Diagnostic Terms

BUILT FROM WORD PARTS

The following terms can be translated using definitions of word parts. Further explanation is provided within parentheses as needed.

DIAGNOSTIC IMAGING

TERM	DEFINITION
1. cholangiogram (kō-LAN-jē-ō-gram)	radiographic image of the bile ducts
2. cholangiography (kō-*lan*-jē-OG-ra-fē)	radiographic imaging of the bile ducts (after administration of contrast agents to outline the ducts)
3. CT colonography (C-T) (*kō*-lon-OG-ra-fē)	radiographic imaging of the colon (using computed tomography) (also called **virtual colonoscopy**)
4. esophagogram (e-SOF-a-gō-gram)	radiographic image of the esophagus (and pharynx) (also called **esophagram** and **barium swallow**)

OPERATIVE CHOLANGIOGRAPHY is performed during surgery to check for residual stones after the removal of the gallbladder. **Postoperative cholangiography**, also called T-tube cholangiography, is performed in the radiology department after a cholecystectomy, to check for residual stones. Both use the injection of contrast agents into the common bile duct.

ESOPHAGOGRAM During an **esophagogram**, a contrast agent, such a barium, is used to study the function and structure of the pharynx and esophagus as they relate to swallowing.

ENDOSCOPY

TERM	DEFINITION
5. capsule endoscopy (KAP-sel) (en-DOS-ko-pē)	(capsule) visual examination within (a hollow organ); (also called **camera endoscopy**) (Fig. 11.13)

CAPSULE ENDOSCOPY records pictures of the gastrointestinal tract and is especially helpful in visualizing the small intestine, which is not easily accessed. The procedure is used to find obscure causes of gastrointestinal bleeding and to help diagnose Crohn disease, celiac disease, and cancer.

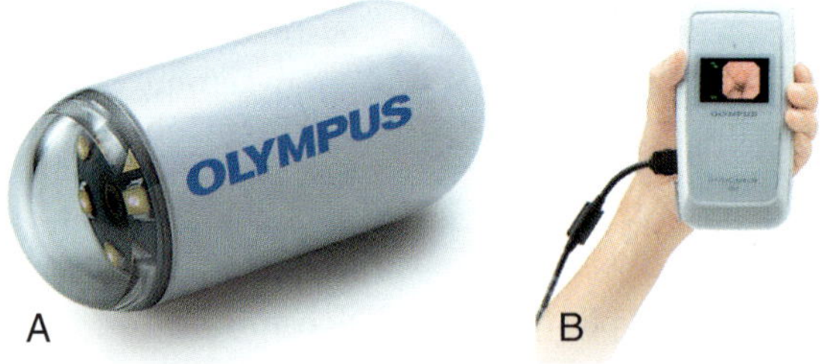

FIG. 11.13 Capsule endoscopy, also known as **camera endoscopy**. **A,** Patients swallow a capsule containing a camera, about the size of a pill. The camera takes pictures as it moves naturally through the gastrointestinal tract, and records thousands of images on a small device worn around the patient's waist. **B,** The recording device is then returned to the physician and the images are transferred to a computer for examination. The video capsule is expelled in the bowel movement and not retrieved.

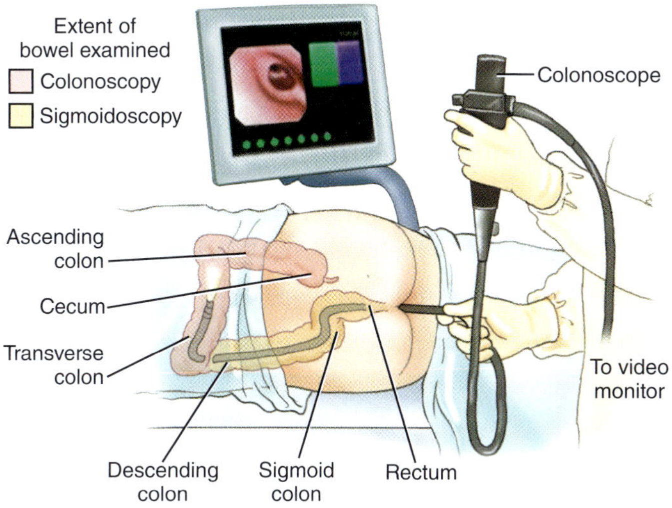

FIG. 11.14 Sigmoidoscopy, colonoscopy.

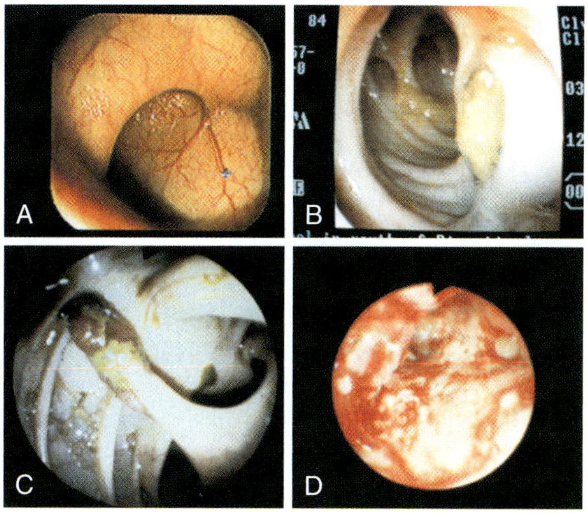

FIG. 11.15 Images obtained during colonoscopy reveal a normal colon **(A),** diverticulosis **(B),** a colon polyp **(C),** and colon cancer **(D).**

TERM	DEFINITION
6. colonoscope (kō-LON-ō-skōp)	instrument used for visual examination of the colon
7. colonoscopy (*kō*-lon-OS-ko-pē)	visual examination of the colon (Figs. 11.14 and 11.15)
8. esophagogastroduodenoscopy (EGD) (*e-sof*-a-gō-*gas*-trō-*dū*-od-e-NOS-ko-pē)	visual examination of the esophagus, stomach, and duodenum
9. esophagoscopy (e-*sof*-a-GOS-ko-pē)	visual examination of the esophagus
10. gastroscope (GAS-trō-skōp)	instrument used for visual examination of the stomach
11. gastroscopy (gas-TROS-ko-pē)	visual examination of the stomach

TERM	DEFINITION
12. laparoscope (LAP-a-rō-skōp)	instrument used for visual examination of the abdominal cavity

LAPAROSCOPES are also used to perform laparoscopic surgery, which is less invasive than open abdominal surgery.

TERM	DEFINITION
13. laparoscopy (*lap*-a-ROS-ko-pē)	visual examination of the abdominal cavity
14. proctoscope (PROK-tō-skōp)	instrument used for visual examination of the rectum
15. proctoscopy (prok-TOS-ko-pē)	visual examination of the rectum
16. sigmoidoscopy (*sig*-moy-DOS-ko-pē)	visual examination of the sigmoid colon (Fig. 11.14)

EXERCISE 18 ■ Pronounce and Spell

Practice pronunciation and spelling on paper and online.

1. Practice on Paper

a. **Pronounce:** Read the phonetic spelling and say aloud the terms listed in the previous table. Refer to the pronunciation key on p. 20 as necessary.
b. **Spell:** Have a study partner read the terms aloud. Write the spelling of the terms on a separate sheet of paper.

2. Practice Online

a. **Access** online learning resources. Go to evolve.elsevier.com > Evolve Resources > Student Resources.
b. **Pronounce:** Select Audio Glossary > Chapter 11 > Exercise 18. Select a term to hear its pronunciation and repeat aloud.
c. **Spell:** Select Activities > Chapter 11 > Spell Terms > Exercise 18. Select the audio icon and type the correct spelling of the term.

❑ Check the box when complete.

EXERCISE 19 ■ Analyze and Define

Analyze and define the following terms.

1. proctoscope
____
____
2. proctoscopy
____
____
3. sigmoidoscopy
____
____
4. cholangiography
____
____
5. colonoscope
____
____
6. laparoscope
____
____
7. laparoscopy
____
____
8. esophagogram
____
____

EXERCISE 20 ■ Build

A Fill In

Build diagnostic terms for the following definitions by using the word parts you have learned.

1. visual examination of the esophagus
________ / __ / ________
WR / CV / S

2. radiographic image of the bile ducts
________ / __ / ________
WR / CV / S

3. visual examination of the esophagus, stomach, and duodenum
____ / __ / ____ / __ / ____ / __ / ____
WR / CV / WR / CV / WR / CV / S

B Label

Build terms pictured by writing word parts above definitions.

1.

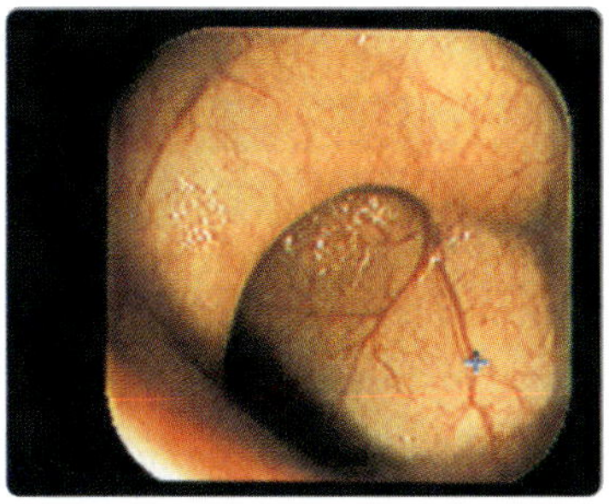

_______ / ____ / ___________
colon CV visual examination

2.

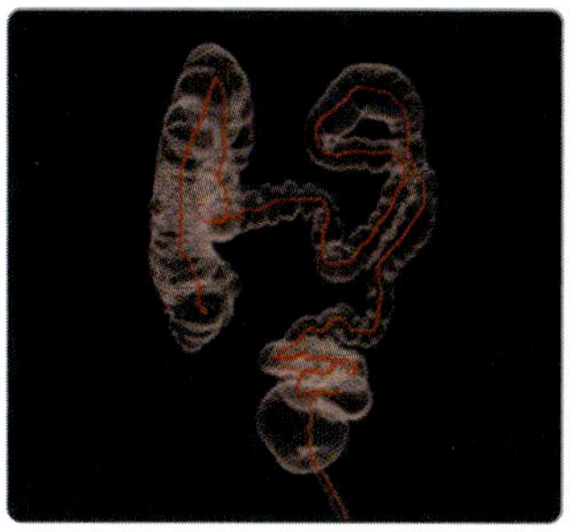

CT _______ / ____ / ___________
colon CV radiographic imaging

3.

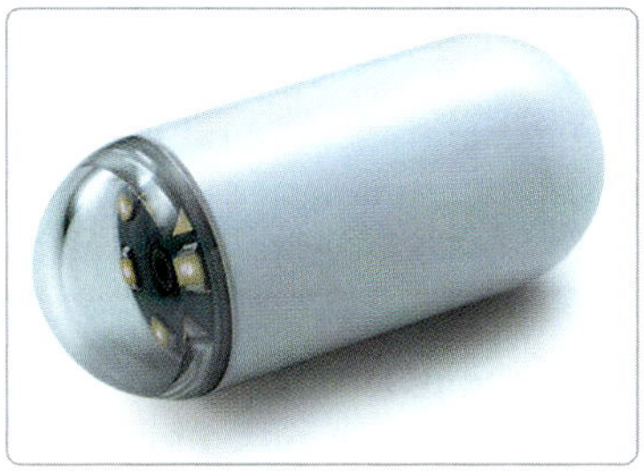

capsule ___________ / ___________
within (hollow organ) visual examination

4.

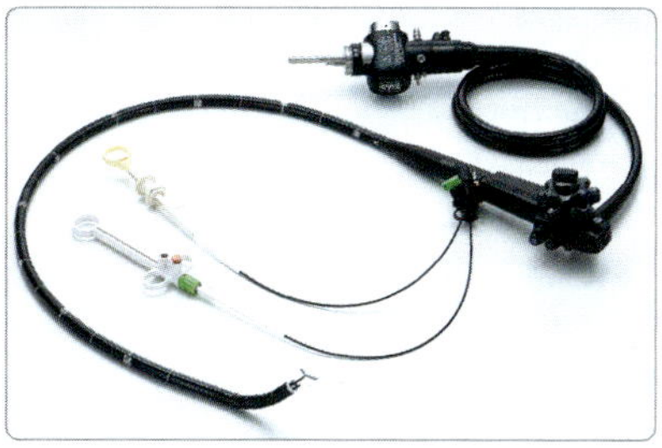

_______ / ____ / ___________
stomach CV instrument used for visual examination

5.

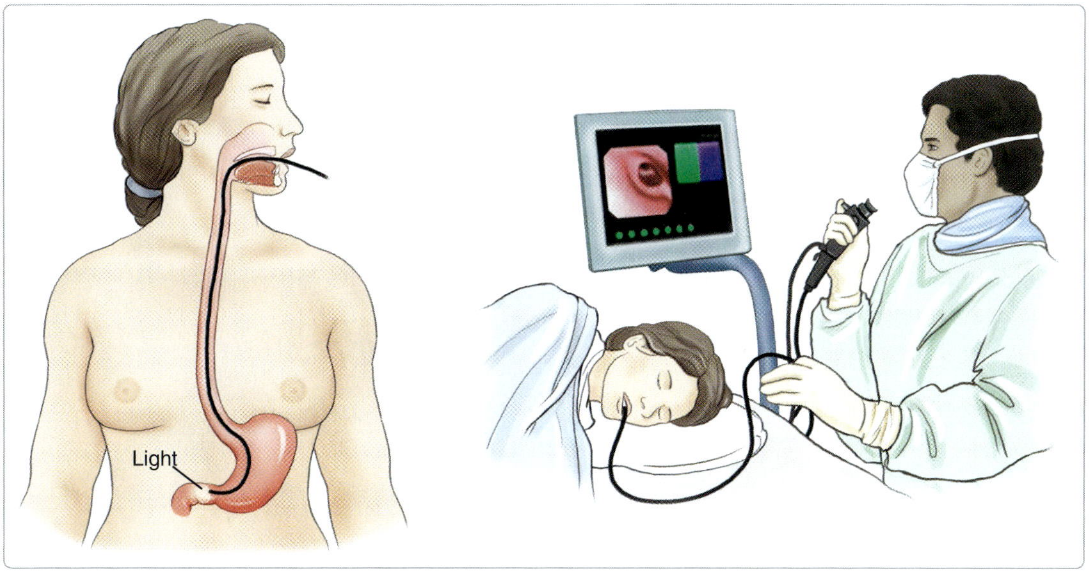

_______ / ____ / ___________
stomach CV visual examination

Diagnostic Terms

NOT BUILT FROM WORD PARTS

Word parts may be present in the following terms; however, their full meanings cannot be translated using definitions of word parts alone.

DIAGNOSTIC IMAGING

TERM	DEFINITION
1. **abdominal sonography** (ab-DOM-i-nal) (so-NOG-ra-fē)	ultrasound scanning of the abdominal cavity in which the size and structure of organs such as the aorta, liver, gallbladder, bile ducts, and pancreas can be visualized (Table 11.2)
2. **barium enema (BE)** (BAR-ē-um) (EN-e-ma)	series of radiographic images taken of the large intestine after the contrast agent barium has been administered rectally (also called **lower GI series**) (Fig. 11.16)
3. **endoscopic retrograde cholangiopancreatography (ERCP)** (*en*-dō-SKOP-ic) (RET-rō-grād) (kō-*lan*-jē-ō-*pan*-krē-a-TOG-rah-fē)	procedure using an endoscope to visualize the biliary and pancreatic ducts, introduce contrast agents, and record x-ray images (fluoroscopy); used to evaluate obstructions, strictures, and some diseases of the liver and pancreas. Stone removal, biopsy, and stenting may be performed during the procedure for treatment.
4. **endoscopic ultrasound (EUS)** (*en*-dō-SKOP-ic) (UL-tra-sound)	procedure using an endoscope fitted with an ultrasound probe that provides images of the esophageal and gastric linings, as well as the walls of the small and large intestines; used to detect tumors and cystic growths and for staging of malignant tumors
5. **upper GI series** (UP-per) (G-Ī) (SE-rēz)	series of radiographic images taken of the pharynx, esophagus, stomach, and duodenum after the contrast agent barium has been administered orally (also called **upper gastrointestinal series**)

TABLE 11.2 Abdominal Sonography

AREAS VISUALIZED AND POSSIBLE FINDINGS

- **Liver**—cysts, abscess, tumors, hepatitis, fatty infiltration, cirrhosis, hepatomegaly
- **Gallbladder and bile ducts**—cholelithiasis, choledocholithiasis, inflammation, obstruction, tumors (including polyps)
- **Pancreas**—inflammation, tumors, abscess, pseudocysts, obstruction
- **Kidney**—calculi, cysts, tumors, hydronephrosis, malformations, abscess, inflammation, scarring, atrophy
- **Aorta**—aneurysm, dissection, atherosclerosis

IMAGE

Abdominal ultrasound showing cholelithiasis.
GB, Gallbladder; *St*, stone

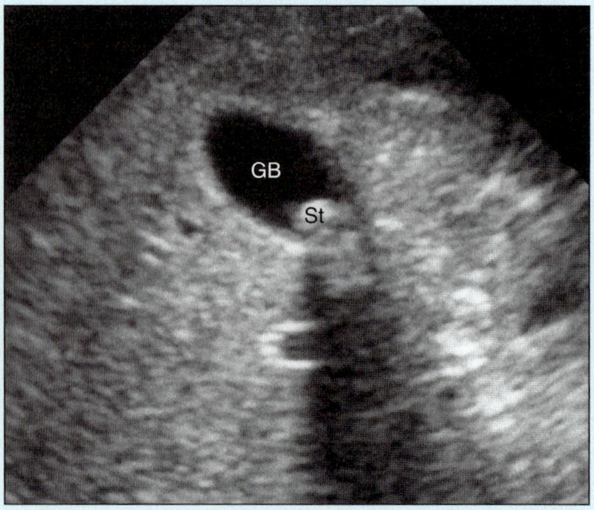

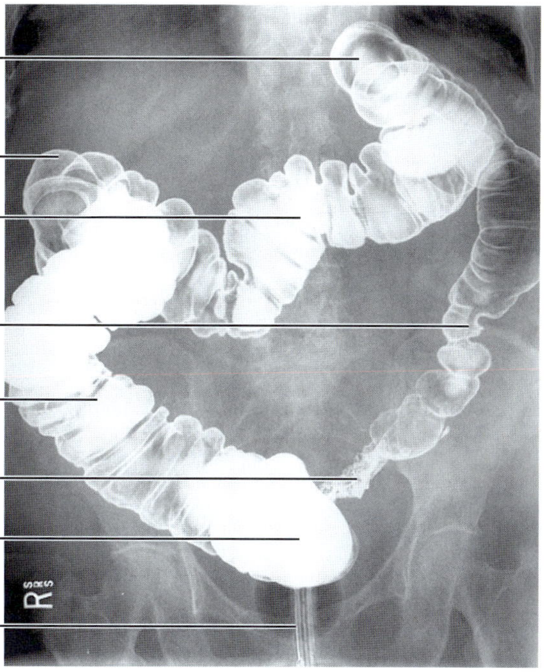

FIG. 11.16 Barium enema (BE); also called a **lower GI series.**

LABORATORY

TERM	DEFINITION
6. fecal occult blood test (FOBT) (FĒ-kl) (o-KULT) (blud) (test)	examination of a stool sample to detect blood not directly visible. Occult blood refers to blood that is present but can only be detected by chemical testing or by microscope. The test is used to screen for colon cancer or polyps.

FECAL IMMUNOCHEMICAL TEST (FIT) for occult blood is currently the standard stool test for screening for colorectal cancer and large polyps that may become cancerous. The FIT test requires only one stool specimen and is specific for occult blood in the lower gastrointestinal tract.

TERM	DEFINITION
7. *Helicobacter pylori (H. pylori)* stool antigen (*hel*-i-kō-BAK-ter) (pī-LŌ-rē) (stul) (AN-ti-jen)	chemical test on a fecal sample to determine the presence of the bacteria *(H. pylori)* that can cause peptic ulcers

HELICOBACTER PYLORI TESTING refers to various tests used to determine the presence of *Helicobacter pylori (H. pylori)* bacteria, which can cause peptic ulcers. Testing may be performed on a biopsy specimen during endoscopy (such as esophagogastroduodenoscopy), or via noninvasive testing, such as stool antigen or urea breath tests.

EXERCISE 21 ■ Pronounce and Spell

Practice pronunciation and spelling on paper and online.

1. Practice on Paper

a. **Pronounce:** Read the phonetic spelling and say aloud the terms listed in the previous table. Refer to the pronunciation key on p. 20 as necessary.
b. **Spell:** Have a study partner read the terms aloud. Write the spelling of the terms on a separate sheet of paper.

2. Practice Online

a. **Access** online learning resources. Go to evolve.elsevier.com > Evolve Resources > Student Resources.
b. **Pronounce:** Select Audio Glossary > Chapter 11 > Exercise 21. Select a term to hear its pronunciation and repeat aloud.
c. **Spell:** Select Activities > Chapter 11 > Spell Terms > Exercise 21. Select the audio icon and type the correct spelling of the term.

❑ Check the box when complete.

EXERCISE 22 ■ Match

Match the diagnostic terms in the first column with their correct definitions in the second column.

_____ 1. fecal occult blood test	a. used to identify bacteria that can cause peptic ulcers
_____ 2. barium enema	b. radiographic images of the pharynx, esophagus, stomach, and duodenum
_____ 3. *Helicobacter pylori* stool antigen	c. provides images of esophageal and gastric linings, and also walls of the intestines
_____ 4. upper GI series	d. detects blood in a stool sample
_____ 5. endoscopic retrograde cholangiopancreatography	e. radiographic imaging of biliary and pancreatic ducts
_____ 6. abdominal sonography	f. radiographic images of the large intestine
_____ 7. endoscopic ultrasound	g. ultrasound to visualize a portion of the aorta, liver, gallbladder, bile ducts, and pancreas

EXERCISE 23 ■ Fill In

A Label

Write the diagnostic terms pictured and defined.

1. ______________________________
____
procedure using an endoscope to visualize the biliary and pancreatic ducts, introduce contrast agents, and record x-ray images

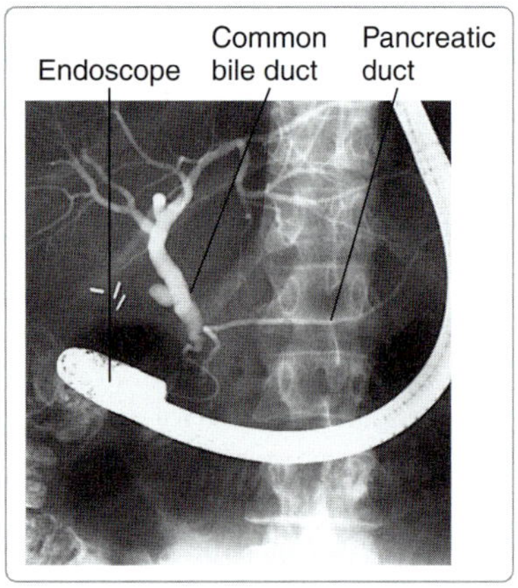

2. ______________________________
____
series of radiographic images taken of the large intestine afer the contrast agent barium has been administered rectally

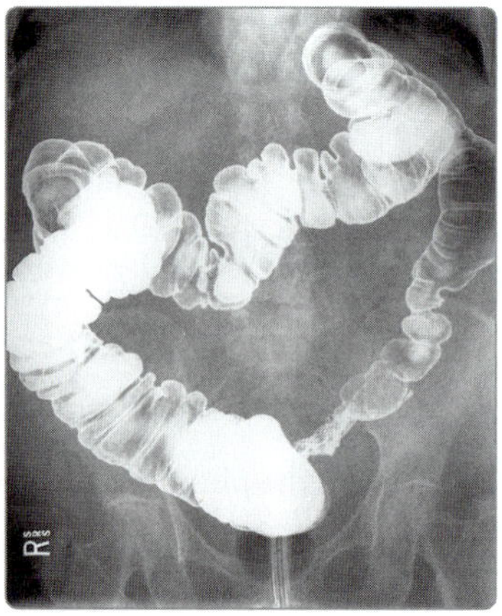

B Identify

Write the term for each of the following definitions.

1. chemical test on a fecal sample to determine the presence of the bacteria that can be found in the lining of the stomach and can cause peptic ulcers ______
2. examination of a stool sample to detect blood not directly visible ______
3. ultrasound scanning of the abdominal cavity to visualize the organs within ______
4. procedure using an endoscope fitted with an ultrasound probe that provides images of the esophageal and gastric linings, as well as the walls of the small and large intestines ______
5. series of radiographic images taken of the pharynx, esophagus, stomach, and duodenum after the contrast agent barium has been administered orally ______

EXERCISE 24 ■ Review of Diagnostic Terms

Can you define, pronounce, and spell the following terms?

abdominal sonography
abdominocentesis
barium enema (BE)
capsule endoscopy
cholangiography
colonoscope
colonoscopy
CT colonography
endoscopic retrograde cholangiopancreatography (ERCP)
endoscopic ultrasound (EUS)
esophagogastroduodenoscopy (EGD)
esophagogram
esophagoscopy
fecal occult blood test (FOBT)
gastroscope
gastroscopy
Helicobacter pylori stool antigen
laparoscope
laparoscopy
proctoscope
proctoscopy
sigmoidoscopy
upper GI series

Complementary Terms

BUILT FROM WORD PARTS

The following terms can be translated using definitions of word parts. Further explanation is provided within parentheses as needed.

SIGNS AND SYMPTOMS

TERM	DEFINITION
1. aphagia (a-FĀ-ja)	without swallowing (the inability to)
2. dyspepsia (dis-PEP-sē-a)	difficult digestion (often used to describe GI symptoms, such as abdominal pain and bloating)
3. dysphagia (dis-FĀ-ja)	difficult swallowing
4. hepatomegaly (*hep*-a-tō-MEG-a-lē)	enlargement of the liver
5. steatorrhea (*stē*-a-tō-RĒ-a)	discharge of fat (excessive amount of fat in the stool, causing frothy, foul-smelling fecal matter usually associated with the malabsorption of fat in conditions such as chronic pancreatitis and celiac disease)
6. steatosis (*stē*-a-TŌ-sis)	abnormal condition of fat (increased fat at the cellular level often affecting the liver)

Complementary Terms—cont'd

BUILT FROM WORD PARTS

MEDICAL SPECIALTIES

TERM	DEFINITION
7. **gastroenterologist** (*gas*-trō-*en*-ter-OL-o-jist)	physician who studies and treats diseases of the stomach and intestines (GI tract and accessory organs)
8. **gastroenterology** (*gas*-trō-*en*-ter-OL-o-jē)	study of the stomach and intestines (branch of medicine that deals with treating diseases of the GI tract and accessory organs)

DESCRIPTIVE TERMS

TERM	DEFINITION
9. **anal** (Ā-nal)	pertaining to the anus
10. **celiac** (SĒ-lē-ak)	pertaining to the abdomen
11. **colorectal** (*kō*-lō-REK-tal)	pertaining to the colon and rectum
12. **duodenal** (dū-OD-e-nal)	pertaining to the duodenum
13. **esophageal** (e-*sof*-a-JĒ-al)	pertaining to the esophagus
14. **ileocecal** (*il*-ē-ō-SĒ-kal)	pertaining to the ileum and cecum
15. **nasogastric** (*nā*-zō-GAS-trik)	pertaining to the nose and stomach
16. **oral** (OR-al)	pertaining to the mouth
17. **palatal** (PAL-a-tal)	pertaining to the palate
18. **pancreatic** (*pan*-krē-AT-ik)	pertaining to the pancreas
19. **peritoneal** (*per*-i-tō-NĒ-al)	pertaining to the peritoneum
20. **rectal** (REK-tal)	pertaining to the rectum
21. **sublingual** (sub-LING-gwal)	pertaining to under the tongue

EXERCISE 25 ■ Pronounce and Spell

Practice pronunciation and spelling on paper and online.

1. Practice on Paper

a. **Pronounce:** Read the phonetic spelling and say aloud the terms listed in the previous table. Refer to the pronunciation key on p. 20 as necessary.
b. **Spell:** Have a study partner read the terms aloud. Write the spelling of the terms on a separate sheet of paper.

2. Practice Online

a. **Access** online learning resources. Go to evolve.elsevier.com > Evolve Resources > Student Resources.
b. **Pronounce:** Select Audio Glossary > Chapter 11 > Exercise 25. Select a term to hear its pronunciation and repeat aloud.
c. **Spell:** Select Activities > Chapter 11 > Spell Terms > Exercise 25. Select the audio icon and type the correct spelling of the term.

❑ Check the box when complete.

EXERCISE 26 ■ Analyze and Define

Analyze and define the following complementary terms.

1. rectal
____
____
2. dyspepsia
____
____
3. palatal
____
____
4. esophageal
____
____
5. steatorrhea
____
____
6. duodenal
____
____
7. oral
____
____
8. gastroenterologist
____
____
9. steatosis
____
____
10. pancreatic
____
____

EXERCISE 27 ■ Build

Build complementary terms for the following definitions by using the word parts you have learned.

1. enlargement of the liver ______ / ______ / ______
WR / CV / S
2. without swallowing (the inability to) ______ / ______
P / S(WR)
3. pertaining to under the tongue ______ / ______ / ______
P / WR / S
4. pertaining to the nose and the stomach ______ / ______ / ______ / ______
WR / CV / WR / S
5. pertaining to the mouth and the stomach ______ / ______ / ______ / ______
WR / CV / WR / S
6. pertaining to the anus ______ / ______
WR / S

7. pertaining to the peritoneum ______ / ______
WR / S

8. pertaining to the abdomen ______ / ______
WR / S

9. difficult swallowing ______ / ______
P / S(WR)

10. pertaining to the ileum and cecum ______ / ______ / ______ / ______
WR / CV / WR / S

11. pertaining to the colon and rectum ______ / ______ / ______ / ______
WR / CV / WR / S

Complementary Terms

NOT BUILT FROM WORD PARTS

Word parts may be present in the following terms; however, their full meanings cannot be translated using definitions of word parts alone.

SIGNS AND SYMPTOMS

TERM	DEFINITION
1. ascites (a-SĪ-tēz)	abnormal collection of fluid in the peritoneal cavity
2. diarrhea (dī-a-RĒ-a)	frequent discharge of liquid stool
DIARRHEA contains the prefix **dia-**, meaning **through**, and the suffix **-rrhea**, meaning **flow**.	
3. emesis (EM-e-sis)	expelling matter from the stomach through the mouth (also called **vomiting**)
4. flatus (FLĀ-tus)	gas in the gastrointestinal tract or expelled through the anus
5. hematemesis (*hē*-ma-TEM-e-sis)	vomiting of blood
6. hematochezia (*hē*-ma-tō-KĒ-zha)	passage of visibly bloody feces
7. malabsorption (*mal*-ab-SORP-shun)	impaired digestion or intestinal absorption of nutrients
8. melena (me-LĒ-na)	black, tarry stool that contains digested blood; usually a result of bleeding in the upper GI tract
9. nausea (NAW-zē-a)	urge to vomit
10. reflux (RĒ-fluks)	abnormal backward flow. In esophageal reflux, the stomach contents flow back into the esophagus.

TREATMENTS

TERM	DEFINITION
11. gastric lavage (GAS-trik) (la-VOZH)	washing out of the stomach

OTHER TERMS	
TERM	**DEFINITION**
12. feces (FĒ-sēz)	waste from the gastrointestinal tract expelled through the anus (also called **stool** or **fecal matter**)
13. palpate (PAL-pāt)	to examine by hand; to feel
14. stoma (STŌ-ma)	surgical opening between an organ and the surface of the body, such as the opening established in the abdominal wall by colostomy, ileostomy, or a similar operation. Stoma may also refer to an opening created between body structures or between portions of the intestines.

Refer to **Appendix E** for pharmacology terms related to the digestive system.

EXERCISE 28 ■ Pronounce and Spell

Practice pronunciation and spelling on paper and online.

1. Practice on Paper

a. **Pronounce:** Read the phonetic spelling and say aloud the terms listed in the previous table. Refer to the pronunciation key on p. 20 as necessary.
b. **Spell:** Have a study partner read the terms aloud. Write the spelling of the terms on a separate sheet of paper.

2. Practice Online

a. **Access** online learning resources. Go to evolve.elsevier.com > Evolve Resources > Student Resources.
b. **Pronounce:** Select Audio Glossary > Chapter 11 > Exercise 28. Select a term to hear its pronunciation and repeat aloud.
c. **Spell:** Select Activities > Chapter 11 > Spell Terms > Exercise 28. Select the audio icon and type the correct spelling of the term.

❑ Check the box when complete.

EXERCISE 29 ■ Match

Match the definitions in the first column with their correct terms in the second column.

_____	1. abnormal collection of fluid in the peritoneal cavity	a. hematemesis
_____	2. expelling matter from the stomach	b. flatus
_____	3. to examine by hand	c. gastric lavage
_____	4. washing out of the stomach	d. reflux
_____	5. urge to vomit	e. emesis
_____	6. frequent discharge of liquid stool	f. stoma
_____	7. waste expelled through the anus	g. melena
_____	8. vomiting of blood	h. palpate
_____	9. abnormal backward flow	i. diarrhea
_____	10. impaired digestion or intestinal absorption	j. malabsorption
_____	11. gas expelled through the anus	k. feces
_____	12. passage of visibly bloody feces	l. nausea
_____	13. black, tarry stools	m. ascites
_____	14. surgical opening between an organ and the surface of the body	n. hematochezia

EXERCISE 30 ■ Fill In

A Label

Write the medical terms pictured and defined.

1. ______________________________
surgical opening between an organ and the surface of the body

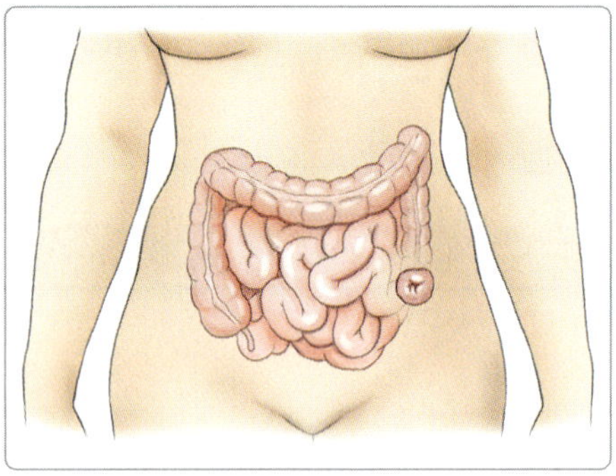

2. ______________________________
to examine by hand; to feel

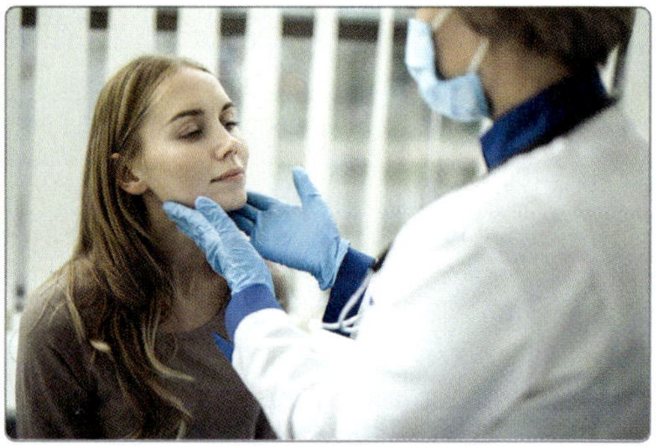

3. ______________________________
abnormal backward flow

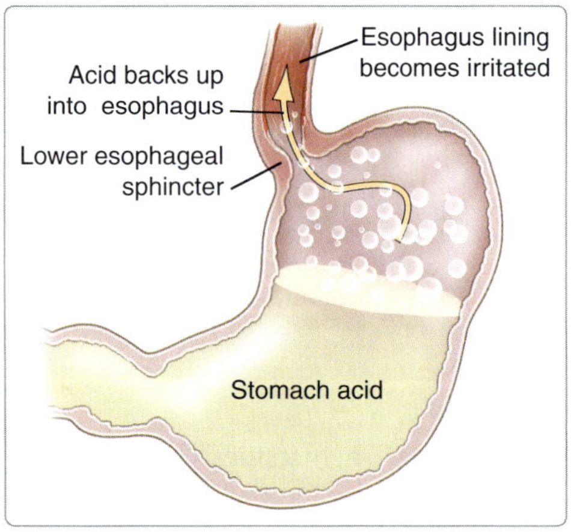

4. ______________________________
abnormal collection of fluid in the peritoneal cavity

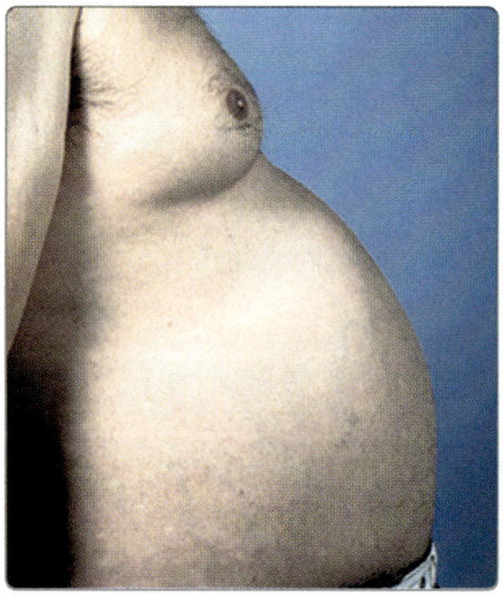

B Identify

Write the term for each of the following definitions.

1. also called stool ______________________________
2. frequent discharge of liquid stool ______________________________
3. washing out of the stomach ______________________________
4. also called vomiting ______________________________
5. passage of visibly bloody feces ______________________________
6. black, tarry stool that contains digested blood ______________________________
7. urge to vomit ______________________________
8. impaired digestion or intestinal absorption of nutrients ______________________________
9. vomiting of blood ______________________________
10. gas in the gastrointestinal tract or expelled through the anus ______________________________

EXERCISE 31 ■ Review of Complementary Terms

Can you define, pronounce, and spell the following terms?

anal	emesis	hepatomegaly	pancreatic
aphagia	esophageal	ileocecal	peritoneal
ascites	feces	malabsorption	rectal
celiac	flatus	melena	reflux
colorectal	gastric lavage	nasogastric	steatorrhea
diarrhea	gastroenterologist	nausea	steatosis
duodenal	gastroenterology	oral	stoma
dyspepsia	hematemesis	palatal	sublingual
dysphagia	hematochezia	palpate	

Abbreviations

DISEASE AND DISORDER

ABBREVIATION	TERM	ABBREVIATION	TERM
IBS	irritable bowel syndrome	**UC**	ulcerative colitis
GERD	gastroesophageal reflux disease		

DIAGNOSTIC

ABBREVIATION	TERM	ABBREVIATION	TERM
BE	barium enema	**EUS**	endoscopic ultrasound
EGD	esophagogastroduodenoscopy	**FIT**	fecal immunochemical test
ERCP	endoscopic retrograde cholangiopancreatography	**FOBT**	fecal occult blood test

TREATMENT

ABBREVIATION	TERM	ABBREVIATION	TERM
APR	abdominoperineal resection	**UPPP**	uvulopalatopharyngoplasty
PEG	percutaneous endoscopic gastrostomy		

DESCRIPTIVE

ABBREVIATION	TERM	ABBREVIATION	TERM
GI	gastrointestinal	**UGI**	upper gastrointestinal

OTHER

ABBREVIATION	TERM	ABBREVIATION	TERM
H. pylori	*Helicobacter pylori* (bacteria that can cause pectic ulcers)	**N&V**	nausea and vomiting

Refer to **Appendix D** for a complete list of abbreviations.

EXERCISE 32 ■ Abbreviations

Write abbreviations for the terms listed below.

1. upper gastrointestinal ____________
2. *Helicobacter pylori* (bacteria that can cause pectic ulcers) ____________
3. nausea and vomiting ____________
4. endoscopic retrograde cholangiopancreatography ____________
5. gastrointestinal ____________
6. uvulopalatopharyngoplasty ____________
7. gastroesophageal reflux disease ____________
8. ulcerative colitis ____________
9. barium enema ____________
10. irritable bowel syndrome ____________
11. esophagogastroduodenoscopy ____________
12. percutaneous endoscopic gastrostomy ____________
13. endoscopic ultrasound ____________
14. abdominoperineal resection ____________
15. fecal occult blood test ____________
16. fecal immunochemical test ____________

PRACTICAL APPLICATION

EXERCISE 33 ■ Case Study: Translate Between Everyday Language and Medical Language

CASE STUDY: Ruth Clifton

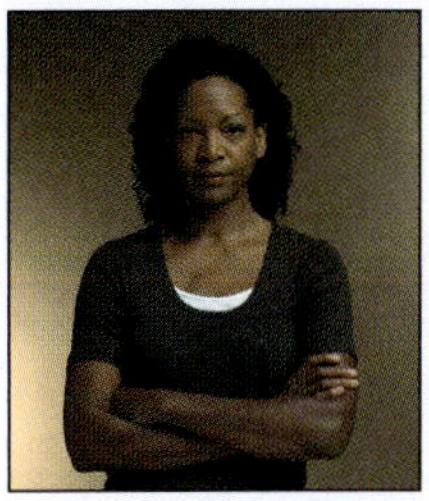

Ruth is worried about her stomach. She has been having pain on and off for about 3 months. At first it was just once in a while but now it seems to be every day. Her pain seems to be worse when she hasn't eaten for a while, and after she eats something bland it usually gets a bit better. She bought some antacids at the pharmacy and chewing those also seems to help. Lately the pain in her stomach has been waking her up at night. A glass of milk usually helps with that. The last few days, however, she has felt sick to her stomach, has been throwing up, and is finding it difficult to eat. Her friend recommends that she see a stomach doctor, who helped her when she had similar problems.

Now that you have worked through Chapter 11 on the digestive system, consider the medical terms that might be used to describe Ruth Clifton's experience. See the Chapter at a Glance section at the end of this chapter for a list of terms that might apply.

A. *Underline phrases in the case study that could be substituted with medical terms.*

B. *Write the medical term and its definition for three of the phrases you underlined.*

MEDICAL TERM	DEFINITION
1. ______________	______________
2. ______________	______________
3. ______________	______________

DOCUMENTATION: Excerpt from Endoscopic Procedure Report

Ms. Clifton made an appointment with a gastroenterologist. He recommended an endoscopic procedure; a portion of the report is documented below.

ENDOSCOPY REPORT: Procedure: Esophagogastroduodenoscopy

The patient was given 2 mg of intravenous midazolam along with lidocaine spray to the pharynx. After she was placed in the left lateral decubitus position, the gastroscope was passed into the pharynx without difficulty. No abnormalities were noted in the esophagus or in the cardia and the body of the stomach. A biopsy of the gastric mucosa was obtained for *Helicobacter pylori* testing. In the distal antrum, some mild erythematous changes were noted. The pylorus appeared normal, but a single 1-cm ulceration of the proximal duodenum, a peptic ulcer, was observed.

C. *Underline medical terms presented in Chapter 11 in the previous excerpt from Ms. Clifton's medical record. See the Chapter at a Glance section at the end of the chapter for a complete list.*

D. *Select and define three of the medical terms you underlined. To check your answers, go to Appendix A.*

MEDICAL TERM	DEFINITION
1. ______________	______________
2. ______________	______________
3. ______________	______________

EXERCISE 34 ■ Interact with Medical Documents

A

Read the report and complete it by writing medical terms on answer lines within the document. Definitions of terms to be written appear after the document.

01182003 JOHNSON, Sylvia

File Patient Navigate Custom Fields Help

Chart Review | Encounters | Notes | Labs | Imaging | Procedures | Rx | Documents | Referrals | Scheduling | Billing

Name: **Sylvia Johnson** MR#: **01182003** DOB: **11/03/19xx** Gender: **F** Age: **63** Allergies: **None known** PCP: **Chambers, Jacqueline DO**

Gastroenterology Consultation Note

Sylvia Johnson is a 63-year-old female who was referred by her PCP for evaluation of 1. ______________________. She reports this has been occurring for the last 3 weeks. She also reports a change in bowel habits with alternating constipation and 2. ______________________ over the last 3 months. She denies 3. ______________________ or 4. ______________________. She has a history of 5. ______________________ and was tested for 6. ______________________ approximately 8 years ago. She denies any history of 7. ______________________, 8. ______________________, or 9. ______________________. Her family history is significant for 10. ______________________ cancer in her father, who died at age 70, and 11. ______________________ in her mother, who died of other causes at age 88.

On exam, she is a thin African American female, pleasant and in no acute distress. Vital signs are normal. Abdominal exam reveals normal bowel sounds, nontender to palpation with no 12. ______________________ or 13. ______________________. Rectal exam reveals normal tone, external 14. ______________________, and no stool.

Impression and Plan: Hematochezia in a 63-year-old female with several risk factors for colon cancer. We will schedule her for a 15. ______________________ as soon as possible.

Abdul Ismail, MD
Gastroenterologist

Start | Log On/Off | Print | Edit

Definitions of Medical Terms to Complete the Document

Write the medical terms defined on corresponding answer lines in the document.

1. discharge of visibly bloody feces
2. frequent discharge of liquid stool
3. urge to vomit
4. expelling matter from the stomach through the mouth
5. abnormal backward flow of the gastrointestinal contents into the esophagus
6. test on a fecal sample to determine the presence of a bacteria found in the lining of the stomach that can cause peptic ulcers
7. erosion of the mucous membrane of the stomach or duodenum
8. chronic inflammation of the intestinal tract characterized by cobblestone ulcerations and the formation of scar tissue that may lead to intestinal obstruction
9. disease characterized by inflammation of the colon with the formation of ulcers, which can cause bloody diarrhea
10. pertaining to the colon and rectum
11. inflammation of the esophagus
12. abnormal collection of fluid in the peritoneal cavity
13. enlargement of the liver
14. swollen or distended veins in the rectum or anus
15. visual examination of the colon

B

Read the medical report and answer the questions below it.

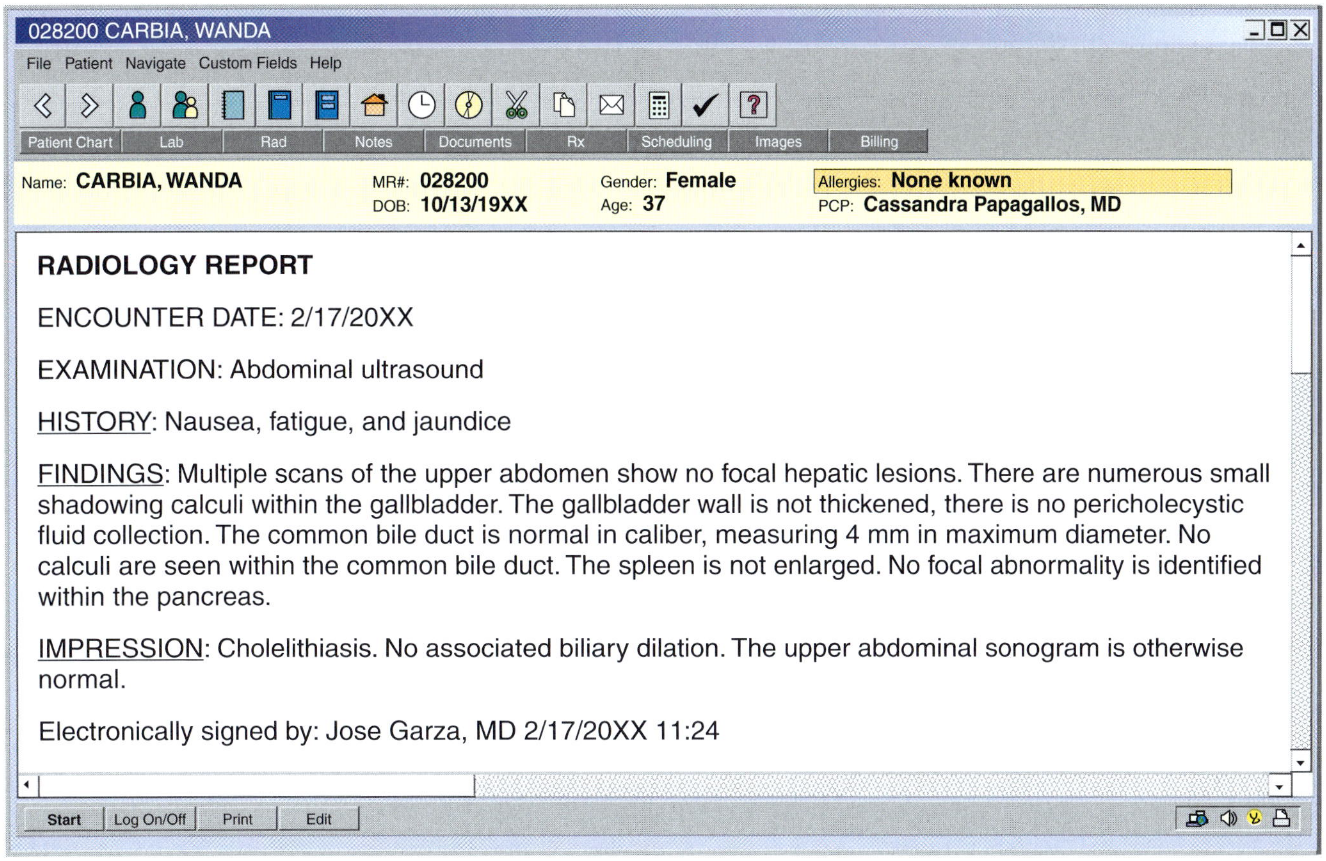

028200 CARBIA, WANDA

File Patient Navigate Custom Fields Help

Patient Chart | Lab | Rad | Notes | Documents | Rx | Scheduling | Images | Billing

Name: **CARBIA, WANDA** MR#: **028200** DOB: **10/13/19XX** Gender: **Female** Age: **37** Allergies: **None known** PCP: **Cassandra Papagallos, MD**

RADIOLOGY REPORT

ENCOUNTER DATE: 2/17/20XX

EXAMINATION: Abdominal ultrasound

HISTORY: Nausea, fatigue, and jaundice

FINDINGS: Multiple scans of the upper abdomen show no focal hepatic lesions. There are numerous small shadowing calculi within the gallbladder. The gallbladder wall is not thickened, there is no pericholecystic fluid collection. The common bile duct is normal in caliber, measuring 4 mm in maximum diameter. No calculi are seen within the common bile duct. The spleen is not enlarged. No focal abnormality is identified within the pancreas.

IMPRESSION: Cholelithiasis. No associated biliary dilation. The upper abdominal sonogram is otherwise normal.

Electronically signed by: Jose Garza, MD 2/17/20XX 11:24

Start | Log On/Off | Print | Edit

Use the medical report above to answer the questions.

1. The exam included which diagnostic procedure:
   a. radiographic imaging of the colon with computerized tomography
   b. radiographic imaging of the bile ducts after administration of contrast agents
   c. use of an endoscope fitted with an ultrasound probe to obtain images of layers of the intestinal wall
   d. recording images of organs with sound waves produced by a transducer placed directly on the skin
2. The patient's symptoms included:
   a. expelling matter from the stomach through the mouth
   b. urge to vomit
   c. passage of visibly bloody feces
   d. vomiting of blood
3. The examination revealed the presence of:
   a. stones within the gallbladder
   b. stones within the common bile duct
   c. lesions in the liver
   d. inflammation of the pancreas
4. "Biliary dilation" would most likely refer to:
   a. inflammation of the pancreas
   b. the presence of fluid in the upper abdomen
   c. choledocholithiasis
   d. widening of the bile ducts or gallbladder

EXERCISE 35 ■ Use Medical Language in Online Electronic Health Records

Select the correct medical terms to complete three medical records in one patient's electronic file.

Access online resources at evolve.elsevier.com > Evolve Resources > Student Resources > Activities > Chapter 11 > Electronic Health Records

Topic: Bowel Obstruction
Record 1: Office Visit
Record 2: Radiology Report
Record 3: Colonoscopy Report

❑ Check the box when complete.

EXERCISE 36 ■ Pronounce Medical Terms in Use

Practice pronunciation of terms by reading aloud the following paragraphs. Use the phonetic spellings following medical terms from the chapter to assist with pronunciation. The script also contains medical terms not presented in the chapter. If interested, research their meanings in a medical dictionary or a reliable online source.

COLORECTAL CANCER

Colorectal (kō-lō-REK-tal) cancer begins in the colon or rectum and is the second leading cause of cancer deaths in the United States. Most are adenocarcinomas that originate as a benign, adenomatous **polyp** (POL-ip).

Many people have no symptoms until the tumor is quite advanced, and symptoms vary depending on the location of the tumor. Warning signs are altered bowel habits, **rectal** (REK-tal) bleeding, abdominal cramps, **flatus** (FLĀ-tus) and bloating, iron deficiency anemia, and weight loss.

Screening and diagnostic tests for colorectal cancer include digital rectal examination, **fecal occult blood test** (FĒ-kl) (o-KULT) (blud) (test) or other stool testing, **sigmoidoscopy** (*sig*-moy-DOS-ko-pē), **colonoscopy** (kō-lon-OS-ko-pē), and **barium enema** (BAR-ē-um) (EN-e-ma). As well as being an important diagnostic tool, colonoscopy may be used for biopsy and for the removal of pedunculated **polyps** (POL-ips). To perform a **polypectomy** (*pol*-i-PEK-to-mē), a braided wire snare is inserted into the **colonoscope** (kō-LON-ō-skōp). A snare loop is placed around the stem of the polyp. With electrosurgical power attached to the snare, the polyp is detached. The polyp is removed from the colon for histologic examination.

For cancer beyond the early stage, conventional surgery is the main treatment. The type of surgery depends on the location and stage of the tumor. Types of surgeries performed are left or right-sided **hemicolectomy** (*hem*-ē-kō-LEK-to-mē) with **anastomosis** (a-*nas*-to-MŌ-sis), sigmoid **colectomy** (kō-LEK-to-mē), and **abdominoperineal resection** (ab-*dom*-i-nō-per-i-NĒ-el) (rē-SEK-shun) with **colostomy** (ko-LOS-to-mē). Currently, colorectal surgeons can sometimes perform low anterior resection (LAR), which preserves the anal sphincter and prevents the need for a colostomy.

CHAPTER REVIEW

EXERCISE 37 ■ Chapter Content Quiz

Test your understanding of terms and abbreviations introduced in this chapter. Circle the letter for the medical term or abbreviation related to the words in italics.

1. Mr. Gomez was tentatively diagnosed with *gallstones*, or
   a. cholelithiasis
   b. cholecystitis
   c. choledocholithiasis
2. An abdominal ultrasound confirmed the diagnosis, and Mr. Gomez is now scheduled for a laparoscopic *excision of the gallbladder*, or
   a. cholecystostomy
   b. cholecystectomy
   c. colectomy
3. After prior surgeries to remove portions of his intestines due to Crohn disease, Mr. Kipling was able to have *connections created by surgically joining two structures* when his disease went into remission. (hint: plural form)
   a. anastomoses
   b. anastomosis
   c. anastomosices
4. Mrs. Marshall was having symptoms of bloody diarrhea, abdominal pain and cramping, and fatigue. She was eventually diagnosed with *disease characterized by inflammation of the colon with the formation of ulcers, which can cause bloody diarrhea.*
   a. UC
   b. UPPP
   c. UGI
5. As an infant, Cameron Liu had an episode of *prolapse of one part of the intestine inside the part next to it*, which was diagnosed and treated by a barium enema.
   a. irritable bowel syndrome
   b. ileum
   c. intussusception
6. Because of her frequent heartburn, Mrs. Patel had a(n) *series of radiographic images taken of the pharynx, esophagus, stomach, and duodenum after the contrast agent barium has been administered orally*.
   a. upper GI series
   b. endoscopic ultrasound
   c. barium enema
7. After years of taking medication for peptic ulcers with no relief, it was recommended that Mr. Ezaki have *cutting of certain branches of the vagus nerve* to help treat his symptoms.
   a. gastrectomy
   b. pyloroplasty
   c. vagotomy
8. Mrs. Schwartz found that she *experienced difficult digestion, (such as abdominal pain and bloating)*, shortly after taking her osteoporosis medication.
   a. dyspepsia
   b. diarrhea
   c. dysphagia
9. During the colonoscopy, Dr. Mostafa found it difficult to visualize the colon all the way to the *pertaining to the ileum and cecum* valve.
   a. esophageal
   b. ileocecal
   c. peritoneal
10. After multiple surgeries for various gynecologic and gastrointestinal problems, Ms. Harding developed *abnormal growing together of two peritoneal surfaces that normally are separated.*
    a. hemorrhoids
    b. celiac disease
    c. adhesions
11. Mrs. Palmeri had an abdominal ultrasound that revealed *enlargement of the liver*, which was thought to be due to steatosis.
    a. hepatitis
    b. hepatoma
    c. hepatomegaly
12. A percutaneous endoscopic *creation of an artificial opening into the stomach (PEG)* tube was used for Mrs. McKee after her stroke.
    a. gastrostomy
    b. gastrectomy
    c. gastrotomy
13. John Begay saw his doctor because of right upper quadrant pain after eating fatty foods. An abdominal ultrasound revealed a stone in the common bile duct. A(n) *procedure using an endoscope to visualize the biliary and pancreatic ducts, introduce contrast agents, and record x-ray images* was performed and the stone was removed.
    a. ERCP
    b. EUS
    c. EGD
14. Mrs. Martinez, who was morbidly obese, was diagnosed with diabetes and hypertension. Her physician referred her for *a surgical reduction of gastric capacity to treat morbid obesity, a condition which can cause serious illness.*
    a. abdominocentesis
    b. bariatric surgery
    c. abdominoperineal resection

15. After his last episode of diverticulitis, Mr. Small developed *inflammation of the peritoneum*.
    a. cholecystitis
    b. pancreatitis
    c. peritonitis

16. As a result of her Parkinson disease, Mrs. Borders developed *difficult swallowing*.
    a. dysphagia
    b. aphagia
    c. dysentery

17. Laura Schmidt complained of *discharge of fat (excessive amount of fat in the stool, causing frothy, foul-smelling fecal matter)* which later led to her diagnosis of celiac disease.
    a. steatohepatitis
    b. steatosis
    c. steatorrhea

18. Many years ago, Jaime Garza had *excision of the uvula* for treatment of his sleep apnea.
    a. gingivectomy
    b. uvulectomy
    c. uvulopalatopharyngoplasty

19. Indu Deshmukh was born with cleft palate and cleft lip. She had palatoplasty and *surgical repair of the lip* during her childhood.
    a. pyloroplasty
    b. cheiloplasty
    c. gastroplasty

20. After eating very spicy Vietnamese food, Johan Johanssen developed *inflammation of the tongue*.
    a. gingivitis
    b. cheilitis
    c. glossitis

CHAPTER AT A GLANCE Word Parts New to This Chapter

COMBINING FORMS

abdomin/o
an/o
antr/o
append/o
appendic/o
cec/o
celi/o
cheil/o
chol/e
cholangi/o
choledoch/o
col/o
colon/o
cyst/o
diverticul/o
duoden/o
enter/o
gastr/o
gingiv/o
gloss/o
hepat/o
herni/o
ile/o
jejun/o
lapar/o
lingu/o
or/o
palat/o
pancreat/o
peritone/o
polyp/o
proct/o
rect/o
sial/o
sigmoid/o
steat/o
stomat/o
uvul/o

PREFIX

hemi-

SUFFIXES

-ac
-pepsia
-y

CHAPTER AT A GLANCE Digestive System Terms Built from Word Parts

DISEASE AND DISORDER

appendicitis
cheilitis
cholangioma
cholecystitis
choledocholithiasis
cholelithiasis
colitis
dysentery
diverticulitis
diverticulosis
enteritis
enteropathy
esophagitis
gastritis
gastroenteritis
gingivitis
glossitis
hepatitis
hepatoma
pancreatitis
peritonitis
polyposis
proctitis
rectocele
sialolith
steatohepatitis
stomatitis
uvulitis

SURGICAL

abdominocentesis
abdominoplasty
anoplasty
antrectomy
appendectomy
cheiloplasty
cholecystectomy
choledocholithotomy
colectomy
colostomy
diverticulectomy
enterorrhaphy
esophagogastroplasty
gastrectomy
gastrojejunostomy
gastroplasty
gastrostomy
gingivectomy
glossorrhaphy
hemicolectomy
herniorrhaphy
ileostomy
laparotomy
palatoplasty
pancreatectomy
polypectomy
pyloroplasty
uvulectomy
uvulopalatopharyngoplasty (UPPP)

DIAGNOSTIC
capsule endoscopy
cholangiogram
cholangiography
colonoscope
colonoscopy
CT colonography
esophagogastroduodenoscopy (EGD)
esophagogram
esophagoscopy
gastroscope
gastroscopy
laparoscope
laparoscopy
proctoscope
proctoscopy
sigmoidoscopy

COMPLEMENTARY
anal
aphagia
celiac
colorectal
duodenal
dyspepsia
dysphagia
esophageal
gastroenterologist
gastroenterology
hepatomegaly
ileocecal
nasogastric
oral
palatal
pancreatic
peritoneal
rectal
steatorrhea
steatosis
sublingual

CHAPTER AT A GLANCE Digestive System Terms *NOT* Built from Word Parts

DISEASE AND DISORDER
adhesion
celiac disease
cirrhosis
Crohn disease
gastroesophageal reflux disease (GERD)
hemochromatosis
hemorrhoids
ileus
intussusception
irritable bowel syndrome (IBS)
obesity
peptic ulcer
polyp
ulcerative colitis (UC)
volvulus

SURGICAL
abdominoperineal resection (APR)
anastomosis (*pl.* anastomoses)
bariatric surgery
hemorrhoidectomy
vagotomy

DIAGNOSTIC
abdominal sonography
barium enema (BE)
endoscopic retrograde cholangiopancreatography (ERCP)
endoscopic ultrasound (EUS)
fecal occult blood test (FOBT)
Helicobacter pylori stool antigen
upper GI series

COMPLEMENTARY
ascites
diarrhea
emesis
feces
flatus
gastric lavage
hematemesis
hematochezia
malabsorption
melena
nausea
palpate
reflux
stoma

Chapter 12 Eye

Objectives

Upon completion of this chapter, you will be able to:

1. Pronounce organs and anatomic structures of the eye.
2. Define and spell word parts related to the eye.
3. Define, pronounce, and spell disease and disorder terms related to the eye.
4. Define, pronounce, and spell surgical terms related to the eye.
5. Define, pronounce, and spell diagnostic terms related to the eye.
6. Define, pronounce, and spell complementary terms related to the eye.
7. Interpret the meaning of abbreviations related to the eye.
8. Apply medical language in clinical contexts.

Outline

ANATOMY

Function

The eyes are organs of vision and are located in a bony protective cavity of the skull called the orbit. Only a small portion of the eye is visible from the exterior (Figs. 12.1 and 12.2).

Organs and Anatomic Structures of the Eye

TERM	DEFINITION
eye (ī)	organ of vision
sclera (SKLER-ah)	outer protective layer of the eye; the portion seen on the anterior portion of the eyeball is referred to as the **white of the eye**
cornea (KŌR-nē-a)	transparent anterior part of the sclera, which is anterior to the aqueous humor and lies over the iris. It allows the light rays to enter the eye.
uvea (Ū-vē-a)	layer of tissue beneath the sclera and cornea; contains the choroid, iris, and ciliary body
choroid (KŌR-oid)	middle layer of the eye, which is interlaced with many blood vessels that supply nutrients to the eye
iris (Ī-ris)	pigmented muscular structure that regulates the amount of light entering the eye by controlling the size of the pupil
IRIS was the special messenger of the Queen of Heaven according to Greek mythology. In this role she passed from heaven to earth over the rainbow while dressed in rainbow hues. Her name was applied to the **circular eye muscle** because of its varied colors.	
ciliary body (SIL-ē-*ar*-ē) (BOD-ē)	connects the choroid to the iris; produces aqueous humor and helps change the shape of the lens for focusing
pupil (PŪ-pil)	opening in the center of the iris
lens (lenz)	lies directly behind the pupil; its function is to focus and bend light
retina (RET-i-nah)	innermost layer of the eye, which contains the vision receptors (Fig. 12.3)
macula (MAC-ū-la)	small portion of the retina at the back of the eye; responsible for detailed central vision
optic nerve (OP-tik) (nurv)	carries visual impulses from the retina to the brain
aqueous humor (Ā-kwē-us) (HŪ-mor)	watery liquid found in the anterior cavity of the eye. It provides nourishment to nearby structures and maintains shape in the anterior part of the eye.
vitreous humor (VIT-rē-us) (HŪ-mor)	jellylike substance found behind the lens in the posterior cavity of the eye that maintains its shape
meibomian glands (mī-BŌ-mē-an) (glans)	oil glands found in the upper and lower edges of the eyelids that help lubricate the eye (also called **tarsal glands**)
lacrimal apparatus (LAK-ri-mal) (*ap*-ah-RAT-us)	network of glands, ducts, canals, and sacs that produce and drain tears; the lacrimal gland produces tears, which then flow through the lacrimal ducts to cover the surface of the eye. Tears drain into lacrimal canals, flow into the lacrimal sac (tear sac) and then into the nasolacrimal duct, which opens into the nasal cavity. (Fig. 12.1C)
conjunctiva (kon-JUNK-ti-vah)	mucous membrane lining the eyelids and covering the anterior portion of the sclera

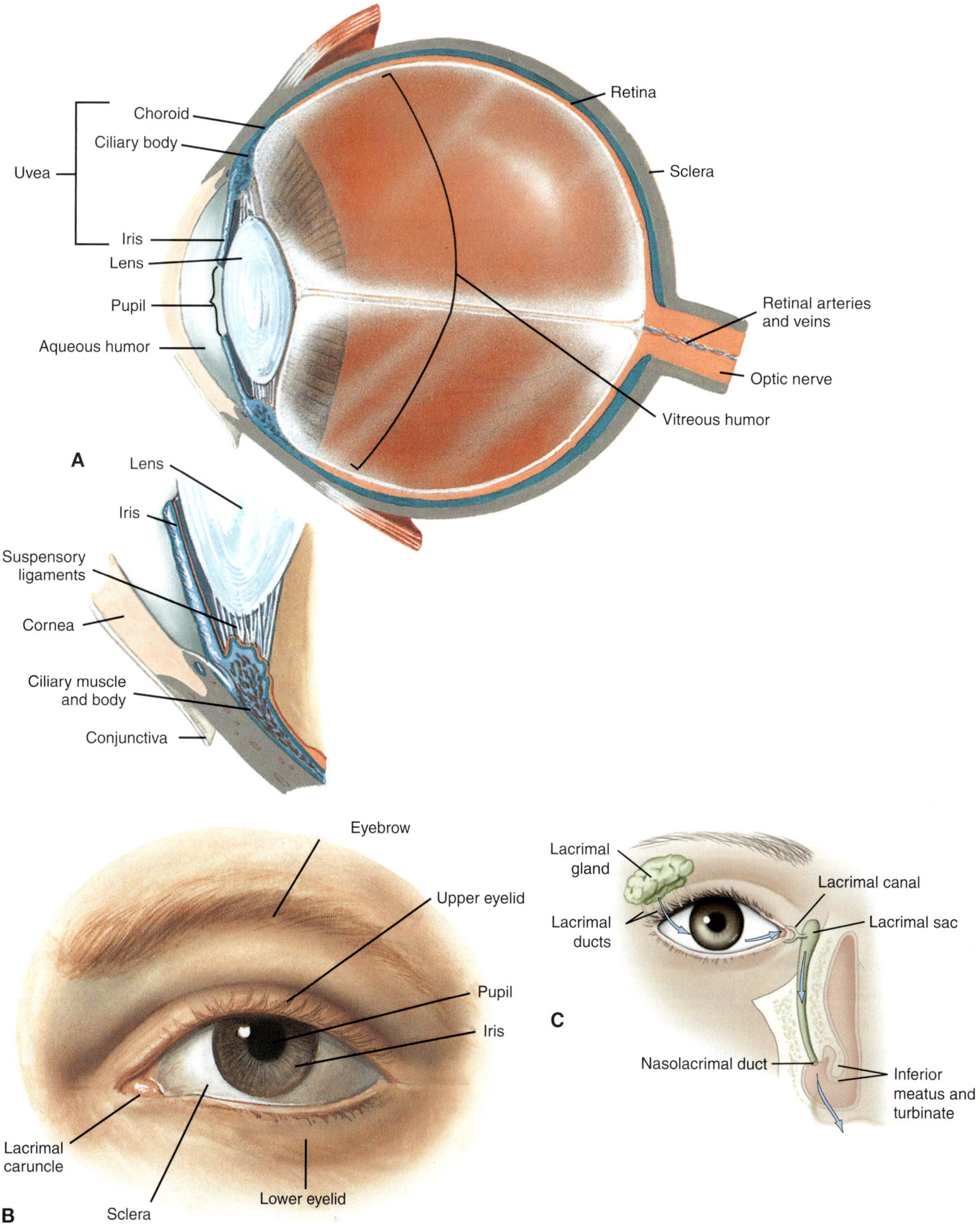

FIG. 12.1 **A,** Anatomy of the eye. **B,** Visible surface of the eye. **C,** Lacrimal apparatus.

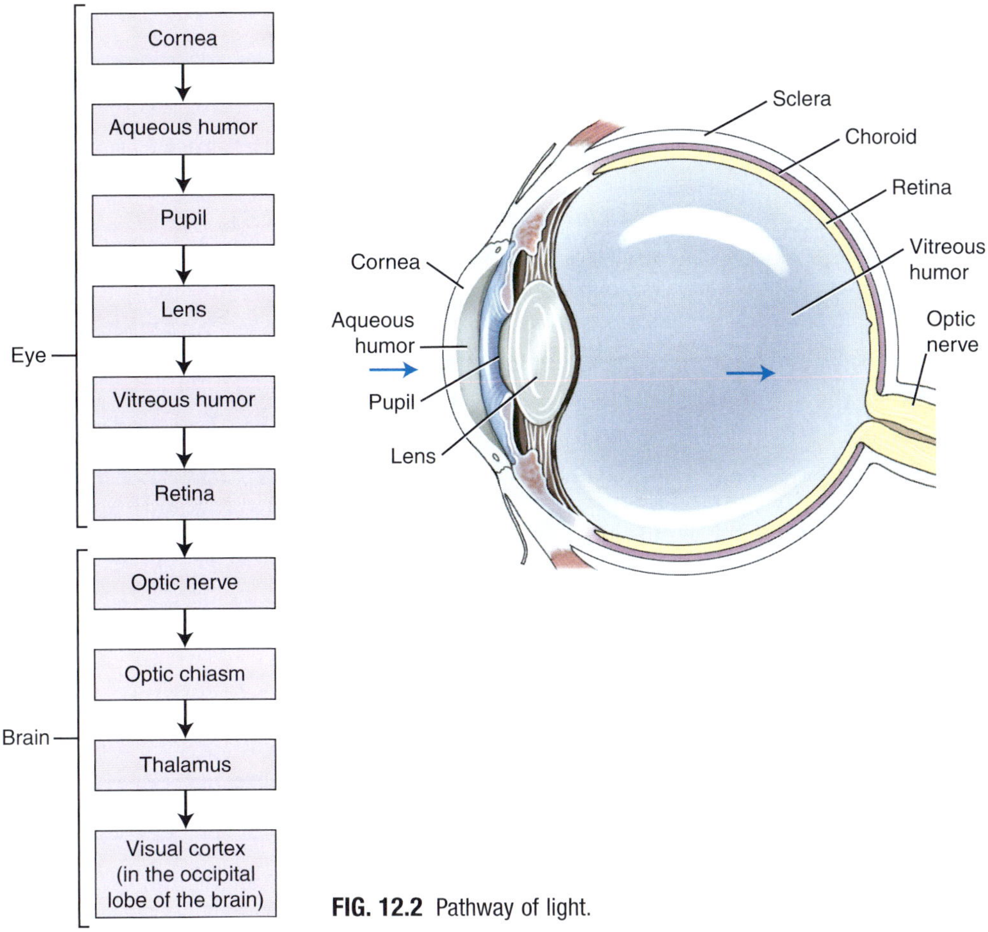

FIG. 12.2 Pathway of light.

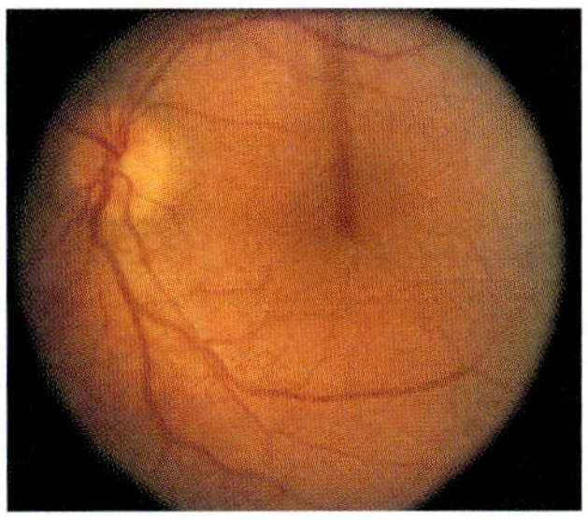

FIG. 12.3 Ophthalmoscopic view of the retina.

PRONOUNCE ANATOMIC STRUCTURES

Practice saying aloud each of the organs and specific structures on the previous pages.

To hear the terms, go to Evolve Resources at www.evolve.elsevier.com and select: Student Resources > Audio Glossary > Chapter 12 > Anatomic Structures.

❑ Check the box when complete.

WORD PARTS

1 ■ Combining Forms of the Eye

Use paper flashcards or electronic flashcards on Evolve to memorize word parts used to analyze, define, and build medical terms in this chapter. To reinforce learning, study one section of the Word Parts Table at a time, then complete the corresponding exercises on the following pages.

COMBINING FORM	DEFINITION
blephar/o	eyelid
conjunctiv/o	conjunctiva
cor/o	pupil
corne/o	cornea
dacry/o	tear(s)
ir/o	iris

COMBINING FORM	DEFINITION
irid/o	iris
kerat/o	cornea
KERAT/O refers to horny tissue (keratin) or hard texture when used with dermatology terms.	
lacrim/o	tear(s)
ocul/o	eye

1 ■ Combining Forms of the Eye—cont'd

COMBINING FORM	DEFINITION	COMBINING FORM	DEFINITION
ophthalm/o	eye	**phak/o**	lens
SPELLING OPHTHALM Look closely at the spelling of the word root **ophthalm**. Medical terms containing **ophthalm** are often misspelled by omitting the first h; **ph** gives the **f** sound followed by the sound of **thal**. Think pronunciation when spelling terms that contain **ophthalm**, as in ophthalmology (of[ph]-thal-MOL-o-jē).		**pupill/o**	pupil *(Note: pupil has one l; the combining form has two ls.)*
		retin/o	retina (Fig. 12.3)
		scler/o	sclera
opt/o	vision	**uve/o**	uvea
phac/o	lens		

2 ■ Combining Forms Used with Eye Terms

COMBINING FORM	DEFINITION	COMBINING FORM	DEFINITION
angi/o	vessel(s); blood vessel(s)	**is/o**	equal
blast/o	developing cell, germ cell	**leuk/o**	white
cry/o	cold	**myc/o**	fungus
cyst/o	bladder, sac *(Note: In terms describing the eye, the definition "sac" is used.)*	**nas/o**	nose
DACRY/O + CYST/O When the combining forms **dacry/o** and **cyst/o** appear together, the medical term refers to the lacrimal sac (directly translated as the "tear sac").		**phot/o**	light
		pseud/o	false
		rhin/o	nose
dipl/o	two, double	**ton/o**	tension, pressure
		xer/o	dry, dryness

3 ■ Prefixes

PREFIXES	DEFINITION	PREFIXES	DEFINITION
a-, an-	absence of, without	**endo-**	within
bin-	two	**intra-**	within

4 ■ Suffixes

SUFFIXES	DEFINITION	SUFFIXES	DEFINITION
-al	pertaining to	**-meter**	instrument used to measure
-algia	pain	**-metry**	measurement
-ar	pertaining to	**-oma**	tumor, swelling
-ary	pertaining to	**-opia**	vision
-eal	pertaining to	**-osis**	abnormal condition
-ectomy	excision, surgical removal	**-pathy**	disease
-graphy	process of recording, radiographic imaging	**-pexy**	surgical fixation
		-phobia	abnormal fear or aversion
-ia	diseased or abnormal state, condition of	**-plasty**	surgical repair
		-plegia	paralysis
-ic	pertaining to	**-ptosis**	drooping, sagging, prolapse
-itis	inflammation	**-scope**	instrument used for visual examination
-logist	one who studies and treats (specialist, physician)	**-scopy**	visual examination
-logy	study of	**-stomy**	creation of an artificial opening
-malacia	softening	**-tomy**	cut into, incision

Refer to **Appendix B** and **Appendix C** for a complete listing of word parts.

EXERCISE 1 ■ Combining Forms of the Eye

Refer to the first section of the word parts table.

A Label

Fill in the blanks with combining forms to label this diagram of the eye. *To check your answers, go to Appendix A at the back of the textbook.*

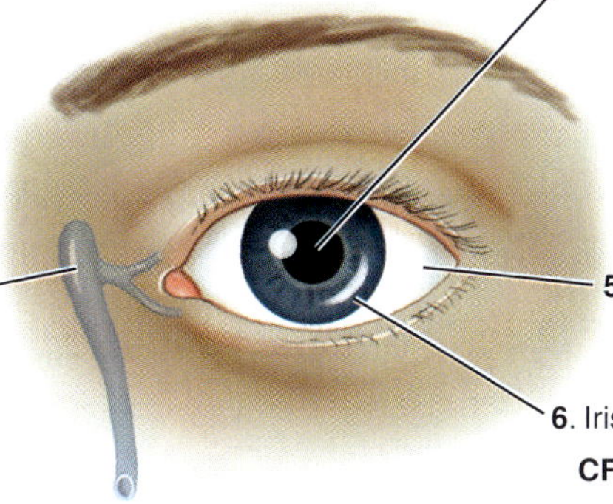

1. Eye

CF: ____________________

CF: ____________________

2. Eyelid

CF: ____________________

3. Lacrimal (**tear**) sac

CF: ____________________

CF: ____________________

4. Pupil

CF: ____________________

CF: ____________________

5. Sclera

CF: ____________________

6. Iris

CF: ____________________

CF: ____________________

7. Vision

CF: ____________________

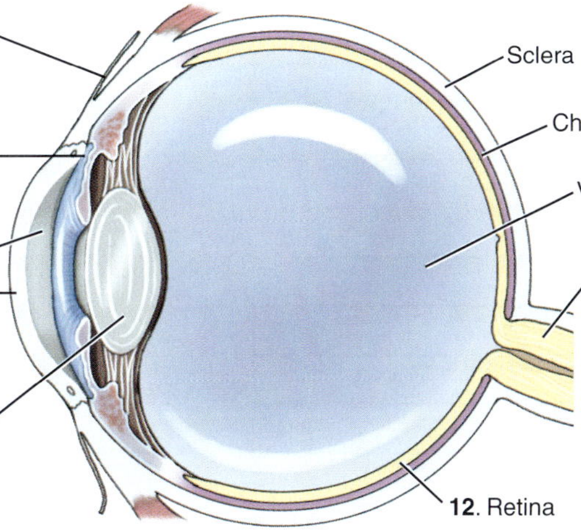

8. Conjunctiva

CF: ____________________

9. Uvea

CF: ____________________

10. Cornea

CF: ____________________

CF: ____________________

11. Lens

CF: ____________________

CF: ____________________

12. Retina

CF: ____________________

B Define and Match

Step 1: Write the definitions after the following combining forms.
Step 2: Match the descriptions on the right with the combining forms and definitions. Answers may be used more than once; no answer line appears for those not described in a lettered item.

_____ 1. scler/o, ______________________
_____ 2. cor/o, ______________________
_____ 3. corne/o, ______________________
_____ 4. conjunctiv/o, ______________________
_____ 5. lacrim/o, ______________________
_____ 6. uve/o, ______________________
_____ 7. phac/o, phak/o, ______________________
_____ 8. ocul/o, ______________________
_____ 9. ir/o, irid/o, ______________________
_____ 10. pupill/o, ______________________
_____ 11. kerat/o, ______________________
_____ 12. ophthalm/o, ______________________
_____ 13. dacry/o, ______________________
_____ 14. retin/o, ______________________
15. blephar/o, ______________________
16. opt/o, ______________________

a. opening in the center of the iris
b. lies directly behind the pupil; focuses and bends light
c. organ of vision
d. pigmented muscular structure regulating the amount of light entering the eye
e. outer protective layer of the eye
f. produced by and drained by the lacrimal apparatus
g. innermost layer of the eye containing vision receptors
h. mucous membrane lining the eyelids and the anterior portion of the sclera
i. transparent anterior part of the sclera
j. layer that contains the choroid, iris, and ciliary body

EXERCISE 2 ■ Combining Forms Used with Eye Terms

Refer to the second section of the word parts table.

A Define

Write the definitions of the following combining forms.

1. ton/o ______________________
2. phot/o ______________________
3. cry/o ______________________
4. dipl/o ______________________
5. is/o ______________________
6. cyst/o ______________________
7. xer/o ______________________
8. angi/o ______________________
9. rhin/o ______________________
10. myc/o ______________________
11. blast/o ______________________
12. leuk/o ______________________
13. pseud/o ______________________
14. nas/o ______________________

B Identify

Write the combining form for each of the following definitions.

1. cold ______________________
2. tension, pressure ______________________
3. bladder, sac ______________________
4. two, double ______________________
5. light ______________________
6. equal ______________________
7. white ______________________
8. false ______________________
9. developing cell, germ cell ______________________
10. fungus ______________________
11. dry, dryness ______________________
12. vessel(s), blood vessel(s) ______________________
13. nose a. ______________________
b. ______________________

EXERCISE 3 ■ Prefixes

Refer to the third section of the word parts table.

A Define

Write the definitions of the following prefixes.

1. intra- ____________________
2. an- ____________________
3. endo- ____________________
4. a- ____________________
5. bin- ____________________

B Identify

Write the prefixes for the following definitions.

1. two ____________________
2. without a. ____________________
   b. ____________________
3. within a. ____________________
   b. ____________________

EXERCISE 4 ■ Suffixes

Refer to the fourth section of the word parts table.

A Identify

Write the suffixes that mean "pertaining to."

1. ____________________
2. ____________________
3. ____________________
4. ____________________
5. ____________________

B Match

Match the suffixes in the first column with their correct definitions in the second column.

_____	1. -stomy	a. disease
_____	2. -graphy	b. instrument used to measure
_____	3. -osis	c. drooping, sagging, prolapse
_____	4. -scope	d. one who studies and treats (specialist, physician)
_____	5. -algia	e. excision, surgical removal
_____	6. -logist	f. abnormal condition
_____	7. -ectomy	g. creation of an artificial opening
_____	8. -meter	h. process of recording, radiographic imaging
_____	9. -ptosis	i. instrument used for visual examination
_____	10. -pathy	j. pain

C Label

Write the suffixes pictured and defined.

1. ______________________
vision

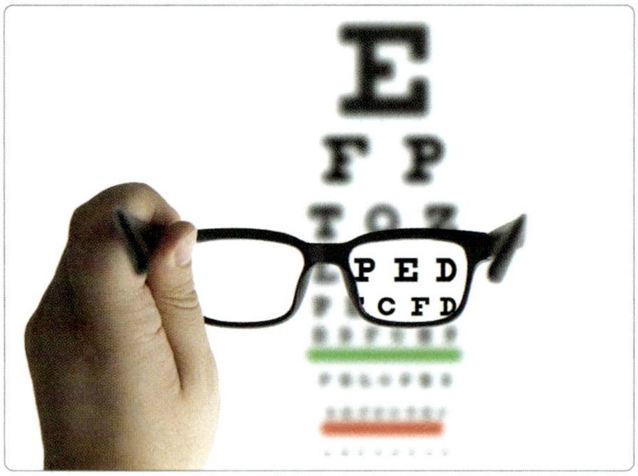

2. ______________________
abnormal fear or aversion

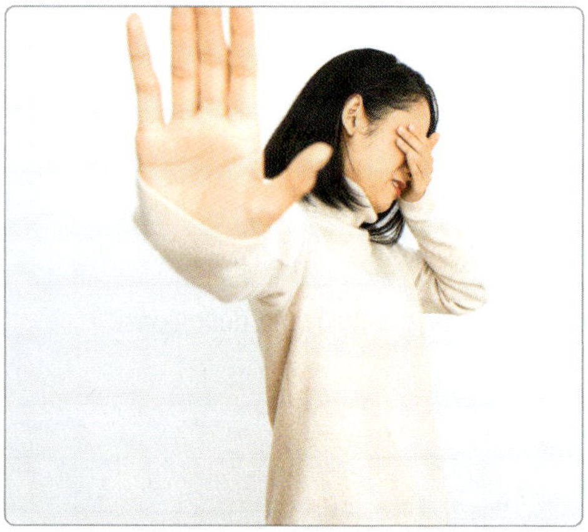

3. ______________________
paralysis

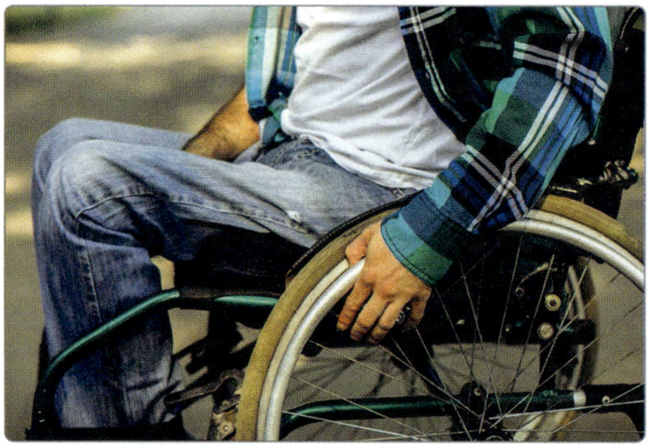

D Define

Write the definitions of the following suffixes.

1. -scopy ______________________
2. -itis ______________________
3. -malacia ______________________
4. -plasty ______________________

E Identify

Write the suffix for each of the following definitions.

1. study of ______________________
2. measurement ______________________
3. cut into, incision ______________________
4. tumor, swelling ______________________
5. surgical fixation ______________________
6. diseased or abnormal state, condition of ______________________

MEDICAL TERMS

Medical terms relevant to this chapter have been grouped by topics, such as Disease and Disorder, and are listed in tables designated as Built from Word Parts or *NOT* Built from Word Parts. The exercises following each table assist with learning term definitions, pronunciations, and spellings.

Disease and Disorder Terms

BUILT FROM WORD PARTS

The following terms can be translated using definitions of word parts. Further explanation is provided within parentheses as needed.

TERM	DEFINITION	TERM	DEFINITION
1. **aphakia** (a-FĀ-kē-a)	condition of without a lens (may be congenital, though often is the result of extraction of a cataract without the placement of an intraocular lens)	12. **leukocoria** (*lū*-kō-KŌ-rē-a)	condition of white pupil
2. **blepharitis** (*blef*-a-RĪ-tis)	inflammation of the eyelid	13. **oculomycosis** (*ok*-ū-lō-mī-KŌ-sis)	abnormal condition of the eye caused by a fungus
3. **blepharoptosis** (*blef*-ar-op-TŌ-sis)	drooping of the eyelid (also called **ptosis**)	14. **ophthalmalgia** (*of-thal*-MAL-ja)	pain in the eye
4. **conjunctivitis** (kon-*junk*-ti-VĪ-tis)	inflammation of the conjunctiva (also called **pink eye**)	15. **ophthalmopathy** (*of*-thal-MOP-a-thē)	(any) disease of the eye
5. **dacryocystitis** (*dak*-rē-ō-sis-TĪ-tis)	inflammation of the tear (lacrimal) sac	16. **ophthalmoplegia** (of-thal-mō-PLĒ-ja)	paralysis of the eye (muscle)
6. **diplopia** (di-PLŌ-pē-a)	double vision	17. **phacomalacia** (*fāk*-ō-ma-LĀ-sha)	softening of the lens
7. **endophthalmitis** (*en*-dof-thal-MĪ-tis)	inflammation within the eye *(Note: the* o *in the prefix endo- is dropped.)*	18. **retinoblastoma** (*ret*-i-nō-blas-TŌ-ma)	tumor arising from a developing retinal cell (malignant, may be congenital; occurs mainly in children)
8. **iridoplegia** (*ir*-i-dō-PLĒ-ja)	paralysis of the iris	19. **retinopathy** (*ret*-i-NOP-a-thē)	(any noninflammatory) disease of the retina (such as **diabetic retinopathy**)
9. **iritis** (*ī*-RĪ-tis)	inflammation of the iris	20. **scleritis** (skle-RĪ-tis)	inflammation of the sclera
10. **keratitis** (*ker*-a-TĪ-tis)	inflammation of the cornea	21. **scleromalacia** (*sklĕr*-ō-ma-LĀ-sha)	softening of the sclera
11. **keratomalacia** (*ker*-a-tō-ma-LĀ-sha)	softening of the cornea (usually a bilateral condition associated with vitamin A deficiency)	22. **uveitis** (*ū*-vē-Ī-tis)	inflammation of the uvea
		23. **uveoscleritis** (*ū*-vē-ō-sklē-RĪ-tis)	inflammation of the uvea and sclera
		24. **xerophthalmia** (*zēr*-of-THAL-mē-a)	condition of dry eye (conjunctiva and cornea)

EXERCISE 5 ■ Pronounce and Spell

Practice pronunciation and spelling on paper and online.

1. Practice on Paper

a. **Pronounce:** Read the phonetic spelling and say aloud the terms listed in the previous table. Refer to the pronunciation key on p. 20 as necessary.
b. **Spell:** Have a study partner read the terms aloud. Write the spelling of the terms on a separate sheet of paper.

2. Practice Online

a. **Access** online learning resources. Go to evolve.elsevier.com > Evolve Resources > Student Resources.
b. **Pronounce:** Select Audio Glossary > Chapter 12 > Exercise 5. Select a term to hear its pronunciation and repeat aloud.
c. **Spell:** Select Activities > Chapter 12 > Spell Terms > Exercise 5. Select the audio icon and type the correct spelling of the term.

❑ Check the box when complete.

EXERCISE 6 ■ Analyze and Define

Analyze and define the following terms.

1. scleritis
____
____

2. ophthalmoplegia
____
____

3. retinopathy
____
____

4. endophthalmitis
____
____

5. xerophthalmia
____
____

6. aphakia
____
____

7. ophthalmopathy
____
____

8. scleromalacia
____
____

9. uveitis
____
____

10. keratomalacia
____
____

EXERCISE 7 ■ Build

A Label

Build terms pictured by writing word parts above definitions.

1.

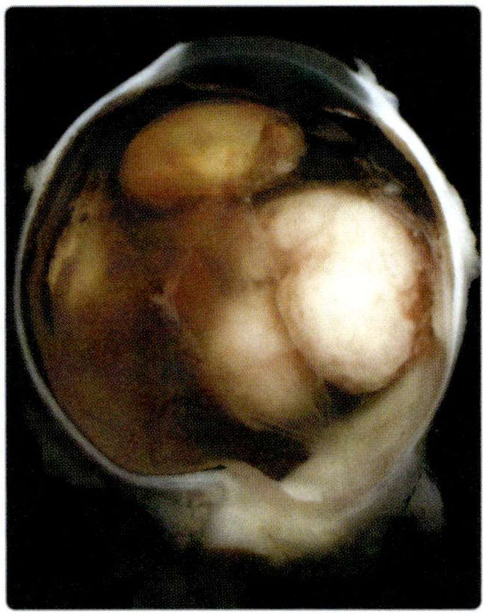

_______ /_______ /__________ /__________
retina CV developing cell tumor

2.

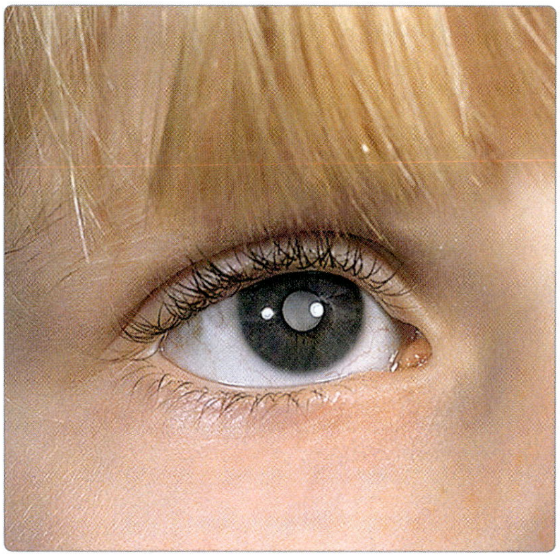

_______ /_______ /_________ /__________
white CV pupil condition of

3.

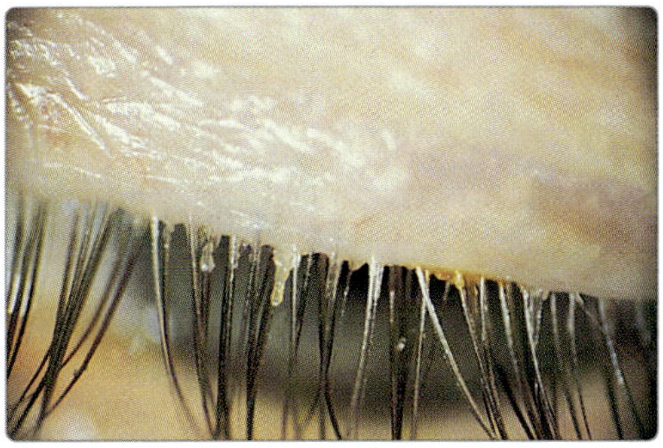

______________ /________________
eyelid inflammation

4.

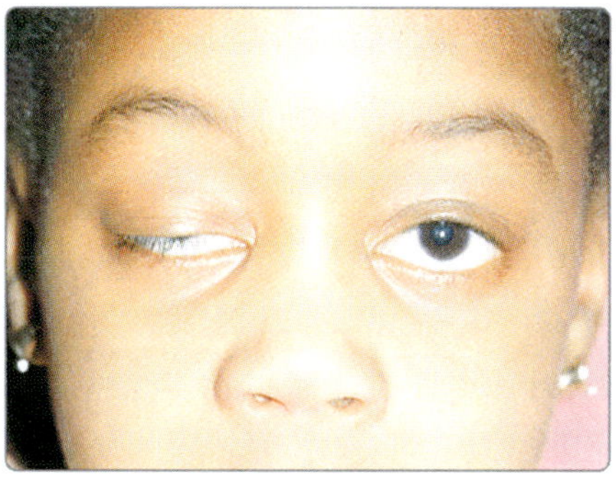

_________ /____ /______________
eyelid CV drooping

5.

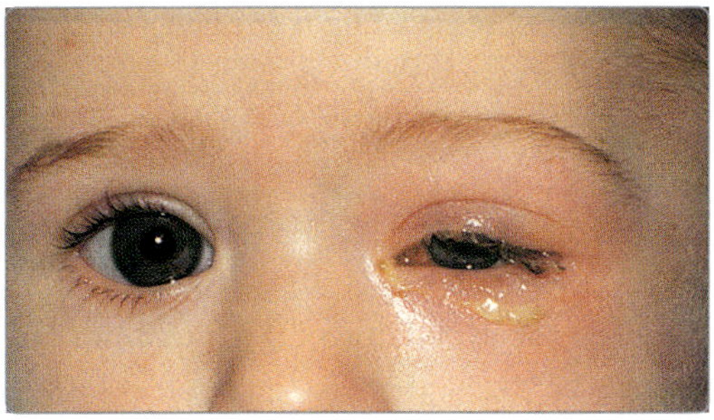

______________ /________________
conjunctiva inflammation

6.

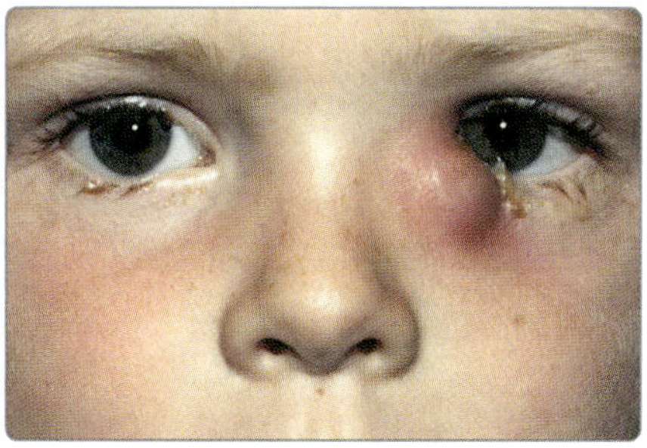

________ /____ /________ /______________
tear CV sac inflammation

B Fill In

Build disease and disorder terms for the following definitions by using the word parts you have learned.

1. inflammation of the iris ______ / ______ (WR / S)
2. abnormal condition of the eye caused by a fungus ______ / ______ / ______ / ______ (WR / CV / WR / S)
3. pain in the eye ______ / ______ (WR / S)
4. double vision ______ / ______ (WR / S)
5. inflammation of the cornea ______ / ______ (WR / S)
6. inflammation of the uvea and sclera ______ / ______ / ______ / ______ (WR / CV / WR / S)
7. paralysis of the iris ______ / ______ / ______ (WR / CV / S)
8. softening of the lens ______ / ______ / ______ (WR / CV / S)

Disease and Disorder Terms

NOT BUILT FROM WORD PARTS

Word parts may be present in the following terms; however, their full meanings cannot be translated using definitions of word parts alone.

TERM	DEFINITION
1. amblyopia (*am*-blē-Ō-pē-a)	reduced vision in one eye caused by disuse or misuse associated with strabismus, unequal refractive errors, or otherwise impaired vision. The brain suppresses images from the impaired eye to avoid double vision. (also called **lazy eye**)
2. anisometropia (an-*i*-sō-ma-TRŌ-pē-a)	significant unequal refractive error between two eyes
3. astigmatism (Ast) (a-STIG-ma-tizm)	blurred vision caused by irregular curvature of the cornea or lens. Light refracts improperly, resulting in diffused, rather than points of light focusing on the retina. (Fig. 12.5C)
4. cataract (KAT-a-rakt)	clouding of the lens of the eye (Fig. 12.4)
CATARACT is derived from the Greek **kato**, meaning **down**, and **raktos**, meaning **precipice**. Together, the words were interpreted as **waterfall**. The individual with a cataract sees things as through a watery veil of mist or waterfall.	
5. chalazion (ka-LĀ-zē-on)	noninfected obstruction of an oil gland of the eyelid (also called **meibomian cyst**)
6. drusen (DRŪ-zen)	yellowish deposits located under the retina; commonly associated with aging and macular degeneration

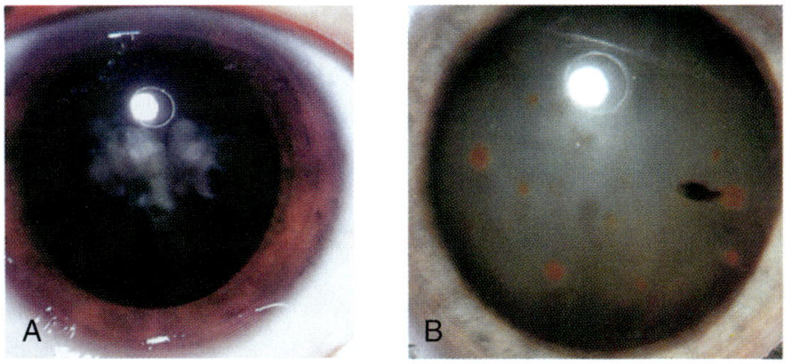

FIG. 12.4 **A,** Snowflake cataract. **B,** Senile cataract.

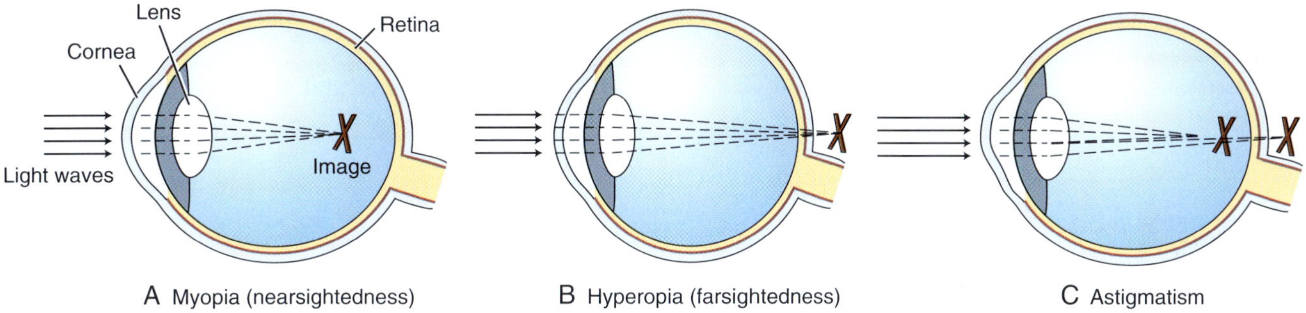

FIG. 12.5 Refraction errors. **A,** Myopia, nearsightedness. **B,** Hyperopia, farsightedness. **C,** Astigmatism.

TERM	DEFINITION
7. glaucoma (glaw-KŌ-ma)	eye disorder characterized by increase of intraocular pressure (IOP). If left untreated may progress to optic nerve damage and visual impairment or loss.
GLAUCOMA is composed of the Greek **glaukos**, meaning **blue-gray** or **sea green**, and **oma**, meaning a morbid condition. The term was given to any condition in which gray or green replaced the black in the pupil.	
8. hyperopia (*hī*-per-Ō-pē-a)	farsightedness (Fig. 12.5B)
9. hyphema (hī-FĒ-ma)	hemorrhage within the anterior chamber of the eye; most often caused by blunt trauma (also called **hyphemia**)
10. macular degeneration (MAC-ū-lar) (dē-*gen*-e-RĀ-shun)	progressive deterioration of the portion of the retina called the **macula**, resulting in loss of central vision (Fig. 12.6). Age-related macular degeneration (AMD) is the leading cause of legal blindness in persons older than 65 years; onset occurs between the ages of 50 and 60.
11. myopia (mī-Ō-pē-a)	nearsightedness (Fig. 12.5A)
12. nyctalopia (*nik*-ta-LŌ-pē-a)	poor vision at night or in faint light (also called **night blindness**)
13. nystagmus (nis-TAG-mus)	involuntary, jerking movements of the eyes
14. pinguecula (ping-GWEH-kū-la)	yellowish mass on the conjunctiva that may be related to long-term exposure to ultraviolet light, dry climates, and dust. A pinguecula that spreads onto the cornea becomes a **pterygium.**
15. presbyopia (*pres*-bē-Ō-pē-a)	impaired vision as a result of aging
16. pterygium (te-RIJ-ē-um)	thin tissue growing onto the cornea from the conjunctiva, usually caused by sun exposure

Disease and Disorder Terms—cont'd

NOT BUILT FROM WORD PARTS

TERM	DEFINITION
17. retinal detachment (RET-in-al) (dē-TACH-ment)	separation of the retina from the choroid in the posterior portion of the eye resulting in a disruption of vision that may be permanent if treatment is delayed; onset may be gradual or sudden and is not painful (Fig. 12.7)
18. retinitis pigmentosa (*ret*-i-NĪ-tis) (*pig*-men-TŌ-sa)	hereditary, progressive disease marked by night blindness with atrophy and retinal pigment changes
19. strabismus (stra-BIZ-mus)	condition in which the eyes look in different directions; caused by dysfunction of the external eye muscles or an uncorrected refractive error (called **cross-eyed** when one eye turns in)
20. sty (stī)	infection of an oil gland of the eyelid (also spelled **stye** and also called **hordeolum**)

EXERCISE 8 ■ Pronounce and Spell

Practice pronunciation and spelling on paper and online.

1. Practice on Paper

a. **Pronounce:** Read the phonetic spelling and say aloud the terms listed in the previous table. Refer to the pronunciation key on p. 20 as necessary.
b. **Spell:** Have a study partner read the terms aloud. Write the spelling of the terms on a separate sheet of paper.

2. Practice Online

a. **Access** online learning resources. Go to evolve.elsevier.com > Evolve Resources > Student Resources.
b. **Pronounce:** Select Audio Glossary > Chapter 12 > Exercise 8. Select a term to hear its pronunciation and repeat aloud.
c. **Spell:** Select Activities > Chapter 12 > Spell Terms > Exercise 8. Select the audio icon and type the correct spelling of the term.

❑ Check the box when complete.

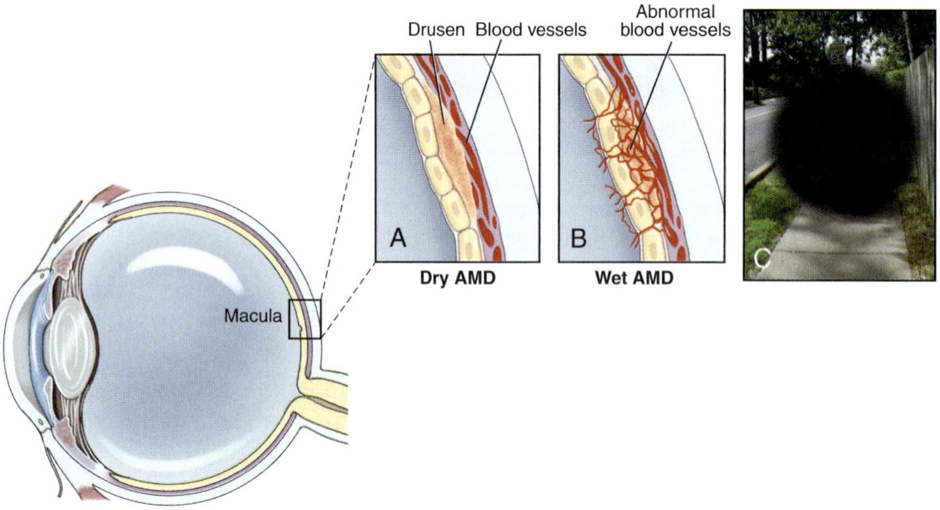

FIG. 12.6 Age-related macular degeneration (AMD). **A, Dry macular degeneration,** where blood vessels under the macula become brittle and yellow deposits called drusen form, is the most common form of age-related macular degeneration (AMD). **B, Wet macular degeneration,** where new abnormal blood vessels form under the macula, is less common though more likely to cause legal blindness. **C, Central vision loss** as may be experienced in AMD.

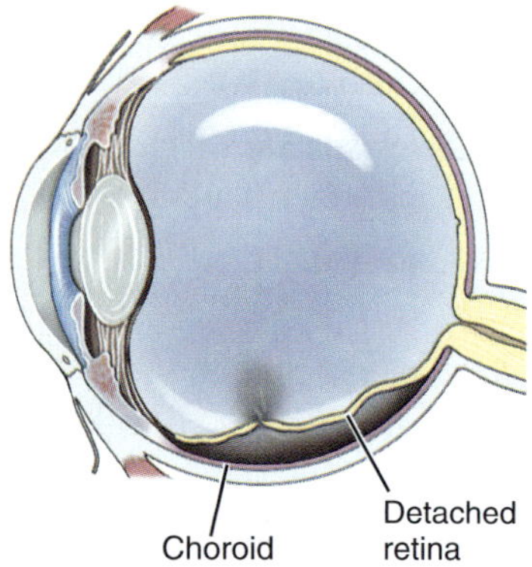

FIG. 12.7 Retinal detachment. Vitreous fluid has seeped through a tear in the retina, causing the retina to separate from the choroid.

EXERCISE 9 ■ Fill In

A Identify

Fill in the blanks with the correct terms.

1. Another name for nearsightedness is ______________________________.
2. Impaired vision as a result of aging is ______________________________.
3. Significant unequal refractive error between two eyes is ______________________________.
4. Irregular curvature of the cornea or lens causes a condition known as ______________________________.
5. ______________________________ is the name given to involuntary, jerking movements of the eye.
6. Eye disorder characterized by the increase of intraocular pressure is ______________________________.
7. Another name for farsightedness is ______________________________.
8. ______________________________ is a hereditary, progressive disease causing night blindness with retinal pigment changes and atrophy.
9. Another name for night blindness is ______________________________.
10. Another name for lazy eye is ______________________________.

B Label

Write the medical terms pictured and defined.

1. ______________________________
yellowish deposits located under the retina

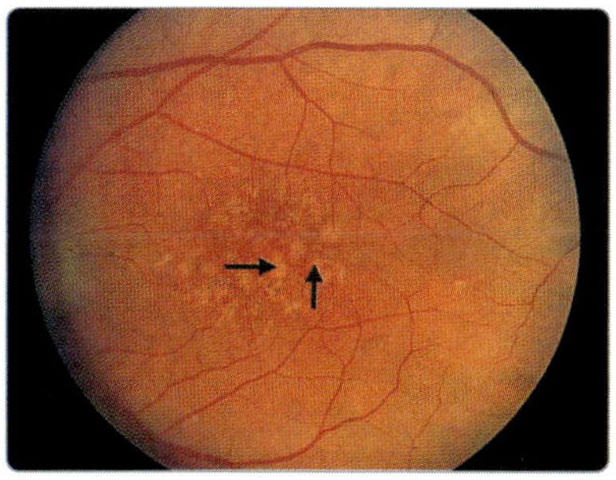

2. ______________________________
progressive deterioration of the portion of the retina called the macula, resulting in loss of central vision

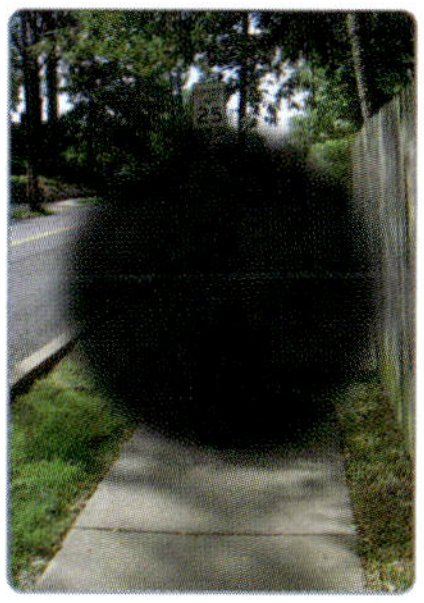

3. ______________________________
thin tissue growing onto the cornea from the conjunctiva, usually caused by sun exposure

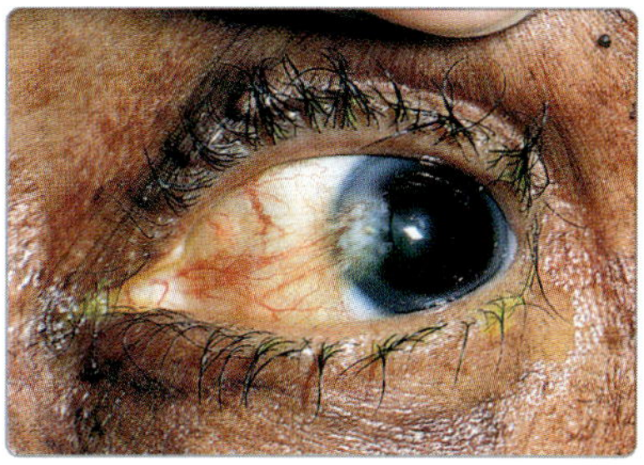

4. ______________________________
yellowish mass on the conjunctiva that may be related to long-term exposure to ultraviolet light, dry climates, and dust

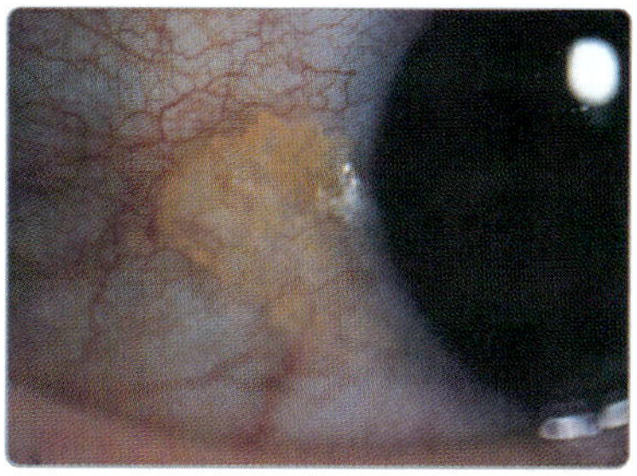

5. ______________________________
noninfected obstruction of an oil gland of the eyelid

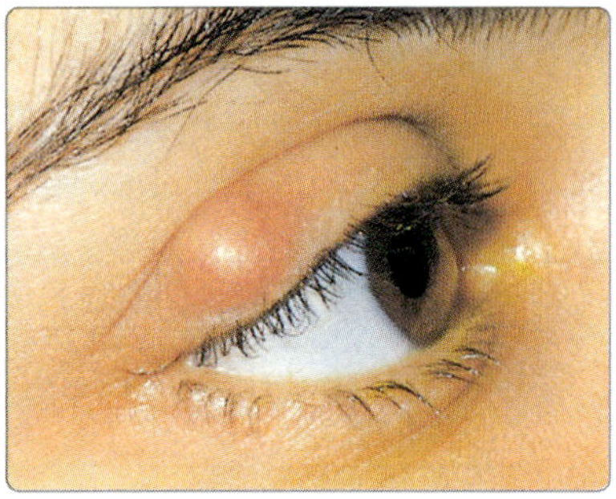

6. ______________________________
infection of an oil gland of the eyelid

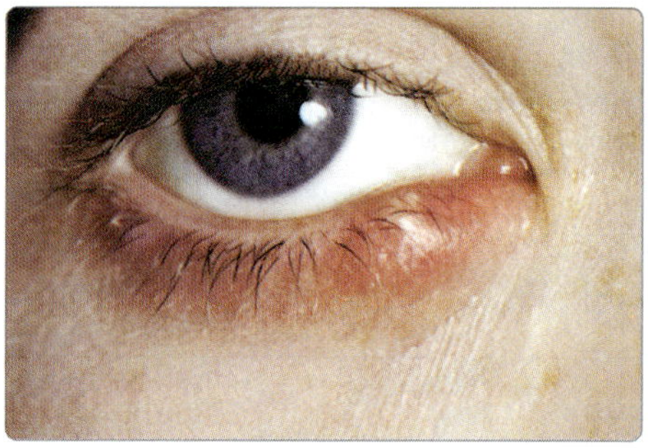

7. ______________________________
clouding of the lens of the eye

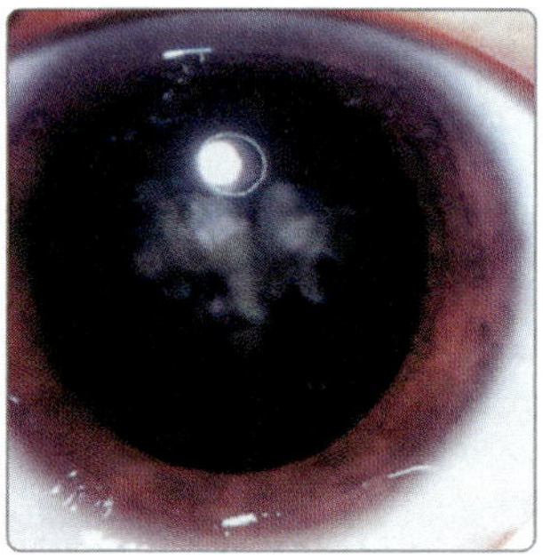

8. ______________________________
hemorrhage within the anterior chamber of the eye; most often caused by blunt trauma

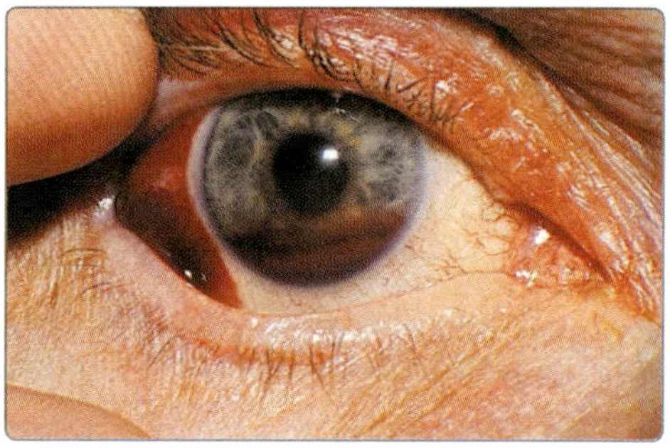

9. ______________________________
condition in which the eyes look in different directions

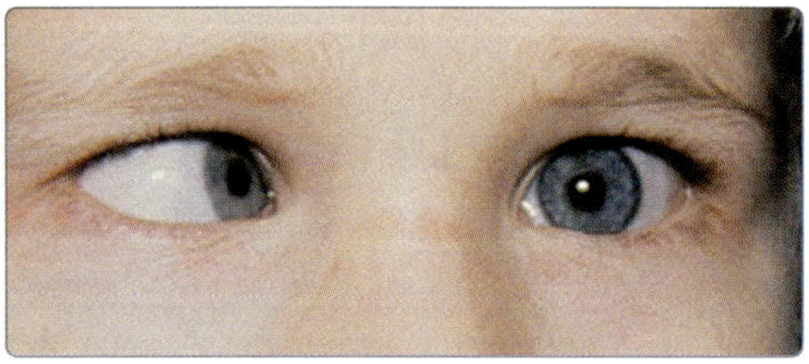

10. ______________________________
separation of the retina from the choroid in the posterior portion of the eye

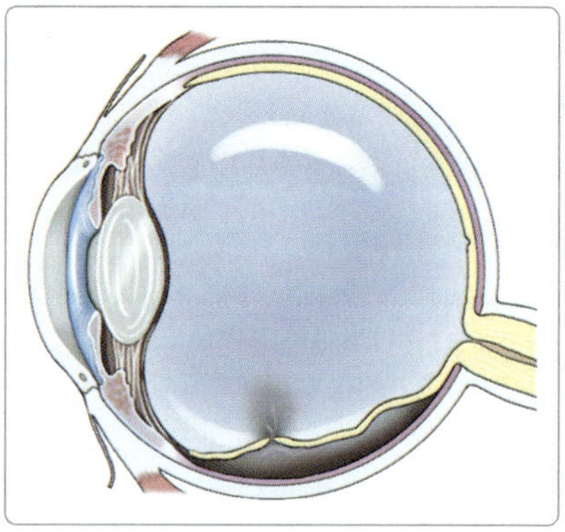

C Match

Match the terms in the first column with their correct definitions in the second column.

_____ 1. hyphema	a. significant unequal refractive error between two eyes
_____ 2. pterygium	b. characterized by increase of intraocular pressure
_____ 3. anisometropia	c. also called meibomian cyst
_____ 4. sty	d. disease marked by night blindness with atrophy and retinal pigment changes
_____ 5. glaucoma	e. thin tissue growing onto the cornea from the conjunctiva
_____ 6. chalazion	f. irregular curvature of the cornea or lens
_____ 7. myopia	g. also called hordeolum
_____ 8. retinitis pigmentosa	h. hemorrhage within the anterior chamber of the eye
_____ 9. astigmatism	i. yellowish mass on the conjunctiva
_____ 10. pinguecula	j. nearsightedness

D Match

Match the terms in the first column with their correct definitions in the second column.

_____ 1. nyctalopia	a. called cross-eyed when one eye turns in
_____ 2. drusen	b. yellowish deposits located under the retina
_____ 3. retinal detachment	c. impaired vision as a result of aging
_____ 4. amblyopia	d. results in loss of central vision
_____ 5. strabismus	e. involuntary, jerking movements of the eyes
_____ 6. presbyopia	f. disruption of vision caused by separation of the retina from the choroid
_____ 7. macular degeneration	g. clouding of the lens of the eye
_____ 8. hyperopia	h. also called lazy eye
_____ 9. nystagmus	i. also called night blindness
_____ 10. cataract	j. farsightedness

EXERCISE 10 ■ Review of Disease and Disorder Terms

Can you define, pronounce, and spell the following terms?

amblyopia
anisometropia
aphakia
astigmatism (Ast)
blepharitis
blepharoptosis
cataract
chalazion
conjunctivitis
dacryocystitis
diplopia
drusen
endophthalmitis
glaucoma
hyperopia
hyphema
iridoplegia
iritis
keratitis
keratomalacia
leukocoria
macular degeneration
myopia
nyctalopia
nystagmus
oculomycosis
ophthalmalgia
ophthalmopathy
ophthalmoplegia
phacomalacia
pinguecula
presbyopia
pterygium
retinal detachment
retinitis pigmentosa
retinoblastoma
retinopathy
scleritis
scleromalacia
strabismus
sty
uveitis
uveoscleritis
xerophthalmia

Surgical Terms

BUILT FROM WORD PARTS AND *NOT* BUILT FROM WORD PARTS

The first portion of the table contains Surgical Terms that can be translated using definitions of word parts. The second portion of the table contains Surgical Terms that cannot be fully understood using the definitions of word parts.

Built from Word Parts

TERM	DEFINITION
1. blepharoplasty (BLEF-a-rō-*plas*-tē)	surgical repair of the eyelid
2. cryoretinopexy (*krī*-ō-RE-tin-ō-*pek*-sē)	surgical fixation of the retina by using extreme cold (carbon dioxide)
3. dacryocystorhinostomy (*dak*-rē-ō-sis-tō-rī-NOS-to-mē)	creation of an artificial opening between the tear (lacrimal) sac and the nose (to restore drainage into the nose when the nasolacrimal duct is obstructed or obliterated)
4. iridectomy (*ir*-i-DEK-to-mē)	excision (of part) of the iris
5. iridotomy (*ir*-i-DOT-o-mē)	incision into the iris
6. keratoplasty (KER-a-tō-*plas*-tē)	surgical repair of the cornea (corneal transplant)
7. sclerotomy (skle-ROT-o-mē)	incision into the sclera

NOT Built from Word Parts

TERM	DEFINITION
1. enucleation (ē-*nū*-klē-Ā-shun)	surgical removal of the eyeball (also, excision of a whole organ or mass without cutting into it)
2. LASIK (laser-assisted in situ keratomileusis) (LĀ-sik) (*ker*-a-tō-mi-LOO-sis)	laser procedure that reshapes the corneal tissue beneath the surface of the cornea to correct astigmatism, hyperopia, and myopia. It differs from photorefractive keratectomy (PRK) in that it reshapes corneal tissue beneath the surface rather than on the surface (Fig. 12.8B).
3. phacoemulsification (PHACO) (*fa*-kō-ē-*mul*-si-fi-KĀ-shun)	method to remove cataracts in which an ultrasonic needle probe breaks up the lens, which is then aspirated
4. photorefractive keratectomy (PRK) (*fō*-tō-rē-FRAK-tiv) (*ker*-a-TEK-to-mē)	procedure for the treatment of astigmatism, hyperopia, and myopia in which a laser is used to reshape (flatten) the corneal surface by removing a portion of the cornea (Fig. 12.8A)
5. retinal photocoagulation (RET-in-al) (*fō*-tō-kō-*ag*-ū-LĀ-shun)	intense beam of light from a laser condenses retinal tissue to seal leaking blood vessels, to destroy abnormal tissue or lesions, or to bond the retina to the back of the eye. Used to treat retinal tears, diabetic retinopathy, wet macular degeneration, glaucoma, and intraocular tumors.
6. scleral buckling (SKLER-al) (BUK-ling)	procedure to repair retinal detachment in which a piece of silicone is applied to the abnormal part of the sclera. This pushes in, or "buckles" the sclera toward the middle of the eye, decreasing the traction on the retina. For larger detachments, an entire band may encircle the eyeball. Cryoretinopexy is often used to repair the hole in the retina prior to the buckling procedure. (Fig. 12.9)
7. trabeculectomy (tra-*bek*-ū-LEK-to-mē)	surgical creation of an opening that allows aqueous humor to drain out of the eye to underneath the conjunctiva where it is absorbed; used to treat glaucoma by reducing intraocular pressure. (Laser trabeculoplasty may also be used.)
8. vitrectomy (vi-TREK-to-mē)	surgical removal of all or part of the vitreous humor (to provide access to interior structures of the eye; used to treat diabetic retinopathy, retinal detachment, or a hole in the macula)

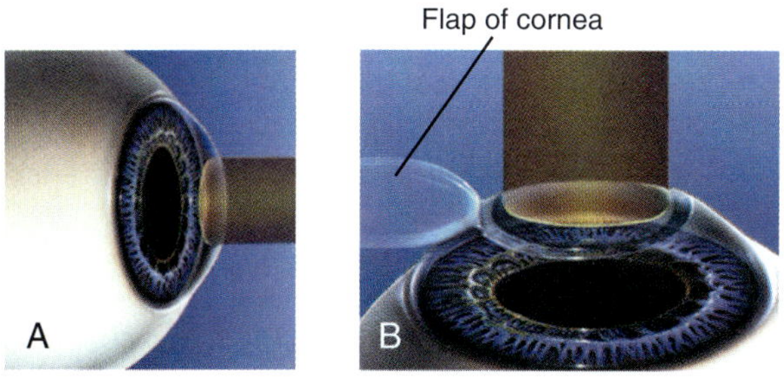

FIG. 12.8 Laser treatments for near-sightedness. **A, Photorefractive keratectomy** (PRK) removes tissue from the surface of the cornea. **B, LASIK** (laser-assisted in situ keratomileusis) reshapes corneal tissue below the surface of the cornea. The excimer laser was invented in the early 1980s. It is a computer-controlled ultraviolet beam of light that reshapes the cornea. It has replaced **RK** (radial keratotomy), a surgery in which spokelike incisions are made to reshape the cornea.

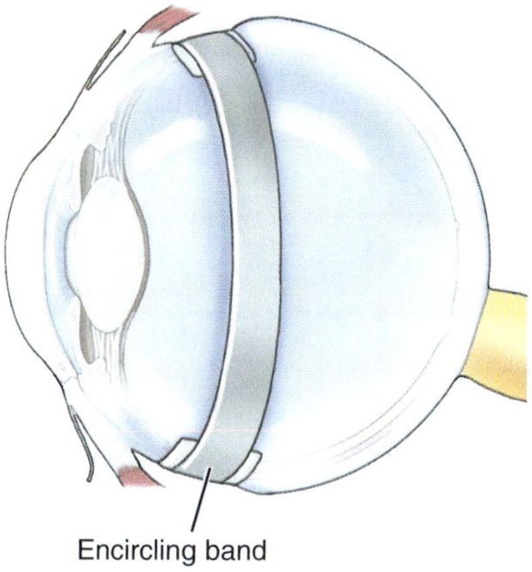

FIG. 12.9 Scleral buckling. A surgical procedure to repair a detached retina.

EXERCISE 11 ■ Pronounce and Spell

Practice pronunciation and spelling on paper and online.

1. Practice on Paper

a. **Pronounce:** Read the phonetic spelling and say aloud the terms listed in the previous table. Refer to the pronunciation key on p. 20 as necessary.
b. **Spell:** Have a study partner read the terms aloud. Write the spelling of the terms on a separate sheet of paper.

2. Practice Online

a. **Access** online learning resources. Go to evolve.elsevier.com > Evolve Resources > Student Resources.
b. **Pronounce:** Select Audio Glossary > Chapter 12 > Exercise 11. Select a term to hear its pronunciation and repeat aloud.
c. **Spell:** Select Activities > Chapter 12 > Spell Terms > Exercise 11. Select the audio icon and type the correct spelling of the term.

❑ Check the box when complete.

EXERCISE 12 ■ Surgical Terms Built from Word Parts

A Analyze and Define

Analyze and define the following surgical terms.

1. keratoplasty

____
____

2. sclerotomy

____
____

3. cryoretinopexy

____
____

4. blepharoplasty

____
____

5. iridectomy

____
____

6. dacryocystorhinostomy

____
____

7. iridotomy

____
____

B Label

Build terms pictured by writing word parts above definitions.

1.

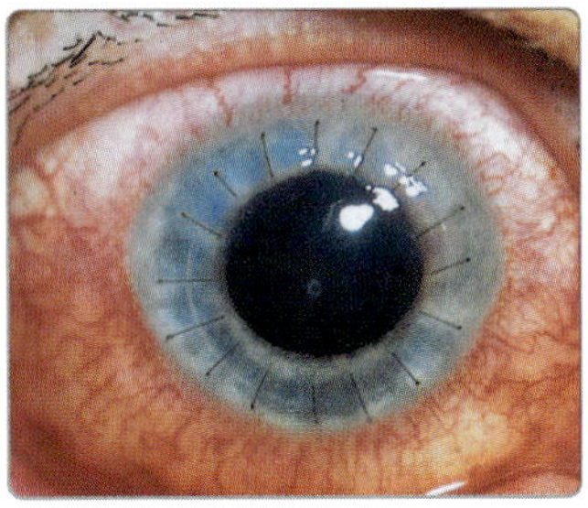

Appearance of the eye after
_____ / _____ / _____
cornea CV surgical repair

2.

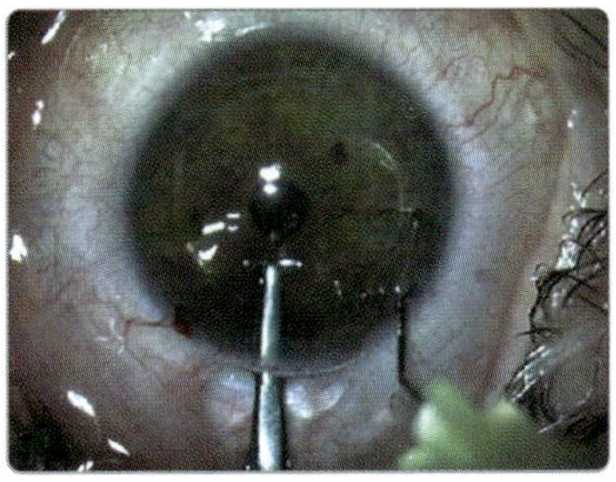

_____ / _____ / _____
iris CV incision

3.

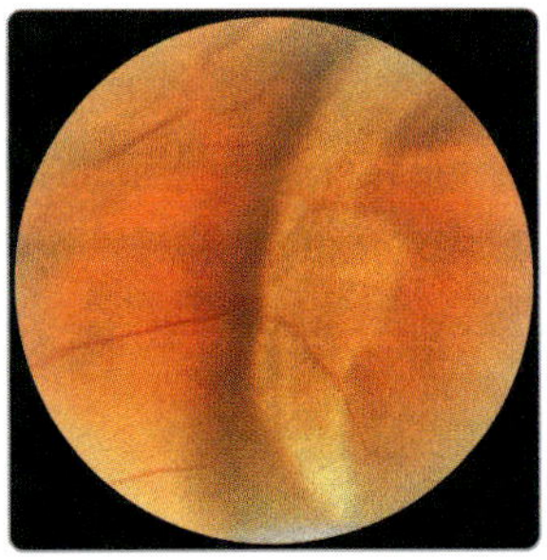

Retina after _____ / _____ / _____ / _____ / _____
cold CV retina CV surgical fixation

C Fill In

Build surgical terms for the following definitions by using the word parts you have learned.

1. creation of an artificial opening between the tear (lacrimal) sac and the nose
_____ / _____ / _____ / _____ / _____ / _____ / _____
WR / CV / WR / CV / WR / CV / S

2. excision (of part) of the iris
_____ / _____
WR / S

3. incision into the sclera ______ / ______ / ______
WR / CV / S

4. surgical repair of the eyelid ______ / ______ / ______
WR / CV / S

EXERCISE 13 ■ Surgical Terms *NOT* Built from Word Parts

A Label

Write the surgical terms pictured and defined.

1. ______________________
procedure in which a laser is used to reshape (flatten) the corneal surface by removing a portion of the cornea

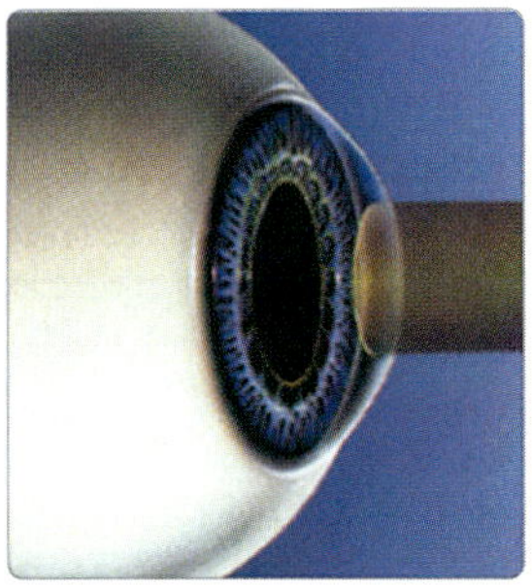

2. ______________________
laser procedure that reshapes the corneal tissue beneath the surface of the cornea to correct astigmatism, hyperopia, and myopia

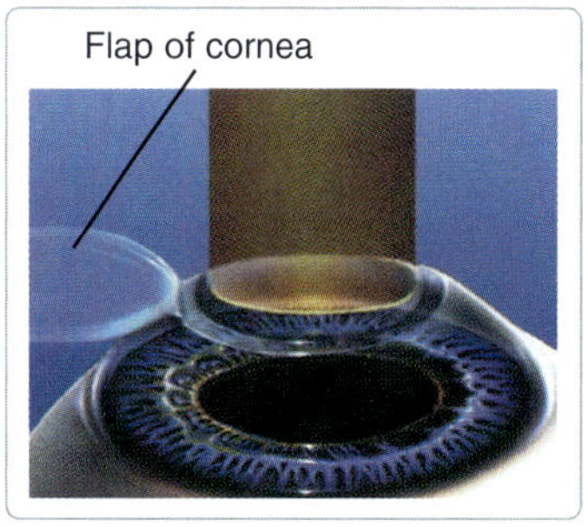

3. ______________________
procedure to repair retinal detachment in which a piece of silicone is applied to the abnormal part of the sclera.

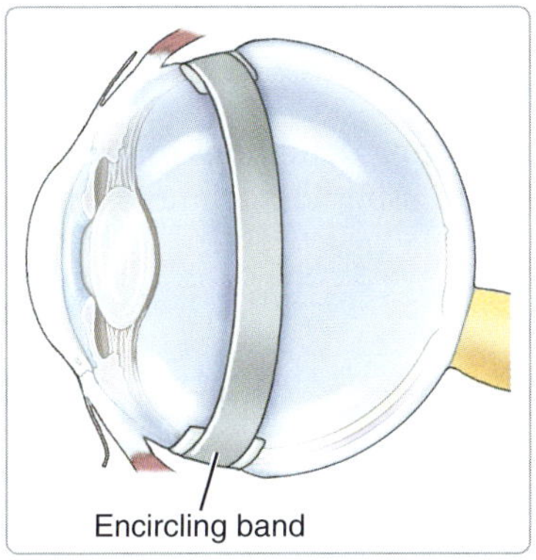

4. ______________________
method to remove cataracts in which an ultrasonic needle probe breaks up the lens, which is then aspirated

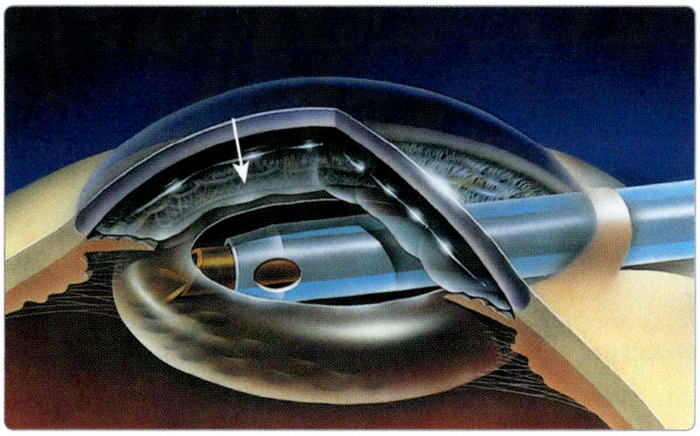

B Identify

Fill in the blanks with the correct terms.

1. ______________ ______________ is the use of a laser beam to condense retinal tissue to seal leaking blood vessels, destroy abnormal tissue, or bond the retina to the back of the eye.

2. Surgical removal of an eyeball is called a(n) ______________________.
3. ______________________ is the surgical creation of an opening that allows aqueous humor to drain out of the eye to reduce intraocular pressure.
4. Surgery to remove vitreous humor from the eye is called ______________________.

C Match

Match the terms in the first column with their correct definitions in the second column.

_____ 1. LASIK
_____ 2. enucleation
_____ 3. trabeculectomy
_____ 4. retinal photocoagulation
_____ 5. phacoemulsification
_____ 6. scleral buckling
_____ 7. vitrectomy
_____ 8. photorefractive keratectomy

a. use of a laser beam to repair retinal tears and detachment, as well as other retinopathies
b. surgical creation of an opening to reduce intraocular pressure
c. procedure for the treatment of astigmatism, hyperopia, and myopia in which a laser is used to reshape the corneal surface by removing the outermost layer of the cornea
d. procedure in which the lens is broken up by ultrasound and aspirated
e. procedure used to correct astigmatism, nearsightedness, and farsightedness by reshaping tissue beneath the corneal surface
f. surgical removal of an eyeball
g. surgical removal of vitreous humor
h. procedure to repair retinal detachment in which a piece of silicone is applied to the abnormal part of the sclera

EXERCISE 14 ■ Review of Surgical Terms

Can you define, pronounce, and spell the following terms?

blepharoplasty
cryoretinopexy
dacryocystorhinostomy
enucleation
iridectomy
iridotomy
keratoplasty
LASIK (laser-assisted in situ keratomileusis)
phacoemulsification (PHACO)
photorefractive keratectomy (PRK)
retinal photocoagulation
scleral buckling
sclerotomy
trabeculectomy
vitrectomy

Diagnostic Terms

BUILT FROM WORD PARTS AND *NOT* BUILT FROM WORD PARTS

The first portion of the table contains Diagnostic Terms that can be translated using definitions of word parts. The second portion of the table contains Diagnostic Terms that cannot be fully understood using the definitions of word parts.

■ Built From Word Parts

TERM	DEFINITION	TERM	DEFINITION
DIAGNOSTIC IMAGING		**3. ophthalmoscope** (of-THAL-mō-skōp)	instrument used for visual examination (of the interior) of the eye
1. fluorescein angiography (FA) (flō-RES-ēn) (*an*-jē-OG-ra-fē)	radiographic imaging of blood vessels (of the eye with fluorescing dye)	**4. ophthalmoscopy** (*of*-thal-MOS-ko-pē)	visual examination of the eye
OPHTHALMIC EVALUATION		**5. optometry** (op-TOM-e-trē)	measurement of vision (also measurement of the eye and visual processing system)
2. keratometer (*ker*-a-TOM-e-ter)	instrument used to measure (the curvature of) the cornea (used for fitting contact lenses)	**6. pupillometer** (*pū*-pil-OM-e-ter)	instrument used to measure (the diameter of) the pupil

TERM	DEFINITION	TERM	DEFINITION
7. pupilloscope (pū-PIL-ō-skōp)	instrument used for visual examination of the pupil	**9. tonometer** (tō-NOM-e-ter)	instrument used to measure pressure (within the eye, used to diagnose glaucoma)
8. retinoscopy (*ret*-i-NOS-ko-pē)	visual examination of the retina	**10. tonometry** (tō-NOM-e-trē)	measurement of pressure (within the eye)

NOT Built from Word Parts

TERM	DEFINITION
DIAGNOSTIC IMAGING	
1. optical coherence tomography (OCT) (OP-ti-kul)(kō-HĒR-entz) (tō-MOG-rah-fē)	noninvasive test that uses light waves to take cross-sectional images of the retina; used to detect many eye conditions including macular degeneration, glaucoma, retinopathy, and optic nerve damage.
OPHTHALMIC EVALUATION	
2. slit lamp (slit) (lamp)	horizontally mounted binocular microscope that uses a very narrow vertical beam of light (slit) to examine the eye in great detail. It is especially useful for viewing the conjunctiva, cornea, lens, and vitreous humor.

EXERCISE 15 ■ Pronounce and Spell

Practice pronunciation and spelling on paper and online.

1. Practice on Paper

a. **Pronounce:** Read the phonetic spelling and say aloud the terms listed in the previous table. Refer to the pronunciation key on p. 20 as necessary.
b. **Spell:** Have a study partner read the terms aloud. Write the spelling of the terms on a separate sheet of paper.

2. Practice Online

a. **Access** online learning resources. Go to evolve.elsevier.com > Evolve Resources > Student Resources.
b. **Pronounce:** Select Audio Glossary > Chapter 12 > Exercise 15. Select a term to hear its pronunciation and repeat aloud.
c. **Spell:** Select Activities > Chapter 12 > Spell Terms > Exercise 15. Select the audio icon and type the correct spelling of the term.

❑ Check the box when complete.

EXERCISE 16 ■ Diagnostic Terms Built from Word Parts

A Fill In

Build diagnostic terms for the following definitions by using the word parts you have learned.

1. measurement of pressure (within the eye) ______ / ______ / ______
WR / CV / S

2. instrument used to measure (the curvature of) the cornea ______ / ______ / ______
WR / CV / S

3. measurement of vision _______ / ___ / _______
WR CV S

4. instrument used to measure pressure (within the eye) _______ / ___ / _______
WR CV S

5. instrument used for visual examination of the pupil _______ / ___ / _______
WR CV S

6. visual examination of the retina _______ / ___ / _______
WR CV S

B Label

Build terms pictured by writing word parts above definitions.

1.

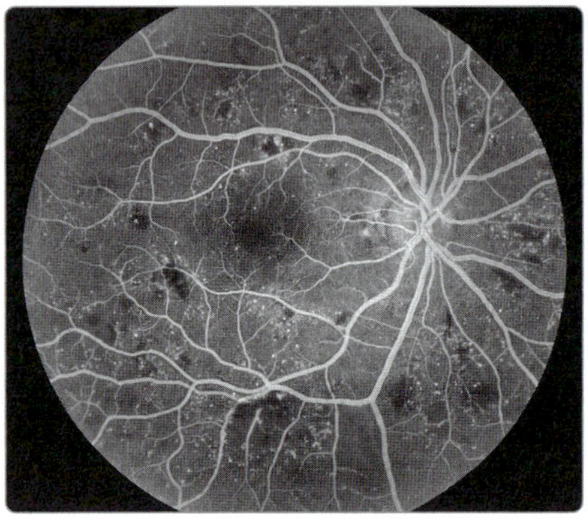

fluorescein _______ / ___ / _______
blood vessel CV radiographic imaging

2.

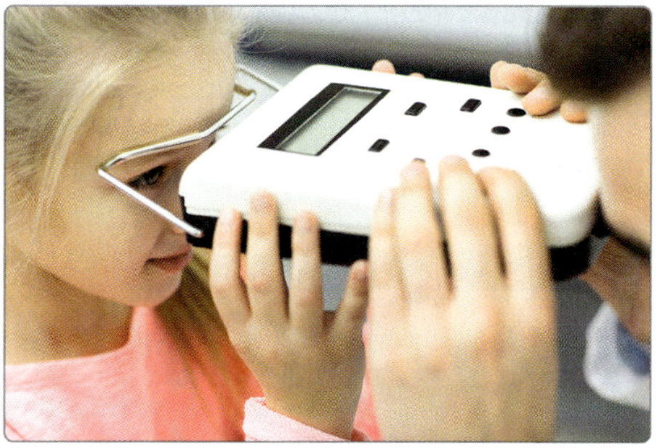

_______ / ___ / _______
pupil CV instrument used to measure

3.

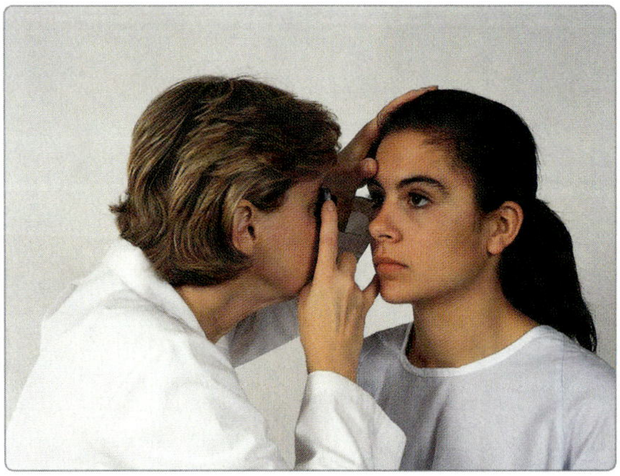

_______ / ___ / _______
eye CV visual examination

4.

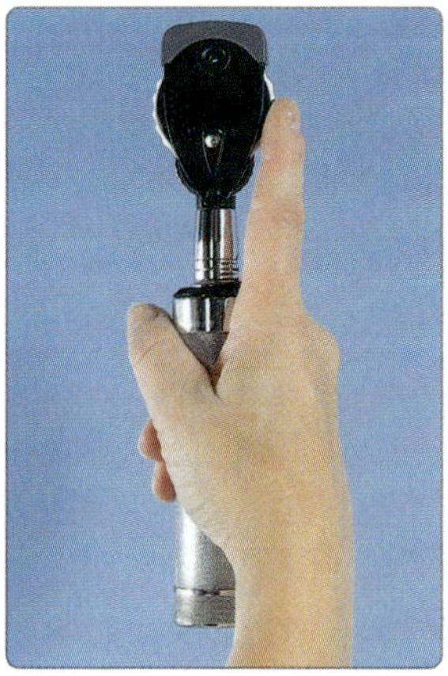

_______ / ___ / _______
eye CV instrument used for visual examination

C Analyze and Define

Analyze and define the following diagnostic terms.

1. pupilloscope
____
____

2. optometry
____
____

3. ophthalmoscope
____
____

4. tonometry
____
____

5. pupillometer
____
____

6. tonometer
____
____

7. keratometer
____
____

8. ophthalmoscopy
____
____

9. (fluorescein) angiography
____
____

10. retinoscopy
____
____

EXERCISE 17 ■ Diagnostic Terms *NOT* Built from Word Parts

A Label

Write the diagnostic terms pictured and defined.

1. ______________________________
microscope that sees a very narrow beam of light to examine the eye in great detail

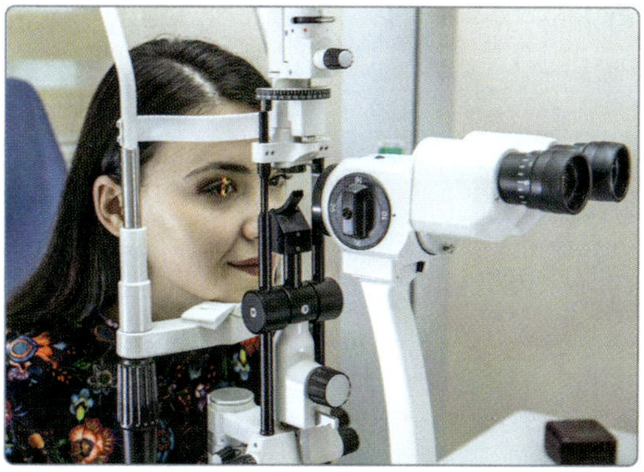

2. ______________________________
noninvasive test that uses light waves to take cross-sectional images of the retina.

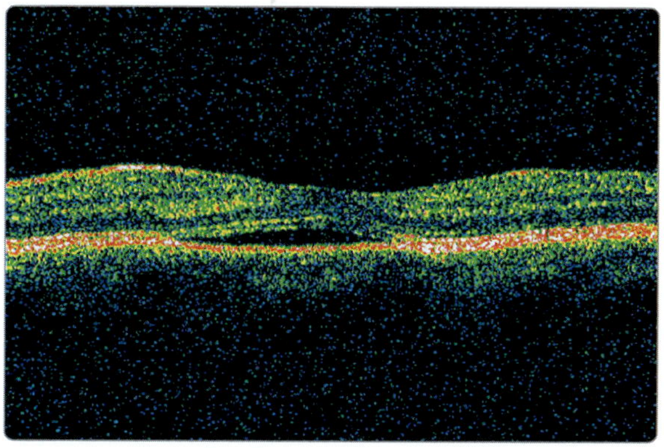

B Identify

Fill in the blanks with the correct terms.

1. ______________________ ______________________ ______________________ is used to detect many eye conditions, including retinopathy and optic nerve damage.
2. A binocular microscope, mounted horizontally, that uses a vertical beam of light, or ______________________ ______________________, is especially useful for viewing structures in the front of the eye, including the conjunctiva, cornea, and lens.

EXERCISE 18 ■ Review of Diagnostic Terms

Can you define, pronounce, and spell the following terms?

fluorescein angiography (FA)	ophthalmoscopy	optometry	slit lamp
keratometer	optical coherence tomography (OCT)	pupillometer	tonometer
ophthalmoscope		pupilloscope	tonometry
		retinoscopy	

Complementary Terms

BUILT FROM WORD PARTS AND *NOT* BUILT FROM WORD PARTS

The first portion of the table contains Eye Complementary Terms that can be translated using definitions of word parts. The second portion of the table contains Eye Complementary Terms that cannot be fully understood using the definitions of word parts.

■ Built from Word Parts

SIGNS AND SYMPTOMS

TERM	DEFINITION	TERM	DEFINITION
1. anisocoria (an-ī-sō-KŌR-ē-a)	condition of absence of equal pupil (size) (unequal size of pupils)	**3. photophobia** (*fō*-tō-FŌ-bē-a)	abnormal fear of (sensitivity to) light
2. isocoria (ī-sō-KŌR-ē-a)	condition of equal pupil (size)	**4. pseudophakia** (*soo*-dō-FĀ-ke-a)	condition of false lens (placement of an intraocular lens during surgery to treat cataracts)

MEDICAL SPECIALTIES

TERM	DEFINITION	TERM	DEFINITION
5. ophthalmologist (*of*-thal-MOL-o-jist)	physician (surgeon) who studies and treats diseases of the eye	**6. ophthalmology (Ophth)** (*of*-thal-MOL-o-jē)	study of the eye (branch of medicine that treats diseases of the eye)

DESCRIPTIVE TERMS

TERM	DEFINITION	TERM	DEFINITION
7. binocular (bin-OK-ū-lar)	pertaining to two or both eyes	**9. intraocular** (*in*-tra-OK-ū-lar)	pertaining to within the eye
8. corneal (KOR-nē-al)	pertaining to the cornea	**10. lacrimal** (LAK-ri-mal)	pertaining to tear(s)

TERM	DEFINITION	TERM	DEFINITION
11. nasolacrimal (*nā*-zō-LAK-ri-mal)	pertaining to the nose and tear (ducts)	**14. pupillary** (PŪ-pi-lar-ē)	pertaining to the pupil
12. ophthalmic (of-THAL-mik)	pertaining to the eye	**15. retinal** (RET-i-nal)	pertaining to the retina
13. optic (OP-tik)	pertaining to vision		

NOT Built from Word Parts

SIGNS AND SYMPTOMS

TERM	DEFINITION
1. emmetropia (Em) (*em*-e-TRŌ-pē-a)	normal refractive condition of the eye
2. visual acuity (VA) (VIZH-ū-al) (a-KŪ-i-tē)	sharpness of vision for either distance or near

MEDICAL SPECIALTIES

TERM	DEFINITION
3. optician (op-TISH-in)	specialist who fills prescriptions for lenses (cannot prescribe lenses)
4. optometrist (op-TOM-e-trist)	health professional who diagnoses, treats, and manages diseases and disorders of the eyes and visual processing system; doctor of optometry (OD)

OPTOMETRIST is derived from the Greek **optikos**, meaning **sight**, and **metron**, meaning **measure**. Literally, an optometrist is a person who measures sight.

TREATMENTS

TERM	DEFINITION
5. intraocular lens (IOL) (*in*-tra-OK-ū-lar) (lenz)	artificial lens implanted within the eye during cataract surgery
6. miotic (mī-OT-ik)	agent that constricts the pupil
7. mydriatic (*mid*-rē-AT-ik)	agent that dilates the pupil

Refer to **Appendix E** for pharmacology terms related to the eye.

EXERCISE 19 ■ Pronounce and Spell

Practice pronunciation and spelling on paper and online.

1. Practice on Paper

a. **Pronounce:** Read the phonetic spelling and say aloud the terms listed in the previous table. Refer to the pronunciation key on p. 20 as necessary.

b. **Spell:** Have a study partner read the terms aloud. Write the spelling of the terms on a separate sheet of paper.

2. Practice Online

a. **Access** online learning resources. Go to evolve.elsevier.com > Evolve Resources > Student Resources.
b. **Pronounce:** Select Audio Glossary > Chapter 12 > Exercise 19. Select a term to hear its pronunciation and repeat aloud.
c. **Spell:** Select Activities > Chapter 12 > Spell Terms > Exercise 19. Select the audio icon and type the correct spelling of the term.

❑ Check the box when complete.

EXERCISE 20 ■ Complementary Terms Built from Word Parts

A Analyze and Define

Analyze and define the following complementary terms.

1. ophthalmology
____
____

2. binocular
____
____

3. lacrimal
____
____

4. pupillary
____
____

5. ophthalmologist
____
____

6. corneal
____
____

7. ophthalmic
____
____

8. nasolacrimal
____
____

9. optic
____
____

10. intraocular
____
____

11. retinal
____
____

12. photophobia
____
____

13. isocoria

____

____

14. anisocoria

____

____

15. pseudophakia

____

____

B Label

Build terms pictured by writing word parts above definitions.

1.

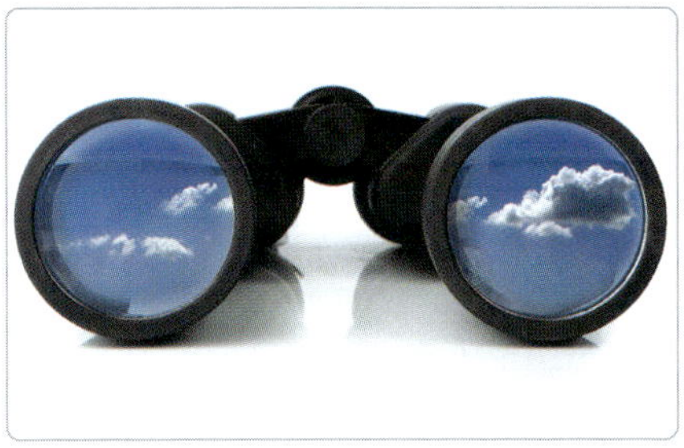

_______ /_______ /_______

two / eye / pertaining to

2.

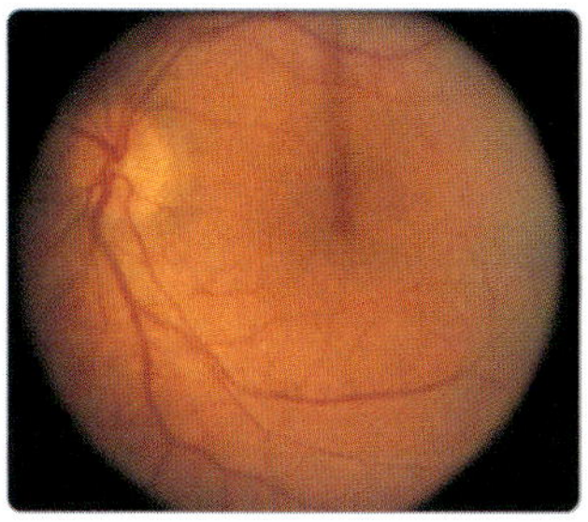

_______ /_______

retina / pertaining to

3.

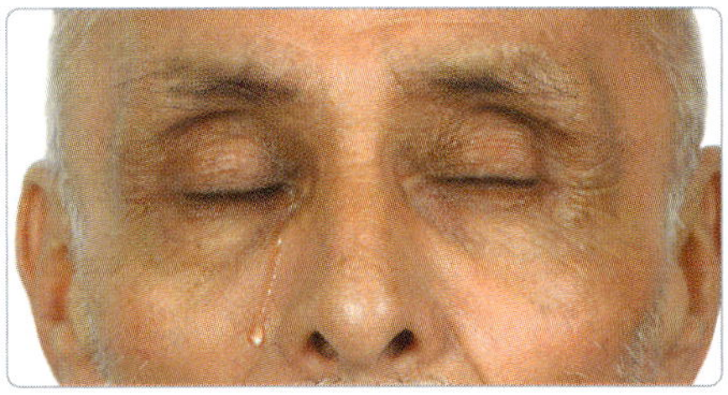

_______ /_______

tears / pertaining to

4.

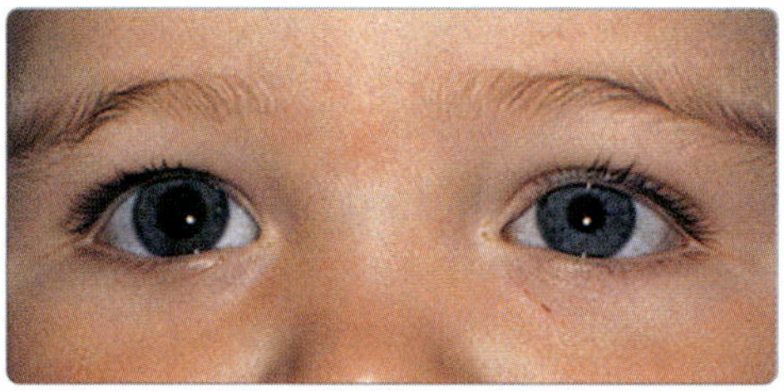

_______ /_______ /_______ /_______ /_______

absence of / equal / CV / pupil / condition of

5.

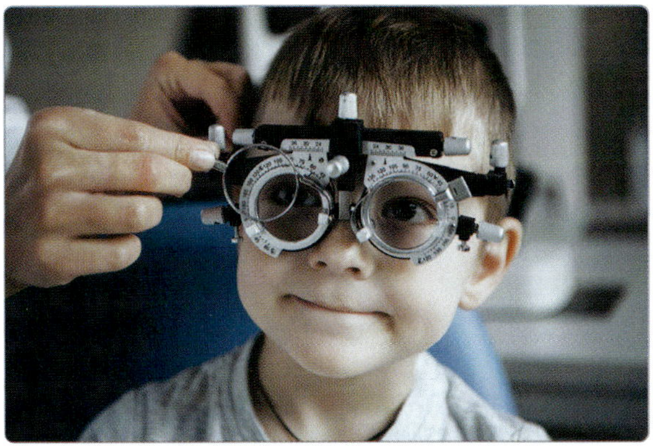

_______ /_______

vision / pertaining to

6.

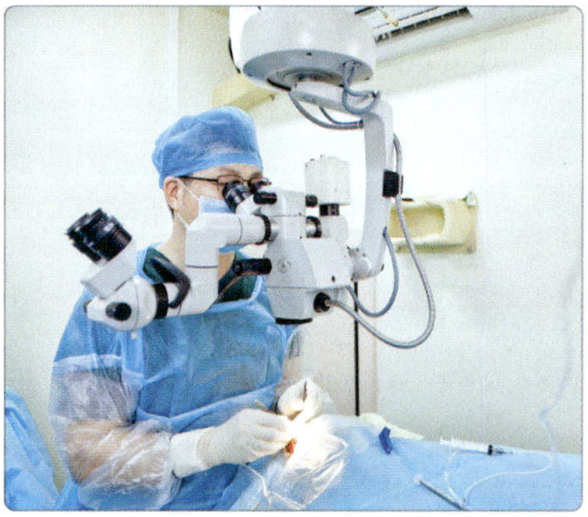

_______ /_______ /_______

eye / CV / physician who studies and treats

C Fill In

Build complementary terms for the following definitions by using the word parts you have learned.

1. study of the eye ________ WR / CV / ________ S
2. condition of false lens ________ WR / CV / ________ WR / ________ S
3. condition of equal pupil (size) ________ WR / CV / ________ WR / ________ S
4. pertaining to within the eye ________ P / ________ WR / ________ S
5. abnormal fear of (sensitivity to) light ________ WR / CV / ________ S
6. pertaining to the pupil ________ WR / ________ S
7. pertaining to the eye ________ WR / ________ S
8. pertaining to the cornea ________ WR / ________ S
9. pertaining to the nose and tear (ducts) ________ WR / CV / ________ WR / ________ S

EXERCISE 21 ■ Complementary Terms *NOT* Built from Word Parts

A Label

Write the complementary terms pictured and defined.

1. ________________________
agent that dilates the pupil

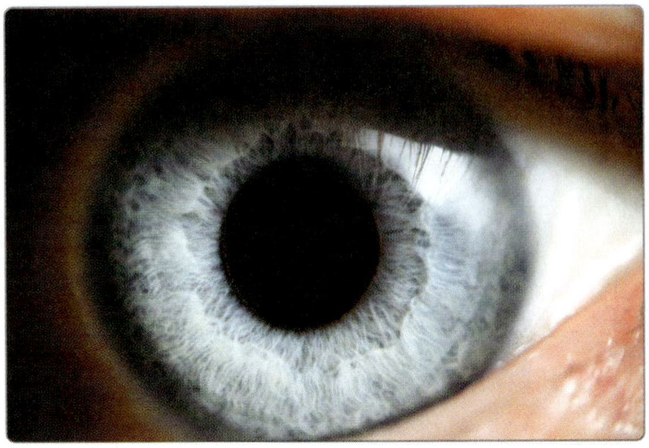

2. ________________________
agent that constricts the pupil

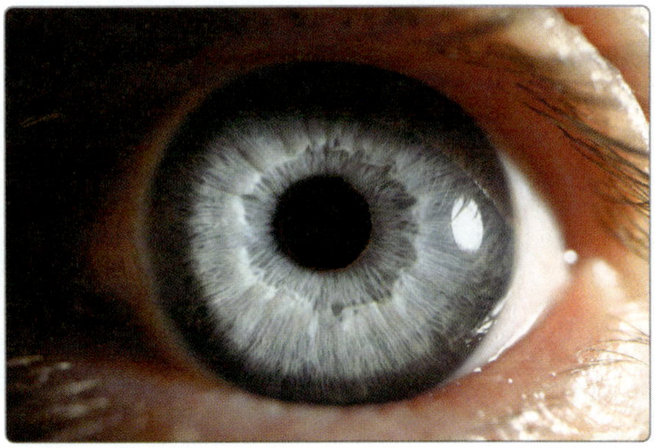

3. ________________________________
artificial lens implanted within the eye during cataract surgery

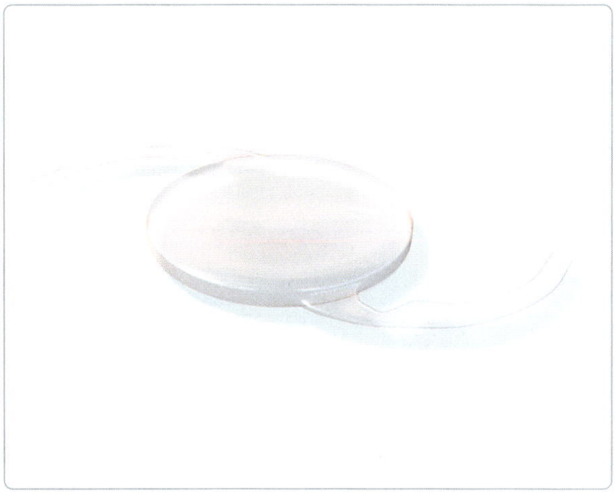

4. ________________________________
sharpness of vision for either distance or near

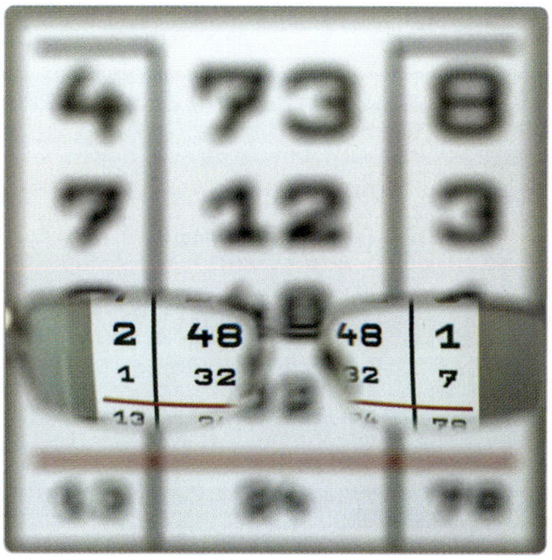

B Identify

Fill in the blanks with the correct terms.

1. Health professional who diagnoses, treats, and manages diseases and disorders of the eyes and visual processing system is a(n) ________________________________.
2. Specialist who fills prescriptions for lenses but who cannot prescribe lenses is a(n) ________________.
3. Normal refractive condition of the eye is called ________________.

C Match

Match the terms in the first column with their correct definitions in the second column.

______ 1. optician	a. sharpness of vision for either distance or near
______ 2. intraocular lens	b. health professional who diagnoses, treats, and manages diseases and disorders of the eyes and visual processing system
______ 3. visual acuity	c. agent that constricts the pupil
______ 4. mydriatic	d. specialist who fills prescriptions for lenses (cannot prescribe lenses)
______ 5. emmetropia	e. artificial lens implanted within the eye during cataract surgery
______ 6. optometrist	f. agent that dilates the pupil
______ 7. miotic	g. normal refractive condition of the eye

EXERCISE 22 ■ Review of Complementary Terms

Can you define, pronounce, and spell the following terms?

anisocoria	isocoria	optic	pseudophakia
binocular	lacrimal	optician	pupillary
corneal	miotic	ophthalmologist	retinal
emmetropia (Em)	mydriatic	ophthalmology (Ophth)	visual acuity (VA)
intraocular	nasolacrimal	optometrist	
intraocular lens (IOL)	ophthalmic	photophobia	

Abbreviations

DISEASE AND DISORDER

ABBREVIATION	TERM	ABBREVIATION	TERM
AMD	age-related macular degeneration	**Ast**	astigmatism

SIGNS AND SYMPTOMS

ABBREVIATION	TERM	ABBREVIATION	TERM
Em	emmetropia	**VA**	visual acuity
IOP	intraocular pressure		

DIAGNOSTIC

ABBREVIATION	TERM	ABBREVIATION	TERM
FA	fluorescein angiography	**OCT**	optical coherence tomography

TREATMENTS

ABBREVIATION	TERM	ABBREVIATION	TERM
LASIK	laser-assisted in situ keratomileusis	**PRK**	photorefractive keratectomy
PHACO	phacoemulsification	**IOL**	intraocular lens

MEDICAL SPECIALTY

ABBREVIATION	TERM
Ophth	ophthalmology

EXERCISE 23 ■ Abbreviations

Write the terms abbreviated.

1. Diagnostic tests related to the eye include **FA** __________ ______________ and **OCT** _________ __________ __________. Both tests can be used to assess the severity of **AMD** _____-_________ __________ ____________.
2. Cataracts, if left untreated, can lead to a decrease in **VA** ___________ ____________. **PHACO** ______________ is one type of treatment for this condition; an **IOL** __________ ________ is inserted during the same procedure.
3. **PRK** ______________________ _____________ and **LASIK** ________-__________ ___ ________ _________ are both used to correct **Ast** _______________, hyperopia, and myopia, with the goal of establishing **Em** ___________.
4. Patients with glaucoma have increased **IOP** ______________ ________________. Treatment involves medications and/or surgery. Frequent **Ophth** ___________________ follow up is required.

PRACTICAL APPLICATION

EXERCISE 24 ■ Case Study: Translate Between Everyday Language and Medical Language

CASE STUDY: Anjit Singh

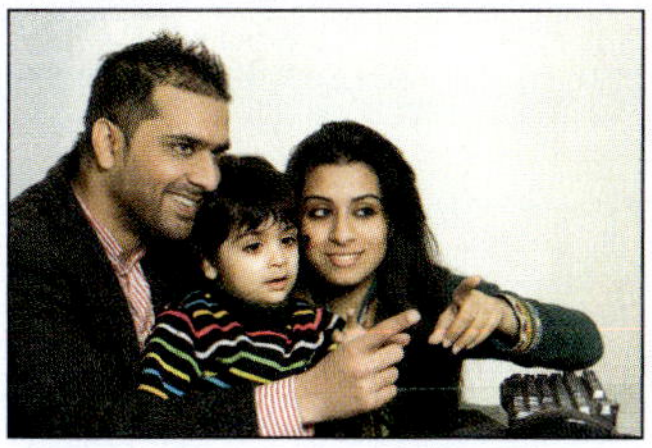

Anjit Singh, a 2-year-old boy, was brought by his parents to the pediatrician for his well-child examination. His mother noted that lately he seemed to be having trouble seeing things that he could identify previously and that one of his eyes seemed to move more slowly and to look in a different direction. Also, the white part of the same eye seemed to be irritated and looked red and inflamed. She also noticed that on a recent flash photograph that she took of her son, one pupil had a typical "red eye" look, but the other pupil looked white. The pediatrician agreed that there was a problem and sent Anjit to an eye physician for further work-up.

Now that you have worked through Chapter 12, consider the medical terms that might be used to describe Anjit's experience. See the Chapter at a Glance section at the end of the chapter for a list of terms that might apply.

A. *Underline phrases in the case study that could be substituted with medical terms.*

B. *Write the medical term and its definition for three of the phrases you underlined.*

MEDICAL TERM	DEFINITION
1. ______________	______________
2. ______________	______________
3. ______________	______________

DOCUMENTATION: Excerpt From Ophthalmology Visit

Anjit was examined by an ophthalmologist; an excerpt from the medical record is documented below.

Anjit Singh is a 2-year-old male referred by his pediatrician for issues related to his left eye. He is accompanied by his mother and father. History is significant for leukocoria, strabismus with resultant amblyopia, and scleritis. There is no family history of eye disease. Ophthalmoscopy reveals the absence of a red reflex on the left, with confirmation of leukocoria in that eye. The left eye also deviates outward on extraocular motor testing, and visual acuity is markedly decreased on the left. Retinal exam reveals a normal right eye and a mass suspicious for retinoblastoma in the left.

C. *Underline medical terms presented in Chapter 12 used in the previous excerpt from Anjit's medical record. See the Chapter at a Glance section at the end of the chapter for a complete list.*

D. *Select and define three of the medical terms you underlined. To check your answers, go to Appendix A.*

MEDICAL TERM	DEFINITION
1. ______________	______________
2. ______________	______________
3. ______________	______________

EXERCISE 25 ■ Interact With Medical Documents

A

Read the report and complete it by writing medical terms on answer lines within the document. Definitions of terms to be written appear after the document.

763217 GRAVES, William

File Patient Navigate Custom Fields Help

Chart Review | Encounters | Notes | Labs | Imaging | Procedures | Rx | Documents | Referrals | Scheduling | Billing

Name: **GRAVES, William** MR#: 763217 DOB: 6/27/19XX Sex: M Age: 66 **Allergies:** None known **PCP:** Murphy, Clara MD

Ophthalmology Clinic Visit
Date: 03 April 20XX 10:15

Subjective: Mr. Graves is a 66-year-old male here today for his annual 1.____________________ exam. He has no current complaint. He has a family history of 2.____________________ in his brother. He has a history of hypertension and type 2 diabetes mellitus. A 3.________________ was removed from his right eye 5 years ago.

Medications: Glyburide 5 mg bid and metoprolol 50 mg bid.

Objective:
Visual Acuities: Aided: right eye 20/25 left eye 20/30-1 both eyes 20/25
Unaided: right eye 20/100 left eye 20/80-1 both eyes 20/80

Externals: 2 mm 4.____, right eye.
PERLA (pupils equal and reactive to light and accommodation).
EOMI (extraocular movements intact).

Ophthalmoscopic:
Lens: left eye showed early cortical spokes
Disk: margins normal
Cup-to-disk ratio: 0.2 both eyes
Fundus: scattered microaneurysms bilaterally, with dot and blot hemorrhages noted in all four quadrants of both eyes
Refraction: right eye 1.00-0.50 x 90 20/20, left eye 1.25-0.25 x 90 20/20
Tonometry: 14 mm Hg/right eye, 13 mm Hg/left eye

Visual Field: Full

Assessment: Patient has compound myopic 5.__________________________ and 6.____________________________ with diabetic 7.________________ and grade 2 hypertension. He also shows an early 8.__________________________________ in the left eye.

Plan: Provide prescription for corrective lenses. See patient for follow-up visit in 6 months to reevaluate diabetic retinopathy and cataract. Counseled patient to report any sudden changes in vision.

Electronically signed: Rwabunihi, Anella MD on 05 April 20XX 14:00

Start | Log On/Off | Print | Edit

Definitions of Medical Terms to Complete the Document

Write the medical terms defined on corresponding answer lines in the document.

1. study of the eye
2. eye disorder characterized by the increase of intraocular pressure
3. thin tissue growing into the cornea from the conjunctiva
4. drooping of the eyelid
5. irregular curvature of the cornea or lens
6. impaired vision as a result of aging
7. (any noninflammatory) disease of the retina
8. clouding of the lens of the eye

B

Read the patient profile and answer the questions below it.

Patient Profile

This 70-year-old woman was admitted for surgical treatment of chronic, poorly controlled **glaucoma** and for **cataract** extraction.

Subjective: The patient reported a progressive loss of **visual acuity** in her right eye; she complained of headaches and problems with glare (particularly at night) and said she perceives halos around lights.

Objective: Vision testing and physical examination (i.e., **ophthalmoscopy, slit lamp** microscopy, and **tonometry**) revealed acuity (unaided) of 10/100 for the right eye and 20/60 for the left eye. Opacification of right lens was evident, as was moderate **corneal** edema. **Intraocular** pressure measurements were 28 mm Hg in the right eye and 21 mm Hg in the left eye.

Therapeutic Management: After a **mydriatic** agent was applied to the right pupil, a combined procedure **phacoemulsification** of the cataract and **trabeculectomy** with releasable sutures (to minimize **IOP**) was performed with the patient under local anesthesia. The patient tolerated the procedure well and returned to her room wearing a 12-hour collagen shield on the treated eye.

Use the patient profile above to answer the questions.

1. Vision testing and physical examination of the patient revealed opacification of the right lens, confirming the need for:
   a. PRK
   b. phacoemulsification
   c. scleral buckling
   d. enucleation
2. Application of a mydriatic agent would:
   a. reduce tears
   b. produce tears
   c. constrict the pupil
   d. dilate the pupil
3. A trabeculectomy was performed because the patient had a history of:
   a. condition of crossed eyes
   b. disorder characterized by increased intraocular pressure
   c. nearsightedness
   d. progressive deterioration of a portion of the retina
4. The abbreviation IOP stands for:
   a. both eyes
   b. normal vision
   c. intraocular pressure
   d. iris outer pupil

EXERCISE 26 ■ Use Medical Language in Online Electronic Health Records

Select the correct medical terms to complete three medical records in one patient's electronic file.

Access online resources at evolve.elsevier.com > Evolve Resources > Student Resources > Activities > Chapter 12 > Electronic Health Records

Topic: Glaucoma
Record 1: New Patient Evaluation
Record 2: Consultation Letter to PCP
Record 3: Operative Note

❏ Check the box when complete.

EXERCISE 27 ■ Pronounce Medical Terms in Use

Practice pronunciation of terms by reading aloud the following paragraphs. Use the phonetic spellings to assist with pronunciation. The script also contains medical terms not presented in the chapter. If interested, research their meanings in a medical dictionary or a reliable online source.

An elderly gentleman visited his **ophthalmologist** (*of*-thal-MOL-o-jist) because of decreased vision. A **tonometry** (tō-NOM-e-trē) examination showed borderline readings. **Visual acuity** (VIZH-ū-al) (a-KŪ-i-tē) measurement indicated a mild degree of **myopia** (mī-Ō-pē–a) and **presbyopia** (*pres*-bē-Ō-pē-a). A diagnosis of **glaucoma** (glaw-KŌ-ma) was suspected in this case and timolol eye drops were prescribed, one drop daily.

A **cataract** (KAT-a-rakt) of the right eye was found. Lens implant surgery, which places an **intraocular lens** (in-tra-OK-ū-lar) (lenz), will be performed when the cataract matures sufficiently. Approximately 5 years ago the patient had a **retinal detachment** (RET-in-al) (dē-TACH-ment) of the left eye. A **scleral buckling** (SKLER-al) (BUK-ling) procedure was performed and was successful in halting the progression of retinal detachment.

CHAPTER REVIEW

EXERCISE 28 ■ Chapter Content Quiz

Test your understanding of terms and abbreviations introduced in this chapter. Circle the letter for the medical term or abbreviation related to the words in italics.

1. Before the exam, a medication to *dilate the pupils* was placed in the patient's eyes using a dropper.
   a. miotic
   b. mydriatic
   c. myopia

2. A person with an *irregular curvature of the cornea or lens* of the eye has:
   a. astigmatism
   b. glaucoma
   c. strabismus

3. To *measure the pressure within the patient's eye*, the optometrist used a:
   a. pupillometer
   b. tonometer
   c. keratometer

4. A patient with an *involuntary jerking movement of the eyes* has a condition known as:
   a. astigmatism
   b. anisometropia
   c. nystagmus

5. The ophthalmologist ordered a *radiographic imaging of the blood vessels of the eye with a dye* to assess the progression of the patient's diabetic retinopathy.
   a. fluorescein angiography
   b. tonometry
   c. ophthalmoscopy

6. A person who is *farsighted* has:
   a. hyperopia
   b. myopia
   c. diplopia

7. *Health professionals who diagnose, treat, and manage diseases and disorders of the eyes and visual processing system* are licensed by the state and have earned doctorate degrees abbreviated as OD.
   a. optician
   b. optometrist
   c. ophthalmologist

8. *Inflammation of the white of the eye* can be very painful and may be associated with an underlying autoimmune disorder, such as rheumatoid arthritis and systemic lupus erythematosus.
   a. scleritis
   b. scleromalacia
   c. conjunctivitis

9. The surgery schedule indicated the patient being treated for cataracts would undergo right eye *PHACO* with IOL.
   a. photorefractive keratectomy
   b. photocoagulation
   c. phacoemulsification

10. During cataract surgery, an intraocular lens was placed in the patient's right eye, which would now be described as having *condition of false lens*.
    a. anisocoria
    b. aphakia
    c. pseudophakia
11. *Progressive deterioration of the retina, resulting in loss of central vision* may be described as dry, where the blood vessels become thin and brittle, or wet, where new abnormal vessels develop under the macula.
    a. retinitis pigmentosa
    b. macular degeneration
    c. presbyopia
12. The patient explained that she experienced an *abnormal sensitivity to light* before her migraine.
    a. photophobia
    b. nyctalopia
    c. isocoria
13. In hopes of giving up her glasses, the patient elected to have *a laser procedure to reshape her corneal tissue beneath the surface of the cornea* to treat nearsightedness.
    a. PRK
    b. LASIK
    c. IOP
14. In a surgical procedure, *retinal tissue was condensed using an intense beam of light* to repair retinal tears in the patient's left eye and prevent retinal detachment.
    a. retinal photocoagulation
    b. phacoemulsification
    c. scleral buckling
15. *Inflammation of the tear sac* is an infection of the lacrimal sac, which may be acute or chronic.
    a. blepharitis
    b. endophthalmitis
    c. dacryocystitis
16. The *instrument used to measure the diameter of the pupil* may be used as a part of a neurological examination to provide an objective measure of pupillary response.
    a. tonometer
    b. pupillometer
    c. keratometer
17. Macular degeneration may be detected by *noninvasive test that uses light waves to take cross-sectional images of the retina*.
    a. fluorescein angiography
    b. tonometry
    c. optical coherence tomography
18. A corneal abrasion might be diagnosed using a *horizontally mounted binocular microscope that uses a very narrow vertical beam of light to examine the eye in great detail.*
    a. slit lamp
    b. keratometer
    c. pupilloscope
19. Autoimmune disorders such as rheumatoid arthritis and lupus may cause *inflammation of the uvea and sclera*.
    a. uveitis
    b. uveoscleritis
    c. scleritis
20. A patient with retinal detachment might require *surgical removal of all or part of the vitreous humor.*
    a. retinal photocoagulation
    b. scleral buckling
    c. vitrectomy

CHAPTER AT A GLANCE Word Parts New to This Chapter

COMBINING FORMS				PREFIX	SUFFIXES
blephar/o	dipl/o	ocul/o	pupill/o	bin-	-opia
conjunctiv/o	ir/o	ophthalm/o	retin/o		-phobia
cor/o	irid/o	opt/o	scler/o		-plegia
corne/o	is/o	phac/o	ton/o		
cry/o	kerat/o	phak/o	uve/o		
dacry/o	lacrim/o	phot/o			

CHAPTER AT A GLANCE Eye Terms Built from Word Parts

DISEASE AND DISORDER
aphakia
blepharitis
blepharoptosis
conjunctivitis
dacryocystitis
diplopia
endophthalmitis
iridoplegia
iritis
keratitis
keratomalacia
leukocoria
oculomycosis
ophthalmalgia
ophthalmopathy
ophthalmoplegia
phacomalacia
retinoblastoma
retinopathy
scleritis
scleromalacia
uveitis
uveoscleritis
xerophthalmia

SURGICAL
blepharoplasty
cryoretinopexy
dacryocystorhinostomy
iridectomy
iridotomy
keratoplasty
sclerotomy

DIAGNOSTIC
fluorescein angiography (FA)
keratometer
ophthalmoscope
ophthalmoscopy
optometry
pupillometer
pupilloscope
retinoscopy
tonometer
tonometry

COMPLEMENTARY
anisocoria
binocular
corneal
intraocular
isocoria
lacrimal
nasolacrimal
ophthalmic
ophthalmologist
ophthalmology (Ophth)
optic
photophobia
pseudophakia
pupillary
retinal

CHAPTER AT A GLANCE Eye Terms *NOT* Built from Word Parts

DISEASE AND DISORDER
amblyopia
anisometropia
astigmatism (Ast)
cataract
chalazion
drusen
glaucoma
hyperopia
hyphema
macular degeneration
myopia
nyctalopia
nystagmus
pinguecula
presbyopia
pterygium
retinal detachment
retinitis pigmentosa
strabismus
sty

SURGICAL
enucleation
LASIK (laser-assisted in situ keratomileusis)
phacoemulsification (PHACO)
photorefractive keratectomy (PRK)
retinal photocoagulation
scleral buckling
trabeculectomy
vitrectomy

DIAGNOSTIC
optical coherence tomography (OCT)
slit lamp

COMPLEMENTARY
emmetropia (Em)
intraocular lens (IOL)
miotic
mydriatic
optician
optometrist
visual acuity (VA)

Chapter 13
Ear

Outline

Objectives

Upon completion of this chapter, you will be able to:

1. Pronounce organs and anatomic structures of the ear.
2. Define and spell word parts related to the ear.
3. Define, pronounce, and spell disease and disorder terms related to the ear.
4. Define, pronounce, and spell surgical terms related to the ear.
5. Define, pronounce, and spell diagnostic terms related to the ear.
6. Define, pronounce, and spell complementary terms related to the ear.
7. Interpret the meaning of abbreviations related to the ear.
8. Apply medical language in clinical contexts.

ANATOMY

Function

The two functions of the ear are to hear and to provide the sense of balance. The ear is made up of three parts: the **external ear**, the **middle ear**, and the **inner ear** (Figs. 13.1 and 13.2). The process of hearing begins with the **auricles** directing sound waves into the **external auditory canal.** As the sound waves ripple through the external ear, the **tympanic membrane** vibrates. The **ossicles** in the middle ear carry the vibration to the inner ear, where the stimulus is transmitted by the cochlear nerve to the brain and is interpreted as sound.

Balance is a function of the **inner ear** and is maintained through a series of complex processes. The vestibular nerve transmits information about motion and body position from the semicircular canals and the vestibule to the brain for interpretation.

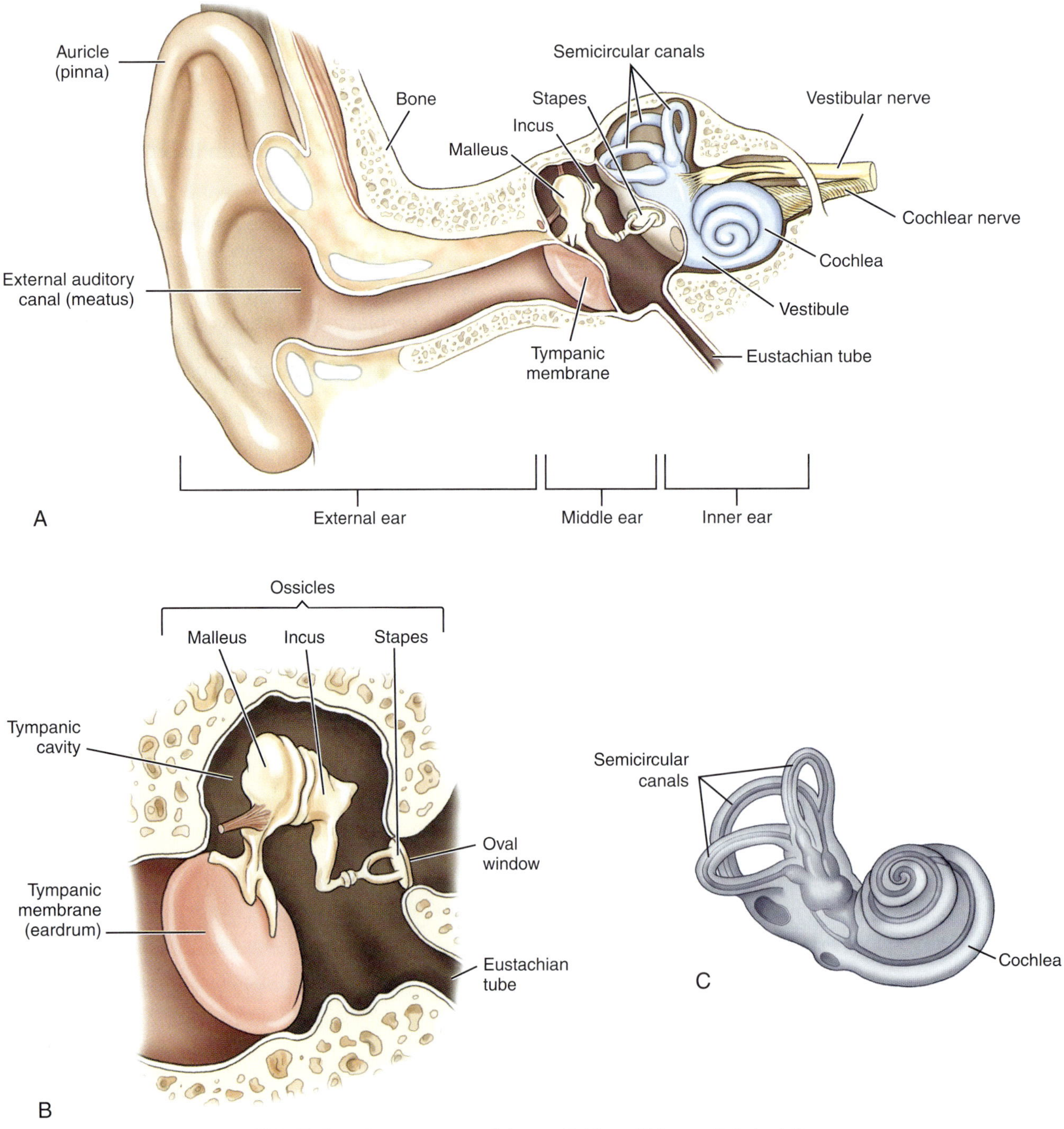

FIG. 13.1 **A,** Gross anatomy of the ear. **B,** The middle ear. **C,** Labyrinth.

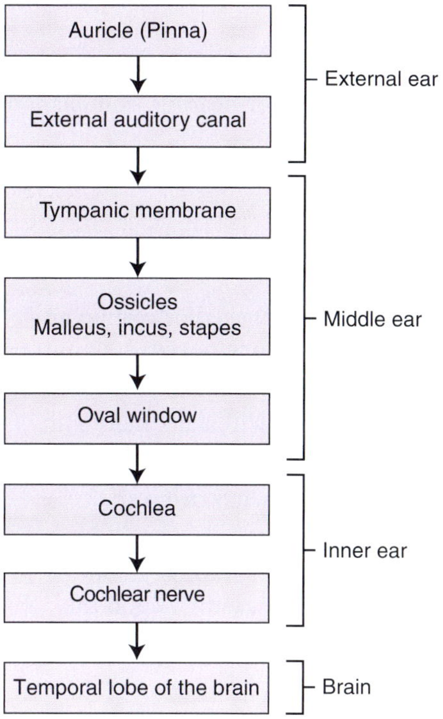

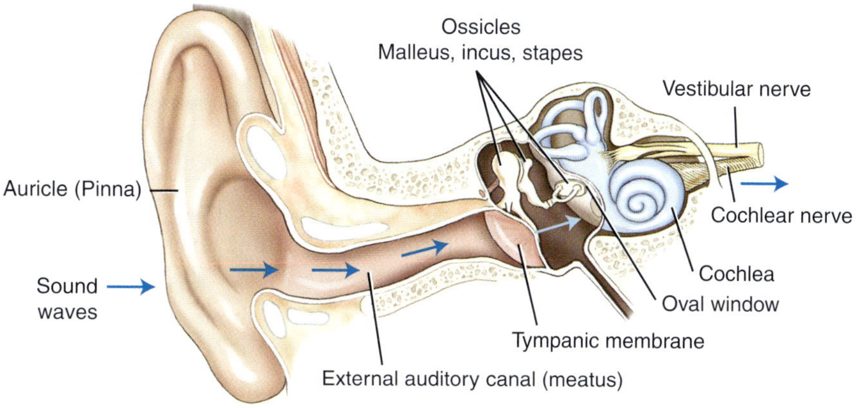

FIG. 13.2 Perception of sound.

Organs and Anatomic Structures of the Ear

TERM	DEFINITION
ear (ēr)	organ of hearing and balance; includes the external ear, middle ear, and labyrinth or inner ear
external ear (ek-STER-nal) (ēr)	consists of the auricle and external auditory canal (meatus)
auricle (AW-ri-kl)	external, visible part of the ear located on both sides of the head; directs sound waves into the external auditory canal (also called **pinna**)
external auditory canal (ek-STER-nal) (AW-di-tor-ē) (kah-NAL)	short tube that ends at the tympanic membrane. The inner part lies within the temporal bone of the skull and contains the glands that secrete earwax (cerumen). (also called **external auditory meatus**)
middle ear (MID-l) (ēr)	consists of the tympanic membrane and the tympanic cavity containing the ossicles
tympanic membrane (tim-PAN-ik) (MEM-brān)	semitransparent membrane that separates the external auditory canal and the middle ear cavity. The tympanic membrane transmits sound vibrations to the ossicles. (also called **eardrum**)
TYMPANIC MEMBRANE is derived from the Greek **tympanon**, meaning **drum**, because of its resemblance to a drum or tambourine.	
ossicles (OS-i-kalz)	bones of the middle ear that carry sound vibrations. The ossicles are composed of the **malleus** (hammer), **incus** (anvil), and **stapes** (stirrup). The stapes connects to the **oval window**, which transmits the sound vibrations to the cochlea of the inner ear.
STAPES is Latin for **stirrup**. The anatomic stapes was so named for its stirrup-like shape.	
eustachian tube (yū-STĀ-shan) (toob)	passage between the middle ear and the pharynx; equalizes air pressure on both sides of the tympanic membrane
inner ear (IN-ar) (ēr)	consists of the labyrinth and connectors of the vestibular and the cochlear nerves
labyrinth (LAB-e-rinth)	bony spaces within the temporal bone of the skull made up of three distinct parts, the cochlea, the semicircular canals, and the vestibule. The cochlea facilitates hearing. The semicircular canals and the vestibule facilitate equilibrium and balance.

Organs and Anatomic Structures of the Ear—cont'd

TERM	DEFINITION
cochlea (KŌK-lē-ah)	coiled portion of the inner ear containing the sensory organ for hearing; connects to the oval window in the middle ear
semicircular canals and vestibule (*sem*-ī-SUR-kū-lar) (kah-NALS), (VES-ti-būl)	sensory organs of balance; contain receptors and endolymph that provide sensory information about the body's position to maintain equilibrium
vestibulocochlear nerves (ves-*tib*-ū-lō-KOK-lē-ar) (nurvz)	paired cranial nerves responsible for hearing and balance; composed of vestibular fibers and cochlear fibers (also called **acoustic nerve** or **auditory nerve**)
vestibular nerve (ves-TIB-ū-lar) (nurv)	conveys information about position and balance from the semicircular canals and vestibule to the brain
cochlear nerve (KOK-lē-ar) (nurve)	conveys information about sound, including volume and frequency, from the cochlea to the brain
mastoid bone (MAS-toid) (bōn)	portion of the temporal bone of the skull posterior and inferior to each auditory canal; contains mastoid air cells that drain into the middle ear cavity behind the external auditory canal (also called **mastoid process**)

PRONOUNCE ANATOMIC STRUCTURES

Practice saying aloud each of the organs and specific structures on the previous pages.

To hear the terms, go to Evolve Resources at www.evolve.elsevier.com and select:

Student Resources > Audio Glossary > Chapter 13 > Anatomic Structures.

❑ Check the box when complete.

WORD PARTS

Use paper flashcards or electronic flashcards on Evolve to memorize word parts used to analyze, define, and build medical terms in this chapter. To reinforce learning, study one section of the Word Parts Table at a time, then complete the corresponding exercise on the following pages.

1 ■ Combining Forms of the Ear

COMBINING FORM	DEFINITION	COMBINING FORM	DEFINITION
audi/o	hearing	**myring/o**	tympanic membrane (eardrum)
aur/i	ear	**ot/o**	ear
cochle/o	cochlea	**staped/o**	stapes
labyrinth/o	labyrinth	**tympan/o**	middle ear
mastoid/o	mastoid bone	**vestibul/o**	vestibule

2 ■ Combining Forms Used with Ear Terms

COMBINING FORM	DEFINITION	COMBINING FORM	DEFINITION
electr/o	electricity, electrical activity	**py/o**	pus
myc/o	fungus		

3 ■ Suffixes

SUFFIX	DEFINITION	SUFFIX	DEFINITION
-al	pertaining to	**-metry**	measurement
-algia	pain	**-osis**	abnormal condition (means increase when used with blood cell word roots)
-ar	pertaining to	**-plasty**	surgical repair
-ectomy	excision, surgical removal	**-rrhea**	flow, discharge
-gram	the record, radiographic image	**-sclerosis**	hardening
-graphy	process of recording, radiographic imaging	**-scope**	instrument used for visual examination
-itis	inflammation	**-scopy**	visual examination
-logist	one who studies and treats (specialist, physician)	**-stomy**	creation of an artificial opening
-logy	study of	**-tomy**	cut into, incision
-meter	instrument used to measure		

Refer to **Appendix B** and **Appendix C** for a complete list of word parts.

EXERCISE 1 ■ Combining Forms of the Ear

Refer to the first section of the word parts table.

A Label

Fill in the blanks with combining forms to label this diagram of the ear. *To check your answers, go to Appendix A at the the back of the textbook.*

1. Ear

CF: ______________________

CF: ______________________

2. Hearing

CF: ______________________

3. Middle ear

CF: ______________________

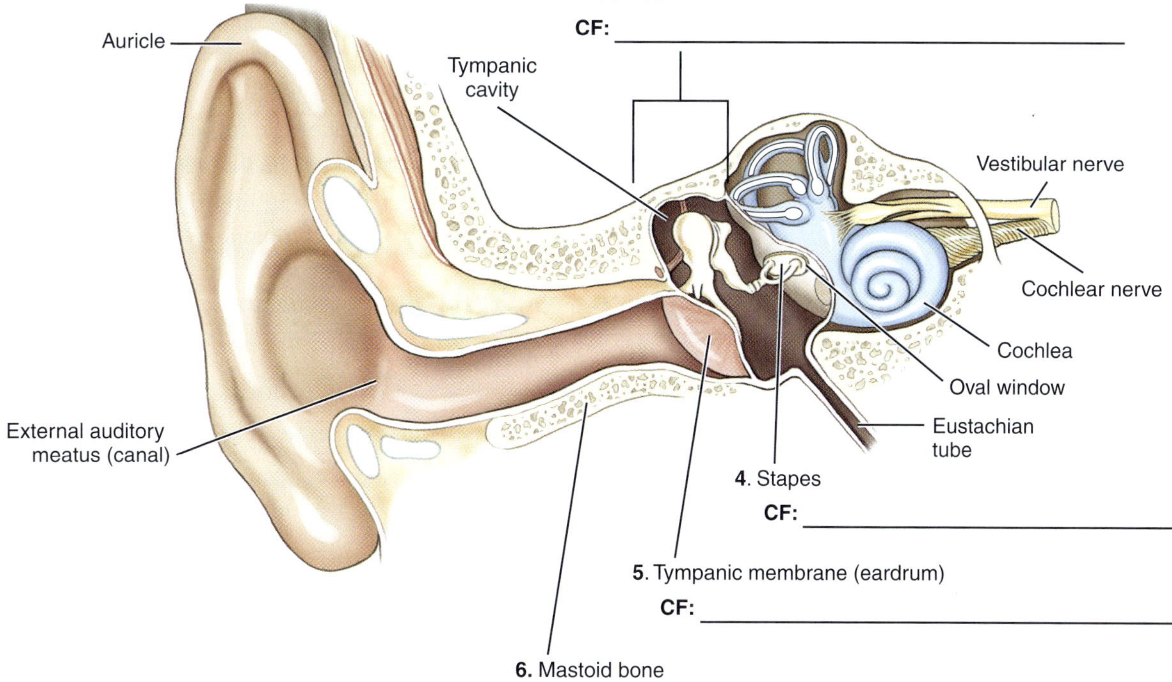

4. Stapes

CF: ______________________

5. Tympanic membrane (eardrum)

CF: ______________________

6. Mastoid bone

CF: ______________________

B Label

Fill in the blanks with combining forms of the ear.

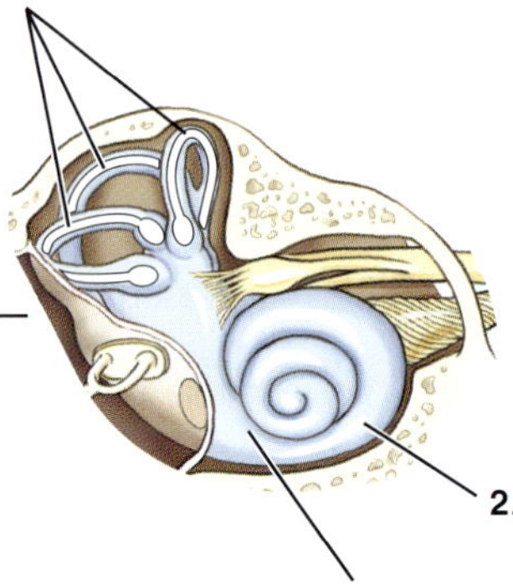

C Define and Match

Step 1: Write the definitions after the following combining forms.
Step 2: Match the descriptions on the right with the combining forms and definitions. Answers may be used more than once; no answer line appears for those not described in a lettered item.

_____ 1. staped/o, ______________________
_____ 2. vestibul/o, ______________________
_____ 3. aur/i, ______________________
_____ 4. cochle/o, ______________________
_____ 5. labyrinth/o, ______________________
_____ 6. myring/o, ______________________
_____ 7. tympan/o, ______________________
_____ 8. ot/o, ______________________
_____ 9. mastoid/o, ______________________
10. audi/o, ______________________

a. organ of hearing and balance
b. semitransparent membrane that separates the external auditory canal and the middle ear cavity
c. portion of the temporal bone of the skull posterior and inferior to each auditory canal
d. sensory organ of balance containing receptors and endolymph
e. bony spaces within the temporal bone of the skull made up of three distinct parts, the cochlea, the semicircular canals, and the vestibule
f. coiled portion of the inner ear containing the sensory organ for hearing
g. one of three bones of the middle ear; shaped like a stirrup and connected to the oval window
h. portion of the ear containing the tympanic membrane and the tympanic cavity

EXERCISE 2 ■ Combining Forms Used with Ear Terms

Refer to the second section of the word parts table.

A Define

Write the definitions of the following combining forms.

1. myc/o ______________________
2. py/o ______________________
3. electr/o ______________________

B Identify

Write the combining form for each of the following.

1. electricity, electrical activity ______
2. fungus ______
3. pus ______

EXERCISE 3 ■ Suffixes

Refer to the third section of the word parts table.

A Match

Match the suffixes in the first column with their definitions in the second column.

______	1. -plasty	a. excision, surgical removal
______	2. -meter	b. one who studies and treats
______	3. -ectomy	c. abnormal condition
______	4. -rrhea	d. surgical repair
______	5. -osis	e. flow, discharge
______	6. -tomy	f. pain
______	7. -algia	g. instrument used to measure
______	8. -logist	h. instrument used for visual examination
______	9. -scope	i. hardening
______	10. -sclerosis	j. cut into, incision

B Define

Write definitions for the following suffixes.

1. -stomy ______
2. -scopy ______
3. -metry ______
4. -logy ______

C Identify

Write the suffix for each of the following.

1. process of recording, radiographic imaging ______
2. inflammation ______
3. pertaining to a. ______
   b. ______
4. the record, radiographic image ______

MEDICAL TERMS

Medical terms relevant to this chapter have been grouped by topics, such as Disease and Disorder, and are listed in tables designated as Built from Word Parts or *NOT* Built from Word Parts. The exercises following each table assist with learning term definitions, pronunciations, and spellings.

Disease and Disorder Terms

BUILT FROM WORD PARTS

The following terms can be translated using definitions of word parts. Further explanation is provided within parentheses as needed.

TERM	DEFINITION
1. **labyrinthitis** (*lab*-i-rin-THĪ-tis)	inflammation of the labyrinth
2. **mastoiditis** (*mas*-toyd-Ī-tis)	inflammation of the mastoid bone
3. **myringitis** (*mir*-in-JĪ-tis)	inflammation of the tympanic membrane (eardrum)
4. **otalgia** (ō-TAL-ja)	pain in the ear
5. **otomycosis** (*ō*-tō-mī-KŌ-sis)	abnormal condition of fungus in the ear (usually affects the external auditory canal)
6. **otopyorrhea** (*ō*-tō-*pī*-ō-RĒ-a)	discharge of pus from the ear
7. **otorrhea** (*ō*-tō-RĒ-a)	discharge from the ear (may be serous, bloody, consisting of pus, or containing cerebrospinal fluid)
8. **otosclerosis** (*ō*-tō-skle-RŌ-sis)	hardening of the ear (stapes) (caused by irregular bone development and resulting in hearing loss)

EXERCISE 4 ▪ Pronounce and Spell

Practice pronunciation and spelling on paper and online.

1. Practice on Paper

a. **Pronounce:** Read the phonetic spelling and say aloud the terms listed in the previous table. Refer to the pronunciation key on p. 20 as necessary.

b. **Spell:** Have a study partner read the terms aloud. Write the spelling of the terms on a separate sheet of paper.

2. Practice Online

a. **Access** online learning resources. Go to evolve.elsevier.com > Evolve Resources > Student Resources.

b. **Pronounce:** Select Audio Glossary > Chapter 13 > Exercise 4. Select a term to hear its pronunciation and repeat aloud.

c. **Spell:** Select Activities > Chapter 13 > Spell Terms > Exercise 4. Select the audio icon and type the correct spelling of the term.

❑ Check the box when complete.

EXERCISE 5 ▪ Analyze and Define

Analyze and define the following terms.

1. otomycosis

____

____

2. otalgia

____

____

3. labyrinthitis

____

____

4. myringitis

____

____

5. otosclerosis

____

____

6. mastoiditis

____

____

7. otopyorrhea

____

____

8. otorrhea

____

____

EXERCISE 6 ■ Build

A Label

Build terms pictured by writing word parts above definitions.

1.

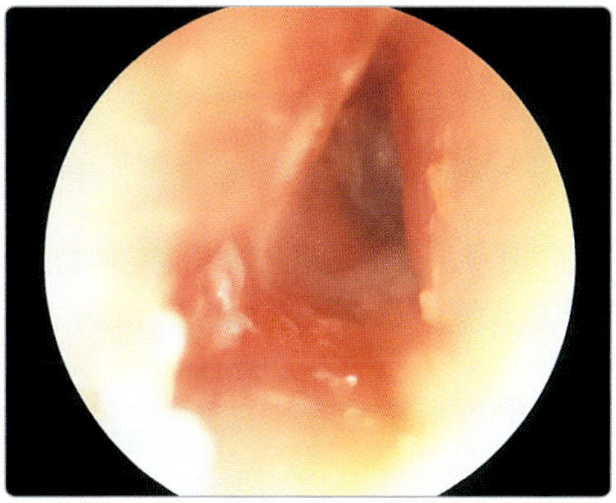

_______ / ___ / _______ / ___ / _______
ear CV pus CV discharge

2.

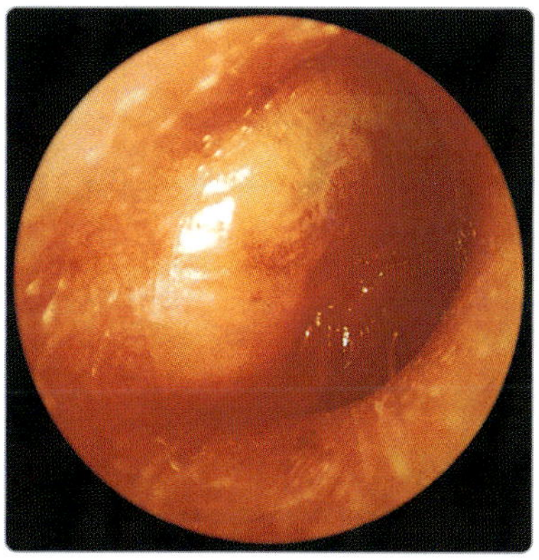

__________ / __________
tympanic membrane inflammation

B Fill In

Build disease and disorder terms for the following definitions by using the word parts you have learned.

1. inflammation of the mastoid bone ______ / ______
WR S

2. pain in the ear ______ / ______
WR S

3. hardening of the ear (stapes) ______ / ___ / ______
WR CV S

4. abnormal condition of fungus in the ear ______ WR / CV / WR / S

5. inflammation of the labyrinth ______ WR / S

6. discharge from the ear ______ WR / CV / S

Disease and Disorder Terms

NOT BUILT FROM WORD PARTS

Word parts may be present in the following terms; however, their full meanings cannot be translated using definitions of word parts alone.

TERM	DEFINITION
1. **acoustic neuroma** (a-KOOS-tik) (nū-RŌ-ma)	benign tumor within the internal auditory canal growing from the acoustic nerve; may cause hearing loss and may damage structures of the cerebellum as it grows
2. **cholesteatoma** (*ko*-le-stē-a-TŌ-ma)	cystlike mass composed of epithelial cells and cholesterol occurring in the middle ear; may be associated with chronic otitis media
3. **Ménière disease** (me-NYĀR) (di-ZĒZ)	chronic disease of the inner ear characterized by a sensation of spinning motion (vertigo), ringing in the ear (tinnitus), aural fullness, and fluctuating hearing loss; symptoms are related to a change in volume or composition of fluid within the labyrinth
4. **otitis externa (OE)** (ō-TĪ-tis) (eks-TER-na)	inflammation of the outer ear
5. **otitis media (OM)** (ō-TĪ-tis) (MĒ-dē-a)	inflammation of the middle ear (Fig. 13.3A)
6. **ototoxicity** (*ō*-tō-tok-SIS-i-tē)	adverse pharmocological reaction causing damage to the vestibulocochlear nerve; results in abnormalities of hearing and balance
7. **presbycusis** (*prez*-bi-KŪ-sis)	hearing impairment occurring with age
8. **tinnitus** (tin-NĪ-tus)	ringing in the ears (*Note:* the ending is **itus** and not **itis**, the usual ending for inflammation)
9. **vertigo** (VER-ti-gō)	sense that either one's own body (subjective vertigo) or the environment (objective vertigo) is revolving; may indicate inner ear disease

BENIGN PAROXYSMAL POSITIONAL VERTIGO (BPPV) is characterized by brief episodes of vertigo associated with a change in the position of the head, such as turning over in bed or sitting up in the morning. In BPPV, normal calcium carbonate crystals called otoconia break loose and shift within the labyrinth, triggering an episode of vertigo.

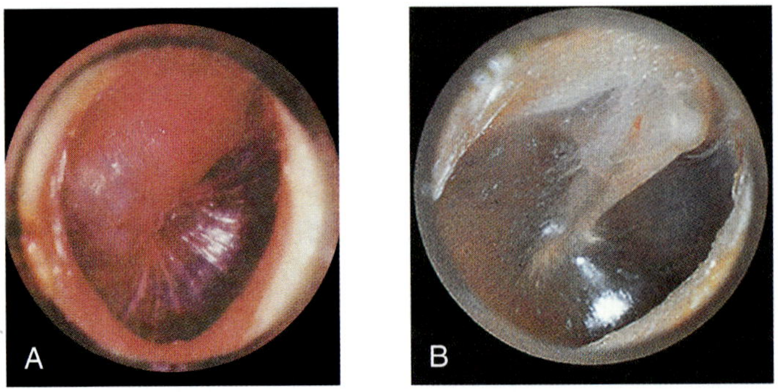

FIG. 13.3 Otitis media. Signs include bulging, perforated, reddened, or retracted tympanic membrane. **A,** Tympanic membrane demonstrating **acute otitis media (AOM)**. **B,** Normal tympanic membrane.

EXERCISE 7 ■ Pronounce and Spell

Practice pronunciation and spelling on paper and online.

1. Practice on Paper

a. **Pronounce:** Read the phonetic spelling and say aloud the terms listed in the previous table. Refer to the pronunciation key on p. 20 as necessary.
b. **Spell:** Have a study partner read the terms aloud. Write the spelling of the terms on a separate sheet of paper.

2. Practice Online

a. **Access** online learning resources. Go to evolve.elsevier.com > Evolve Resources > Student Resources.
b. **Pronounce:** Select Audio Glossary > Chapter 13 > Exercise 7. Select a term to hear its pronunciation and repeat aloud.
c. **Spell:** Select Activities > Chapter 13 > Spell Terms > Exercise 7. Select the audio icon and type the correct spelling of the term.

❑ Check the box when complete.

EXERCISE 8 ■ Fill In

A Identify

Fill in the blanks with the correct terms.

1. The patient reported a sense that her body seemed to be revolving, or ______________________________, and ringing in the ears, or ______________________________.
2. A chronic ear disease characterized by vertigo, tinnitus, aural fullness, and fluctuating hearing loss is called ______________________________ disease.
3. ______________________________ is hearing impairment occurring with age.
4. An adverse reaction causing damage to the vestibulocochlear nerve that results in abnormalities of hearing and balance is ______________________________.

B Label

Write the medical terms pictured and defined.

1. ______________________________
inflammation of the outer ear

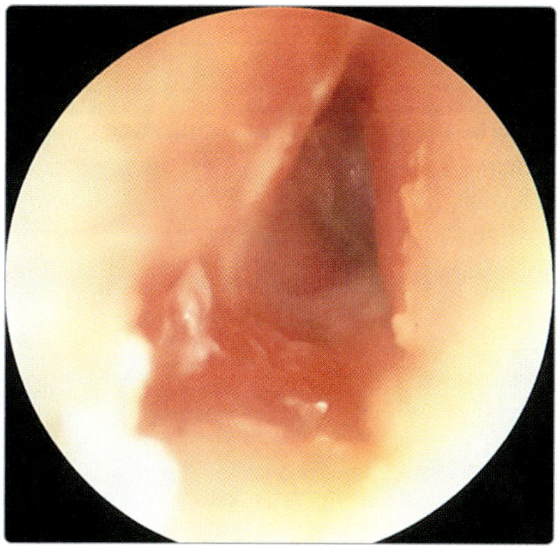

2. ______________________________
inflammation of the middle ear

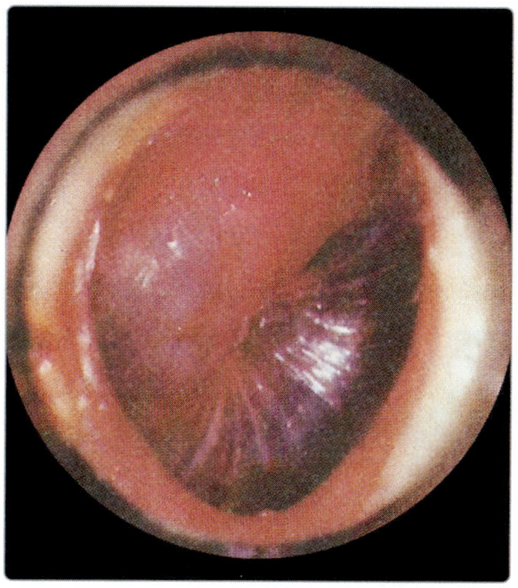

3. ______________________________
cystlike mass composed of epithelial cells and cholesterol occurring in the middle ear

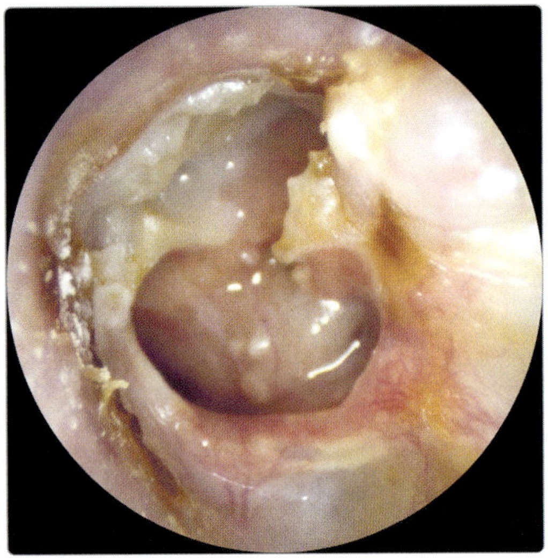

4. ______________________________
benign tumor within the internal auditory canal growing from the acoustic nerve

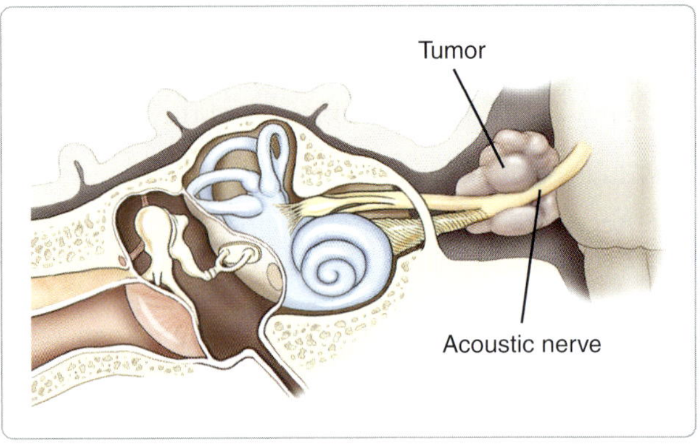

EXERCISE 9 ■ Match

Match the terms in the first column with their correct definitions in the second column.

_____ 1. vertigo	a. inflammation of the middle ear
_____ 2. tinnitus	b. adverse pharmocological reaction causing damage to the vestibulocochlear nerve
_____ 3. Ménière disease	c. benign tumor arising from the acoustic nerve
_____ 4. otitis externa	d. sense of revolving of one's own body or the environment
_____ 5. acoustic neuroma	e. ringing in the ears
_____ 6. otitis media	f. inflammation of the outer ear
_____ 7. presbycusis	g. hearing impairment occurring with age
_____ 8. cholesteatoma	h. mass composed of epithelial cells and cholesterol
_____ 9. ototoxicity	i. chronic ear problem characterized by vertigo, tinnitus, and fluctuating hearing loss

EXERCISE 10 ■ Review of Disease and Disorder Terms

Can you define, pronounce, and spell the following terms?

acoustic neuroma
cholesteatoma
labyrinthitis
mastoiditis
Ménière disease
myringitis
otalgia
otitis externa (OE)
otitis media (OM)
otomycosis
otopyorrhea
otorrhea
otosclerosis
ototoxicity
presbycusis
tinnitus
vertigo

Surgical Terms

BUILT FROM WORD PARTS

The following terms can be translated using definitions of word parts. Further explanation is provided within parentheses as needed.

TERM	DEFINITION
1. **cochlear implant** (KŌK-lē-ar) (IM-plant)	pertaining to the cochlea implant (surgically inserted electronic device that converts sound into electrical impulses. The impulses stimulate the auditory nerve to carry the signal to the brain which learns to interpret the signal as sound. The damaged part of the ear is bypassed.)
COCHLEAR IMPLANTS are fitted in adults and children who are deaf or severely hard of hearing.	
2. **labyrinthectomy** (*lab*-i-rin-THEK-to-mē)	excision of the labyrinth
3. **mastoidectomy** (*mas*-toy-DEK-to-mē)	excision of the mastoid bone
4. **mastoidotomy** (*mas*-toy-DOT-o-mē)	incision into the mastoid bone
5. **myringoplasty** (mi-RING-gō-*plas*-tē)	surgical repair of the tympanic membrane
6. **myringotomy** (*mir*-ing-GOT-o-mē)	incision into the tympanic membrane (performed to relieve pressure in the middle ear by releasing pus or fluid and for the placement of tubes)
7. **otoplasty** (Ō-tō-*plas*-tē)	surgical repair of the (outer) ear
8. **stapedectomy** (*stā*-pe-DEK-to-mē)	excision of the stapes (performed to restore hearing in cases of otosclerosis; the stapes is replaced by a prosthesis) (Fig. 13.4)
9. **tympanoplasty** (TIM-pa-nō-*plas*-tē)	surgical repair (of the hearing mechanism) of the middle ear (including the tympanic membrane and the ossicles)
10. **tympanostomy** (*tim*-pa-NOS-to-mē)	creation of an artificial opening into the middle ear

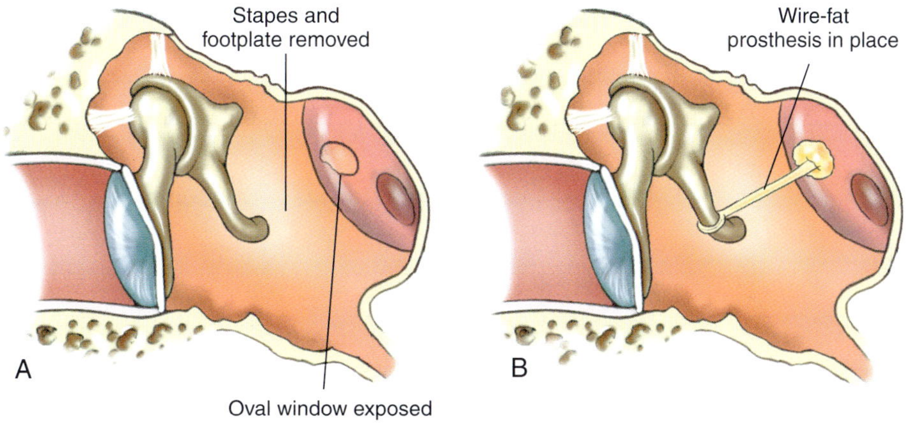

FIG. 13.4 Stapedectomy. **A,** Stapes is removed. **B,** Prosthesis is in place.

EXERCISE 11 ■ Pronounce and Spell

Practice pronunciation and spelling on paper and online.

1. Practice on Paper

a. **Pronounce:** Read the phonetic spelling and say aloud the terms listed in the previous table. Refer to the pronunciation key on p. 20 as necessary.
b. **Spell:** Have a study partner read the terms aloud. Write the spelling of the terms on a separate sheet of paper.

2. Practice Online

a. **Access** online learning resources. Go to evolve.elsevier.com > Evolve Resources > Student Resources.
b. **Pronounce:** Select Audio Glossary > Chapter 13 > Exercise 11. Select a term to hear its pronunciation and repeat aloud.
c. **Spell:** Select Activities > Chapter 13 > Spell Terms > Exercise 11. Select the audio icon and type the correct spelling of the term.

❑ Check the box when complete.

EXERCISE 12 ■ Analyze and Define

Analyze and define the following surgical terms.

1. mastoidectomy
____
____

2. myringotomy
____
____

3. labyrinthectomy
____
____

4. mastoidotomy
____
____

5. tympanoplasty
____
____

6. myringoplasty
____
____

7. stapedectomy
____
____

8. cochlear (implant)
____
____

9. otoplasty
____
____

10. tympanostomy
____
____

EXERCISE 13 ■ Build

A Fill In

Build surgical terms for the following definitions by using the word parts you have learned.

1. incision into the mastoid bone ________ / __ / ________
WR / CV / S

2. excision of the labyrinth ________ / ________
WR / S

3. surgical repair (of the hearing mechanism) of the middle ear ________ WR / CV / S

4. excision of the mastoid bone ________ WR / S

5. surgical repair of the (outer) ear ________ WR / CV / S

6. surgical repair of the tympanic membrane ________ WR / CV / S

B Label

Build terms pictured by writing word parts above definitions.

1.

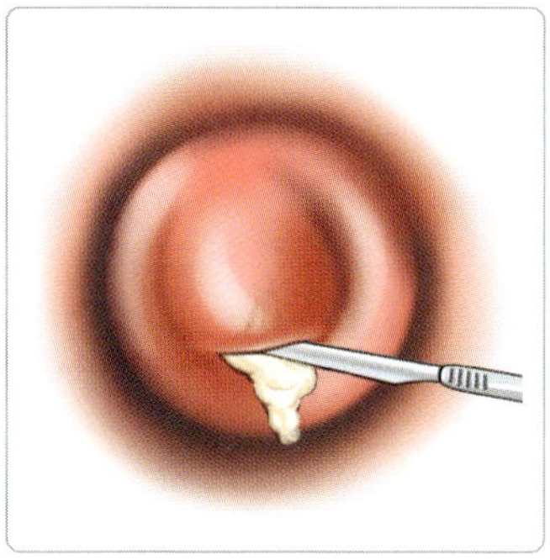

______ / ____ / ______
tympanic membrane / CV / incision

2.

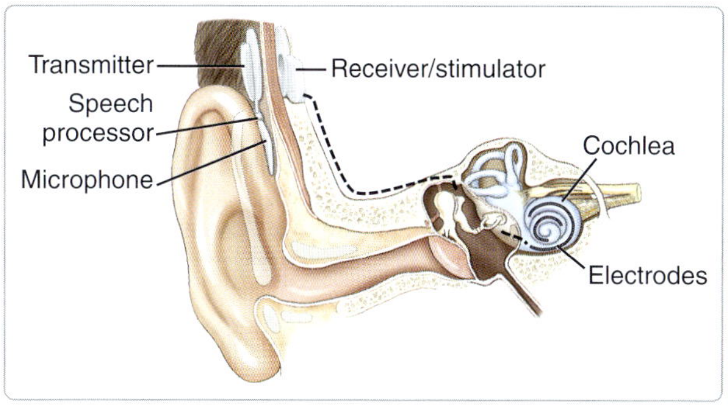

______ / ______ implant
cochlea / pertaining to

3.

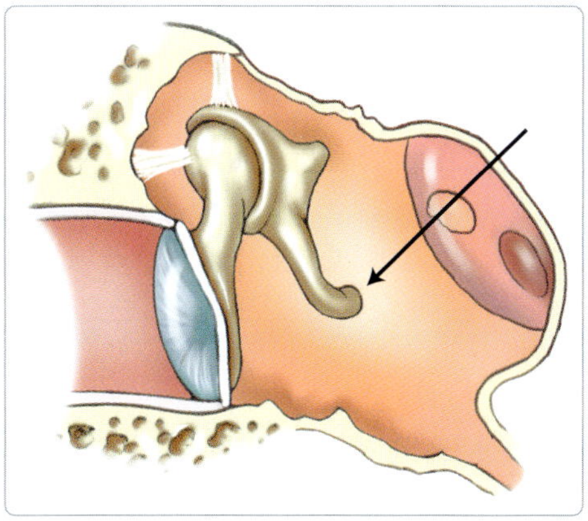

______ / ______
stapes / excision

4.

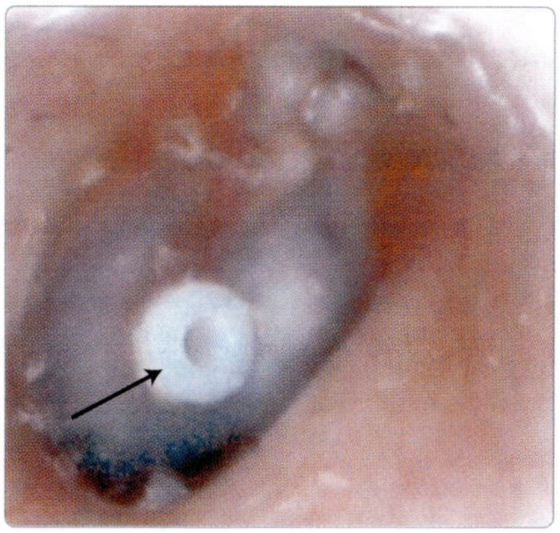

______ / ____ / ______
middle ear / CV / creation of an artificial opening

EXERCISE 14 ■ Review of Surgical Terms

Can you define, pronounce, and spell the following terms?

cochlear implant	mastoidotomy	otoplasty	tympanoplasty
labyrinthectomy	myringoplasty	stapedectomy	tympanostomy
mastoidectomy	myringotomy		

Diagnostic Terms

BUILT FROM WORD PARTS

The following terms can be translated using definitions of word parts. Further explanation is provided within parentheses as needed.

TERM	DEFINITION	TERM	DEFINITION
1. audiogram (AW-dē-ō-*gram*)	(graphic) record of hearing	**5. otoscope** (Ō-tō-skōp)	instrument used for visual examination of the ear
2. audiometer (*aw*-dē-OM-e-ter)	instrument used to measure hearing	**6. otoscopy** (ō-TOS-ko-pē)	visual examination of the ear
3. audiometry (*aw*-dē-OM-e-trē)	measurement of hearing	**7. tympanometer** (*tim*-pa-NOM-e-ter)	instrument used to measure middle ear (function)
4. electrocochleography (ē-*lek*-trō-*kok*-lē-OG-ra-fē)	process of recording the electrical activity in the cochlea (in response to sound)	**8. tympanometry** (*tim*-pa-NOM-e-trē)	measurement of middle ear (function)

EXERCISE 15 ■ Pronounce and Spell

Practice pronunciation and spelling on paper and online.

1. Practice on Paper

a. **Pronounce:** Read the phonetic spelling and say aloud the terms listed in the previous table. Refer to the pronunciation key on p. 20 as necessary.
b. **Spell:** Have a study partner read the terms aloud. Write the spelling of the terms on a separate sheet of paper.

2. Practice Online

a. **Access** online learning resources. Go to evolve.elsevier.com > Evolve Resources > Student Resources.
b. **Pronounce:** Select Audio Glossary > Chapter 13 > Exercise 15. Select a term to hear its pronunciation and repeat aloud.
c. **Spell:** Select Activities > Chapter 13 > Spell Terms > Exercise 15. Select the audio icon and type the correct spelling of the term.

❑ Check the box when complete.

EXERCISE 16 ■ Analyze and Define

Analyze and define the following diagnostic terms.

1. otoscope

____

____

2. audiometry

____

____

3. audiogram

____

____

4. otoscopy

____

____

5. audiometer

____

____

6. tympanometry

____

____

7. tympanometer

____

____

8. electrocochleography

____

____

EXERCISE 17 ■ Build

A Label

Build terms pictured by writing word parts above definitions.

1.

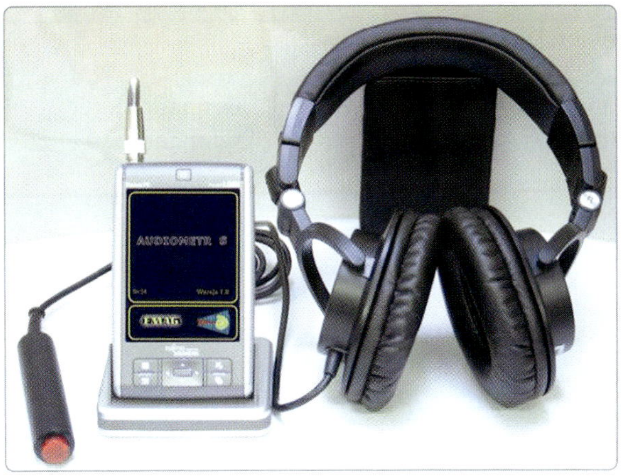

__________ / ____ / __________
hearing / CV / instrument used to measure

2.

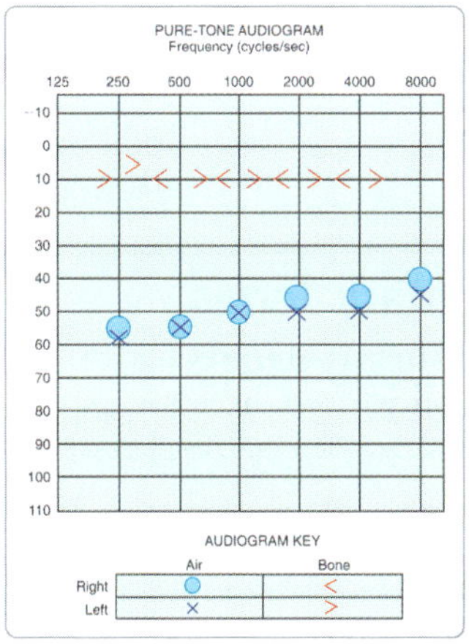

__________ / ____ / __________
hearing / CV / (graphic) record

3.

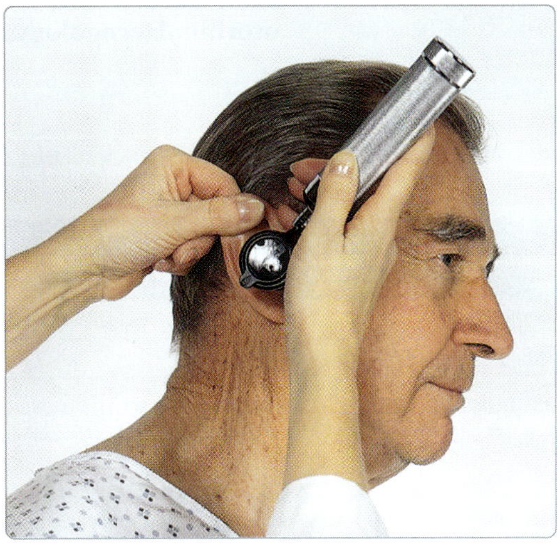

__________ / ____ / __________
ear / CV / visual examination

4.

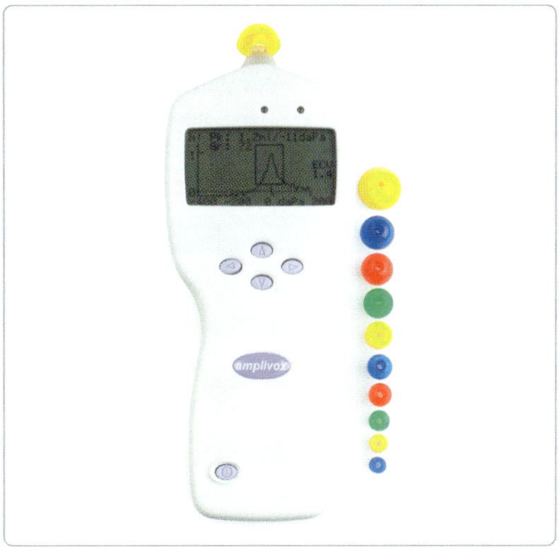

__________ / ____ / __________
middle ear / CV / instrument used to measure

B Fill In

Build diagnostic terms for the following definitions by using the word parts you have learned.

1. measurement of middle ear (function) _______ WR / CV / _______ S
2. instrument used for visual examination of the ear _______ WR / CV / _______ S
3. measurement of hearing _______ WR / CV / _______ S
4. process of recording the electrical activity in the cochlea _______ WR / CV / _______ WR / CV / _______ S

EXERCISE 18 ■ Review of Diagnostic Terms

Can you define, pronounce, and spell the following terms?

audiogram	audiometry	otoscope	tympanometer
audiometer	electrocochleography	otoscopy	tympanometry

Complementary Terms

BUILT FROM WORD PARTS

The following terms can be translated using definitions of word parts. Further explanation is provided within parentheses as needed.

MEDICAL SPECIALTIES

TERM	DEFINITION	TERM	DEFINITION
1. audiologist (*aw*-dē-OL-o-jist)	one who studies and specializes in hearing	**4. otolaryngology** (*ō*-tō-*lar*-ing-GOL-o-jē)	study of the ear, (nose), and larynx (throat) (branch of medicine that treats diseases of the ear, nose, and throat); (also called **otorhinolaryngology**)
2. audiology (*aw*-dē-OL-o-jē)	study of hearing		
3. otolaryngologist (ENT) (*ō*-tō-*lar*-ing-GOL-o-jist)	physician who studies and treats diseases of the ear, (nose), and larynx (throat); (also called **otorhinolaryngologist**)		

DESCRIPTIVE TERMS

TERM	DEFINITION	TERM	DEFINITION
5. aural (AW-rul)	pertaining to the ear	**7. vestibular** (ves-TIB-ū-lar)	pertaining to the vestibule
6. cochlear (KOK-lē-ar)	pertaining to the cochlea	**8. vestibulocochlear** (ves-*tib*-ū-lō-KOK-lē-ar)	pertaining to the vestibule and the cochlea

Refer to **Appendix E** for pharmacology terms related to the ear.

EXERCISE 19 ■ Pronounce and Spell

Practice pronunciation and spelling on paper and online.

1. Practice on Paper

a. **Pronounce:** Read the phonetic spelling and say aloud the terms listed in the previous table. Refer to the pronunciation key on p. 20 as necessary.
b. **Spell:** Have a study partner read the terms aloud. Write the spelling of the terms on a separate sheet of paper.

2. Practice Online

a. **Access** online learning resources. Go to evolve.elsevier.com > Evolve Resources > Student Resources.
b. **Pronounce:** Select Audio Glossary > Chapter 13 > Exercise 19. Select a term to hear its pronunciation and repeat aloud.
c. **Spell:** Select Activities > Chapter 13 > Spell Terms > Exercise 19. Select the audio icon and type the correct spelling of the term.

❑ Check the box when complete.

EXERCISE 20 ■ Analyze and Define

Analyze and define the following complementary terms.

1. otolaryngology

____

____

2. audiologist

____

____

3. otolaryngologist

____

____

4. audiology

____

____

5. aural

____

____

6. cochlear

____

____

7. vestibular

____

____

8. vestibulocochlear

____

____

EXERCISE 21 ■ Build

A Label

Build terms pictured by writing word parts above definitions.

1.

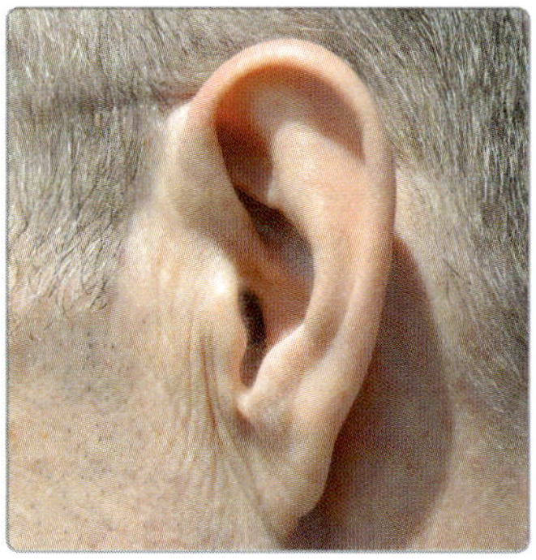

_______ / _______
ear pertaining to

2.

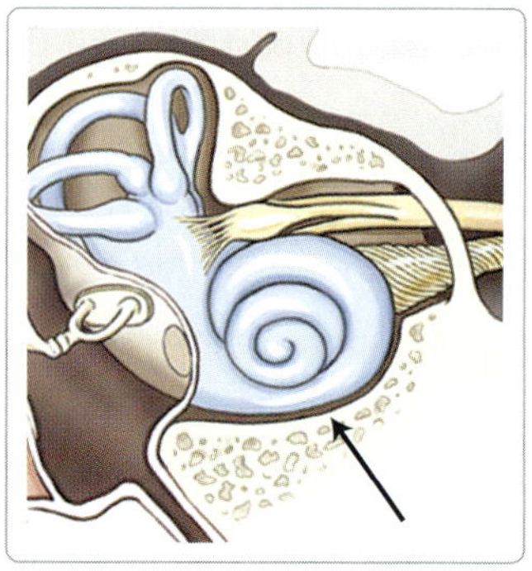

_______ / _______
cochlea pertaining to

3.

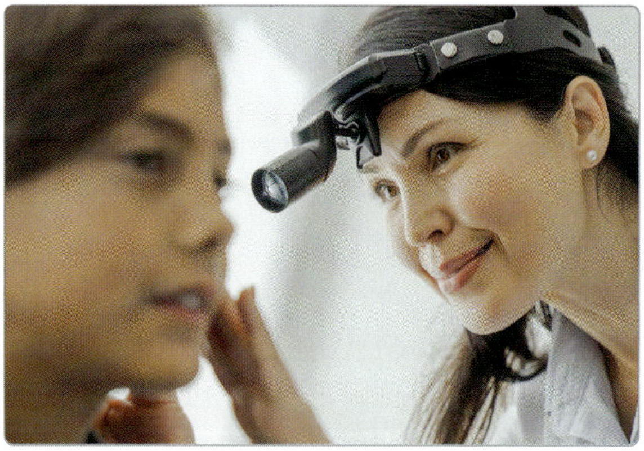

____ / ____ / ____ / ____ / ____
ear CV larynx CV physician who studies and treats

4.

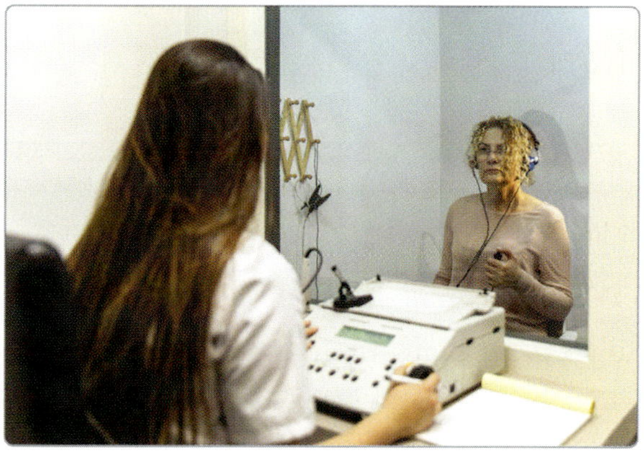

_______ / ____ / _______
hearing CV one who studies and specializes

B Fill In

Build complementary terms for the following definitions by using the word parts you have learned.

1. study of hearing ____ / ____ / ____ (WR / CV / S)

2. study of the ear, (nose), and larynx (throat) ____ / ____ / ____ / ____ / ____ (WR / CV / WR / CV / S)

3. pertaining to the vestibule and the cochlea ____ / ____ / ____ / ____ (WR / CV / WR / S)

4. pertaining to the vestibule ____ / ____ (WR / S)

EXERCISE 22 ■ Review of Complementary Terms

Can you define, pronounce, and spell the following terms?

audiologist	aural	otolaryngologist (ENT)	vestibular
audiology	cochlear	otolaryngology	vestibulocochlear

Abbreviations

DISEASES AND DISORDERS

ABBREVIATION	TERM	ABBREVIATION	TERM
AOM	acute otitis media	**OE**	otitis externa
BPPV	benign paroxysmal positional vertigo	**OM**	otitis media

MEDICAL SPECIALTIES

ABBREVIATION	TERM
ENT	ears, nose, throat; otolaryngologist

DESCRIPTIVE

ABBREVIATION	TERM
HOH	hard of hearing

EXERCISE 23 ■ Abbreviations

Write the terms abbreviated.

1. **OM** ________ ________ may be acute, abbreviated as **AOM** ________ ________ ________, or chronic.
2. **BPPV** ________ ________ ________ ________ symptoms may include dizziness, vertigo, nausea, or vomiting. Symptoms generally come and go, but patients with prolonged or worsening episodes may need referral to an **ENT** ________ ________ ________ doctor or ________________.
3. **OE** ________ ________ is sometimes called "swimmer's ear" because repeated exposure to water can make the ear canal more prone to inflammation.
4. **HOH** ________ ________ ________ generally describes a person with mild to moderate hearing loss.

PRACTICAL APPLICATION

EXERCISE 24 ■ Case Study: Translate Between Everyday Language and Medical Language

CASE STUDY: Marisol Montoya

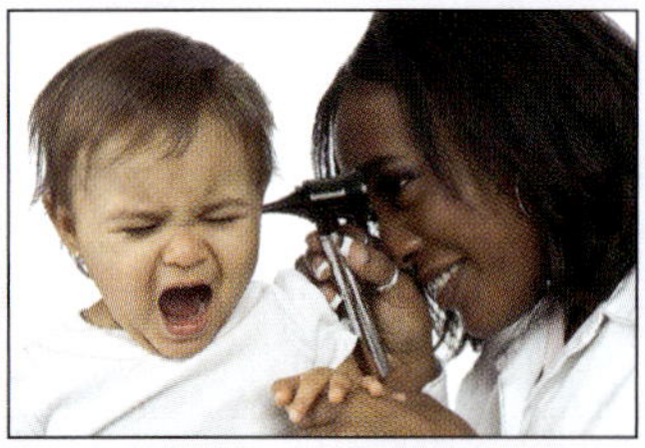

Marisol Montoya is only 13 months old, and she has already had five episodes of middle ear infections (inflammation). For the last few days she has had a fever and she keeps pulling on her ear as if it is painful. Today her mother noticed a pus-like liquid coming out of her left ear. Now her mother is seeing redness and swelling on her skull behind Marisol's earlobe. She calls her pediatrician, who arranges an immediate referral to an ear, nose, and throat physician.

Now that you have worked through Chapter 13, consider the medical terms that might be used to describe Marisol's experience. See the Chapter at a Glance section at the end of the chapter for a list of terms that might apply.

A. *Underline phrases in the case study that could be substituted with medical terms.*

B. *Write the medical term and its definition for three of the phrases you underlined.*

MEDICAL TERM	DEFINITION
1. ______________________	______________________________________
2. ______________________	______________________________________
3. ______________________	______________________________________

DOCUMENTATION: Excerpt from Otolaryngology Visit

Marisol was examined by an otolaryngologist; an excerpt from the medical record is documented below.

Marisol Montoya is a 13-month-old female referred by her pediatrician for possible mastoiditis. Her mother reports a history of frequent episodes of otitis media, and she currently has symptoms of fever, otalgia, and otopyorrhea. Today her mother noted inflammation in the left mastoid region. Physical exam reveals an unhappy child with a temperature of 101.7°F. Otoscopy is difficult due to pain but shows both otitis externa in the left ear and otitis media bilaterally. Tympanometry shows evidence of poor mobility and suggests a collection of fluid and pressure in the middle ear. Examination of the left mastoid region reveals erythema, edema, and severe tenderness. My impression is that this child has acute mastoiditis. We will perform bilateral myringotomies and send the fluid for cultures. In the meantime, we will start antibiotics and obtain a CT scan of the affected area. If she worsens or does not improve, mastoidectomy will be considered.

C. *Underline medical terms presented in Chapter 13 used in the previous excerpt from Marisol's medical record. See the Chapter at a Glance section at the end of the chapter for a complete list.*

D. *Select and define three of the medical terms you underlined. To check your answers, go to Appendix A.*

MEDICAL TERM	DEFINITION
1. ______________________	______________________________________
2. ______________________	______________________________________
3. ______________________	______________________________________

EXERCISE 25 ■ Interact with Medical Documents

A

Read the report and complete it by writing medical terms on answer lines within the document. Definitions of terms to be written appear after the document.

99665-AUD TOHE, Jimmy

File Patient Navigate Custom Fields Help

Chart Review | Encounters | Notes | Labs | Imaging | Procedures | Rx | Documents | Referrals | Scheduling | Billing

Name: TOHE, Jimmy | MR#: 99665-AUD | Gender: M | Allergies: Demerol
DOB: 03/09/19XX | Age: 62 | PCP: Unknown

ENT Clinic Visit
Date: 04 September 20XX 10:00

Subjective: Jimmy Tohe is a 62-year-old male, appearing younger than his stated age. He was brought into the 1. ______________________ clinic by his daughter, who states that he is unable to hear what is being said to him by family members. She states that this problem has existed for at least 30 years but that it appears to be getting markedly worse. The patient states he had several episodes of ear infections as a child and young adult. He denies any 2. ______________________ or 3.______________________.

Objective: Temperature, 99.4. Pulse, 72. Respirations, 20. Blood pressure, 136/76 mm Hg. Weight, 162 pounds. Patient ambulates without difficulty. Alert and oriented x3. 4. ________________ reveals scarring of the tympanic membranes bilaterally. Auditory canals appear normal bilaterally.

Assessment:
1. Mild loss of hearing bilaterally, probably caused by 5.________________________ as a child.
2. Recent exacerbation of hearing loss most likely attributable to 6. _________________.

Plan:
1. Patient referred to 7. ___________________________ for complete 8. __________________________ workup.

Electronically signed: McKeegan, Bridey MD, 09/04/20XX 10:30

Start | Log On/Off | Print | Edit

Definitions of Medical Terms to Complete the Document

Write the medical terms defined on corresponding answer lines in the document.

1. abbreviation for ears, nose, and throat
2. ringing in the ears
3. sense of one's own body or the environment revolving
4. visual examination of the ear
5. inflammation of the middle ear
6. hearing impairment occurring with age
7. one who studies and specializes in hearing
8. measurement of hearing

EXERCISE 25 ■ Interact with Medical Documents—cont'd

B

Read the medical report and answer the questions below it.

028464 MARIEB, PAULINA

File Patient Navigate Custom Fields Help

Patient Chart | Lab | Rad | Notes | Documents | Rx | Scheduling | Images | Billing

Name: **MARIEB, PAULINA** MR#: **028464** DOB: **3/24/19XX** Gender: **Female** Age: **65** Allergies: **None known** PCP: **Tamika Jefferson, MD**

CLINICAL NOTES REPORT

ENCOUNTER DATE: 1/7/20XX
PURPOSE OF VISIT: Referred by Dr. Tamika Jefferson for itching ears.

HISTORY: The patient is a 65-year-old female who has had about 6 months difficulty with itching in her outer ears. She was seen by an internist who has given her Cortaid cream to use in this area. She denies otorrhea or otalgia or aural fullness, congestion, vertigo, or hearing changes. She denies any ear surgeries or previous ear infections.

PHYSICAL EXAMINATION: Under the operating microscope, the left ear was examined. The external ear shows no edema, no involvement of cartilage. No chondritis noted, but along the conchal bowl there is some dry scaling of the skin. There was some cerumen which was removed with suction. Inspection of the right ear revealed more of the same. There are no fissures forming. There was no postauricular dermatitis noted on either ear. There was no lymphadenopathy or adenopathy.

IMPRESSION: Chronic otitis externa.

PLAN: Continue with the cream twice a day until itching symptoms resolve and then to use the cream once a day. The patient has been educated as to the importance of keeping her ears dry. We would be happy to see her back as needed if her symptoms worsen or persist.

Electronically signed by: David Lee, MD 1/7/20XX 16:24

Start | Log On/Off | Print | Edit

Use the medical report above to answer the questions.

1. The patient has been experiencing:
   a. pruritus
   b. hearing loss
   c. otalgia
   d. vertigo
2. In the patient's left ear, suction removed:
   a. scaling
   b. cerumen
   c. chondritis
   d. otorrhea
3. The patient's condition has been diagnosed as chronic:
   a. abnormal condition of fungus in the ear
   b. inflammation of the tympanic membrane
   c. hardening of the stapes
   d. inflammation of the outer ear

EXERCISE 26 ■ Use Medical Language in Online Electronic Health Records

Select the correct medical terms to complete three medical records in one patient's electronic file.

Access online resources at evolve.elsevier.com > Evolve Resources > Student Resources > Activities > Chapter 13 > Electronic Health Records

Topic: Acoustic Neuroma
Record 1: Audiology Assessment
Record 2: Urgent Care Clinic Note
Record 3: Office Visit

❏ Check the box when complete.

EXERCISE 27 ■ Pronounce Medical Terms in Use

Practice pronunciation of terms by reading aloud the following paragraph. Use the phonetic spellings to assist with pronunciation. The script also contains medical terms not presented in the chapter. If interested, research their meanings in a medical dictionary or a reliable online source.

ACUTE OTITIS MEDIA

Acute **otitis media** (ō-TĪ-tis) (MĒ-dē-a) is one of the most common pediatric infections. Most middle ear infections are caused by bacteria, and some by viruses. Symptoms include **otalgia** (ō-TAL-ja), **otorrhea** (ō-tō-RĒ-a), ear pulling, and irritability. The tympanic membrane will be bulging, red in color, with a thickened appearance and reduced translucency. Antibiotics may be ordered if the infection does not resolve on its own. If unresponsive to antibiotic treatment, a **myringotomy** (*mir*-ing-GOT-o-mē) may be performed to identify the causative pathogen, allowing for the appropriate antibiotic treatment to be prescribed.

CHAPTER REVIEW

EXERCISE 28 ■ Chapter Content Quiz

Test your understanding of terms and abbreviations introduced in this chapter. Circle the letter for the medical term or abbreviation related to the words in italics.

1. The vestibular nerve and the auditory nerve are branches of the *pertaining to the vestibule and the cochlea* nerve.
   a. aural
   b. cochlear
   c. vestibulocochlear
2. The abbreviation *ENT*, meaning "ears, nose, and throat," can also refer to the following:
   a. otolaryngologist
   b. audiologist
   c. otoscopy
3. A person who studies and specializes in hearing is a(n):
   a. otolaryngology
   b. otolaryngologist
   c. audiologist
4. The patient reported being bothered by *ringing in the ears* for the last three weeks.
   a. tinnitus
   b. vertigo
   c. presbycusis
5. Vertigo, tinnitus, and fluctuating hearing loss in *chronic disease of the inner ear* usually occur in episodes that can last for several days.
   a. mastoiditis
   b. presbycusis
   c. Ménière disease
6. *Process of recording electrical activity in the cochlea in response to sound*, may be used in the diagnosis of Ménière disease.
   a. electrocochleography
   b. tympanometry
   c. audiometry
7. Thought to be caused by a viral infection, labyrinthitis may cause sudden intense *sensation of revolving*, nausea, vomiting, and imbalance.
   a. tinnitus
   b. vertigo
   c. aural fullness
8. A *cystlike mass composed of epithelial cells and cholesterol* may destroy adjacent bones, including the ossicles.
   a. cholesteatoma
   b. otosclerosis
   c. otitis media
9. Manifestations of *benign tumor within the auditory canal growing from the vestibulocochlear nerve* often begin with tinnitus and gradual hearing loss.
   a. otitis externa
   b. mastoiditis
   c. acoustic neuroma
10. Typical presentation of *abnormal condition of fungus in the ear* is with inflammation, pruritus, scaling, and extreme discomfort.
    a. otomycosis
    b. otalgia
    c. otopyorrhea
11. Mild *hardening of the ear* may be treated with a hearing aid.
    a. otalgia
    b. otomycosis
    c. otosclerosis
12. A(n) *instrument used to measure middle ear function* changes the air pressure in the ear causing the eardrum to move back and forth.
    a. tympanometer
    b. audiometer
    c. otoscope
13. *Surgical repair of the middle ear* may include placement of a graft to close perforation of the eardrum and improve hearing.
    a. myringotomy
    b. myringoplasty
    c. tympanoplasty
14. A *surgically implanted electronic device that converts sound into electrical impulses* has internal and external components.
    a. cochlear implant
    b. audiogram
    c. electrocochleography
15. The abbreviation for *inflammation of the outer ear* is
    a. OM
    b. OE
    c. AOM
16. Gentamicin is a powerful antibiotic that may cause *adverse pharmocological reaction causing damage to the vestibulocochlear nerve.*
    a. acoustic neuroma
    b. ototoxicity
    c. cholesteatoma

17. Children with multiple episodes of otitis media may require *creation of an artificial opening in the middle ear* for the placement of tubes.
   a. stapedectomy
   b. myringotomy
   c. tympanostomy

18. *Surgical repair of the (outer) ear* is usually performed for cosmetic reasons and involves changing the shape, position, or size of the ears.
   a. otoplasty
   b. tympanoplasty
   c. myringoplasty

19. *Visual examination of the ear* would be the best method for determining the presence of a foreign body in the ear canal.
   a. audiometry
   b. tympanometry
   c. otoscopy

20. Hearing aids may be prescribed for people who have *hearing impairment occurring with age.*
   a. tinnitus
   b. presbycusis
   c. cochlear implant

CHAPTER AT A GLANCE Word Parts New to This Chapter

COMBINING FORMS

audi/o
aur/i
cochle/o
labyrinth/o
mastoid/o
myring/o
ot/o
staped/o
tympan/o
vestibul/o

CHAPTER AT A GLANCE Ear Terms Built from Word Parts

DISEASE AND DISORDER

labyrinthitis
mastoiditis
myringitis
otalgia
otomycosis
otopyorrhea
otorrhea
otosclerosis

SURGICAL

cochlear implant
labyrinthectomy
mastoidectomy
mastoidotomy
myringoplasty
myringotomy
otoplasty
stapedectomy
tympanoplasty
tympanostomy

DIAGNOSTIC

audiogram
audiometer
audiometry
electrocochleography
otoscope
otoscopy
tympanometer
tympanometry

COMPLEMENTARY

audiologist
audiology
aural
cochlear
otolaryngologist (ENT)
otolaryngology
vestibular
vestibulocochlear

CHAPTER AT A GLANCE Ear Terms NOT Built from Word Parts

DISEASE AND DISORDER

acoustic neuroma
cholesteatoma
Ménière disease
otitis externa (OE)
otitis media (OM)
ototoxicity
presbycusis
tinnitus
vertigo

Chapter 14 Musculoskeletal System

Objectives

Upon completion of this chapter, you will be able to:

1 Pronounce anatomic structures of the musculoskeletal system.

2 Define and spell word parts related to the musculoskeletal system.

3 Define, pronounce, and spell disease and disorder terms related to the musculoskeletal system.

4 Define, pronounce, and spell surgical terms related to the musculoskeletal system.

5 Define, pronounce, and spell diagnostic terms related to the musculoskeletal system.

6 Define, pronounce, and spell complementary terms related to the musculoskeletal system.

7 Interpret the meaning of abbreviations related to the musculoskeletal system.

8 Apply medical language in clinical contexts.

Outline

ANATOMY

The musculoskeletal system consists of muscles, bones, bone marrow, joints, cartilage, tendons, ligaments, and bursae. The adult human skeleton contains 206 bones and more than 600 muscles. Joints form the union between bones and often allow for movement, although some do not. Most of the joints in the skeleton are freely moving and contain cartilage and bursae.

Function

The functions of the muscular system are movement, posture, joint stability, and heat production. The functions of the skeletal system are to provide a framework for the body, protect the soft body parts such as the brain, store calcium, and support and protect bone marrow (where blood cells are produced). The organs and structures of the musculoskeletal system work together to protect, support, and move the body.

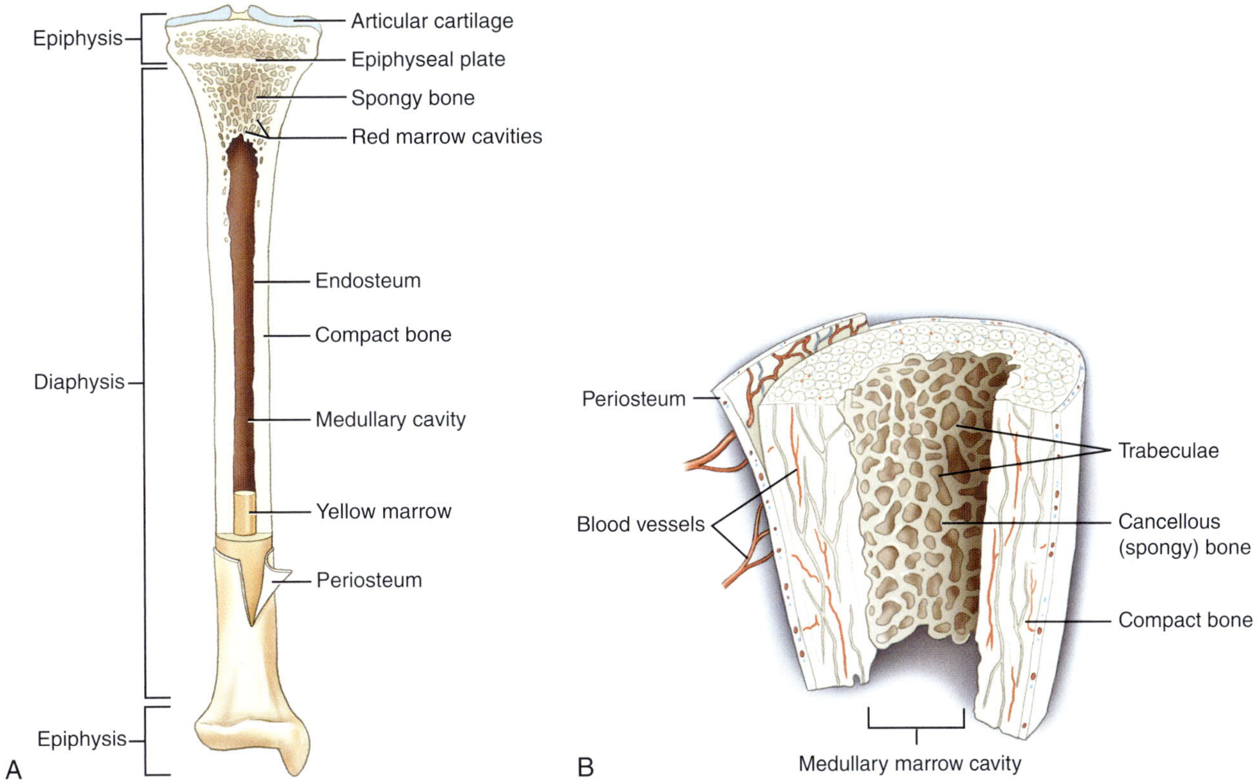

FIG. 14.1 **A,** Bone structure. **B,** Magnified view of bone structure.

Bone Structure

TERM	DEFINITION
bone (bōn)	organ made up of hard connective tissue with a dense outer layer and spongy inner layer
periosteum (*per*-ē-OS-tē-um)	outermost layer of the bone, made up of fibrous tissue
PERIOSTEUM is composed of the prefix **peri-**, meaning **surrounding**, and the word root **oste**, meaning **bone**.	
compact bone (KOM-pakt) (bōn)	dense, hard layers of bone tissue that lie underneath the periosteum
cancellous bone (KAN-sel-us) (bōn)	contains little spaces like a sponge and is encased in the layers of compact bone (also called **spongy bone**)
endosteum (en-DOS-tē-um)	membranous lining of the hollow cavity of the bone
ENDOSTEUM is composed of the prefix **endo-**, meaning **within**, and the word root **oste**, meaning **bone**.	

Bone Structure—cont'd

TERM	DEFINITION
diaphysis (dī-AF-i-sis)	shaft of the long bones (Fig. 14.1)
DIAPHYSIS comes from the Greek **diaphusis**, meaning state of growing between.	
epiphysis (*pl.* epiphyses) (e-PIF-i-sis), (e-PIF-i-sēz)	end of each long bone (Fig. 14.1)
EPIPHYSIS has been used in the English language since the 1600s and retains the meaning given to it by a Greco-Roman physician. It means a **portion of bone attached for a time to another bone** by cartilage, but that later combines with the principal bone. During the period of growth, the epiphysis is separated from the main portion of the bone by cartilage.	
bone marrow (bōn) (MAR-ō)	material found in the cavities of bones
red marrow (red) (MAR-ō)	thick, bloodlike material found in flat bones and the ends of long bones; location of blood cell formation
yellow marrow (YEL-ō) (MAR-ō)	soft, fatty material found in the medullary cavity of long bones

Skeletal Bones

TERM	DEFINITION
maxilla (mak-SIL-a)	upper jawbone
mandible (MAN-di-bul)	lower jawbone

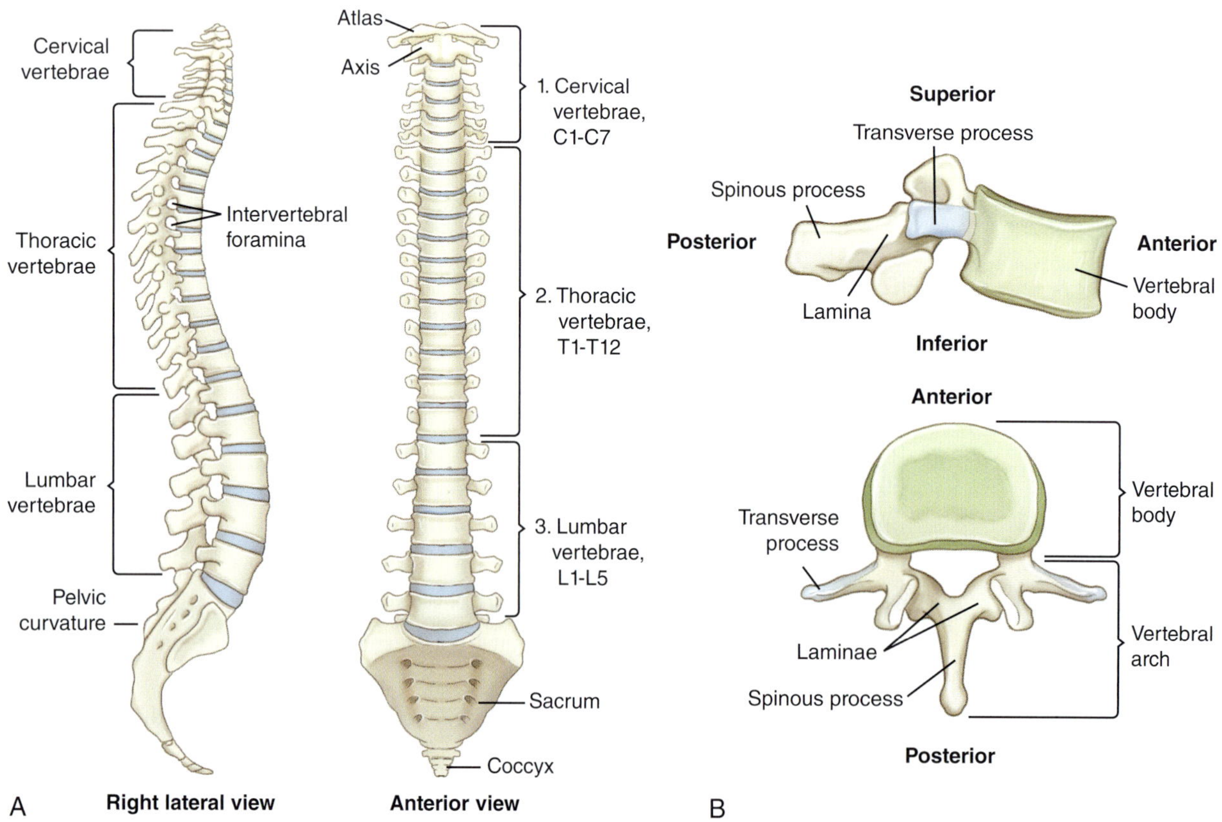

FIG. 14.2 A, Vertebral column, right lateral view and anterior view. **B,** A typical vertebra, lateral view and transverse view.

TERM	DEFINITION
vertebral column (ver-TĒ-brel) (KOL-em)	made up of bones called vertebrae *(pl.)* or vertebra *(s.)* through which the spinal cord runs. The vertebral column protects the spinal cord, supports the head, and provides points of attachment for ribs and muscles. (Fig. 14.2)
cervical vertebrae (C1 to C7) (SUR-vi-kal) (VER-te-bray)	first set of seven vertebrae, forming the neck
thoracic vertebrae (T1 to T12) (tha-RAS-ik) (VER-te-bray)	second set of 12 vertebrae. They articulate with the 12 pairs of ribs to form the outward curve of the spine.
lumbar vertebrae (L1 to L5) (LUM-bar) (VER-te-brāy)	third set of five larger vertebrae, which forms the inward curve of the spine
sacrum (SĀ-krum)	next five vertebrae, which fuse together to form a triangular bone positioned between the two hip bones, forming joints called the sacroiliac joints
coccyx (KOK-siks)	four vertebrae fused together to form the tailbone
laminae (*s.* lamina) (LAM-i-nā) (LAM-i-na)	flat plates of bone that form the vertebral arch, the posterior portion of the spinal canal
clavicle (KLAV-i-kul)	collarbone
scapula (SKAP-ū-la)	shoulder blade
acromion process (a-KRŌ-mē-on) (PRA-ses)	extension of the scapula, which forms the superior point of the shoulder
sternum (STUR-num)	breastbone
xiphoid process (ZĪ-foid) (PRA-ses)	lower portion of the sternum
humerus (HŪ-mer-us)	upper arm bone
ulna and radius (UL-na), (RĀ-dē-us)	lower arm bones
olecranon process (ō-LEK-ra-non) (PRA-ses)	projection at the proximal end of the ulna that forms the bony point of the elbow
carpal bones (KAR-pal) (bōnz)	wrist bones
metacarpal bones (*met*-a-KAR-pal) (bōnz)	hand bones (also called **metacarpus**)

METACARPUS is composed of the prefix **meta-**, meaning **beyond**, and **carpus**, meaning **wrist**.

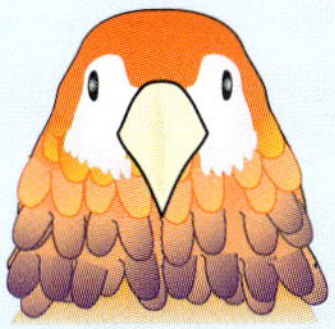

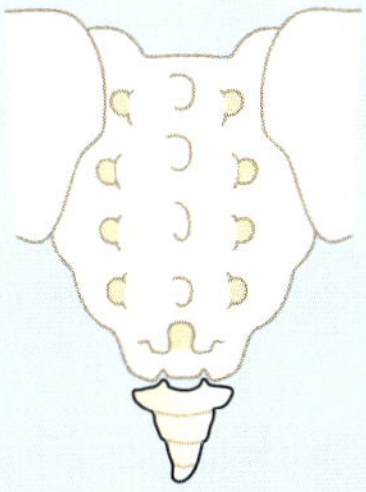

Coccyx is derived from the Greek word *cuckoo* because of its resemblance to a cuckoo's beak.

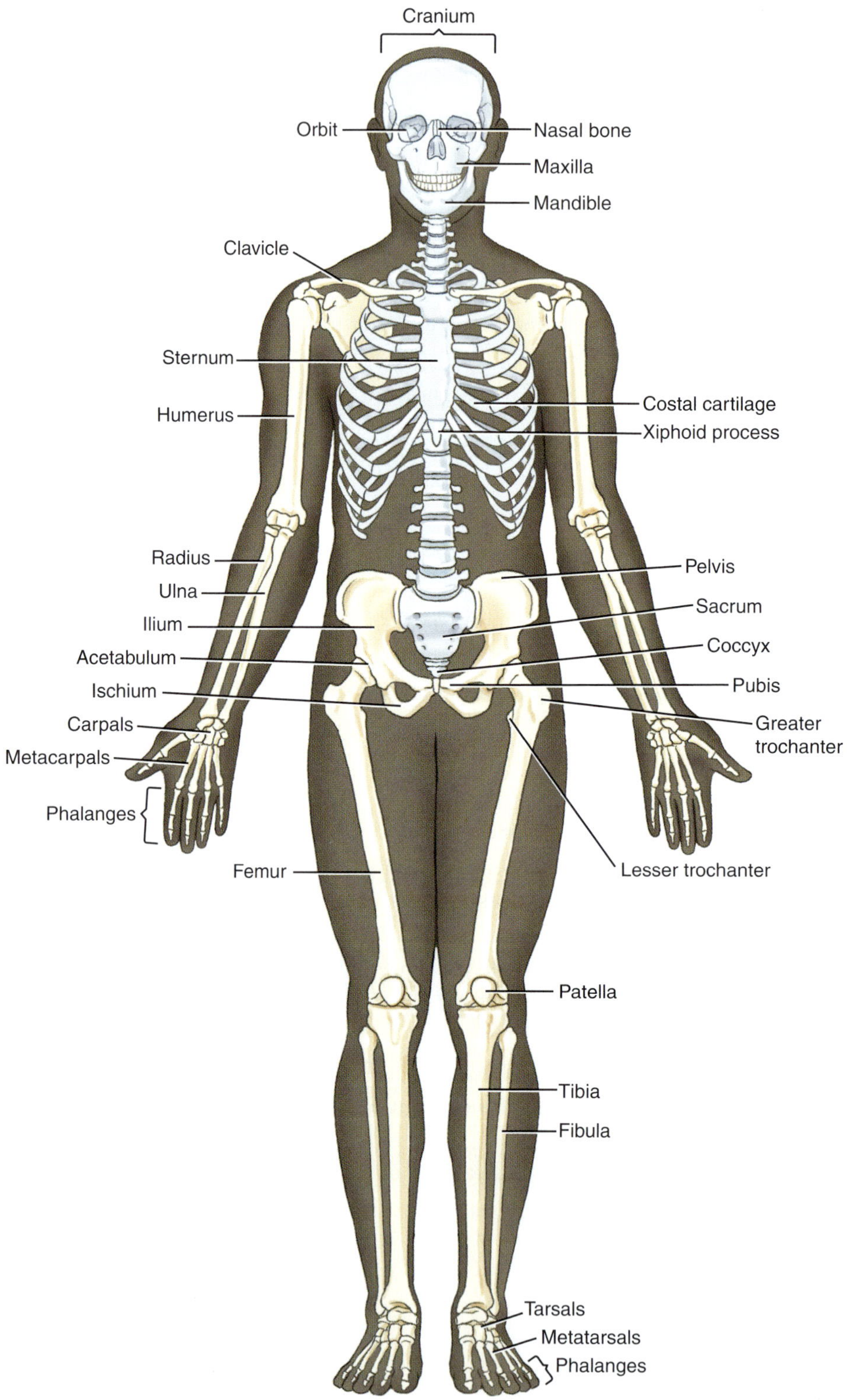

FIG. 14.3 Anterior view of the skeleton.

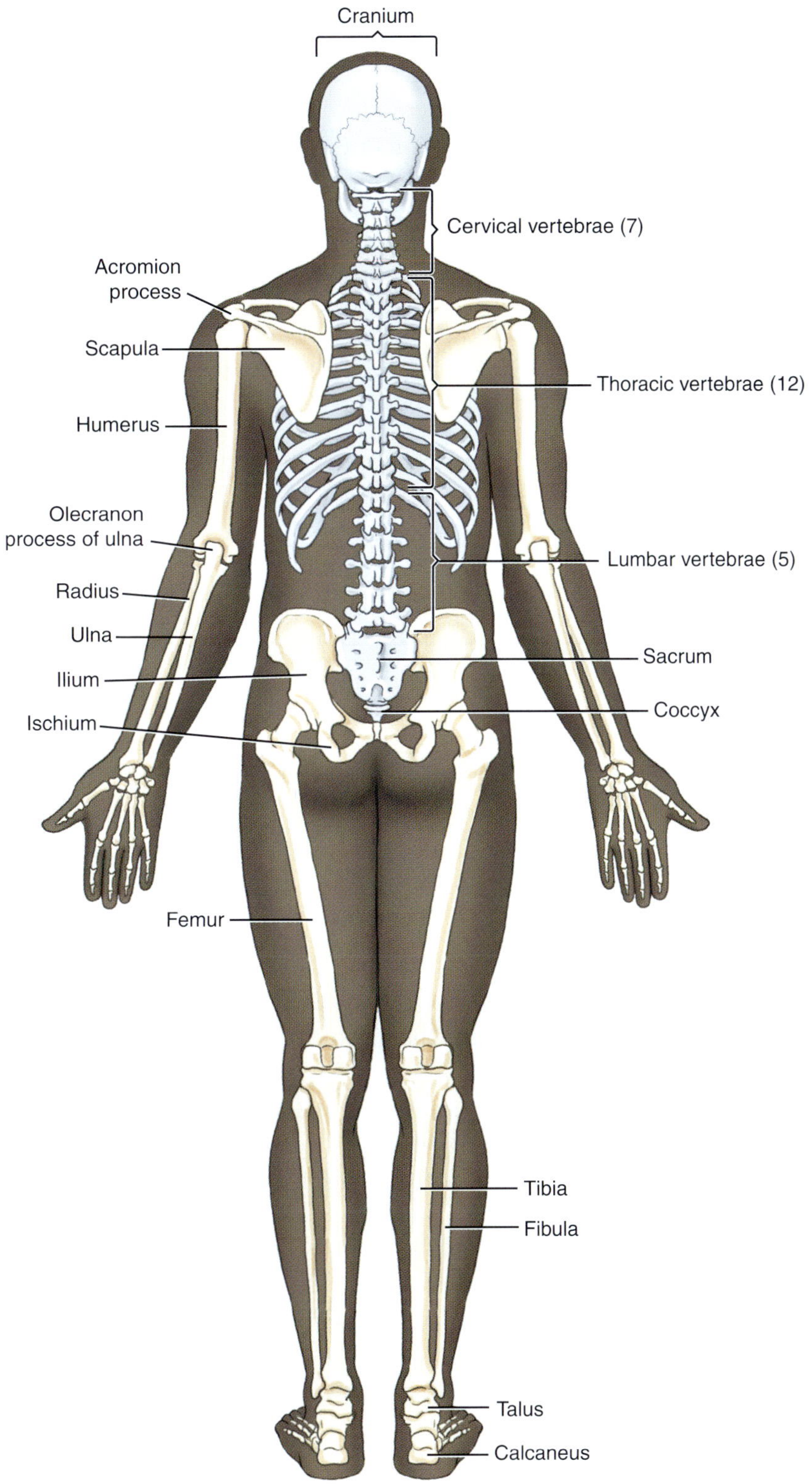

FIG. 14.4 Posterior view of the skeleton.

Skeletal Bones—cont'd

TERM	DEFINITION
phalanx (*pl.* phalanges) (FĀ-lanks) (fa-LAN-jēz)	finger and toe bones
pelvis (PEL-vis)	made up of three bones fused together (also called **pelvic bones** and **hip bones**)
ischium (IS-kē-um)	lower, posterior portion of the pelvis on which one sits
ilium (IL-ē-um)	upper, wing-shaped part on each side of the pelvis
pubis (PŪ-bis)	anterior portion of the pelvis
acetabulum (*as*-a-TAB-ū-lum)	large socket in the pelvis for the head of the femur
femur (FĒ-mer)	upper leg bone
tibia and fibula (TIB-ē-a), (FIB-ū-la)	lower leg bones
patella (*pl.* patellae) (pa-TEL-a) (pa-TEL-ē)	kneecap
tarsal bones (TAR-sal) (bōnz)	ankle bones
calcaneus (kal-KĀ-nē-us)	heel bone
metatarsal bones (*met*-a-TAHR-sal) (bōnz)	foot bones

Joints

TERM	DEFINITION
joint (joint)	junction of two or more bones, which often allows for movement of these bones (also called **articulation**) (Fig. 14.5)
cartilage (KAR-ti-lej)	firm connective tissue primarily found in joints. Articular cartilage covers the contacting surfaces of bones.
meniscus (me-NIS-kus)	crescent-shaped cartilage found in some joints, including the knee
intervertebral disk (*in*-ter-VUR-tē-bral) (disk)	cartilaginous pad found between the vertebrae in the spine
pubic symphysis (PŪ-bik) (SIM-fi-sis)	cartilaginous joint at which two pubic bones come together anteriorly at the midline
synovia (si-NŌ-vē-a)	fluid secreted by the synovial membrane and found in joint cavities, bursae, and around tendons
bursa (*pl.* bursae) (BUR-sa) (BUR-sā)	fluid-filled sac that allows for easy movement of one part of a joint over another

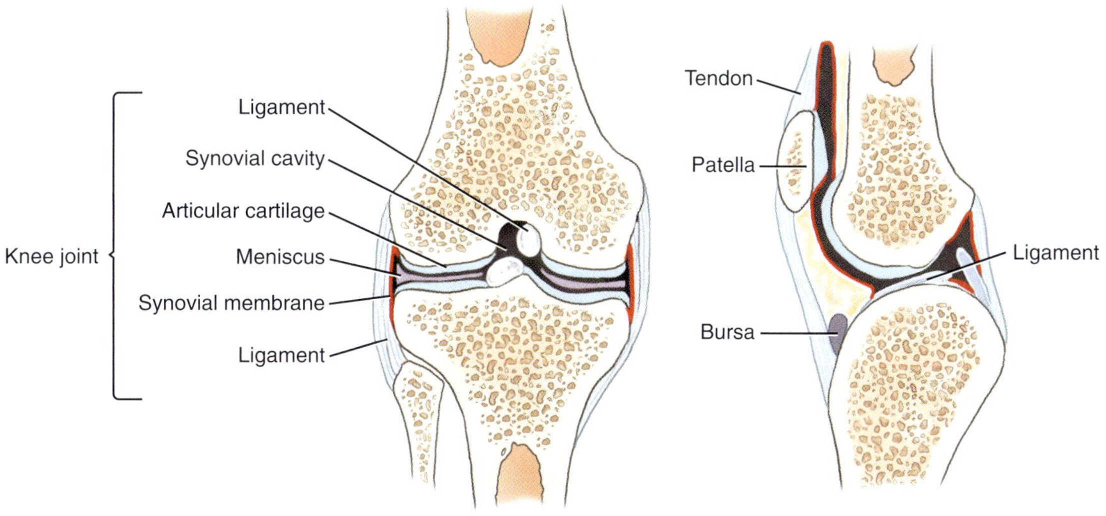

FIG. 14.5 Knee joint.

TERM	DEFINITION
ligament (LIG-a-ment)	flexible, tough band of fibrous connective tissue that attaches one bone to another at a joint
tendon (TEN-don)	band of fibrous connective tissue that attaches muscle to bone
aponeurosis (*ap*-ō-noo-RŌ-sis)	strong sheet of tissue that acts as a tendon to attach muscles to bone

Muscles

TERM	DEFINITION
muscle (MUS-el)	tissue composed of specialized cells with the ability to contract to produce movement; the three types of muscle tissue are skeletal, smooth, and cardiac
fascia (FASH-uh)	band or sheet of connective tissue that encloses muscles and separates their layers
skeletal muscles (SKEL-e-tal) (MUS-els)	attached to bones by tendons and make body movement possible. Skeletal muscles produce action by pulling and by working in pairs. They are also known as voluntary muscles because we have control over these muscles. Alternating dark and light bands create striations (stripes). (also called **striated muscles**) (Figs. 14.6. 14.7, and 14.8A)
smooth muscles (smooth) (MUS-els)	located in internal organs such as the walls of blood vessels and the digestive tract. They are also known as involuntary muscles because they respond to impulses from the autonomic nerves and are not controlled voluntarily. (also called **unstriated muscles**) (Fig. 14.8B)
cardiac muscle (KAR-dē-ak) (MUS-el)	forms most of the wall of the heart. Its involuntary contraction produces the heartbeat. (also called **myocardium**) (Fig. 14.8C)

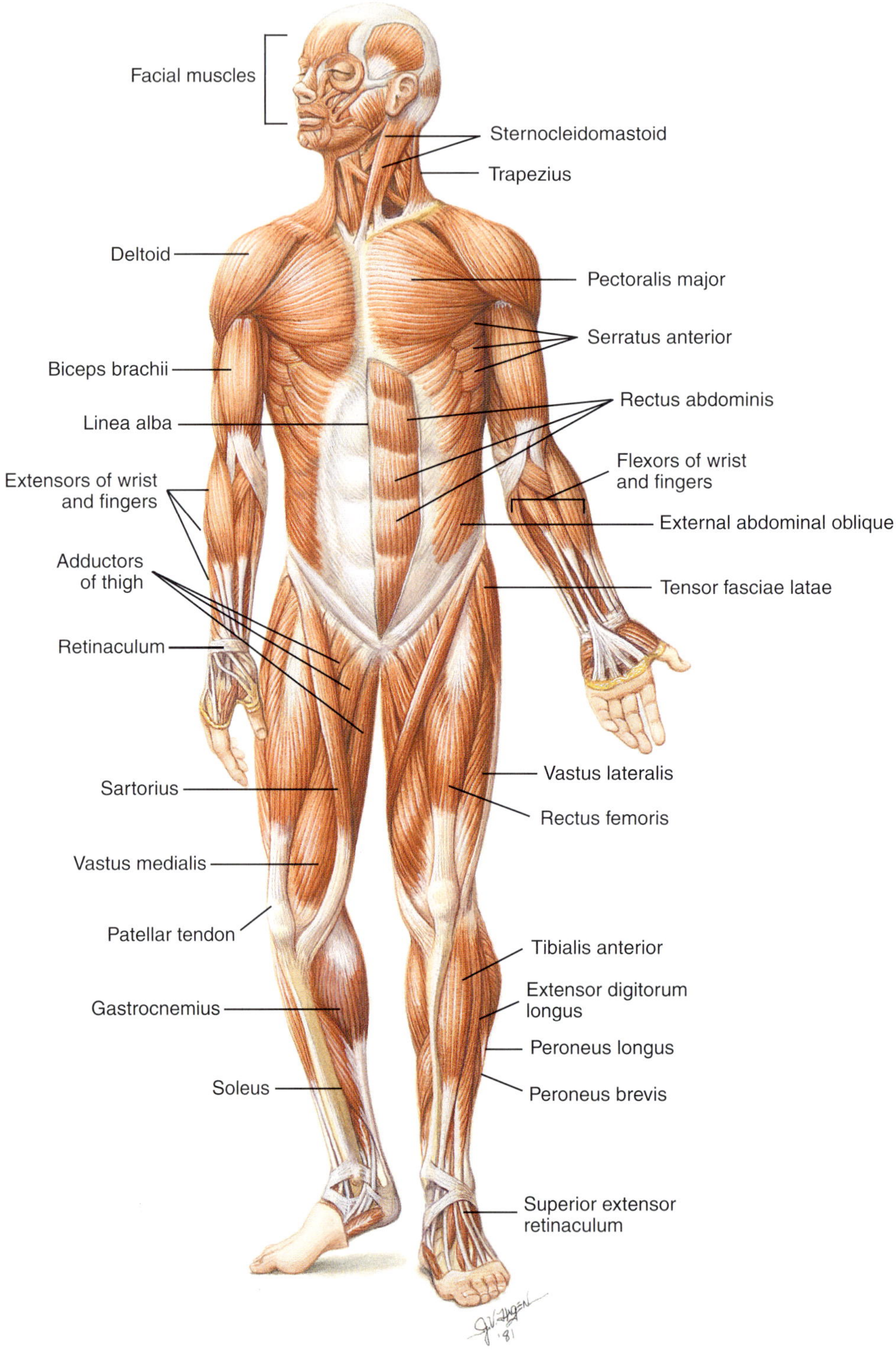

FIG. 14.6 Anterior view of the muscular system.

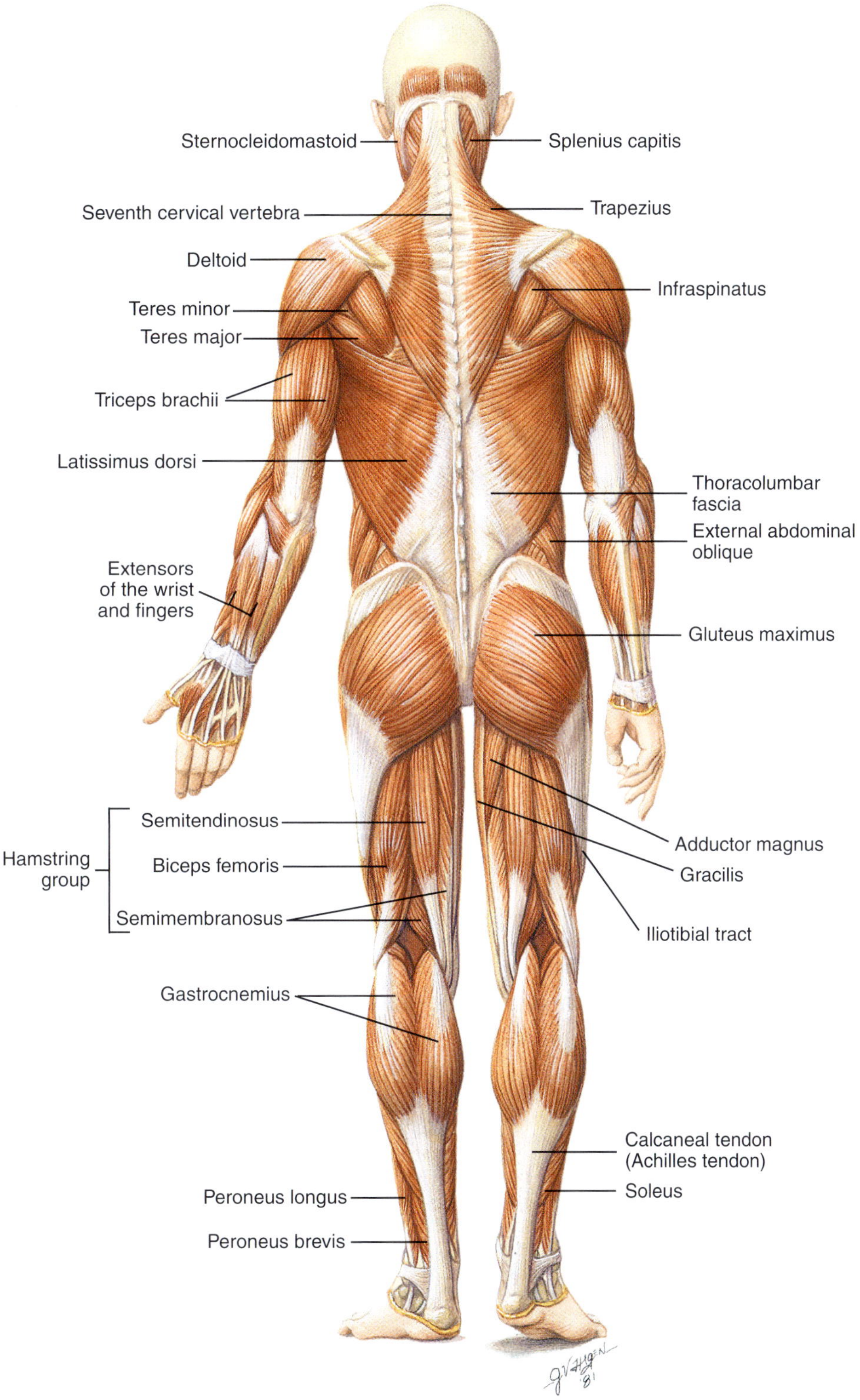

FIG. 14.7 Posterior view of the muscular system.

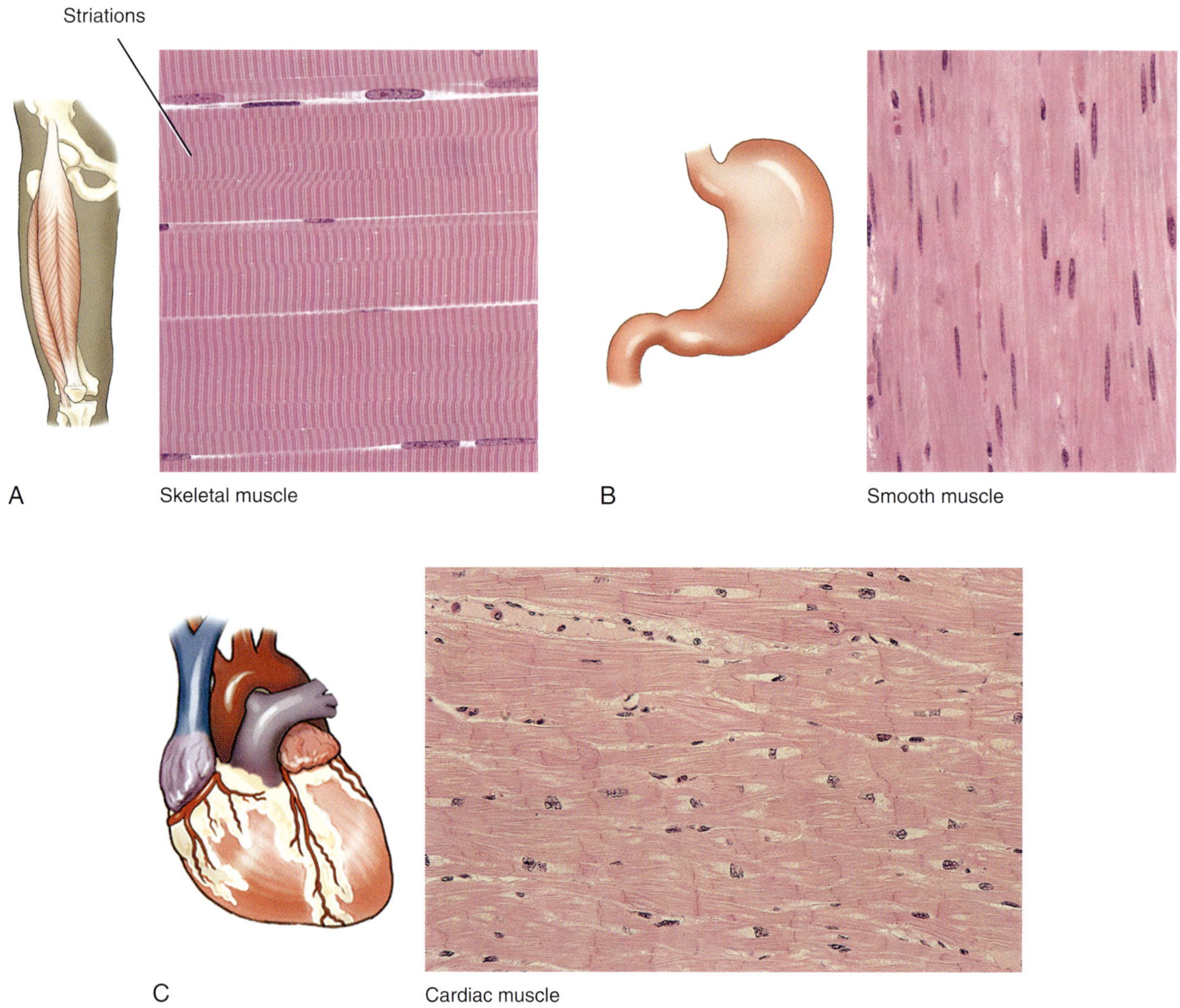

FIG. 14.8 Types of muscle tissue, with their related histology views.

PRONOUNCE ANATOMIC STRUCTURES

Practice saying aloud each of the organs and specific structures on the previous pages.

To hear the terms, go to Evolve Resources at www.evolve.elsevier.com and select:
Student Resources > Chapter 14 > Audio Glossary > Anatomic Structures

❑ Check the box when complete.

WORD PARTS

Use paper flashcards or electronic flashcards on Evolve to memorize word parts used to analyze, define, and build medical terms in this chapter. To reinforce learning, study one section of the Word Parts Table at a time, then complete the corresponding exercise on the following pages.

1 ■ Bone Combining Forms

COMBINING FORM	DEFINITION
carp/o	carpals (wrist)
clavicul/o	clavicle (collarbone)
cost/o	rib
crani/o	cranium (skull)
femor/o	femur (upper leg bone) *(Note: The* u *in femur changes to an* o *in the word root femor/.)*
fibul/o	fibula (lower leg bone)
humer/o	humerus (upper arm bone)
ili/o	ilium (upper winged-shaped portion of the pelvis)
ischi/o	ischium (lower posterior portion of the pelvis)
lumb/o	loin, lumbar region of the spine
mandibul/o	mandible (lower jawbone)
maxill/o	maxilla (upper jawbone)
myel/o	bone marrow
oste/o	bone
patell/o	patella (kneecap)
pelv/i	pelvis, pelvic cavity
phalang/o	phalanx (*pl.* phalanges) (any bone of the fingers or toes)
pub/o	pubis (anterior portion of the pelvis)
rachi/o	vertebra (*pl.* vertebrae), spine, vertebral column
radi/o	radius (lower arm bone)
sacr/o	sacrum (lower portion of the spine forming the posterior pelvic wall)
scapul/o	scapula (shoulder blade)
spondyl/o	vertebra (*pl.* vertebrae), spine, vertebral column
stern/o	sternum (breastbone)
tars/o	tarsals (ankle bones)
tibi/o	tibia (lower leg bone)
uln/o	ulna (lower arm bone)
vertebr/o	vertebra (*pl.* vertebrae), spine, vertebral column

ILIUM VS. ILEUM Compare the combining form for ilium, **ili/o**, the portion of the pelvis, with the combining form for ileum, **ile/o**, the distal portion of the intestine. The pronunciation is the same. Think of **i**lium with an **i** and intestin**e** with an **e** to help distinguish the word roots.

2 ■ Muscle and Joint Combining Forms

COMBINING FORM	DEFINITION
arthr/o	joint
burs/o	bursa (cavity)
chondr/o	cartilage
disc/o	intervertebral disk
fasci/o	fascia (connective tissue enclosing and separating muscle layers)
lamin/o	lamina (thin, flat plate or layer)
menisc/o	meniscus (crescent)
my/o	muscle
myos/o	muscle
synovi/o	synovia, synovial membrane
tendin/o	tendon
ten/o	tendon

3 ■ Combining Forms Used with Musculoskeletal System Terms

COMBINING FORM	DEFINITION
ankyl/o	stiff, bent
electr/o	electricity, electrical activity
hem/o	blood
kinesi/o	movement, motion
kyph/o	hump (increased convexity of the spine)
lord/o	bent forward (increased concavity of the spine)
necr/o	death (cells, body)
rhabd/o	rod-shaped, striated
petr/o	stone *(Note:* lith/o, *also a combining form for* stone, *was introduced in Chapter 6.)*
sarc/o	flesh, connective tissue
scoli/o	(lateral) curved (spine)

SARC When **sarc** appears with **oma** in a term, the suffix **-sarcoma** is used rather than the combining form **sarc/o**.

4 ■ Prefixes

PREFIX	DEFINITION
a-	absence of, without
brady-	slow
dys-	painful, abnormal, difficult, labored
hyper-	above, excessive
inter-	between
intra-	within
micro-	small
poly-	many, much
sub-	under, below
supra-	above
syn-	together, joined

5 ■ Suffixes

SUFFIX	DEFINITION
-a	noun suffix, no meaning
-ac	pertaining to
-al	pertaining to
-algia	pain
-ar	pertaining to
-ary	pertaining to
-asthenia	weakness
-centesis	surgical puncture to aspirate fluid (with a sterile needle)
-desis	surgical fixation, fusion
-eal	pertaining to
-ectomy	excision, surgical removal
-gram	the record, radiographic image
-graphy	process of recording, radiographic imaging
-ia	diseased or abnormal state, condition of
-ic	pertaining to
-is	noun suffix, no meaning
-itis	inflammation
-malacia	softening
-oma	tumor, swelling
-osis	abnormal condition (means increase when used with blood cell word roots)
-penia	abnormal reduction in number
-plasty	surgical repair
-rrhaphy	suturing, repairing
-sarcoma	malignant tumor
-schisis	split, fissure
-scopy	visual examination
-tomy	cut into, incision
-trophy	nourishment, development

Refer to **Appendix B** and **Appendix C** for alphabetical lists of word parts and their meanings.

EXERCISE 1 ■ Bone Combining Forms

Refer to the first section of the word parts table.

A Label

Fill in the blanks with combining forms in this diagram of the skeleton, anterior view. *To check your answers, go to Appendix A.*

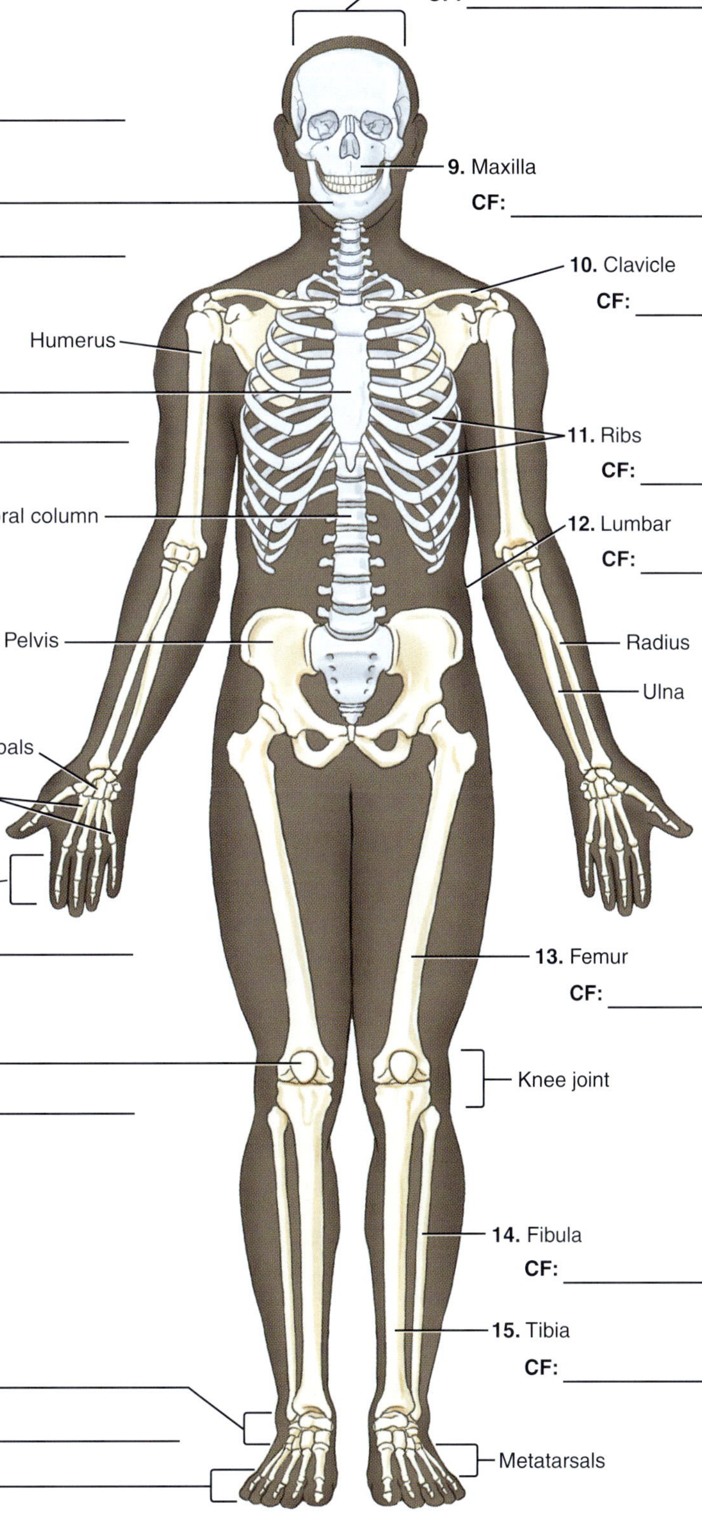

8. Cranium
CF: ____________________

1. Bone
CF: ____________________

9. Maxilla
CF: ____________________

2. Mandible
CF: ____________________

10. Clavicle
CF: ____________________

3. Sternum
CF: ____________________

11. Ribs
CF: ____________________

12. Lumbar
CF: ____________________

4. Phalanges
CF: ____________________

13. Femur
CF: ____________________

5. Patella
CF: ____________________

14. Fibula
CF: ____________________

15. Tibia
CF: ____________________

6. Tarsals
CF: ____________________

7. Phalanges
CF: ____________________

B Label

Fill in the blanks with combining forms in this diagram of the skeleton, posterior view, and the pelvis.

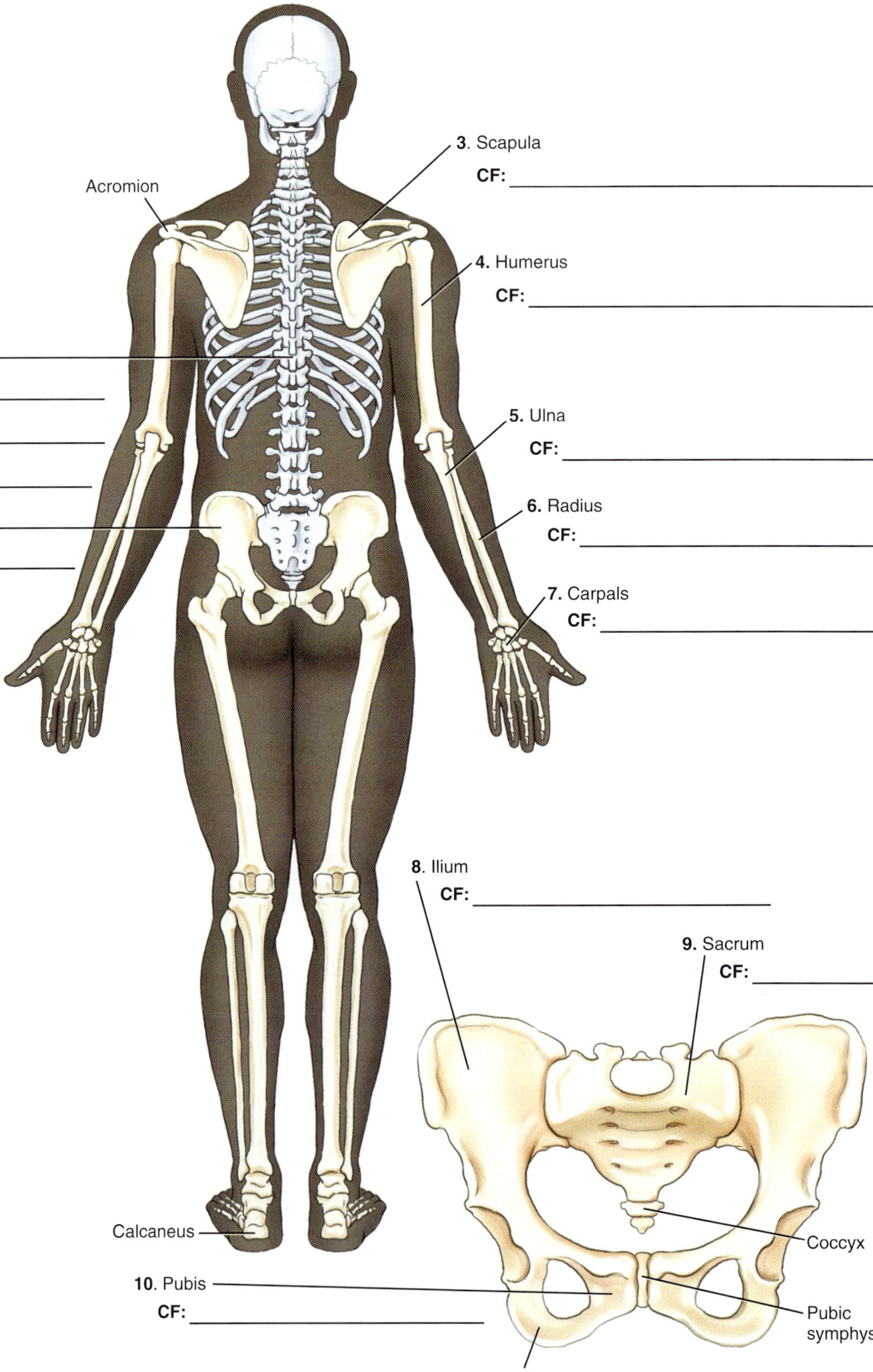

C Define and Match

Step 1: Write the definitions after the following combining forms.
Step 2: Match the descriptions on the right with the combining forms and definitions.

_____ 1. rachi/o, _____________	a. upper jawbone
_____ 2. patell/o, _____________	b. finger and toe bones
_____ 3. maxill/o, _____________	c. wrist bones
_____ 4. phalang/o, _____________	d. kneecap
_____ 5. carp/o, _____________	e. upper arm bone
_____ 6. humer/o, _____________	f. made up of bones called vertebrae through which the spinal cord runs

D Define and Match

Step 1: Write the definitions after the following combining forms.
Step 2: Match the descriptions on the right with the combining forms and definitions.

_____ 1. lumb/o, _____________	a. anterior portion of the pelvis
_____ 2. ischi/o, _____________	b. made up of bones called vertebrae through which the spinal cord runs
_____ 3. pub/o, _____________	c. ankle bones
_____ 4. spondyl/o, _____________	d. third set of five larger vertebrae
_____ 5. scapul/o, _____________	e. lower, posterior portion of the pelvis on which one sits
_____ 6. tars/o, _____________	f. shoulder blade
_____ 7. pelv/i, _____________	g. made up of three bones fused together

E Define and Match

Step 1: Write the definitions after the following combining forms.
Step 2: Match the descriptions on the right with the combining forms and definitions.

_____ 1. mandibul/o, _____________	a. upper leg bone
_____ 2. sacr/o, _____________	b. upper, wing-shaped part on each side of the pelvis
_____ 3. femor/o, _____________	c. lower jawbone
_____ 4. clavicul/o, _____________	d. made up of bones called vertebrae through which the spinal cord runs
_____ 5. ili/o, _____________	e. breastbone
_____ 6. vertebr/o, _____________	f. collarbone
_____ 7. stern/o, _____________	g. five vertebrae, which fuse together to form a triangular bone positioned between the two hip bones

F Identify

Write the combining form for each of the following terms.

1. rib ______
2. radius (lower arm bone) ______
3. tibia (lower leg bone) ______
4. fibula (lower leg bone) ______
5. ulna (lower arm bone) ______
6. cranium (skull) ______
7. bone ______
8. bone marrow ______

EXERCISE 2 ■ Muscle and Joint Combining Forms

Refer to the second section of the word parts table.

A Label

Fill in the blanks with combining forms on these diagrams of the knee joint and vertebra.

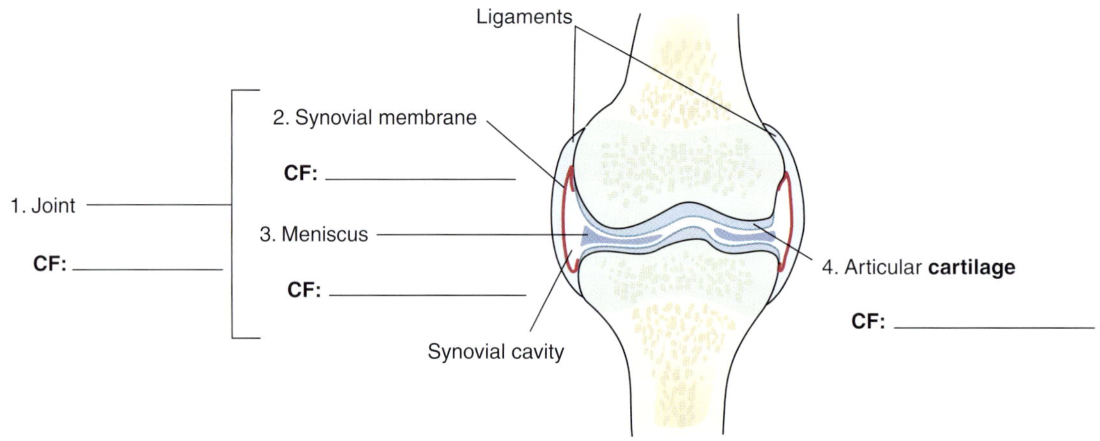

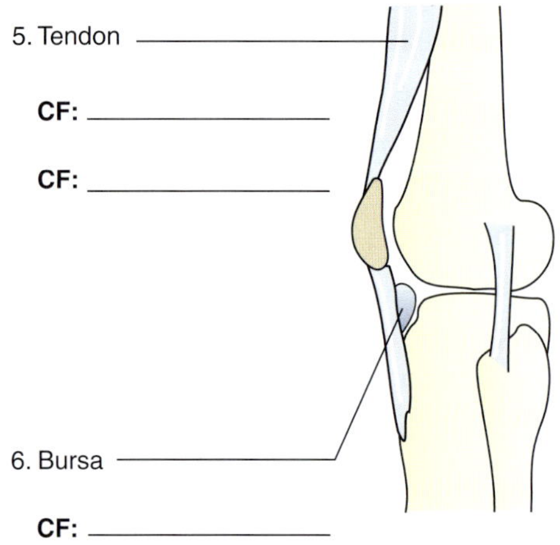

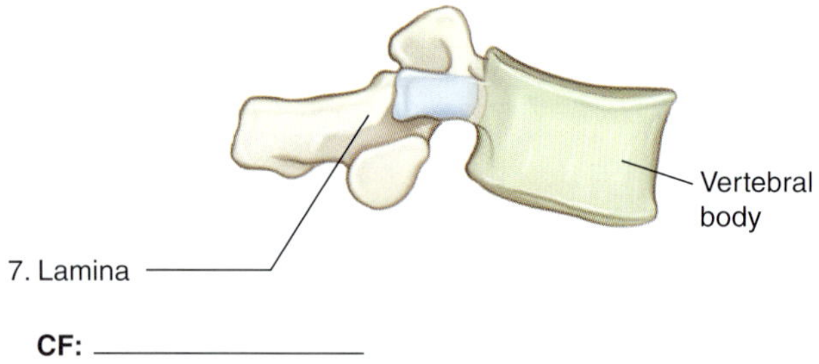

B Define and Match

Step 1: Write the definitions after the following combining forms.
Step 2: Match the descriptions on the right with the combining forms and definitions.

_____ 1. disc/o, ______________________
_____ 2. synovi/o, ______________________
_____ 3. fasci/o, ______________________
_____ 4. ten/o, ______________________
_____ 5. arthr/o, ______________________

a. band of fibrous connective tissue that attaches muscle to bone
b. junction of two or more bones, which often allows for movement of these bones
c. cartilaginous pad found between the vertebrae in the spine
d. fluid secreted by the synovial membrane
e. connective tissue enclosing and separating muscle layers

C Define and Match

Step 1: Write the definitions after the following combining forms.
Step 2: Match the descriptions on the right with the combining forms and definitions. Answers may be used more than once.

_____ 1. myos/o, ______________________
_____ 2. tendin/o, ______________________
_____ 3. burs/o, ______________________
_____ 4. menisc/o, ______________________
_____ 5. chondr/o, ______________________
_____ 6. my/o, ______________________

a. firm connective tissue primarily found in joints
b. band of fibrous connective tissue that attaches muscle to bone
c. fluid-filled sac that allows for easy movement of one part of a joint over another
d. crescent-shaped cartilage found in some joints, including the knee
e. tissue composed of specialized cells with the ability to contract

EXERCISE 3 ■ Combining Forms Used with Musculoskeletal System Terms

Refer to the third section of the word parts table.

A Define

Write the definitions of the following combining forms.

1. rhabd/o ______________________
2. petr/o ______________________
3. kinesi/o ______________________
4. necr/o ______________________
5. hem/o ______________________
6. electr/o ______________________
7. kyph/o ______________________
8. ankyl/o ______________________
9. scoli/o ______________________
10. lord/o ______________________
11. sarc/o ______________________

B Identify

Write the combining form for each of the following.

1. electricity, electrical activity ______________________
2. stone ______________________
3. movement, motion ______________________
4. rod-shaped, striated ______________________

5. blood ______
6. death (cells, body) ______
7. hump (increased convexity of the spine) ______
8. stiff, bent ______
9. (lateral) curved (spine) ______
10. bent forward (increased concavity of the spine) ______
11. flesh, connective tissue ______

EXERCISE 4 ■ Prefixes

Refer to the fourth section of the word parts table.

A Define

Write the definitions of the following prefixes.

1. supra- ______
2. syn- ______
3. inter- ______

B Identify

Write the prefix for each of the following definitions.

1. together, joined ______
2. between ______
3. above ______
4. under, below ______
5. absence of, without ______
6. many, much ______
7. slow ______
8. small ______
9. above, excessive ______
10. within ______
11. painful, abnormal, difficult, labored______

EXERCISE 5 ■ Suffixes

Refer to the fifth section of the word parts table.

A Define

Write the definitions of the following suffixes.

1. -desis ______
2. -schisis ______
3. -asthenia ______
4. -trophy ______
5. -ac, -al, -ar, -ary, -eal, -ic, ______

B Identify

Write the suffix for each of the following definitions.

1. weakness ______
2. surgical fixation, fusion ______
3. split, fissure ______
4. nourishment, development ______
5. noun suffix, no meaning ______

C Match

Match the suffixes in the first column with their correct definitions in the second column.

______ 1. -algia	a. diseased or abnormal state, condition of
______ 2. -penia	b. tumor, swelling
______ 3. -oma	c. softening
______ 4. -malacia	d. abnormal condition
______ 5. -osis	e. malignant tumor
______ 6. -itis	f. pain
______ 7. -sarcoma	g. inflammation
______ 8. -ia	h. abnormal reduction in number

D Match

Match the suffixes in the first column with their correct definitions in the second column.

______ 1. -centesis	a. surgical fixation, fusion
______ 2. -ectomy	b. cut into, incision
______ 3. -plasty	c. excision, surgical removal
______ 4. -rrhaphy	d. surgical puncture to aspirate fluid (with a sterile needle)
______ 5. -tomy	e. surgical repair
______ 6. -desis	f. suturing, repairing
______ 7. -scopy	g. process of recording, radiographic imaging
______ 8. -graphy	h. visual examination
______ 9. -gram	i. the record, radiographic image

MEDICAL TERMS

Medical terms relevant to this chapter have been grouped by topics, such as Disease and Disorder, and are listed in tables designated as Built from Word Parts or *NOT* Built from Word Parts. The exercises following each table assist with learning term definitions, pronunciations, and spellings.

Disease and Disorder Terms

BUILT FROM WORD PARTS

The following terms can be translated using definitions of word parts. Further explanation is provided within parentheses as needed.

TERM	DEFINITION
1. ankylosis (*ang*-ki-LŌ-sis)	abnormal condition of stiffness (often referring to fusion of a joint, such as the result of chronic rheumatoid arthritis)
2. arthritis (ar-THRĪ-tis)	inflammation of a joint (The most common forms of arthritis are osteoarthritis and rheumatoid arthritis.) (Fig. 14.9)
3. bursitis (ber-SĪ-tis)	inflammation of a bursa
4. chondromalacia (*kon*-drō-ma-LĀ-sha)	softening of cartilage
5. chondrosarcoma (*kon*-dro-sar-KŌ-ma)	malignant tumor of cartilage
6. cranioschisis (*krā*-nē-OS-ki-sis)	fissure (split) of the cranium (congenital)
7. discitis (dis-KĪ-tis)	inflammation of an intervertebral disk

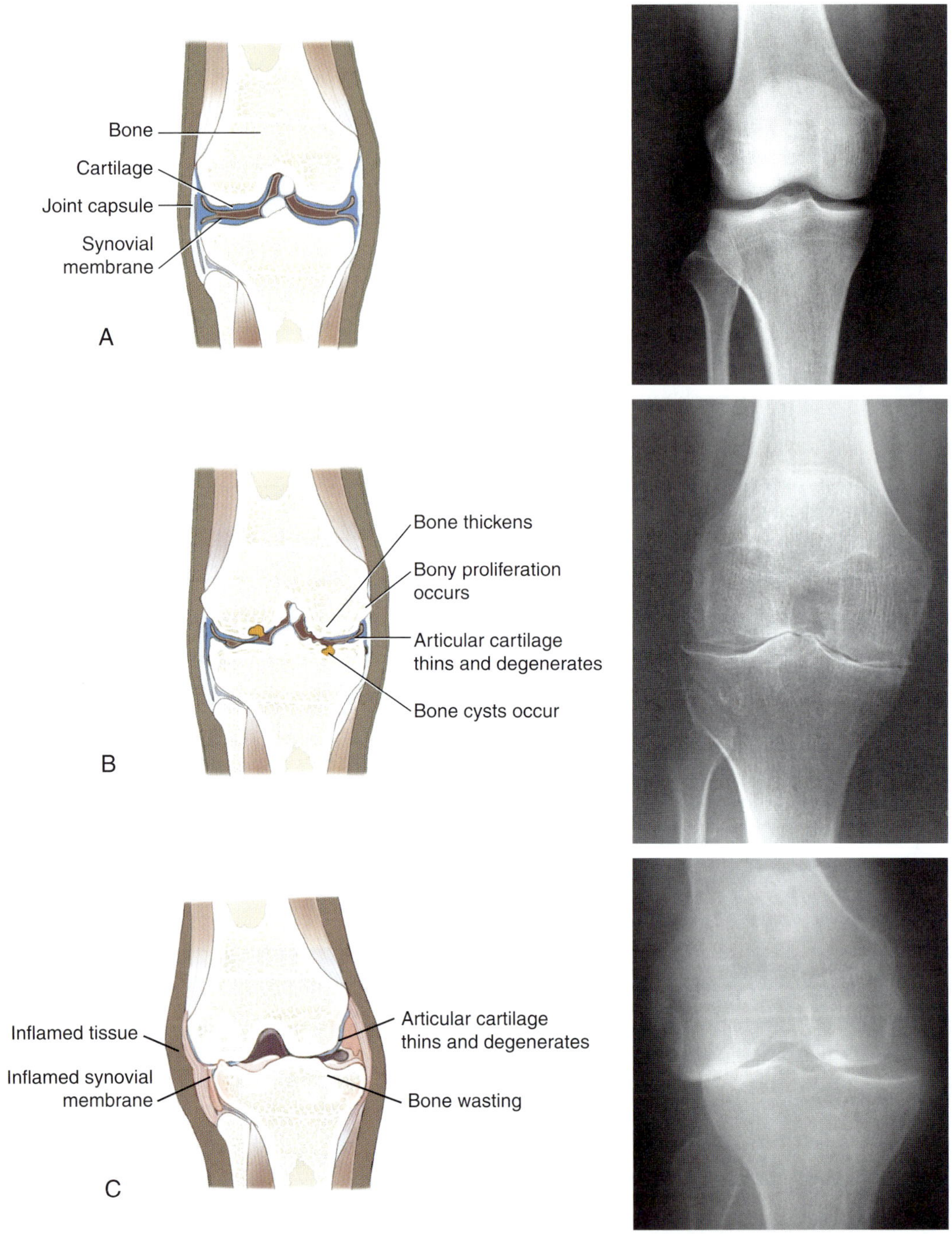

FIG. 14.9 Normal and arthritic knee joints. **A,** Normal knee joint, illustration and radiograph. **B,** Osteoarthritis of the knee joint, illustration and radiograph. **C,** Rheumatoid arthritis of the knee joint, illustration and radiograph.

Disease and Disorder Terms—cont'd

BUILT FROM WORD PARTS

TERM	DEFINITION	TERM	DEFINITION
8. **fasciitis** (*fa*-shē-Ī-tis)	inflammation of the fascia (connective tissue enclosing and separating muscle layers)	9. **fibromyalgia** (*fī*-brō-mī-AL-ja)	pain in the fibrous tissues and muscles (a common condition characterized by widespread pain and stiffness of muscles, fatigue, and disturbed sleep)

TERM	DEFINITION
10. kyphosis (kī-FŌ-sis)	abnormal condition of a hump (in the thoracic spine) (also called **hunchback** or **humpback**)
11. lordosis (lōr-DŌ-sis)	abnormal condition of bending forward (in the lumbar spine) (also called **swayback**)
12. meniscitis (*men*-i-SĪ-tis)	inflammation of a meniscus
13. myasthenia (*mī*-as-THĒ-nē-a)	muscle weakness
14. myeloma (*mī*-e-LŌ-ma)	tumor of the bone marrow (malignant)
15. osteitis (*os*-tē-Ī-tis)	inflammation of the bone
16. osteoarthritis (OA) (*os*-tē-ō-ar-THRĪ-tis)	inflammation of the bone and joint (Fig. 14.9B)
17. osteochondritis (*os*-tē-ō-kon-DRĪ-tis)	inflammation of the bone and cartilage
18. osteochondroma (*os*-tē-ō-kon-DRŌ-ma)	tumor composed of bone and cartilage (benign)
19. osteomalacia (*os*-tē-ō-ma-LĀ-sha)	softening of bone
20. osteomyelitis (*os*-tē-ō-*mī*-e-LĪ-tis)	inflammation of the bone and bone marrow (caused by bacterial infection)
21. osteonecrosis (*os*-tē-ō-ne-KRŌ-sis)	abnormal condition of bone death (due to lack of blood supply)
22. osteopenia (*os*-tē-ō-PĒ-nē-a)	abnormal reduction of bone mass (caused by inadequate replacement of bone lost to normal bone lysis and can lead to osteoporosis)
23. osteopetrosis (*os*-tē-ō-pe-TRŌ-sis)	abnormal condition of stonelike bones (very dense bones caused by defective resorption of bone)
24. osteosarcoma (*os*-tē-ō-sar-KŌ-ma)	malignant tumor of the bone
25. polymyositis (PM) (*pol*-ē-*mī*-ō-SĪ-tis)	inflammation of many muscles
26. rachischisis (ra-KIS-ki-sis)	fissure (split) of the vertebral column (congenital) (also called **spina bifida**)
27. rhabdomyolysis (*rab*-dō-mī-OL-i-sis)	dissolution of striated muscle (caused by trauma, extreme exertion, or drug toxicity; in severe cases renal failure can result)
28. sarcopenia (*sar*-kō-PĒ-nē-a)	abnormal reduction of connective tissue (such as loss of skeletal muscle mass in the elderly)
29. scoliosis (*skō*-lē-Ō-sis)	abnormal condition of (lateral) curved (spine) (Fig. 14.10)
30. spondylarthritis (*spon*-dil-ar-THRĪ-tis)	inflammation of the vertebral joints (also called **spondyloarthritis**)
31. spondylosis (*spon*-di-LŌ-sis)	abnormal condition of the vertebrae (a general term used to describe changes to the spine from osteoarthritis or ankylosis)
32. synoviosarcoma (si-*nō*-vē-ō-sar-KŌ-ma)	malignant tumor of the synovial membrane
33. tendinitis (*ten*-di-NĪ-tis)	inflammation of a tendon (also spelled **tendonitis**)
34. tenosynovitis (*ten*-ō-sin-ō-VĪ-tis)	inflammation of the tendon and synovial membrane *(Note: the* i *in* synovi *is dropped because the suffix begins with an* i.*)*

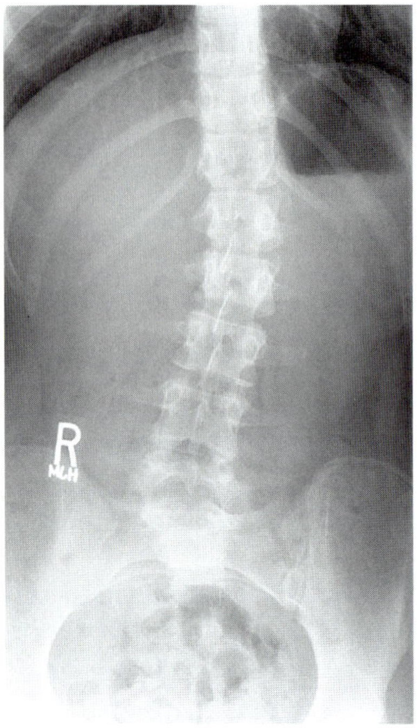

FIG. 14.10 AP lumbar spine radiograph demonstrating congenital scoliosis.

EXERCISE 6 ■ Pronounce and Spell

Practice pronunciation and spelling on paper and online.

1. Practice on Paper

a. **Pronounce:** Read the phonetic spelling and say aloud the terms listed in the previous table. Refer to the pronunciation key on p. 20 as necessary.
b. **Spell:** Have a study partner read the terms aloud. Write the spelling of the terms on a separate sheet of paper.

2. Practice Online

a. **Access** online learning resources. Go to evolve.elsevier.com > Evolve Resources > Student Resources.
b. **Pronounce:** Select Audio Glossary > Chapter 14 > Exercise 6. Select a term to hear its pronunciation and repeat aloud.
c. **Spell:** Select Activities > Chapter 14 > Spell Terms > Exercise 6. Select the audio icon and type the correct spelling of the term.

❑ Check the box when complete.

EXERCISE 7 ■ Analyze and Define

Analyze and define the following disease and disorder terms.

1. osteitis

____

____

2. tenosynovitis

____

____

3. osteopetrosis

4. osteomalacia

5. chondrosarcoma

6. osteochondroma

7. discitis

8. osteonecrosis

9. sarcopenia

10. synoviosarcoma

11. myasthenia

12. spondylosis

13. cranioschisis

14. chondromalacia

15. ankylosis

16. meniscitis

17. fibromyalgia

18. fasciitis

EXERCISE 8 ■ Build

A Label

Build terms pictured by writing word parts above definitions.

1.

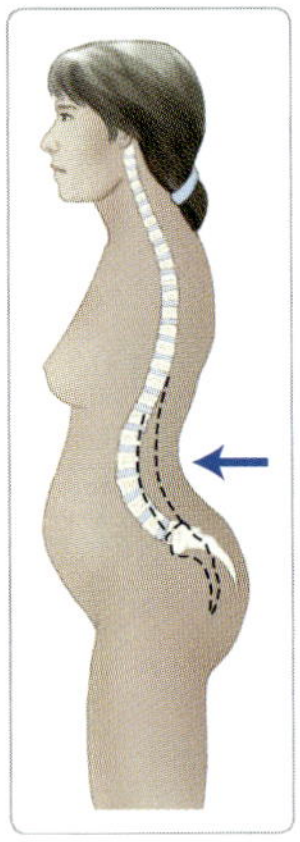

_______ / _______
bent forward (lumbar spine) / abnormal condition

2.

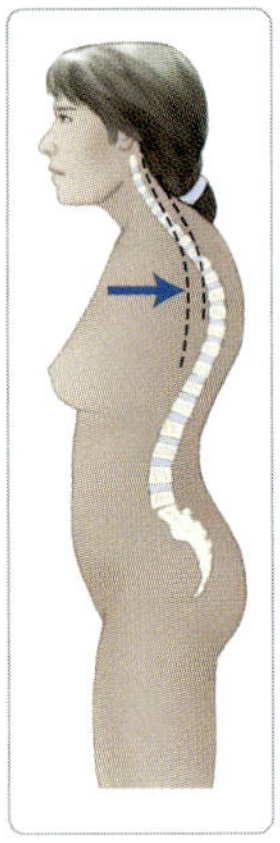

_______ / _______
hump / abnormal condition

3.

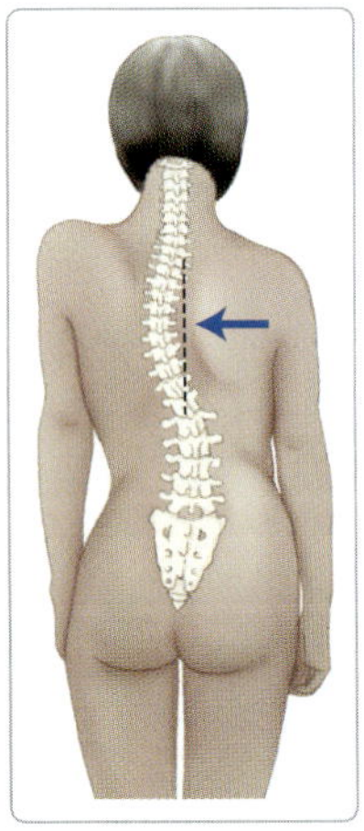

_______ / _______
(lateral) curved / abnormal condition

4.

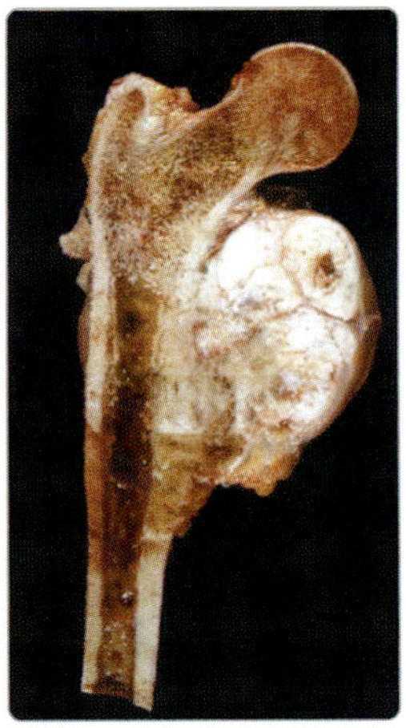

_______ / ___ / _______
bone / CV / malignant tumor

5.

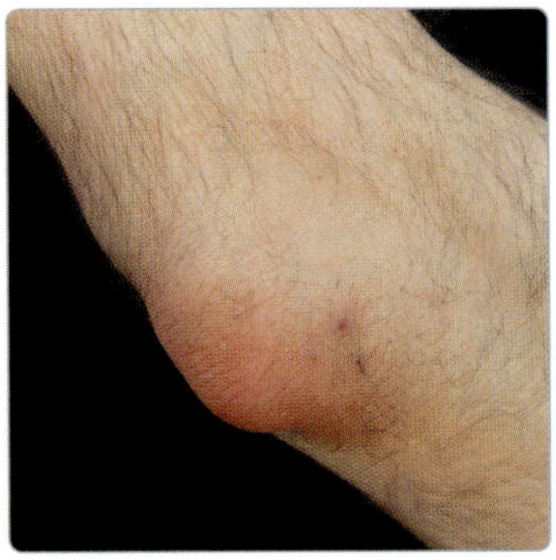

Olecranon (elbow) _______ / _______
bursa / inflammation

6.

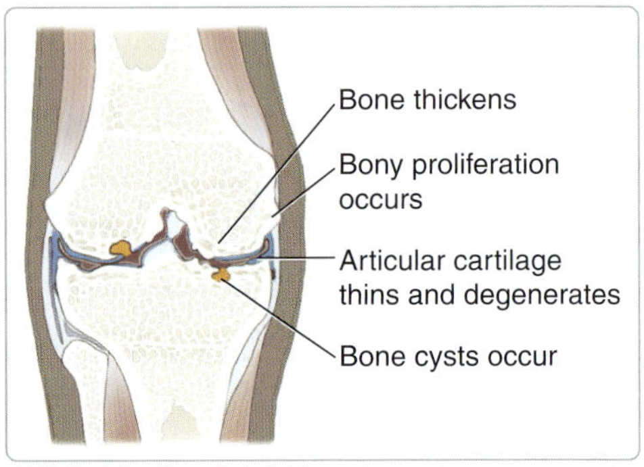

_______ / ___ / _______ / _______
bone / CV / joint / inflammation

B Fill In

Build disease and disorder terms for the following definitions with the word parts you have learned.

1. inflammation of the bone and cartilage ______ / ______ / ______ / ______
   WR / CV / WR / S
2. inflammation of the bone and bone marrow ______ / ______ / ______ / ______
   WR / CV / WR / S
3. inflammation of a joint ______ / ______
   WR / S
4. dissolution of striated muscle ______ / ______ / ______ / ______ / ______
   WR / CV / WR / CV / S
5. tumor of the bone marrow ______ / ______
   WR / S
6. inflammation of a tendon ______ / ______
   WR / S
7. abnormal condition of the vertebrae ______ / ______
   WR / S
8. abnormal reduction of bone mass ______ / ______ / ______
   WR / CV / S
9. fissure (split) of the vertebral column (congenital) ______ / ______
   WR / S
10. inflammation of the vertebral joints ______ / ______ / ______
   WR / WR / S

Disease and Disorder Terms

NOT BUILT FROM WORD PARTS

Word parts may be present in the following terms; however, their full meanings cannot be translated using definitions of word parts alone.

TERM	DEFINITION
1. ankylosing spondylitis (*ang*-ki-LŌ-sing) (*spon*-di-LĪ-tis)	form of arthritis that first affects the spine and adjacent structures and that, as it progresses, causes a forward bend of the spine (also called **Strümpell-Marie arthritis** or **disease,** or **rheumatoid spondylitis**)
ANKYLOSING SPONDYLITIS was first described in 1884 by Adolf von Strümpell (1853–1925). It became known as **Strümpell-Marie disease** after von Strümpell and French physician Pierre Marie.	
2. bunion (BUN-yun)	abnormal prominence of the joint at the base of the great toe, the metatarsal-phalangeal joint. It is a common problem, often hereditary or caused by poorly fitted shoes. (also called **hallux valgus**)
3. carpal tunnel syndrome (CTS) (KAR-pl) (TUN-el) (SIN-drōm)	common nerve entrapment disorder of the wrist caused by compression of the median nerve; symptoms include pain and tingling in portions of the hand and fingers
4. compartment syndrome (kom-PART-ment) (SIN-drōm)	painful condition caused by increased pressure within a muscle that can lead to ischemia; acute compartment syndrome is a medical emergency and is caused by severe injury

Disease and Disorder Terms—cont'd

NOT BUILT FROM WORD PARTS

TERM	DEFINITION
5. dislocation (*dis*-lō-KĀ-shun)	displacement of bones in a joint from their normal alignment (also called **luxation**)
6. exostosis (*ek*-sos-TŌ-sis)	abnormal benign growth on the surface of a bone (also called **spur**)
7. fracture (fx) (FRAK-chūr)	broken bone
8. ganglion cyst (GANG-glē-on) (sist)	collection of jellylike fluid forming a benign mass arising from joints, most commonly appearing in the wrist, hand, and ankle
9. gout (gowt)	disease in which an excessive amount of uric acid in the blood causes sodium urate crystals (tophi) to be deposited in the joints, producing arthritis. The great toe is frequently affected.
10. herniated disk (HER-nē-*āt*-ed) (disk)	rupture of the intervertebral disk cartilage, which allows the contents to protrude through it, putting pressure on the spinal nerve roots (also called **slipped disk, ruptured disk, herniated intervertebral disk,** or **herniated nucleus pulposus [HNP]**)
11. Lyme disease (līm) (di-ZĒZ)	infection caused by a bite from a deer tick infected with *Borrelia burgdorferi.* This bacterium provokes an immune response in the body, the symptoms of which can mimic several musculoskeletal diseases. Patients may experience fever, headache, and joint pain. A rash (target lesion) may initially arise at the site of the tick bite.
LYME DISEASE was first reported in Lyme, Connecticut, in 1975.	
12. muscular dystrophy (MD) (MUS-kū-lar) (DIS-tro-fē)	group of hereditary diseases characterized by degeneration of muscle and weakness
13. myasthenia gravis (MG) (*mī*-as-THĒ-nē-a) (GRA-vis)	chronic disease characterized by muscle weakness and thought to be caused by a defect in the transmission of impulses from nerve to muscle cell. The face, larynx, and throat are frequently affected; no true paralysis of the muscles exists.
14. osteoporosis (*os*-tē-ō-po-RŌ-sis)	abnormal loss of bone density that may lead to an increase in fractures of the ribs, thoracic and lumbar vertebrae, hips, and wrists after slight trauma (occurs predominantly in postmenopausal women)
15. plantar fasciitis (PLAN-tar) (fas-ē-Ī-tis)	inflammation of the connective tissue of the sole of the foot (plantar fascia) due to repetitive injury; common cause of heel pain
16. repetitive strain injury (RSI) (rē-PET-i-tiv) (strān) (IN-ja-rē)	cumulative damage to joint, muscle, or other tissue caused by movements performed over and over again; characterized by pain, swelling, numbness, and lack of strength and flexibility, most commonly affecting the hands, wrists, elbows, and shoulders
REPETITIVE MOTION DISORDERS (RMDS) are a group of musculoskeletal disorders that can lead to repetitive strain injuries. They are caused by overuse and repetitive motions performed in the course of normal work or recreational activities and include **tendinitis, bursitis, tenosynovitis, ganglion cyst,** and **carpal tunnel syndrome**. Incorporating rest breaks, stretching, improved posture or ergonomics, antiinflammatory medications, and physical therapy provide the majority of treatment for RMDs. Surgery may be needed as treatment for permanent injuries.	
17. rheumatoid arthritis (RA) (RŪ-ma-toid) (ar-THRĪ-tis)	chronic systemic disease characterized by autoimmune inflammatory changes in the connective tissue throughout the body (Fig. 14.9C)
18. rotator cuff disease (RŌ-tā-tor) (kuf) (di-ZĒZ)	damage to one or more of the four tendons stabilizing the shoulder joint due to injury or degeneration; symptoms may include pain, limited range of motion, and muscle weakness
19. spinal stenosis (SPĪ-nal) (ste-NŌ-sis)	narrowing of the spinal canal with compression of nerve roots. The condition is either congenital or due to spinal degeneration. Symptoms are pain radiating to the thigh or lower legs and numbness or tingling in the lower extremities.

TERM	DEFINITION
20. spondylolisthesis (*spon*-di-lō-lis-THĒ-sis)	forward slipping of one vertebra over another
21. sprain (sprān)	abnormal stretching or tearing of a ligament that supports a joint
22. strain (strān)	abnormal stretching or tearing of a muscle or tendon
23. subluxation (*sub*-luk-SĀ-shun)	partial dislocation of bones in a joint
24. tarsal tunnel syndrome (TĀR-sl) (TUN-el) (SIN-drōm)	painful foot disorder caused by compression of the posterior tibial nerve as it passes through the ankle

EXERCISE 9 ■ Pronounce and Spell

Practice pronunciation and spelling on paper and online.

1. Practice on Paper

a. **Pronounce:** Read the phonetic spelling and say aloud the terms listed in the previous table. Refer to the pronunciation key on p. 20 as necessary.
b. **Spell:** Have a study partner read the terms aloud. Write the spelling of the terms on a separate sheet of paper.

2. Practice Online

a. **Access** online learning resources. Go to evolve.elsevier.com > Evolve Resources > Student Resources.
b. **Pronounce:** Select Audio Glossary > Chapter 14 > Exercise 9. Select a term to hear its pronunciation and repeat aloud.
c. **Spell:** Select Activities > Chapter 14 > Spell Terms > Exercise 9. Select the audio icon and type the correct spelling of the term.

❑ Check the box when complete.

EXERCISE 10 ■ Match

Match the terms in the first column with their correct definitions in the second column.

_____	1. muscular dystrophy	a. abnormal benign growth on the surface of a bone
_____	2. exostosis	b. form of arthritis that first affects the spine and adjacent structures, eventually causing a forward bend of the spine
_____	3. ankylosing spondylitis	c. group of hereditary diseases characterized by degeneration of muscles and weakness
_____	4. myasthenia gravis	d. chronic disease characterized by muscle weakness and thought to be caused by a defect in the transmission of impulses from nerve to muscle cell
_____	5. tarsal tunnel syndrome	e. foot disorder caused by compression of the posterior tibial nerve as it passes through the ankle
_____	6. sublaxation	f. abnormal stretching or tearing of a ligament that supports a joint
_____	7. strain	g. condition caused by increased pressure within a muscle that can lead to ischemia
_____	8. repetitive strain injury	h. cumulative damage to joint, muscle, or other tissue caused by movements performed over and over again
_____	9. compartment syndrome	i. partial dislocation of bones in a joint
_____	10. sprain	j. abnormal stretching or tearing of a muscle or tendon

EXERCISE 11 ■ Label

Write the medical terms pictured and defined.

1. ______________________
rupture of the intervertebral disk cartilage, which allows the contents to protrude through it, putting pressure on the spinal nerve roots

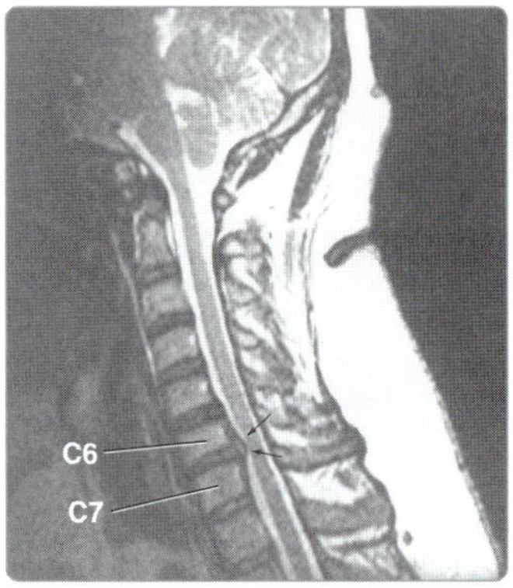

2. ______________________
chronic systemic disease characterized by autoimmune inflammatory changes in the connective tissue throughout the body

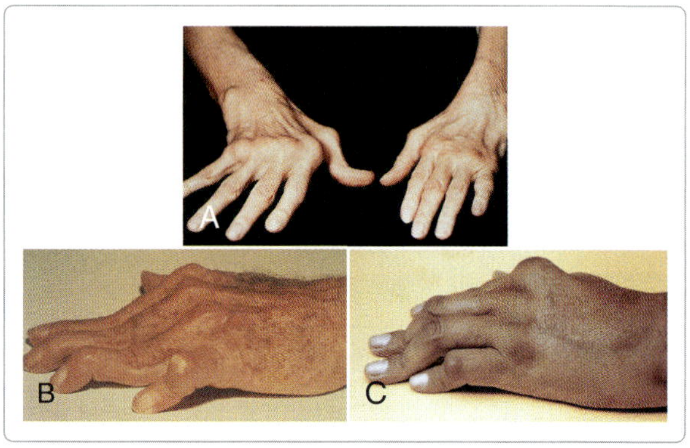

3. ______________________
common nerve entrapment disorder of the wrist caused by compression of the median nerve

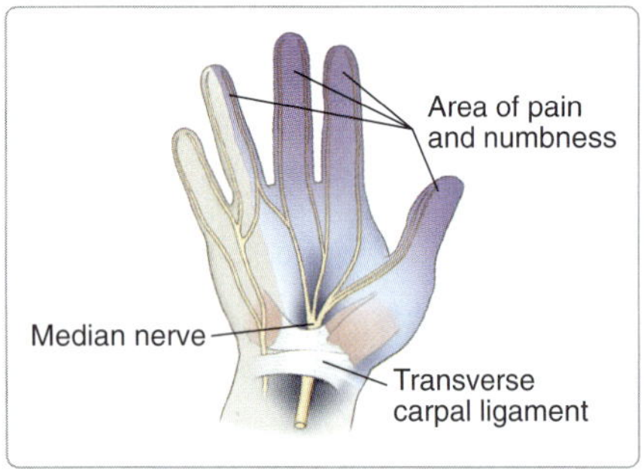

4. ______________________
forward slipping of one vertebra over the other

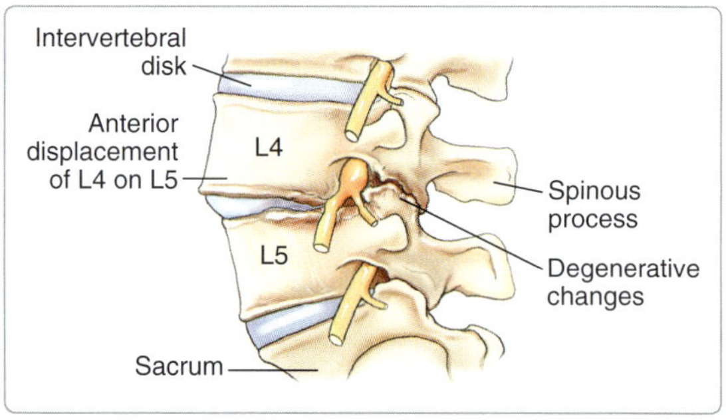

5. ______________________
disease in which an excessive amount of uric acid in the blood causes sodium urate crystals (tophi) to be deposited in the joints

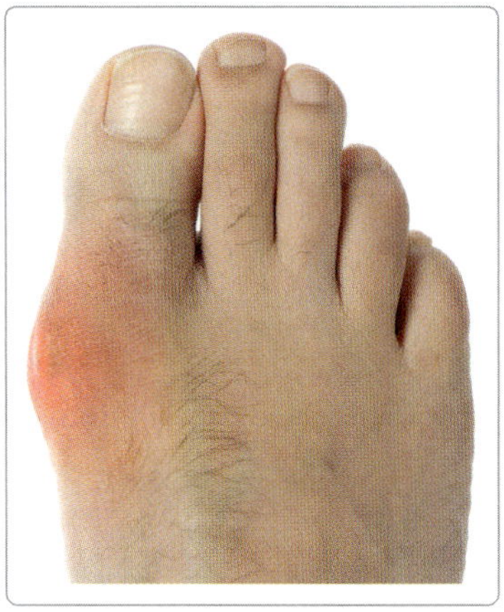

6. ______________________
abnormal loss of density that may lead to an increase in fractures

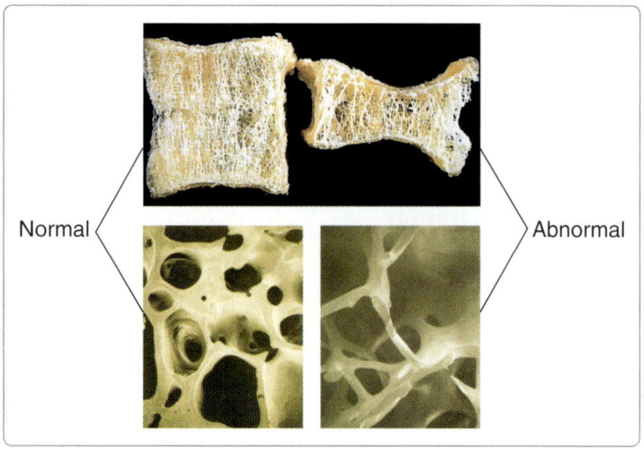

7. ____________________
broken bone

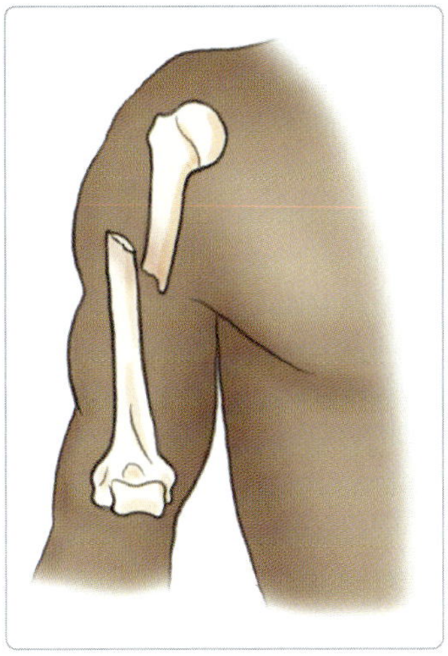

8. ____________________
infection caused by a bite from an infected deer tick, which provokes an immune response that can mimic several musculoskeletal diseases. A rash (target lesion) may be found at the site of the tick bite.

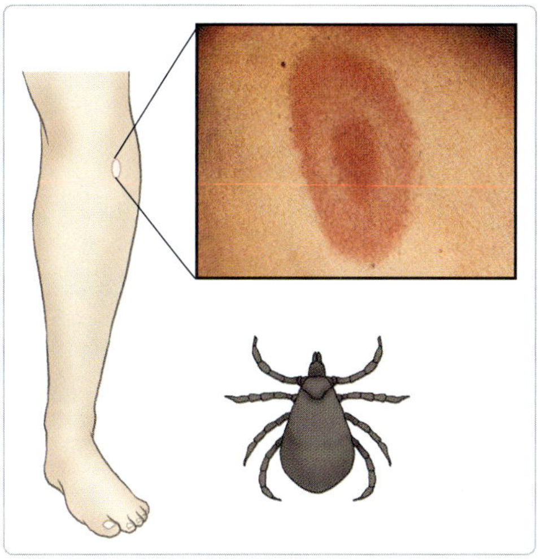

9. ____________________
abnormal prominence of the joint at the base of the great toe, the metatarsal-phalangeal joint

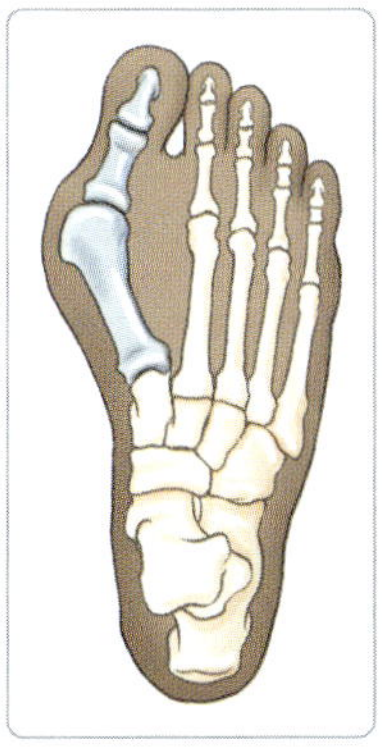

10. ____________________
narrowing of the spinal canal with compression of nerve roots

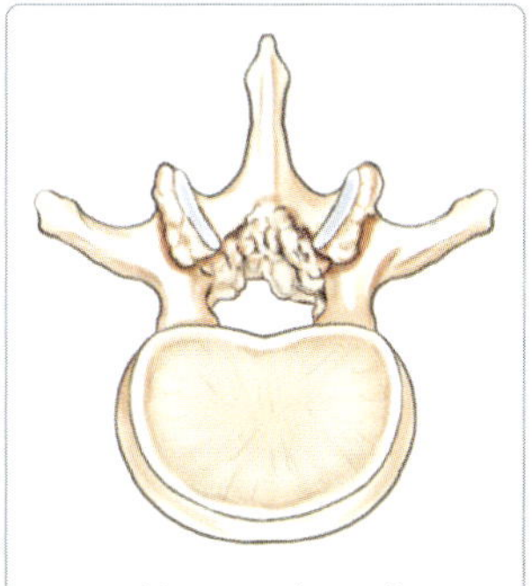

11. ____________________
inflammation of the connective tissue of the sole of the foot, common cause of heel pain

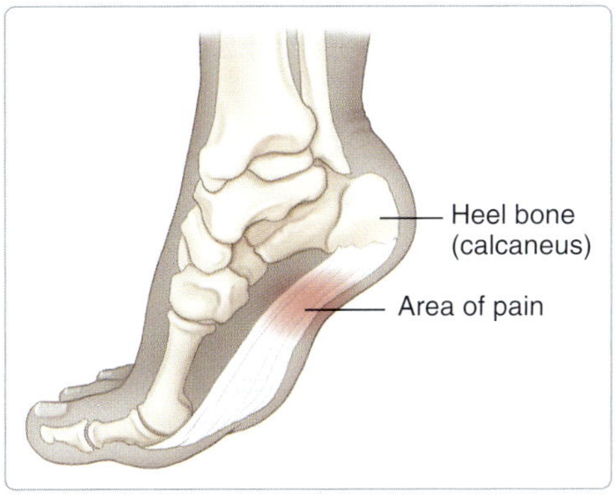

12. ____________________
collection of jellylike fluid forming a benign mass arising from joints

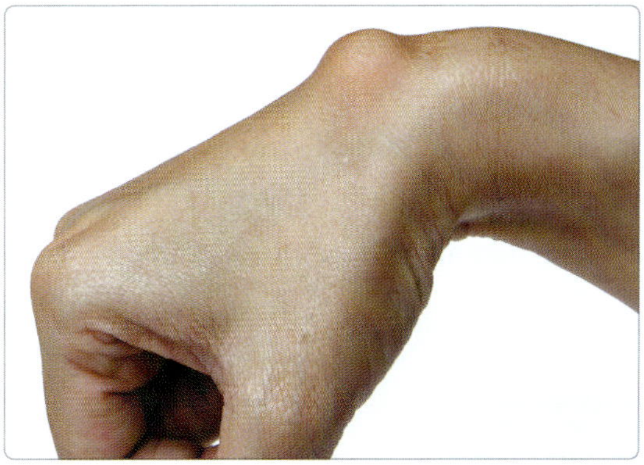

13. ______________________________
damage to one or more of the four tendons stabilizing the shoulder joint due to injury or degeneration

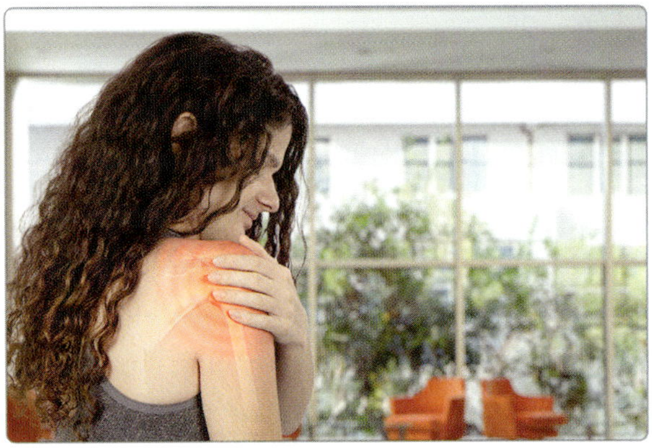

14. ______________________________
displacement of bones in a joint from their normal alignment

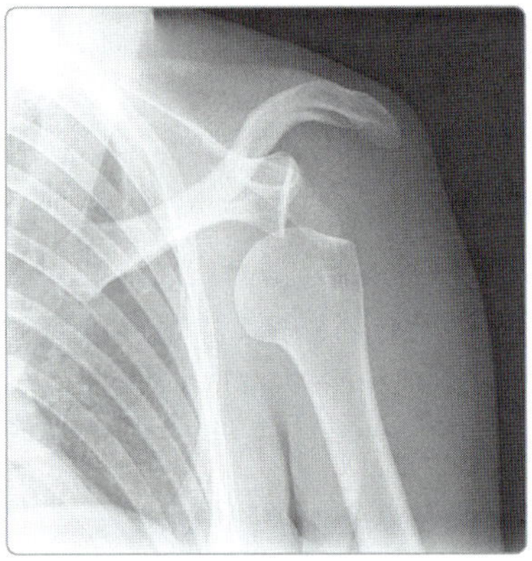

EXERCISE 12 ■ Identify

Write the medical terms defined.

1. Conditions affecting the spine:
   a. forward slipping of one vertebra over another ______________________________
   b. rupture of the intervertebral disk cartilage, which allows the contents to protrude through it, putting pressure on the spinal nerve roots ______________________________
   c. form of arthritis that first affects the spine and adjacent structures and that, as it progresses, causes a forward bend of the spine ______________________________
   d. narrowing of the spinal canal with compression of nerve roots ______________________________
2. Conditions involving joints:
   a. abnormal prominence of the joint at the base of the great toe, the metatarsal-phalangeal joint ______________________________
   b. painful foot disorder caused by compression of the posterior tibial nerve as it passes through the ankle ______________________________
   c. common nerve entrapment disorder of the wrist caused by compression of the median nerve ______________________________
   d. collection of jellylike fluid forming a benign mass arising from joints, most commonly appearing in the wrist, hand, and ankle ______________________________
   e. disease in which an excessive amount of uric acid in the blood causes sodium urate crystals (tophi) to be deposited in the joints, producing arthritis. The great toe is frequently affected. ______________________________
   f. infection caused by a bite from a deer tick infected with *Borrelia burgdorferi*. This bacterium provokes an immune response in the body, the symptoms of which include joint pain. ______________________________
   g. chronic systemic disease characterized by autoimmune inflammatory changes in the connective tissue throughout the body, including joint linings causing painful swelling ______________________________
   h. displacement of bones in a joint from their normal alignment (also called luxation) ______________________________

i. partial dislocation of bones in a joint ______
j. cumulative damage to joint, muscle, or other tissue caused by movements performed over and over again; characterized by pain, swelling, numbness, and lack of strength and flexibility, most commonly affecting the hands, wrists, elbows, and shoulders ______

3. Conditions affecting bone:
a. abnormal benign growth on the surface of a bone (also called spur) ______
b. broken bone ______
c. abnormal loss of bone density that may lead to an increase in fractures of the ribs, thoracic and lumbar vertebrae, hips, and wrists after slight trauma ______

4. Conditions affecting muscle:
a. damage to one or more of the four tendons stabilizing the shoulder joint due to injury or degeneration; symptoms may include pain, limited range of motion, and muscle weakness ______
b. abnormal stretching or tearing of a muscle or tendon ______
c. abnormal stretching or tearing of a ligament that supports a joint ______
d. painful condition caused by increased pressure within a muscle that can lead to ischemia ______
e. inflammation of the connective tissue of the sole of the foot due to repetitive injury; common cause of heel pain ______
f. chronic disease characterized by muscle weakness and thought to be caused by a defect in the transmission of impulses from nerve to muscle cell ______
g. group of hereditary diseases characterized by degeneration of muscle and weakness ______

EXERCISE 13 ■ Review of Disease and Disorder Terms

Can you define, pronounce, and spell the following terms?

ankylosing spondylitis
ankylosis
arthritis
bunion
bursitis
carpal tunnel syndrome (CTS)
chondromalacia
chondrosarcoma
compartment syndrome
cranioschisis
discitis
dislocation
exostosis
fasciitis
fibromyalgia
fracture (fx)
ganglion cyst
gout
herniated disk
kyphosis
lordosis
Lyme disease
meniscitis
muscular dystrophy (MD)
myasthenia
myasthenia gravis (MG)
myeloma
osteitis
osteoarthritis (OA)
osteochondritis
osteochondroma
osteomalacia
osteomyelitis
osteonecrosis
osteopenia
osteopetrosis
osteoporosis
osteosarcoma
plantar fasciitis
polymyositis (PM)
rachischisis
repetitive strain injury (RSI)
rhabdomyolysis
rheumatoid arthritis (RA)
rotator cuff disease
sarcopenia
scoliosis
spinal stenosis
spondylarthritis
spondylolisthesis
spondylosis
sprain
strain
subluxation
synoviosarcoma
tarsal tunnel syndrome
tendinitis
tenosynovitis

Surgical Terms

BUILT FROM WORD PARTS

The following terms can be translated using definitions of word parts. Further explanation is provided within parentheses as needed.

TERM	DEFINITION
1. **arthrocentesis** (*ar*-thrō-sen-TĒ-sis)	surgical puncture to aspirate fluid from a joint
2. **arthrodesis** (*ar*-thrō-DĒ-sis)	surgical fixation of a joint (also called **joint fusion**)
3. **arthroplasty** (AR-thrō-*plas*-tē)	surgical repair of a joint (Table 14.1)
4. **bursectomy** (bur-SEK-to-mē)	excision of a bursa
5. **carpectomy** (kar-PEK-to-mē)	excision of a carpal bone
6. **chondrectomy** (kon-DREK-to-mē)	excision of cartilage
7. **chondroplasty** (KON-drō-*plas*-tē)	surgical repair of cartilage
8. **costectomy** (kos-TEK-to-mē)	excision of a rib
9. **cranioplasty** (KRĀ-nē-ō-*plas*-tē)	surgical repair of the skull
10. **craniotomy** (*krā*-nē-OT-o-mē)	incision into the cranium (as for surgery of the brain)
11. **discectomy** (dis-KEK-to-mē)	excision of an intervertebral disk (a portion of the herniated disk is removed to relieve pressure on nerve roots; uses a larger incision than microdiscectomy)
12. **fasciotomy** (*fash*-ē-OT-o-mē)	incision into fascia (to relieve tension or pressure)
13. **laminectomy** (*lam*-i-NEK-to-mē)	excision of a lamina (often performed to relieve pressure on the nerve roots in the lower spine caused by a herniated disk and other conditions)
14. **maxillectomy** (*mak*-si-LEK-to-mē)	excision of the maxilla
15. **meniscectomy** (*men*-i-SEK-to-mē)	excision of a meniscus (performed for a torn cartilage)
16. **microdiscectomy** (*mī*-kro-dis-KEK-to-mē)	small excision of an intervertebral disk (minimally invasive surgery to remove a portion of the herniated disk to relieve pressure on nerve roots)

MICROENDOSCOPIC DISCECTOMY (MED) uses a fluoroscope and special dilating instrumentation to create a small tunnel to the affected disk area. An endoscopic tool allows the surgeon to visualize and remove the thick, sticky nucleus of the herniated disk. The disk then softens and contracts, relieving severe low back and leg pain. Recovery time is significantly less than open discectomy because of a small incision and less trauma to surrounding tissues.

TERM	DEFINITION
17. **myorrhaphy** (mī-OR-a-fē)	suturing of a muscle
18. **osteotomy** (*os*-tē-OT-o-mē)	incision into a bone
19. **phalangectomy** (*fal*-an-JEK-to-mē)	excision of a finger or toe bone
20. **rachiotomy** (*rā*-kē-OT-o-mē)	incision into the vertebral column
21. **spondylosyndesis** (*spon*-di-lō-sin-DĒ-sis)	fusing together of the vertebrae (also called **spinal fusion**) *(Note: the prefix* syn- *appears in the middle of the term.)*
22. **synovectomy** (*sin*-ō-VEK-to-mē)	excision of the synovial membrane (of a joint) *(Note: the i in* synovi *is dropped because the suffix begins with a vowel.)*
23. **tarsectomy** (tar-SEK-to-mē)	excision of (one or more) tarsal bones
24. **tenomyoplasty** (*ten*-ō-MĪ-ō-*plas*-tē)	surgical repair of the tendon and muscle
25. **tenorrhaphy** (te-NOR-a-fē)	suturing of a tendon
26. **vertebroplasty** (VER-te-brō-*plas*-tē)	surgical repair of a vertebra (usually performed for compression fractures due to osteoporosis) (Table 14.2)

TABLE 14.1 Types of Arthroplasty

Total hip arthroplasty (THA) is indicated for degenerative joint disease or rheumatoid arthritis. The operation originally involved replacement of the hip joint with a metallic femoral head and a plastic-coated acetabulum. More recently, however, many different materials have been used in an attempt to prevent the artificial joint from wearing out too quickly. These materials include joints composed of metal, ceramics, polyethylene (plastic), and combinations of each.

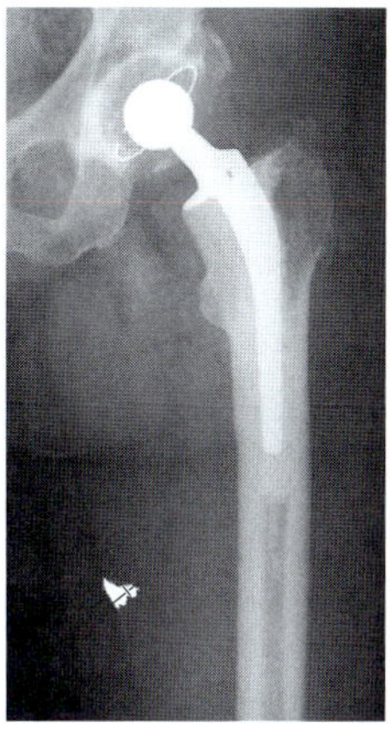
Total hip arthroplasty

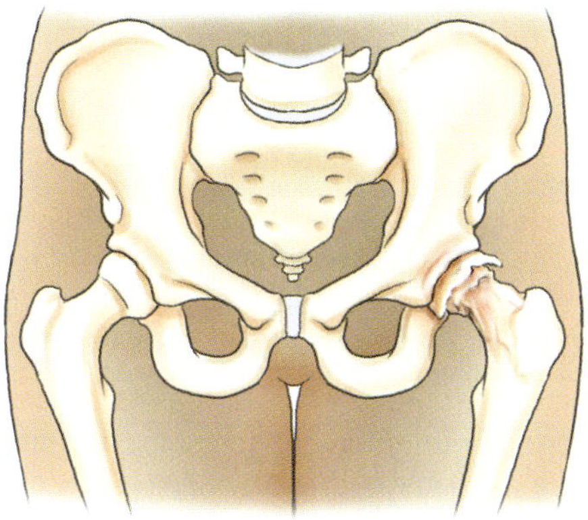
Normal hip joint
Hip joint damaged by osteoarthritis

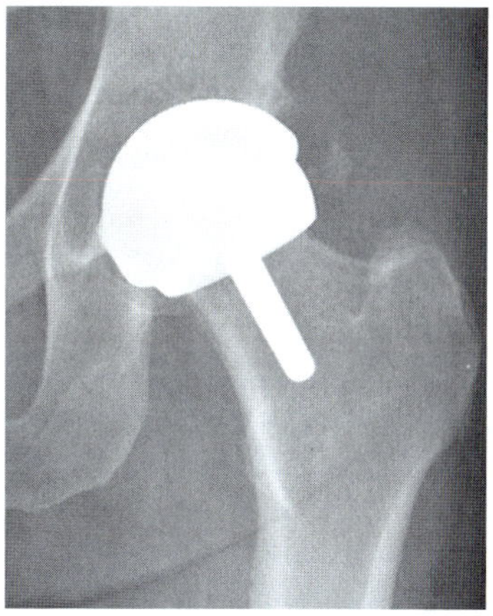
Hip resurfacing arthroplasty

Hip resurfacing arthroplasty (HRA) is a procedure that provides an option for younger, active patients needing a total hip arthroplasty. The procedure requires the removal of a few millimeters of bone from the femoral head instead of the removal of the entire femoral head required in total hip arthroplasty. A metal cap is then placed on top of the femur, and smooth metal is placed in the acetabulum. The risk of fracture of the neck of the femur is increased when smaller diameter components are used, making HRA less appropriate for women.

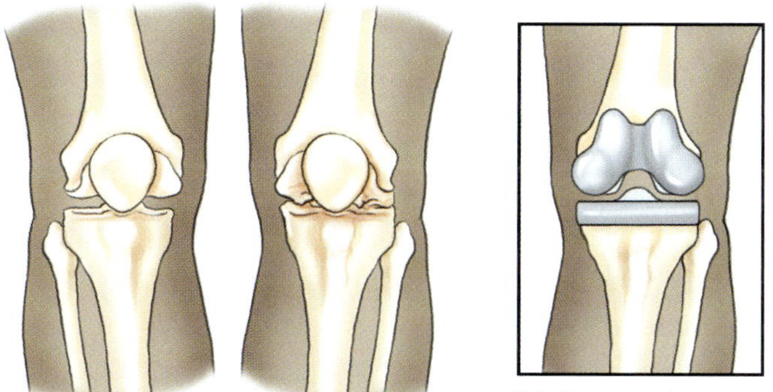
Normal knee joint
Knee joint damaged by osteoarthritis
Total knee replacement

Total knee arthroplasty (TKA) is designed to replace worn surfaces of the knee joint. Various prostheses (artificial parts) are used.

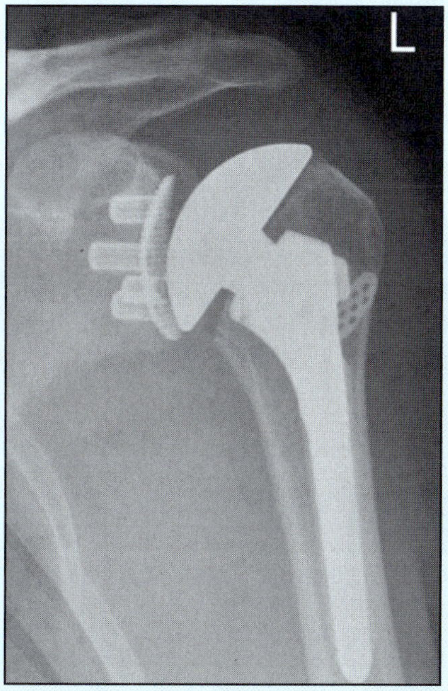

Shoulder arthroplasty is a procedure that restores the major functions of this ball and socket joint: motion, stability, strength, and smoothness. Prostheses are applied to the head of the humerus and the glenoid cavity (part of the scapula). Osteoarthritis, rheumatoid arthritis, and severe rotator cuff tears are some of the most common reasons for this surgery.

TABLE 14.2 Procedures for Treatment of Compression Fractures Caused by Osteoporosis

Percutaneous vertebroplasty (PV) is a minimally invasive operation in which an interventional radiologist places a needle through the skin into the damaged vertebra. A special liquid cement is injected into the area through the needle to fill the holes left by osteoporosis.

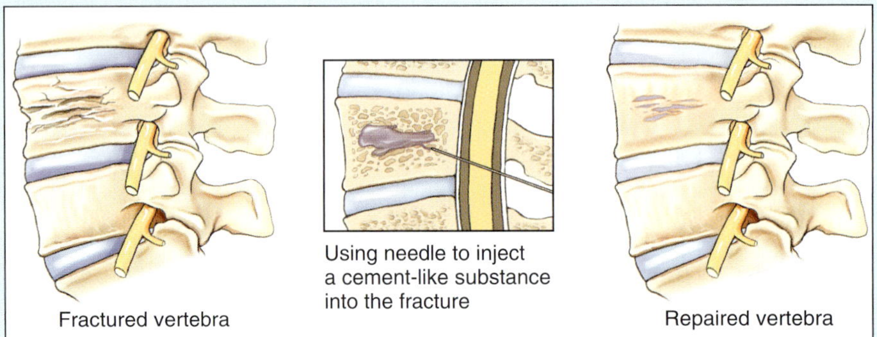

Percutaneous vertebroplasty

Kyphoplasty is similar to vertebroplasty except a balloonlike device is used to expand the compressed vertebra before the cement is injected. Recent studies have generated controversy as to whether these procedures are better than non-surgical management, such as pain medication and physical therapy. In either case, it is important to treat the underlying osteoporosis, to prevent future fractures.

EXERCISE 14 ■ Pronounce and Spell

Practice pronunciation and spelling on paper and online.

1. Practice on Paper

a. **Pronounce:** Read the phonetic spelling and say aloud the terms listed in the previous table. Refer to the pronunciation key on p. 20 as necessary.
b. **Spell:** Have a study partner read the terms aloud. Write the spelling of the terms on a separate sheet of paper.

2. Practice Online

a. **Access** online learning resources. Go to evolve.elsevier.com > Evolve Resources > Student Resources.
b. **Pronounce:** Select Audio Glossary > Chapter 14 > Exercise 14. Select a term to hear its pronunciation and repeat aloud.
c. **Spell:** Select Activities > Chapter 14 > Spell Terms > Exercise 14. Select the audio icon and type the correct spelling of the term.

❑ Check the box when complete.

EXERCISE 15 ■ Analyze and Define

Analyze and define the following surgical terms.

1. vertebroplasty
____
____

2. tarsectomy
____
____

3. arthrodesis
____
____

4. laminectomy
____
____

5. synovectomy

____

____

6. fasciotomy

____

____

7. rachiotomy

____

____

8. bursectomy

____

____

9. discectomy

____

____

10. arthrocentesis

____

____

11. maxillectomy

____

____

12. cranioplasty

____

____

13. carpectomy

____

____

14. phalangectomy

____

____

EXERCISE 16 ■ Build

A Label

Build terms pictured by writing word parts above definitions.

1.

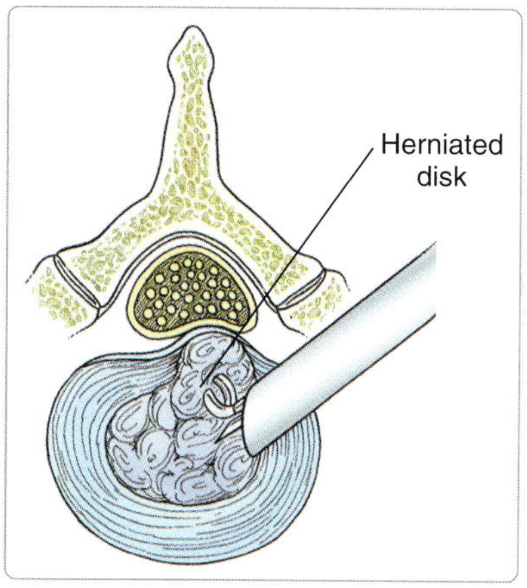

_______ / _______ / _______
small / invertebral disk / excision

2.

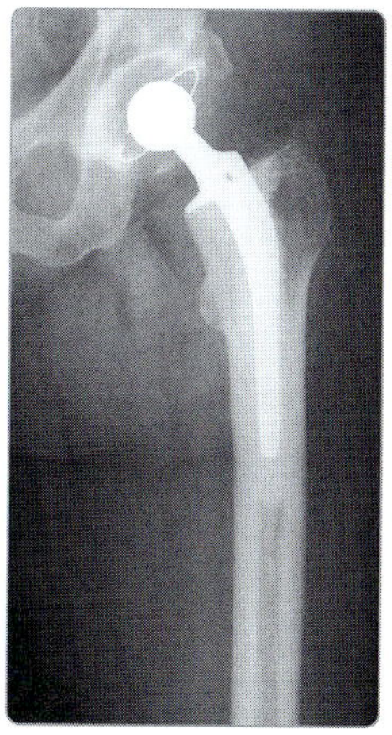

total hip _______ / _______ / _______
joint / CV / surgical repair

3.

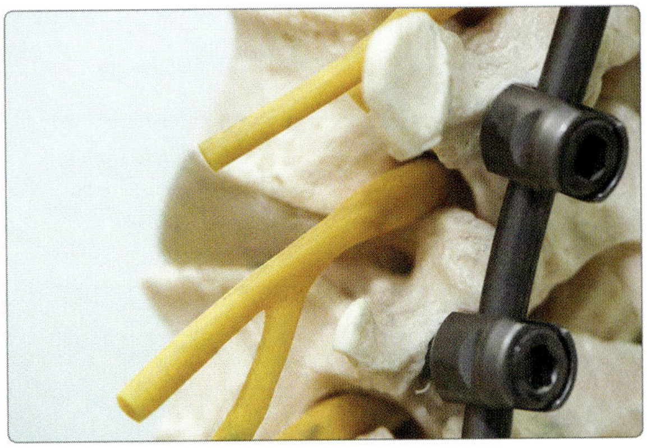

_______ / ___ / syn / _______
vertebra CV together fusion

4.

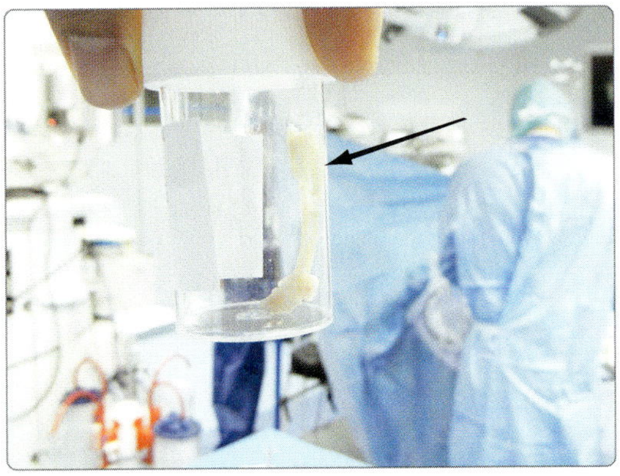

_______ / _______
meniscus excision

5.

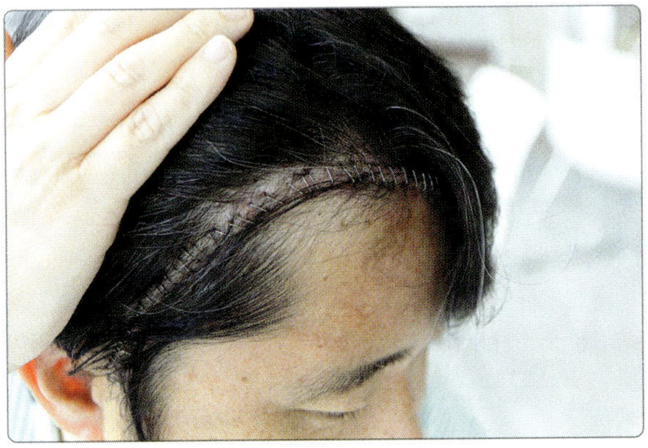

_______ / ___ / _______
cranium CV incision

6.

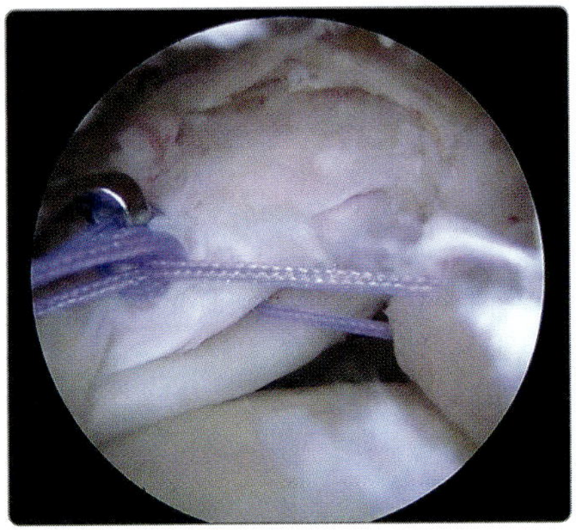

_______ / ___ / _______
tendon CV suturing

B Fill In

Build surgical terms for the following definitions by using the word parts you have learned.

1. incision into a bone _______ WR / CV / _______ S
2. excision of cartilage _______ WR / _______ S
3. surgical repair of cartilage _______ WR / CV / _______ S
4. suturing of a muscle _______ WR / CV / _______ S
5. surgical repair of a tendon and muscle _______ WR / CV / _______ WR / CV / _______ S
6. excision of a rib _______ WR / _______ S

EXERCISE 17 ■ Review of Surgical Terms

Can you define, pronounce, and spell the following terms?

arthrocentesis	costectomy	meniscectomy	synovectomy
arthrodesis	cranioplasty	microdiscectomy	tarsectomy
arthroplasty	craniotomy	myorrhaphy	tenomyoplasty
bursectomy	discectomy	osteotomy	tenorrhaphy
carpectomy	fasciotomy	phalangectomy	vertebroplasty
chondrectomy	laminectomy	rachiotomy	
chondroplasty	maxillectomy	spondylosyndesis	

Diagnostic Terms

BUILT FROM WORD PARTS AND *NOT* BUILT FROM WORD PARTS

The first portion of the table contains Diagnostic Terms that can be translated using definitions of word parts. The second portion of the table contains Diagnostic Terms that cannot be fully understood using the definitions of word parts.

■ Built from Word Parts

DIAGNOSTIC IMAGING

TERM	DEFINITION
1. **arthrography** (ar-THROG-ra-fē)	radiographic imaging of a joint (with contrast media)

MAGNETIC RESONANCE (MR) has mostly replaced conventional **arthrography** as the imaging technique for joints such as the knee, wrist, hip, and shoulder. Many of the remaining arthrograms are performed in conjunction with MR. A conventional arthrogram might be used in situations in which a patient cannot undergo MR, such as a person with a cardiac pacemaker.

TERM	DEFINITION
2. **myelography** (*mī*-e-LOG-ra-fē)	radiographic imaging of the spinal cord (with contrast media)

ENDOSCOPY

TERM	DEFINITION
3. **arthroscopy** (ar-THROS-ko-pē)	visual examination of a joint

OTHER

TERM	DEFINITION
4. **electromyogram (EMG)** (ē-*lek*-trō-MĪ-ō-gram)	record of the (intrinsic) electrical activity in a (skeletal) muscle

■ *NOT* Built from Word Parts

DIAGNOSTIC IMAGING

TERM	DEFINITION
1. **dual x-ray absorptiometry (DXA)** (du-al) (EKS-rā) (ab-*sorp*-shē-OM-e-trē)	radiographic imaging, usually of the lumbar spine and hips, to measure bone loss and bone mineral density; the procedure utilizes low doses of radiation and is used in the diagnosis of osteoporosis and monitoring of treatment (also called **dual-energy x-ray absorptiometry [DEXA], bone densitometry,** and **bone density test**) (Fig. 14.11)

TABLE 14.3 Diagnostic Imaging Procedures Used for the Musculoskeletal System

In addition to **arthrography**, the following diagnostic imaging procedures are commonly used for diagnosing diseases, fractures, strains, and other conditions of the musculoskeletal system.

Bone densitometry is a method of determining the density of bone by radiographic techniques used to diagnose osteoporosis. **Dual X-ray absorptiometry (DXA)** is commonly used for this test. (Fig. 14.11)

Bone scan (nuclear medicine test) is used to detect the presence of metastatic disease of the bone and to monitor degenerative bone disease. (Fig. 14.13)

Magnetic resonance (MR) is used to evaluate the bones and soft tissue of the shoulders, hips, elbows, knees, ankles, feet, and spinal cord for stenosis, spinal cord defects, and degenerative disk changes. (Fig. 14.12)

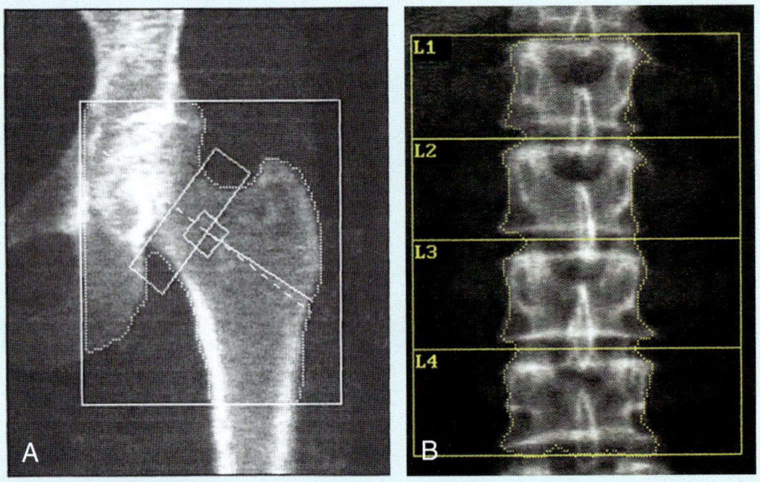

FIG. 14.11 DXA images of the (A) left hip and (B) spine.

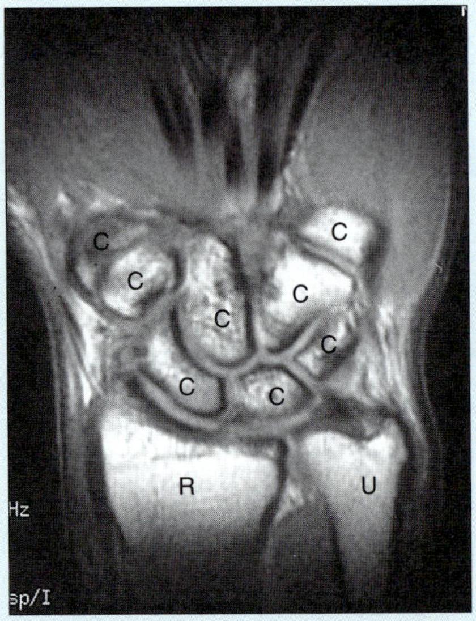

FIG. 14.12 Coronal MR scan of the wrist. Marrow within the carpal bones (C), radius (R), and ulna (U).

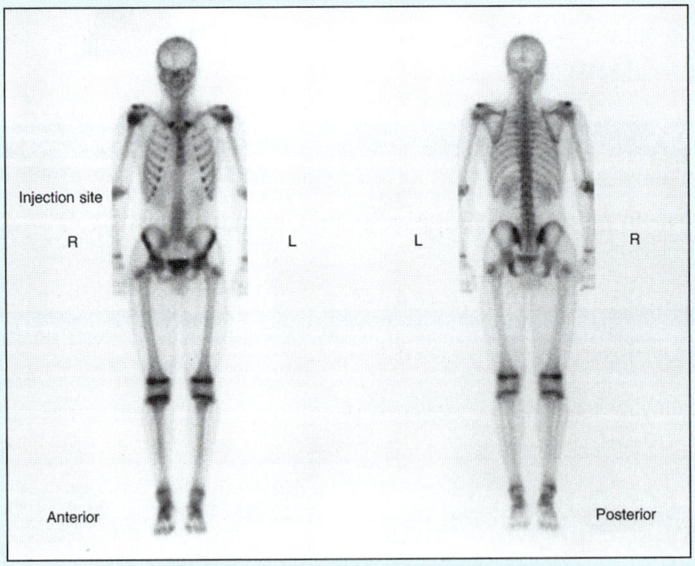

FIG. 14.13 Whole body nuclear medicine bone scan.

Radiography (radiographic imaging) of the bones and joints is used to identify fractures or tumors, monitor healing, or identify abnormal structures.

Single-photon emission computed tomography (SPECT) of the bone is an even more sensitive nuclear method for detecting bone abnormalities.

Diagnostic Terms—cont'd

BUILT FROM WORD PARTS AND *NOT* BUILT FROM WORD PARTS

NOT Built from Word Parts

LABORATORY

TERM	DEFINITION
2. bone markers (bōn) (MAR-krs)	blood and urine tests to determine the rate of bone turnover (resorption and formation); often used with DXA to diagnose and monitor treatment of osteoporosis and other bone disorders
3. muscle biopsy (MUS-el) (BĪ-op-sē)	removal of muscle tissue using a needle or small incision; used to assess musculoskeletal abnormalities involving weakness or pain such as muscular dystrophy, myasthenia gravis, and polymyositis

EXERCISE 18 ■ Pronounce and Spell

Practice pronunciation and spelling on paper and online.

1. Practice on Paper

a. **Pronounce:** Read the phonetic spelling and say aloud the terms listed in the previous table. Refer to the pronunciation key on p. 20 as necessary.
b. **Spell:** Have a study partner read the terms aloud. Write the spelling of the terms on a separate sheet of paper.

2. Practice Online

a. **Access** online learning resources. Go to evolve.elsevier.com > Evolve Resources > Student Resources.
b. **Pronounce:** Select Audio Glossary > Chapter 14 > Exercise 18. Select a term to hear its pronunciation and repeat aloud.
c. **Spell:** Select Activities > Chapter 14 > Spell Terms > Exercise 18. Select the audio icon and type the correct spelling of the term.

❑ Check the box when complete.

EXERCISE 19 ■ Diagnostic Terms Built from Word Parts

A Analyze and Define

Analyze and define the following diagnostic terms.

1. electromyogram

____

____

2. arthrography

____

____

3. arthroscopy

____

____

4. myelography

____

____

B Build

Build diagnostic terms for the following definitions using word parts you have learned.

1. radiographic imaging of a joint ______ WR / CV / ______ S

2. radiographic imaging of the spinal cord ______ WR / CV / ______ S

C Label

Build terms pictured by writing word parts above definitions.

1.

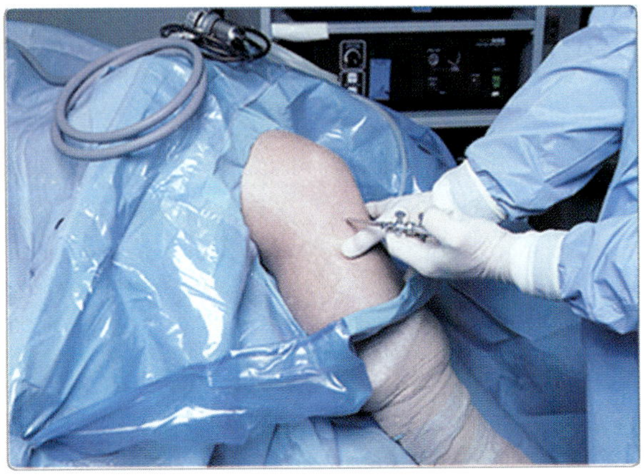

______ / ______ / ______
joint CV visual examination

2.

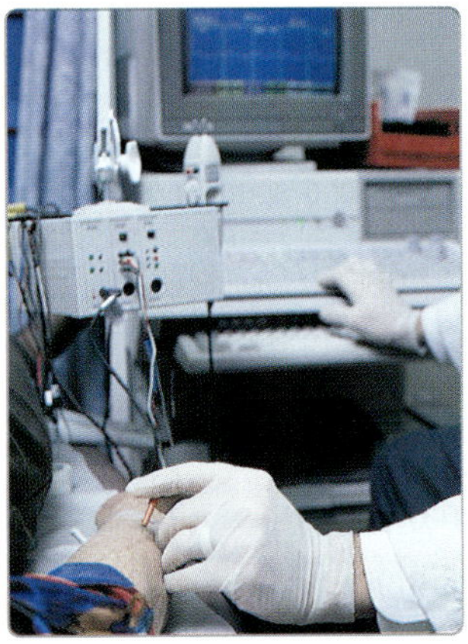

______ / ____ / ______ / ____ / ______
electrical activity CV muscle CV record

EXERCISE 20 ■ Diagnostic Terms *NOT* Built from Word Parts

A Match

Select the term described. Answers may be used more than once.

_____ 1. often used with DXA
_____ 2. also called bone density test
_____ 3. used to assess musculoskeletal abnormalities involving weakness or pain
_____ 4. collects a sample using a needle or small incision
_____ 5. determines the rate of bone turnover
_____ 6. measures bone loss and bone mineral density

a. dual x-ray absorptiometry
b. bone markers
c. muscle biopsy

B Label

Write the medical terms pictured and defined.

1. ____________________
radiographic imaging, usually of the lumbar spine and hips, to measure bone loss and bone mineral density

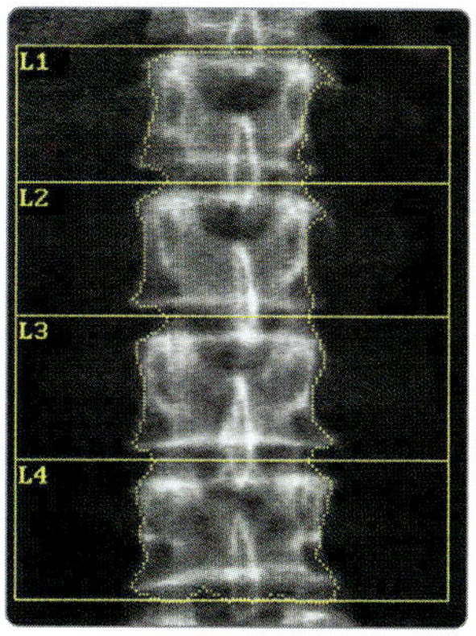

2. ____________________
removal of muscle tissue using a needle or small incision used to assess musculoskeletal abnormalities involving weakness or pain

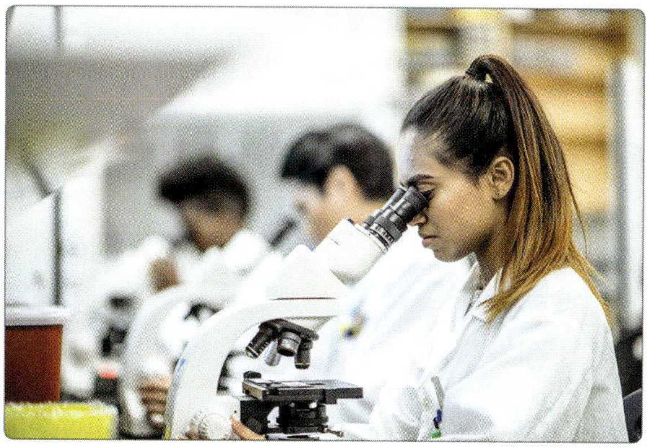

3. ____________________
blood and urine tests to determine the rate of bone turnover (resorption and formation)

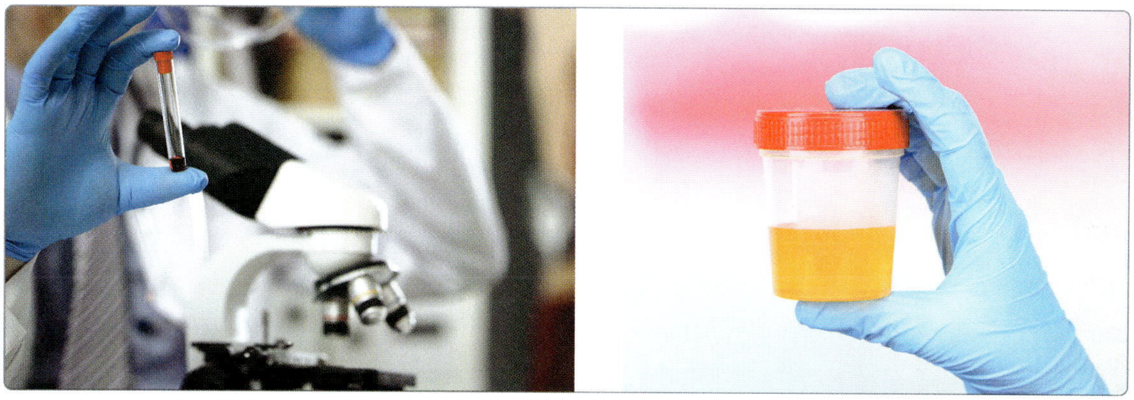

EXERCISE 21 ■ Review of Diagnostic Terms

Can you define, pronounce, and spell the following terms?

arthrography
arthroscopy
bone markers
dual x-ray absorptiometry (DXA)
electromyogram (EMG)
muscle biopsy
myelography

Complementary Terms

BUILT FROM WORD PARTS

The following terms can be translated using definitions of word parts. Further explanation is provided within parentheses as needed.

SIGNS AND SYMPTOMS

TERM	DEFINITION
1. arthralgia (ar-THRAL-ja)	joint pain
2. atrophy (AT-ro-fē)	without development (process of wasting away)
3. bradykinesia (*brad*-ē-ki-NĒ-zha)	slow movement
4. dyskinesia (*dis*-ki-NĒ-zha)	difficult movement
5. dystrophy (DIS-tro-fē)	abnormal development
6. hemarthrosis (*hē*-mar-THRŌ-sis)	abnormal condition of blood in the joint
7. hyperkinesia (*hī*-per-ki-NĒ-zha)	excessive movement (hyperactive)
8. hypertrophy (hī-PER-tro-fē)	excessive development
9. myalgia (mī-AL-ja)	muscle pain

MOVEMENT DISORDERS are impairments in voluntary movement and are also known as **dyskinesias**. **Bradykinesia** is characterized by slowness of all voluntary movement and speech, while **hyperkinesia** describes excessive or involuntary movements. Parkinson disease and Tourette syndrome are some examples of movement disorders.

DESCRIPTIVE TERMS

TERM	DEFINITION
10. carpal (CAR-pal)	pertaining to the carpals (wrist)
11. clavicular (kla-VIK-ū-lar)	pertaining to the clavicle (collarbone)
12. cranial (KRĀ-nē-al)	pertaining to the cranium (skull)
13. femoral (FEM-or-al)	pertaining to the femur (upper leg bone)
14. fibular (FIB-ū-lar)	pertaining to the fibula (lower leg bone)
15. humeral (HŪ-mer-al)	pertaining to the humerus (upper arm bone)
16. iliac (IL-ē-ak)	pertaining to the ilium (upper winged-shaped portion of the pelvis)
17. intercostal (*in*-ter-KOS-tal)	pertaining to between the ribs
18. intervertebral (*in*-ter-VER-te-bral)	pertaining to between the vertebrae
19. intracranial (*in*-tra-KRĀ-nē-al)	pertaining to within the cranium (skull)
20. ischial (IS-kē-al)	pertaining to the ischium (lower posterior portion of the pelvis)
21. lumbar (LUM-bar)	pertaining to the loins (the part of the back between the thorax and pelvis)
22. patellar (pa-TEL-lar)	pertaining to the patella (kneecap)
23. patellofemoral (pa-*tel*-ō-FEM-or-al))	pertaining to the patella and femur
24. phalangeal (fa-LAN-jē-al)	pertaining to the phalanx (*pl.* phalanges) (any bone of the fingers or toes)
25. pubic (PŪ-bik)	pertaining to the pubis (anterior portion of the pelvis)
26. radial (RĀ-dē-al)	pertaining to the radius (lower arm bone)
27. sacral (SĀ-kral)	pertaining to the sacrum (lower portion of the spine forming the posterior pelvic wall)
28. scapular (SKAP-ū-lar)	pertaining to the scapula (shoulder blade)
29. sternal (STER-nal)	pertaining to the sternum (breastbone)

TERM	DEFINITION	TERM	DEFINITION
30. submandibular (*sub*-man-DIB-ū-lar)	pertaining to below the mandible (lower jaw bone)	**35. tarsal** (TAR-sal)	pertaining to the tarsals (ankle bones)
31. submaxillary (sub-MAK-si-*lar*-ē)	pertaining to below the maxilla (upper jaw bone)	**36. tibial** (TIB-ē-al)	pertaining to the tibia (lower leg bone)
32. substernal (sub-STER-nal)	pertaining to under the sternum (breastbone)	**37. ulnar** (UL-nar)	pertaining to the ulna (lower arm bone)
33. supraclavicular (*sū*-pra-kla-VIK-ū-lar)	pertaining to above the clavicle (collarbone)	**38. vertebral** (VER-te-bral), (ver-TĒ-bral)	pertaining to the vertebrae
34. suprapatellar (*sū*-pra-pa-TEL-ar)	pertaining to above the patella (kneecap)		

EXERCISE 22 ■ Pronounce and Spell

Practice pronunciation and spelling on paper and online.

1. Practice on Paper

a. **Pronounce:** Read the phonetic spelling and say aloud the terms listed in the previous table. Refer to the pronunciation key on p. 20 as necessary.

b. **Spell:** Have a study partner read the terms aloud. Write the spelling of the terms on a separate sheet of paper.

2. Practice Online

a. **Access** online learning resources. Go to evolve.elsevier.com > Evolve Resources > Student Resources.

b. **Pronounce:** Select Audio Glossary > Chapter 14 > Exercise 22. Select a term to hear its pronunciation and repeat aloud.

c. **Spell:** Select Activities > Chapter 14 > Spell Terms > Exercise 22. Select the audio icon and type the correct spelling of the term.

❑ Check the box when complete.

EXERCISE 23 ■ Analyze and Define

Analyze and define the following complementary terms describing signs and symptoms.

1. myalgia

____

____

2. arthralgia

____

____

3. hypertrophy

____

____

4. atrophy

____

____

5. hyperkinesia

6. dyskinesia

7. bradykinesia

8. hemarthrosis

9. dystrophy

EXERCISE 24 ■ Build

A Fill In

Build complementary descriptive terms for the following definitions by using the word parts you have learned.

1. pertaining to above the collarbone ____ / ____ / ____ (P / WR / S)
2. pertaining to above the kneecap ____ / ____ / ____ (P / WR / S)
3. pertaining to between the vertebrae ____ / ____ / ____ (P / WR / S)
4. pertaining to below the upper jaw bone ____ / ____ / ____ (P / WR / S)
5. pertaining to below the lower jaw bone ____ / ____ / ____ (P / WR / S)
6. pertaining to under the breastbone ____ / ____ / ____ (P / WR / S)
7. pertaining to within the cranium ____ / ____ / ____ (P / WR / S)
8. pertaining to between the ribs ____ / ____ / ____ (P / WR / S)
9. pertaining to the patella and femur ____ / ____ / ____ / ____ (WR / CV / WR / S)

B Label

Build terms for the following definitions. Write the corresponding word parts above the abbreviations as shown in number 1.

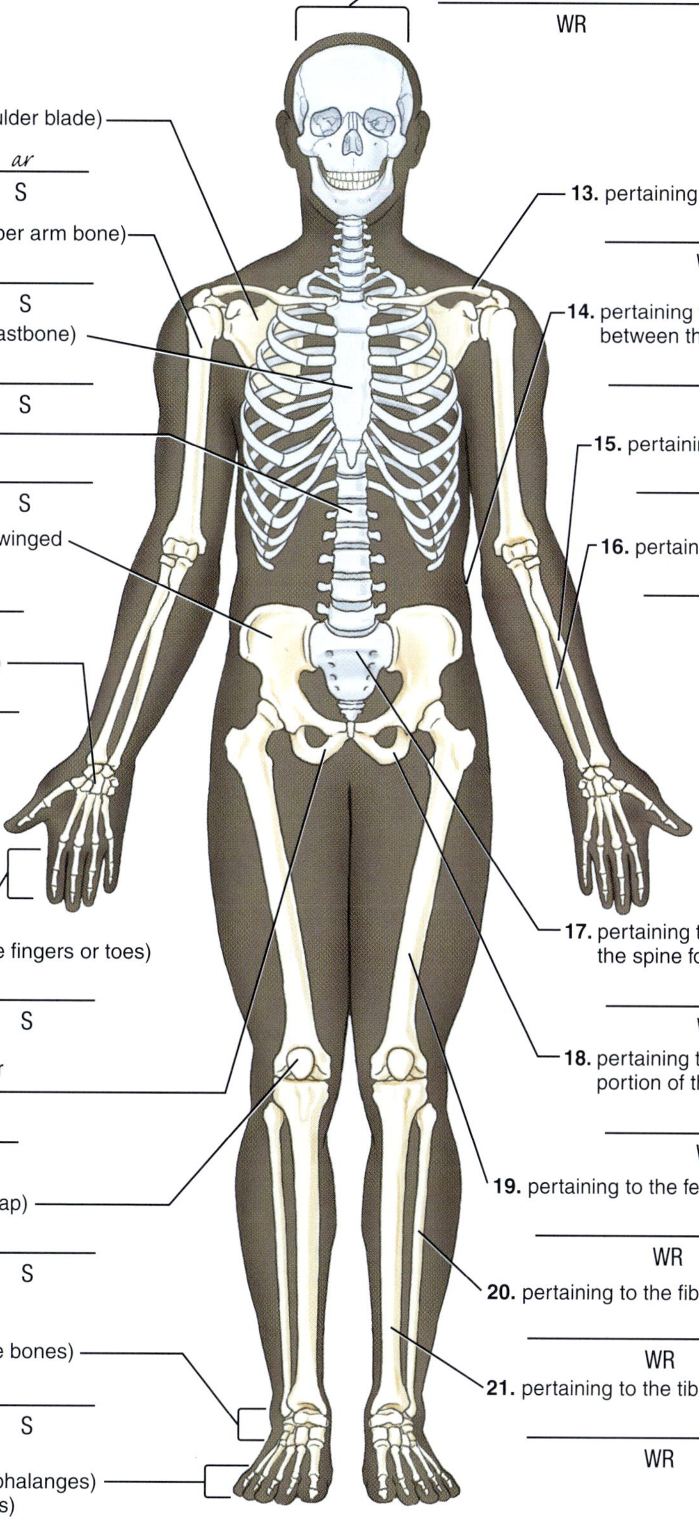

1. pertaining to the scapula (shoulder blade)

scapul / *ar*
WR S

2. pertaining to the humerus (upper arm bone)

______ / ______
WR S

3. pertaining to the sternum (breastbone)

______ / ______
WR S

4. pertaining to the vertebrae

______ / ______
WR S

5. pertaining to the ilium (upper winged shaped portion of the pelvis)

______ / ______
WR S

6. pertaining to the carpals (wrist)

______ / ______
WR S

7. pertaining to the phalanx (*pl.* phalanges) (any bone of the fingers or toes)

______ / ______
WR S

8. pertaining to the pubis (anterior portion of the pelvis)

______ / ______
WR S

9. pertaining to the patella (kneecap)

______ / ______
WR S

10. pertaining to the tarsals (ankle bones)

______ / ______
WR S

11. pertaining to the phalanx (*pl.* phalanges) (any bone of the fingers or toes)

______ / ______
WR S

12. pertaining to the cranium (skull)

______ / ______
WR S

13. pertaining to the clavicle (collarbone)

______ / ______
WR S

14. pertaining to the loins (the part of the back between the thorax and pelvis)

______ / ______
WR S

15. pertaining to the radius (lower arm bone)

______ / ______
WR S

16. pertaining to the ulna (lower arm bone)

______ / ______
WR S

17. pertaining to the sacrum (lower portion of the spine forming the posterior pelvic wall)

______ / ______
WR S

18. pertaining to the ischium (lower posterior portion of the pelvis)

______ / ______
WR S

19. pertaining to the femur (upper leg bone)

______ / ______
WR S

20. pertaining to the fibula (lower leg bone)

______ / ______
WR S

21. pertaining to the tibia (lower leg bone)

______ / ______
WR S

Complementary Terms

NOT BUILT FROM WORD PARTS

Word parts may be present in the following terms; however, their full meanings cannot be translated using definitions of word parts alone.

SIGNS & SYMPTOMS

TERM	DEFINITION
1. **crepitus** (KREP-i-tus)	crackling sensation heard or felt when two bones rub against each other or grating caused by the rubbing together of dry surfaces of a joint (also called **crepitation**)

CREPITUS is also used to describe the crackling sounds heard during auscultation of the lungs (with a stethoscope) in patients with pneumonia.

EQUIPMENT

TERM	DEFINITION
2. **prosthesis (*pl.* prostheses)** (pros-THĒ-sis), (pros-THĒ-sēz)	artificial substitute for a missing body part such as a limb, joint, or eye

MEDICAL SPECIALTIES

TERM	DEFINITION
3. **chiropractic** (*kī*-rō-PRAK-tik)	system of treatment that consists of manipulation of the vertebral column
4. **chiropractor (DC)** (KĪ-rō-*prak*-tor)	specialist in manipulation of the vertebral column (chiropractic)
5. **orthopedics (Ortho)** (*or*-thō-PĒ-diks)	branch of medicine dealing with the study and treatment of diseases and abnormalities of the musculoskeletal system
6. **orthopedist** (*or*-thō-PĒ-dist)	physician who specializes in the study and treatment of diseases and abnormalities of the musculoskeletal system
7. **orthotics** (or-THOT-iks)	making and fitting of orthopedic appliances used to support, align, prevent, or treat musculoskeletal deformities; examples of appliances include braces, splints, and arch supports
8. **orthotist** (or-THOT-ist)	specialist in making and fitting appliances used to support, align, prevent or treat musculoskeletal deformities
ORTHOSIS the Greek word meaning **make straight** refers to the orthopedic appliance. The plural form is orthoses.	
9. **osteopath (DO)** (OS-tē-ō-*path*)	physician who specializes in a system of medicine placing emphasis on the relation between organs and the musculoskeletal system (osteopathy)
10. **osteopathy** (*os*-tē-OP-a-thē)	system of medicine that uses the usual forms of diagnosis and treatment but places greater emphasis on the relation between body organs and the musculoskeletal system; manipulation may be used in addition to other treatments
11. **podiatrist** (pō-DĪ-a-trist)	specialist in treating and diagnosing diseases and disorders of the foot, including medical and surgical treatment
12. **rheumatologist** (*roo*-ma-TOL-ō-jist)	physician who specializes in the study and treatment of musculoskeletal disorders characterized by inflammation and degeneration of structures (rheumatic diseases)
13. **rheumatology** (*roo*-ma-TOL-ō-jē)	study and treatment of musculoskeletal disorders characterized by inflammation and degeneration of structures (rheumatic diseases)

RHEUMATOLOGY AND ORTHOPEDICS: WHAT IS THE DIFFERENCE? While both medical specialties focus on the diagnosis and treatment of disease and disorders of the musculoskeletal system, **rheumatology** focuses on medical management for chronic conditions while **orthopedics** focuses on surgical treatment for acute or chronic conditions. For example, a patient with **rheumatoid arthritis** would see a **rheumatologist** for medications to manage symptoms of the disease and would be referred to an **orthopedist** if joint replacement surgery was warranted.

TYPES OF BODY MOVEMENT (FIG. 14.14)	
TERM	**DEFINITION**
14. abduction (ab-DUK-shun)	moving away from the midline
15. adduction (ad-DUK-shun)	moving toward the midline
16. inversion (in-VER-zhun)	turning inward
17. eversion (ē-VER-zhun)	turning outward
18. extension (ek-STEN-shun)	movement in which a limb is placed in a straight position, increasing the angle between the bone and the joint
19. flexion (FLEK-shun)	movement in which a limb is bent, decreasing the angle between the bone and the joint
20. pronation (prō-NĀ-shun)	movement that turns the palm down
21. supination (*sū*-pi-NĀ-shun)	movement that turns the palm up
22. rotation (rō-TĀ-shun)	turning around its own axis

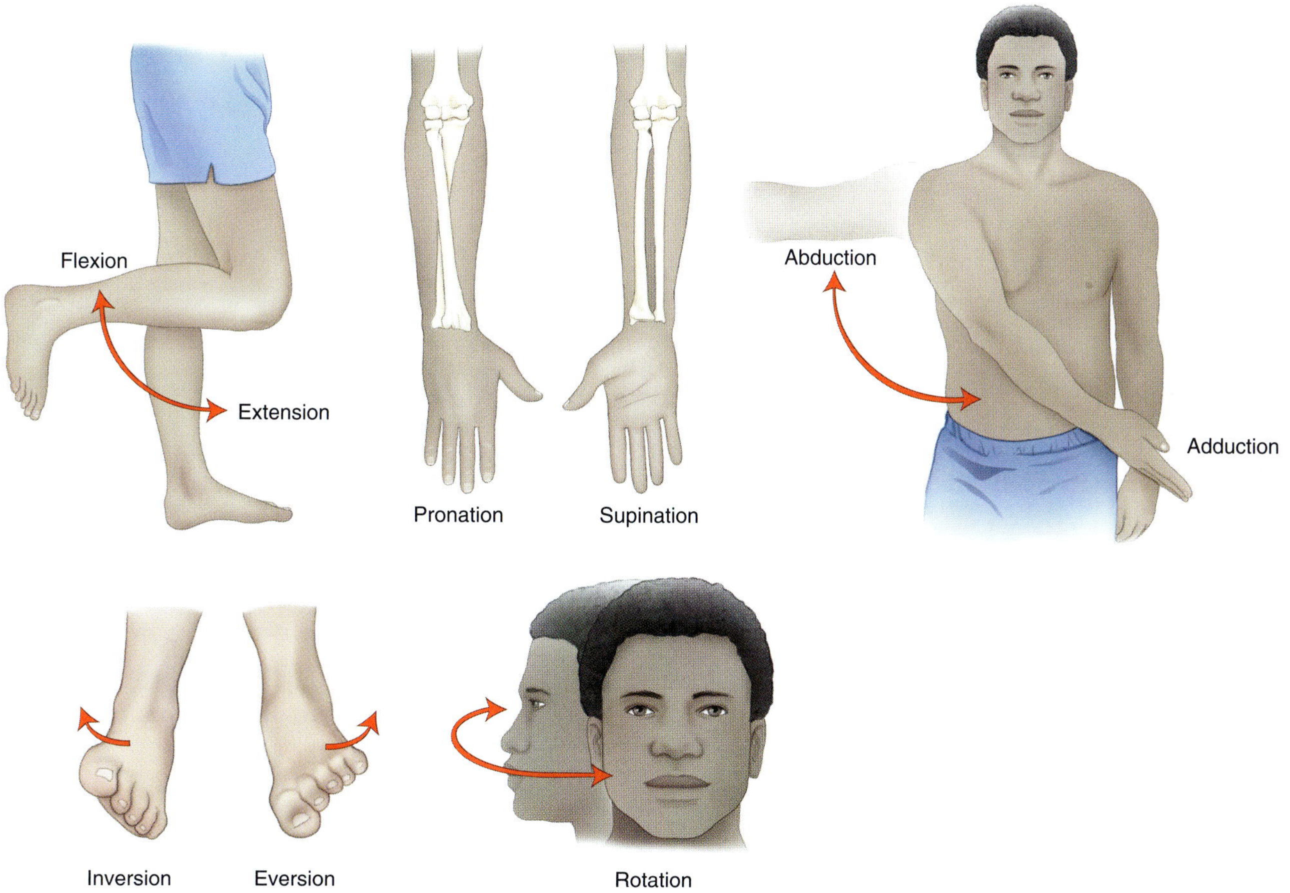

FIG. 14.14 Types of body movements.

MIDLINE VS. MIDDLE The two terms are synonyms, both describing an imaginary line that separates the body, or body part, into equal halves. In medical language, *midline* is the preferred term and is used as a common reference point.

Refer to **Appendix E** for pharmacology terms related to the musculoskeletal system.

EXERCISE 25 ■ Pronounce and Spell

Practice pronunciation and spelling on paper and online.

1. Practice on Paper

a. **Pronounce:** Read the phonetic spelling and say aloud the terms listed in the previous table. Refer to the pronunciation key on p. 20 as necessary.
b. **Spell:** Have a study partner read the terms aloud. Write the spelling of the terms on a separate sheet of paper.

2. Practice Online

a. **Access** online learning resources. Go to evolve.elsevier.com > Evolve Resources > Student Resources.
b. **Pronounce:** Select Audio Glossary > Chapter 14 > Exercise 25. Select a term to hear its pronunciation and repeat aloud.
c. **Spell:** Select Activities > Chapter 14 > Spell Terms > Exercise 25. Select the audio icon and type the correct spelling of the term.

❑ Check the box when complete.

EXERCISE 26 ■ Fill In

A Identify

Fill in the blanks with the correct terms.

1. The study and treatment of musculoskeletal disorders characterized by inflammation and degeneration of structures is the medical specialty called ______________________________.
2. The making and fitting of appliances used to support, align, prevent, or treat musculoskeletal deformities (examples include braces, splints, and arch supports) is called __________________________.
3. The crackling sensation heard or felt when two bones rub against each other or grating caused by the rubbing together of dry surfaces of a joint is called __________________________.
4. The system of treatment that consists of manipulation of the vertebral column is called ______________________.
5. The branch of medicine dealing with the study and treatment of diseases and abnormalities of the musculoskeletal system is called ____.
6. The system of medicine that uses the usual forms of diagnosis and treatment, considers the relation between body organs and the musculoskeletal system, and may use manipulation of the musculoskeletal system in addition to other treatments is called ______________________.
7. An artificial substitute for a missing body part such as limb, joint, or eye is called a ____________________________.

B Label

Write the medical terms pictured and defined.

1. ______________________________
physician who specializes in the study and treatment of diseases and abnormalities of the musculoskeletal system

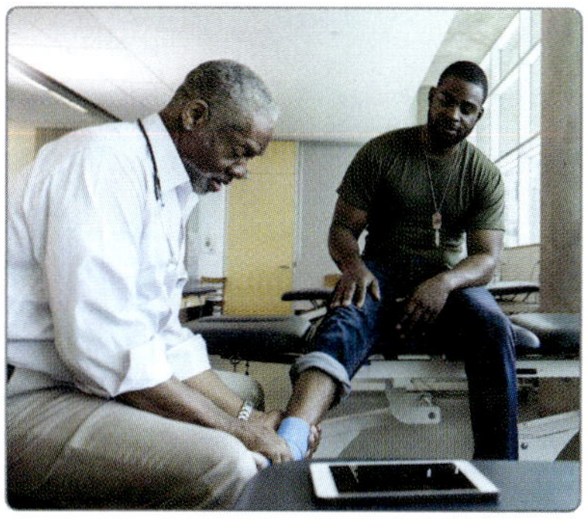

2. ______________________________
physician who specializes in the study and treatment of musculoskeletal disorders characterized by inflammation and degeneration of structures

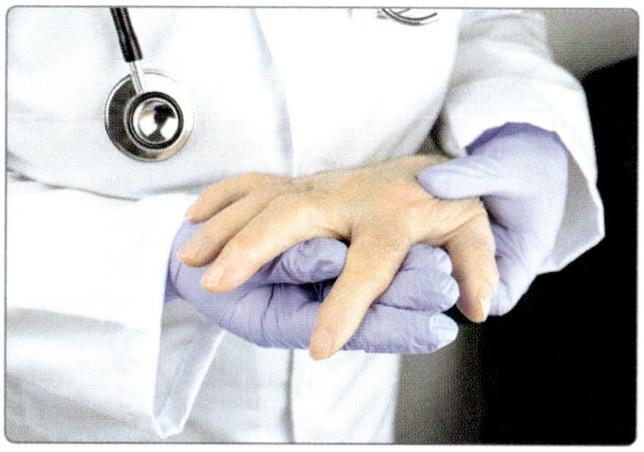

3. ______________________________
specialist in treating and diagnosing diseases and disorders of the foot, including medical and surgical treatment

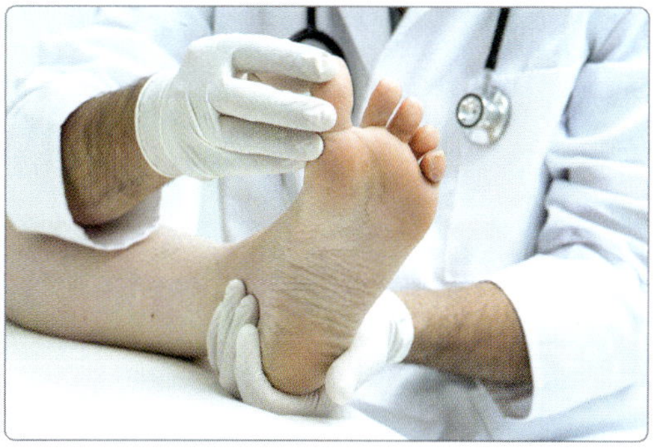

4. ______________________________
specialist in making and fitting appliances used to support, align, prevent or treat musculoskeletal deformities

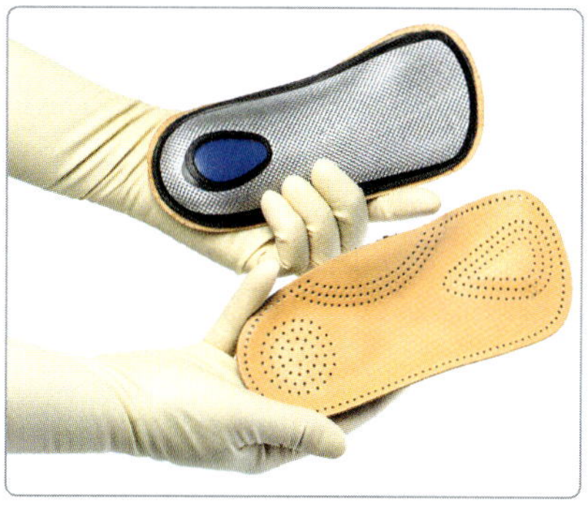

5. ______________________________
specialist in the manipulation of the vertebral column

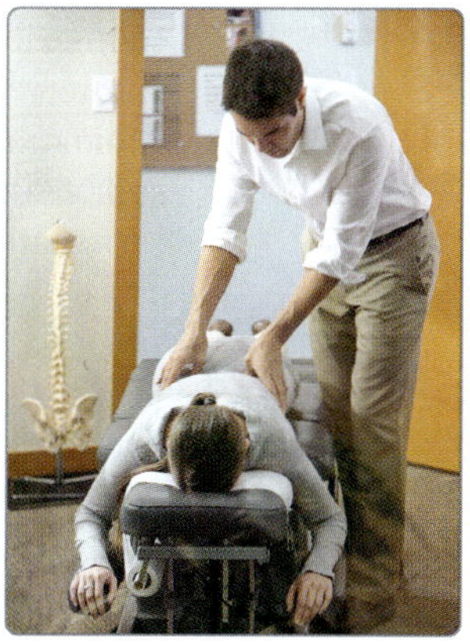

6. ______________________________
physician specializing in a system of medicine placing emphasis on the relation between organs and the musculoskeletal system; manipulation may be used in addition to other treatments

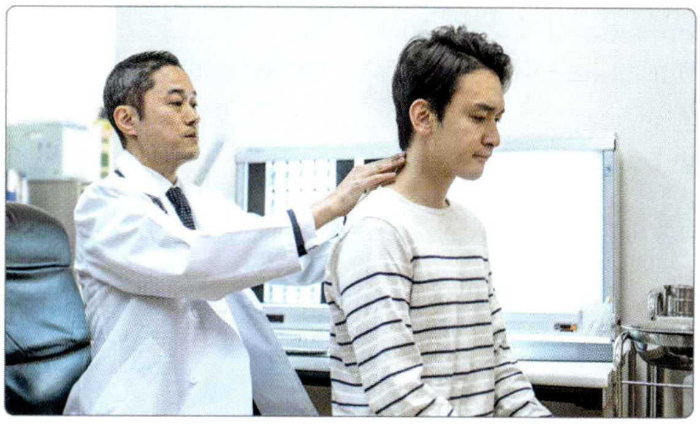

EXERCISE 27 ▪ Match

Match the descriptions in the first column with the correct terms in the second column.

_____ 1. replaces a body part
_____ 2. the making of supports for body parts responsible for motion
_____ 3. manages the treatment of RA
_____ 4. performs joint replacement surgery
_____ 5. performs foot surgery
_____ 6. physician trained in manipulation of the musculoskeletal system as well as allopathic treatment and diagnosis
_____ 7. trained in the manipulation of the vertebral column and is not a physician
_____ 8. crackling sensation or sound

a. rheumatologist
b. chiropractor
c. osteopath
d. prosthesis
e. crepitus
f. orthopedist
g. podiatrist
h. orthotics

EXERCISE 28 ▪ Types of Body Movement

Match the terms in the first column with their correct definitions in the second column.

_____ 1. abduction
_____ 2. adduction
_____ 3. pronation
_____ 4. rotation
_____ 5. eversion
_____ 6. extension
_____ 7. flexion
_____ 8. inversion
_____ 9. supination

a. movement in which a limb is placed in a straight position
b. movement that turns the palm up
c. turning outward
d. moving toward the midline
e. turning around its own axis
f. turning inward
g. movement in which a limb is bent
h. moving away from the midline
i. movement that turns the palm down

EXERCISE 29 ▪ Review of Complementary Terms

Can you define, pronounce, and spell the following terms?

abduction
adduction
arthralgia
atrophy
bradykinesia
carpal
chiropractic
chiropractor (DC)
clavicular
cranial
crepitus
dyskinesia
dystrophy
eversion
extension
femoral
fibular
flexion
hemarthrosis
humeral
hyperkinesia
hypertrophy
iliac
intercostal
intervertebral
intracranial
inversion
ischial
lumbar
myalgia
orthopedics (Ortho)
orthopedist
orthotics
orthotist
osteopath (DO)
osteopathy
patellar
patellofemoral
phalangeal
podiatrist
pronation
prosthesis
(*pl.* prostheses)
pubic
radial
rheumatologist
rheumatology
rotation
sacral
scapular
sternal
submandibular
submaxillary
substernal
supination
supraclavicular
suprapatellar
tarsal
tibial
ulnar
vertebral

Abbreviations

DISEASE AND DISORDER

ABBREVIATION	TERM	ABBREVIATION	TERM
CTS	carpal tunnel syndrome	**OA**	osteoarthritis
fx	fracture	**PM**	polymyositis
HNP	herniated nucleus pulposus	**RA**	rheumatoid arthritis
MD	muscular dystrophy	**RSI**	repetitive strain injury
MG	myasthenia gravis		

DIAGNOSTIC

ABBREVIATION	TERM	ABBREVIATION	TERM
DEXA	dual-energy x-ray absorptiometry (bone density test)	**DEXA AND DXA** are spoken as a whole word and pronounced as (de-ksa).	
DXA	dual x-ray absorptiometry (bone density test)	**EMG**	electromyogram

TREATMENT

ABBREVIATION	TERM	ABBREVIATION	TERM
THA	total hip arthroplasty	**TKA**	total knee arthroplasty

MEDICAL SPECIALTIES

ABBREVIATION	TERM	ABBREVIATION	TERM
DC	Doctor of Chiropractic	**Ortho**	orthopedics
DO	Doctor of Osteopathy		

DESCRIPTIVE

ABBREVIATION	TERM	ABBREVIATION	TERM
C1-C7	cervical vertebrae	**T1-T12**	thoracic vertebrae
L1-L5	lumbar vertebrae		

Refer to **Appendix D** for a complete list of abbreviations.

EXERCISE 30 ■ Abbreviations

Write the terms abbreviated.

1. Vertebrae make up the bones of the spinal column. **C1 to C7** ____________ ____________ are the first set that form the neck. The second set **T1 to T12** ____________ ____________ articulate with the 12 pairs of ribs that form the outward curve of the spine. **L1 to L5** ____________ ____________, the third set, are larger and form the inward curve of the spine.
2. Patients with **RA** ____________ ____________ may experience muscle atrophy and weakness because of inactivity.
3. Water exercise or gentle movement, such as Tai Chi, is recommended for many patients with **OA** ________________________, the most common joint disease.
4. **MG** ____________ ____________ most often affects women and the onset occurs at any age. It is an acquired autoimmune disorder.

5. **EMG** ______________________ is used to evaluate patients with localized or diffuse muscle weakness, such as **PM** ______________________.
6. **CTS** __________ __________ __________ is a common condition in which, for various reasons, the median nerve in the wrist becomes compressed, causing numbness and pain. A patient with symptoms of CTS that didn't improve with splints and physical therapy might be referred to **Ortho** ______________ for possible surgery.
7. Nine types of **MD** __________ __________ have been identified. Because symptoms of the disease are similar to other muscular disorders, diagnosis is often difficult.
8. **HNP** __________ __________ __________ may also be referred to as slipped disk, ruptured disk, or herniated intervertebral disk.
9. **THA** __________ __________ __________ is used to treat severe osteoarthritis of the hip joints.
10. Taking a holistic view of medicine, the **DO** __________ ______ ______________ evaluates the patient's musculoskeletal system in relation to overall health.
11. Knee replacement surgery, also called **TKA** __________ __________ ______________, is used in patients that have disabling pain due to arthritis.
12. Movements performed over and over again may lead to **RSI**, __________ __________ ______________, the cumulative damage to a joint, muscle, or other tissue.
13. Various **fx** ______________ types describe the nature of the break and include transverse, spiral, oblique, comminuted, and compression.
14. **DXA** ______________ __________ ______________ and **DEXA** ______________ ______________ __________ name the same diagnostic procedure measuring bone loss and bone mineral density.
15. A **DC** ______________ __ __________ is not a medical doctor, but has received graduate-level training in the treatment of some musculoskeletal disorders with a primary focus on pain reduction.

PRACTICAL APPLICATION

EXERCISE 31 ■ Case Study: Translate Between Everyday Language and Medical Language

CASE STUDY: Shanti Mehra

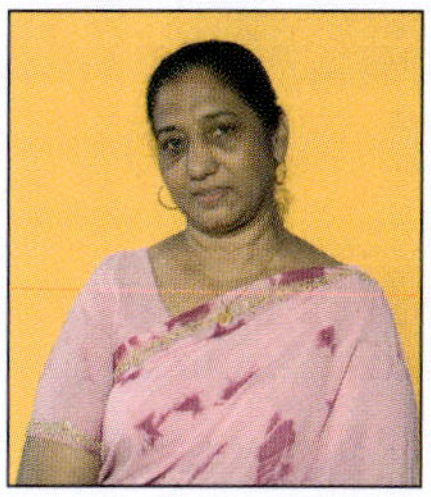

Shanti Mehra was walking to the store to buy more cigarettes. It was cold and icy and unfortunately, she slipped on some ice on the pavement. Her hand and wrist buckled under her when she fell. Now she is worried she may have broken some finger or wrist bones. She goes to the emergency department and an x-ray is done. She is told that she has broken one of her lower arm bones and is referred to a musculoskeletal specialist. She is also told that her bones are not dense enough and that she needs to have additional tests done.

Now that you have worked through Chapter 14, consider the medical terms that might be used to describe Mrs. Mehra's experience. See the Chapter at a Glance Section at the end of the chapter for a list of terms that might apply.

A. *Underline phrases in the case study that could be substituted with medical terms.*

B. *Write the medical term and its definition for three of the phrases you underlined.*

MEDICAL TERM	DEFINITION
1. ______________	______________
2. ______________	______________
3. ______________	______________

DOCUMENTATION: Excerpt from Orthopedic Clinic Visit

Mrs. Mehra made an appointment with an orthopedist; a portion of the report is documented below.

Progress Note

Physical Examination: *She has prominent dorsal kyphosis in the thoracic vertebral column. AP and lateral radiographs of the right wrist reveal a distal radial fracture. Her bones show evidence of osteoporosis.*

Assessment and Plan: *A DXA test is recommended to assess bone mineral density. She was advised to continue immobilization of the radio-carpal joint for at least 4 weeks.*

C. *Underline medical terms presented in Chapter 14 used in the previous excerpt from Mrs. Mehra's medical record. See the Chapter at a Glance Section at the end of the chapter for a complete list.*

D. *Select and define three of the medical terms you underlined. To check your answers, go to Appendix A.*

MEDICAL TERM	DEFINITION
1. ______________	______________
2. ______________	______________
3. ______________	______________

EXERCISE 32 ■ Interact With Medical Documents

A

Read the report and complete it by writing medical terms on answer lines within the document. Definitions of terms to be written appear after the document.

10003-MKL McBRIDE, William

File Patient Navigate Custom Fields Help

Chart Review | Encounters | Notes | Labs | Imaging | Procedures | Rx | Documents | Referrals | Scheduling | Billing

Name: **McBRIDE, William** MR#: **10003-MKL** DOB: 12/04/19XX Gender: M Age: 55 **Allergies:** Penicillin, Promethazine **PCP:** Annie Morocco, MD

Operative Report:

History: William McBride is a 55-year-old male who reports pain in his left knee when walking and golfing. He states that his knees have "been painful" for many years since he quit playing semiprofessional hockey, but the pain has become much more severe in the last 6 months. He was admitted to the Medical Center's Outpatient 1.________________ Center for an 2.____________________ of his left knee.

Preoperative Diagnosis: Degenerative 3. __________________ of the left knee, with possible tear of the 4. _________________ meniscus.

Operative Report: After induction of spinal anesthetic, the patient was positioned on the operating table, and a tourniquet was applied over the upper left thigh. After positioning the leg in a circumferential holder, the end of the table was flexed to allow the leg to hang freely. The patient's left leg was prepped and draped in the usual manner. After exsanguination of the leg with an Esmarch bandage, the tourniquet was inflated to 300 mm Hg. The knee was inspected by anterolateral and anteromedial parapatellar portholes.

Findings: The synovium in the 5. _______________________ pouch showed moderate to severe inflammatory changes with villi formation and hyperemia. The undersurface of the patella showed loss of normal articular cartilage on the lateral patellar facet with exposed bone in that area and moderate to severe 6. _____________________________ of the medial facet. Similar changes were noted in the intercondylar groove. In the medial compartment, the patient had smooth articular cartilage on the femur and moderate chondromalacia of the tibial plateau. The medial meniscus appeared normal with no evidence of tears and a smooth articular surface on the femoral condyle. No additional 7. _______________________ was identified.

The tourniquet was then released and the knee flushed with lactated Ringer solution until the bleeding slowed. The wounds were Steri-Stripped closed, a sterile bandage with an external Ace wrap applied, and the patient returned to the postoperative recovery area in stable condition. The patient tolerated the procedure well.

Postoperative Diagnosis: Degenerative arthritis with mild chondromalacia of the left knee.

Electronically signed: Martin Spencer, DO 02/13/20XX 07:59

Start | Log On/Off | Print | Edit

Definitions of Medical Terms to Complete the Document

Write the medical terms defined on corresponding answer lines in the document.

1. branch of medicine dealing with the study and treatment of diseases and abnormalities of the musculoskeletal system
2. visual examination of a joint
3. inflammation of a joint
4. toward the middle or midline
5. pertaining to above the patella
6. softening of cartilage
7. study of (body changes caused by) disease

B

Read the medical report and answer the questions below it.

011107 TAFT, Grace

File Patient Navigate Custom Fields Help

Chart Review | Encounters | Notes | Labs | Imaging | Procedures | Rx | Documents | Referrals | Scheduling | Billing

Name: **TAFT, Grace** MR#: 011107 DOB: 10/17/19xx Gender: F **Allergies: Penicillin** **PCP:** Gidget Thomas, APRN

RHEUMATOLOGY CLINIC NOTE
ENCOUNTER DATE: 04/02/20XX

HISTORY: This 61-year-old female is being seen today for follow up of her rheumatoid arthritis. She is taking methotrexate with some relief but continues to have pain and swelling in her fingers and toes. She is also noticing some pain in both wrists, with numbness along the distribution of the medial nerve.

PHYSICAL EXAMINATION: The patient is 5'5" tall and weighs 117 pounds. Examination of the hands reveals deviation of the phalanges to the ulnar side, with rheumatoid nodules noted over the metacarpophalangeal joints bilaterally. There is also carpal tenderness and warmth.

Impression: Progressive rheumatoid arthritis with arthralgia at the phalangeal, carpal, and ulnoradial joints bilaterally.

Plan: Consider adding a short course of steroids to help with this most recent flare of rheumatoid arthritis. CTS splints for night time use. A synovectomy may be required if symptoms worsen or do not improve.

Start | Log On/Off | Print | Edit

Use the medical report above to answer the questions.

1. Pain and numbness in the wrist with compression of the medial nerve could indicate
   a. ankylosing spondylitis
   b. gout
   c. carpal tunnel syndrome
   d. plantar fasciitis

2. The patient is exhibiting tenderness and warmth over the
   a. ankles
   b. wrists
   c. elbows
   d. knees

EXERCISE 33 ■ Use Medical Language in Online Electronic Health Records

Select the correct medical terms to complete three medical records in one patient's electronic file.

Access online resources at evolve.elsevier.com > Evolve Resources > Student Resources > Activities > Chapter 14 > Electronic Health Records

Topic: Fracture, Parkinson Disease
Record 1: Admission Note
Record 2: Radiology Report
Record 3: Neurology Consultation

❏ Check the box when complete.

EXERCISE 34 ■ Pronounce Medical Terms in Use

Practice pronunciation of terms by reading aloud the following sentences. Use the phonetic spellings to assist with pronunciation. The script also contains medical terms not presented in the chapter. If interested, research their meanings in a medical dictionary or a reliable online source.

1. The **orthopedist** (or-thō-PĒ-dist) recommended Mr. Shah have an **arthrodesis** (*ar*-thrō-DĒ-sis) to reduce pain caused from an ankle **fracture** (FRAK-chur) he sustained several years ago.
2. Mrs. Diaz severed a tendon by accidentally walking through a glass patio door. A **tenorrhaphy** (te-NOR-a-fē) was performed to repair the tendon.
3. An **electromyogram** (e-*lek*-trō-MĪ-ō-gram) can assist the physician in diagnosing **muscular dystrophy** (MUS-kū-lar) (DIS-trō-fē). **Atrophy** (AT-rō-fē) frequently occurs in patients with this disease.
4. Adjective forms of medical terms are used by health professionals to indicate areas of the body that describe anatomic locations, areas of pain, sites of injections, locations of lesions, and so forth. Below are some examples.
   a. **cranial** (KRĀ-nē-al) laceration
   b. **intercostal** (*in*-ter-KOS-tal) muscles
   c. pain in the **supraclavicular** (*sū*-pra-kla-VIK-ū-lar) region
   d. herniation of an **intervertebral** (*in*-ter-VER-te-bral) disk
   e. **intracranial** (*in*-tra-KRĀ-nē-al) pressure
   f. **femoral** (FEM-or-al) artery
   g. strain of the **patellofemoral** (pa-*tel*-ō-FEM-or-al) ligament
   h. degenerative disease of the **vertebral** (ver-TĒ-bral) joints

EXERCISE 35 ■ Use Plural Endings

Circle the correct singular or plural term to match the context of the sentence.

1. The (**epiphysis, epiphyses**) are the enlarged ends of the long bone.
2. The distal (**phalanx, phalanges**) of the ring finger was fractured.
3. Osteoporosis was present in four lumbar (**vertebrae, vertebra**).
4. A (**prosthesis, prostheses**) was implanted in the left hip.
5. Many synovial joints contain (**bursa, bursae**).
6. Two (**lamina, laminae**) make up the vertebral arch in a single vertebrae.

CHAPTER REVIEW

EXERCISE 36 ■ Chapter Content Quiz

Test your understanding of terms and abbreviations introduced in this chapter. Circle the letter for the medical term or abbreviation related to the words in italics.

1. Jessie Steinbach was diagnosed with *an infection caused by a bite from a deer tick infected with Borrelia burgdorferi*, after noting symptoms of fever, headache and joint pain. Her symptoms started after a camping trip last summer.
   a. rheumatoid arthritis
   b. Lyme disease
   c. rhabdomyolysis

2. Tommy John surgery, named after the first professional baseball player to have it performed, involves *suturing of a tendon* of the ulnar collateral ligament, usually with a graft from a different tendon in the body.
   a. tenomyoplasty
   b. myorrhaphy
   c. tenorrhaphy

3. Orthopedists may perform *visual examination of a joint* to diagnose and sometimes treat problems in the knee, shoulder, or elbow.
   a. arthroscopy
   b. arthrography
   c. arthrocentesis

4. Ever since his initial diagnosis of ankylosing spondylitis, James Montoya has been seeing a *physician who specializes in the study and treatment of rheumatic diseases*.
   a. podiatrist
   b. rheumatologist
   c. chiropractor

5. Dr. Lu ordered an electromyogram (EMG) for Mr. Borunda when he suspected *chronic disease characterized by muscle weakness and thought to be caused by a defect in the transmission of impulses from nerve to muscle*.
   a. muscular dystrophy
   b. meniscitis
   c. myasthenia gravis

6. A total hip *surgical repair of a joint* was recommended for Mrs. Jiang, when she could no longer tolerate the pain from her osteoarthritis.
   a. arthrodesis
   b. arthroplasty
   c. chondroplasty

7. Ayaz Ismail noticed ulnoradial pain whenever he was asked to put his forearm into *movement that turns the palm up*.
   a. pronation
   b. eversion
   c. supination

8. While training for the National Guard, Jayla experienced unusual achy, cramping pain in her lower legs that increased as she ran. She also felt a tingling sensation and noticed swelling in both legs. She was diagnosed with chronic exertional *condition caused by increased pressure within a muscle that can lead to ischemia* and fasciotomy was performed when nonsurgical treatments did not provide relief.
   a. repetitive strain injury
   b. myasthenia gravis
   c. compartment syndrome

9. A(n) *excision of a lamina* was performed on Mr. Lopez, who had been experiencing spinal stenosis for many years.
   a. laminectomy
   b. synovectomy
   c. vertebroplasty

10. Dawn Labenz met with a *specialist in making and fitting of appliances used to support, align, prevent, or treat musculoskeletal deformities* to have arch supports made for her shoes after experiencing plantar fasciitis for the second time.
    a. orthopedist
    b. osteopath
    c. orthotist

11. Mr. O'Rourke had a radiograph of his knee to determine how much *inflammation of the bone and joint* was present.
    a. OA
    b. RA
    c. DO

12. Mrs. Jerue developed *abnormal condition of bone death* of the jaw after a rather difficult tooth extraction.
    a. osteomalacia
    b. osteopetrosis
    c. osteonecrosis

13. Natalie Pageau experienced *pertaining to under the sternum* pain after eating; she was relieved to find indigestion to be the cause rather than angina.
    a. supraclavicular
    b. substernal
    c. submandibular

14. Mr. Sadowsky's symptoms of *slow movement* worsened as his Parkinson disease progressed.
    a. bradykinesia
    b. hyperkinesia
    c. hypertrophy

15. After his fall from a ladder, Adam Murphy had an emergency *incision into the cranium* to relieve intracranial pressure.
    a. cranioplasty
    b. craniotomy
    c. rachiotomy

16. Two-year-old Joshia presented to Urgent Care crying and refusing to use his left arm. Prior to the injury, his teenage brother was swinging him around in a circle holding both wrists. Examination revealed radial head *partial dislocation of bones in a joint*, which was quickly treated with a gentle maneuver to slip the bone back in place.
    a. subluxation
    b. hemarthrosis
    c. sprain

17. Mr. Cohen complained of chronic wrist *pain in the joint*. A plain radiograph showed soft tissue swelling along with erosions in the carpal bones. Arthrocentesis revealed monosodium urate crystals and confirmed the diagnosis of gout.
    a. atrophy
    b. arthralgia
    c. myalgia

18. An osteotomy or partial phalangectomy may be required during *abnormal prominence of the joint at the base of the great toe* surgery to realign the metatarsal-phalangeal joint.
    a. carpal tunnel syndrome
    b. exostosis
    c. bunion

19. Lily Chakraborty developed severe *abnormal condition of (lateral) curved (spine)* as a teen; a partial costectomy and other corrective surgery was performed with good results.
    a. scoliosis
    b. kyphosis
    c. lordosis

20. Dr. Nair advised Melanie Chua to increase her calcium and vitamin D intake after radiographs showed *abnormal reduction of bone mass* at the distal radial portion of her wrist.
    a. osteosarcoma
    b. osteopetrosis
    c. osteopenia

CHAPTER AT A GLANCE Word Parts New to This Chapter

COMBINING FORMS

ankyl/o
arthr/o
burs/o
carp/o
chondr/o
clavicul/o
cost/o
crani/o
disc/o
fasci/o
femor/o
fibul/o
humer/o
ili/o
ischi/o
kinesi/o
kyph/o
lamin/o
lord/o
lumb/o
mandibul/o
maxill/o
menisc/o
myos/o
oste/o
patell/o
petr/o
phalang/o
pub/o
rachi/o
radi/o
sacr/o
scapul/o
scoli/o
spondyl/o
stern/o
synovi/o
tars/o
ten/o
tendin/o
tibi/o
uln/o
vertebr/o

PREFIXES

inter-
supra-
syn-

SUFFIXES

-asthenia
-schisis
-trophy

CHAPTER AT A GLANCE Musculoskeletal System Terms Built From Word Parts

DISEASE AND DISORDER

ankylosis
arthritis
bursitis
chondromalacia
chondrosarcoma
cranioschisis
discitis
fibromyalgia
fasciitis
kyphosis
lordosis
meniscitis
myasthenia
myeloma
osteitis
osteoarthritis (OA)
osteochondritis
osteochondroma
osteomalacia
osteomyelitis
osteonecrosis
osteopenia
osteopetrosis
osteosarcoma
polymyositis (PM)
rachischisis
rhabdomyolysis
sarcopenia
scoliosis
spondylarthritis
spondylosis
synoviosarcoma
tendinitis
tenosynovitis

SURGICAL

arthrocentesis
arthrodesis
arthroplasty
bursectomy
carpectomy
chondrectomy
chondroplasty
costectomy
cranioplasty
craniotomy
discectomy
fasciotomy
laminectomy
maxillectomy
meniscectomy
microdiscectomy
myorrhaphy
osteotomy
phalangectomy
rachiotomy
spondylosyndesis
synovectomy
tarsectomy
tenomyoplasty
tenorrhaphy
vertebroplasty

DIAGNOSTIC

arthroscopy
arthrography
electromyogram (EMG)
myelography

COMPLEMENTARY

arthralgia
atrophy
bradykinesia
carpal
clavicular
cranial
dyskinesia
dystrophy
femoral
fibular
hemarthrosis
humeral
hyperkinesia
hypertrophy
iliac
intercostal
intervertebral
intracranial
ischial
lumbar
myalgia
patellar
patellofemoral
phalangeal
pubic
radial
sacral
scapular
sternal
submandibular
submaxillary
substernal
supraclavicular
suprapatellar
tarsal
tibial
ulnar
vertebral

CHAPTER AT A GLANCE Musculoskeletal System Terms *NOT* Built from Word Parts

DISEASE AND DISORDER

ankylosing spondylitis
bunion
carpal tunnel syndrome (CTS)
compartment syndrome
dislocation
exostosis
fracture (fx)
ganglion cyst
gout
herniated disk
Lyme disease
muscular dystrophy (MD)
myasthenia gravis (MG)
osteoporosis
plantar fasciitis
repetitive strain injury (RSI)
rheumatoid arthritis (RA)
rotator cuff disease
spinal stenosis
spondylolisthesis
sprain
strain
subluxation
tarsal tunnel syndrome

DIAGNOSTIC

dual x-ray absorptiometry (DXA)
bone markers
muscle biopsy

COMPLEMENTARY

chiropractic
chiropractor (DC)
crepitus
orthopedics (Ortho)
orthopedist
orthotics
orthotist
osteopath (DO)
osteopathy
podiatrist
prosthesis (*pl.* prostheses)
rheumatologist
rheumatology

TYPES OF BODY MOVEMENT

abduction
adduction
inversion
eversion
extension
flexion
pronation
supination
rotation

Chapter 15 Nervous System and Behavioral Health

Objectives

Upon completion of this chapter, you will be able to:

1. Pronounce organs and anatomic structures of the nervous system.
2. Define and spell word parts related to the nervous system.
3. Define, pronounce, and spell disease and disorder terms related to the nervous system.
4. Define, pronounce, and spell surgical terms related to the nervous system.
5. Define, pronounce, and spell diagnostic terms related to the nervous system.
6. Define, pronounce, and spell complementary terms related to the nervous system.
7. Define, pronounce, and spell behavioral health terms.
8. Interpret the meaning of abbreviations related to the nervous system and behavioral health.
9. Apply medical language in clinical contexts.

Outline

ANATOMY

The nervous system consists of the brain, spinal cord, and nerves and may be divided into two parts: the **central nervous system** (CNS) and the **peripheral nervous system** (PNS). The central nervous system consists of the brain and spinal cord. The peripheral nervous system is the collection of spinal and cranial nerves, whose branches infiltrate virtually all parts of the body, conveying messages to and from the CNS. (Figs. 15.1 and 15.2)

Function

The nervous system forms a complex communication system allowing for the coordination of body functions and activities. The nervous system can also be divided into two parts from a functional standpoint. The somatic nervous system is responsible for sending signals to the skeletal (voluntary) muscles and receives input from the senses. The autonomic nervous system generally operates on a "subconscious" level, meaning it governs itself without our conscious knowledge. It sends signals to the "involuntary" tissues, which include smooth muscles, cardiac muscles, glands, and fat. These tissues have receptors that send autonomic signals back to the brain and spinal cord. As a whole, the nervous system is designed to detect changes inside and outside the body, to evaluate this sensory information, and to send directions to muscles or glands in response. This system also provides for mental activities such as thought, memory, and emotions.

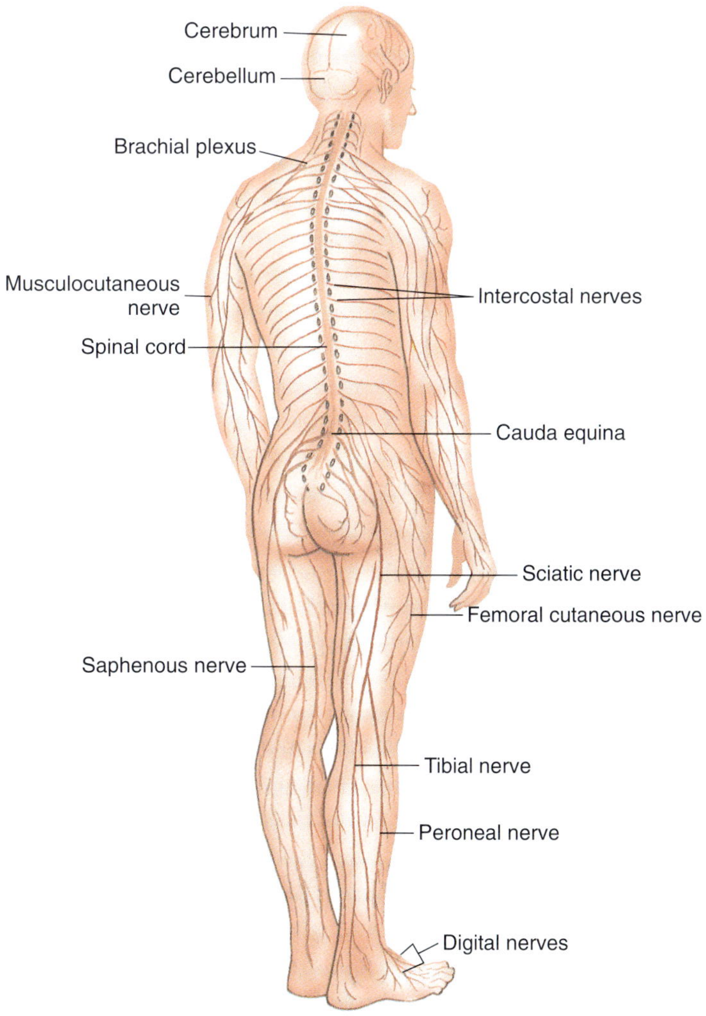

FIG. 15.1 Simplified view of the nervous system.

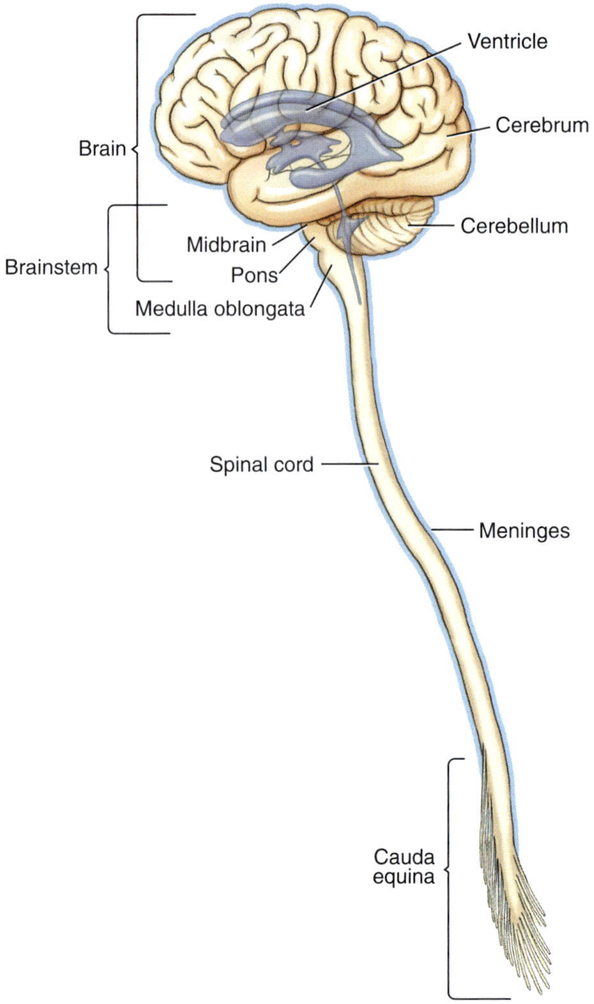

FIG. 15.2 Brain and spinal cord.

Organs and Anatomic Structures of the Nervous System

TERM	DEFINITION
brain (brān)	contained within the cranium, the center for coordinating body activities and comprises the cerebrum, cerebellum, and brainstem (Fig. 15.2).
cerebrum (se-RĒ-brum)	largest portion of the brain, divided into left and right hemispheres. The cerebrum controls the skeletal muscles, interprets general senses (such as temperature, pain, and touch), and contains centers for sight and hearing. Intellect, memory, and emotional reactions also take place in the cerebrum.
gray matter (grā) (MAT-ur)	outer portion of the cerebrum, contains neuron cell bodies that collect and process information. Gray matter forms the inner portion of the spinal cord (Fig 15.3).
white matter (wīt) (MAT-ur)	inner portion of the cerebrum, contains axons, long cords that extend from neurons; conveys information to different parts of the brain. White matter forms the outer portion of the spinal cord (Fig. 15.3).
ventricles (VEN-tri-kulz)	cavities (spaces) within the brain that contain **cerebrospinal fluid (CSF)**. The cerebrospinal fluid flows through the subarachnoid space around the brain and spinal cord.

TERM	DEFINITION
cerebellum (*ser*-a-BEL-um)	located under the posterior portion of the cerebrum; assists in the coordination of skeletal muscles to maintain balance (also called **hindbrain**)

CEREBELLUM was named in the third century BC by Erasistratus, who also named the cerebrum. **Cerebellum** literally means **little brain** and is the diminutive of **cerebrum**, meaning **brain**. Although it was named long ago, its function was not understood until the nineteenth century.

TERM	DEFINITION
brainstem (BRĀN-stem)	stemlike portion of the brain that connects with the spinal cord; contains centers that control respiration and heart rate. Three structures comprise the brainstem: pons, medulla oblongata, and midbrain.
pons (ponz)	literally means **bridge**. It connects the cerebrum with the cerebellum and brainstem.
medulla oblongata (ma-DŪL-a) (*ob*-long-GAH-ta)	located between the pons and spinal cord. It contains centers that control respiration, heart rate, and the muscles in the blood vessel walls, which assist in determining blood pressure.
midbrain (MID-brān)	most superior portion of the brainstem
cerebrospinal fluid (CSF) (*ser*-ē-brō-SPĪ-nal) (FLOO-id)	clear, colorless fluid contained in the ventricles that flows through the subarachnoid space around the brain and spinal cord. It cushions the brain and spinal cord from shock, transports nutrients, and clears metabolic waste.
spinal cord (SPĪ-nal) (kord)	passes through the vertebral canal extending from the medulla oblongata to the level of the second lumbar vertebra. The spinal cord conducts nerve impulses to and from the brain and initiates reflex action to sensory information without input from the brain.
meninges (me-NIN-jēz)	three layers of membrane that cover the brain and spinal cord (Fig. 15.3)

MENINGES were first named by a Persian physician in the tenth century. When translated into Latin, they became **dura mater**, meaning **hard mother** (because it is a tough membrane), and **pia mater**, meaning **soft mother** (because it is a delicate membrane). **Mater** was used because the Arabians believed that the meninges were the mother of all other body membranes.

TERM	DEFINITION
dura mater (DUR-a) (MĀ-ter)	tough outer layer of the meninges
arachnoid (a-RAK-noid)	delicate middle layer of the meninges. The arachnoid membrane is loosely attached to the pia mater by weblike fibers, which allow for the **subarachnoid space**.
pia mater (PĒ-a) (MĀ-ter)	thin inner layer of the meninges

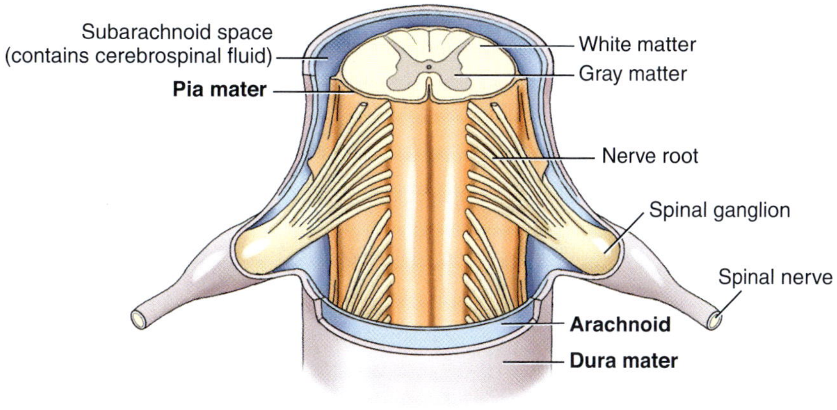

FIG. 15.3 Layers of meninges.

Organs and Anatomic Structures of the Nervous System—cont'd

TERM	DEFINITION
nerve (nurv)	cordlike structure made up of fibers that carries impulses from one part of the body to another. There are 12 pairs of cranial nerves and 31 pairs of spinal nerves. (Figs. 15.1 and 15.4)
ganglion (*pl.* ganglia) (GANG-glē-on) (GANG-glē-a)	group of nerve cell bodies located outside the central nervous system
glia (GLĒ-a)	specialized cells located throughout the nervous system that support and nourish nervous tissue. Some cells assist in the secretion of cerebrospinal fluid and others assist with phagocytosis. They do not conduct impulses. (also called **neuroglia**)

GLIA the Greek word for **glue**, were named in 1856 by the pathologist Rudolph Virchow. These gelatinous cells were originally credited with holding the nerves together. Today we know that they perform many more tasks in the brain and spinal cord.

TERM	DEFINITION
neuron (NŪR-on)	nerve cell that conducts impulses to carry out the function of the nervous system. Destroyed neurons in the central nervous system cannot be replaced.

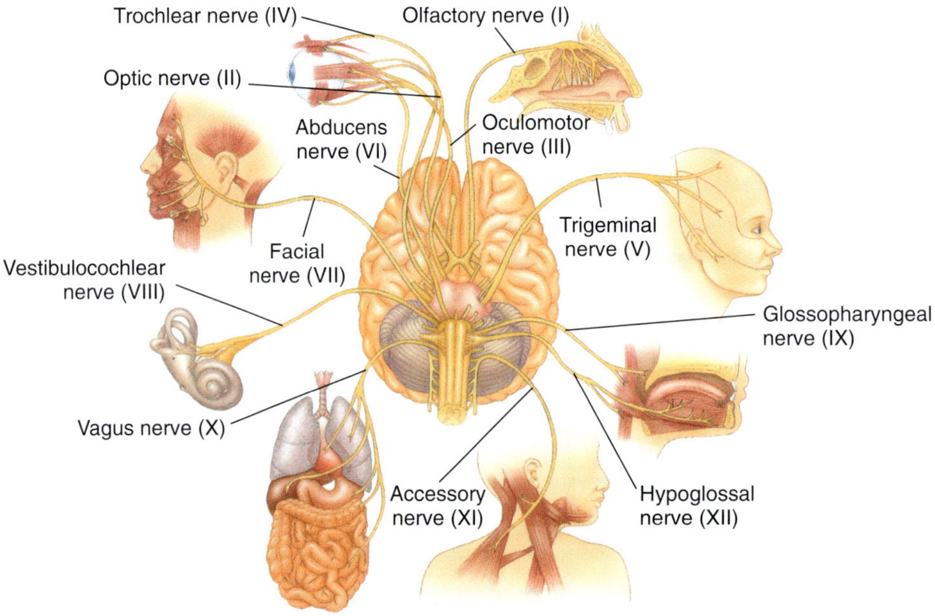

FIG. 15.4 Cranial nerves.

PRONOUNCE ANATOMIC STRUCTURES

Practice saying aloud each of the organs and specific structures on the previous pages.

To hear the terms, go to Evolve Resources at www.evolve.elsevier.com and select:
Student Resources > Audio Glossary > Chapter 15 > Anatomic Structures

❑ Check the box when complete.

WORD PARTS

Use paper flashcards or electronic flashcards on Evolve to memorize word parts used to analyze, define, and build medical terms in this chapter. To reinforce learning, study one section of the Word Parts Table at a time, then complete the corresponding exercise on the following pages.

1 ■ Combining Forms of the Nervous System

COMBINING FORM	DEFINITION
cerebell/o	cerebellum
cerebr/o	cerebrum, brain
dur/o	hard, dura mater
encephal/o	brain
gangli/o	ganglion
ganglion/o	ganglion
gli/o	glia
mening/o	meninges
meningi/o	meninges
myel/o	spinal cord
MYEL/O refers to bone marrow when used with musculoskeletal terms.	
neur/o	nerve
poli/o	gray matter
radicul/o	nerve root (proximal end of a peripheral nerve, closest to the spinal cord)
rhiz/o	nerve root (proximal end of a peripheral nerve, closest to the spinal cord)

2 ■ Combining Forms Used With Nervous System Terms

COMBINING FORM	DEFINITION
angi/o	vessel(s); blood vessel(s)
blast/o	developing cell, germ cell
cephal/o	head
crani/o	cranium (skull)
embol/o	plug
esthesi/o	sensation, sensitivity, feeling
hem/o	blood
hemat/o	blood
hydr/o	water
ment/o	mind
mon/o	one, single
phas/o	speech
psych/o	mind
quadr/i	four *(Note: an i is the combining vowel in quadr/i.)*
thromb/o	blood clot

3 ■ Prefixes

PREFIX	DEFINITION
a-	absence of, without
an-	absence of, without
dys-	painful, abnormal, difficult, labored
hemi-	half
hyper-	above, excessive
inter-	between
intra-	within
para-	beside, beyond, around, abnormal
poly-	many, much
post-	after
pre-	before
sub-	under, below

4 ■ Suffixes

SUFFIX	DEFINITION	SUFFIX	DEFINITION
-a	noun suffix, no meaning	**-logy**	study of
-al	pertaining to	**-lysis**	loosening, dissolution, separating
-algia	pain	**-malacia**	softening
-cele	hernia, protrusion	**-oma**	tumor, swelling
-ectomy	excision, surgical removal	**-osis**	abnormal condition (means increase when used with blood cell word roots)
-genic	producing, originating, causing	**-paresis**	slight paralysis
-graphy	process of recording, radiographic imaging	**-pathy**	disease
-ia	diseased or abnormal state, condition of	**-plasty**	surgical repair
-iatrist	specialist, physician	**-plegia**	paralysis
-iatry	treatment, specialty	**-rrhage**	excessive flow
-ictal	seizure, attack	**-rrhaphy**	suturing, repairing
-ism	state of	**-tomy**	cut into, incision
-itis	inflammation	**-us**	noun suffix, no meaning
-logist	one who studies and treats (specialist, physician)		

Refer to **Appendix B** and **Appendix C** for a complete list of word parts.

EXERCISE 1 ■ Nervous System Combining Forms

Refer to the first section of the word parts table.

A Label

Fill in the blanks with combining forms in this diagram of the brain and spinal cord. *To check your answers, go to Appendix A.*

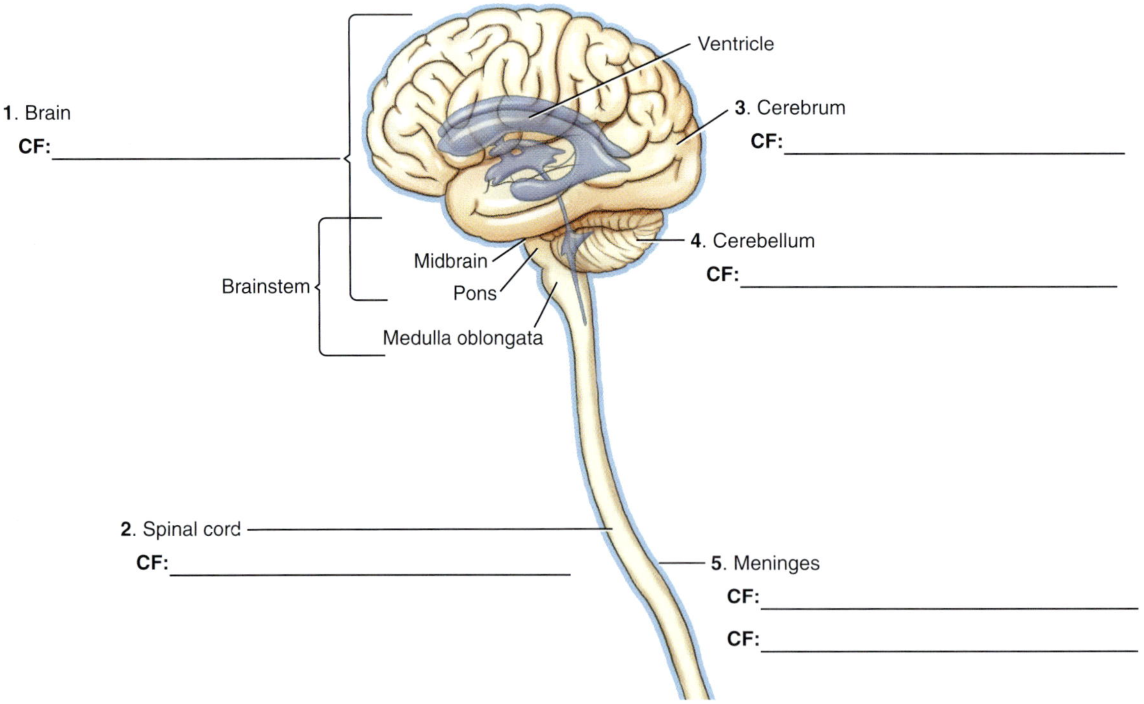

B Identify

Write the combining form for each of the following definitions.

1. glia ____________
2. nerve ____________

C Label

Fill in the blanks with combining forms in this diagram of the spinal cord and layers of meninges.

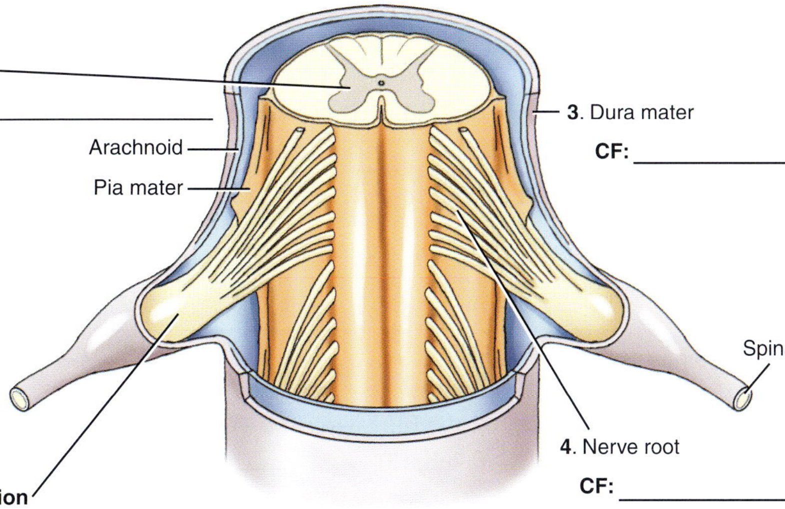

D Define and Match

Step 1: Write the definitions after the following combining forms.
Step 2: Match the descriptions on the right with the combining forms and definitions.

_____ 1. gangli/o, ______________________
_____ 2. dur/o, ______________________
_____ 3. encephal/o, ______________________
_____ 4. cerebell/o, ______________________
_____ 5. meningi/o, ______________________
_____ 6. neur/o, ______________________

a. assists in the coordination of skeletal muscles to maintain balance
b. cordlike structure made up of fibers that carries impulses from one part of the body to another
c. contained within the cranium, the center for coordinating body activities
d. tough outer layer of the meninges
e. group of nerve cell bodies located outside the central nervous system
f. three layers of membrane that cover the brain and spinal cord

E Define and Match

Step 1: Write the definitions after the following combining forms.
Step 2: Match the descriptions on the right with the combining forms and definitions.

_____ 1. gli/o, ______________________
_____ 2. ganglion/o, ______________________
_____ 3. mening/o, ______________________
_____ 4. cerebr/o, ______________________
_____ 5. myel/o, ______________________
_____ 6. poli/o, ______________________

a. conducts impulses to and from the brain and initiates reflex action to sensory information
b. specialized cells that support and nourish nervous tissue
c. outer portion of cerebrum, inner portion of spinal cord; processes information
d. group of nerve cell bodies located outside the central nervous system
e. three layers of membrane that cover the brain and spinal cord
f. largest portion of the brain, divided into left and right hemispheres

F Identify

Write the combining forms for the following term.

1. nerve root
   a. ______
   b. ______

EXERCISE 2 ■ Combining Forms Used with Nervous System Terms

Refer to the second section of the word parts table.

A Define

Write the definitions of the following combining forms new to this chapter.

1. mon/o ______
2. psych/o ______
3. quadr/i ______
4. ment/o ______
5. phas/o ______
6. esthesi/o ______

B Match

Match the combining forms in the first column with their correct definitions in the second column. Answers may be used more than once.

______ 1. thromb/o	a. blood
______ 2. hydr/o	b. blood clot
______ 3. hemat/o	c. skull
______ 4. hem/o	d. developing cell, germ cell
______ 5. embol/o	e. head
______ 6. crani/o	f. plug
______ 7. cephal/o	g. vessel(s); blood vessel(s)
______ 8. blast/o	h. water
______ 9. angi/o	

EXERCISE 3 ■ Prefixes

Refer to the third section of the word parts table. Match the prefixes in the first column with their correct definitions in the second column.

______ 1. sub-	a. above, excessive
______ 2. pre-	b. absence of, without
______ 3. post-	c. after
______ 4. poly-	d. before
______ 5. intra-	e. between
______ 6. inter-	f. half
______ 7. hyper-	g. beside, beyond, around, abnormal
______ 8. hemi-	h. painful, abnormal, difficult, labored
______ 9. dys-	i. under, below
______ 10. a-, an-	j. within
______ 11. para-	k. many, much

EXERCISE 4 ■ Suffixes

Refer to the fourth section of the word parts table.

A Define

Write the definitions of the following suffixes new to this chapter.

1. -paresis ____________________
2. -iatry ____________________
3. -ictal ____________________
4. -iatrist ____________________

B Match

Match the suffixes in the first column with their correct definitions in the second column.

_____	1. -al	a. suturing, repairing
_____	2. -ectomy	b. surgical repair
_____	3. -graphy	c. noun suffix, no meaning
_____	4. -genic	d. process of recording, radiographic imaging
_____	5. -logy	e. pertaining to
_____	6. -lysis	f. one who studies and treats (specialist, physician)
_____	7. -plasty	g. loosening, dissolution, separating
_____	8. -rrhaphy	h. excision, surgical removal
_____	9. -tomy	i. cut into, incision
_____	10. -a, -us	j. study of
_____	11. -logist	k. producing, originating, causing

C Match

Match the suffixes in the first column with their correct definitions in the second column.

_____	1. -algia	a. tumor, swelling
_____	2. -cele	b. state of
_____	3. -ia	c. softening
_____	4. -ism	d. paralysis
_____	5. -itis	e. pain
_____	6. -oma	f. inflammation
_____	7. -osis	g. hernia, protrusion
_____	8. -pathy	h. excessive flow
_____	9. -malacia	i. diseased or abnormal state, condition of
_____	10. -plegia	j. disease
_____	11. -rrhage	k. abnormal condition (means increase when used with blood cell word roots)

MEDICAL TERMS

Medical terms relevant to this chapter have been grouped by topics, such as Disease and Disorder, and are listed in tables designated as Built from Word Parts or *NOT* Built from Word Parts. The exercises following each table assist with learning term definitions, pronunciations, and spellings.

Disease and Disorder Terms

BUILT FROM WORD PARTS

The following terms can be translated using definitions of word parts. Further explanation is provided within parentheses as needed.

TERM	DEFINITION
1. **cerebellitis** (*ser*-e-bel-Ī-tis)	inflammation of the cerebellum
2. **cerebral embolism** (se-RĒ-bral) (EM-bō-lizm)	pertaining to the cerebrum, state of a plug (clot or piece of plaque from a distant site lodged in a cerebral artery, causing sudden blockage of blood supply to the brain tissue)
3. **cerebral thrombosis** (se-RĒ-bral) (throm-BŌ-sis)	pertaining to the cerebrum, abnormal condition of a blood clot (onset of symptoms may appear from minutes to days after an obstruction of a blood vessel in the brain)

CEREBRAL EMBOLISM and **THROMBOSIS** are both causes of ischemic stroke, which results from blocked vessels.

TERM	DEFINITION
4. **duritis** (dū-RĪ-tis)	inflammation of the dura mater
5. **encephalitis** (en-*sef*-a-LĪ-tis)	inflammation of the brain
6. **encephalomalacia** (en-*sef*-a-lō-ma-LĀ-sha)	softening of the brain
7. **encephalopathy** (en-*sef*-a-LOP-a-thē)	disease of the brain
8. **encephalomyeloradiculitis** (en-*sef*-a-lō-*mī*-e-lō-ra-*dik*-ū-LĪ-tis)	inflammation of the brain, spinal cord, and nerve roots
9. **gangliitis** (*gang*-glē-Ī-tis)	inflammation of a ganglion
10. **glioblastoma** (*glī*-ō-blas-TŌ-ma)	tumor composed of developing glia (the most malignant primary tumor of the brain)
11. **glioma** (glī-Ō-ma)	tumor composed of glia

GLIOMA is a general term referring to brain and spinal cord tumors developing from any of the types of glial cells or their developing cells. **Glioblastoma** is the most aggressive form of glioma.

TERM	DEFINITION
12. **hydrocephalus** (*hī*-drō-SEF-a-lus)	water (increased amount of cerebrospinal fluid) in the head (brain)

HYDROCEPHALUS may be congenital or acquired and is caused by obstructed circulation of cerebrospinal fluid, which results in dilated cerebral ventricles and impaired brain function. For infants, hydrocephalus can cause enlargement of the cranium. The condition was first described around 30 AD in the book De Medicina.

TERM	DEFINITION
13. **intracerebral hemorrhage** (*in*-tra-SER-e-bral) (HEM-o-rij)	pertaining to within the brain, excessive flow of blood (bleeding into the brain as a result of a ruptured blood vessel within the brain)

INTRACEREBRAL HEMORRHAGE symptoms often develop suddenly and vary depending on the location of the hemorrhage; acute symptoms include dyspnea, dysphagia, aphasia, diminished level of consciousness, and hemiparesis. Intracerebral hemorrhage is a cause of hemorrhagic stroke and is frequently associated with high blood pressure.

TERM	DEFINITION
14. **meningioma** (me-*nin*-jē-Ō-ma)	tumor of the meninges (usually benign and slow growing; most common tumor originating in the brain and surrounding tissues)
15. **meningitis** (*men*-in-JĪ-tis)	inflammation of the meninges
16. **meningocele** (me-NING-gō-sēl)	protrusion of the meninges (through a defect in the skull or vertebral arch)
17. **meningomyelocele** (me-*ning*-gō-MĪ-e-lō-*sēl*)	protrusion of the meninges and spinal cord (through a neural arch defect in the vertebral column) (also called **myelomeningocele**) (see Fig. 9.7)

TERM	DEFINITION
18. mononeuropathy (*mon*-ō-nū-ROP-a-thē)	disease affecting a single nerve (such as carpal tunnel syndrome)
19. myelitis (*mī*-e-LĪ-tis)	inflammation of the spinal cord
20. myelomalacia (*mī*-e-lō-ma-LĀ-sha)	softening of the spinal cord
21. neuralgia (nū-RAL-ja)	nerve pain
22. neuritis (nū-RĪ-tis)	inflammation of a nerve
23. poliomyelitis (*pō*-lē-ō-*mī*-e-LĪ-tis)	inflammation of the gray matter of the spinal cord (This infectious disease, commonly referred to as *polio*, is caused by one of three polio viruses.)
24. polyneuritis (*pol*-ē-nū-RĪ-tis)	inflammation of many nerves
25. polyneuropathy (*pol*-ē-nū-ROP-a-thē)	disease of many nerves

POLYNERUOPATHY most often occurs as a complication of diabetes mellitus, but may also occur as a result of drug therapy, critical illness such as sepsis, or carcinoma; symptoms include weakness, distal sensory loss, and burning.

TERM	DEFINITION
26. radiculitis (ra-*dik*-ū-LĪ-tis)	inflammation of the nerve roots
27. radiculopathy (ra-*dik*-ū-LOP-a-thē)	disease of the nerve roots

PERIPHERAL NEUROPATHY refers to disorders of the peripheral nervous system, including **radiculopathy**, **mononeuropathy**, and **polyneuropathy**. (Fig. 15.5)

TERM	DEFINITION
28. rhizomeningomyelitis (*rī*-zō-me-*ning*-gō-*mī*-e-LĪ-tis)	inflammation of the nerve root, meninges, and spinal cord
29. subdural hematoma (sub-DŪ-ral) (*hē*-ma-TŌ-ma)	pertaining to below the dura mater, tumor of blood (collection of blood that has leaked out of a broken vessel)

HEMATOMA, though translated as *tumor of blood* from the meaning of its word parts, is a collection of blood resulting from a broken blood vessel.

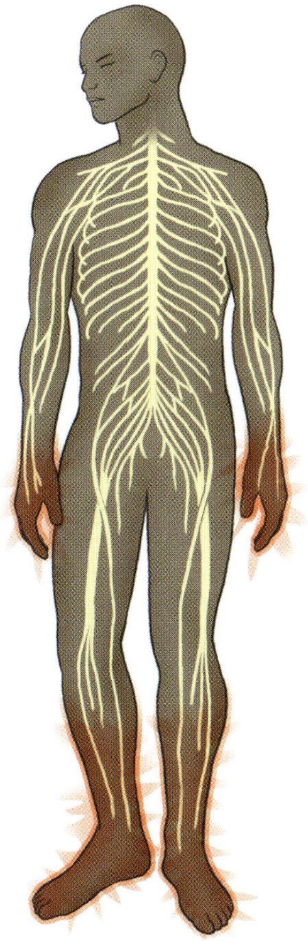

FIG. 15.5 Peripheral neuropathy.

EXERCISE 5 ■ Pronounce and Spell

Practice pronunciation and spelling on paper and online.

1. Practice on Paper

a. **Pronounce:** Read the phonetic spelling and say aloud the terms listed in the previous table. Refer to the pronunciation key on p. 20 as necessary.
b. **Spell:** Have a study partner read the terms aloud. Write the spelling of the terms on a separate sheet of paper.

2. Practice Online

a. **Access** online learning resources. Go to evolve.elsevier.com > Evolve Resources > Student Resources.
b. **Pronounce:** Select Audio Glossary > Chapter 15 > Exercise 5. Select a term to hear its pronunciation and repeat aloud.
c. **Spell:** Select Activities > Chapter 15 > Spell Terms > Exercise 5. Select the audio icon and type the correct spelling of the term.

❑ Check the box when complete.

EXERCISE 6 ■ Analyze and Define

Analyze and define the following terms.

1. myelitis
____
____

2. hydrocephalus
____
____

3. poliomyelitis
____
____

4. radiculopathy
____
____

5. encephalopathy
____
____

6. encephalitis
____
____

7. rhizomeningomyelitis
____
____

8. cerebral thrombosis
____
____

9. meningocele
____
____

10. myelomalacia
____
____

11. radiculitis

____

____

12. gangliitis

____

____

13. duritis

____

____

14. polyneuritis

____

____

EXERCISE 7 ■ Build

A Label

Build terms pictured by writing word parts above definitions.

1. 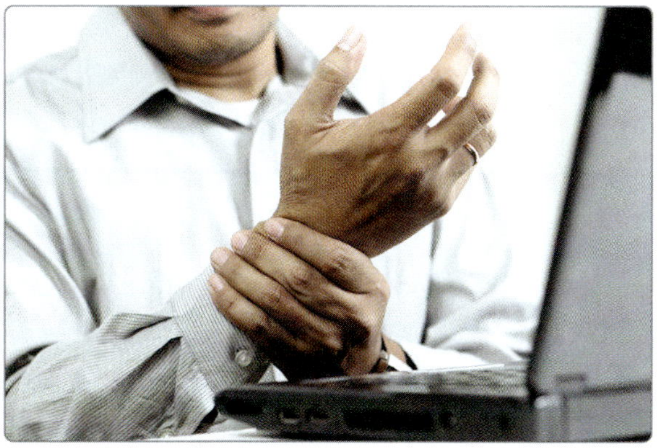

_____ / _____ / _____ / _____ / _____
single CV nerve CV disease

2. 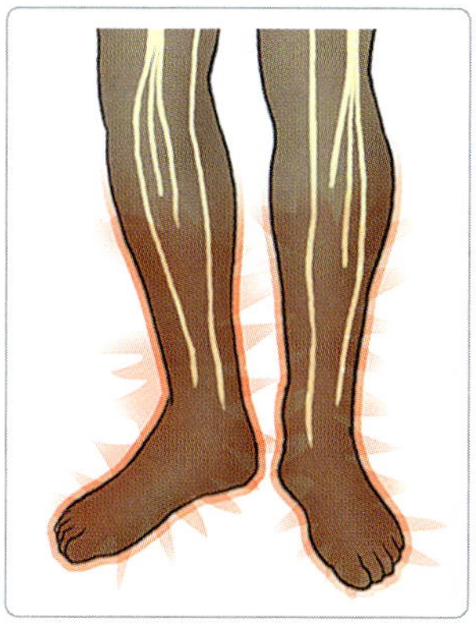

_____ / _____ / _____ / _____
many nerve CV disease

3. 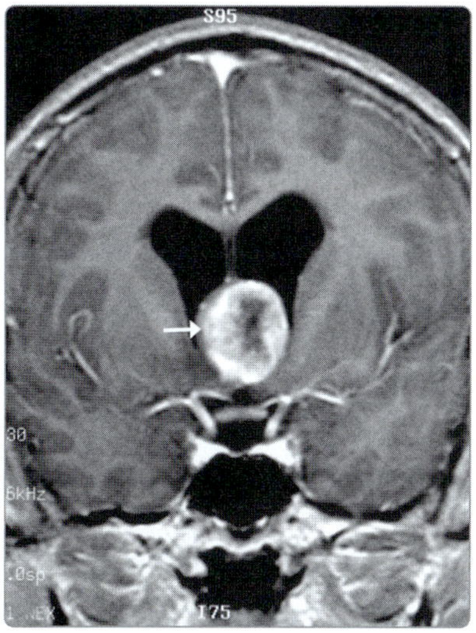

MR image of brain demonstrating

_____ / _____ / _____ / _____
glia CV developing cell tumor

4. 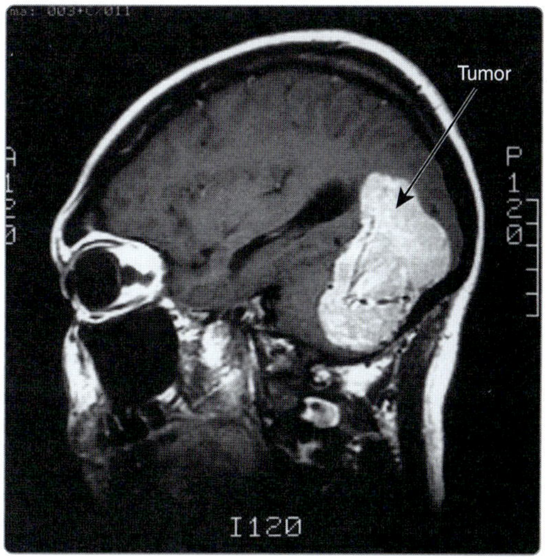

_____ / _____
meninges tumor

5.

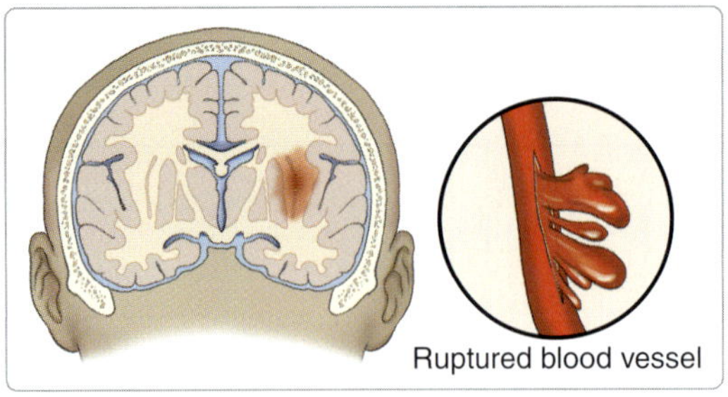

_____ / _____ / _________   _____ / ____ / _______

within   brain   pertaining to   blood   CV   excessive flow

6.

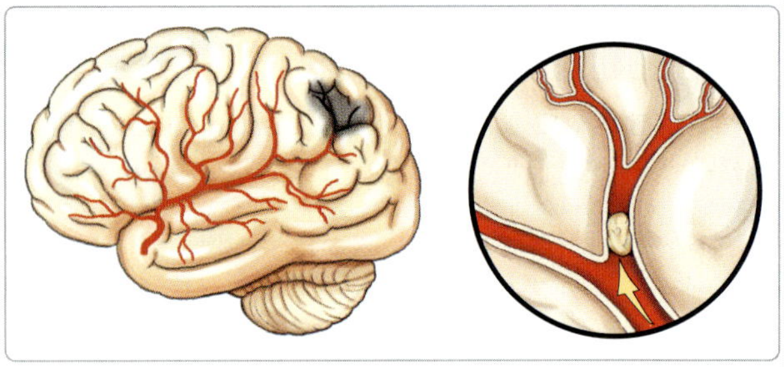

_________ / _________   _______ / _________

cerebrum   pertaining to   plug   state of

7.

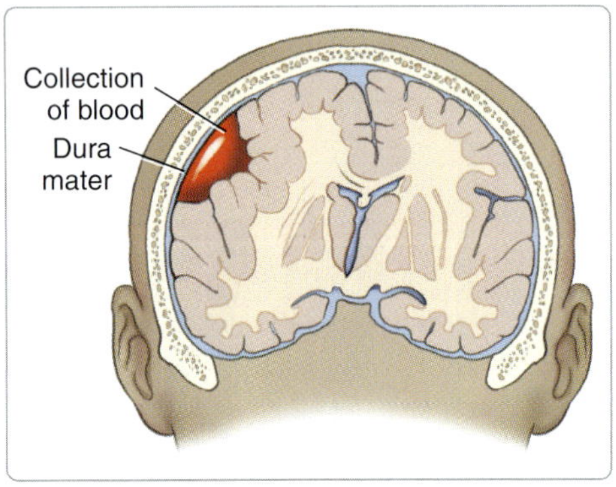

_____ / ____ / _________   _______ / _____

below   dura   pertaining to   blood   tumor

8.

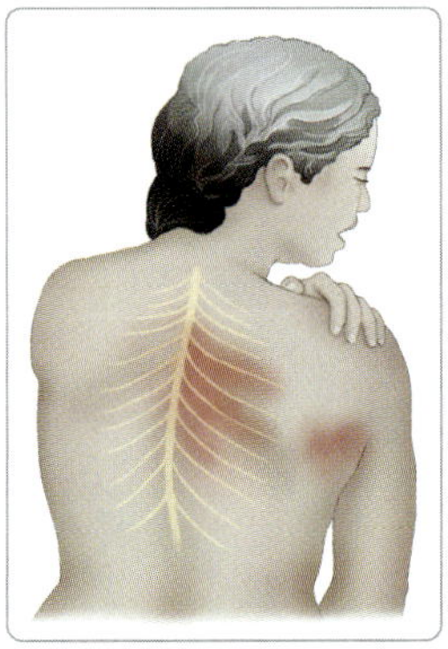

postherpetic _________ / _________

nerve   pain

B Fill In

Build disease and disorder terms for the following definitions by using the word parts you have learned.

1. inflammation of the nerve _______ / _______
   WR / S
2. tumor composed of glia _______ / _______
   WR / S
3. softening of the brain _______ / ___ / _______
   WR / CV / S
4. inflammation of the cerebellum _______ / _______
   WR / S
5. inflammation of the brain, spinal cord, and nerve roots ____ / __ / ____ / __ / ____ / ____
   WR / CV / WR / CV / WR / S
6. inflammation of the meninges _______ / _______
   WR / S
7. protrusion of the meninges and spinal cord (through the vertebral column) ____ / __ / ____ / __ / ____
   WR / CV / WR / CV / S

Disease and Disorder Terms

NOT BUILT FROM WORD PARTS

Word parts may be present in the following terms; however, their full meanings cannot be translated using definitions of word parts alone.

TERM	DEFINITION
1. **Alzheimer disease (AD)** (AWLTZ-hī-mer) (di-ZĒZ)	type of dementia that occurs more frequently after the age of 65, but can begin at any age. The brain shrinks dramatically as nerve cells die and tissues atrophy. The disease is slowly progressive and usually results in profound dementia in 5 to 10 years. A prominent feature of AD is the inability to remember the recent past, while memories of the distant past remain intact.
2. **amyotrophic lateral sclerosis (ALS)** (ā-*mī*-ō-TRŌ-fik) (LAT-er-al) (skle-RŌ-sis)	progressive muscle atrophy caused by degeneration and scarring of neurons along the lateral columns of the spinal cord that control muscles (also called **Lou Gehrig disease**)
3. **Bell palsy** (bel) (PAWL-zē)	paralysis of muscles on one side of the face caused by inflammation or compression of the facial nerve, cranial nerve VII. Signs include a sagging mouth on the affected side and nonclosure of the eyelid; paralysis is usually temporary.
4. **botulism** (BOCH-e-liz-um)	serious illness caused by a bacterial toxin that interferes with nerve conduction, causing skeletal muscle paralysis. Initial symptoms may include trouble seeing and muscle weakness leading to difficulty swallowing and breathing. Foodborne botulism, wound botulism, and infant botulism are types of the illness, all of which can be fatal and are medical emergencies.
5. **cerebral aneurysm** (se-RĒ-bral) (AN-ū-rizm)	ballooning of a weakened portion of an arterial wall (aneurysm) in the cerebrum. It is usually asymptomatic until it ruptures, which can be very serious and can result in death.
6. **cerebral palsy (CP)** (se-RĒ-bral) (PAWL-zē)	condition characterized by lack of muscle control and partial paralysis, caused by a brain defect or lesion present at birth or shortly after
7. **chronic traumatic encephalopathy (CTE)** (KRON-ik) (tra-MAT-ik) (en-*sef*-a-LOP-a-thē)	progressive degenerative disease of the brain which generally appears years or decades after repeated head trauma. Originally diagnosed in boxers (dementia pugilistica), it has now been found in other professional athletes who experienced repeated head trauma, such as football, ice hockey, soccer, wrestling, and basketball players. Signs and symptoms include memory loss, aggression, confusion, attention deficits, poor judgment, anxiety, and depression. Currently, CTE can only be definitively diagnosed after death by brain autopsy, but in the future, diagnostic imaging, chemical biomarkers, and neuropsychological tests may be helpful.
8. **dementia** (de-MEN-sha)	cognitive impairment characterized by loss of intellectual brain function. Patients have difficulty in various ways, including difficulty in performing complex tasks, reasoning, learning and retaining new information, orientation, word finding, and behavior. Dementia has several causes and is not considered part of normal aging. (Table 15.1)
9. **epilepsy** (EP-i-lep-sē)	condition characterized by recurrent seizures; a general term given to a group of neurologic disorders, all characterized by abnormal electrical activity in the brain

EPILEPSY was written about by Hippocrates, in 400 BC, in a book titled **Sacred Disease**. It was believed at one time that epilepsy was a punishment for offending the gods. The Greek **epilepsia** meant **seizure** and is derived from **epi**, meaning upon, and **lambanein**, meaning **to seize**. The term literally means **seized upon** (by the gods).

TERM	DEFINITION
10. **multiple sclerosis (MS)** (MUL-ti-pl) (skle-RŌ-sis)	chronic degenerative disease characterized by sclerotic patches along the brain and spinal cord; signs and symptoms fluctuate over the course of the disease; more common symptoms include fatigue, balance and coordination impairments, numbness, and vision problems
11. **Parkinson disease (PD)** (PAR-kin-sun) (di-ZĒZ)	chronic degenerative disease of the central nervous system. Signs and symptoms include resting tremors of the hands and feet, rigidity, expressionless face, shuffling gait, and eventually dementia. It usually occurs after the age of 50 years (also called **parkinsonism**).

PARKINSON DISEASE was first described by James Parkinson, an English professor, in his **Essay on the Shaking Palsy** in 1817.

TABLE 15.1 Types of Dementia

COMMON TYPES OF DEMENTIA	
Alzheimer disease	most common type of dementia, responsible for 60% to 80% of all cases. The disease, which appears to be due to a variety of causes, is a progressive neurodegenerative disorder characterized by diffuse brain atrophy and the presence of senile plaques and neurofibrillary tangles within the brain cortex. Women are affected more than men, possibly because women tend to live longer, and because the chances of having AD double with every 5 additional years of life after age 65.
Vascular or multiple infarct dementia	affects approximately 10% of patients with dementia. It is secondary to cerebrovascular disease and usually occurs in older patients. Dementia usually worsens in a step-wise fashion, and other neurological findings (like paralysis or cranial nerve abnormalities) are often present.
Lewy body dementia	usually a rapidly progressive form of dementia which is responsible for approximately 10% of all dementias. Lewy body dementia is characterized by hallucinations, fluctuations in severity, sleep disorders, and Parkinson symptoms, the latter of which occur less than 1 year before the dementia.
Parkinson dementia	generally does not develop until patients have advanced Parkinson disease; similar to Lewy body dementia
Frontotemporal dementia (Pick disease)	affects the anterior portions of the brain; most common symptoms are personality changes, disinhibition, and impulsiveness. Atrophy may be observed on brain CT or MR.
LESS COMMON FORMS OF DEMENTIA	
Normal pressure hydrocephalus	imbalance of cerebrospinal fluid in the brain leads to a triad of dementia, urinary incontinence, and gait instability. Sometimes caused by trauma or subarachnoid hemorrhage; can be treated with a ventricular peritoneal shunt
Wernicke-Korsakoff syndrome	form of dementia found with chronic alcoholism; caused by thiamine deficiency and poor nutritional status
Infections	including Creutzfeldt-Jakob disease, HIV infection, syphilis, and tuberculosis
Tumors and chronic subdural hematomas	space-occupying lesions that prevent normal brain function

Disease and Disorder Terms—cont'd

NOT BUILT FROM WORD PARTS

TERM	DEFINITION
12. sciatica (sī-AT-i-ka)	inflammation of the sciatic nerve, causing pain that travels from the thigh through the leg to the foot and toes; can be caused by injury, infection, arthritis, herniated disk, or from prolonged pressure on the nerve from sitting for long periods
13. shingles (SHING-gelz)	viral disease that affects the peripheral nerves and causes blisters on the skin that follow the course of the affected nerves (also called **herpes zoster**)

POSTHERPETIC NEURALGIA is a complication of **shingles** (herpes zoster) and is caused by damage to the nerve fibers. Severe pain and hyperesthesia persist after the skin lesions disappear and may last months or even years.

TERM	DEFINITION
14. stroke (strōk)	interruption of blood supply to a region of the brain, depriving nerve cells in the affected area of oxygen and nutrients. The cells cannot perform and may be damaged or die within minutes. The parts of the body controlled by the involved cells will experience dysfunction. Speech, movement, memory, and other CNS functions may be affected in varying degrees. **Ischemic stroke** is a result of a blocked blood vessel. **Hemorrhagic stroke** is a result of bleeding (also called **cerebrovascular accident [CVA]** or **brain attack**).

TERM	DEFINITION
15. subarachnoid hemorrhage (SAH) (*sub*-e-RAK-noid) (HEM-o-rij)	bleeding between the pia mater and arachnoid layers of the meninges (subarachnoid space), caused by a ruptured blood vessel (usually a cerebral aneurysm). The patient may experience an intense, sudden headache accompanied by nausea, vomiting, and neck pain. SAH is a critical condition which must be recognized and treated immediately to prevent permanent brain damage or death (a cause of **hemorrhagic stroke**).
16. transient ischemic attack (TIA) (TRAN-sē-ent) (is-KĒ-mik) (a-TAK)	sudden deficient supply of blood to the brain lasting a short time. The symptoms may be similar to those of stroke, but with TIA the symptoms are temporary and the usual outcome is complete recovery. TIAs are often warning signs for eventual occurrence of a stroke.

EXERCISE 8 ■ Pronounce and Spell

Practice pronunciation and spelling on paper and online.

1. Practice on Paper

a. **Pronounce:** Read the phonetic spelling and say aloud the terms listed in the previous table. Refer to the pronunciation key on p. 20 as necessary.
b. **Spell:** Have a study partner read the terms aloud. Write the spelling of the terms on a separate sheet of paper.

2. Practice Online

a. **Access** online learning resources. Go to evolve.elsevier.com > Evolve Resources > Student Resources.
b. **Pronounce:** Select Audio Glossary > Chapter 15 > Exercise 8. Select a term to hear its pronunciation and repeat aloud.
c. **Spell:** Select Activities > Chapter 15 > Spell Terms > Exercise 8. Select the audio icon and type the correct spelling of the term.

❑ Check the box when complete.

EXERCISE 9 ■ Match

Match the terms in the first column with their definitions in the second column.

_____ 1. multiple sclerosis
_____ 2. epilepsy
_____ 3. cerebral palsy
_____ 4. Parkinson disease
_____ 5. amyotrophic lateral sclerosis
_____ 6. dementia
_____ 7. botulism
_____ 8. chronic traumatic encephalopathy

a. condition characterized by lack of muscle control and partial paralysis, caused by a brain defect or a lesion present at birth or shortly after
b. progressive muscle atrophy caused by degeneration and scarring of neurons along the lateral columns of the spinal cord
c. cognitive impairment characterized by loss of intellectual brain function; not considered part of normal aging
d. progressive degenerative disease of the brain which generally appears years or decades after repeated head trauma
e. serious illness caused by a bacterial toxin that interferes with nerve conduction, causing skeletal muscle paralysis
f. chronic degenerative disease of the central nervous system, characterized by resting tremors of the hands and feet, rigidity, expressionless face, shuffling gait, and dementia
g. condition characterized by recurrent seizures
h. chronic degenerative disease characterized by sclerotic patches along the brain and spinal cord

EXERCISE 10 ■ Label

Write the medical terms pictured and defined.

1. ____________________
inflammation of the sciatic nerve, causing pain that travels from the thigh through the leg to the foot and toes

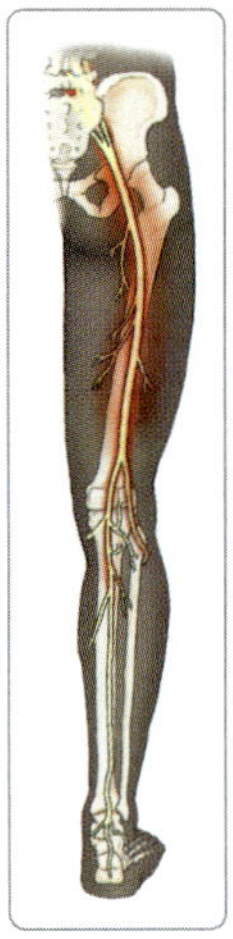

2. ____________________
type of dementia that occurs more frequently after the age of 65; the brain shrinks dramatically

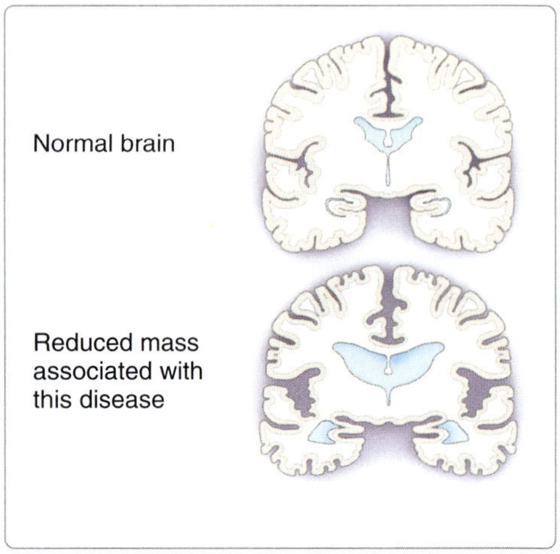

3. ____________________
viral disease that affects the peripheral nerves and causes blisters on the skin that follow the course of the affected nerves

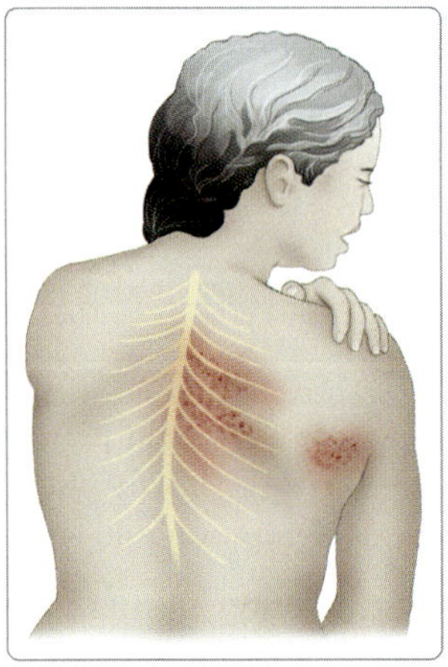

4. ____________________
ballooning of a weakened portion of an arterial wall in the cerebrum

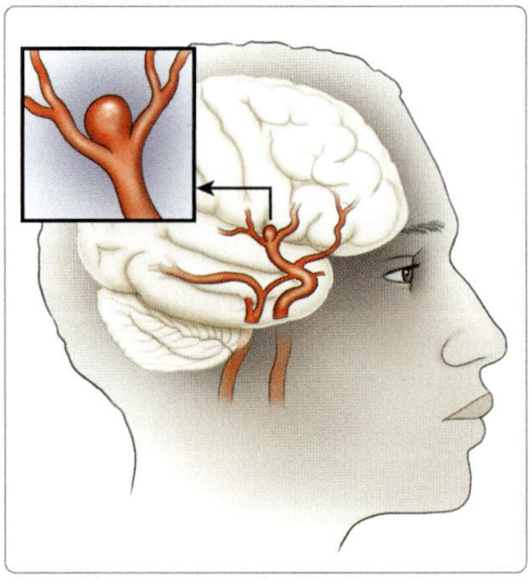

5. ____________________
bleeding between the pia mater and arachnoid layers of the meninges caused by a ruptured blood vessel

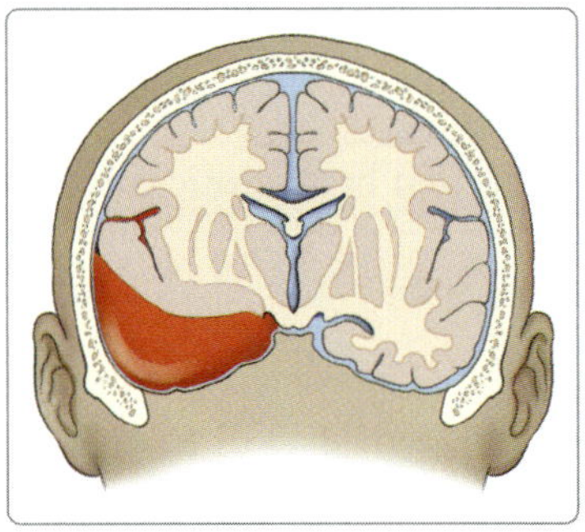

6. ____________________
interruption of blood supply to a region of the brain, depriving nerve cells in the affected area of oxygen and nutrients

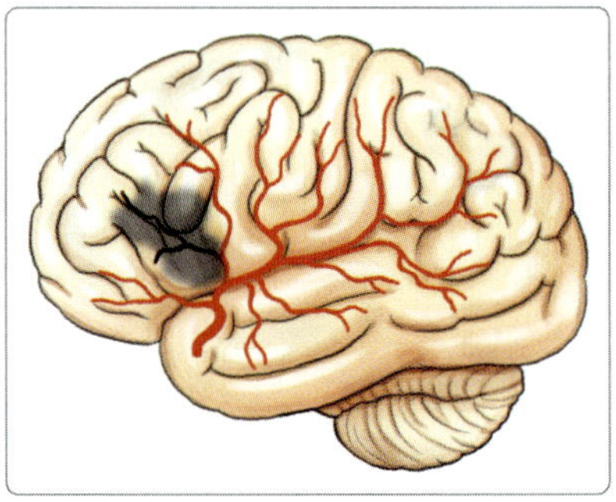

7. ______________________________
sudden deficient supply of blood to the brain lasting a short time

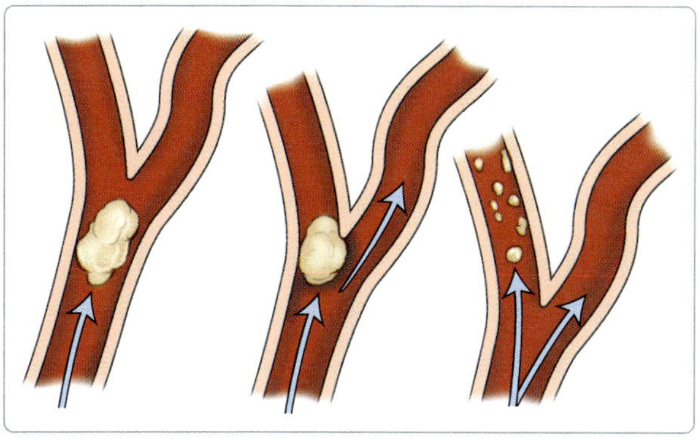

8. ______________________________
paralysis of muscles on one side of the face caused by inflammation or compression of the facial nerve

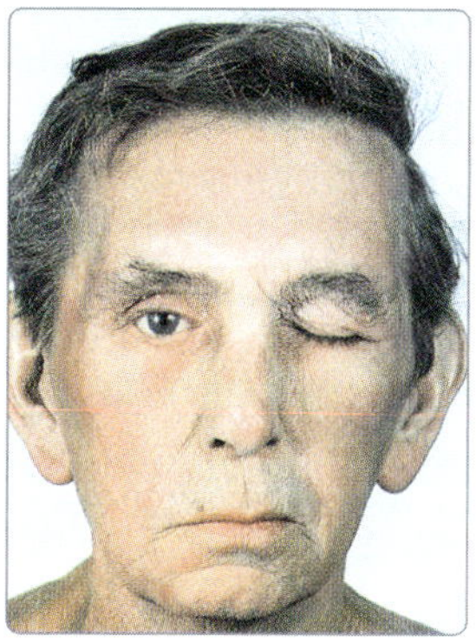

EXERCISE 11 ■ Review of Disease and Disorder Terms

Can you define, pronounce, and spell the following terms?

Alzheimer disease (AD)
amyotrophic lateral sclerosis (ALS)
Bell palsy
botulism
cerebellitis
cerebral aneurysm
cerebral embolism
cerebral palsy (CP)
cerebral thrombosis
chronic traumatic encephalopathy (CTE)
dementia
duritis
encephalitis
encephalomalacia
encephalomyeloradiculitis
encephalopathy
epilepsy
gangliitis
glioblastoma
glioma
hydrocephalus
intracerebral hemorrhage
meningioma
meningitis
meningocele
meningomyelocele
mononeuropathy
multiple sclerosis (MS)
myelitis
myelomalacia
neuralgia
neuritis
Parkinson disease (PD)
poliomyelitis
polyneuritis
polyneuropathy
radiculitis
radiculopathy
rhizomeningomyelitis
sciatica
shingles
stroke
subarachnoid hemorrhage (SAH)
subdural hematoma
transient ischemic attack (TIA)

Surgical Terms

BUILT FROM WORD PARTS

The following terms can be translated using definitions of word parts. Further explanation is provided within parentheses as needed.

TERM	DEFINITION
1. ganglionectomy (*gang*-glē-o-NEK-to-mē)	excision of a ganglion (also called **gangliectomy**)

GANGLIONECTOMY may be performed to treat ganglion cysts that are painful, limit movement, or cause nerve entrapment.

TERM	DEFINITION
2. neurectomy (nū-REK-to-mē)	excision of a nerve
3. neurolysis (nū-ROL-i-sis)	loosening, separating a nerve (to release it from surrounding tissues)
4. neuroplasty (NŪR-ō-*plas*-tē)	surgical repair of a nerve
5. neurorrhaphy (nū-ROR-a-fē)	suturing of a nerve
6. neurotomy (nū-ROT-o-mē)	incision into a nerve
7. rhizotomy (rī-ZOT-o-mē)	incision into a nerve root

EXERCISE 12 ■ Pronounce and Spell

Practice pronunciation and spelling on paper and online.

1. Practice on Paper

a. **Pronounce:** Read the phonetic spelling and say aloud the terms listed in the previous table. Refer to the pronunciation key on p. 20 as necessary.
b. **Spell:** Have a study partner read the terms aloud. Write the spelling of the terms on a separate sheet of paper.

2. Practice Online

a. **Access** online learning resources. Go to evolve.elsevier.com > Evolve Resources > Student Resources.
b. **Pronounce:** Select Audio Glossary > Chapter 15 > Exercise 12. Select a term to hear its pronunciation and repeat aloud.
c. **Spell:** Select Activities > Chapter 15 > Spell Terms > Exercise 12. Select the audio icon and type the correct spelling of the term.

❑ Check the box when complete.

EXERCISE 13 ■ Analyze and Define

Analyze and define the following surgical terms.

1. neurectomy

____
____

2. neurorrhaphy

____
____

3. ganglionectomy

____
____

4. neurotomy

____
____

5. neurolysis

____
____

6. neuroplasty

____
____

7. rhizotomy

____
____

EXERCISE 14 ■ Build

A Fill In

Build surgical terms for the following definitions by using the word parts you have learned.

1. excision of a nerve ______ / ______
WR / S

2. suturing of a nerve ______ / ___ / ______
WR / CV / S

3. incision into a nerve ________ WR / CV / ________ S

4. loosening, separating a nerve (to release it from surrounding tissue) ________ WR / CV / ________ S

5. surgical repair of a nerve ________ WR / CV / ________ S

B Label

Build terms pictured by writing word parts above definitions.

1.

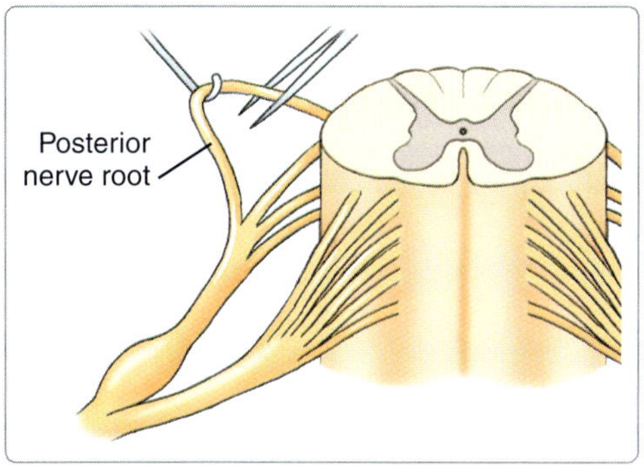

________ / ____ / ________
nerve root CV incision

2.

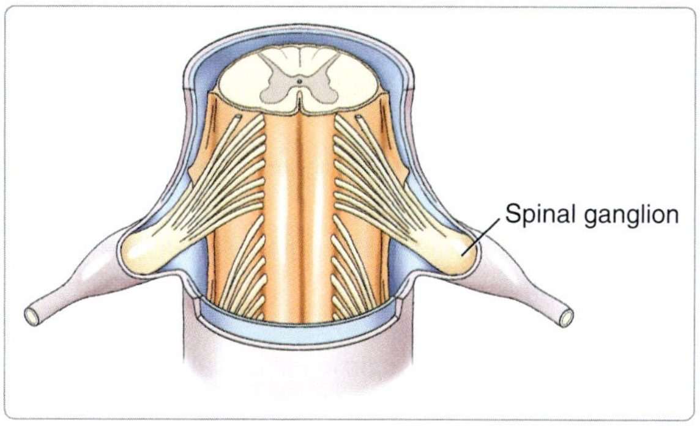

________ / ________
ganglion surgical removal

EXERCISE 15 Review of Surgical Terms

Can you define, pronounce, and spell the following terms?

ganglionectomy
neurectomy
neurolysis
neuroplasty
neurorrhaphy
neurotomy
rhizotomy

Diagnostic Terms

BUILT FROM WORD PARTS AND *NOT* BUILT FROM WORD PARTS

The first portion of the table contains nervous system diagnostic terms that can be translated using definitions of word parts. The second portion of the table contains terms that cannot be fully understood using the definitions of word parts.

Terms Built from Word Parts

DIAGNOSTIC IMAGING

TERM	DEFINITION	TERM	DEFINITION
1. **cerebral angiography** (se-RĒ-bral) (*an*-jē-OG-ra-fē)	process of recording (scan of) the blood vessels of the cerebrum (after an injection of a contrast agent)	2. **CT myelography** (C-T) (*mī*-e-LOG-ra-fē)	process of recording (scan of) the spinal cord (after an injection of a contrast agent into the subarachnoid space by lumbar puncture; size, shape, and position of the spinal cord and nerve roots are demonstrated)
		CT is the abbreviation for computed tomography.	

Diagnostic Terms—cont'd

BUILT FROM WORD PARTS AND *NOT* BUILT FROM WORD PARTS

Terms Built from Word Parts

NEURODIAGNOSTIC PROCEDURES

TERM	DEFINITION
3. **electroencephalogram (EEG)** (ē-*lek*-trō-en-SEF-a-lō-gram)	record of electrical activity of the brain
4. **electroencephalograph** (ē-*lek*-trō-en-SEF-a-lō-graf)	instrument used to record electrical activity of the brain
5. **electroencephalography** (ē-*lek*-trō-en-*sef*-a-LOG-ra-fē)	process of recording the electrical activity of the brain

NOT Built from Word Parts

DIAGNOSTIC IMAGING

TERM	DEFINITION
1. **positron emission tomography (PET) scan** (POZ-i-tron) (ē-MISH-un) (tō-MOG-rah-fē) (skan)	nuclear medicine procedure creating computerized images of chemical changes, such as sugar metabolism in brain tissue. Radioactive materials called tracers are bound to molecules used in metabolism. Areas that are more active, such as cancers, will use more of these molecules, and the PET scan will detect higher activity there. PET is usually combined with CT imaging, which shows precise anatomic location of the abnormality.

NEURODIAGNOSTIC PROCEDURES

TERM	DEFINITION
2. **evoked potential studies (EP studies)** (i-VŌKD) (pō-TEN-shal) (STUD-ēz)	group of diagnostic tests that measure changes and responses in brain waves elicited by visual, auditory, or somatosensory stimuli
3. **deep tendon reflexes (DTR)** (dēp) (TEN-don) (RĒ-flek-suhs)	portion of the physical examination where gentle strikes at specific locations are performed to assess the possibility of potential neurological abnormalities (also called **muscle stretch reflexes [MSR]**)

OTHER

TERM	DEFINITION
4. **lumbar puncture (LP)** (LUM-bar) (PUNK-chur)	diagnostic procedure performed by insertion of a needle into the subarachnoid space usually between the third and fourth lumbar vertebrae; performed for many reasons, including the removal of cerebrospinal fluid (also called **spinal tap**)

EXERCISE 16 ■ Pronounce and Spell

Practice pronunciation and spelling on paper and online.

1. Practice on Paper

a. **Pronounce:** Read the phonetic spelling and say aloud the terms listed in the previous table. Refer to the pronunciation key on p. 20 as necessary.

b. **Spell:** Have a study partner read the terms aloud. Write the spelling of the terms on a separate sheet of paper.

2. Practice Online

a. **Access** online learning resources. Go to evolve.elsevier.com > Evolve Resources > Student Resources.

b. **Pronounce:** Select Audio Glossary > Chapter 15 > Exercise 16. Select a term to hear its pronunciation and repeat aloud.

c. **Spell:** Select Activities > Chapter 15 > Spell Terms > Exercise 16. Select the audio icon and type the correct spelling of the term.

❑ Check the box when complete.

EXERCISE 17 ■ Diagnostic Terms Built from Word Parts

A Analyze and Define

Analyze and define the following diagnostic terms.

1. electroencephalogram

____

____

2. electroencephalograph

____

____

3. electroencephalography

____

____

4. CT myelography

____

____

5. cerebral angiography

____

____

B Label

Build terms pictured by writing word parts above definitions.

1.

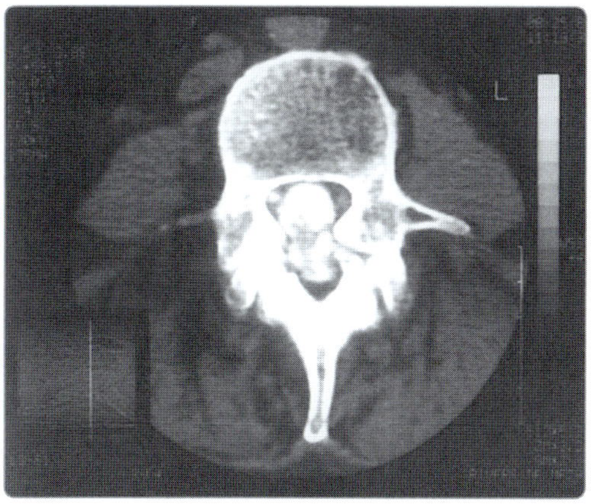

CT ____________ / ____ / ________________

spinal cord / CV / process of recording

2.

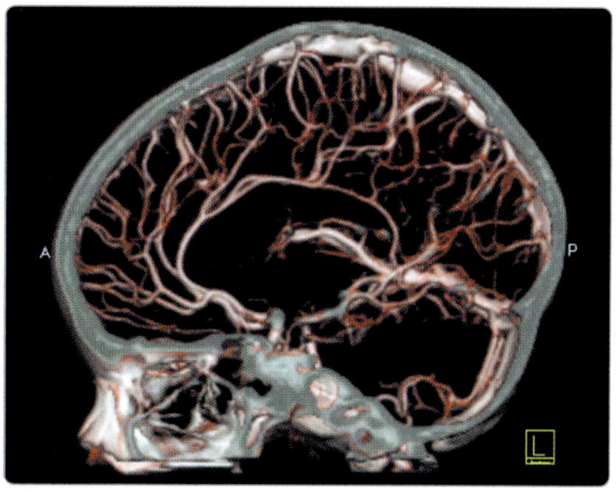

________ / ________ / ______ / ___ / ________

cerebrum / pertaining to / blood vessels / CV / process of recording

C Fill In

Build diagnostic terms that correspond to the following definitions by using the word parts you have learned.

1. record of electrical activity of the brain ______ / ______ / ______ / ______ / ______
   WR / CV / WR / CV / S

2. instrument used to record electrical activity of the brain ______ / ______ / ______ / ______ / ______
   WR / CV / WR / CV / S

3. process of recording the electrical activity of the brain ______ / ______ / ______ / ______ / ______
   WR / CV / WR / CV / S

EXERCISE 18 ■ Diagnostic Terms NOT Built from Word Parts

A Match

Match the diagnostic terms in the first column with their correct definitions in the second column.

______ 1. evoked potential studies
______ 2. positron emission tomography scan
______ 3. lumbar puncture
______ 4. deep tendon reflexes

a. diagnostic procedure performed by insertion of a needle into the subarachnoid space usually between the third and fourth lumbar vertebrae
b. portion of the physical examination where gentle strikes at specific locations are performed to assess the possibility of potential neurological abnormalities
c. group of diagnostic tests that measure changes and responses in brain waves elicited by visual, auditory, or somatosensory stimuli
d. nuclear medicine procedure creating computerized images of chemical changes, such as sugar metabolism in brain tissue

B Label

Write the diagnostic terms pictured and defined.

1. ____

group of diagnostic tests that measure changes and responses in brain waves elicited by visual, auditory, or somatosensory stimuli

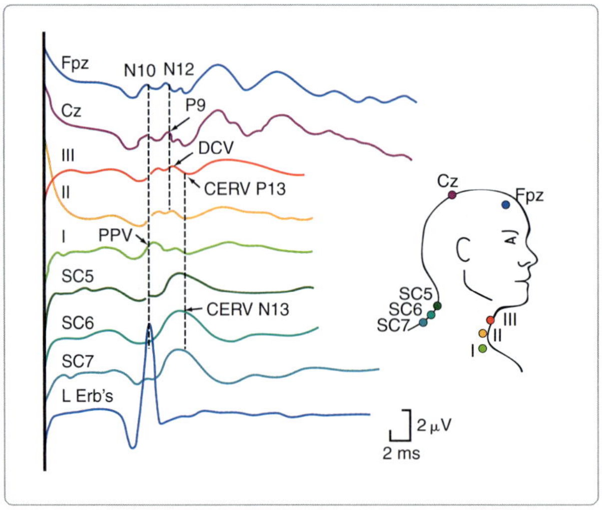

2. ____

diagnostic procedure performed by insertion of a needle into the subarachnoid space

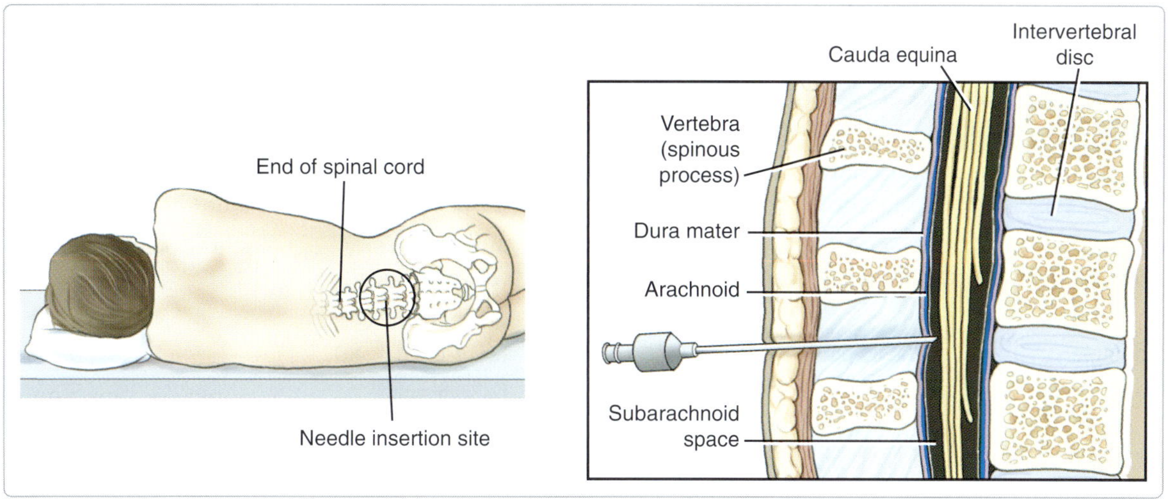

3. ____

portion of the physical examination where gentle strikes at specific locations are performed to assess the possibility of potential neurological abnormalities

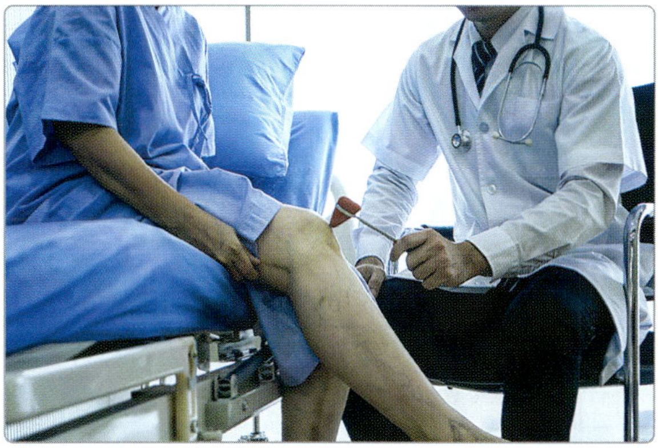

4. ____

nuclear medicine procedure creating computerized images of chemical changes; areas that are more active, such as cancers, will use more of these molecules and higher activity will be detected there

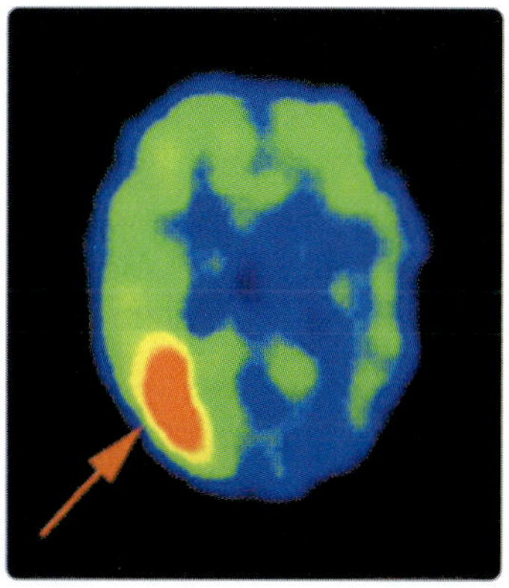

EXERCISE 19 ■ Review of Diagnostic Terms

Can you define, pronounce, and spell the following terms?

- cerebral angiography
- CT myelography
- deep tendon reflexes (DTR)
- electroencephalogram (EEG)
- electroencephalograph
- electroencephalography
- evoked potential studies (EP studies)
- lumbar puncture (LP)
- positron emission tomography (PET) scan

Complementary Terms

BUILT FROM WORD PARTS

The following terms can be translated using definitions of word parts. Further explanation is provided within parentheses as needed.

SIGNS & SYMPTOMS

TERM	DEFINITION
1. anesthesia (*an*-es-THĒ-zha)	without (loss of) feeling or sensation
2. aphasia (a-FĀ-zha)	condition of without speaking (loss or impairment of the ability to speak)
3. cephalgia (sef-AL-ja)	head pain (headache) *(NOTE: the* al *is dropped from the combining form cephal/o)*
4. dysphasia (dis-FĀ-zha)	condition of difficulty speaking
5. hemiparesis (*hem*-ē-pa-RĒ-sis)	slight paralysis of half (right or left side of the body)
6. hemiplegia (*hem*-ē-PLĒ-ja)	paralysis of half (right or left side of the body; stroke is the most common cause of hemiplegia)
7. hyperesthesia (*hī*-per-es-THĒ-zha)	excessive sensitivity (to stimuli)
8. monoparesis (*mon*-ō-pa-RĒ-sis)	slight paralysis of one (limb)
9. monoplegia (*mon*-ō-PLĒ-ja)	paralysis of one (limb)
10. paresthesia (*par*-es-THĒ-zha)	abnormal sensation (such as burning, prickling, or tingling sensation, often in the extremities; may be caused by nerve damage or peripheral neuropathy) *(Note: the* a *is dropped from the prefix para.)*
11. quadriplegia (*kwod*-ri-PLĒ-ja)	paralysis of four (limbs)

MIGRAINE, tension headache, and cluster headaches account for nearly 90% of all headaches.

MEDICAL SPECIALTIES

TERM	DEFINITION
12. neurologist (nū-ROL-o-jist)	physician who studies and treats diseases of the nervous system
13. neurology (nū-ROL-o-jē)	study of nerves (branch of medicine dealing with diseases of the nervous system)

DESCRIPTIVE TERMS

TERM	DEFINITION
14. craniocerebral (*krā*-nē-ō-su-RĒ-bral)	pertaining to the cranium and cerebrum
15. dysesthesia (dis-es-THĒ-zha)	painful sensation
16. interictal (*in*-ter-IK-tal)	(occurring) between seizures or attacks
17. mental (MEN-tel)	pertaining to the mind
18. postictal (pōst-IK-tal)	(occurring) after a seizure or attack
19. preictal (prē-IK-tal)	(occurring) before a seizure or attack

EXERCISE 20 ■ Pronounce and Spell

Practice pronunciation and spelling on paper and online.

1. Practice on Paper

a. **Pronounce:** Read the phonetic spelling and say aloud the terms listed in the previous table. Refer to the pronunciation key on p. 20 as necessary.
b. **Spell:** Have a study partner read the terms aloud. Write the spelling of the terms on a separate sheet of paper.

2. Practice Online

a. **Access** online learning resources. Go to evolve.elsevier.com > Evolve Resources > Student Resources.
b. **Pronounce:** Select Audio Glossary > Chapter 15 > Exercise 20. Select a term to hear its pronunciation and repeat aloud.
c. **Spell:** Select Activities > Chapter 15 > Spell Terms > Exercise 20. Select the audio icon and type the correct spelling of the term.

❑ Check the box when complete.

EXERCISE 21 ■ Analyze and Define

Analyze and define the following complementary terms.

1. preictal

____

____

2. paresthesia

____

____

3. mental

____

____

4. interictal

____

____

5. monoparesis

____

____

6. dysesthesia

____

____

EXERCISE 22 ■ Build

A Label

Build terms pictured by writing word parts above definitions.

1.

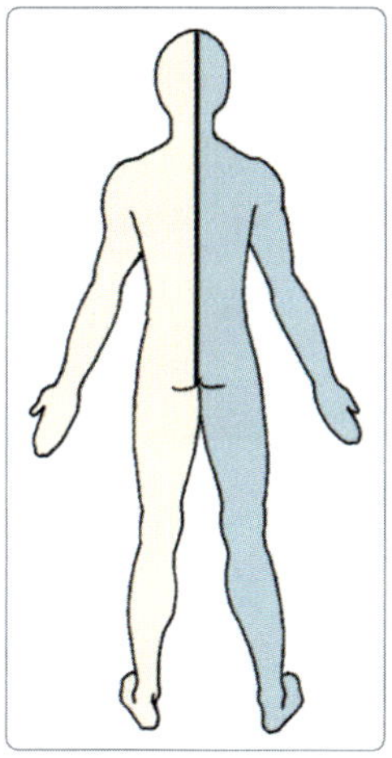

________ / ________
half paralysis

2.

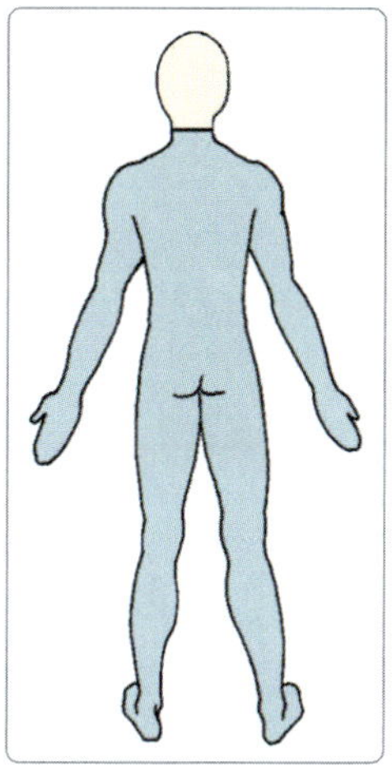

________ / ________ / ________
four CV paralysis

3.

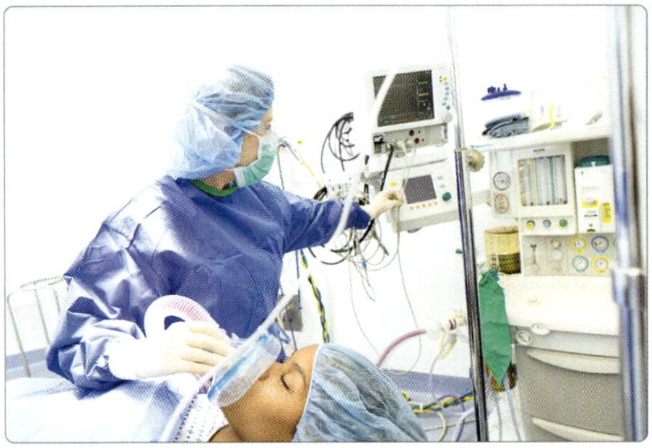

______________ / ______________ / a
without sensation

4.

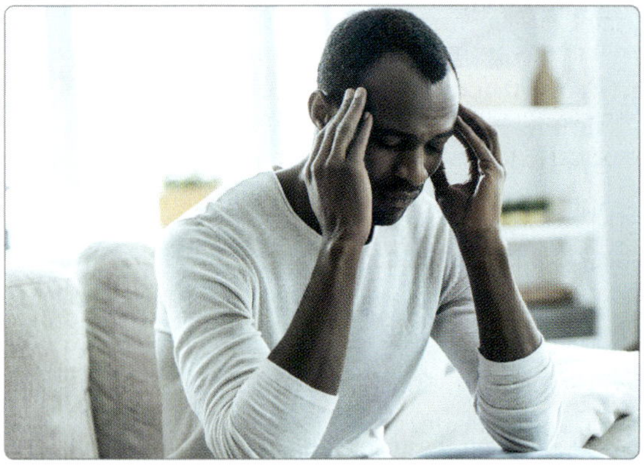

______________ / ______________
head pain

5.

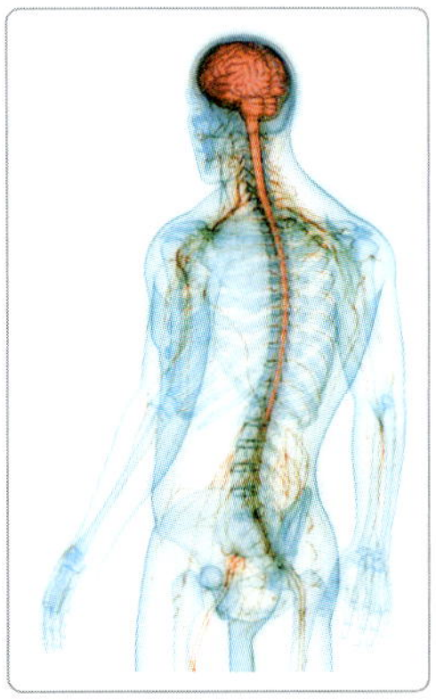

__________ / ______ / __________
nerves CV study of

6.

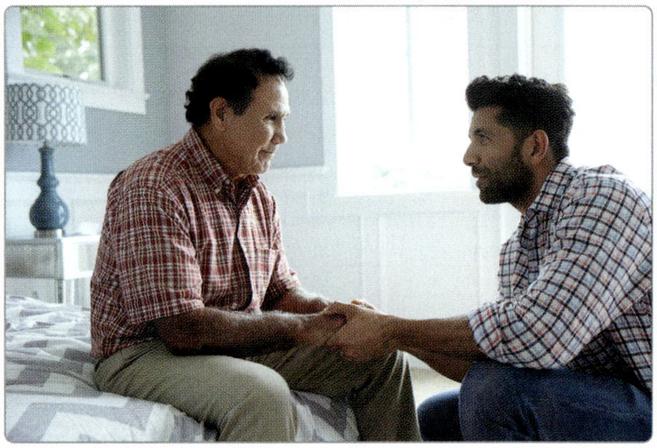

____________ / ____________ / ____________
without speaking condition of

B Fill In

Build complementary terms for the following definitions by using the word parts you have learned.

1. slight paralysis of half (right or left side of the body)
   ______ / ______
   P S(WR)

2. condition of difficulty speaking
   ______ / ______ / ______
   P WR S

3. excessive sensitivity (to stimuli)
   ______ / ______ / ______
   P WR S

4. pertaining to the cranium and cerebrum
   ______ / ______ / ______ / ______
   WR CV WR S

5. slight paralysis of one (limb)
   ______ / ______ / ______
   WR CV S

6. (occurring) after a seizure or attack

_______ P _______ / _______ S(WR) _______

7. physician who studies and treats diseases of the nervous system

_______ WR _______ / CV / _______ S _______

Complementary Terms

NOT BUILT FROM WORD PARTS

Word parts may be present in the following terms; however, their full meanings cannot be translated using definitions of word parts alone.

SIGNS AND SYMPTOMS

TERM	DEFINITION
1. ataxia (a-TAK-sē-a)	lack of muscle coordination
2. coma (KŌ-ma)	state of profound unconsciousness
3. concussion (kon-KUSH-un)	injury to the brain caused by minor or major head trauma; symptoms include vertigo, headache, and possible loss of consciousness

CONCUSSION is a common type of **traumatic brain injury (TBI)**, an umbrella term used to describe mild to severe damage to the brain sustained by a wide range of injuries. Falls, motor vehicle accidents, sports injuries, combat-related injuries or violence may all cause TBI.

TERM	DEFINITION
4. convulsion (kun-VUL-zhun)	sudden, involuntary contraction of a group of muscles; may be present during a seizure
5. disorientation (dis-*or*-ē-en-TĀ-shun)	state of mental confusion as to time, place, or identity
6. dysarthria (dis-AR-thrē-a)	inability to use speech that is distinct and connected because of a loss of muscle control after damage to the peripheral or central nervous system
7. paraplegia (*par*-a-PLĒ-ja)	paralysis from the waist down caused by damage to the lower level of the spinal cord

PARAPLEGIA is composed of the Greek **para**, meaning **beside**, and **plegia**, meaning **paralysis**. It has been used since Hippocrates' time and at first meant paralysis of any limb or side of the body. Since the nineteenth century, it has been used to mean paralysis from the waist down.

TERM	DEFINITION
8. seizure (SĒ-zher)	sudden, abnormal surge of electrical activity in the brain, resulting in involuntary body movements or behaviors
9. spasticity (spa-STIS-i-tē)	continued contraction of certain muscles due to damage of the brain or spinal cord controlling voluntary movement and causing tightness and stiffness that can interfere with normal movement, speech, and gait; associated with cerebral palsy, multiple sclerosis, and other neurological disorders

SPASTICITY derives from the Greek word **spastikos** meaning *to pull.*

TERM	DEFINITION
10. syncope (SINK-o-pē)	fainting or sudden loss of consciousness caused by lack of blood supply to the cerebrum
11. unconsciousness (un-KON-shus-nes)	state of being unaware of surroundings and incapable of responding to stimuli as a result of injury, shock, illness, or drugs

EQUIPMENT

TERM	DEFINITION
12. shunt (shunt)	tube implanted in the body to redirect the flow of a fluid

TABLE 15.2 Types of Cognitive Impairment

Mild cognitive impairment (MCI)	presence of significant memory changes when adjusted for age-related norms. The patient usually has little difficulty performing activities of daily living. This condition may be an early manifestation of Alzheimer disease or other forms of dementia.
Age-associated memory impairment	refers to a normal aging process in which the speed of mental processing and the performance of tasks decreases, and recent memory and learning are more difficult. Verbal intelligence is preserved, and this condition is not a forerunner of dementia.
Delirium	potentially reversible acute disturbance of consciousness with impairment of cognition. A number of conditions can cause delirium by interfering with brain metabolism. Drugs, alcohol, systemic infections, head trauma, hypoglycemia, and electrolyte disturbances are common examples.
Pseudodementia	behavioral disorder resembling dementia but is not caused by brain tissue abnormalities. This can be found in mental illness, such as major depression, and can be reversible with treatment.

Complementary Terms—cont'd

NOT BUILT FROM WORD PARTS

DESCRIPTIVE TERMS

TERM	DEFINITION
13. cognitive (COG-ni-tiv)	pertaining to the mental processes of comprehension, judgment, memory, and reason (Table 15.2)
14. conscious (KON-shus)	awake, alert, aware of one's surroundings
15. gait (gāt)	manner or style of walking
16. incoherent (*in*-kō-HĒR-ent)	unable to express one's thoughts or ideas in an orderly, intelligible manner

EXERCISE 23 ■ Pronounce and Spell

Practice pronunciation and spelling on paper and online.

1. Practice on Paper

a. **Pronounce:** Read the phonetic spelling and say aloud the terms listed in the previous table. Refer to the pronunciation key on p. 20 as necessary.
b. **Spell:** Have a study partner read the terms aloud. Write the spelling of the terms on a separate sheet of paper.

2. Practice Online

a. **Access** online learning resources. Go to evolve.elsevier.com > Evolve Resources > Student Resources.
b. **Pronounce:** Select Audio Glossary > Chapter 15 > Exercise 23. Select a term to hear its pronunciation and repeat aloud.
c. **Spell:** Select Activities > Chapter 15 > Spell Terms > Exercise 23. Select the audio icon and type the correct spelling of the term.

❑ Check the box when complete.

EXERCISE 24 ■ Fill In

A Label

Write the medical terms pictured and defined.

1. ______________________________
paralysis from the waist down caused by damage to the lower level of the spinal cord

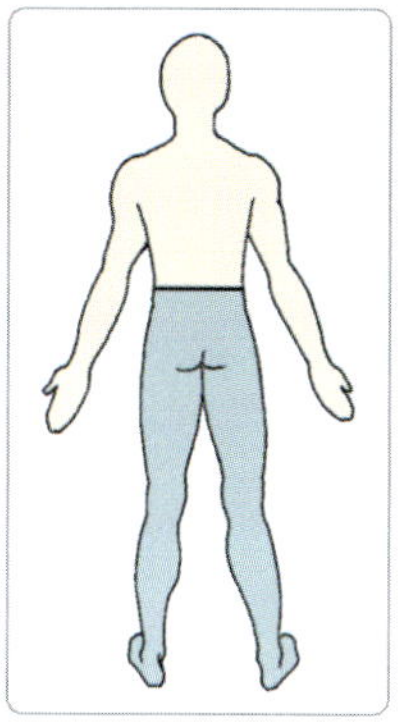

2. ______________________________
injury to the brain caused by minor or major head trauma; symptoms include vertigo, headache, and possible loss of consciousness

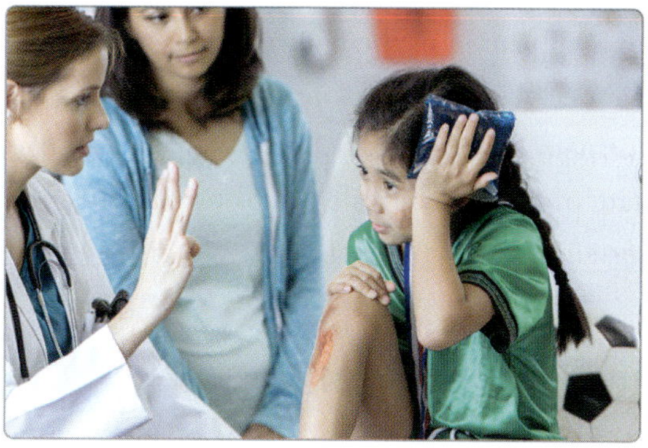

3. ______________________________
fainting or sudden loss of consciousness caused by lack of blood supply to the cerebrum

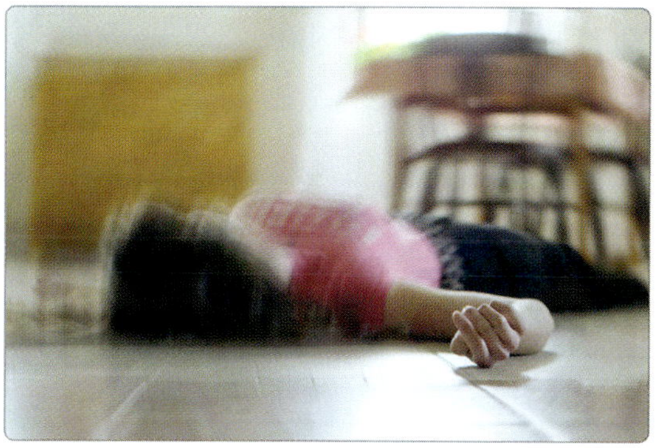

4. ______________________________
lack of muscle coordination

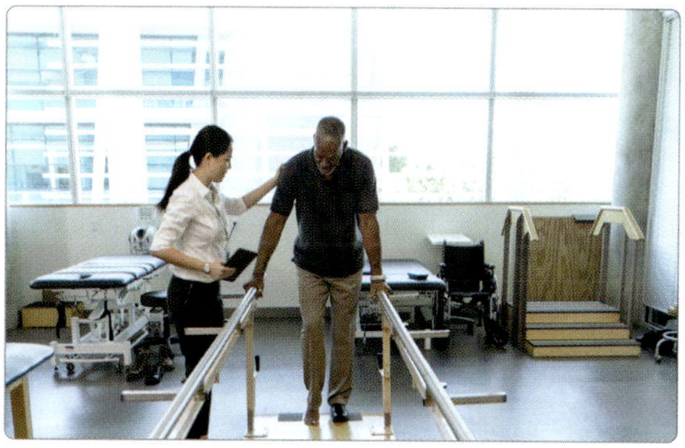

5. ______________________________
inability to use speech that is distinct and connected because of a loss of muscle control after damage to the peripheral or central nervous system

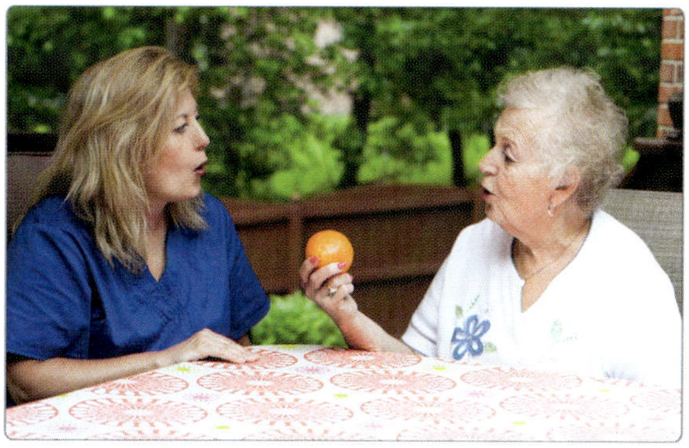

6. ______________________________
state of profound unconsciousness

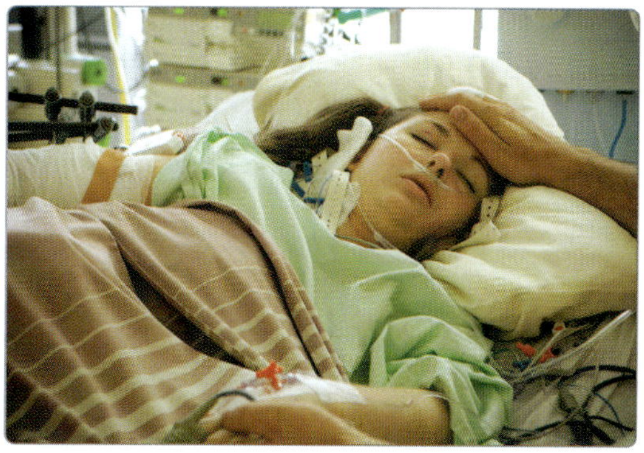

B Identify

Write the term for each of the following definitions.

1. continued contraction of certain muscles due to damage of the brain or spinal cord ____________________
2. state of being unaware of surroundings and incapable of responding to stimuli as a result of injury, shock, illness, or drugs ____________________
3. awake, alert, aware of one's surroundings ____________________
4. sudden, abnormal surge of electrical activity in the brain ____________________
5. sudden, involuntary contraction of a group of muscles ____________________
6. tube implanted in the body to redirect the flow of a fluid ____________________
7. manner or style of walking ____________________
8. unable to express one's thoughts or ideas in an orderly, intelligible manner ____________________
9. state of mental confusion as to time, place, or identity ____________________
10. pertaining to the mental processes of comprehension, judgment, memory, and reason ____________________

EXERCISE 25 ■ Match

Match the definitions in the first column with the correct terms in the second column.

	Definitions		Terms
______	1. state of profound unconsciousness	a.	shunt
______	2. fainting or sudden loss of consciousness	b.	paraplegia
______	3. paralysis from the waist down caused by damage to the lower level of the spinal cord	c.	coma
		d.	concussion
______	4. lack of muscle coordination	e.	unconsciousness
______	5. tube implanted in the body to redirect the flow of a fluid	f.	conscious
______	6. manner or style of walking	g.	seizure
______	7. inability to use speech that is distinctive and connected because of a loss of muscle control	h.	convulsion
		i.	syncope
______	8. sudden, abnormal surge of electrical activity in the brain	j.	ataxia
______	9. unable to express one's thoughts or ideas in an orderly, intelligible manner	k.	dysarthria
______	10. awake, alert, aware of one's surroundings	l.	gait
______	11. continued contraction of certain muscles due to damage of the brain or spinal cord controlling voluntary movement	m.	cognitive
		n.	disorientation
______	12. state of being unaware of surroundings and incapable of responding to stimuli as a result of injury, shock, illness, or drugs	o.	incoherent
______	13. pertaining to the mental processes of comprehension, judgment, memory, and reason	p.	spasticity
______	14. injury to the brain caused by head trauma		
______	15. state of mental confusion as to time, place, or identity		
______	16. sudden, involuntary contraction of a group of muscles		

EXERCISE 26 ■ Review of Complementary Terms

Can you define, pronounce, and spell the following terms?

anesthesia	craniocerebral	incoherent	postictal
aphasia	disorientation	interictal	preictal
ataxia	dysarthria	mental	quadriplegia
cephalgia	dysesthesia	monoparesis	seizure
cognitive	dysphasia	monoplegia	shunt
coma	gait	neurologist	spasticity
concussion	hemiparesis	neurology	syncope
conscious	hemiplegia	paraplegia	unconsciousness
convulsion	hyperesthesia	paresthesia	

Behavioral Health Terms

Although the terms below are listed as behavioral health terms, medications, physical changes, substance abuse, and illness may contribute to these conditions.

BUILT FROM WORD PARTS

The following terms can be translated using definitions of word parts. Further explanation is provided within parentheses as needed.

TERM	DEFINITION
1. **psychiatrist** (sī-KĪ-a-trist)	physician who studies and treats disorders of the mind (Psychiatrists have additional training and experience in prevention, diagnosis, and treatment of mental, emotional, and behavioral disorders. Psychiatrists often prescribe medications for patients with these disorders.)
2. **psychiatry** (sī-KĪ-a-trē)	specialty of the mind (branch of medicine that deals with the treatment of mental disorders)
3. **psychogenic** (sī-*kō*-JEN-ik)	originating in the mind
4. **psychologist** (sī-KOL-o-jist)	specialist of the mind (Clinical psychologists have graduate training in clinical psychology, administer psychological tests, and treat individuals with disturbances of mental, emotional, and behavioral disorders by counseling therapy.)
5. **psychology** (sī-KOL-o-jē)	study of the mind (a profession that involves dealing with the mind and mental processes in relation to human behavior)
6. **psychopathy** (sī-KOP-a-thē)	(any) disease of the mind
7. **psychosis** (***pl.*** **psychoses**) (sī-KO-sis), (sī-KO-sēz)	abnormal condition of the mind (major mental disorder characterized by extreme derangement, often with delusions and hallucinations)
8. **psychosomatic** (*sī*-kō-sō-MAT-ik)	pertaining to the mind and body (interrelations of)

EXERCISE 27 ■ Pronounce and Spell

Practice pronunciation and spelling on paper and online.

1. Practice on Paper

a. **Pronounce:** Read the phonetic spelling and say aloud the terms listed in the previous table. Refer to the pronunciation key on p. 20 as necessary.
b. **Spell:** Have a study partner read the terms aloud. Write the spelling of the terms on a separate sheet of paper.

2. Practice Online

a. **Access** online learning resources. Go to evolve.elsevier.com > Evolve Resources > Student Resources.
b. **Pronounce:** Select Audio Glossary > Chapter 15 > Exercise 27. Select a term to hear its pronunciation and repeat aloud.
c. **Spell:** Select Activities > Chapter 15 > Spell Terms > Exercise 27. Select the audio icon and type the correct spelling of the term.

❏ Check the box when complete.

EXERCISE 28 ■ Analyze and Define

Analyze and define the following terms.

1. psychosomatic

____

____

2. psychopathy

____

____

3. psychology

____

____

4. psychiatry

____

____

5. psychologist

____

____

6. psychogenic

____

____

7. psychiatrist

____

____

8. psychosis

____

____

EXERCISE 29 ■ Build

Build behavioral health terms for the following definitions by using the word parts you have learned.

1. specialty of the mind (branch of medicine that deals with the treatment of mental disorders)

_______ / _______
WR / S

2. abnormal condition of the mind

_______ / _______
WR / S

3. study of the mind (a profession that involves dealing with the mind and mental processes in relation to human behavior)
   WR / CV / S

4. originating in the mind
   WR / CV / S

5. physician who studies and treats disorders of the mind
   WR / S

6. specialist of the mind
   WR / CV / S

7. pertaining to the mind and body
   WR / CV / WR / S

8. (any) disease of the mind
   WR / CV / S

Behavioral Health Terms

NOT BUILT FROM WORD PARTS

Word parts may be present in the following terms; however, their full meanings cannot be translated using definitions of word parts alone.

TERM	DEFINITION
1. anorexia nervosa (*an*-ō-REK-sē-a) (ner-VŌ-sa)	eating disorder characterized by a disturbed perception of body image resulting in failure to maintain body weight, intensive fear of gaining weight, pronounced desire for thinness, and, in females, amenorrhea
2. anxiety disorder (ang-ZĪ-e-tē) (dis-OR-der)	disorder characterized by feelings of apprehension, tension, or uneasiness arising typically from the anticipation of unreal or imagined danger
3. attention deficit/hyperactivity disorder (ADHD) (a-TEN-shun) (DEF-i-sit) (*hī*-per-ak-TIV-i-tē) (dis-OR-der)	disorder of learning and behavioral problems characterized by marked inattention, distractibility, impulsiveness, and hyperactivity
4. autism (AW-tizm)	spectrum of mental disorders, the features of which include onset during infancy or childhood, preoccupation with subjective mental activity, inability to interact socially, and impaired communication (also referred to as **autism spectrum disorders [ASD]**)
5. bipolar disorder (bī-PŌ-lar) (dis-OR-der)	major psychological disorder typified by a disturbance in mood. The disorder is manifested by manic (elevated or irritated mood, excessive energy, impulsiveness) and depressive episodes that may alternate; or elements of both may occur simultaneously.
6. bulimia nervosa (bū-LĒ-mē-a) (ner-VŌ-sa)	eating disorder characterized by uncontrolled binge eating followed by purging (induced vomiting)
7. major depression (MĀ-jor) (dē-PRESH-un)	mood disturbance characterized by feelings of sadness, despair, discouragement, hopelessness, lack of joy, altered sleep patterns, and difficulty with decision making and daily function. Depression ranges from normal feelings of sadness (resulting from and proportional to personal loss or tragedy), through dysthymia (chronic depressive neurosis), to major depression. (also referred to as **clinical depression, mood disorder**)

Behavioral Health Terms—cont'd

NOT BUILT FROM WORD PARTS

TERM	DEFINITION
8. obsessive-compulsive disorder (OCD) (ob-SES-iv) (kom-PUL-siv) (dis-OR-der)	disorder characterized by intrusive, unwanted thoughts that result in the tendency to perform repetitive acts or rituals (compulsions), usually as a means of releasing tension or anxiety
9. panic attack (PAN-ik) (a-TAK)	episode of sudden onset of acute anxiety, occurring unpredictably, with feelings of acute apprehension, dyspnea, dizziness, sweating, and/or chest pain, depersonalization, paresthesia and fear of dying, loss of mind or control
10. phobia (FŌ-bē-a)	marked and persistent fear that is excessive or unreasonable cued by the presence or anticipation of a specific situation or object (such as claustrophobia, the abnormal fear of being in enclosed spaces)
11. pica (PĪ-ka)	compulsive eating of nonnutritive substances such as clay or ice. This condition may be a result of an iron deficiency. When iron deficiency is the cause of pica the condition will disappear in 1 or 2 weeks when treated with iron therapy.
12. posttraumatic stress disorder (PTSD) (*pōst*-tra-MAT-ik) (stres) (dis-OR-der)	significant behavioral health disorder in which some people exposed to a traumatic event go on to develop a series of symptoms related to it. These include mentally re-experiencing the event, increased autonomic arousal (the fight-flight-freeze response), avoidance of thoughts or activities that are reminders of the trauma, social withdrawal, and difficulty making emotional contacts with family and friends.
13. schizophrenia (*skit*-sō-FRĒ-nē-a)	any one of a large group of psychotic disorders characterized by gross distortions of reality, disturbance of language and communication, withdrawal from social interaction, and the disorganization and fragmentation of thought, perception, and emotional reaction
14. somatoform disorders (sō-MAT-ō-form) (dis-OR-derz)	disorders characterized by physical symptoms for which no known physical cause exists

Refer to **Appendix E** for pharmacology terms related to the nervous system and behavioral health.

EXERCISE 30 ■ Pronounce and Spell

Practice pronunciation and spelling on paper and online.

1. Practice on Paper

a. **Pronounce:** Read the phonetic spelling and say aloud the terms listed in the previous table. Refer to the pronunciation key on p. 20 as necessary.
b. **Spell:** Have a study partner read the terms aloud. Write the spelling of the terms on a separate sheet of paper.

2. Practice Online

a. **Access** online learning resources. Go to evolve.elsevier.com > Evolve Resources > Student Resources.
b. **Pronounce:** Select Audio Glossary > Chapter 15 > Exercise 30. Select a term to hear its pronunciation and repeat aloud.
c. **Spell:** Select Activities > Chapter 15 > Spell Terms > Exercise 30. Select the audio icon and type the correct spelling of the term.

❑ Check the box when complete.

EXERCISE 31 ■ Match

Match the definitions in the first column with the correct terms in the second column.

_____ 1. manifested by manic and depressive episodes
_____ 2. episode of acute anxiety, occurs unpredictably
_____ 3. characterized by feelings of apprehension and tension
_____ 4. disorder of learning and behavioral problems with distractibility
_____ 5. mood disturbance characterized by feelings of sadness, despair, and discouragement
_____ 6. marked and persistent fear that is excessive or unreasonable
_____ 7. binge eating followed by purging
_____ 8. physical symptoms for which no known physical cause exists
_____ 9. eating of nonnutritive substances, such as ice
_____ 10. disturbed perception of body image with failure to maintain body weight
_____ 11. characterized by gross distortions of reality and disturbance of language and communication
_____ 12. preoccupation with subjective mental activity, inability to interact socially, and impaired communication
_____ 13. mentally re-experiencing a traumatic event; avoidance of thoughts or activities that are reminders of the trauma
_____ 14. intrusive unwanted thoughts that result in rituals and/or repetitive acts

a. phobia
b. anxiety disorder
c. attention deficit/hyperactivity disorder
d. somatoform disorders
e. schizophrenia
f. anorexia nervosa
g. bulimia nervosa
h. pica
i. bipolar disorder
j. major depression
k. obsessive-compulsive disorder
l. posttraumatic stress disorder
m. panic attack
n. autism

EXERCISE 32 ■ Review of Behavioral Health Terms

Can you define, pronounce, and spell the following terms?

anorexia nervosa
anxiety disorder
attention deficit/hyperactivity disorder (ADHD)
autism
bipolar disorder
bulimia nervosa
major depression
obsessive-compulsive disorder (OCD)
panic attack
phobia
pica
posttraumatic stress disorder (PTSD)
psychiatrist
psychiatry
psychogenic
psychologist
psychology
psychopathy
psychosis (*pl.* psychoses)
psychosomatic
schizophrenia
somatoform disorders

Abbreviations

DISEASES AND DISORDERS

ABBREVIATION	TERM	ABBREVIATION	TERM
AD	Alzheimer disease	**OCD**	obsessive-compulsive disorder
ADHD	attention deficit/hyperactivity disorder	**PD**	Parkinson disease
ALS	amyotrophic lateral sclerosis	**PTSD**	posttraumatic stress disorder
CP	cerebral palsy	**SAH**	subarachnoid hemorrhage
CTE	chronic traumatic encephalopathy	**TBI**	traumatic brain injury
CVA	cerebrovascular accident	**TIA**	transient ischemic attack
MS	multiple sclerosis		

Abbreviations—cont'd

DIAGNOSTIC			
ABBREVIATION	**TERM**	**ABBREVIATION**	**TERM**
DTR	deep tendon reflexes	**LP**	lumbar puncture
EEG	electroencephalogram	**PET**	positron emission tomography
EP studies	evoked potential studies		

DESCRIPTIVE			
ABBREVIATION	**TERM**	**ABBREVIATION**	**TERM**
CNS	central nervous system	**PNS**	peripheral nervous system
CSF	cerebrospinal fluid		

Refer to **Appendix D** for a complete list of abbreviations.

EXERCISE 33 ■ Fill In

Write the terms abbreviated.

1. **DTR** _______ _______ _______ provide an objective sign of neurological abnormality.
2. Diagnostic tests used to diagnose patients with diseases of the nervous system include **EEG** _______ _______, CT, MR, **PET** _______ _______ _______, **EP studies** _______ _______ _______, and **LP** _______ _______.
3. Diseases that affect the nervous system are **AD** _______ _______, **ALS** _______ _______ _______, **CP** _______ _______, **MS** _______ _______, and **PD** _______ _______.
4. Stroke is the disruption of normal blood supply to the brain; it often occurs suddenly. Because of this, Hippocrates used the term *apoplexy*, which literally means *struck down*, to describe the condition. The term *stroke* grew out of the term *apoplexy*. The term *brain attack* is used to signify that a stroke is in progress and an emergency situation exists. **CVA** _______ _______ is also used to describe a stroke. An ischemic stroke, which is caused by a thrombosis or embolus, is frequently preceded by a **TIA** _______ _______ _______. A ruptured cerebral aneurysm is the most common cause of **SAH** _______ _______, a type of hemorrhagic stroke.
5. The examination of **CSF** _______ _______ may assist in the diagnosis of cerebral hemorrhage, meningitis, encephalitis, and other diseases.
6. Two common psychiatric disorders are **OCD** _______-_______ _______, and **ADHD** _______ _______ / _______ _______.
7. The nervous system may be divided into the **CNS** _______ _______ _______, and the **PNS** _______ _______ _______.
8. Psychiatric disorders related to trauma include **PTSD** _______ _______ _______ and **CTE** _______ _______ _______.
9. A concussion is a mild form of **TBI** _______ _______ _______. More severe TBI can lead to serious physical and psychological symptoms, coma, and death.

PRACTICAL APPLICATION

EXERCISE 34 ■ Case Study: Translate Between Everyday Language and Medical Language

CASE STUDY: Koji Kaneshiro

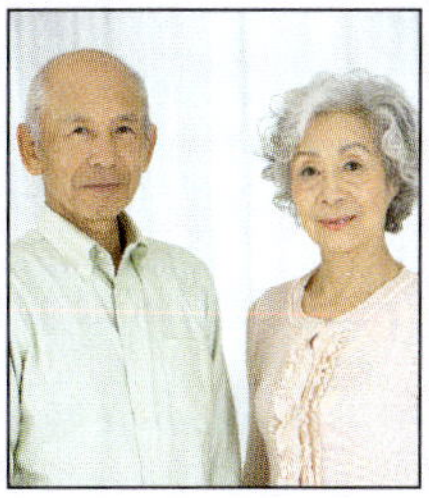

Kazuno Kaneshiro is worried about her husband, Koji. He was eating breakfast with her when he suddenly stopped speaking and dropped his spoon onto the table. "He never does that!" she thought. He seemed to be unable to speak. Also, his right arm was hanging limply by his side. She noticed that the left side of his face was also droopy. She had seen a billboard about strokes and was afraid he might be having one. She remembered the billboard saying that every minute counts, so she called 911 immediately.

Now that you have worked through Chapter 15, consider the medical terms that might be used to describe Mr. Kaneshiro's experience. See the Chapter at a Glance Section at the end of the chapter for a list of terms that might apply.

A. *Underline phrases in the case study that could be substituted with medical terms.*

B. *Write the medical term and its definition for three of the phrases you underlined.*

MEDICAL TERM	DEFINITION
1. ______________________	______________________________________
2. ______________________	______________________________________
3. ______________________	______________________________________

DOCUMENTATION: Excerpt from Emergency Department Visit

Mr. Kaneshiro was evaluated in the local emergency department; an excerpt from the medical record is documented below.

This 78-year-old male presented to the emergency department after the sudden onset of aphasia, right hemiplegia, and facial droop. Physical exam reveals an elderly male who is alert and oriented x3, but shows evidence of dysphasia. Focused neurologic exam is significant for right-sided facial drooping with paralysis of the seventh cranial nerve. The rest of the cranial nerves appear normal. Motor exam reveals hemiparesis on the right. Paresthesias are also present on the right. Cerebellar exam is normal, though difficult to test on the right. Gait is not assessed due to the patient's weakness. A CT of the head without contrast indicates no evidence of cerebral or subarachnoid hemorrhage. The patient appears to be experiencing a CVA. We will start him on the stroke protocol.

C. *Underline medical terms presented in Chapter 15 used in the previous excerpt from Mr. Kaneshiro's medical record. See the Chapter at a Glance Section at the end of the chapter for a complete list.*

D. *Select and define three of the medical terms you underlined. To check your answers, go to Appendix A.*

MEDICAL TERM	DEFINITION
1. ______________________	______________________________________
2. ______________________	______________________________________
3. ______________________	______________________________________

EXERCISE 35 ■ Interact with Medical Documents

A

Read the report and complete it by writing medical terms on answer lines within the document. Definitions of terms to be written appear after the document.

71086-NUR DRAKE, Eldon

File Patient Navigate Custom Fields Help

Chart Review | Encounters | Notes | Labs | Imaging | Procedures | Rx | Documents | Referrals | Scheduling | Billing

Name: **DRAKE, Eldon** MR#: 71086-NUR DOB: 08/12/19XX Gender: M Age: 85 **Allergies:** NKDA **PCP:** Maggie Alcott, APRN

History: Eldon Drake is an 85-year-old male who was admitted to the hospital on 01/02/20XX for fever and confusion. Mr. Drake was in his usual state of good health until 3 days before admission, when he began to show signs of confusion and 1.________________ accompanied by a fever of 38.5°C. His fever continued, and he showed a steady decline in 2. ________________ function. He developed expressive 3. ________________.

Objective Findings: On physical examination the patient was 4. ________________ and alert but disoriented to time and place. Blood pressure was 160/80 mm Hg. Pulse, 96. Respirations, 20. Temperature 38.8° C. There were no focal neurologic deficits. Chest radiograph, urinalysis, and blood cultures were negative. A 5. ________________ consultation was obtained. MR of the brain was performed, which disclosed 6.________________. An 7. ________________ was markedly abnormal for his age.

Treatment Summary: The patient was given acyclovir by intravenous infusion. On the second hospital day, the patient developed a generalized 8. ________________. He was placed on intravenous phenytoin and lorazepam. He later lapsed into a semicomatose state. He responded to tactile and verbal stimuli but was completely 9. ________________.
A nasogastric tube was placed, and enteral feedings were begun. After 14 days of IV acyclovir, the patient slowly began to improve and by the third week of his illness, he was talking normally and taking nourishment.

Electronically signed: Rashid Maitryi MD 01/23/20XX 11:18

Start | Log On/Off | Print | Edit

Definitions of Medical Terms to Complete the Document

Write the medical terms defined on corresponding answer lines in the document.

1. a state of mental confusion as to time, place, or identity
2. pertaining to the mental processes of comprehension, judgment, memory, and reason
3. loss of the ability to speak
4. awake, alert, and aware of one's surroundings
5. study of nerves (branch of medicine dealing with diseases of the nervous system)
6. inflammation of the brain
7. record of electrical impulses of the brain
8. sudden, abnormal surge of electrical activity in the brain
9. unable to express one's thoughts or ideas in an orderly, intelligible manner

B

Read the medical report and answer the questions below it.

32463 CASTILLA, ALANZE

File Patient Navigate Custom Fields Help

Patient Chart | Lab | Rad | Notes | Documents | Rx | Scheduling | Images | Billing

Name: **CASTILLA, ALANZE** MR#: **32463** Gender: **F** Allergies: **Sulfonamides**
DOB: **04/11/19XX** PCP: **Mei Shang, MD**

NEUROLOGY CONSULTATION

ENCOUNTER DATE: 06/04/20XX

HISTORY: The patient is a 63-year-old female referred to Neurology because of persistent low back and right leg pain and paresthesias of 6 months, duration. The pain is described as dull and aching and is rated 6/10. The discomfort is worse when standing and intensifies after walking about a block. The pain improves when the patient is sitting or when bending over. Her general health is good and there has been no weight loss.

NEUROLOGIC EXAM: The gait is somewhat wide based. Balance is normal. No muscle atrophy is present. Muscle strength is normal for age. The right Achilles reflex is absent. Sensation to pinprick is diminished over the right S1 dermatome.

LAB AND IMAGING: CBC and sed rate are normal. Fasting blood sugar is 106 mg/dL. A lumbosacral spine radiograph shows spondylosis and spondylolisthesis of L5 over S1. A CT scan shows a moderate degree of facet joint arthropathy and bulging discs at L2-3 and L4-5 levels along with narrowing of the spinal canal at these levels.

IMPRESSION: Lumbar spinal stenosis with radiculopathy of the S1 nerve root.

RECOMMENDATION: Referral to Neuroanesthesia for a series of epidural steroid injections. Physical therapy is also advised. Surgical referral is not necessary at this time.

Electronically signed by: Susan Rand, MD 06/04/20XX 18:15

Start | Log On/Off | Print | Edit

Use the medical report above to answer the questions.

1. Spinal stenosis causes compression of nerve roots demonstrated by which of the following symptoms for the patient?
   a. total paralysis
   b. abnormal sensation of burning, prickling, or tingling
   c. paralysis of one limb
   d. slight paralysis

2. The patient's diagnosis is spinal stenosis with:
   a. disease of the nerve roots
   b. disease of peripheral nerves
   c. disease affecting a single nerve
   d. disease of many nerves

EXERCISE 36 ■ Use Medical Language in Online Electronic Health Records

Select the correct medical terms to complete three medical records in one patient's electronic file.

Access online resources at evolve.elsevier.com > Evolve Resources > Student Resources > Activities > Chapter 15 > Electronic Health Records

Topic: Migraine
Record 1: Office Visit Report
Record 2: Emergency Department Report
Record 3: Diagnostic Imaging Report

❑ Check the box when complete.

EXERCISE 37 ■ Pronounce Medical Terms in Use

Practice pronunciation of terms by reading aloud the following paragraph. Use the phonetic spellings to assist with pronunciation. The script also contains medical terms not presented in the chapter. If interested, research their meanings in a medical dictionary or a reliable online source.

A 36-year-old right-handed female presents to the emergency department for an episode of **monoparesis** (*mon*-ō-pa-RĒ-sis) of the right leg, which started earlier in the day. She has a history of **major depression** (MĀ-jor) (dē-PRESH-un), for which she sees a **psychiatrist** (sī-KĪ-a-trist), and is treated with medication. About 6 months ago, she had an episode of optic **neuritis** (nū-RĪ-tis), which was treated with steroids. She denies any history of **seizures** (SĒ-zherz). On examination, she was noted to have **gait** (gāt) difficulties due to the weakness of her right leg. There was no evidence of **paresthesia** (*par*-es-THĒ-zha) or **cognitive** (COG-ni-tiv) impairment. Because of her age, a diagnosis of **stroke** (strōk) or **TIA** (T-I-A) is unlikely. A **subdural hematoma** (sub-DŪ-ral) (*hē*-ma-TŌ-ma) or intracranial lesion, such as **meningioma** (me-*nin*-jē-Ō-ma) or **glioblastoma** (*glī*-ō-blas-TŌ-ma), must be ruled out. Her symptoms are suggestive of **multiple sclerosis** (MUL-ti-pl) (skle-RŌ-sis). We will order an MR of the brain with contrast to see if any characteristic lesions are present. If not, we will consider a **lumbar puncture** (LUM-bar) (PUNK-chur) and refer her to a **neurologist** (nū-ROL-o-jist) for **evoked potential studies** (i-VŌKD) (pō-TEN-shal) (STUD-ēz).

CHAPTER REVIEW

EXERCISE 38 ■ Chapter Content Quiz

Test your understanding of terms and abbreviations introduced in this chapter. Circle the letter for the medical term or abbreviation related to the words in italics.

1. Jack Cheng was in a serious motorcycle accident that resulted in *paralysis of all four limbs.*
   a. quadriplegia
   b. monoplegia
   c. hemiplegia

2. During her stroke, Mrs. Delgado had *inability to speak.*
   a. dysarthria
   b. aphasia
   c. dysphasia

3. Jacob Mamula experienced a brief period of being *unaware of his or her surroundings and unable to respond to stimuli* after suffering a concussion from a hard hit during the football game.
   a. convulsion
   b. incoherent
   c. unconsciousness

4. The newborn had *protrusion of the meninges* through a defect in his skull.
   a. myelomalacia
   b. myelomeningocele
   c. meningocele

5. Gabriella Moreno was advised to schedule an appointment with the *physician who studies and treats disorders of the mind* when she was diagnosed with bipolar disorder.
   a. neurologist
   b. psychologist
   c. psychiatrist

6. *Chronic degenerative disease characterized by sclerotic patches along the brain and spinal cord* is more common in women, and frequently presents in the fourth or fifth decade of life.
   a. multiple sclerosis
   b. schizophrenia
   c. amyotrophic lateral sclerosis

7. The *process of recording of electrical activity of the brain* was scheduled for Caleb Cook when he started experiencing seizures.
   a. electroencephalogram
   b. electroencephalography
   c. electroencephalograph

8. *Abnormal condition of a clot in the cerebrum* was the cause of the TIA that Mr. Hernandez experienced.
   a. cerebral thrombosis
   b. cerebral aneurysm
   c. cerebral embolism

9. Mrs. Patel was having headaches and blurred vision. Her doctor was concerned about a meningioma. She ordered a *diagnostic procedure to examine blood flow and metabolic activity.*
   a. evoked potential studies
   b. positron emission tomography
   c. lumbar puncture

10. Misha Sanov was diagnosed with *viral disease that affects the peripheral nerves and causes blisters on the skin that follow the course of the affected nerves* over her upper abdomen.
    a. shingles
    b. sciatica
    c. epilepsy

11. Because of scarring from a burn injury to her right hand, Emma Sammani had *loosening, separating a nerve to release it from surrounding tissues* to provide pain relief.
    a. neurolysis
    b. neuralgia
    c. rhizotomy

12. Mr. Rosenthal was taking medication to try to prevent rapid progression of his *type of dementia that occurs more frequently after the age of 65, with dramatic brain shrinkage.*
    a. PD
    b. CP
    c. AD

13. After his military service ended, Brandon O'Rourke experienced *significant behavioral disorder in which some people exposed to a traumatic event go on to develop a series of symptoms related to it.*
    a. somatoform disorder
    b. panic attacks
    c. posttraumatic stress disorder

14. James Robbins had poliomyelitis as a child, and was left with *slight paralysis of one (limb)*, which made it difficult for him to walk without assistance.
    a. monoparesis
    b. monoplegia
    c. hemiparesis

15. The physician assistant thought that Mrs. Ng's complaints of headaches and abdominal pain, which started after she lost her job, might be *pertaining to the mind and body.*
    a. psychopathy
    b. psychogenic
    c. psychosomatic

16. Corrine Pageau was brought to the emergency department after experiencing a seizure. She was eventually diagnosed with herpes simplex *inflammation of the brain.*
    a. meningitis
    b. encephalitis
    c. radiculitis

17. Daniel Roth lost consciousness after complaining of severe cephalgia; a CT scan revealed *bleeding between the pia mater and arachnoid layers of the meninges caused by a ruptured blood vessel.*
    a. subarachnoid hemorrhage
    b. subdural hematoma
    c. hydrocephalus

18. Malia Williams has been receiving therapy in the psychology department for her *disorder characterized by intrusive, unwanted thoughts that result in the tendency to perform repetitive acts or rituals.*
    a. attention deficit/hyperactivity disorder
    b. bipolar disorder
    c. obsessive-compulsive disorder

19. Kevin, who has primary progressive multiple sclerosis, experiences painful bouts of *continued contraction of certain muscles due to damage of the brain or spinal cord controlling voluntary movement.*
    a. ataxia
    b. spasticity
    c. dysesthesia

20. Causes of transverse *inflammation of the spinal cord* include infections, immune system disorders, and other conditions that damage the insulating substance covering nerves.
    a. myelitis
    b. neuritis
    c. meningitis

CHAPTER AT A GLANCE Word Parts New to This Chapter

COMBINING FORMS

cerebell/o
cerebr/o
dur/o
encephal/o
esthesi/o
gangli/o
ganglion/o
gli/o
mening/o
meningi/o
ment/o
mon/o
myel/o
phas/o
poli/o
psych/o
quadr/i
radicul/o
rhiz/o

SUFFIXES

-iatrist
-iatry
-ictal
-paresis

CHAPTER AT A GLANCE Nervous System Terms Built from Word Parts

DISEASE AND DISORDER

cerebellitis
cerebral embolism
cerebral thrombosis
duritis
encephalitis
encephalomalacia
encephalopathy
encephalomyeloradiculitis
gangliitis
glioblastoma
glioma
hydrocephalus
intracerebral hemorrhage
meningioma
meningitis
meningocele
meningomyelocele
mononeuropathy
myelitis
myelomalacia
neuralgia
neuritis
poliomyelitis
polyneuritis
polyneuropathy
radiculitis
radiculopathy
rhizomeningomyelitis
subdural hematoma

SURGICAL

ganglionectomy
neurectomy
neurolysis
neuroplasty
neurorrhaphy
neurotomy
rhizotomy

DIAGNOSTIC

cerebral angiography
CT myelography
electroencephalogram (EEG)
electroencephalograph
electroencephalography

COMPLEMENTARY

anesthesia
aphasia
cephalgia
craniocerebral
dysesthesia
dysphasia
hemiparesis
hemiplegia
hyperesthesia
interictal
mental
monoparesis
monoplegia
neurologist
neurology
paresthesia
postictal
preictal
quadriplegia

BEHAVIORAL HEALTH

psychiatrist
psychiatry
psychogenic
psychologist
psychology
psychopathy
psychosis (*pl.* psychoses)
psychosomatic

CHAPTER AT A GLANCE Nervous System Terms *NOT* Built from Word Parts

DISEASE AND DISORDER

Alzheimer disease (AD)
amyotrophic lateral sclerosis (ALS)
Bell palsy
botulism
cerebral aneurysm
cerebral palsy (CP)
chronic traumatic encephalopathy (CTE)
dementia
epilepsy
multiple sclerosis (MS)
Parkinson disease (PD)
sciatica
shingles
stroke
subarachnoid hemorrhage (SAH)
transient ischemic attack (TIA)

DIAGNOSTIC

deep tendon reflexes (DTR)
evoked potential studies (EP studies)
lumbar puncture (LP)
positron emission tomography (PET) scan

COMPLEMENTARY

ataxia
cognitive
coma
concussion
conscious
convulsion
disorientation
dysarthria
gait
incoherent
paraplegia
seizure
shunt
spasticity
syncope
unconsciousness

BEHAVIORAL HEALTH

anorexia nervosa
anxiety disorder
attention deficit/hyperactivity disorder (ADHD)
autism
bipolar disorder
bulimia nervosa
major depression
obsessive-compulsive disorder (OCD)
panic attack
phobia
pica
posttraumatic stress disorder (PTSD)
schizophrenia
somatoform disorders

Chapter 16 Endocrine System

Outline

Objectives

Upon completion of this chapter, you will be able to:

1. Pronounce glands and hormones of the endocrine system.
2. Define and spell word parts related to the endocrine system.
3. Define, pronounce, and spell disease and disorder terms related to the endocrine system.
4. Define, pronounce, and spell surgical terms related to the endocrine system.
5. Define, pronounce, and spell diagnostic terms related to the endocrine system.
6. Define, pronounce, and spell complementary terms related to the endocrine system.
7. Interpret the meaning of abbreviations related to the endocrine system.
8. Apply medical language in clinical contexts.

ANATOMY

The endocrine system is composed of endocrine glands distributed throughout the body. The endocrine glands are: pituitary, thyroid, parathyroid, adrenal, pancreas, gonads (ovaries and testes), and thymus.

Function

The endocrine system regulates body activities through the use of chemical messengers called **hormones**, which when released into the bloodstream influence metabolic activities, growth, and development (Fig. 16.1). The nervous system also regulates body activities by receiving electrical impulses that convey information about the state of the body, and then activating glandular secretions in response. Hormones secreted by the **endocrine glands** that make up the endocrine system go directly into the bloodstream and are transported throughout the body. They are referred to as **ductless glands** because they do not have ducts to carry their secretions. In contrast, the **exocrine** or **duct glands** have ducts that carry their secretions from the producing gland to other parts of the body. An example is the parotid gland, which produces saliva that flows through the parotid duct into the mouth. Only those terms related to the major endocrine glands—pituitary, thyroid, parathyroids, adrenals, and the islets of Langerhans in the pancreas—are presented in this chapter. The thymus primarily functions as part of the lymphatic system and was presented in Chapter 10. The male and female sex glands were also presented in previous chapters.

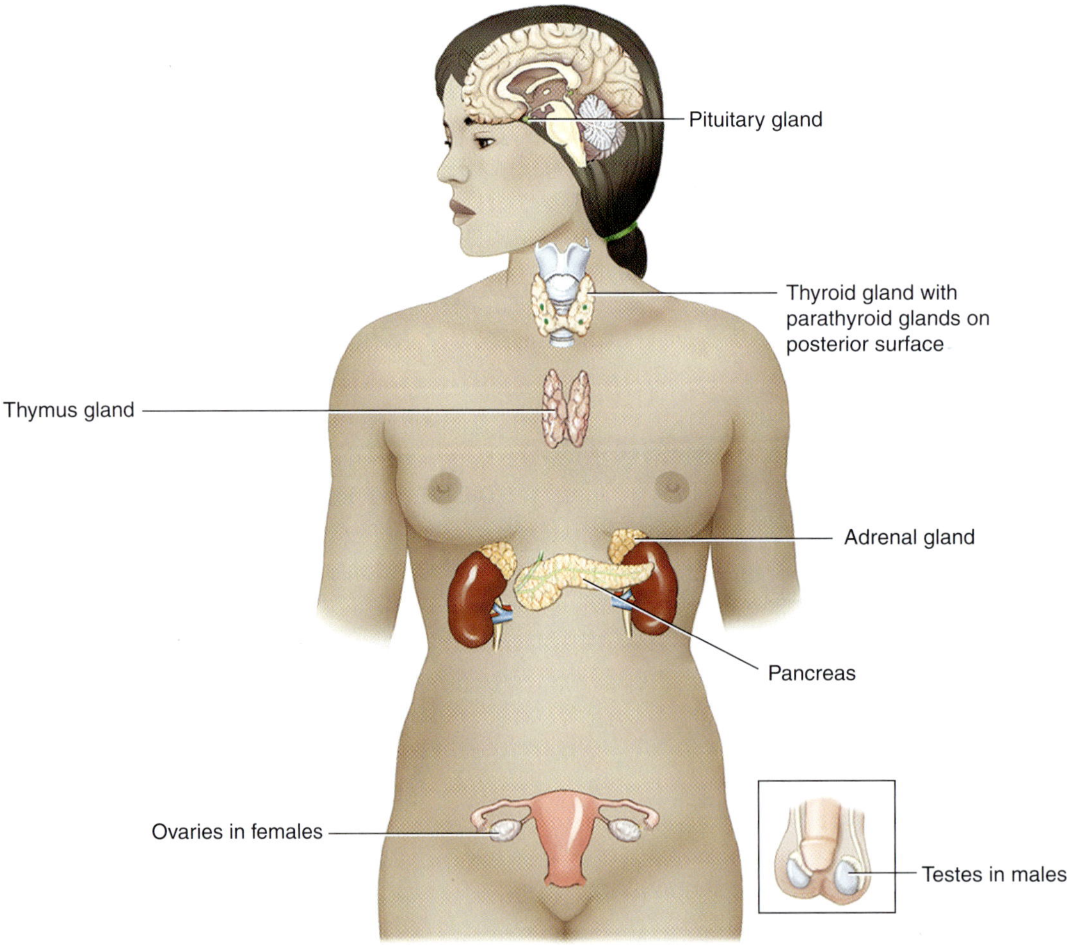

FIG. 16.1 The endocrine system.

Endocrine Glands and Hormones

TERM	DEFINITION
pituitary gland (pi-TOO-i-*tar*-ē) (gland)	approximately the size of a pea and located at the base of the brain. The pituitary is divided into two lobes. It is often referred to as the master gland because it produces hormones that stimulate the function of other endocrine glands. (also called **hypophysis cerebri**) (Fig. 16.2 and Fig. 16.3A)
anterior lobe (ān-TĒR-ē-er) (lōb)	produces and secretes the following hormones (also called **adenohypophysis**):
growth hormone (GH) (grohth) (HŌR-mōn)	regulates the growth of the body
adrenocorticotropic hormone (ACTH) (a-*drē*-nō-*kōr*-ti-kō-TRŌ-pik) (HŌR-mōn)	stimulates the adrenal cortex
thyroid-stimulating hormone (TSH) (THĪ-royd) (STIM-yuh-lāt-ing) (HŌR-mōn)	stimulates the thyroid gland
gonadotropic hormones (*gō-na*-dō-TRŌ-pik) (HŌR-mōns)	stimulate the gonads (the testes in males and ovaries in females). **Follicle-stimulating hormone** (FSH) and **luteinizing hormone** (LH) are the gonadotropic hormones released from the adenohypophysis.
prolactin (PRL) (prō-LAK-tin)	promotes development of glandular tissue during pregnancy and produces milk after birth of an infant
posterior lobe (po-STĒR-ē-er) (lōb)	stores and releases antidiuretic hormone and oxytocin (also called **neurohypophysis**)
antidiuretic hormone (ADH) (*an*-tē-*dī*-ū-RET-ik) (HŌR-mōn)	stimulates the kidney to reabsorb water and constricts blood vessels to help maintain blood pressure (also called **vasopressin**)
oxytocin (*ok*-sē-TŌ-sin)	stimulates uterine contractions during labor and postpartum, and milk let down by the breasts postpartum

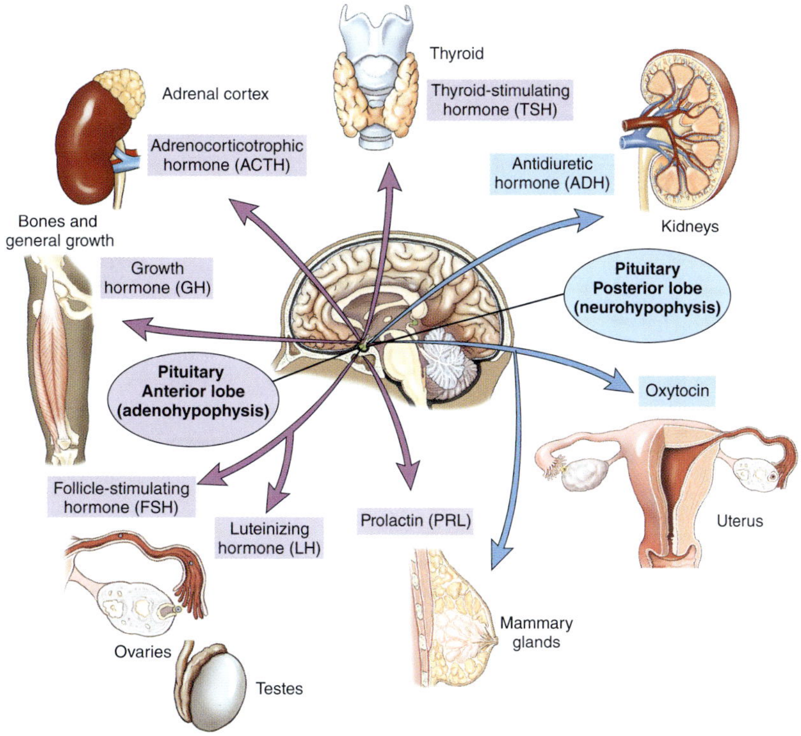

FIG. 16.2 Pituitary gland, hormones secreted, and target organs.

Endocrine Glands and Hormones—cont'd

TERM	DEFINITION
hypothalamus (*hī*-pō-THAL-a-mus)	located superior to the pituitary gland in the brain. The hypothalamus secretes "releasing" hormones that function to stimulate or inhibit the release of pituitary gland hormones.
thyroid gland (THĪ-royd) (gland)	largest endocrine gland. It is located anteriorly in the neck below the larynx and comprises bilateral lobes connected by an isthmus (Fig. 16.3C). The thyroid gland secretes the hormones triiodothyronine (T_3) and thyroxine (T_4), which require iodine for their production. Thyroxine is necessary for body cell metabolism.
parathyroid glands (*par*-a-THĪ-royd) (glans)	four small bodies embedded in the posterior aspect of the lobes of the thyroid gland (Fig. 16.3D). Parathyroid hormone (PTH), the hormone produced by the glands, helps maintain the level of calcium in the blood by its effects on bone and kidneys.
islets of Langerhans (Ī-lets) (LAHNG-er-hahnz)	clusters of endocrine tissue found throughout the pancreas, made up of different cell types that secrete various hormones, including insulin and glucagon. Non-endocrine cells found throughout the pancreas produce enzymes that facilitate digestion (Fig. 16.4).
adrenal glands (a-DRĒ-nal) (glans)	paired glands, one of which is located superior to each kidney. The outer portion is called the **adrenal cortex,** and the inner portion is called the **adrenal medulla.** The following hormones are secreted by the adrenal glands:
cortisol (KOR-ti-sol)	secreted by the adrenal cortex. It aids the body during stress by increasing glucose levels to provide energy (also called **hydrocortisone**).
aldosterone (al-DOS-ter-ōn)	secreted by the adrenal cortex. Electrolytes (mineral salts) that are necessary for normal body function are regulated by this hormone.
epinephrine, norepinephrine (*ep*-i-NEF-rin), (*nor*-ep-i-NEF-rin)	secreted by the adrenal medulla. These hormones help the body to deal with stress by increasing the blood pressure, heartbeat, and respirations. (also called **adrenaline** and **noradrenaline**, respectively)

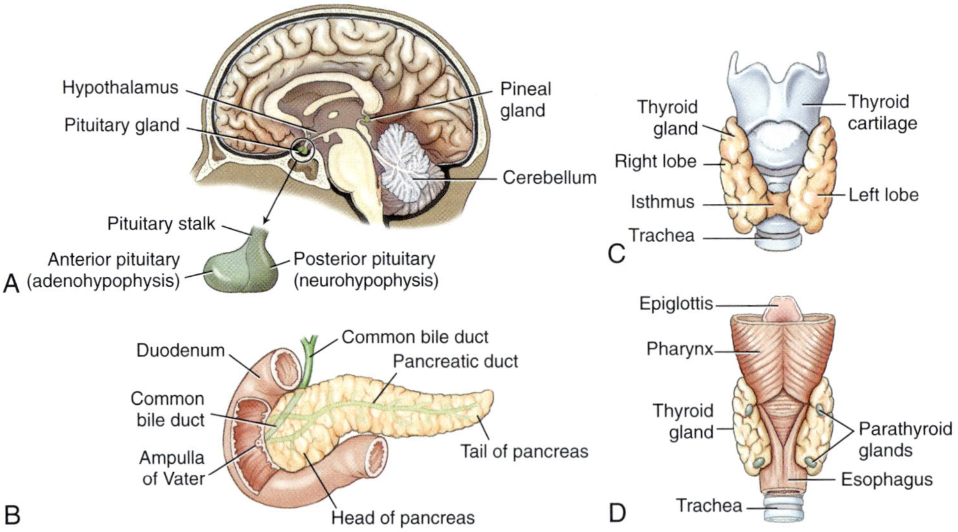

FIG. 16.3 A, Pituitary and pineal glands. **B,** Pancreas. **C,** Thyroid gland. **D,** Parathyroid glands, posterior view.

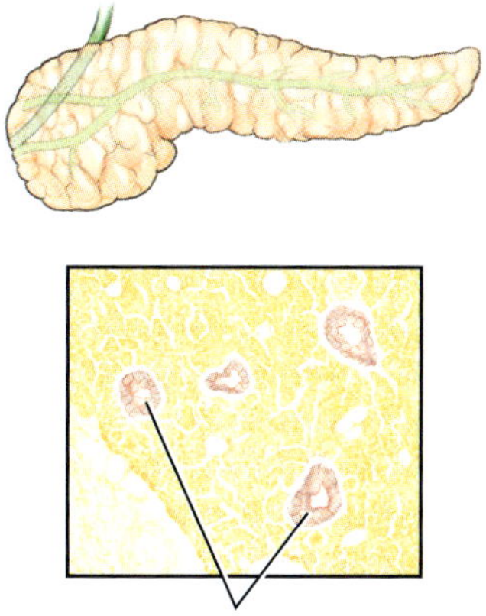

FIG. 16.4 Pancreas, with islets of Langerhans.

PRONOUNCE ANATOMIC STRUCTURES

Practice saying aloud each of the organs and specific structures on the previous pages.

To hear the terms, go to Evolve Resources at www.evolve.elsevier.com and select:

Student Resources > Audio Glossary > Chapter 16 > Anatomic Structures

❑ Check the box when complete.

WORD PARTS

Use paper flashcards or electronic flashcards on Evolve to memorize word parts used to analyze, define, and build medical terms in this chapter. To reinforce learning, study one section of the Word Parts Table at a time, then complete the corresponding exercises on the following pages.

1 ■ Endocrine System Combining Forms

COMBINING FORM	DEFINITION	COMBINING FORM	DEFINITION
adren/o	adrenal glands	**endocrin/o**	endocrine
adrenal/o	adrenal glands	**parathyroid/o**	parathyroid glands
cortic/o	cortex (the outer layer of a body organ)	**pituitar/o**	pituitary gland
		thyroid/o	thyroid gland

2 ■ Combining Forms Used with Endocrine System Terms

COMBINING FORM	DEFINITION	COMBINING FORM	DEFINITION
acr/o	extremities, height	**glyc/o**	sugar
calc/i	calcium *(Note: the combining vowel is* i.*)*	**kal/i**	potassium *(Note: the combining vowel is* i.*)*
dips/o	thirst	**natr/o**	sodium

3 ■ Prefixes

PREFIX	DEFINITION	PREFIX	DEFINITION
eu-	normal, good	**pan-**	all, total
hyper-	above, excessive	**poly-**	many, much
hypo-	below, incomplete, deficient, under	**syn-**	together, joined

4 ■ Suffixes

SUFFIX	DEFINITION	SUFFIX	DEFINITION
-al	pertaining to	**-logist**	one who studies and treats (specialist, physician)
-drome	run, running	**-logy**	study of
-ectomy	excision, surgical removal	**-megaly**	enlargement
-emia	in the blood	**-oma**	tumor, swelling
-ia	diseased or abnormal state, condition of	**-pathy**	disease
-ism	state of	**-plasia**	condition of formation, development, growth
-itis	inflammation		

Refer to **Appendix B** and **Appendix C** for a complete list of word parts.

EXERCISE 1 ■ Endocrine System Combining Forms

Refer to the first section of the word parts table.

A Label

Fill in the blanks with combining forms in this diagram of the endocrine glands. *To check your answers, go to Appendix A* at the back of the textbook.

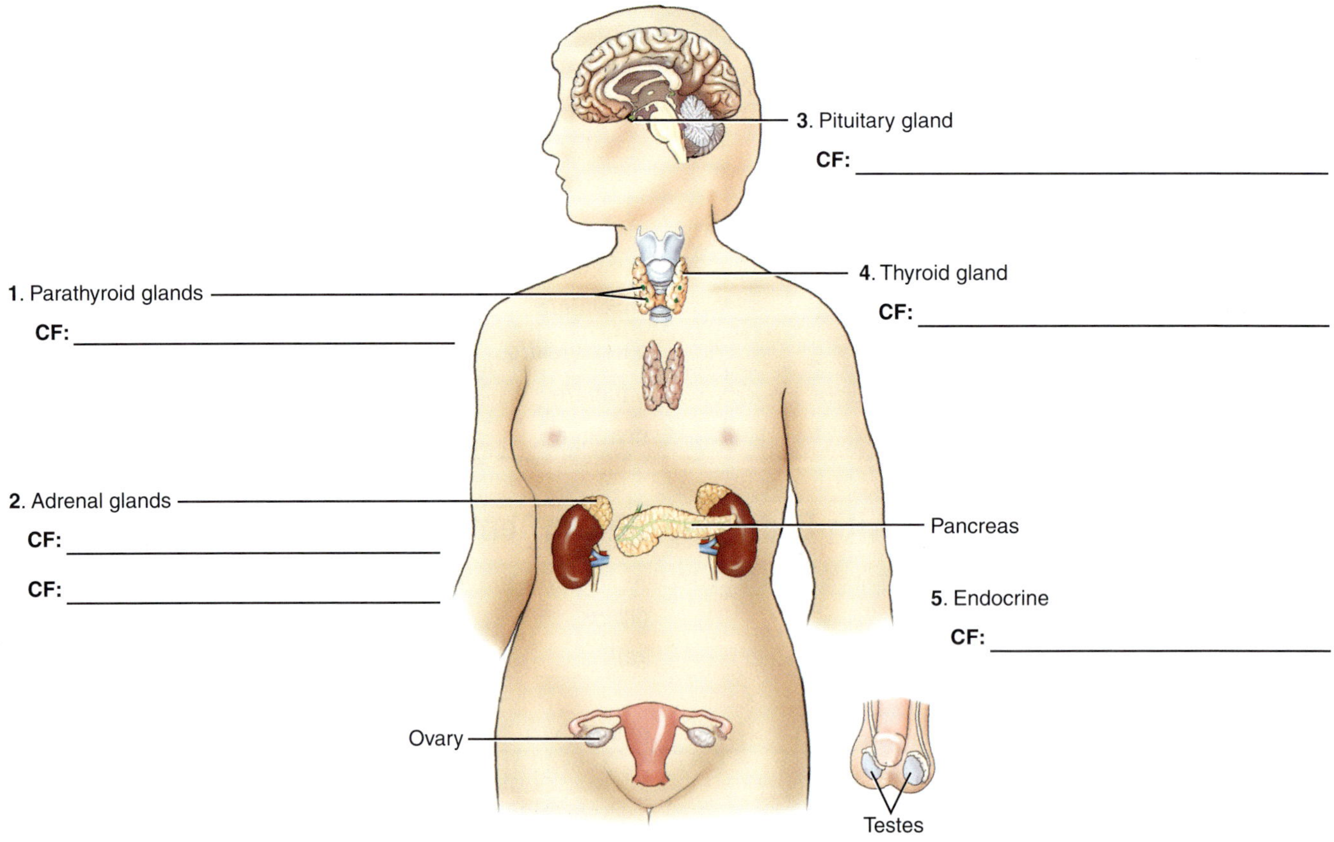

B Label

Fill in the blank with the combining form in this diagram of adrenal glands (with transverse cross-sectional view).

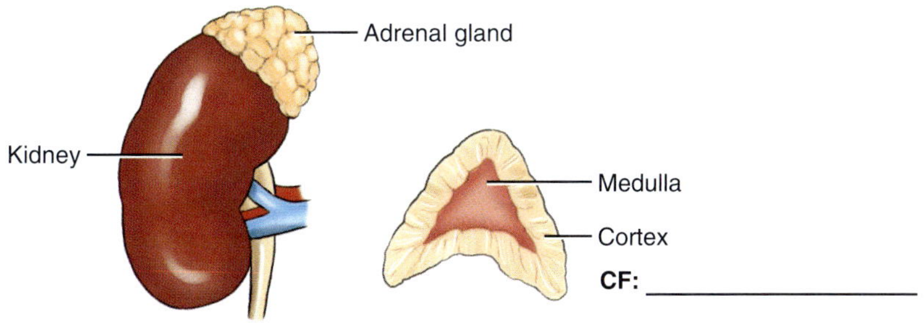

C Define and Match

Step 1: Write the definitions after the following combining forms.
Step 2: Match the descriptions on the right with the combining forms and definitions. Answers may be used more than once; no answer line appears for those not described in a lettered item.

_____ 1. adrenal/o, ___________________

_____ 2. pituitar/o, ___________________

_____ 3. cortic/o, ___________________

_____ 4. parathyroid/o, ___________________

_____ 5. adren/o, ___________________

_____ 6. thyroid/o, ___________________

7. endocrin/o, ___________________

a. referred to as the master gland because it produces hormones that stimulate the function of other endocrine glands

b. four small bodies embedded in the posterior aspect of the lobes of the thyroid gland

c. largest endocrine gland, secretes triiodothyronine (T_3) and thyroxine (T_4)

d. paired glands, one of which is located above each kidney

e. outer portion of adrenal gland

EXERCISE 2 ■ Combining Forms Used with Endocrine System Terms

Refer to the second portion of the word parts table.

A Define

Write the definitions of the following combining forms.

1. dips/o ___________________
2. kal/i ___________________
3. calc/i ___________________
4. acr/o ___________________
5. natr/o ___________________
6. glyc/o ___________________

B Identify

Write the combining form for each of the following.

1. extremities, height ___________________
2. calcium ___________________
3. thirst ___________________
4. sugar ___________________
5. potassium ___________________
6. sodium ___________________

EXERCISE 3 ■ Prefixes

Refer to the third section of the word parts table.

A Define

Write the definitions of the following prefixes.

1. syn- ____________________
2. hypo- ____________________
3. pan- ____________________
4. eu- ____________________
5. poly- ____________________
6. hyper- ____________________

B Identify

Write the prefix for each of the following.

1. all, total ____________________
2. normal, good ____________________
3. many, much ____________________
4. above, excessive ____________________
5. together, joined ____________________
6. below, incomplete, deficient, under ____________________

EXERCISE 4 ■ Suffixes

Refer to the fourth section of the word parts table.

A Identify

Write the suffix for each of the following.

1. state of ____________________
2. enlargement ____________________
3. in the blood ____________________
4. pertaining to ____________________
5. disease ____________________
6. one who studies and treats (specialist, physician) ____________________

B Label

Write the suffix pictured and defined.

1. ____________________
run, running

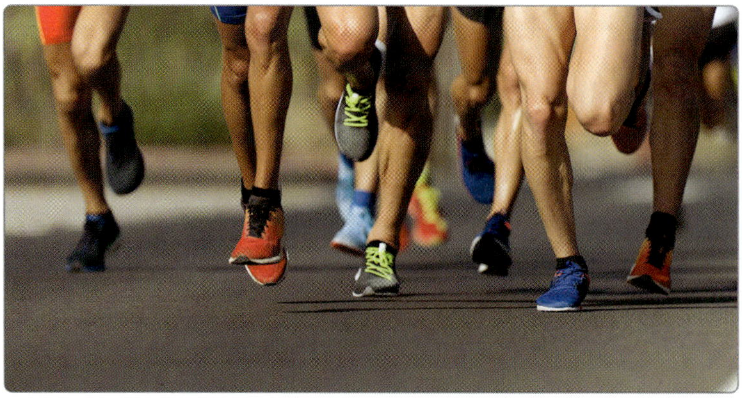

C Define

Write definitions for the following suffixes

1. -oma ______
2. -ectomy ______
3. -plasia ______
______
4. -logy ______
5. -itis ______
6. -drome ______
7. -ia ______
______

MEDICAL TERMS

Medical terms relevant to this chapter have been grouped by topics, such as Disease and Disorder, and are listed in tables designated as Built from Word Parts or *NOT* Built from Word Parts. The exercises following each table assist with learning term definitions, pronunciations, and spellings.

Disease and Disorder Terms

BUILT FROM WORD PARTS

The following terms can be translated using definitions of word parts. Further explanation is provided within parentheses as needed.

TERM	DEFINITION
1. acromegaly (*ak*-rō-MEG-a-lē)	enlargement of the extremities (and face due to increased soft tissue, bone, and cartilage; caused by excessive production of the growth hormone by the pituitary gland after puberty)
2. adrenalitis (a-*drē*-nal-Ī-tis)	inflammation of the adrenal glands
3. adrenomegaly (a-*drē*-nō-MEG-a-lē)	enlargement (of one or both) of the adrenal glands
4. endocrinopathy (*en*-dō-kri-NOP-a-thē)	(any) disease of the endocrine (system)
5. hypercalcemia (*hī*-per-kal-SĒ-mē-a)	excessive calcium in the blood
6. hyperglycemia (*hī*-per-glī-SĒ-mē-a)	excessive sugar in the blood
7. hyperkalemia (*hī*-per-ka-LĒ-mē-a)	excessive potassium in the blood
8. hyperparathyroidism (*hī*-per-*par*-a-THĪ-royd-izm)	state of excessive parathyroid gland activity (resulting in hypercalcemia and leading to osteoporosis, as well as symptoms of muscle weakness, abdominal pain, nausea, vomiting, and drowsiness)
9. hyperpituitarism (*hī*-per-pi-TOO-i-ta-*rizm*)	state of excessive pituitary gland activity (characterized by excessive secretion of pituitary hormones)
10. hyperthyroidism (*hī*-per-THĪ-royd-izm)	state of excessive thyroid gland activity (characterized by excessive secretion of thyroid hormones; signs and symptoms include tachycardia, weight loss, irritability, and heat intolerance)
11. hypocalcemia (*hī*-pō-kal-SĒ-mē-a)	deficient calcium in the blood
12. hypoglycemia (*hī*-pō-glī-SĒ-mē-a)	deficient sugar in the blood
13. hypokalemia (*hī*-pō-ka-LĒ-mē-a)	deficient potassium in the blood
14. hyponatremia (*hī*-pō-na-TRĒ-mē-a)	deficient sodium in the blood

Disease and Disorder Terms—cont'd

BUILT FROM WORD PARTS

TERM	DEFINITION
15. hypopituitarism (*hī*-pō-pi-TŪ-i-ta-*rizm*)	state of deficient pituitary gland activity (characterized by decreased secretion of one or more of the pituitary hormones, which can affect the function of the target endocrine gland; for example, hypothyroidism can result from decreased secretion of thyroid-stimulating hormone by the pituitary gland)
16. hypothyroidism (*hī*-pō-THĪ-royd-izm)	state of deficient thyroid gland activity (characterized by decreased secretion of thyroid hormones; signs and symptoms include fatigue, weight gain, and cold intolerance)

HYPOTHYROIDISM results in decreased production of the thyroid hormone called thyroxine. A severe form of hypothyroidism in adults is called **myxedema** and in infants is called **congenital hypothyroidism**.

TERM	DEFINITION
17. panhypopituitarism (pan-*hī*-pō-pi-TŪ-i-ta-*rizm*)	state of total deficient pituitary gland activity (characterized by decreased secretion of all the anterior pituitary hormones; this is a more serious condition than hypopituitarism in that it affects the function of all the other endocrine glands)

PANHYPOPITUITARISM contains two prefixes, **pan-** meaning total and **hypo-** meaning *deficient.*

TERM	DEFINITION
18. parathyroidoma (*par*-a-*thī*-royd-Ō-ma)	tumor of a parathyroid gland
19. thyroiditis (*thī*-royd-Ī-tis)	inflammation of the thyroid gland

EXERCISE 5 ■ Pronounce and Spell

Practice pronunciation and spelling on paper and online.

1. Practice on Paper

a. **Pronounce:** Read the phonetic spelling and say aloud the terms listed in the previous table. Refer to the pronunciation key on p. 20 as necessary.
b. **Spell:** Have a study partner read the terms aloud. Write the spelling of the terms on a separate sheet of paper.

2. Practice Online

a. **Access** online learning resources. Go to evolve.elsevier.com > Evolve Resources > Student Resources.
b. **Pronounce:** Select Audio Glossary > Chapter 16 > Exercise 5. Select a term to hear its pronunciation and repeat aloud.
c. **Spell:** Select Activities > Chapter 16 > Spell Terms > Exercise 5. Select the audio icon and type the correct spelling of the term.

❑ Check the box when complete.

EXERCISE 6 ■ Analyze and Define

Analyze and define the following terms.

1. adrenalitis

____

____

2. hypocalcemia

____

____

3. hyperthyroidism

____

____

4. hyperkalemia

____

____

5. hyperpituitarism

____

____

6. adrenomegaly

____

____

7. endocrinopathy

____

____

8. hyponatremia

____

____

9. parathyroidoma

____

____

10. panhypopituitarism

____

____

EXERCISE 7 ■ Build

A Label

Build terms pictured by writing word parts above definitions.

1.

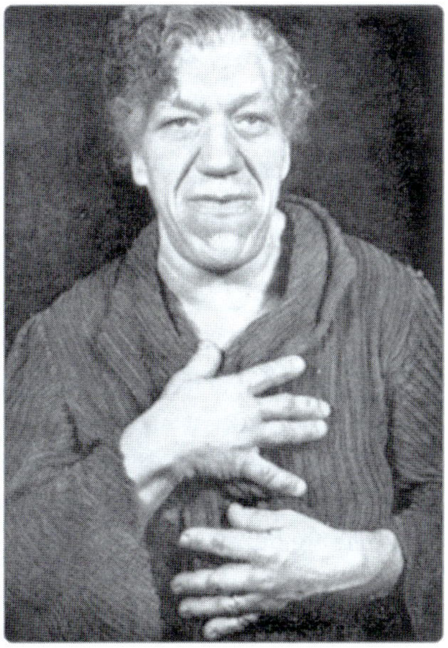

_______ / ___ / _______
extremities CV enlargement

2.

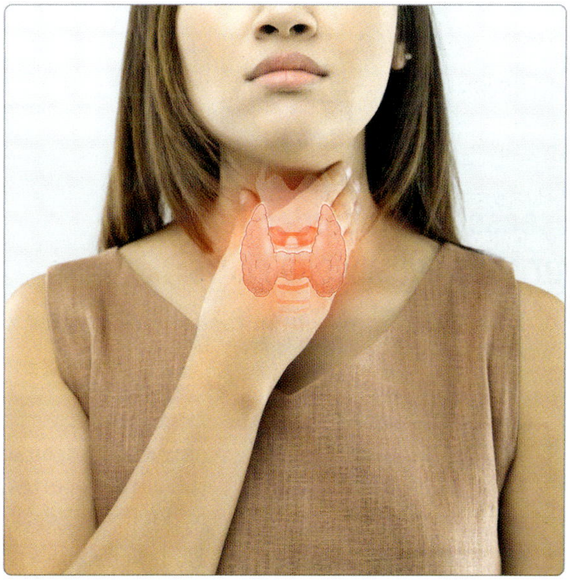

_______ / _______
thyroid inflammation

3.

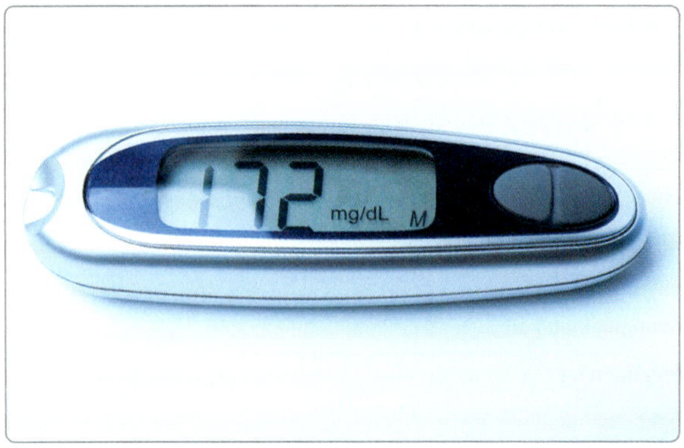

_________ / _________ / _________
excessive sugar in the blood

4.

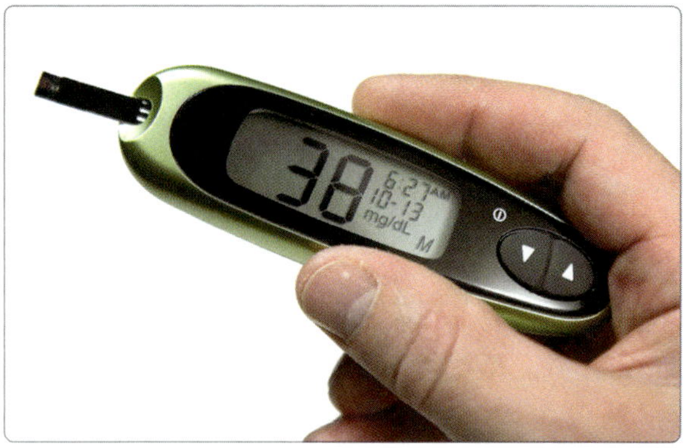

_________ / _________ / _________
deficient sugar in the blood

B Fill In

Build disease and disorder terms for the following definitions by using the word parts you have learned.

1. state of deficient thyroid gland activity _________ / _________ / _________ (P / WR / S)

2. deficient potassium in the blood _________ / _________ / _________ (P / WR / S)

3. state of excessive parathyroid gland activity _________ / _________ / _________ (P / WR / S)

4. state of deficient pituitary gland activity _________ / _________ / _________ (P / WR / S)

5. excessive calcium in the blood _________ / _________ / _________ (P / WR / S)

Disease and Disorder Terms

NOT BUILT FROM WORD PARTS

Word parts may be present in the following terms; however, their full meanings cannot be translated using definitions of word parts alone.

TERM	DEFINITION
1. Addison disease (AD-i-sun) (di-ZĒZ)	chronic syndrome resulting from a deficiency in the hormonal secretion of the adrenal cortex. Signs and symptoms may include weakness, weight loss, hypotension, darkening of skin, and loss of appetite.
ADDISON DISEASE was named in **1855** for **Thomas Addison**, an English physician and pathologist. He described the disease as a "morbid state with feeble heart action, anemia, irritability of the stomach, and a peculiar change in the color of the skin."	
2. congenital hypothyroidism (kon-JEN-i-tal) (hī-pō-THĪ-royd-izm)	condition caused by congenital absence or atrophy (wasting away) of the thyroid gland, resulting in hypothyroidism. The disease is characterized by puffy features, mental deficiency, large tongue, and short stature.

TERM	DEFINITION
3. **Cushing syndrome** (KOOSH-ing) (SIN-drōm)	group of signs and symptoms attributed to the excessive production of cortisol by the adrenal cortices (*pl.* of cortex). This syndrome may be the result of a pituitary tumor that produces ACTH or a primary adrenal cortex hypersecretion. Signs include abnormally pigmented skin, "moon face," pads of fat on the chest and abdomen, "buffalo hump" (fat on the upper back), wasting away of muscle, and hypertension.

CUSHING SYNDROME was named for an American neurosurgeon, **Harvey Williams Cushing** (1869-1939), after he described adrenocortical hyperfunction.

TERM	DEFINITION
4. **diabetes insipidus (DI)** (*dī*-a-BĒ-tēz) (in-SIP-i-dus)	result of decreased secretion of antidiuretic hormone by the posterior lobe of the pituitary gland. Symptoms include excessive thirst (polydipsia), large amounts of urine (polyuria), and water being excreted from the body.
5. **diabetes mellitus (DM)** (*dī*-a-BĒ-tēz) (MEL-li-tus)	chronic disease involving a disorder of carbohydrate metabolism caused by under-activity of the insulin-producing islets of Langerhans and characterized by elevated blood sugar (hyperglycemia). DM can cause chronic renal disease, retinopathy, and neuropathy. In extreme cases the patient may develop ketosis, acidosis, and finally coma (Table 16.1).
6. **gigantism** (jī-GAN-tizm)	condition brought about by hypersecretion of growth hormone by the pituitary gland before puberty

GIGANTISM AND ACROMEGALY are both caused by overproduction of growth hormone. **Gigantism** occurs before puberty and before the growing ends of the bones have closed. If untreated, an individual may reach 8 feet tall in adulthood. **Acromegaly** occurs after puberty. The body parts most affected are those in the hands, feet, and jaw.

TERM	DEFINITION
7. **Graves disease** (grāvz) (di-ZĒZ)	autoimmune disorder of the thyroid gland characterized by the production of more thyroid hormone than the body needs (hyperthyroidism), goiter, and exophthalmos (abnormal protrusion of the eyeballs)
8. **Hashimoto thyroiditis** (*hah*-she-MŌ-tō) (*thī*-royd-Ī-tis)	disease in which thyroid gland cells are destroyed by autoimmune processes. Characterized by hypothyroidism and goiter; more common in females.
9. **ketoacidosis** (*kē*-tō-*as*-i-DŌ-sis)	serious condition resulting from uncontrolled diabetes mellitus in which acid ketones accumulate from fat metabolism in the absence of adequate insulin. If not promptly controlled by adequate insulin and hydration, can progress to coma and death.
10. **metabolic syndrome** (*met*-a-BOL-ik) (SIN-drōm)	group of signs and symptoms including insulin resistance, obesity characterized by excessive fat around the area of the waist and abdomen, hypertension, hyperglycemia, elevated triglycerides, and low levels of the "good" cholesterol HDL. Risks include development of type 2 diabetes mellitus, coronary heart disease, or stroke (also called **syndrome X** and **insulin resistance syndrome**).
11. **myxedema** (*mik*-se-DĒ-ma)	condition resulting from an extreme deficiency of the thyroid hormone thyroxine; a severe form of hypothyroidism in an adult. Signs include puffiness of the face and hands, coarse and thickened skin, enlarged tongue, slow speech, and anemia.
12. **neuroblastoma** (*nū*-rō-blas-TŌ-ma)	malignant cancer that often starts in the adrenal medulla, composed of immature nerve cells. Primarily affects children.
13. **pheochromocytoma** (*fē*-ō-*krō*-mō-sī-TŌ-ma)	tumor of the adrenal medulla, which is usually non-malignant and characterized by hypertension, headaches, palpitations, diaphoresis, chest pain, and abdominal pain. Surgical removal of the tumor is the most common treatment. Though usually curable with early detection, it can be fatal if untreated.
14. **thyrotoxicosis** (*thī*-rō-*tok*-si-KŌ-sis)	condition caused by excessive thyroid hormones

TABLE 16.1 Diabetes Mellitus

Two major forms of diabetes mellitus are **type 1,** previously called insulin-dependent diabetes mellitus (IDDM) or juvenile-onset diabetes, and **type 2,** previously called noninsulin-dependent diabetes mellitus (NIDDM) or adult-onset diabetes mellitus (AODM). Type 2 diabetes mellitus has reached epidemic proportions and is a major cause of cardiovascular disease.

TYPE 1 DIABETES MELLITUS	
Cause	autoimmune disease in which the beta cells of the pancreas that produce insulin are destroyed and eventually no insulin is produced
Characteristics	abrupt onset, occurs primarily in childhood or adolescence; patients often are thin
Signs and Symptoms	polyuria, polydipsia, weight loss, and hyperglycemia; these are present if blood sugar is not controlled and can progress to ketoacidosis if not promptly treated
Treatment	insulin injections and diet
TYPE 2 DIABETES MELLITUS	
Cause	resistance of body cells to the action of insulin, coupled with a decrease in the ability of the pancreas to make sufficient insulin to overcome this resistance
Characteristics	slow onset, usually occurs in middle-aged or elderly adults; most patients are obese
Signs and Symptoms	fatigue, blurred vision, thirst, and hyperglycemia; these may be present if blood sugar is not controlled
Treatment	diet, exercise, oral or injected medication, and sometimes insulin

LONG-TERM COMPLICATIONS OF DIABETES MELLITUS

MACROVASCULAR COMPLICATIONS

- coronary artery disease → myocardial infarction
- cerebrovascular disease → stroke
- peripheral artery disease → leg pain when walking (intermittent vascular claudication)

MICROVASCULAR COMPLICATIONS

- diabetic retinopathy → loss of vision
- diabetic nephropathy → chronic renal disease, kidney failure
- neuropathy → loss of feeling in the distal extremities (feet, hands), which can lead to amputation

EXERCISE 8 ■ Pronounce and Spell

Practice pronunciation and spelling on paper and online.

1. Practice on Paper

a. **Pronounce:** Read the phonetic spelling and say aloud the terms listed in the previous table. Refer to the pronunciation key on p. 20 as necessary.
b. **Spell:** Have a study partner read the terms aloud. Write the spelling of the terms on a separate sheet of paper.

2. Practice Online

a. **Access** online learning resources. Go to evolve.elsevier.com > Evolve Resources > Student Resources.
b. **Pronounce:** Select Audio Glossary > Chapter 16 > Exercise 8. Select a term to hear its pronunciation and repeat aloud.
c. **Spell:** Select Activities > Chapter 16 > Spell Terms > Exercise 8. Select the audio icon and type the correct spelling of the term.

❑ Check the box when complete.

EXERCISE 9 ■ Match

Match the terms in the first column with their correct definitions in the second column.

_____ 1. diabetes insipidus
_____ 2. neuroblastoma
_____ 3. pheochromocytoma
_____ 4. thyrotoxicosis
_____ 5. diabetes mellitus
_____ 6. ketoacidosis
_____ 7. Graves disease

a. serious condition resulting from uncontrolled diabetes mellitus in which acid ketones accumulate from fat metabolism in the absence of adequate insulin
b. tumor of the adrenal medulla, characterized by hypertension, headaches, palpitations, diaphoresis, chest pain, and abdominal pain
c. result of decreased secretion of antidiuretic hormone by the posterior lobe of the pituitary gland
d. condition caused by excessive thyroid hormones
e. autoimmune disorder characterized by hyperthyroidism, goiter, and exophthalmos
f. chronic disease involving a disorder of carbohydrate metabolism characterized by elevated blood sugar (hyperglycemia)
g. childhood cancer that often starts in the adrenal medulla

EXERCISE 10 ■ Match

Match the terms in the first column with their correct definitions in the second column.

_____ 1. metabolic syndrome
_____ 2. congenital hypothyroidism
_____ 3. myxedema
_____ 4. Addison disease
_____ 5. gigantism
_____ 6. Cushing syndrome
_____ 7. Hashimoto thyroiditis

a. severe form of hypothyroidism in an adult
b. excessive production of cortisol by the adrenal cortices
c. condition brought about by hypersecretion of growth hormone by the pituitary gland before puberty
d. condition caused by absence or atrophy (wasting away) of the thyroid gland in childhood
e. also called syndrome X and insulin resistance syndrome
f. autoimmune disease characterized by hypothyroidism and goiter
g. associated with weakness, weight loss, hypotension, darkening of skin, and loss of appetite.

EXERCISE 11 ■ Fill In

A Identify

Fill in the blanks with the correct terms

1. _______________ is a malignant cancer that often starts in the adrenal medulla.
2. A condition caused by excessive thyroid hormones, or _______________, can become a medical emergency.
3. A disease in which thyroid gland cells are destroyed by autoimmune processes, or _______________ _______________, differs from Graves disease in that it usually presents with hypothyroidism.
4. _______________ _______________ is associated with excessive thirst and excessive urine output.
5. If not promptly controlled by insulin and hydration, _______________ can progress to coma and death.
6. A chronic disease involving a disorder of carbohydrate metabolism, _______________ _______________, can cause renal disease, retinopathy, and neuropathy.

B Label

Write the medical terms pictured and defined.

1. ______________________________
condition brought about by hypersecretion of growth hormone by the pituitary gland before puberty

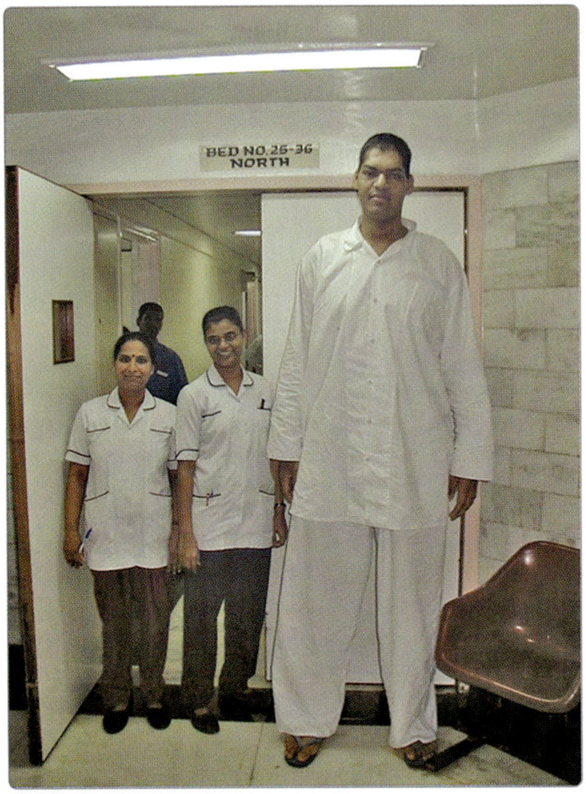

2. ______________________________
chronic syndrome resulting from a deficiency in the hormonal secretion of the adrenal cortex with symptoms of weight loss, hypotension, and skin darkening

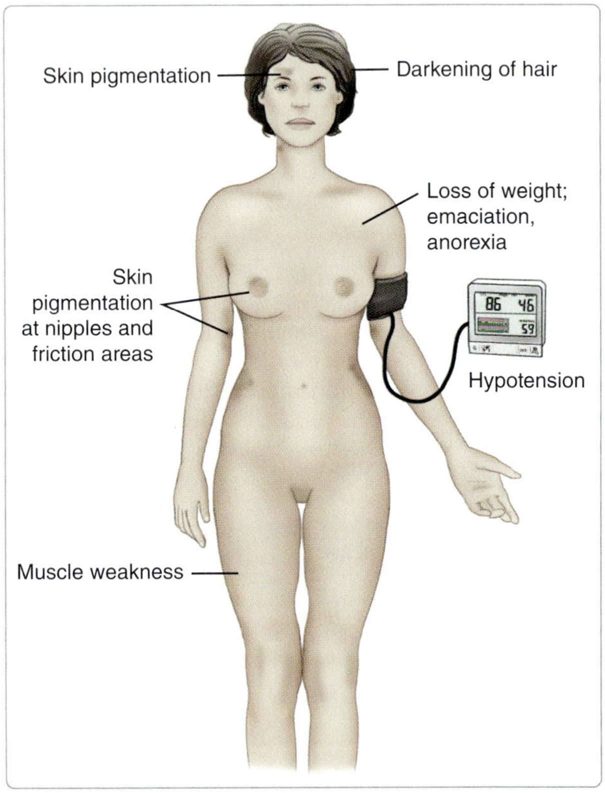

3. ______________________________
A. condition caused by congenital absence or atrophy of the thyroid gland, resulting in hypothyroidism; characterized by puffy features, mental deficiency, large tongue, and short stature
B. same child after treatment for this condition

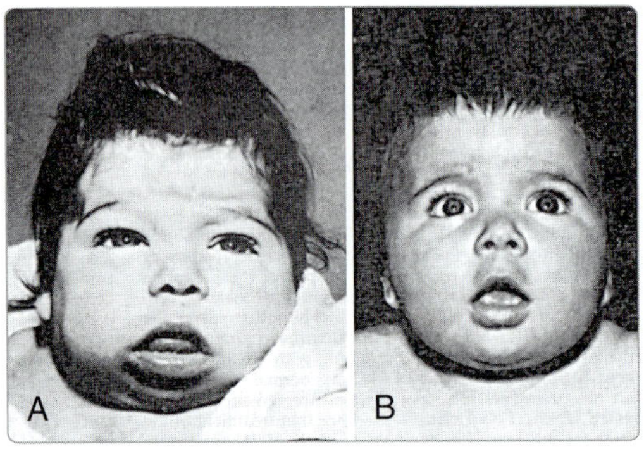

4. ______________________________
condition resulting from a deficiency of the thyroid hormone thyroxine; a severe form of hypothyroidism in an adult, characterized by puffiness of the face and hands, coarse and thickened skin, enlarged tongue, slow speech, and anemia

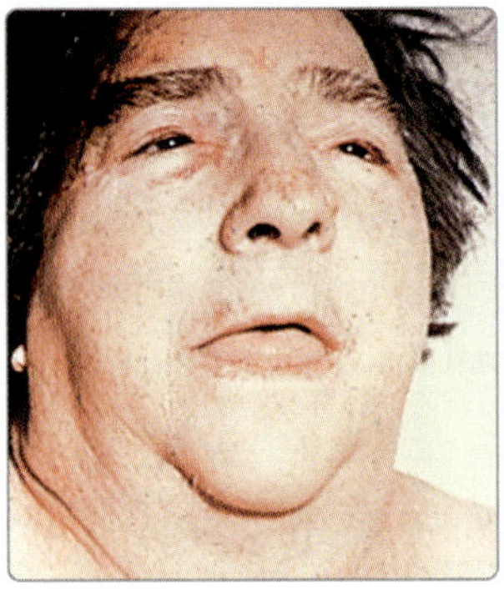

5. ____________________

A. group of signs and symptoms attributed to the excessive production of cortisol by the adrenal cortices

B. same child after treatment for this condition

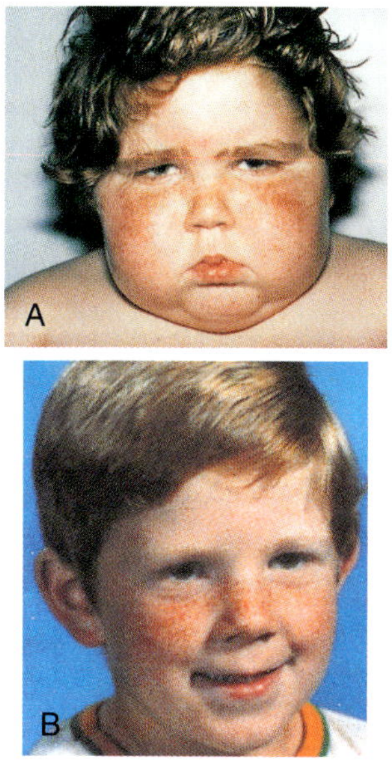

6. ____________________

group of signs and symptoms including insulin resistance, obesity characterized by excessive fat around the area of the waist, hypertension, hyperglycemia, elevated triglycerides, and low levels of the "good" cholesterol HDL

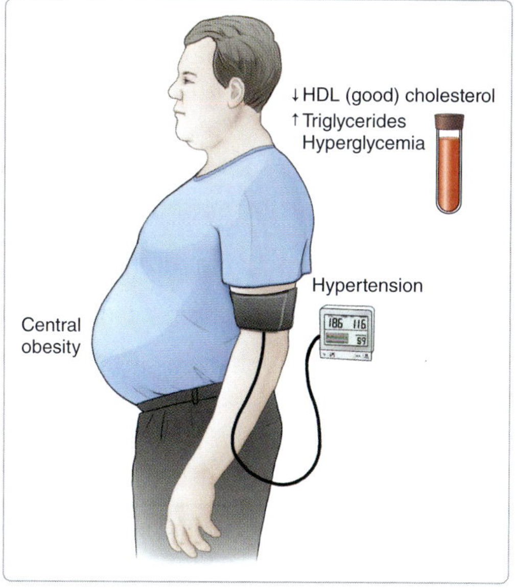

7. ____________________

tumor of the adrenal medulla characterized by hypertension, headaches, palpitations, and other symptoms

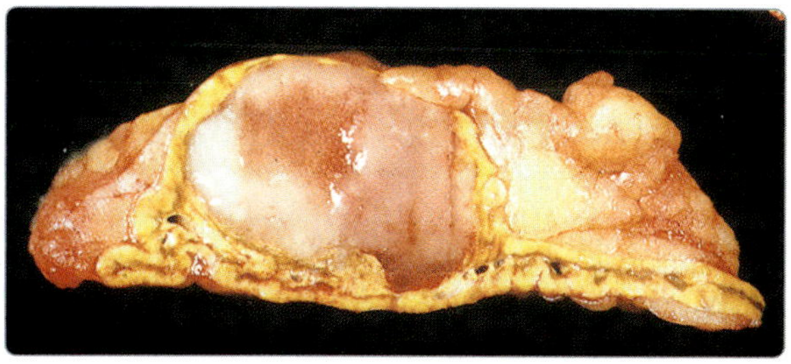

8. ____________________

autoimmune disorder of the thyroid gland characterized by hyperthyroidism, goiter, and protrusion of the eyeballs

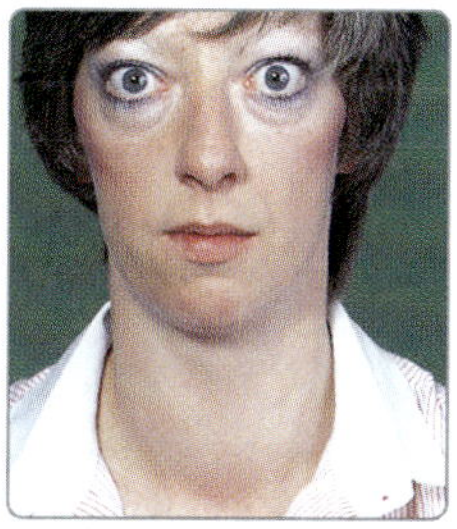

EXERCISE 12 ■ Review of Disease and Disorder Terms

Can you define, pronounce, and spell the following terms?

acromegaly
Addison disease
adrenalitis
adrenomegaly
congenital hypothyroidism
Cushing syndrome
diabetes insipidus (DI)
diabetes mellitus (DM)
endocrinopathy
gigantism
Graves disease
Hashimoto thyroiditis
hypercalcemia
hyperglycemia
hyperkalemia
hyperparathyroidism
hyperpituitarism
hyperthyroidism
hypocalcemia
hypoglycemia
hypokalemia
hyponatremia
hypopituitarism
hypothyroidism
ketoacidosis
metabolic syndrome
myxedema
neuroblastoma
panhypopituitarism
parathyroidoma
pheochromocytoma
thyroiditis
thyrotoxicosis

Surgical Terms

BUILT FROM WORD PARTS

The following terms can be translated using definitions of word parts. Further explanation is provided within parentheses as needed.

TERM	DEFINITION
1. adrenalectomy (ad-*rē*-nal-EK-to-mē)	excision of (one or both) adrenal glands
2. parathyroidectomy (*par*-a-*thī*-royd-EK-to-mē)	excision of (one or more) parathyroid glands
3. thyroidectomy (thī-royd-EK-to-mē)	excision of the thyroid gland

EXERCISE 13 ■ Pronounce and Spell

Practice pronunciation and spelling on paper and online.

1. Practice on Paper

a. **Pronounce:** Read the phonetic spelling and say aloud the terms listed in the previous table. Refer to the pronunciation key on p. 20 as necessary.
b. **Spell:** Have a study partner read the terms aloud. Write the spelling of the terms on a separate sheet of paper.

2. Practice Online

a. **Access** online learning resources. Go to evolve.elsevier.com > Evolve Resources > Student Resources.
b. **Pronounce:** Select Audio Glossary > Chapter 16 > Exercise 13. Select a term to hear its pronunciation and repeat aloud.
c. **Spell:** Select Activities > Chapter 16 > Spell Terms > Exercise 13. Select the audio icon and type the correct spelling of the term.

❏ Check the box when complete.

EXERCISE 14 ■ Analyze and Define

Analyze and define the following terms.

1. adrenalectomy

____

____

2. thyroidectomy

____

____

3. parathyroidectomy

____

____

EXERCISE 15 ■ Build

Build surgical terms for the following definitions by using the word parts you have learned.

1. excision of the thyroid gland __________ / __________
WR / S

2. excision of (one or both) adrenal glands ______ / ______
WR S

3. excision of (one or more) parathyroid glands ______ / ______
WR S

EXERCISE 16 ■ Review of Surgical Terms

Can you define, pronounce, and spell the following terms?

adrenalectomy
parathyroidectomy
thyroidectomy

Diagnostic Terms

NOT BUILT FROM WORD PARTS

Word parts may be present in the following terms; however, their full meanings cannot be translated using definitions of word parts alone.

DIAGNOSTIC IMAGING

TERM	DEFINITION
1. radioactive iodine uptake (RAIU) (*rā*-dē-ō-AK-tiv) (Ī-ō-dīn) (UP-tāk)	nuclear medicine scan that measures thyroid function, particularly when distinguishing different causes of hyperthyroidism. Radioactive iodine is given to the patient orally, after which the amount of its uptake into the thyroid gland is measured. Images of the gland can also be obtained using this procedure.
2. sestamibi parathyroid scan (*ses*-ta-MIB-ē) (*par*-a-THĪ-royd) (skan)	nuclear medicine procedure used to localize hyperactive parathyroid glands. The glands that take up an abnormal amount of radioactive substance are identified and selected for surgical removal; the other parathyroid glands may be left in place.
3. thyroid sonography (THĪ-royd) (so-NOG-ra-fē)	ultrasound test of the thyroid gland used to help determine whether a thyroid nodule is likely benign or possibly malignant, including whether it is cystic or solid. Also used to help guide a fine needle aspiration (FNA) biopsy.

LABORATORY

TERM	DEFINITION
4. fasting blood sugar (FBS) (FAST-ing) (blud) (SHOOG-er)	blood test to determine the amount of glucose (sugar) in the blood after fasting for 8 to 10 hours. Elevation may indicate diabetes mellitus.
5. fine needle aspiration (FNA) (FĪN) (NĒ-del) (*as*-pi-RĀ-shen)	biopsy technique that uses a narrow hollow needle to obtain tiny amounts of tissue for pathologic examination. Thyroid nodules are frequently biopsied using FNA.
6. glycosylated hemoglobin (HbA1c) (glī-KŌ-sa-*lāt*-ad) (HĒ-mō-*glō*-bin)	blood test used to diagnose diabetes and monitor its treatment by measuring the amount of glucose (sugar) bound to hemoglobin in the blood. HbA1c provides an indication of blood sugar level over the past three months, covering the 120-day lifespan of the red blood cell (also called **glycated hemoglobin, hemoglobin A1c, and A1c test**).
7. thyroid-stimulating hormone level (TSH) (THĪ-royd) (STIM-yuh-lāt-ing) (HŌR-mōn) (LEV-el)	blood test that measures the amount of thyroid-stimulating hormone in the blood; used to diagnose thyroid disorders and to monitor patients on thyroid replacement therapy
8. thyroxine level (T_4) (thī-ROK-sin) (LEV-el)	blood test that gives the direct measurement of the amount of thyroxine in the patient's blood. A greater-than-normal amount indicates hyperthyroidism; a less-than-normal amount indicates hypothyroidism.

EXERCISE 17 ■ Pronounce and Spell

Practice pronunciation and spelling on paper and online.

1. Practice on Paper

a. **Pronounce:** Read the phonetic spelling and say aloud the terms listed in the previous table. Refer to the pronunciation key on p. 20 as necessary.
b. **Spell:** Have a study partner read the terms aloud. Write the spelling of the terms on a separate sheet of paper.

2. Practice Online

a. **Access** online learning resources. Go to evolve.elsevier.com > Evolve Resources > Student Resources.
b. **Pronounce:** Select Audio Glossary > Chapter 16 > Exercise 17. Select a term to hear its pronunciation and repeat aloud.
c. **Spell:** Select Activities > Chapter 16 > Spell Terms > Exercise 17. Select the audio icon and type the correct spelling of the term.

❑ Check the box when complete.

EXERCISE 18 ■ Fill In

A Label

Write the diagnostic terms pictured and defined.

1. ______________________________
ultrasound test of the thyroid gland used to help determine whether a thyroid nodule is likely benign or possibly malignant

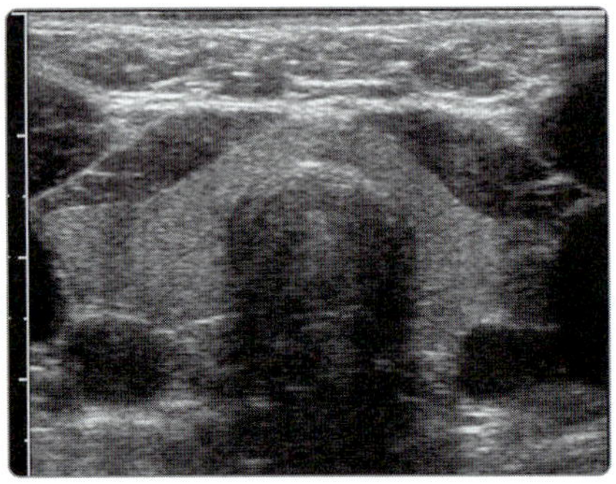

2. ______________________________
nuclear medicine scan that measures thyroid function, particularly when distinguishing different causes of hyperthyroidism

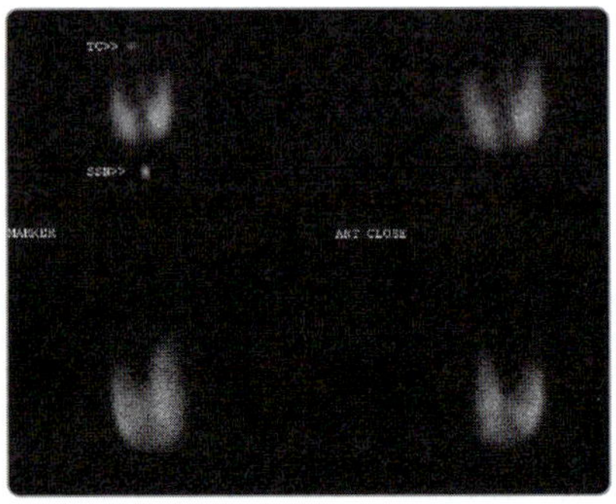

3. ______________________________
nuclear medicine procedure used to localize hyperactive parathyroid glands

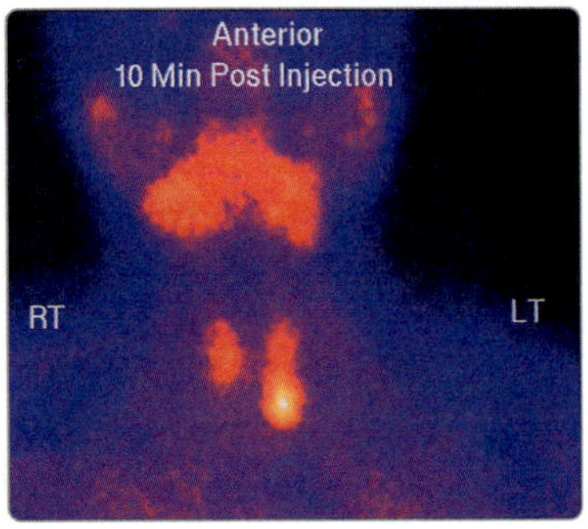

4. ______________________________
biopsy technique that uses a narrow hollow needle to obtain tiny amounts of tissue for pathologic examination

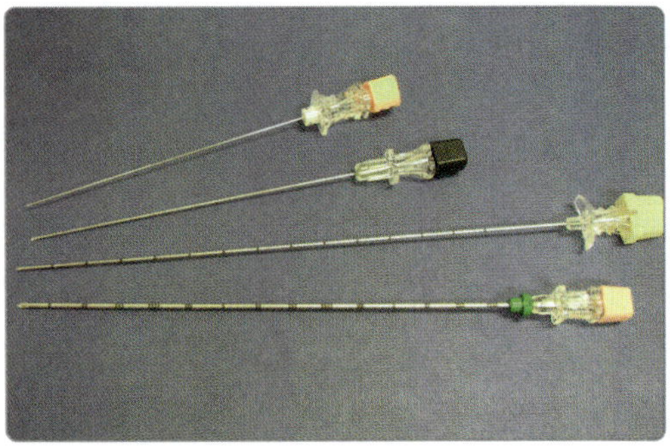

B Identify

Fill in the blanks with the correct terms

1. ____________________ ____________________ is a blood test that measures the direct amount of that hormone in the blood; higher than normal values represent hyperthyroidism.
2. A glucometer is a device that is frequently used to measure the amount of glucose in the blood after not eating for 8-10 hours, referred to as ____________________ ____________________ ____________________.
3. A test that provides an idea of blood sugar levels over the past three months, or ____________________ ____________________, is related to the lifespan of red blood cells, about 120 days.
4. A blood test that is used to diagnose thyroid disorders and to monitor patients on thyroid replacement therapy is called ____________________-____________________ ____________________ ____________________.

EXERCISE 19 ■ Match

Match the terms in the first column with their correct definitions in the second column.

_____ 1. fasting blood sugar	a. nuclear medicine procedure used to localize hyperactive parathyroid glands
_____ 2. sestamibi parathyroid scan	b. determines the amount of glucose in the blood after fasting for 8 to 10 hours
_____ 3. thyroxine level	c. uses a hollow needle to obtain tiny amounts of tissue for pathologic examination
_____ 4. radioactive iodine uptake	d. uses radioactive iodine to measure thyroid function
_____ 5. thyroid-stimulating hormone level	e. used to indicate whether a thyroid nodule is likely benign or possibly malignant
_____ 6. glycosylated hemoglobin	f. used to diagnose thyroid disorders and to monitor thyroid replacement therapy
_____ 7. thyroid sonography	g. measures the amount of thyroxine in the blood
_____ 8. fine needle aspiration	h. provides an indication of blood sugar level over the past 3 months

EXERCISE 20 ■ Review of Diagnostic Terms

Can you define, pronounce, and spell the following terms?

fasting blood sugar (FBS)	glycosylated hemoglobin (HbA1c)	sestamibi parathyroid scan	thyroid-stimulating hormone level (TSH)
fine needle aspiration (FNA)	radioactive iodine uptake (RAIU)	thyroid sonography	thyroxine level (T_4)

Complementary Terms

BUILT FROM WORD PARTS AND *NOT* BUILT FROM WORD PARTS

■ Built from Word Parts

The first portion of the table contains Endocrine System Complementary Terms that can be translated using definitions of word parts. The second portion of the table contains Endocrine System Complementary Terms that cannot be fully understood using the definitions of word parts.

SIGNS AND SYMPTOMS

TERM	DEFINITION	TERM	DEFINITION
1. adrenocorticohyperplasia (a-*drē*-nō-*kōr*-ti-kō-*hī*-per-PLĀ-zha)	excessive development of the adrenal cortex *(Note: hyper, a prefix, appears within this term.)*	**2. euglycemia** (*ū*-glī-SĒ-mē-a)	normal (level of) sugar in the blood (within normal range)

Complementary Terms—cont'd

BUILT FROM WORD PARTS AND *NOT* BUILT FROM WORD PARTS

Built From Word Parts

SIGNS AND SYMPTOMS—CONT'D

TERM	DEFINITION	TERM	DEFINITION
3. **euthyroid** (ū-THĪ-royd)	normal thyroid gland activity	5. **polydipsia** (*pol*-ē-DIP-sē-a)	abnormal state of much thirst
4. **glycemia** (glī-SĒ-mē-a)	sugar in the blood		

MEDICAL SPECIALTIES

TERM	DEFINITION	TERM	DEFINITION
6. **endocrinologist** (*en*-dō-kri-NOL-o-jist)	physician who studies and treats diseases of the endocrine (system)	7. **endocrinology** (*en*-dō-kri-NOL-o-jē)	study of the endocrine (system) (a branch of medicine dealing with diseases of the endocrine system)

DESCRIPTIVE TERMS

TERM	DEFINITION
8. **cortical** (KŌR-ti-kal)	pertaining to the cortex

OTHER

TERM	DEFINITION
9. **syndrome** (SIN-drōm)	run together (signs and symptoms occurring together that are characteristic of a specific disorder)

NOT Built from Word Parts

SIGNS AND SYMPTOMS

TERM	DEFINITION
1. **exophthalmos** (*ek*-sof-THAL-mos)	abnormal protrusion of the eyeball
2. **goiter** (GOY-ter)	enlargement of the thyroid gland. May be caused by autoimmune diseases of the thyroid (Graves disease or Hashimoto thyroiditis), iodine deficiency, or the presence of multiple nodules.
3. **tetany** (TET-a-nē)	condition affecting nerves causing muscle spasms as a result of low amounts of calcium in the blood caused by a deficiency of the parathyroid hormone

OTHER

TERM	DEFINITION
4. **hormone** (HOR-mōn)	chemical substance secreted by an endocrine gland that is carried in the blood to a target tissue
5. **incretins** (in-KRĒ-tins)	a group of hormones produced by the gastrointestinal system that stimulate the release of insulin from the pancreas and help preserve the beta cells. *Incretin mimetics* are medications that copy this action and help control blood sugar in patients with type 2 diabetes mellitus.
6. **metabolism** (me-TAB-ō-*lizm*)	sum total of all the chemical processes that take place in a living organism

EXERCISE 21 ■ Pronounce and Spell

Practice pronunciation and spelling on paper and online.

1. Practice on Paper

a. **Pronounce:** Read the phonetic spelling and say aloud the terms listed in the previous table. Refer to the pronunciation key on p. 20 as necessary.
b. **Spell:** Have a study partner read the terms aloud. Write the spelling of the terms on a separate sheet of paper.

2. Practice Online

a. **Access** online learning resources. Go to evolve.elsevier.com > Evolve Resources > Student Resources.
b. **Pronounce:** Select Audio Glossary > Chapter 16 > Exercise 21. Select a term to hear its pronunciation and repeat aloud.
c. **Spell:** Select Activities > Chapter 16 > Spell Terms > Exercise 21. Select the audio icon and type the correct spelling of the term.

❑ Check the box when complete.

EXERCISE 22 ■ Complementary Terms Built from Word Parts

A Analyze and Define

Analyze and define the following terms.

1. syndrome

____

____

2. endocrinologist

____

____

3. polydipsia

____

____

4. euglycemia

____

____

5. adrenocorticohyperplasia

____

____

6. euthyroid

____

____

7. cortical

____

____

8. endocrinology

____

____

9. glycemia

____

____

B Label

Build terms pictured by writing word parts above definitions.

1.

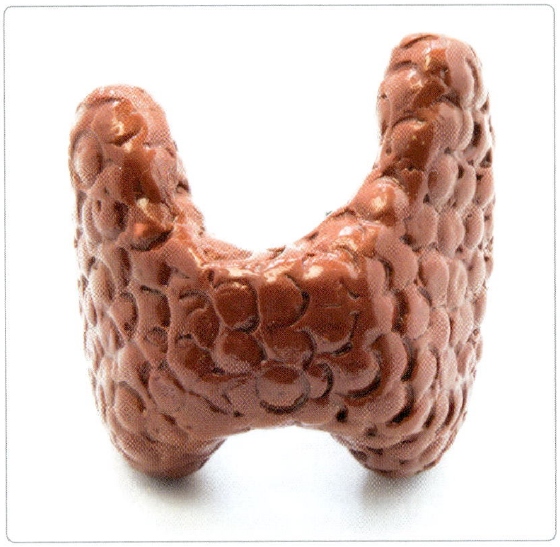

_______ / _______________

normal / thyroid gland (activity)

2.

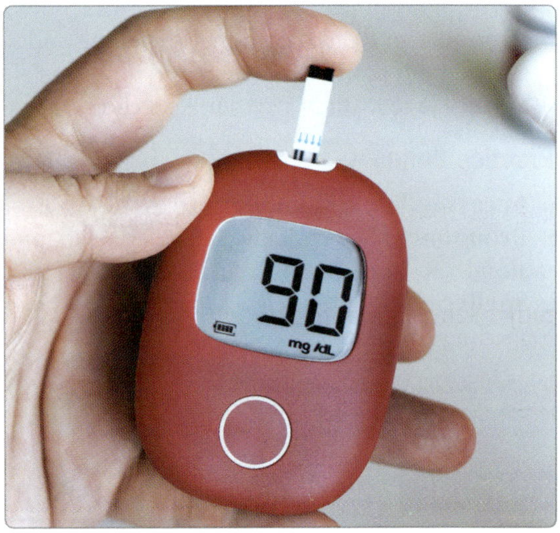

_______ / _______ / _______

normal / (level of) sugar / in the blood

3.

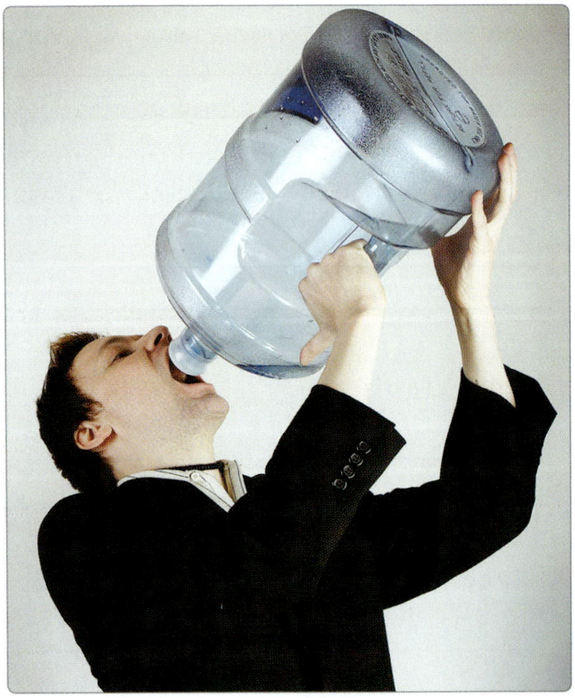

_______ / _______ / _______

much / thirst / abnormal state

4.

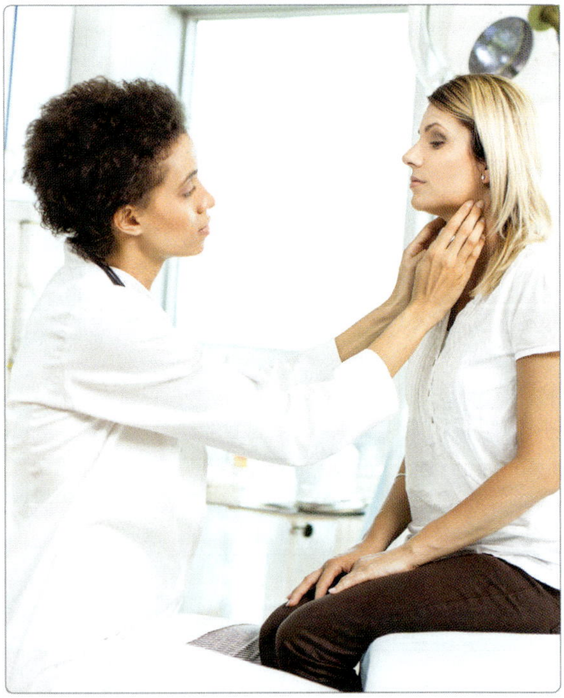

_______ / ___ / _______________

endocrine (system) / CV / physician who studies and treats

C Fill In

Build complementary terms for the following definitions by using the word parts you have learned.

1. sugar in the blood ______ / ______
   WR / S
2. run together (signs and symptoms occurring together) ______ / ______
   P / S(WR)
3. excessive development of the adrenal cortex ______ / ______ / ______ / ______ / ______ / ______
   WR / CV / WR / CV / P / S
4. study of the endocrine (system) ______ / ______ / ______
   WR / CV / S
5. pertaining to the cortex ______ / ______
   WR / S

EXERCISE 23 ■ Complementary Terms *NOT* Built from Word Parts

A Match

Match the terms in the first column with their correct definitions in the second column

______ 1. tetany
______ 2. incretins
______ 3. goiter
______ 4. exophthalmos
______ 5. metabolism
______ 6. hormone

a. chemical substance secreted by an endocrine gland that is carried in the blood to a target tissue
b. nerve condition causing muscle spasms due to low amounts of calcium in the blood
c. sum total of all the chemical processes that take place in a living organism
d. may be caused by autoimmune diseases of the thyroid, iodine deficiency or multiple nodules
e. abnormal protrusion of the eyeball
f. group of hormones that stimulate the release of insulin from the pancreas and help preserve the beta cells

B Label

Write the terms pictured and defined.

1. ______________________
enlargement of the thyroid gland

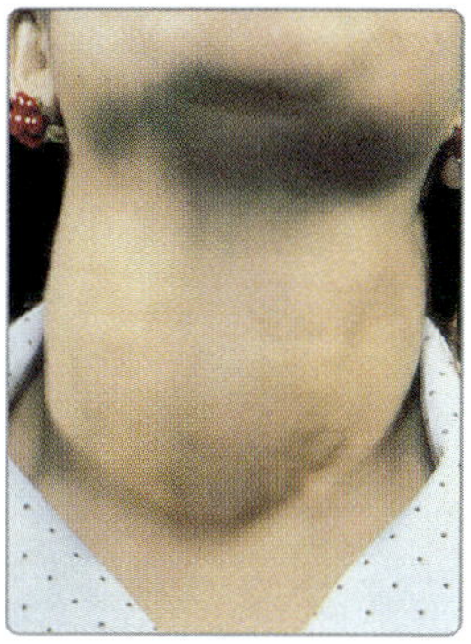

2. ______________________
abnormal protrusion of the eyeball

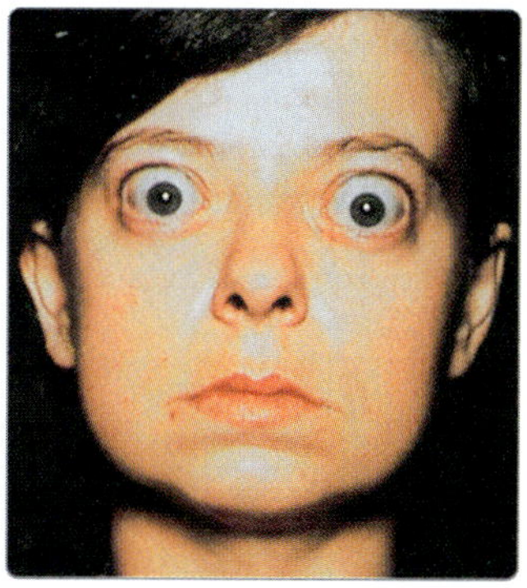

C Identify

Fill in the blanks with the correct terms.

1. The sum total of all the chemical processes that take place in a living organism is called its ______________.
2. A chemical substance secreted by an endocrine gland is called a(n) ______________.
3. ______________ describes muscle spasms that result from low calcium due to parathroid hormone deficiency.
4. Hormones produced by the gastrointestinal system that stimulate insulin release are called ______________.

EXERCISE 24 ■ Review of Complementary Terms

Can you define, pronounce, and spell the following terms?

adrenocorticohyperplasia
endocrinologist
endocrinology
exophthalmos
cortical
euglycemia
euthyroid
goiter
glycemia
hormone
incretins
metabolism
polydipsia
syndrome
tetany

Abbreviations

DISEASE AND DISORDERS

ABBREVIATION	TERM	ABBREVIATION	TERM
DI	diabetes insipidus	**T1DM**	type 1 diabetes mellitus (also abbreviated **T1D**)
DKA	diabetic ketoacidosis	**T2DM**	type 2 diabetes mellitus (also abbreviated **T2D**)
DM	diabetes mellitus		
SIADH	syndrome of inappropriate ADH (secretion)		

DIAGNOSTIC

ABBREVIATION	TERM	ABBREVIATION	TERM
ACTH	adrenocorticotropic hormone	**LH**	luteinizing hormone
ADH	antidiuretic hormone	**PRL**	prolactin
FBS	fasting blood sugar	**PTH**	parathyroid hormone
FNA	fine needle aspiration	**RAIU**	radioactive iodine uptake
FSH	follicle-stimulating hormone	**TSH**	thyroid-stimulating hormone
GH	growth hormone	**T_4**	thyroxine level
HbA1c	glycosylated hemoglobin		

Refer to **Appendix D** for a complete list of abbreviations.

EXERCISE 25 ▪ Abbreviations

Write the terms abbreviated.

1. **DM** ___________ _____________ is a chronic disease characterized by elevated blood sugar. **T1DM** ______ _______ ___________ ____________ is an autoimmune disease that generally starts in childhood or adolescence. It is important to monitor **FBS** ________ ____________ __________, as episodes of severe hyperglycemia can lead to **DKA** ________ __________, which can be fatal.
2. **T2DM** ________ __________ ___________ ____________ has a slower onset, and is associated with obesity. **HbA1c** ____________ ____________ is used for both diagnosis and monitoring treatment.
3. Patients presenting with Graves disease will likely have a high T_4 ______________ ______________ and a low **TSH** __________-__________ ___________. **RAIU** __________ __________ __________ testing can help differentiate this from other forms of thyrotoxicosis. **FNA** ________ ________ _____________ of the thyroid may be needed if ultrasound reveals any nodules. If thyroidectomy is required, it is important to try to leave at least one parathyroid gland intact. A low **PTH** __________ ______________ can reveal inadvertent removal of all four glands.
4. In addition to a semen analysis for men, an infertility work-up in women would include **FSH** ___________- __________ ____________ and **LH** ____________ ____________ levels.
5. **ADH** ____________ ___________ evaluation may be performed along with other blood and urine tests to help diagnose **DI** ____________ _____________, which results from too little ADH (or a lack of response to it), and **SIADH** ________ of ___________ ____________ (secretion), which results from too much ADH.
6. Functional pituitary tumors most commonly cause overproduction of specific hormones, including **GH** _________ _____________, which leads to acromegaly, **ACTH** _________________________ ___________, which causes Cushing syndrome, and **PRL** _____________, which can cause galactorrhea, infertility, and menstrual irregularities in women.

PRACTICAL APPLICATION

EXERCISE 26 ■ Case Study: Translate Between Everyday Language and Medical Language

CASE STUDY: Lily Macabal

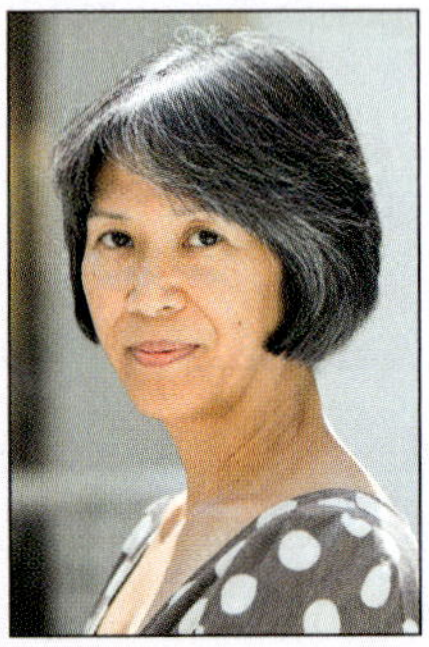

Lily Macabal has not been feeling well. She feels restless all the time and feels more irritable. Her appetite is increased, but she has been losing weight. She seems to always feel warm, and sometimes her heart races. Her hair seems thin and brittle. Recently she has noticed a lump in the front of her neck, and her husband says that her eyes seem to stick out more than they used to. She remembers her mother having a condition caused by too much thyroid hormone, and she wonders if she is going through the same thing. She sees her family doctor, who recommends a referral to an endocrine specialist.

Now that you have worked through Chapter 16 on the endocrine system, consider the medical terms that might be used to describe Mrs. Macabal's experience. See the Chapter at a Glance section at the end of the chapter for a list of terms that might apply.

A. *Underline phrases in the case study that could be substituted with medical terms.*

B. *Write the medical term and its definition for three of the phrases you underlined.*

MEDICAL TERM	DEFINITION
1. ______________________	______________________________________
2. ______________________	______________________________________
3. ______________________	______________________________________

DOCUMENTATION: Excerpt from Emergency Department Visit

Mrs. Macabal saw an endocrinologist; an excerpt from her medical record is presented below.

This 56-year-old female was referred by her PCP for evaluation of a thyroid endocrinopathy. She has had multiple symptoms of hyperthyroidism and appears to be experiencing thyrotoxicosis. Her exophthalmos is suggestive of Graves disease. Thyroid sonography performed in our office showed no discrete nodules, with increased vascularity and diffuse hypoechoic tissue throughout. We have ordered a TSH and free T_4 level to assess her thyroid function. A radioactive iodine uptake test will be performed to assess her thyroid function. We will consider treatment with either radioiodine therapy or near-total thyroidectomy, with the understanding that either treatment may result in hypothyroidism and require thyroid hormone replacement therapy.

C. *Underline medical terms presented in Chapter 16 used in the previous excerpt from Mrs. Macabal's medical record. See the Chapter at a Glance section at the end of the chapter for a complete list.*

D. *Select and define three of the medical terms you underlined. To check your answers, go to Appendix A.*

MEDICAL TERM	DEFINITION
1. ______________________	______________________________________
2. ______________________	______________________________________
3. ______________________	______________________________________

EXERCISE 27 ■ Interact with Medical Documents

A

Read the report and complete it by writing medical terms on answer lines within the document. Definitions of terms to be written appear after the document.

021286 BLACKWATER, Josephina

File Patient Navigate Custom Fields Help

Chart Review | Encounters | Notes | Labs | Imaging | Procedures | Rx | Documents | Referrals | Scheduling | Billing

Name: **BLACKWATER, Josephina** MR#: 021286 DOB: 05/21/19xx Gender: F **Allergies: NKDA** **PCP:** Julius Netou, PA-C

DATE: 06/20/20XX

HISTORY AND PHYSICAL

CHIEF COMPLANT: Josephina Blackwater is a 51-year-old female complaining of excessive urination, excessive thirst, and fatigue for approximately 1 month.

HISTORY OF PRESENT ILLNESS: For the past 4 weeks, she has been having polyuria and 1. ____________________, drinking 3 to 4 quarts of water daily for the past 10 days. This has also resulted in nocturia, getting up 2 to 3 times each night to void. She also reports fatigue, which has been present for at least 4 weeks. She denies anorexia, nausea, vomiting, hematemesis, or any abdominal pain. She denies blurred vision.

MEDICAL HISTORY: No known allergies. No previous hospitalizations. She has had no recent illness.

FAMILY HISTORY: Her mother died of a stroke at age 63. Her father is still living at the age of 78 but has had 2. __________ ______________ for 20 years. She has two brothers, both in good health, and no sisters.

SOCIAL HISTORY: She is married with 3 children . She does not smoke and does not use alcohol or other drugs.

REVIEW OF SYSTEMS: She denies fever, chills, headache, palpitations, chest pain, or edema.

PHYSICAL EXAM: Temperature, 98.9°F. Pulse, 80. Respirations, 24. Her blood pressure is 125/80 mm Hg. Her height is 5 ft. 3 inches, weight is 186 pounds, and BMI is 33 (obese). HEENT: Normal, no evidence of 3. ________________ . CHEST: Clear to auscultation and percussion. HEART: Regular rhythm. No murmurs or extra heart sounds. ABDOMEN: Soft, nontender, bowel sounds normal, without evidence of organomegaly. RECTAL: Unremarkable. EXTREMITIES: No clubbing, cyanosis, or edema. Pedal pulses are intact. NEUROLOGIC: Alert and oriented to time, person, and place. Cranial nerves 2 through 12 are grossly intact.

LABORATORY FINDINGS: 4. ____________ _________ ________ was discovered to be 200 mg/dL. Urinalysis showed moderate proteinuria. 5. ______________ _________________ was 9.2%.

ASSESSMENT: Newly diagnosed 6. __________ __________ _____________ ___________.

PLAN:

1. Since her fasting glucose and hemoglobin A1C are quite elevated, we will immediately institute a regimen of metformin 500 mg at bedtime, with increase to 500 mg bid as tolerated. She will be given a glucometer and test strips so that she can monitor her sugars at home. She is already familiar with this after caring for her diabetic father for many years.
2. The patient was educated about her diagnosis and the relationship between strict control of 7. ________________ and the reduction of diabetes-related complications. She was also educated about the risks of 8. ________________. She will schedule appointments with the diabetes educator and nutritionist for further management of her condition.
3. Consider a(n) 9.__________________ consult if she does not respond to lifestyle changes and metformin.

Christina Kraemer, MD
CK/mcm

Start | Log On/Off | Print | Edit

Definitions of Medical Terms to Complete the Document

Write the medical terms defined on corresponding answer lines in the document.

1. excessive thirst
2. chronic disease involving a disorder of carbohydrate metabolism and characterized by elevated blood sugar
3. abnormal protrusion of the eyeball
4. blood test to determine the amount of glucose (sugar) in the blood after fasting for 8 to 10 hours
5. the test measuring the amount of hemoglobin coated in sugar over the lifespan of the red blood cell
6. T2DM
7. excessive sugar in the blood
8. deficient sugar in the blood
9. study of the endocrine (system)

EXERCISE 27 ■ Interact with Medical Documents—cont'd

B

Read the medical report and answer the questions below it.

029210 GOMEZ, RUTH

File Patient Navigate Custom Fields Help

Patient Chart | Lab | Rad | Notes | Documents | Rx | Scheduling | Images | Billing

Name: **GOMEZ, RUTH** MR#: **029210** DOB: **5/11/19XX** Gender: **Female** Age: **39** Allergies: **None known** PCP: **Anna Tang, MD**

DATE OF OPERATION: April 10, 20XX

SURGERY PERFORMED: Right laparoscopic adrenalectomy

PREOPERATIVE DIAGNOSIS: Primary hyperaldosteronism (Conn syndrome), adrenal adenoma.

INDICATIONS: The patient is a 39-year-old woman who has a history of hypertension and hypokalemia seen on referral from her endocrinologist. The patient complained of headache and muscle weakness. She underwent a 24-hour urine collection, a general metastatic workup, and evaluation for Cushing syndrome. Laboratory studies indicated elevated plasma and urinary aldosterone levels. CT scan revealed the presence of a 3.5-cm right adrenal mass, and adrenal biopsy confirmed that it was an aldosterone-producing adenoma.

PROCEDURE: The procedure was performed with the patient under general endotracheal anesthesia and with an arterial line, a Foley catheter, and a central venous pressure line in place. A Veress needle was inserted into the abdominal cavity between the midclavicular and anterior axillary lines. The abdominal cavity was then insufflated with CO_2. A 10- to 11-mm trocar was placed at the site of the Veress needle, and a 30-degree videotelescope was inserted. A third 10- to 11-mm port was placed 3 to 4 cm behind the posterior axillary line, and a fourth port inserted after mobilization of the right lobe of the liver. The superior pole and lateral border of the adrenal gland were mobilized first, with the dissection proceeding carefully along the lateral edge of the inferior vena cava. The right adrenal vein was ligated with endoscopic clips and divided, freeing the adrenal gland from its surrounding attachments. The gland was placed in an impermeable entrapment sac and removed from the most anterior port site. After evacuation of CO_2, all ports were removed, and the incisions were closed with absorbable sutures.

POSTOPERATIVE DIAGNOSIS: Aldosteronoma

Electronically signed by: Merriam Fitch, MD 4/11/20XX 11:24

Start | Log On/Off | Print | Edit

Use the medical report above to answer the questions.

1. Which procedure was performed during surgery:
   a. excision of a parathyroid gland
   b. surgical repair of the thyroid gland
   c. excision of an adrenal gland
   d. surgical repair of the thymus
2. The patient had a history of:
   a. excessive sugar in the blood
   b. deficient potassium in the blood
   c. deficient sodium in the blood
   d. deficient calcium in the blood
3. The patient was evaluated for a:
   a. group of symptoms from the excessive production of cortisol
   b. condition caused by congenital absence of the thyroid gland
   c. syndrome caused by deficient secretion from the adrenal cortex
   d. condition causing muscle spasms resulting from low amounts of calcium

EXERCISE 28 ▪ Use Medical Language in Online Electronic Health Records

Select the correct medical terms to complete three medical records in one patient's electronic file.

Access online resources at evolve.elsevier.com > Evolve Resources > Student Resources > Activities > Chapter 16 > Electronic Health Records

Topic: Hyperparathyroidism
Record 1: Preoperative Note
Record 2: Nuclear Medicine Report
Record 3: Office Visit Report

❑ Check the box when complete.

EXERCISE 29 ▪ Pronounce Medical Terms in Use

Practice pronunciation of terms by reading aloud the following paragraph. Use the phonetic spellings to assist with pronunciation. The script also contains medical terms not presented in the chapter. If interested, research their meanings in a medical dictionary or a reliable online source.

A 65-year-old female patient presented to her doctor because of a 10-pound weight gain, fatigue, hair loss, dry skin, and cold intolerance. She was referred to an **endocrinologist** (*en*-dō-kri-NOL-o-jist) who established a diagnosis of **hypothyroidism** (*hī*-pō-THĪ-royd-izm) after test results indicated an elevated **thyroid-stimulating hormone level** (THĪ-royd) (STIM-yuh-lāt-ing) (HŌR-mōn) (LEV-el) and a low **thyroxine level** (thī-ROK-sin) (LEV-el). Approximately 20 years ago she had a painless thyroid nodule. At that time, **thyroid sonography** (THĪ-royd) (so-NOG-ra-fē) and **fine needle aspiration** (FĪN) (NĒ-del) (*as*-pi-RĀ-shen) were performed; a diagnosis of thyroid cancer was confirmed, but it had not spread beyond the gland. She underwent a **thyroidectomy** (*thī*-royd-EK-to-mē) and received thyroid hormone replacement therapy thereafter. She remained in a **euthyroid** (ū-THĪ-royd) state until she stopped taking the medication 6 months ago. Consequently, she became hypothyroid and could have easily developed **myxedema** (*mik*-se-DĒ-ma) if she had not sought treatment.

CHAPTER REVIEW

EXERCISE 30 ▪ Chapter Content Quiz

Test your understanding of terms and abbreviations introduced in this chapter. Circle the letter for the medical term or abbreviation related to the words in italics.

1. Inez Villalvazo was diagnosed with Hashimoto thyroiditis after she presented to her doctor with *enlargement of the thyroid gland.*
   a. myxedema
   b. tetany
   c. goiter

2. An episode of *serious condition resulting from uncontrolled diabetes mellitus in which acid ketones accumulate* resulted in admission to the intensive care unit for Mr. Khalile.
   a. ketoacidosis
   b. tetany
   c. euglycemia

3. Diana Worthington complained of weight loss and muscle aches, as well as darkening of her skin. She was diagnosed with *chronic syndrome resulting from a deficiency in hormonal secretion from the adrenal cortex.*
   a. Cushing syndrome
   b. Graves disease
   c. Addison disease

4. Malini Sobel noticed polydipsia and polyuria and found herself drinking a lot of water. This was related to *decreased secretion of antidiuretic hormone by the posterior lobe of the pituitary gland.*
   a. diabetes mellitus
   b. diabetes insipidus
   c. diabetic retinopathy

5. Ryan McAvoy had *condition brought about by hypersecretion of growth hormone by the pituitary gland before puberty* and was over 6 feet tall as an 11-year-old.
   a. gigantism
   b. acromegaly
   c. metabolic syndrome

6. *Deficient sodium in the blood* and *excessive potassium in the blood* are two laboratory findings in Addison disease.
   a. hypoglycemia and hypercalcemia
   b. hyponatremia and hyperkalemia
   c. hypocalcemia and hyperglycemia

7. A(n) *excision of (one or both) adrenal glands* was performed on Mr. Rockov after a tumor was discovered.
   a. thyroidectomy
   b. adrenalectomy
   c. parathyroidectomy

8. Mrs. Lucio has been working hard to help control her diabetes mellitus with diet and exercise. Her recent *blood test used to diagnose diabetes and monitor its treatment by measuring the amount of glucose (sugar) bound to hemoglobin in the blood* showed marked improvement since the last test 3 months ago.
   a. FSH
   b. FBS
   c. HbA1c

9. Dr. Chen told Mrs. Onwubiko that weight loss, regular exercise, and healthy eating are central in the treatment and prevention of *a group of health problems including insulin resistance, obesity, hypertension, hyperglycemia, elevated triglycerides, and low levels of HDL.*
   a. metabolic syndrome
   b. Cushing syndrome
   c. irritable bowel syndrome

10. Congenital hypothyroidism is a(n) *any disease of the endocrine system* that is characterized by puffy features, mental deficiency, large tongue, and short stature.
    a. adrenopathy
    b. neuropathy
    c. endocrinopathy

11. Dr. Turecki performed a *biopsy technique that uses a narrow hollow needle to obtain tiny amounts of tissue for pathologic examination* on the patient who had been found to have a multinodular goiter on thyroid sonography.
    a. thyroid-stimulating hormone level (TSH)
    b. thyroxine level (T_4)
    c. fine needle aspiration (FNA)

12. *Excessive development of the adrenal cortex* was the cause of Cushing syndrome in Mr. Lim when he presented with "moon face," "buffalo hump," and hypertension.
    a. pheochromocytoma
    b. thyrotoxicosis
    c. adrenocorticohyperplasia

13. The pharmacist told Mrs. Tranh that her new diabetes medication acted in the same way as *a group of hormones produced by the gastrointestinal system that stimulate the release of insulin from the pancreas.*
    a. hormones
    b. incretins
    c. corticoids

14. Mrs. Webber had *nuclear medicine scan that measures thyroid function using radioactive iodine* and was diagnosed with Graves disease. Since she had her thyroid removed, she has been on thyroid hormone replacement therapy and had periodic measurements of her *blood test that measures the amount of thyroid-stimulating hormone in the blood.*
    a. thyroid scan, T_4
    b. RAIU, TSH
    c. thyroid sonography, LH

15. Dr. Nair performed a parathyroidectomy on Mrs. Chaugary to treat her *state of excessive parathyroid gland activity*.
    a. hyperpituitarism
    b. hyperthyroidism
    c. hyperparathyroidism

16. Rodrigo Garcia was diagnosed during infancy with *malignant cancer that often starts in the adrenal medulla, composed of immature nerve cells;* luckily, it had not metastasized.
    a. neuroblastoma
    b. pheochromocytoma
    c. parathyroidoma

17. Jianna Roberts had a goiter and a high TSH level; she was eventually diagnosed with *disease in which thyroid gland cells are destroyed by autoimmune processes.*
    a. Graves disease
    b. Hashimoto thyroiditis
    c. Cushing syndrome

18. *Result of decreased secretion of antidiuretic hormone by the posterior lobe of the pituitary gland* was the cause of Max Mazet's polydipsia.
    a. DI
    b. SIADH
    c. DKA

19. Sheehan syndrome is a rare cause of *state of total deficient pituitary gland activity* that results from severe blood loss or low blood pressure during pregnancy or delivery.
    a. hypopituitarism
    b. panhypopituitarism
    c. hypothyroidism

20. *Nuclear medicine procedure used to localize hyperactive parathyroid glands* would be useful in diagnosing a parathyroidoma.
    a. parathyroidectomy
    b. sestamibi parathyroid scan
    c. fine needle aspiration

CHAPTER AT A GLANCE Word Parts New to This Chapter

COMBINING FORMS

acr/o
adren/o
adrenal/o
calc/i
cortic/o
dips/o
endocrin/o
glyc/o
kal/i
natr/o
parathyroid/o
pituitar/o
thyroid/o

SUFFIXES

-drome

CHAPTER AT A GLANCE Endocrine System Terms Built from Word Parts

DISEASE AND DISORDER

acromegaly
adrenalitis
adrenomegaly
endocrinopathy
hypercalcemia
hyperglycemia
hyperkalemia
hyperparathyroidism
hyperpituitarism
hyperthyroidism
hypocalcemia
hypoglycemia
hypokalemia
hyponatremia
hypopituitarism
hypothyroidism
panhypopituitarism
parathyroidoma
thyroiditis

SURGICAL

adrenalectomy
parathyroidectomy
thyroidectomy

COMPLEMENTARY

adrenocorticohyperplasia
cortical
endocrinologist
endocrinology
euglycemia
euthyroid
glycemia
polydipsia
syndrome

CHAPTER AT A GLANCE Endocrine System Terms *NOT* Built from Word Parts

DISEASE AND DISORDER

Addison disease
congenital hypothyroidism
Cushing syndrome
diabetes insipidus (DI)
diabetes mellitus (DM)
gigantism
Graves disease
Hashimoto thyroiditis
ketoacidosis
metabolic syndrome
myxedema
neuroblastoma
pheochromocytoma
thyrotoxicosis

DIAGNOSTIC

fasting blood sugar (FBS)
fine needle aspiration (FNA)
glycosylated hemoglobin (HbA1c)
radioactive iodine uptake (RAIU)
sestamibi parathyroid scan
thyroid sonography
thyroid-stimulating hormone level (TSH)
thyroxine level (T_4)

COMPLEMENTARY

exophthalmos
goiter
hormone
incretins
metabolism
tetany

Appendix A

Answer Key

ANSWERS TO CHAPTER 1 EXERCISES

Exercise 1

1. b
2. a
3. c
4. d
5. a
6. d
7. c
8. b

Exercise 2

Built from Word Parts; NOT Built from Word Parts

Exercise 3

1. a word part that is the core of the word
2. a word part attached to the end of the word root to modify its meaning
3. a word part attached to the beginning of a word root to modify its meaning

Exercise 4

1. a word part, usually an o, used to ease pronunciation
2. used
3. vowel
4. word roots
5. not

Exercise 5

a word root with the combining vowel attached, separated by a slash

Exercise 6

1. b
2. a
3. d
4. e
5. c

Exercise 7

1. *F*, a medical term may begin with the word root and have no prefix.
2. *F*, if the suffix begins with a vowel, the combining vowel is usually not used.
3. *T*
4. *T*
5. *F*, o is the combining vowel most often used.
6. *T*
7. *F*, a combining vowel is used between two word roots or between a word root and a suffix to ease pronunciation.
8. *F*, a combining form is a word root with a combining vowel attached and is not one of the four word parts.
9. *T*

Exercise 8

A

1. Divide the term into word parts.
2. Label each word part.
3. Identify each combining form by underlining the word root and combining vowel, and then writing the abbreviation CF below the underlined combining form.

B

WR CV S
oste/o/pathy
CF

Exercise 9

A

apply the meaning of each word part

B

disease of the bone and joint

Exercise 10

1. WR S
   arthr/itis
   inflammation of a joint
2. WR S
   hepat/itis
   inflammation of the liver
3. P WR S
   sub/hepat/ic
   pertaining to under the liver
4. P WR S
   intra/ven/ous
   pertaining to within the vein
5. WR CV S
   arthr/o/pathy
   CF
   disease of a joint
6. WR S
   oste/itis
   inflammation of the bone
7. WR CV S
   hepat/o/megaly
   CF
   enlargement of the liver
8. WR S
   hepat/ic
   pertaining to the liver

Exercise 11

A

to place word parts together to form terms

B

arthr/o/pathy

Exercise 12

A

oste/o/arthr/itis

B

1. arthr/itis
2. hepat/ic
3. sub/hepat/ic
4. intra/ven/ous
5. oste/itis
6. hepat/itis
7. oste/o/arthr/o/pathy
8. hepat/o/megaly

Exercise 13

Check marks for numbers 2, 3, 4, 5, 7, 8, 10

Copyright © 2022, Elsevier Inc. All rights reserved.

ANSWERS TO CHAPTER 2 EXERCISES

Exercise 1

A *Label*

1. neur/o
2. epitheli/o
3. sarc/o
4. my/o
5. aden/o
6. fibr/o

B *Label*

1. tissue: hist/o
2. cell: cyt/o
3. organ: organ/o
4. system: system/o
5. internal organs: viscer/o

C *Define and Match*

1. d, flesh, connective tissue
2. e, fat
3. c, internal organs
4. f, cell
5. b, tissue
6. a, muscle

D *Define and Match*

1. c, nerve
2. f, organ
3. d, system
4. a, epithelium
5. b, fiber
6. e, gland
7. g, blood

Exercise 2

A *Define*

1. tumor, mass
2. cancer
3. cause (of disease)
4. disease
5. body
6. cancer
7. rod-shaped, striated
8. smooth
9. knowledge
10. physician, medicine
11. life
12. virus
13. self
14. death (cells, body)

B *Identify*

1. path/o
2. onc/o
3. eti/o
4. a. cancer/o
   b. carcin/o
5. somat/o
6. lei/o
7. rhabd/o
8. gno/o
9. iatr/o
10. aut/o
11. vir/o
12. bi/o
13. necr/o

Exercise 3

A *Define*

1. blue
2. red
3. white
4. yellow
5. black

B *Identify*

1. cyan/o
2. erythr/o
3. leuk/o
4. melan/o
5. xanth/o

Exercise 4

A *Define*

1. new
2. above, excessive
3. after, beyond, change
4. below, incomplete, deficient, under
5. painful, abnormal, difficult, labored
6. through, complete
7. before
8. small

B *Identify*

1. neo-
2. hyper-
3. hypo-
4. meta-
5. dys-
6. dia-
7. pro-
8. micro-

Exercise 5

A *Label*

1. -cyte
2. -plasia
3. -logist
4. -logy
5. -megaly
6. -oma

B *Match*

1. g
2. j
3. b
4. c
5. e
6. d
7. f
8. i
9. a
10. h
11. k

C *Define*

1. one who studies and treats (specialist, physician)
2. disease
3. study of
4. pertaining to
5. control, stop, standing
6. cell
7. abnormal condition
8. pertaining to
9. growth, substance, formation
10. pertaining to
11. condition of formation, development, growth
12. resembling
13. substance or agent that produces or causes
14. producing, originating, causing
15. tumor, swelling
16. malignant tumor
17. state of
18. enlargement
19. view of, viewing

Exercise 6

Pronounce and Spell

Exercise 7

1. WR CV S
cyt/o/logy
CF
study of cells
2. WR CV S
hist/o/logy
CF
study of tissue
3. WR S
viscer/al
pertaining to internal organs
4. P S(WR)
hypo/plasia
incomplete development (of an organ or tissues)
5. WR CV S
neur/o/pathy
CF
disease of the nerves
6. WR S
system/ic
pertaining to a (body) system
7. WR S
somat/ic
pertaining to the body
8. WR CV S
somat/o/genic
CF
originating in the body
9. WR S
epitheli/al
pertaining to the epithelium
10. WR CV WR S
erythr/o/cyt/osis
CF
increase in the number of red (blood) cells
11. WR CV WR S
leuk/o/cyt/osis
CF
increase in the number of white (blood) cells
12. WR CV S
my/o/pathy
CF
disease of the muscle

Copyright © 2022, Elsevier Inc. All rights reserved.

13. WR CV S
erythr/o/cyte
CF
red (blood) cell

14. WR CV S
leuk/o/cyte
CF
white (blood) cell

Exercise 8

A *Fill In*

1. neur/o/pathy
2. cyt/o/logy
3. somat/ic
4. my/o/pathy
5. dys/plasia
6. viscer/al
7. somat/o/genic
8. organ/o/megaly
9. lip/oid
10. system/ic

B *Label*

1. leuk/o/cyte
2. hyper/plasia
3. erythr/o/cyte
4. necr/osis

Exercise 9

Review of Body Structure Terms

Exercise 10

Pronounce and Spell

Exercise 11

1. WR S
sarc/oma
tumor composed of connective tissue

2. WR S
melan/oma
black tumor

3. WR S
epitheli/oma
tumor composed of epithelium

4. WR S
lip/oma
tumor composed of fat

5. P S(WR)
neo/plasm
new growth

6. WR S
my/oma
tumor composed of muscle

7. WR S
neur/oma
tumor composed of nerve

8. WR S
carcin/oma
cancerous tumor

9. WR CV WR S
melan/o/carcin/oma
CF
cancerous black tumor

10. WR CV WR CV S
rhabd/o/my/o/sarcoma
CF CF
malignant tumor of striated muscle

11. WR S
aden/oma
tumor composed of glandular tissue (benign)

12. WR CV WR S
rhabd/o/my/oma
CF
tumor composed of striated muscle

13. WR S
fibr/oma
tumor composed of fiber (fibrous tissue)

14. WR CV S
lip/o/sarcoma
CF
malignant tumor of fat

15. WR CV S
fibr/o/sarcoma
CF
malignant tumor of fiber (fibrous tissue)

16. P S(WR)
meta/stasis
beyond control (transfer of disease)

Exercise 12

A *Label*

1. carcin/oma
2. sarc/oma
3. melan/oma
4. rhabd/o/my/o/sarcoma
5. lei/o/my/oma
6. neur/oma

B *Fill In*

1. rhabd/o/my/oma
2. lip/o/sarcoma
3. neo/plasm
4. epitheli/oma
5. fibr/oma
6. melan/o/carcin/oma
7. meta/stasis
8. my/oma
9. fibr/o/sarcoma
10. aden/o/carcin/oma

Exercise 13

Pronounce and Spell

Exercise 14

A *Label*

1. encapsulated
2. radiation therapy (XRT)
3. benign
4. malignant
5. chemotherapy
6. carcinoma in situ

B *Identify*

1. biological therapy
2. palliative
3. remission
4. hospice

C *Match*

1. h	6. j
2. i	7. c
3. g	8. d
4. b	9. e
5. a	10. f

Exercise 15

Review of Oncology Terms

Exercise 16

Pronounce and Spell

Exercise 17

A *Analyze and Define*

1. WR CV WR CV S
cyt/o/path/o/logy
CF CF
study of (changes in) cells in disease

2. WR CV WR CV S
hist/o/path/o/logy
CF CF
study of tissue in disease (study of tissue samples taken from patients)

3. WR CV S
vir/o/logy
CF
study of viruses (branch of microbiology that is concerned with viruses and viral diseases)

4. WR CV WR CV S
micr/o/bi/o/logy
CF CF
study of small life (study of microorganisms, such as bacteria, fungi, viruses and parasites)

5. WR S
aut/opsy
view of self

6. WR S
bi/opsy
view of life

B *Fill In*

1. hist/o/path/o/logy
2. vir/o/logy
3. cyt/o/path/o/logy

Copyright © 2022, Elsevier Inc. All rights reserved.

C *Label*

1. hemat/o/logy
2. aut/opsy
3. micr/o/bi/o/logy
4. bi/opsy

Exercise 18

A *Identify*

1. genetic testing
2. Chemistry panel
3. complete blood count with differential
4. Specimen
5. culture and sensitivity

B *Label*

1. specimen
2. chemistry panel
3. genetic testing
4. culture and sensitivity

Exercise 19

Review of Laboratory Terms

Exercise 20

Pronounce and Spell

Exercise 21

1. WR CV S
   path/o/logy
   CF
   study of disease
2. WR CV S
   path/o/logist
   CF
   physician who studies diseases
3. P WR S
   dia/gno/sis
   state of complete knowledge (the art of identifying a disease based on the patient's signs, symptoms, and test results)
4. WR CV S
   onc/o/genic
   CF
   causing tumors
5. WR CV S
   onc/o/logy
   CF
   study of tumors
6. WR S
   cancer/ous
   pertaining to cancer
7. WR CV S
   carcin/o/genic
   CF
   producing cancer
8. WR S
   cyan/osis
   abnormal condition of blue (bluish discoloration of the skin)
9. WR CV S
   eti/o/logy
   CF
   study of causes (of disease)
10. WR S
    xanth/osis
    abnormal condition of yellow
11. WR S
    carcin/oid
    resembling cancer
12. WR CV S
    carcin/o/gen
    CF
    substance that causes cancer
13. WR CV S
    onc/o/logist
    CF
    physician who studies and treats tumors
14. P WR S
    pro/gno/sis
    state of before knowledge

Exercise 22

A *Label*

1. carcin/o/gen
2. cyan/osis
3. onc/o/logist
4. path/o/logist

B *Fill In*

1. dia/gno/sis
2. iatr/o/genic
3. eti/o/logy
4. onc/o/logy
5. path/o/logy
6. carcin/o/genic
7. xanth/osis
8. onc/o/genic
9. cancer/ous
10. pro/gno/sis

Exercise 23

Pronounce and Spell

Exercise 24

A *Label*

1. febrile
2. virus
3. inflammation
4. bacteria

B *Identify*

1. state of being diseased; incidence of illness in a population
2. organism that feeds by absorbing organic molecules from its surroundings and may cause infection by invading body tissue
3. without fever
4. a form of life that is too small to be seen without a microscope
5. redness
6. invasion of pathogens in body tissue.
7. state of being mortal (death); incidence of the number of deaths in a population
8. pertaining to disease of unknown origin
9. increase in the severity of a disease or its symptoms

Exercise 25

A

1. f	5. b
2. e	6. d
3. a	7. g
4. c	

B

1. f	4. c
2. d	5. a
3. e	6. b

Exercise 26

Review of Complementary Terms

Exercise 27

1. etiologies
2. staphylococci
3. cyanoses
4. bacteria
5. nuclei
6. pharynges
7. sarcomata
8. carcinomata
9. anastomoses
10. pubes
11. prognoses
12. spermatozoa
13. fimbriae
14. thoraces
15. appendices

Exercise 28

1. diverticula
2. bronchus
3. testes
4. melanoma
5. emboli
6. diagnoses
7. metastases

Exercise 29

biopsy; diagnosis; carcinoma; metastases; prognosis; red blood cell; white blood cell; chemotherapy; radiation therapy; complete blood count with differential; culture and sensitivity

Exercise 30

A. disease was identified; cancerous tumor; did not have a fever

Copyright © 2022, Elsevier Inc. All rights reserved.

B. diagnosis; carcinoma; afebrile
C. biopsy, cytology, specimen, dysplasia, inflammation, pathologist, diagnosis, carcinoma
D. Answers may vary and may include biopsy, cytology, specimen, dysplasia, inflammation, pathologist, diagnosis, carcinoma, along with their respective definitions.

Exercise 31

A

1. chemotherapy
2. adenocarcinoma
3. pathology
4. malignant
5. radiation therapy
6. organomegaly
7. cyanosis
8. metastases

B

1. b
2. b
3. d
4. a. prognoses
   b. lipomata
   c. histologies

Exercise 32

Pronunciation Exercise

Exercise 33

1. a
2. b
3. a
4. b
5. c
6. b
7. b
8. a
9. b
10. c
11. b
12. b
13. b
14. c
15. b
16. a
17. c
18. a
19. b
20. a

ANSWERS TO CHAPTER 3 EXERCISES

Exercise 1

A *Define*

1. belly (front)
2. head (upward)
3. side
4. middle
5. below
6. near (the point of attachment of a body part)
7. above
8. away (from the point of attachment of a body part)
9. back
10. tail (downward)
11. front
12. back, behind

B *Label*

1. head: cephal/o
2. back: dors/o
3. back, behind: poster/o
4. tail: caud/o
5. front: anter/o
6. belly (front): ventr/o
7. side: later/o
8. above: super/o
9. middle: medi/o
10. near: proxim/o
11. away: dist/o
12. below: infer/o

Exercise 2

A *Match*

1. c
2. a
3. b

B *Label*

1. tom/o
2. radi/o
3. son/o

Exercise 3

A *Label*

1. uni-
2. bi-

B *Define*

1. two
2. one

Exercise 4

A *Label*

1. -ad
2. -graphy
3. -graph
4. -gram

B *Define*

1. process of recording, radiographic imaging
2. instrument used to record; the record
3. the record, radiographic image
4. pertaining to
5. toward
6. one who studies and treats (specialist, physician)
7. study of
8. pertaining to

Exercise 5

Pronounce and Spell

Exercise 6

1. WR S
   cephal/ad
   toward the head
2. WR S
   proxim/al
   pertaining to near
3. WR S
   later/al
   pertaining to a side
4. P WR S
   uni/later/al
   pertaining to one side
5. WR CV WR S
   anter/o/poster/ior
   CF
   pertaining to the front and to the back
6. WR S
   cephal/ic
   pertaining to the head
7. WR S
   super/ior
   pertaining to above
8. WR S
   anter/ior
   pertaining to the front
9. WR S
   caud/ad
   toward the tail
10. WR S
    dist/al
    pertaining to away
11. WR S
    medi/al
    pertaining to the middle
12. P WR S
    bi/later/al
    pertaining to two sides
13. WR CV WR S
    poster/o/anter/ior
    CF
    pertaining to the back and to the front
14. WR S
    caud/al
    pertaining to the tail
15. WR S
    infer/ior
    pertaining to below
16. WR S
    poster/ior
    pertaining to the back

Copyright © 2022, Elsevier Inc. All rights reserved.

17. WR S
dors/al
pertaining to the back
18. WR S
ventr/al
pertaining to the belly (front)

Exercise 7

A *Label*

1. a. super/ior
b. cephal/ic
c. poster/ior, dors/al
d. infer/ior
e. caud/al
f. anter/ior
g. ventr/al
2. dist/al
3. proxim/al
4. later/al
5. medi/al
6. a. poster/o/anter/ior
b. anter/o/poster/ior

B *Fill In*

1. cephal/ad
2. proxim/al
3. dist/al
4. bi/later/al
5. medi/al
6. caud/ad
7. poster/o/anter/ior
8. medi/o/later/al
9. uni/later/al
10. anter/o/poster/ior

Exercise 8

Review of Directional Terms

Exercise 9

Pronounce and Spell

Exercise 10

A *Label*

1. right hypochondriac
2. right lumbar
3. right iliac
4. hypogastric
5. epigastric
6. left hypochondriac
7. umbilical
8. left lumbar
9. left iliac

B *Match*

1. b
2. d
3. a
4. e
5. c
6. f

Exercise 11

Review of Abdominopelvic Regions Terms

Exercise 12

Pronounce and Spell

Exercise 13

A *Label*

1. coronal
2. axial
3. midsagittal

B *Fill In*

1. axial
2. midsagittal
3. coronal
4. sagittal
5. parasagittal

Exercise 14

Review of Anatomic Planes

Exercise 15

Pronounce and Spell

Exercise 16

A *Match*

1. d
2. a
3. f
4. c
5. b
6. e

B *Label*

1. supine
2. prone
3. orthopnea
4. Trendelenburg
5. lithotomy
6. Sims

Exercise 17

Review of Body Position Terms

Exercise 18

Pronounce and Spell

Exercise 19

A *Analyze and Define*

1. WR CV S
tom/o/graphy
CF
process of recording slices (anatomical cross sections)
2. WR CV S
son/o/gram
CF
record of sound
3. WR CV S
radi/o/graphy
CF
process of recording x-rays
4. WR CV S
son/o/graphy
CF
process of recording sound
5. WR CV S
radi/o/graph
CF
record of x-rays
6. WR CV S
radi/o/logist
CF
physician who specializes in x-rays

B *Label*

1. radi/o/graphy
2. radi/o/graph
3. son/o/graphy
4. son/o/gram

C *Fill In*

1. tom/o/graphy
2. radi/o/logist
3. radi/o/logy

Exercise 20

A *Identify*

1. scan
2. Nuclear medicine
3. fluoroscopy
4. magnetic resonance imaging
5. Computed tomography

B *Label*

1. fluoroscopy
2. computed tomography
3. nuclear medicine
4. magnetic resonance imaging

Exercise 21

Review of Diagnostic Imaging Terms

Exercise 22

A *Fill In*

1. superior
2. anterior
3. inferior
4. posteroanterior
5. anteroposterior
6. medial
7. lateral
8. ultrasonography
9. nuclear medicine
10. magnetic resonance imaging
11. computed tomography
12. magnetic resonance

B *Label*

1. right upper quadrant (RUQ)
2. left upper quadrant (LUQ)
3. right lower quadrant (RLQ)
4. left lower quadrant (LLQ)

Copyright © 2022, Elsevier Inc. All rights reserved.

Exercise 23

A. near (her shoulder); belly near the navel; lower back near her waist; on her back facing upward, x-ray department, x-ray doctors, cross sections.
B. Answers will vary and may include proximal, ventral, umbilical region, lumbar region, supine, recumbent, radiology, radiologist, and computed tomography, along with their respective definitions.
C. medial, lateral, proximal, radiograph, AP, CT.
D. Answers will vary and may include medial, lateral, proximal, radiograph, AP, and CT, along with their respective definitions.

Exercise 24

A

1. anteroposterior
2. lateral
3. posterior (dorsal is used for head, trunk, and surfaces of hand and foot)
4. medial
5. anterior
6. radiology

B

1. b
2. a
3. a
4. answers may vary: the upper surface of the foot; the surface opposite the sole; the top of the foot

Exercise 25

Pronunciation Exercise

Exercise 26

Chapter Content Quiz

1. c
2. a
3. c
4. a
5. c
6. a
7. c
8. a
9. b
10. c
11. a
12. b
13. c
14. a
15. b
16. c
17. b
18. c
19. a
20. a. superior
    b. inferior
    c. medial
    d. lateral

ANSWERS TO CHAPTER 4 EXERCISES

Exercise 1

A *Label*

1. horny tissue: kerat/o
2. skin: cutane/o, derm/o, dermat/o
3. sebum: seb/o
4. hair: trich/o
5. sweat: hidr/o
6. nail: onych/o, ungu/o

B *Define and Match*

1. d, skin
2. b, sebum (oil)
3. c, nail
4. d, skin
5. e, horny tissue (keratin), hard
6. c, nail
7. a, sweat
8. f, hair
9. d, skin

Exercise 2

A *Define*

1. yellow
2. grapelike clusters
3. hidden
4. thick
5. white
6. fungus
7. red
8. hard
9. twisted chains
10. dry, dryness
11. wrinkle
12. gland

B *Identify*

1. myc/o
2. leuk/o
3. xanth/o
4. xer/o
5. pachy/o
6. strept/o
7. rhytid/o
8. staphyl/o
9. erythr/o
10. crypt/o
11. scler/o
12. aden/o

Exercise 3

A *Define*

1. under, below
2. beside, beyond, around, abnormal
3. on, upon, over
4. within
5. through
6. through, across, beyond
7. below, incomplete, deficient, under
8. above, excessive

B *Identify*

1. intra-
2. sub-
3. epi-
4. para-
5. per-
6. trans-
7. hyper-
8. hypo-

Exercise 4

A *Match*

1. e
2. c
3. a
4. b
5. d

B *Label*

1. -coccus
2. -rrhea
3. -malacia
4. -itis
5. -plasty
6. -phagia

C *Define*

1. pertaining to
2. study of
3. pertaining to
4. abnormal condition
5. pertaining to
6. excision, surgical removal

Exercise 5

Pronounce and Spell

Exercise 6

1. WR CV WR S
   scler/o/derm/a
   CF
   hard skin (chronic hardening or induration of the connective tissue of the skin and other organs)
2. WR WR S
   hidr/aden/itis
   inflammation of a sweat gland
3. WR S
   dermat/itis
   inflammation of the skin
4. WR WR S
   pachy/derm/a
   thickening of the skin
5. WR CV S
   onych/o/malacia
   CF
   softening of the nails
6. WR S
   kerat/osis
   abnormal condition (growth) of horny tissue (keratin)
7. WR CV WR S
   dermat/o/fibr/oma
   CF
   fibrous tumor of the skin
8. P WR S
   par/onych/ia
   diseased state around the nail
   Note: the a from para- has been dropped because the following word root begins with a vowel.

Copyright © 2022, Elsevier Inc. All rights reserved.

9. WR CV WR S
onych/o/crypt/osis
CF
abnormal condition of a hidden nail
10. WR CV S
seb/o/rrhea
CF
discharge of sebum (excessive)
11. WR CV S
onych/o/phagia
CF
eating the nails, nail biting
12. WR CV WR S
xer/o/derm/a
CF
dry skin (a mild form of a cutaneous disorder characterized by keratinization and noninflammatory scaling)
13. WR S
xanth/oma
yellow tumor (benign, primarily in the skin)

Exercise 7

A *Label*

1. dermat/itis
2. kerat/osis
3. onych/o/myc/osis
4. par/onych/ia

B *Fill In*

1. pachy/derm/a
2. xer/o/derm/a
3. seb/o/rrhea
4. xanth/oma
5. dermat/o/fibr/oma
6. onych/o/malacia
7. hidr/aden/itis
8. onych/o/crypt/osis
9. scler/o/derm/a
10. onych/o/phagia

Exercise 8

Pronounce and Spell

Exercise 9

A *Identify*

1. systemic lupus erythematosus
2. abrasion
3. pediculosis
4. contusion
5. gangrene
6. carbuncle
7. acne
8. laceration
9. pilonidal cyst
10. pressure injury
11. albinism
12. MRSA infection

B *Label*

1. a. fissure b. eczema
2. cellulitis
3. psoriasis
4. herpes
5. tinea
6. Kaposi sarcoma
7. actinic keratosis
8. furuncle
9. squamous cell carcinoma
10. basal cell carcinoma
11. impetigo
12. scabies
13. urticaria
14. candidiasis
15. vitiligo
16. rosacea
17. measles
18. keloid

Exercise 10

1. d
2. j
3. h
4. l
5. k
6. c
7. n
8. b
9. e
10. i
11. g
12. a
13. f
14. m
15. o

Exercise 11

1. d
2. b
3. f
4. p
5. m
6. l
7. o
8. a
9. n
10. e
11. i
12. g
13. k
14. c
15. j
16. h

Exercise 12

Review of Disease and Disorder Terms

Exercise 13

Pronounce and Spell

Exercise 14

A *Analyze and Define*

1. WR S
rhytid/ectomy
excision of wrinkles
2. WR CV S
dermato/o/plasty
CF
surgical repair of the skin

B *Build*

1. rhytid/ectomy
2. dermat/o/plasty

Exercise 15

A *Fill In*

1. Mohs surgery
2. incision
3. cauterization
4. suturing
5. incision and drainage
6. debridement
7. excision
8. laser surgery
9. cryosurgery
10. dermabrasion
11. skin graft

B *Match*

1. i
2. h
3. g
4. d
5. a
6. e
7. b
8. f
9. j
10. c
11. k

Exercise 16

Review of Surgical Terms

Exercise 17

Pronounce and Spell

Exercise 18

1. WR S
ungu/al
pertaining to the nail
2. P WR S
trans/derm/al
pertaining to through the skin
3. WR CV S
strept/o/coccus
CF
berry-shaped (bacterium) in twisted chains
4. P WR S
hypo/derm/ic
pertaining to under the skin
5. WR CV S
dermat/o/logy
CF
study of the skin

Copyright © 2022, Elsevier Inc. All rights reserved.

6. P WR S
sub/cutane/ous
pertaining to under the skin
7. WR CV S
staphyl/o/coccus
CF
berry-shaped (bacterium) in grapelike clusters
8. WR CV S
kerat/o/genic
CF
producing horny tissue
9. WR CV S
dermat/o/logist
CF
physician who studies and treats skin (diseases)
10. WR S
cutane/ous
pertaining to the skin
11. P WR S
epi/derm/al
pertaining to upon the skin
12. WR CV WR S
xanth/o/derm/a
CF
yellow skin
13. WR CV WR S
erythr/o/derm/a
CF
red skin
14. P WR S
per/cutane/ous
pertaining to through the skin
15. WR S
xer/osis
abnormal condition of dryness
16. P WR S
sub/ungu/al
pertaining to under the nail
17. WR CV WR S
leuk/o/derm/a
CF
white skin
18. P WR S
hyper/trich/osis
abnormal condition of excessive hair (growth)

Exercise 19

A *Label*

1. xanth/o/derm/a
2. leuk/o/derm/a
3. erythr/o/derm/a
4. hyper/trich/osis
5. strept/o/cocci
6. staphl/o/cocci
7. intra/derm/al
8. sub/cutane/ous, hypo/derm/ic
9. trans/derm/al

B *Fill In*

1. dermat/o/logy
2. xer/osis
3. ungu/al
4. cutane/ous
5. dermat/o/logist
6. sub/ungu/al
7. epi/derm/al
8. per/cutane/ous
9. kerat/o/genic

Exercise 20

Pronounce and Spell

Exercise 21

A *Identify*

1. diaphoresis
2. macule
3. jaundice
4. leukoplakia
5. petechiae
6. abscess
7. pallor
8. ecchymosis
9. nodule
10. cyst
11. pruritus
12. purpura
13. papule
14. wheal
15. pustule
16. vesicle
17. induration
18. edema
19. lesion

B *Label*

1. ulcer
2. nevus
3. verruca
4. alopecia

Exercise 22

1. e	6. d
2. a	7. b
3. j	8. c
4. f	9. h
5. g	10. i

Exercise 23

1. d	4. k
2. i	5. j
3. a	6. l
7. b	11. c
8. e	12. g
9. f	13. h
10. m	

Exercise 24

Review of Complementary Terms

Exercise 25

1. basal cell carcinoma
2. split-thickness skin grafts
3. full-thickness skin grafts
4. squamous cell carcinoma
5. systemic lupus erythematosus
6. subcutaneous
7. staphylococcus
8. streptococcus
9. incision and drainage
10. transdermal
11. intradermal
12. dermatology
13. methicillin-resistant *Staphylococcus aureus*, healthcare-associated MRSA infection, community-associated MRSA infection

Exercise 26

A. pale; very itchy; (lips beginning to) swell; (cheeks and arms covered with) different sized red and white bumps
B. Answers will vary and may include pallor, pruritus, edema, erythema, urticaria.
C. pallor, pruritus, edema, urticaria
D. Answers will vary and may include pallor, pruritus, edema, urticaria along with their respective definitions.

Exercise 27

A

1. dermatology
2. nodule
3. medial
4. actinic keratosis
5. eczema
6. lesion
7. Mohs surgery
8. subcutaneous
9. excision
10. pathology
11. dermatologist
12. cauterization
13. suturing
14. basal cell carcinoma

Copyright © 2022, Elsevier Inc. All rights reserved.

B

1. a. s
   b. p
   c. p
   d. s
   e. s
   f. p
   g. s
   h. p
2. b
3. dictionary exercise

Exercise 28

Pronunciation Exercise

Exercise 29

1. b
2. b
3. c
4. b
5. a
6. c
7. a
8. a
9. c
10. b
11. a
12. c
13. c
14. b
15. a
16. b
17. b
18. b
19. a
20. b

ANSWERS TO CHAPTER 5 EXERCISES

Exercise 1

A *Define and Match*

1. d, adenoids
2. h, diaphragm
3. e, epiglottis
4. b, lobe(s)
5. a, nose
6. g, pharynx
7. c, lung, air
8. c, lung, air
9. a, nose
10. f, septum

B *Label*

1. sinus: sinus/o
2. nose: nas/o, rhin/o
3. tonsil: tonsill/o
4. epiglottis: epiglott/o
5. larynx: laryng/o
6. trachea: trache/o
7. pleura: pleur/o
8. lobe: lob/o
9. diaphragm: diaphragmat/o
10. adenoids: adenoid/o
11. pharynx: pharyng/o
12. lung: pneum/o, pneumon/o, pulmon/o
13. thorax, chest, chest cavity: thorac/o
14. bronchus: bronch/o, bronchi/o
15. mediastinum: mediastin/o
16. alveolus: alveol/o

C *Define and Match*

1. h, alveolus *(s.)*, alveoli *(pl.)*
2. j, bronchus *(s.)*, bronchi *(pl.)*
3. c, lung
4. g, larynx
5. d, pleura
6. i, thorax, chest, chest cavity
7. b, trachea
8. e, tonsil(s)
9. f, sinus(es)
10. a, mediastinum

Exercise 2

A *Define*

1. oxygen
2. breathe, breathing
3. mucus
4. imperfect, incomplete
5. straight
6. pus
7. blood
8. sleep
9. carbon dioxide
10. sound, voice
11. cancer
12. fungus
13. dust

B *Identify*

1. spir/o
2. ox/i
3. atel/o
4. orth/o
5. py/o
6. muc/o
7. hem/o
8. somn/o
9. phon/o
10. capn/o
11. coni/o
12. carcin/o
13. myc/o

Exercise 3

A *Define*

1. within
2. absence of, without
3. normal, good
4. many, much
5. fast, rapid
6. painful, abnormal, difficult, labored
7. below, incomplete, deficient, under
8. within
9. above, excessive
10. new

B *Identify*

1. a. endo-
   b. intra-
2. eu-
3. a. a-
   b. an-
4. poly-
5. tachy-
6. neo-
7. hyper-
8. hypo-
9. dys-

Exercise 4

A *Match*

1. g
2. c
3. d
4. e
5. a
6. f
7. i
8. k
9. l
10. b
11. h
12. m
13. j

B *Label*

1. -scope
2. -scopy
3. -tomy
4. -stomy
5. -meter
6. -metry
7. -rrhagia
8. -ptysis
9. -ectomy
10. -emia

C *Define*

1. flow, discharge
2. resembling
3. one who studies and treats (specialist, physician)
4. growth, substance, formation
5. pertaining to
6. tumor, swelling
7. study of
8. surgical repair
9. abnormal condition

Exercise 5

Pronounce and Spell

Exercise 6

1. WR S
   trache/itis
   inflammation of the trachea
2. WR CV WR S
   nas/o/pharyng/itis
   CF
   inflammation of the nose and pharynx
3. WR S
   alveol/itis
   inflammation of the alveoli
4. WR CV S
   py/o/thorax
   CF
   pus in the chest cavity (pleural cavity)

Copyright © 2022, Elsevier Inc. All rights reserved.

5. WR S
atel/ectasis
incomplete expansion (of the lung or portion of the lung)
6. WR CV WR S
rhin/o/myc/osis
CF
abnormal condition of fungus in the nose
7. WR CV S
trache/o/stenosis
CF
narrowing of the trachea
8. WR S
epiglott/itis
inflammation of the epiglottis
9. WR S
laryng/itis
inflammation of the larynx
10. WR S P S(WR)
pulmon/ary neo/plasm
pertaining to (in) the lung, new growth (tumor)
11. WR S
pneumon/ia
diseased state of the lung
12. WR S
rhin/itis
inflammation of the nose (mucous membranes)
13. WR CV WR S
pneum/o/coni/osis
CF
abnormal condition of dust in the lungs
14. WR CV WR S
bronch/o/pneumon/ia
CF
diseased state of bronchi and lungs
15. WR CV WR CV WR S
laryng/o/trache/o/bronch/itis
CF CF
inflammation of the larynx, trachea, and bronchi
16. WR CV S
bronch/o/spasm
CF
spasmodic contraction of the bronchi

Exercise 7
A *Label*
1. bronchi/ectasis
2. hem/o/thorax
3. pneum/o/thorax
4. sinus/itis
5. pleur/itis
6. tonsill/itis

B *Fill In*
1. pharyng/itis
2. bronch/o/genic carcin/oma
3. lob/ar pneumon/ia
4. laryng/o/spasm
5. diaphragmat/o/cele
6. adenoid/itis
7. bronch/itis
8. rhin/o/rrhagia
9. pneumon/itis

Exercise 8
Pronounce and Spell

Exercise 9
A *Identify*
1. Cystic fibrosis
2. influenza
3. chronic obstructive pulmonary disease
4. pertussis
5. Croup
6. pulmonary edema
7. Epistaxis
8. idiopathic pulmonary fibrosis
9. Diphtheria
10. asphyxia
11. tuberculosis
12. Acute respiratory distress syndrome
13. coronavirus disease

B *Label*
1. pulmonary embolism
2. obstructive sleep apnea
3. deviated septum
4. pleural effusion
5. asthma
6. coccidioidomycosis
7. emphysema
8. upper respiratory infection

Exercise 10
1. j
2. i
3. d
4. g
5. f
6. c
7. a
8. e
9. b
10. h

Exercise 11
1. d
2. k
3. c
4. e
5. f
6. g
7. h
8. i
9. a
10. j
11. b

Exercise 12
Review of Disease and Disorder Terms

Exercise 13
Pronounce and Spell

Exercise 14
1. WR CV S
trache/o/plasty
CF
surgical repair of the trachea
2. WR CV S
sept/o/plasty
CF
surgical repair of the septum
3. WR CV S
laryng/o/stomy
CF
creation of an artificial opening into the larynx
4. WR CV S
sinus/o/tomy
CF
incision into a sinus
5. WR CV S
laryng/o/plasty
CF
surgical repair of the larynx
6. WR CV S
thorac/o/tomy
CF
incision into the chest cavity

Exercise 15
A *Label*
1. adenoid/ectomy
2. lob/ectomy
3. pneumon/ectomy
4. trache/o/stomy
5. thora/centesis *(Note: "co" is removed from the combining form in common usage)*
6. trache/o/tomy

B *Fill In*
1. laryng/o/trache/o/tomy
2. pleur/o/desis
3. tonsill/ectomy
4. bronch/o/plasty
5. laryng/ectomy
6. rhin/o/plasty

Exercise 16
Review of Surgical Terms

Exercise 17
Pronounce and Spell

Copyright © 2022, Elsevier Inc. All rights reserved.

Exercise 18

1. WR CV S
   spir/o/meter
   CF
   instrument used to measure breathing
2. WR CV S
   laryng/o/scope
   CF
   instrument used for visual examination of the larynx
3. WR CV S
   capn/o/meter
   CF
   instrument used to measure carbon dioxide
4. WR CV S
   spir/o/metry
   CF
   measurement of breathing
5. WR CV S
   ox/i/meter
   CF
   instrument used to measure oxygen
6. WR CV S
   laryng/o/scopy
   CF
   visual examination of the larynx
7. WR CV S
   bronch/o/scope
   CF
   instrument used for visual examination of the bronchi
8. WR CV S
   thorac/o/scope
   CF
   instrument used for visual examination of the chest cavity
9. P S(WR)
   endo/scope
   instrument used for visual examination within (a hollow organ or body cavity)
10. WR CV S
    thorac/o/scopy
    CF
    visual examination of the chest cavity
11. P S(WR)
    endo/scopic
    pertaining to visual examination within (a hollow organ or body cavity)
12. P S(WR)
    endo/scopy
    visual examination within (a hollow organ or body cavity)
13. P WR CV S
    poly/somn/o/graphy
    CF
    process of recording many (tests) during sleep
14. WR CV S
    mediastin/o/scopy
    CF
    visual examination of the mediastinum

Exercise 19

A *Label*

1. laryng/o/scope
2. spir/o/meter
3. capn/o/meter
4. ox/i/meter
5. poly/somn/o/graphy

B *Fill In*

1. laryng/o/scopy
2. mediastin/o/scopy
3. endo/scopic
4. thorac/o/scopy
5. bronch/o/scopy
6. spir/o/metry
7. bronch/o/scope
8. endo/scopy
9. thorac/o/scope
10. endo/scope

Exercise 20

Pronounce and Spell

Exercise 21

A *Label*

1. PPD (purified protein derivative) skin test
2. peak flow meter
3. arterial blood gas
4. pulse oximetry
5. stethoscope
6. lung ventilation/perfusion scan
7. chest radiograph
8. chest computed tomography (CT) scan
9. auscultation
10. percussion

B *Identify*

1. acid-fast bacilli smear
2. Pulmonary function tests

Exercise 22

1. f
2. e
3. a
4. d
5. b
6. c
7. g
8. h
9. k
10. i
11. j
12. l

Exercise 23

Review of Diagnostic Terms

Exercise 24

Pronounce and Spell

Exercise 25

1. WR S
   mediastin/al
   pertaining to the mediastinum
2. WR CV S
   pulmon/o/logy
   CF
   study of the lung
3. WR S
   muc/ous
   pertaining to mucus
4. P S(WR)
   a/pnea
   absence of breathing
5. P WR S
   hyp/ox/ia
   condition of deficient oxygen (to tissues)
6. WR CV WR S
   nas/o/pharyng/eal
   CF
   pertaining to the nose and pharynx
7. P WR S
   intra/pleur/al
   pertaining to within the pleura
8. P WR S
   a/capn/ia
   condition of absence of carbon dioxide (in the blood)
9. P WR S
   dys/phon/ia
   condition of difficulty in speaking (voice)
10. P WR S
    hyp/ox/emia
    deficient oxygen in the blood
11. WR S
    thorac/ic
    pertaining to the chest
12. WR S
    diaphragmat/ic
    pertaining to the diaphragm
13. WR CV WR S
    bronch/o/alveol/ar
    CF
    pertaining to the bronchi and alveoli
14. P S(WR)
    hypo/pnea
    deficient breathing

Exercise 26

A *Label*

1. hem/o/ptysis
2. orth/o/pnea
3. pulmon/o/logist
4. alveol/ar
5. dys/pnea
6. endo/trache/al

Copyright © 2022, Elsevier Inc. All rights reserved.

B *Fill In*

1. tachy/pnea
2. muc/oid
3. rhin/o/rrhea
4. hyper/capn/ia
5. an/ox/ia
6. hyper/pnea
7. laryng/eal
8. hypo/capn/ia
9. eu/pnea
10. a/phon/ia
11. pulmon/ary
12. sept/al

Exercise 27

Pronounce and Spell

Exercise 28

A *Label*

1. airway
2. bronchodilator
3. nebulizer
4. ventilator

B *Identify*

1. hyperventilation
2. wheeze
3. sputum
4. aspirate
5. stridor
6. rhonchi
7. mucopurulent
8. Hypoventilation
9. nosocomial infection
10. paroxysm
11. patent
12. bronchoconstrictor
13. Effusion
14. crackles

Exercise 29

1. b
2. g
3. c
4. h
5. a
6. d
7. f
8. e
9. i

Exercise 30

1. e
2. g
3. h
4. c
5. i
6. a
7. b
8. d
9. f

Exercise 31

Review of Complementary Terms

Exercise 32

1. chronic obstructive pulmonary disease; pulmonary function tests, chest radiograph, arterial blood gas, venous blood gas
2. shortness of breath
3. A. left upper lobe; left lower lobe
   B. right upper lobe, right middle lobe, right lower lobe
4. acid-fast bacilli; tuberculosis
5. polysomnography; obstructive sleep apnea; continuous positive airway pressure
6. oxygen; carbon dioxide
7. peak flow meter
8. idiopathic pulmonary fibrosis
9. influenza; coronavirus disease; upper respiratory infection
10. hospital-acquired pneumonia
11. lung ventilation/perfusion scan; pulmonary embolism
12. acute respiratory distress syndrome
13. cystic fibrosis
14. laryngotracheobronchitis
15. community-acquired pneumonia

Exercise 33

A. difficulty breathing; runny nose; her throat was very sore; thick yellow mucus; cold

B. Answer will vary and may include dyspnea, rhinorrhea, pharyngitis, sputum, and/or upper respiratory infection.

C. dyspnea, mucoid, sputum, rhinorrhea, auscultation, percussion, crackles, rhonchi

D. Answer will vary and may include dyspnea, mucoid, sputum, rhinorrhea, auscultation, percussion, crackles, and/or rhonchi along with their respective definitions.

Exercise 34

A

1. dyspnea
2. pulmonary
3. rhonchi
4. chest radiograph
5. bronchoscopy
6. arterial blood gas
7. hypoxemia
8. bronchogenic carcinoma
9. pulmonary function tests
10. thoracic

B

1. a
2. F
3. F
4. T

Exercise 35

Online Exercise

Exercise 36

Pronunciation Exercise

Exercise 37

1. b
2. c
3. a
4. c
5. a
6. a
7. b
8. c
9. c
10. b
11. a
12. c
13. b
14. c
15. b
16. c
17. a
18. c
19. c
20. a

ANSWERS TO CHAPTER 6 EXERCISES

Exercise 1

A *Label*

1. kidney: nephr/o, ren/o
2. meatus: meat/o
3. ureter: ureter/o
4. bladder: cyst/o, vesic/o
5. urethra: urethr/o

B *Define and Match*

1. g, kidney
2. a, bladder
3. g, kidney
4. d, glomerulus
5. f, renal pelvis
6. c, ureter
7. a, bladder
8. b, meatus
9. e, urethra

C *Label*

1. renal pelvis: pyel/o
2. glomerulus: glomerul/o

Exercise 2

A *Define*

1. water
2. urea, nitrogen
3. night
4. stone(s), calculus (*pl.* calculi)
5. albumin
6. urine, urinary tract
7. developing cell, germ cell
8. scanty, few

Copyright © 2022, Elsevier Inc. All rights reserved.

9. urine, urinary tract
10. sugar
11. sound
12. blood

B *Identify*

1. glycos/o
2. a. urin/o
   b. ur/o
3. hydr/o
4. blast/o
5. albumin/o
6. noct/i
7. azot/o
8. lith/o
9. olig/o
10. hem/o
11. son/o

Exercise 3

A *Define*

1. painful, abnormal, difficult, labored
2. through, across, beyond
3. absence of, without
4. many, much

B *Identify*

1. trans-
2. a-
3. dys-
4. poly-

Exercise 4

A *Label*

1. -lysis
2. -ptosis
3. -tripsy
4. -lith
5. -pexy
6. -uria

B *Match*

1. f
2. i
3. h
4. a
5. e
6. b
7. d
8. g
9. j
10. c

C *Define*

1. constriction or narrowing
2. inflammation
3. condition
4. study of
5. in the blood
6. the record, radiographic image
7. pertaining to
8. diseased or abnormal state, condition of
9. cut into, incision
10. abnormal condition
11. visual examination

Exercise 5

Pronounce and Spell

Exercise 6

1. WR CV WR S
   nephr/o/blast/oma
   CF
   kidney tumor containing developing cells
2. WR CV S
   ureter/o/stenosis
   CF
   narrowing of the ureter
3. WR S
   ur/emia
   urine (urea nitrogen) in the blood (presence of azotemia and wide range of signs and symptoms associated with chronic kidney disease)
4. WR CV S
   nephr/o/ptosis
   CF
   drooping kidney
5. WR CV S
   cyst/o/cele
   CF
   protrusion of the bladder
6. WR S
   nephr/itis
   inflammation of a kidney
7. WR S
   pyel/itis
   inflammation of the renal pelvis
8. WR CV WR S
   ureter/o/lith/iasis
   CF
   condition of stone(s) in the ureter
9. WR CV WR S
   pyel/o/nephr/itis
   CF
   inflammation of the renal pelvis and the kidney
10. WR S
    ureter/itis
    inflammation of a ureter

Exercise 7

A *Fill In*

1. ureter/o/cele
2. urethr/o/cyst/itis
3. vesic/o/ureter/al reflux
4. glomerul/o/nephr/itis
5. nephr/oma

B *Label*

1. urethr/itis
2. nephr/o/megaly
3. hydr/o/nephr/osis
4. cyst/o/lith
5. cyst/itis
6. nephr/o/lith/iasis

Exercise 8

Pronounce and Spell

Exercise 9

A *Label*

1. hypospadias
2. polycystic kidney disease

B *Identify*

1. renal calculus
2. urinary retention
3. renal hypertension
4. urinary suppression
5. epispadias
6. urinary tract infection
7. chronic kidney disease
8. end-stage renal disease
9. acute kidney injury

Exercise 10

1. i
2. f
3. j
4. h
5. a
6. e
7. b
8. g
9. k
10. d
11. c

Exercise 11

Review of Disease and Disorder Terms

Exercise 12

Pronounce and Spell

Exercise 13

A *Analyze and Define*

1. WR CV S
   ureter/o/stomy
   CF
   creation of an artificial opening into the ureter
2. WR CV WR CV S
   nephr/o/lith/o/tomy
   CF CF
   incision into the kidney to remove stone(s)
3. WR CV S
   nephr/o/stomy
   CF
   creation of an artificial opening into the kidney
4. WR CV S
   nephr/o/lysis
   CF
   separating the kidney (from other body structures)
5. WR S
   cyst/ectomy
   excision of the bladder
6. WR CV WR CV S
   pyel/o/lith/o/tomy
   CF CF
   incision into the renal pelvis to remove stone(s)
7. WR CV S
   nephr/o/pexy
   CF
   surgical fixation of the kidney

Copyright © 2022, Elsevier Inc. All rights reserved.

8. WR CV WR CV S
cyst/o/lith/o/tomy
CF CF
incision into the bladder to remove stone(s)
9. WR S
nephr/ectomy
excision of the kidney
10. WR S
ureter/ectomy
excision of the ureter
11. WR CV S
cyst/o/stomy
CF
creation of an artificial opening into the bladder
12. WR CV S
pyel/o/plasty
CF
surgical repair of the renal pelvis
13. WR CV S
ur/o/stomy
CF
creation of an artificial opening into the urinary system
14. WR CV S
meat/o/tomy
CF
incision into the meatus
15. WR CV S
lith/o/tripsy
CF
surgical crushing of stone(s)
16. WR CV S
urethr/o/plasty
CF
surgical repair of the urethra
17. WR CV WR CV S
nephr/o/lith/o/tripsy
CF CF
surgical crushing of stone(s) in the kidney (using shock waves)
18. WR CV WR S
vesic/o/urethr/al suspension
CF
suspension pertaining to the bladder and urethra

B *Build*

1. cyst/o/stomy
2. nephr/o/stomy
3. pyel/o/lith/o/tomy
4. nephr/o/lith/o/tomy
5. lith/o/tripsy

C *Build*

1. ureter/o/stomy
2. nephr/ectomy
3. nephr/o/lith/o/tripsy
4. ur/o/stomy
5. nephr/o/lysis
6. pyel/o/plasty
7. urethr/o/plasty
8. cyst/ectomy
9. meat/o/tomy
10. nephr/o/pexy
11. ureter/ectomy
12. cyst/o/lith/o/tomy
13. vesico/urethr/al (suspension)

Exercise 14

A *Identify*

1. renal transplant
2. fulguration
3. extracorporeal shock wave lithotripsy

B *Match*

1. b
2. a
3. c

Exercise 15

Review of Surgical Terms

Exercise 16

Pronounce and Spell

Exercise 17

A *Analyze and Define*

1. WR CV WR CV S
(voiding) cyst/o/urethr/o/graphy
CF CF
radiographic imaging of the bladder and the urethra
2. WR CV S
cyst/o/graphy
CF
radiographic imaging of the bladder
3. WR CV WR CV S
nephr/o/son/o/graphy
CF CF
process of recording the kidney with sound
4. WR CV S
cyst/o/scope
CF
instrument used for visual examination of the bladder
5. WR CV S
cyst/o/gram
CF
radiographic image of the bladder
6. WR CV S
cyst/o/scopy
CF
visual examination of the bladder
7. WR CV S
ur/o/gram
CF
radiographic image of the urinary tract
8. WR CV S
ren/o/gram
CF
radiographic record of the kidney
9. WR CV S
nephr/o/scopy
CF
visual examination of the kidney
10. WR CV S
ureter/o/scopy
CF
visual examination of the ureter

B *Build*

1. cyst/o/gram
2. (retrograde) ur/o/gram
3. nephr/o/scopy
4. cyst/o/scopy

C *Build*

1. ureter/o/scopy
2. ur/o/gram
3. nephr/o/son/o/graphy
4. cyst/o/scope
5. (voiding) cyst/o/urethr/o/graphy
6. cyst/o/graphy
7. ren/o/gram

Exercise 18

A *Label*

1. blood urea nitrogen
2. urinalysis
3. KUB
4. specific gravity

B *Match*

1. c
2. g
3. d
4. a
5. e
6. b
7. f

Exercise 19

Review of Diagnostic Terms

Exercise 20

Pronounce and Spell

Exercise 21

1. WR S
noct/uria
night urination
2. WR CV S
ur/o/logist
CF
physician who studies and treats diseases of the urinary tract
3. WR S
olig/uria
condition of scanty urine (amount)

Copyright © 2022, Elsevier Inc. All rights reserved.

4. WR CV S
nephr/o/logist
CF
physician who studies and treats diseases of the kidney
5. WR S
hemat/uria
blood in the urine
6. WR CV S
ur/o/logy
CF
study of the urinary tract
7. P S(WR)
poly/uria
much (excessive) urine
8. WR S
albumin/uria
albumin in the urine
9. P S(WR)
an/uria
absence of urine
10. WR S
azot/emia
nitrogen in the blood
11. WR S
py/uria
pus in the urine
12. WR S
urin/ary
pertaining to urine
13. WR S
glycos/uria
sugar in the urine
14. P S(WR)
dys/uria
difficult or painful urination
15. WR CV S
nephr/o/logy
CF
study of the kidney
16. P WR S
intra/vesic/al
pertaining to within the (urinary) bladder
17. WR S
meat/al
pertaining to the meatus
18. P WR S
trans/urethr/al
pertaining to through the urethra

Exercise 22

A *Fill In*

1. noct/uria
2. olig/uria
3. py/uria
4. ur/o/logist
5. poly/uria
6. nephr/o/logy
7. urin/ary
8. azot/emia
9. ur/o/logy
10. trans/urethr/al
11. glycos/uria
12. intra/vesic/al
13. an/uria
14. albumin/uria

B *Label*

1. meat/al
2. nephr/o/logist
3. dys/uria
4. hemat/uria

Exercise 23

Pronounce and Spell

Exercise 24

A *Label*

1. hemodialysis
2. catheter
3. distended
4. enuresis
5. urinal
6. peritoneal dialysis

B *Identify*

1. electrolytes
2. diuretic
3. prolapse
4. urinary incontinence
5. urinary catheterization
6. void
7. stricture

Exercise 25

A

1. d
2. f
3. e
4. a
5. c
6. b

B

1. a
2. d
3. g
4. b
5. f
6. c
7. e

Exercise 26

Review of Complementary Terms

Exercise 27

Fill In

1. kidneys ureters (and) bladder; voiding cystourethrography; vesicoureteral reflux
2. specific gravity; urinalysis
3. blood urea nitrogen
4. extracorporeal shock wave lithotripsy
5. catheterization; urinary tract infection
6. hemodialysis
7. acute renal failure; acute kidney injury; chronic kidney disease, chronic renal failure; end-stage renal disease
8. overactive bladder
9. polycystic kidney disease

Exercise 28

A. blood when he urinated; infection of his bladder; difficulty urinating; physician who treats diseases of the urinary tract
B. Answers will vary and may include hematuria; cystitis; dysuria; urologist
C. and D. hematuria; renal calculi; UTI; end-stage renal disease; hemodialysis along with their respective definitions

Exercise 29

A

1. nephrolithiasis
2. hematuria
3. urology
4. KUB
5. calculi
6. cystoscopy
7. urogram
8. nephrolithotomy
9. catheter

B

1. c
2. d
3. *F*, calculus is singular for stone
4. a. pertaining to the ureter
   b. instrument used for visual examination of the ureter

Exercise 30

Online Exercise

Exercise 31

Pronunciation Exercise

Exercise 32

1. c
2. b
3. c
4. b
5. a
6. a
7. b
8. c
9. b
10. c
11. b
12. c
13. a
14. b
15. b
16. c
17. a
18. a
19. c
20. b

Copyright © 2022, Elsevier Inc. All rights reserved.

ANSWERS TO CHAPTER 7 EXERCISES

Exercise 1

A *Label*

1. male: andr/o
2. seminal vesicle: vesicul/o
3. prostate gland: prostat/o
4. epididymis: epididym/o
5. testis: orch/o, orchi/o, orchid/o
6. vas deferens or ductus deferens: vas/o
7. glans penis: balan/o
8. sperm, spermatozoon: sperm/o, spermat/o

B *Define and Match*

1. g, sperm, spermatozoon
2. a, vessel, duct
3. g, sperm, spermatozoon
4. b, glans penis
5. f, prostate gland
6. d, testis, testicle
7. c, seminal vesicle(s)
8. d, testis, testicle
9. e, epididymis
10. d, testis, testicle
11. male

Exercise 2

A *Define*

1. scanty, few
2. hidden
3. stone(s), calculus (*pl.* calculi)
4. bladder, sac

B *Identify*

1. lith/o
2. cyst/o
3. crypt/o
4. olig/o

Exercise 3

A *Identify*

1. a. an-
   b. a-
2. hyper-

B *Define*

1. above, excessive
2. absence of, without
3. absence of, without

Exercise 4

A *Match*

1. d
2. g
3. f
4. b
5. a
6. e
7. c

B *Match*

1. g
2. f
3. c
4. e
5. a
6. d
7. b

Exercise 5

Pronounce and Spell

Exercise 6

1. WR CV S
   prostat/o/lith (CF: prostat/o)
   stone(s) in the prostate gland
2. WR S
   balan/itis
   inflammation of the glans penis
3. WR S
   orch/itis
   inflammation of the testis
4. WR CV WR S
   prostat/o/vesicul/itis (CF: prostat/o)
   inflammation of the prostate gland and the seminal vesicles
5. WR CV WR S
   prostat/o/cyst/itis (CF: prostat/o)
   inflammation of the prostate gland and the (urinary) bladder
6. WR WR S
   orchi/epididym/itis
   inflammation of the testis and the epididymis
7. WR CV S
   prostat/o/rrhea (CF: prostat/o)
   discharge from the prostate gland
8. WR S
   epididym/itis
   inflammation of the epididymis
9. WR S P S(WR)
   (benign) prostat/ic hyper/plasia
   excessive development pertaining to the prostate gland
10. WR WR S
    crypt/orchid/ism
    state of hidden testis
11. WR CV S
    balan/o/rrhea (CF: balan/o)
    discharge from the glans penis
12. WR S
    prostat/itis
    inflammation of the prostate gland
13. P WR S
    an/orch/ism
    state of absence of testis (unilateral or bilateral)
14. WR CV S
    andr/o/pathy (CF: andr/o)
    disease of the male

Exercise 7

A *Label*

1. crypt/orchid/ism
2. balan/itis
3. benign prostat/ic hyper/plasia

B *Fill In*

1. prostat/o/cyst/itis
2. prostat/o/lith
3. orch/itis
4. epididym/itis
5. prostat/o/rrhea
6. prostat/o/vesicul/itis
7. an/orch/ism
8. prostat/itis
9. orchi/epididym/itis
10. balan/o/rrhea
11. andr/o/pathy

Exercise 8

Pronounce and Spell

Exercise 9

A *Identify*

1. testicular cancer
2. erectile dysfunction
3. priapism
4. testicular torsion
5. spermatocele
6. infertility

B *Label*

1. prostate cancer
2. phimosis
3. hydrocele
4. varicocele

Exercise 10

1. d
2. c
3. e
4. b
5. j
6. f
7. i
8. h
9. g
10. a

Exercise 11

Review of Disease and Disorder Terms

Exercise 12

Pronounce and Spell

Copyright © 2022, Elsevier Inc. All rights reserved.

Exercise 13

1. WR S
   vas/ectomy
   excision of a duct
2. WR CV WR CV S
   prostat/o/cyst/o/tomy
   CF CF
   incision into the prostate gland and (urinary) bladder
3. WR CV S
   orchi/o/tomy
   CF
   incision into the testis
4. WR S
   epdidym/ectomy
   excision of the epididymis
5. WR CV S
   orchi/o/pexy
   CF
   surgical fixation of the testicle
6. WR CV WR S
   prostat/o/vesicul/ectomy
   CF
   excision of the prostate gland and the seminal vesicles
7. WR CV S
   orchi/o/plasty
   CF
   surgical repair of the testis
8. WR S
   vesicul/ectomy
   excision of the seminal vesicle(s)
9. WR S
   prostat/ectomy
   excision of the prostate gland
10. WR CV S
    balan/o/plasty
    CF
    surgical repair of the glans penis
11. WR CV WR CV S
    vas/o/vas/o/stomy
    CF CF
    creation of artificial openings between ducts
12. WR S
    orchi/ectomy
    excision of the testis

Exercise 14

A *Label*

1. vas/ectomy
2. prostat/ectomy
3. orchi/o/pexy
4. epididym/ectomy

B *Fill In*

1. orchi/ectomy
2. balan/o/plasty
3. prostat/o/cyst/o/tomy
4. vesicul/ectomy
5. prostat/o/lith/o/tomy
6. orchi/o/tomy
7. prostat/o/vesicul/ectomy
8. orchi/o/plasty
9. vas/o/vas/o/stomy

Exercise 15

Pronounce and Spell

Exercise 16

A *Label*

1. robotic surgery
2. transurethral resection of the prostate gland
3. transurethral microwave thermotherapy
4. circumcision
5. enucleation

B *Identify*

1. sterilization
2. ablation
3. hydrocelectomy
4. transurethral incision of the prostate gland
5. laser surgery
6. morcellation

Exercise 17

1. g
2. k
3. h
4. j
5. i
6. f
7. b
8. a
9. d
10. c
11. e

Exercise 18

Review of Surgical Terms

Exercise 19

Pronounce and Spell

Exercise 20

1. digital rectal examination
2. prostate-specific antigen
3. transrectal ultrasound
4. semen analysis
5. multiparametric MRI
6. total testosterone
7. MRI ultrasound fusion biopsy

Exercise 21

1. e
2. d
3. f
4. c
5. g
6. b
7. a

Exercise 22

Review of Diagnostic Terms

Exercise 23

Pronounce and Spell

Exercise 24

A *Analyze and Define*

1. WR S
   orchi/algia
   pain in the testis
2. WR CV WR S
   olig/o/sperm/ia
   CF
   condition of scanty sperm (in the semen)
3. P WR S
   a/sperm/ia
   condition of without sperm (or semen or ejaculation)

B *Build*

1. a/sperm/ia
2. olig/o/sperm/ia
3. orchi/algia

Exercise 25

A *Match*

1. c
2. f
3. b
4. g
5. a
6. e
7. d

B *Match*

1. a
2. g
3. d
4. b
5. c
6. h
7. e
8. f

Exercise 26

Review of Complementary Terms

Exercise 27

1. lower urinary tract symptoms; bladder outlet obstruction
2. digital rectal examination; benign prostatic hyperplasia
3. transurethral incision; transurethral resection; transurethral microwave thermotherapy; photoselective vaporization; holmium laser enucleation
4. human immunodeficiency virus
5. human papillomavirus
6. sexually transmitted infection; sexually transmitted disease
7. prostate-specific antigen
8. radical prostatectomy
9. erectile dysfunction
10. transrectal ultrasound

Copyright © 2022, Elsevier Inc. All rights reserved.

Exercise 28

A. pain in his testicle; twisting of the spermatic cord with decreased blood flow to the testis; surgical fixation of the testis; surgical removal of the testis; reduced or absent ability to achieve pregnancy

B. Answers will vary and may include orchialgia, testicular torsion, orchiopexy, orchiectomy, infertility, and their respective definitions.

C. orchialgia, orchiectomy, infertility, testicular torsion, orchiopexy

D. Answers will vary and may include orchialgia, orchiectomy, infertility, testicular torsion, orchiopexy, and their respective definitions.

Exercise 29

A

1. nocturia
2. hematuria
3. BOO
4. urinary
5. benign prostatic hyperplasia
6. urology

B

1. c
2. b
3. c
4. a

Exercise 30

Online exercise

Exercise 31

Pronunciation Exercise

Exercise 32

1. a
2. b
3. a
4. c
5. a
6. c
7. b
8. a
9. c
10. c
11. b
12. a
13. c
14. a
15. c
16. a
17. b
18. a
19. c
20. b

ANSWERS TO CHAPTER 8 EXERCISES

Exercise 1

A *Label*

1. ovary: oophor/o
2. uterus: hyster/o, metr/o
3. fallopian (uterine) tube: salping/o
4. endometrium: endometri/o
5. cervix: cervic/o, trachel/o
6. vagina: colp/o, vagin/o
7. hymen: hymen/o

B *Label*

1. vulva: episi/o, vulv/o
2. perineum: perine/o

C *Identify*

1. men/o
2. gynec/o
3. mamm/o, mast/o
4. pelv/i

D *Define and Match*

1. f: fallopian tube (uterine tube)
2. e: uterus
3. a: perineum
4. c: cervix
5. b: vagina
6. c: cervix
7. d: breast
8. pelvis, pelvic cavity

E *Define and Match*

1. b: vagina
2. a: hymen
3. d: vulva
4. f: uterus
5. e: breast
6. g: ovary
7. d: vulva
8. c: endometrium
9. men/o: menstruation
10. gynec/o: woman

Exercise 2

A *Define*

1. scanty, few
2. blood
3. muscle
4. white
5. pus
6. water

B *Identify*

1. py/o
2. hydr/o
3. hemat/o
4. my/o
5. olig/o
6. leuk/o

Exercise 3

A *Define*

1. within
2. absence of, without
3. surrounding (outer)
4. painful, abnormal, difficult, labored

B *Identify*

1. dys-
2. endo-
3. a-
4. peri-

Exercise 4

A *Match*

1. c
2. h
3. f
4. a
5. e
6. d
7. b
8. g

B *Define*

1. the record, radiographic image
2. abnormal condition
3. pain
4. flow, discharge
5. visual examination
6. pertaining to
7. excision, surgical removal
8. surgical repair
9. excessive bleeding
10. instrument used for visual examination
11. cut into, incision
12. one who studies and treats (specialist, physician)

C *Label*

1. -salpinx
2. -cleisis

Exercise 5

Pronounce and Spell

Exercise 6

1. WR CV WR CV S
olig/o/men/o/rrhea
CF CF
scanty menstrual flow (infrequent menstrual flow)
2. WR S
cervic/itis
inflammation of the cervix
3. WR S
vagin/osis
abnormal condition of the vagina (caused by a bacterial imbalance)
4. WR CV S
hemat/o/salpinx
CF
blood in the fallopian tube
5. WR CV S
metr/o/rrhagia
CF
excessive bleeding from the uterus (irregular, out-of-cycle bleeding ranging from heavy to light, including spotting)

Copyright © 2022, Elsevier Inc. All rights reserved.

6. WR S
oophor/itis
inflammation of the ovary
7. P WR S
peri/metr/itis
inflammation surrounding the uterus (outer layer)
8. WR CV WR S
vulv/o/vagin/itis
CF
inflammation of the vulva and vagina
9. WR CV S
salping/o/cele
CF
hernia of the fallopian tube
10. WR CV WR CV S
men/o/metr/o/rrhagia
CF CF
excessive bleeding from the uterus at menstruation (and between menstrual cycles; heavy and irregular bleeding)

Exercise 7

A *Label*

1. hydr/o/salpinx
2. mast/itis
3. vagin/osis
4. endometri/osis
5. salping/itis
6. endometr/itis

B *Fill In*

1. my/o/metr/itis
2. men/o/rrhagia
3. py/o/salpinx
4. a/men/o/rrhea
5. dys/men/o/rrhea

Exercise 8

Pronounce and Spell

Exercise 9

1. a
2. d
3. b
4. g
5. c
6. f
7. e

Exercise 10

1. h
2. f
3. b
4. c
5. e
6. g
7. a
8. d

Exercise 11

A *Identify*

1. ovarian cancer
2. Adenomyosis
3. toxic shock syndrome
4. Cervical cancer
5. premenstrual syndrome
6. abnormal uterine bleeding
7. Fibrocystic breast changes

B *Label*

1. uterovaginal prolapse
2. uterine fibroid
3. endometrial cancer
4. breast cancer
5. pelvic inflammatory disease
6. vaginal fistula
7. polycystic ovary syndrome
8. Bartholin cyst

Exercise 12

Review of Disease and Disorder Terms

Exercise 13

Pronounce and Spell

Exercise 14

1. WR CV S
colp/o/plasty
CF
surgical repair of the vagina
2. WR CV S
hymen/o/tomy
CF
incision into the hymen
3. WR S
vulv/ectomy
excision of the vulva
4. WR CV S
perine/o/rrhaphy
CF
suturing of the perineum (tear)
5. WR CV S
salping/o/stomy
CF
creation of an artificial opening in the fallopian tube
6. WR S
oophor/ectomy
excision of the ovary
7. WR CV S
mast/o/pexy
CF
surgical fixation of the breast
8. WR CV WR CV S
colp/o/perine/o/rrhaphy
CF CF
suturing of the vagina and the perineum

Exercise 15

A *Label*

1. hyster/ectomy
2. salping/ectomy
3. salping/o/-oophor/ectomy
4. episi/o/rrhaphy
5. mast/ectomy
6. mamm/o/plasty

B *Fill In*

1. colp/o/rrhaphy
2. trachel/ectomy
3. colp/o/cleisis
4. hyster/o/pexy

Exercise 16

Pronounce and Spell

Exercise 17

A *Label*

1. tubal ligation
2. dilation and curettage
3. endometrial ablation
4. myomectomy

B *Identify*

1. anterior and posterior colporrhaphy
2. uterine artery embolization
3. conization

C *Match*

1. c
2. a
3. b
4. c
5. g
6. c
7. c

Exercise 18

Review of Surgical Terms

Exercise 19

Pronounce and Spell

Exercise 20

A *Analyze and Define*

1. WR CV S
colp/o/scopy
CF
visual examination of the vagina
2. WR CV S
mamm/o/gram
CF
radiographic image of the breast
3. WR CV S
colp/o/scope
CF
instrument used for visual examination of the vagina
4. WR CV S
hyster/o/scopy
CF
visual examination of the uterus
5. WR CV WR CV S
hyster/o/salping/o/gram
CF CF
radiographic image of the uterus and fallopian tubes

Copyright © 2022, Elsevier Inc. All rights reserved.

6. WR CV S
   pelv/i/scopic
   CF
   pertaining to visual examination of the pelvic cavity
7. WR CV S
   pelv/i/scopy
   CF
   visual examination of the pelvic cavity
8. WR CV S
   mamm/o/graphy
   CF
   radiographic imaging of the breast
9. WR CV S
   hyster/o/scope
   CF
   instrument used for visual examination of the uterus
10. WR CV WR CV S
   son/o/hyster/o/graphy
   CF CF
   process of recording the uterus with sound

B *Build*

1. mamm/o/graphy
2. mamm/o/gram
3. colp/o/scope
4. hyster/o/salping/o/gram

C *Build*

1. colp/o/scopy
2. hyster/o/scopy
3. pelv/i/scopic
4. pelv/i/scopy
5. hyster/o/scope
6. son/o/hyster/o/graphy

Exercise 21

A *Label*

1. transvaginal sonography
2. Pap test

B *Match*

1. c
2. d
3. e
4. f
5. a
6. b

C *Identify*

1. Sentinel lymph node biopsy
2. stereotactic breast biopsy
3. CA-125 test
4. HPV test

Exercise 22

Review of Diagnostic Terms

Exercise 23

Pronounce and Spell

Exercise 24

A *Analyze and Define*

1. WR CV S
   gynec/o/logist
   CF
   physician who studies and treats (female reproductive system) women
2. WR CV S
   gynec/o/logy
   CF
   study of women (branch of medicine dealing with health and diseases of the female reproductive system)
3. WR CV WR S
   vulv/o/vagin/al
   CF
   pertaining to the vulva and vagina
4. WR S
   mast/algia
   pain in the breast
5. WR S
   pel/vic
   pertaining to the pelvis
6. WR CV S
   leuk/o/rrhea
   CF
   white discharge (from the vagina)
7. WR CV WR S
   vesic/o/vagin/al
   CF
   pertaining to the (urinary) bladder and the vagina
8. WR S
   vagin/al
   pertaining to the vagina
9. P WR S
   endo/cervic/al
   pertaining to within the cervix

B *Build*

1. leuk/o/rrhea
2. pel/vic
3. mast/algia
4. vulv/o/vagin/al
5. gynec/o/logist
6. gynec/o/logy
7. vesic/o/vagin/al
8. vagin/al
9. endo/cervic/al

Exercise 25

A *Match*

1. g
2. d
3. i
4. b
5. c
6. e
7. a
8. h
9. f

B *Label*

1. speculum
2. contraception

C *Fill In*

1. fistula
2. menarche
3. dyspareunia
4. menopause
5. hormone replacement therapy
6. anovulation
7. oligoovulation

Exercise 26

Review of Complementary Terms

Exercise 27

1. anterior and posterior colporrhaphy
2. total abdominal hysterectomy and bilateral salpingo-oophorectomy; hormone replacement therapy
3. sonohysterography; transvaginal sonography
4. vaginal hysterectomy; laparoscopically assisted vaginal hysterectomy; total laparoscopic hysterectomy
5. dilation and curettage; cervix
6. fibrocystic breast changes
7. pelvic inflammatory disease; gynecology
8. premenstrual syndrome
9. uterine artery embolization
10. intrauterine device; intrauterine system; birth control
11. polycystic ovary syndrome
12. abnormal uterine bleeding

Exercise 28

A. trying for over a year to get pregnant; menstruating is very painful; she bleeds a lot; may have given her a disease; only one of his testicles was down; surgery to fix the other one

B. Answers will vary and may include infertility, dysmenorrhea, menorrhagia, sexually transmitted disease (sexually transmitted infection), cryptorchidism, orchiopexy, along with their respective definitions.

C. infertility, cryptorchidism, orchiopexy, menarche, dysmenorrhea, menorrhagia, Pap test, cervicitis, chlamydia, pelvic inflammatory disease, semen analysis, hysterosalpingogram

D. Answers will vary and may include infertility, cryptorchidism, orchiopexy, menarche, dysmenorrhea, menorrhagia, Pap test, cervicitis, chlamydia, pelvic inflammatory disease, semen analysis, hysterosalpingogram, along with their respective definitions

Copyright © 2022, Elsevier Inc. All rights reserved.

Exercise 29

A

1. mammography
2. carcinoma
3. hysterectomy
4. adenomyosis
5. endometriosis
6. HRT
7. stereotactic breast biopsy
8. mediolateral
9. mastectomy
10. sentinel lymph node biopsy

B

1. c
2. a
3. d

Exercise 30

Use Medical Language in Online Electronic Health Records

Exercise 31

Pronunciation Exercise

Exercise 32

1. a
2. c
3. a
4. c
5. b
6. a
7. b
8. b
9. a
10. a
11. b
12. a
13. c
14. b
15. b
16. a
17. c
18. b
19. a
20. c

ANSWERS TO CHAPTER 9 EXERCISES

Exercise 1

A *Label*

1. umbilicus: omphal/o
2. fetus: fet/o, fet/i
3. amnion, amniotic fluid: amni/o, amnion/o
4. chorion: chori/o

B *Identify*

1. puerper/o
2. a. par/o
   b. part/o
3. gravid/o
4. lact/o
5. nat/o

C *Define and Match*

1. c: amnion, amniotic fluid
2. d: umbilicus, navel
3. c: amnion, amniotic fluid
4. b: fetus, unborn offspring
5. a: chorion

D *Define*

1. milk
2. bear, give birth to, labor, childbirth
3. childbirth
4. pregnancy
5. birth

Exercise 2

A *Define*

1. first
2. scanty, few
3. pylorus, pyloric sphincter
4. water
5. head
6. vulva
7. uterus
8. esophagus
9. cancer
10. false
11. malformations
12. trachea
13. sound
14. pelvis, pelvic cavity

B *Identify*

1. cephal/o
2. olig/o
3. prim/i
4. hyster/o
5. pylor/o
6. pelv/i
7. pseud/o
8. episi/o
9. terat/o
10. esophag/o
11. carcin/o
12. trache/o
13. hydr/o
14. son/o

Exercise 3

A *Define*

1. before
2. small
3. new
4. many
5. after
6. painful, abnormal, difficult, labored
7. before
8. many, much
9. within
10. none

B *Identify*

1. nulli-
2. post-
3. micro-
4. intra-
5. a. ante-
   b. pre-
6. poly-
7. multi-
8. neo-
9. dys-

Exercise 4

A *Define*

1. study of
2. substance or agent that produces or causes
3. tumor, swelling
4. pertaining to
5. cut into, incision
6. one who studies and treats (specialist, physician)
7. hernia, protrusion
8. producing, orginating, causing
9. constriction or narrowing
10. inflammation
11. flow discharge
12. process of recording, radiographic imaging

B *Label*

1. -tocia
2. -rrhexis
3. -cyesis
4. -amnios

C *Identify*

1. -a
2. -e
3. -is
4. -um
5. -us

Exercise 5

Pronounce and Spell

Exercise 6

A *Analyze and Define*

1. WR CV WR S
   chori/o/amnion/itis
   CF
   inflammation of the chorion and amnion
2. WR CV WR S
   chori/o/carcin/oma
   CF
   cancerous tumor of the chorion
3. WR CV S
   pseud/o/cyesis
   CF
   false pregnancy (a woman who believes she is pregnant)
4. WR S
   amnion/itis
   inflammation of the amnion
5. WR CV S
   hyster/o/rrhexis
   CF
   rupture of the uterus
6. WR CV WR S
   olig/o/hydr/amnios
   CF
   scanty amnion water (less than the normal amount of amniotic fluid)
7. P WR S
   poly/hydr/amnios
   much amnion water (more than the normal amount of amniotic fluid)

Copyright © 2022, Elsevier Inc. All rights reserved.

8. P S(WR)
dys/tocia
difficult labor

B *Label*

1. poly/hydr/amnios
2. olig/o/hydr/amnios
3. hyster/o/rrhexis
4. dys/tocia

C *Fill In*

1. chori/o/carcin/oma
2. amnion/itis
3. chori/o/amnion/itis
4. pseud/o/cyesis

Exercise 7

A *Match*

1. d
2. f
3. e
4. b
5. a
6. c

B *Label*

1. ectopic pregnancy
2. abruptio placentae
3. placenta previa

C *Identify*

1. eclampsia
2. abortion
3. preeclampsia

Exercise 8

Review of Obstetric Disease and Disorder Terms

Exercise 9

Pronounce and Spell

Exercise 10

A *Analyze and Define*

1. WR S
pylor/ic (stenosis)
narrowing pertaining to the pyloric sphincter
2. WR CV S
omphal/o/cele
CF
hernia at the umbilicus
3. WR S
omphal/itis
inflammation of the umbilicus
4. P WR S
micro/cephal/us
(fetus with a very) small head
5. WR CV WR S
trache/o/esophag/eal (fistula)
CF
abnormal passageway pertaining to the trachea and the esophagus (between the trachea and esophagus)

B *Label*

1. micro/cephal/us
2. omphal/o/cele

C *Fill In*

1. pylor/ic (stenosis)
2. trache/o/esophag/eal (fistula)
3. omphal/itis

Exercise 11

A *Match*

1. i
2. c
3. j
4. f
5. k
6. b
7. g
8. e
9. h
10. a
11. d

B *Label*

1. esophageal atresia
2. coarctation of the aorta
3. spina bifida
4. gastroschisis

C *Identify*

1. Erythroblastosis fetalis
2. congenital heart disease
3. respiratory distress syndrome
4. congenital cytomegalovirus infection
5. Fetal alcohol syndrome
6. cleft lip or palate
7. Down syndrome

Exercise 12

Review of Neonatology Disease and Disorder Terms

Exercise 13

Pronounce and Spell

Exercise 14

A *Analyze and Define*

1. WR CV S
episi/o/tomy
CF
incision into the vulva (perineum)
2. WR CV S
amni/o/tomy
CF
incision into the amnion (rupture of the fetal membrane to induce labor)

B *Build*

1. amni/o/tomy
1. episi/o/tomy

Exercise 15

A *Label*

1. cervical cerclage
2. in vitro fertilization
3. cesarean section

B *Match*

1. b
2. c
3. a

Exercise 16

Review of Obstetric Surgical Terms

Exercise 17

Pronounce and Spell

Exercise 18

A *Analyze and Define*

1. WR CV S
amni/o/centesis
CF
surgical puncture to aspirate amniotic fluid
2. WR S WR CV S
pelv/ic son/o/graphy
CF
pertaining to the pelvis, process of recording sound

B *Build*

1. pelv/ic son/o/graphy
2. amni/o/centesis

Exercise 19

A *Match*

1. c
2. a
3. d
4. b

B *Identify*

1. Apgar score
2. Chorionic villus sampling
3. quad screen
4. Nuchal translucency screening

Exercise 20

Review of Obstetric and Neonatology Diagnostic Terms

Exercise 21

Pronounce and Spell

Exercise 22

A *Analyze and Define*

1. P WR S
multi/gravid/a
many pregnancies
2. WR CV S
lact/o/rrhea
CF
(spontaneous) discharge of milk
3. WR S
puerper/al
pertaining to (immediately after) childbirth

Copyright © 2022, Elsevier Inc. All rights reserved.

4. WR CV S
amni/o/rrhea
CF
discharge (escape) of amniotic fluid
5. P WR S
nulli/par/a
no births
6. WR CV S
amni/o/rrhexis
CF
rupture of the amnion
7. P WR S
post/part/um
after childbirth
8. WR CV WR S
prim/i/par/a
CF
first birth
9. WR S
gravid/a
pregnant (woman)
10. WR S
puerper/a
childbirth

B *Label*

1. ante/part/um
2. intra/part/um
3. lact/o/genic
4. multi/par/a

C *Fill In*

1. gravid/o/puerper/al
2. prim/i/gravid/a
3. par/a
4. nulli/gravid/a

Exercise 23

A *Identify*

1. parturition
2. Midwifery
3. puerperium
4. Quickening
5. obstetrics (OB)
6. In vivo
7. colostrum
8. Lochia

B *Label*

1. cephalic presentation
2. breech presentation
3. lactation
4. in vitro
5. midwife
6. obstetrician

C *Match*

1. e
2. g
3. a
4. b
5. c
6. d
7. f

D *Match*

1. d
2. f
3. c
4. a
5. b
6. g
7. e

Exercise 24

Review of Obstetric Complementary Terms

Exercise 25

Pronounce and Spell

Exercise 26

A *Analyze and Define*

1. WR CV S
terat/o/genic
CF
producing malformations
2. P WR CV S
neo/nat/o/logy
CF
study of the newborn
3. P WR S
neo/nat/e
new birth
4. WR S
fet/al
pertaining to the fetus
5. P WR S
pre/nat/al
pertaining to before birth (reference to the newborn)
6. WR CV S
terat/o/logy
CF
study of malformations
7. WR S
nat/al
pertaining to birth
8. P WR CV S
neo/nat/o/logist
CF
physician who studies and treats disorders of the newborn
9. WR CV S
terat/o/gen
CF
(any agent) producing malformations (in the developing embryo)
10. P WR S
post/nat/al
pertaining to after birth (reference to the newborn)

B *Label*

1. neo/nat/e
2. neo/nat/o/logist
3. fet/al
4. terat/o/gen

C *Fill In*

1. post/nat/al
2. terat/o/logy
3. neo/nat/o/logy
4. terat/o/genic
5. nat/al
6. pre/nat/al

Exercise 27

A *Identify*

1. congenital anomaly
2. Stillborn
3. meconium

B *Label*

1. gavage
2. premature infant

C *Match*

1. d
2. e
3. c
4. a
5. b

Exercise 28

Review of Neonatology Complementary Terms

Exercise 29

1. expected (estimated) date of delivery, last menstrual period, date of birth
2. obstetrics, newborn
3. primipara, multipara
4. chorionic villus sampling, abortion
5. fetal alcohol syndrome
6. cytomegalovirus
7. respiratory distress syndrome
8. Cesarean section
9. vaginal birth after cesarean
10. in vitro fertilization

Exercise 30

A. pregnant for the third time, born dead, ultrasound test, genetic condition that causes physical and mental problems, needle to take fluid out
B. Answers will vary and may include multigravida, para, stillborn, pelvic sonography, Down syndrome, and amniocentesis, and their respective definitions.
C. gravida, para, EDD, prenatal, Down syndrome, amniocentesis, abortion, congenital anomalies, tracheoesophageal fistula, neonatologist
D. Answers will vary and may include gravida, para, EDD, prenatal, Down syndrome, amniocentesis, abortion, congenital anomalies, tracheoesophageal fistula, neonatologist, and their respective definitions.

Copyright © 2022, Elsevier Inc. All rights reserved.

Exercise 31

A

1. gravida
2. para
3. EDD
4. prenatal
5. pelvic sonography
6. cephalic presentation

B

1. c
2. T
3. F, sonography was used

Exercise 32

Online Exercise

Exercise 33

Pronunciation Exercise

Exercise 34

1. b
2. b
3. a
4. a
5. c
6. b
7. a
8. c
9. b
10. b
11. b
12. a
13. c
14. b
15. a
16. b
17. c
18. a
19. c
20. b

ANSWERS TO CHAPTER 10 EXERCISES

Exercise 1

A *Label*

1. heart: cardi/o
2. muscle: my/o
3. valve: valvul/o
4. ventricle: ventricul/o
5. aorta: aort/o
6. atrium: atri/o

B *Define and Match*

1. d, heart
2. e, atrium
3. a, valve
4. b, ventricle
5. c, aorta
6. f, muscle

C *Label*

1. blood vessel: angi/o
2. vein: phelb/o, ven/o
3. artery: arteri/o
4. blood: hem/o, hemat/o
5. bone marrow: myel/o
6. plasma: plasm/o
7. cells: cyt/o

D *Define and Match*

1. c, artery *(s)*, arteries *(pl)*
2. d, bone marrow
3. a, blood
4. e, vein
5. f, vessel, blood vessel
6. e, vein
7. b, plasma
8. a, blood

E *Label*

1. lymph, lymph tissue: lymph/o
2. thymus gland: thym/o
3. lymph node(s): lymphaden/o
4. spleen: splen/o

F *Define and Match*

1. c, spleen
2. d, lymph
3. b, thymus gland
4. a, lymph node

Exercise 2

A *Define*

1. sound
2. blood clot
3. deficiency, blockage
4. red
5. yellowish, fatty plaque
6. electricity, electrical activity
7. white
8. immune system
9. plug

B *Identify*

1. thromb/o
2. ech/o
3. isch/o
4. ather/o
5. immun/o
6. electr/o
7. embol/o
8. leuk/o
9. erythr/o

Exercise 3

A *Define*

1. slow
2. all, total
3. many, much
4. fast, rapid
5. within
6. surrounding (outer)
7. within

B *Identify*

1. tachy-
2. brady-
3. poly-
4. peri-
5. pan-
6. endo-, intra-

Exercise 4

A *Identify*

1. -rrhage
2. -genic
3. -sclerosis
4. -lysis
5. -penia
6. -stasis
7. -apheresis
8. -logy
9. -logist
10. -us
11. -ar, -ic, -ous

B *Match*

1. f
2. l
3. g
4. i
5. c
6. k
7. j
8. b
9. d
10. a
11. h
12. e

C *Match*

1. d
2. f
3. g
4. a
5. c
6. b
7. e

Exercise 5

Pronounce and Spell

Exercise 6

1. WR CV WR S
   atri/o/ventricul/ar
   CF
   pertaining to the atrium and ventricle
2. WR CV WR CV S
   electr/o/cardi/o/graphy
   CF CF
   process of recording the electrical activity of the heart
3. WR CV S
   cardi/o/logist
   CF
   physician who studies and treats diseases of the heart
4. WR CV S
   aort/o/gram
   CF
   radiographic image of the aorta (after an injection of contrast media)

Copyright © 2022, Elsevier Inc. All rights reserved.

5. WR S
valvul/itis
inflammation of a valve (of the heart)
6. WR S
phleb/ectomy
excision of a vein
7. P WR S
tachy/card/ia
condition of a rapid heart (rate)
8. WR CV S
angi/o/scopy
CF
visual examination (of the inside) of a blood vessel
9. WR CV S
angi/o/graphy
CF
radiographic imaging of a blood vessel
10. WR CV S
cardi/o/genic
CF
originating in the heart
11. WR S
isch/emia
deficiency in blood (flow); (caused by constriction or obstruction of a blood vessel)
12. WR CV WR S
thromb/o/phleb/itis
CF
inflammation of a vein associated with a blood clot
13. WR S
ather/ectomy
excision of fatty plaque
14. WR CV S
valvul/o/plasty
CF
surgical repair of a valve
15. WR S
angi/oma
tumor composed of blood vessels
16. WR CV WR CV S
cardi/o/my/o/pathy
CF CF
disease of the heart muscle

Exercise 7

A *Label*

1. aort/ic stenosis *Note: the suffix -stenosis stands as an independent word in this instance*
2. cardi/o/megaly
3. ather/o/sclerosis
4. endarterectomy *Note: the "o" in the prefix endo- is dropped because the following combining form begins with a vowel.*
5. arteri/o/gram
6. ven/o/gram
7. peri/card/itis *Note: the "i" in cardi/o is dropped because the suffix starts with an "i"*
8. peri/cardi/o/centesis
9. intra/ven/ous
10. ech/o/cardi/o/gram
11. electr/o/cardi/o/gram

B *Fill In*

1. phleb/itis
2. angi/o/plasty
3. endo/card/itis
4. brady/card/ia
5. arteri/o/sclerosis
6. embol/ectomy
7. cardi/o/my/o/pathy
8. angi/o/stenosis
9. poly/arter/itis
10. cardi/o/logy

Exercise 8

Pronounce and Spell

Exercise 9

A *Disease and Disorder Terms*

1. cardiac arrest
2. varicose veins
3. Aneurysm
4. Coronary artery disease
5. Angina pectoris
6. myocardial infarction
7. fibrillation; arrhythmia
8. hypertensive
9. Heart failure
10. Peripheral artery disease
11. Intermittent claudication
12. cardiac tamponade
13. mitral valve stenosis; rheumatic heart disease
14. Deep vein thrombosis
15. Acute coronary syndrome
16. cor pulmonale

B *Surgical Terms*

1. artificial cardiac pacemaker
2. thrombolytic therapy
3. coronary artery bypass graft
4. catheter ablation
5. coronary stent
6. percutaneous transluminal coronary angioplasty
7. automatic implantable cardiac defibrillator
8. femoropopliteal bypass

Exercise 10

A *Label*

1. Doppler ultrasound
2. lipid profile
3. exercise stress test
4. sestamibi test
5. digital subtraction angiography
6. sphygmomanometer
7. cardiac catheterization

B *Fill In*

1. Transesophageal echocardiogram
2. single-photon emission computed tomography
3. creatine phosphokinase
4. C-reactive protein
5. Pulse
6. Troponin
7. blood pressure

Exercise 11

A *Match*

1. j
2. g
3. h
4. b
5. d
6. i
7. a
8. e
9. c
10. f

B *Label*

1. defibrillation
2. cardiopulmonary resuscitation

Exercise 12

Review of Cardiovascular Terms

Exercise 13

Pronounce and Spell

Exercise 14

1. WR CV S
hem/o/stasis
CF
stoppage of bleeding
2. WR CV S
hemat/o/logist
CF
physician who studies and treats diseases of the blood
3. WR CV S
hem/o/lysis
CF
dissolution of blood (cells)
4. WR CV WR S
lymph/o/cyt/osis
CF
increase in the number of lymphocytes
5. P WR CV S
pan/cyt/o/penia
CF
abnormal reduction of all (blood) cells
6. WR CV WR CV S
erythr/o/cyt/o/penia
CF CF
abnormal reduction of red (blood) cells

Copyright © 2022, Elsevier Inc. All rights reserved.

7. WR S
   embol/ism
   state of a plug (blood clot, fat, or air lodged in a blood vessel)
8. WR S
   thromb/us
   blood clot

Exercise 15

A *Fill In*

1. leuk/o/cyt/o/penia
2. hem/o/rrhage
3. thromb/o/lysis
4. thromb/o/cyt/o/penia
5. embol/us *Note: the suffix -us is a noun ending with no meaning*
6. multiple myel/oma

B *Label*

1. phleb/o/tomy
2. plasm/apheresis
3. hemat/oma
4. thromb/osis

Exercise 16

Pronounce and Spell

Exercise 17

1. e
2. g
3. f
4. b
5. d
6. c
7. a

Exercise 18

1. bone marrow aspiration
2. bone marrow biopsy
3. phlebotomist
4. perfusionist

Exercise 19

1. blood dyscrasias
2. anticoagulant
3. venipuncture; extravasation
4. bone marrow transplant; peripheral blood stem cell transplant
5. complete blood count with differential
6. hematocrit; hemoglobin
7. bleeding profile, prothrombin time, activated partial thromboplastin time

Exercise 20

Review of Blood Terms

Exercise 21

Pronounce and Spell

Exercise 22

A *Analyze and Define*

1. WR WR CV S
   lymph/angi/o/graphy
   CF
   radiographic imaging of lymph vessels
2. WR S
   thym/ectomy
   excision of the thymus gland
3. WR CV S
   splen/o/rrhaphy
   CF
   suturing, repairing of the spleen
4. WR CV S
   splen/o/megaly
   CF
   enlargement of the spleen
5. WR S
   lymph/oma
   tumor of lymphatic tissue
6. WR S
   lymphaden/itis
   inflammation of lymph nodes

B *Build*

1. lymph/ang/itis *Note: the "i" in angi/o is dropped because the suffix starts with an "i"*
2. lymphaden/o/pathy
3. thym/oma
4. splen/ectomy

Exercise 23

A *Label*

1. infectious mononucleosis
2. lymphedema

B *Fill in*

1. lymphoma
2. lymphangiography
3. thymoma; thymectomy
4. splenectomy; splenomegaly
5. splenorrhaphy
6. lymphadenopathy
7. lymphadenitis
8. lymphangitis

Exercise 24

Review of Lymphatic Terms

Exercise 25

Pronounce and Spell

Exercise 26

1. WR CV S
   lymph/o/cyte
   CF
   lymph cell
2. WR CV S
   immun/o/logy
   CF
   study of the immune system
3. WR CV S
   immun/o/logist
   CF
   physician who studies and treats diseases of the immune system

Exercise 27

1. e
2. j
3. m
4. f
5. l
6. g
7. d
8. a
9. h
10. c
11. i
12. b
13. k
14. o
15. n

Exercise 28

1. allergen; antigen; antibody
2. anaphylaxis
3. Sarcoidosis
4. erythrocyte sedimentation rate; ESR
5. lymphocyte
6. vaccine; immunity
7. acquired immunodeficiency syndrome; AIDS; opportunistic infections
8. immunosuppression
9. immunology; immunodeficiency; allergy
10. immunologist; autoimmune disease; allergist

Exercise 29

Review of Immune Terms

Exercise 30

1. coronary artery disease; electrocardiogram; single-photon emission computed tomography; echocardiogram
2. deep vein thrombosis
3. complete blood count; differential; red blood cell; white blood cell; hemoglobin; hematocrit
4. coronary artery bypass graft; percutaneous transluminal coronary angioplasty
5. myocardial infarction; coronary care unit
6. blood pressure
7. heart failure
8. cardiopulmonary resuscitation
9. hypertensive heart disease
10. prothrombin time
11. atrioventricular

Copyright © 2022, Elsevier Inc. All rights reserved.

12. acute coronary syndrome
13. peripheral artery disease
14. digital subtraction angiography
15. transesophageal echocardiogram
16. C-reactive protein; creatine phosphokinase
17. atrial fibrillation
18. automatic implantable cardiac defibrillator
19. intravenous
20. hypertension
21. peripheral blood stem cell transplant; bone marrow transplant
22. erythrocyte sedimentation rate

Exercise 31

A. high blood pressure, pain in chest, heart was racing, breathing faster
B. answers will vary and may include hypertension, angina pectoris, tachycardia, tachypnea (from Chapter 5)
C. coronary artery disease, hypertension, hypercholesterolemia, varicose veins, cardiologist, coronary artery bypass grafts, aneurysm, along with their respective definitions
D. answers will vary and may include coronary artery disease, hypertension, hypercholesterolemia varicose veins, cardiologist, coronary artery bypass grafts. aneurysm, along with their respective definitions

Exercise 32

A

1. infectious mononucleosis
2. splenomegaly
3. splenectomy
4. lymphoma
5. vaccine
6. lymphadenopathy
7. arrhythmia
8. lymphoma
9. leukemia
10. bone marrow biopsy
11. hematologist

B

1. b
2. c
3. b
4. F, no indication of hemolysis
5. T

Exercise 33

Online Exercise

Exercise 34

Pronunciation Exercise

Exercise 35

1. c
2. a
3. b
4. c
5. b
6. a
7. b
8. c
9. a
10. b
11. c
12. c
13. c
14. a
15. b
16. a
17. b
18. c
19. a
20. b

ANSWERS TO CHAPTER 11 EXERCISES

Exercise 1

A *Label*

1. mouth: or/o, stomat/o
2. esophagus: esophag/o
3. duodenum: duoden/o
4. colon: col/o, colon/o
5. cecum: cec/o
6. anus: an/o
7. stomach: gastr/o
8. antrum: antr/o
9. jejunum: jejun/o
10. ileum: ile/o
11. sigmoid colon: sigmoid/o
12. rectum: proct/o, rect/o

B *Define and Match*

1. e, jejunum
2. g, anus
3. h, stomach
4. b, rectum
5. a, mouth
6. c, colon
7. f, sigmoid colon
8. d, intestines (usually the small intestine)

C *Define and Match*

1. d, ileum
2. g, mouth
3. h, rectum
4. e, esophagus
5. a, antrum
6. f, colon
7. b, duodenum
8. c, cecum

Exercise 2

A *Identify*

1. peritone/o
2. chol/e
3. herni/o
4. diverticul/o
5. polyp/o
6. steat/o

B *Define*

1. hernia
2. abdomen, abdominal cavity
3. saliva, salivary gland
4. gall, bile
5. diverticulum, *pl.* diverticula (pouch extending from a hollow organ)
6. gum(s)
7. appendix
8. tongue
9. liver
10. lip(s)
11. peritoneum
12. palate
13. pancreas
14. abdomen, abdominal cavity
15. tongue
16. common bile duct
17. pylorus, pyloric sphincter
18. uvula
19. bile duct(s)
20. polyp, small growth
21. abdomen, abdominal cavity
22. fat
23. appendix
24. pharynx
25. bladder, sac

C *Label*

1. palate: palat/o
2. pharynx: pharyng/o
3. uvula: uvul/o
4. tongue: gloss/o, lingu/o
5. gallbladder: chol/e (gall), cyst/o (bladder)
6. pyloric sphincter: pylor/o
7. appendix: append/o, appendic/o
8. gum(s): gingiv/o
9. lip(s): cheil/o
10. salivary glands: sial/o
11. liver: hepat/o
12. bile duct(s): cholangi/o
13. common bile duct: choledoch/o
14. pancreas: pancreat/o
15. abdomen, abdominal cavity: abdomin/o, celi/o, lapar/o

Copyright © 2022, Elsevier Inc. All rights reserved.

Exercise 3

A Define

1. painful, abnormal, difficult, labored
2. half
3. absence of, without

B Identify

1. a-
2. hemi-
3. dys-

Exercise 4

A Define

1. digestion
2. pertaining to
3. noun suffix, no meaning
4. abnormal condition (means increase when used with blood cell word roots)
5. condition
6. diseased or abnormal state, condition of

B Identify

1. -scope
2. -graphy
3. -logist
4. -logy
5. -gram
6. -scopy

C Match

1. c
2. a
3. f
4. b
5. g
6. e
7. d

D Match

1. d
2. c
3. g
4. f
5. a
6. b
7. e

Exercise 5

Pronounce and Spell

Exercise 6

1. WR CV WR S
   steat/o/hepat/itis
   CF
   inflammation of the liver associated with (excess) fat
2. WR S
   diverticul/osis
   abnormal condition of having diverticula
3. WR S
   cholangi/oma
   tumor of the bile duct
4. WR S
   hepat/oma
   tumor of the liver
5. WR S
   uvul/itis
   inflammation of the uvula
6. WR S
   pancreat/itis
   inflammation of the pancreas
7. WR S
   proct/itis
   inflammation of the rectum
8. WR S
   cheil/itis
   inflammation of the lips
9. WR S
   gastr/itis
   inflammation of the stomach
10. WR CV S
    rect/o/cele
    CF
    hernia of the rectum
11. WR CV S
    enter/o/pathy
    CF
    disease of the intestines
12. WR S
    periton/itis
    inflammation of the peritoneum
13. WR S
    enter/itis
    inflammation of the intestines
14. WR S
    gloss/itis
    inflammation of the tongue

Exercise 7

A Label

1. stomat/itis
2. gingiv/itis
3. dys/enter/y
4. appendic/itis
5. chol/e/lith/iasis, choledoch/o/lith/iasis

B Fill in

1. hepat/itis
2. col/itis
3. sial/o/lith
4. esophag/itis
5. diverticul/itis
6. chol/e/cyst/itis
7. polyp/osis
8. gastr/o/enter/itis

Exercise 8

Pronounce and Spell

Exercise 9

1. e
2. g
3. c
4. b
5. f
6. h
7. d
8. a

Exercise 10

1. peptic ulcer
2. volvulus
3. polyp
4. gastroesophageal reflux disease
5. adhesions
6. intussusception
7. hemorrhoids

Exercise 11

Review of Disease and Disorder Terms

Exercise 12

Pronounce and Spell

Exercise 13

1. WR CV S
   herni/o/rrhaphy
   CF
   suturing of a hernia
2. WR CV S
   gastr/o/plasty
   CF
   surgical repair of the stomach
3. P WR S
   hemi/col/ectomy
   excision of half of the colon
4. WR S
   antr/ectomy
   excision of the antrum
5. WR CV S
   enter/o/rrhaphy
   CF
   suturing of the (small) intestine
6. WR S
   uvul/ectomy
   excision of the uvula
7. WR CV WR CV S
   gastr/o/jejun/o/stomy
   CF CF
   creation of an artificial opening between the stomach and the jejunum
8. WR CV WR S
   chol/e/cyst/ectomy
   CF
   excision of the gallbladder
9. WR CV S
   abdomin/o/plasty
   CF
   surgical repair of the abdomen
10. WR S
    pancreat/ectomy
    excision of the pancreas
11. WR CV S
    pylor/o/plasty
    CF
    surgical repair of the pylorus
12. WR CV WR CV S
    choledoch/o/lith/o/tomy
    CF CF
    incision into the common bile duct to remove a stone

Copyright © 2022, Elsevier Inc. All rights reserved.

13. WR CV WR CV WR CV S
uvul/o/palat/o/pharyng/o/plasty
CF CF CF
surgical repair of the uvula, palate, and pharynx

14. WR CV S
abdomin/o/centesis
CF
surgical puncture to aspirate fluid from the abdominal cavity

Exercise 14

A Label

1. append/ectomy
2. col/ectomy
3. palat/o/plasty
4. polyp/ectomy
5. ile/o/stomy
6. col/o/stomy
7. gastr/o/stomy
8. gastr/ectomy

B Fill In

1. gloss/o/rrhaphy
2. esophag/o/gastr/o/plasty
3. diverticul/ectomy
4. gingiv/ectomy
5. lapar/o/tomy
6. an/o/plasty
7. chol/e/cyst/ectomy

Exercise 15

Pronounce and Spell

Exercise 16

1. vagotomy
2. anastomosis
3. abdominoperineal resection
4. bariatric surgery
5. hemorrhoidectomy

Exercise 17

Review of Surgical Terms

Exercise 18

Pronounce and Spell

Exercise 19

1. WR CV S
proct/o/scope
CF
instrument used for visual examination of the rectum

2. WR CV S
proct/o/scopy
CF
visual examination of the rectum

3. WR CV S
sigmoid/o/scopy
CF
visual examination of the sigmoid colon

4. WR CV S
cholangi/o/graphy
CF
radiographic imaging of the bile ducts

5. WR CV S
colon/o/scope
CF
instrument used for visual examination of the colon

6. WR CV S
lapar/o/scope
CF
instrument used for visual examination of the abdominal cavity

7. WR CV S
lapar/o/scopy
CF
visual examination of the abdominal cavity

8. WR CV S
esophag/o/gram
CF
radiographic image of the esophagus

Exercise 20

A Fill In

1. esophag/o/scopy
2. cholangi/o/gram
3. esophag/o/gastr/o/duoden/o/scopy

B Label

1. colon/o/scopy
2. CT colon/o/graphy
3. capsule endo/scopy
4. gastr/o/scope
5. gastr/o/scopy

Exercise 21

Pronounce and Spell

Exercise 22

1. d
2. f
3. a
4. b
5. e
6. g
7. c

Exercise 23

A Label

1. endoscopic retrograde cholangiopancreatography
2. barium enema

B Identify

1. *Helicobacter pylori* stool antigen
2. fecal occult blood test
3. abdominal sonography
4. endoscopic ultrasound
5. upper GI series

Exercise 24

Review of Diagnostic Terms

Exercise 25

Pronounce and Spell

Exercise 26

1. WR S
rect/al
pertaining to the rectum

2. P S(WR)
dys/pepsia
difficult digestion

3. WR S
palat/al
pertaining to the palate

4. WR S
esophag/eal
pertaining to the esophagus

5. WR CV S
steat/o/rrhea
CF
discharge of fat

6. WR S
duoden/al
pertaining to the duodenum

7. WR S
or/al
pertaining to the mouth

8. WR CV WR CV S
gastr/o/enter/o/logist
CF CF
physician who studies and treats diseases of the stomach and intestines

9. WR S
steat/osis
abnormal condition of fat

10. WR S
pancreat/ic
pertaining to the pancreas

Exercise 27

1. hepat/o/megaly
2. a/phagia
3. sub/lingu/al
4. nas/o/gastr/ic
5. or/o/gastr/ic
6. an/al
7. peritone/al
8. celi/ac
9. dys/phagia
10. ile/o/cec/al
11. col/o/rect/al

Exercise 28

Pronounce and Spell

Exercise 29

1. m
2. e
3. h
4. c
5. l
6. i
7. k
8. a
9. d
10. j
11. b
12. n
13. g
14. f

Copyright © 2022, Elsevier Inc. All rights reserved.

Exercise 30

A *Label*

1. stoma
2. palpate
3. reflux
4. ascites

B *Identify*

1. feces
2. diarrhea
3. gastric lavage
4. emesis
5. hematochezia
6. melena
7. nausea
8. malabsorption
9. hematemesis
10. flatus

Exercise 31

Review of Complementary Terms

Exercise 32

1. UGI
2. *H. pylori*
3. N&V
4. ERCP
5. GI
6. UPPP
7. GERD
8. UC
9. BE
10. IBS
11. EGD
12. PEG
13. EUS
14. APR
15. FOBT
16. FIT

Exercise 33

A. felt sick to her stomach, throwing up, difficult to eat, stomach doctor

B. Answers will vary and may include nausea, emesis, dysphagia, and gastroenterologist, along with their respective definitions.

C. Esophagogastroduodenoscopy (EGD), gastroscope, *H. pylori*, peptic ulcer

D. Answers will vary and may include esophagogastroduodenoscopy (EGD), gastroscope, *Helicobacter pylori*, peptic ulcer, along with their respective definitions.

Exercise 34

A

1. hematochezia
2. diarrhea
3. nausea
4. emesis
5. gastroesophageal reflux disease (GERD)
6. *Helicobacter pylori* stool antigen
7. peptic ulcer
8. Crohn disease
9. ulcerative colitis
10. colorectal
11. esophagitis
12. ascites
13. hepatomegaly
14. hemorrhoids
15. colonoscopy

B

1. d
2. b
3. a
4. d

Exercise 35

Online Exercise

Exercise 36

Pronunciation Exercise

Exercise 37

1. a
2. b
3. a
4. a
5. c
6. a
7. c
8. a
9. b
10. c
11. c
12. a
13. a
14. b
15. c
16. a
17. c
18. b
19. b
20. c

ANSWERS TO CHAPTER 12 EXERCISES

Exercise 1

A *Label*

1. eye: ocul/o, ophthalm/o
2. eyelid: blephar/o
3. tear(s): dacry/o, lacrim/o
4. pupil: cor/o, pupill/o
5. sclera: scler/o
6. iris: ir/o, irid/o
7. vision: opt/o
8. conjunctiva: conjunctiv/o
9. uvea: uve/o
10. cornea: corne/o, kerat/o
11. lens: phac/o, phak/o
12. retina: retin/o

B *Define and Match*

1. e, sclera
2. a, pupil
3. i, cornea
4. h, conjunctiva
5. f, tear(s)
6. j, uvea
7. b, lens
8. c, eye
9. d, iris
10. a, pupil
11. i, cornea
12. c, eye
13. f, tear(s)
14. g, retina
15. eyelid
16. vision

Exercise 2

A *Define*

1. tension, pressure
2. light
3. cold
4. two, double
5. equal
6. bladder, sac
7. dry, dryness
8. vessel(s); blood vessel(s)
9. nose
10. fungus
11. developing cell, germ cell
12. white
13. false
14. nose

B *Identify*

1. cry/o
2. ton/o
3. cyst/o
4. dipl/o
5. phot/o
6. is/o
7. leuk/o
8. pseud/o
9. blast/o
10. myc/o
11. xer/o
12. angi/o
13. nas/o, rhin/o

Exercise 3

A *Define*

1. within
2. absence of, without
3. within
4. absence of, without
5. two

B *Identify*

1. bin-
2. a-, an-
3. endo-, intra-

Exercise 4

A *Identify*

1. -al
2. -ar
3. -ary
4. -eal
5. -ic

(answers may be in any order)

B *Match*

1. g
2. h
3. f
4. i
5. j
6. d
7. e
8. b
9. c
10. a

Copyright © 2022, Elsevier Inc. All rights reserved.

C *Label*

1. -opia
2. -phobia
3. -plegia

D *Define*

1. visual examination
2. inflammation
3. softening
4. surgical repair

E *Identify*

1. -logy
2. -metry
3. -tomy
4. -oma
5. -pexy
6. -ia

Exercise 5

Pronounce and Spell

Exercise 6

1. WR S
scler/itis
inflammation of the sclera

2. WR CV S
ophthalm/o/plegia
CF
paralysis of the eye (muscles)

3. WR CV S
retin/o/pathy
CF
disease of the retina

4. P WR S
end/ophthalm/itis
inflammation within the eye *Note: the o in the prefix endo- is dropped*

5. WR WR S
xer/ophthalm/ia
condition of dry eye *Note: the o in the combining form xer/o is dropped*

6. P WR S
a/phak/ia
condition of without a lens

7. WR CV S
ophthalm/o/pathy
CF
disease of the eye

8. WR CV S
scler/o/malacia
CF
softening of the sclera

9. WR S
uve/itis
inflammation of the uvea

10. WR CV S
kerat/o/malacia
CF
softening of the cornea

Exercise 7

A *Label*

1. retin/o/blast/oma
2. leuk/o/cor/ia
3. blephar/itis
4. blephar/o/ptosis
5. conjunctiv/itis
6. dacry/o/cyst/itis

B *Fill In*

1. ir/itis
2. ocul/o/myc/osis
3. ophthalm/algia
4. dipl/opia
5. kerat/itis
6. uve/o/scler/itis
7. irid/o/plegia
8. phac/o/malacia

Exercise 8

Pronounce and Spell

Exercise 9

A *Identify*

1. myopia
2. presbyopia
3. anisometropia
4. astigmatism
5. Nystagmus
6. glaucoma
7. hyperopia
8. Retinitis pigmentosa
9. nyctalopia
10. amblyopia

B *Label*

1. drusen
2. macular degeneration
3. pterygium
4. pinguecula
5. chalazion
6. sty
7. cataract
8. hyphema
9. strabismus
10. retinal detachment

C *Match*

1. h
2. e
3. a
4. g
5. b
6. c
7. j
8. d
9. f
10. i

D *Match*

1. i
2. b
3. f
4. h
5. a
6. c
7. d
8. j
9. e
10. g

Exercise 10

Review of Disease and Disorder Terms

Exercise 11

Pronounce and Spell

Exercise 12

A *Analyze and Define*

1. WR CV S
kerat/o/plasty
CF
surgical repair of the cornea

2. WR CV S
scler/o/tomy
CF
incision into the sclera

3. WR CV WR CV S
cry/o/retin/o/pexy
CF CF
surgical fixation of the retina by using extreme cold

4. WR CV S
blephar/o/plasty
CF
surgical repair of the eyelid

5. WR S
irid/ectomy
excision (of part) of the iris

6. WR CV WR CV WR CV S
dacry/o/cyst/o/rhin/o/stomy
CF CF CF
creation of an artificial opening between the tear (lacrimal) sac and the nose

7. WR CV S
irid/o/tomy
CF
incision into the iris

B *Label*

1. kerat/o/plasty
2. irid/o/tomy
3. cry/o/retin/o/pexy

C *Fill In*

1. dacry/o/cyst/o/rhin/o/stomy
2. irid/ectomy
3. scler/o/tomy
4. blephar/o/plasty

Exercise 13

A *Label*

1. photorefractive keratectomy
2. LASIK
3. scleral buckling
4. phacoemulsification

Copyright © 2022, Elsevier Inc. All rights reserved.

B *Identify*
1. Retinal photocoagulation
2. enucleation
3. Trabeculectomy
4. vitrectomy

C *Match*

1. e	5. d
2. f	6. h
3. b	7. g
4. a	8. c

Exercise 14
Review of Surgical Terms

Exercise 15
Pronounce and Spell

Exercise 16

A *Fill In*
1. ton/o/metry
2. kerat/o/meter
3. opt/o/metry
4. ton/o/meter
5. pupill/o/scope
6. retin/o/scopy

B *Label*
1. fluorescein angi/o/graphy
2. pupill/o/meter
3. ophthalm/o/scopy
4. ophthalm/o/scope

C *Analyze and Define*
1. WR CV S
pupill/o/scope
CF
instrument used for visual examination of the pupil
2. WR CV S
opt/o/metry
CF
measurement of vision
3. WR CV S
ophthalm/o/scope
CF
instrument used for visual examination of the eye
4. WR CV S
ton/o/metry
CF
measurement of pressure (within the eye)
5. WR CV S
pupill/o/meter
CF
instrument used to measure the pupil (diameter)
6. WR CV S
ton/o/meter
CF
instrument used to measure pressure (within the eye)
7. WR CV S
kerat/o/meter
CF
instrument used to measure (the curvature of) the cornea
8. WR CV S
ophthalm/o/scopy
CF
visual examination of the eye
9. WR CV S
(fluorescein) angi/o/graphy
CF
radiographic imaging of the blood vessels (of the eye with fluorescing dye)
10. WR CV S
retin/o/scopy
CF
visual examination of the retina

Exercise 17

A *Label*
1. slit lamp
2. optical coherence tomography

B *Identify*
1. Optical coherence tomography
2. slit lamp

Exercise 18
Review of Diagnostic Terms

Exercise 19
Pronounce and Spell

Exercise 20

A *Analyze and Define*
1. WR CV S
ophthalm/o/logy
CF
study of the eye
2. P WR S
bin/ocul/ar
pertaining to two or both eyes
3. WR S
lacrim/al
pertaining to tears
4. WR S
pupill/ary
pertaining to the pupil
5. WR CV S
ophthalm/o/logist
CF
physician (surgeon) who studies and treats diseases of the eye
6. WR S
corne/al
pertaining to the cornea
7. WR S
ophthalm/ic
pertaining to the eye
8. WR CV WR S
nas/o/lacrim/al
CF
pertaining to the nose and tear (ducts)
9. WR S
opt/ic
pertaining to vision
10. P WR S
intra/ocul/ar
pertaining to within the eye
11. WR S
retin/al
pertaining to the retina
12. WR CV S
phot/o/phobia
CF
abnormal fear of (sensitivity to) light
13. WR CV WR S
is/o/cor/ia
CF
condition of equal pupil (size)
14. P WR CV WR S
an/is/o/cor/ia
CF
condition of absence of equal pupil (size)
15. WR CV WR S
pseud/o/phak/ia
CF
condition of false lens

B *Label*
1. bin/ocul/ar
2. retin/al
3. lacrim/al
4. an/is/o/cor/ia
5. opt/ic
6. ophthalm/o/logist

C *Fill In*
1. ophthalm/o/logy
2. pseud/o/phak/ia
3. is/o/cor/ia
4. intra/ocul/ar
5. phot/o/phobia
6. pupill/ary
7. ophthalm/ic
8. corne/al
9. nas/o/lacrim/al

Copyright © 2022, Elsevier Inc. All rights reserved.

Exercise 21

A *Label*

1. mydriatic
2. miotic
3. intraocular lens
4. visual acuity

B *Identify*

1. optometrist
2. optician
3. emmetropia

C *Match*

1. d
2. e
3. a
4. f
5. g
6. b
7. c

Exercise 22

Review of Complementary Terms

Exercise 23

1. fluorescein angiography, optical coherence tomography, age-related macular degeneration
2. visual acuity, phacoemulsification, intraocular lens
3. photorefractive keratectomy, laser-assisted in situ keratomileusis, astigmatism, emmetropia
4. intraocular pressure, ophthalmology

Exercise 24

A. one of his eyes seemed to move more slowly and to look in a different direction; white part of the same eye seemed to be irritated and looked red and inflamed; pupil looked white; eye physician
B. Answers will vary and may include amblyopia, strabismus, scleritis, leukocoria, and ophthalmologist along with their respective definitions.
C. ophthalmologist; leukocoria; strabismus; amblyopia; scleritis; ophthalmoscopy; visual acuity; retinal; retinoblastoma
D. Answers will vary and may include ophthalmologist, leukocoria, strabismus, amblyopia, scleritis, ophthalmoscopy, visual acuity, retinal, and retinoblastoma along with their respective definitions.

Exercise 25

A

1. ophthalmology
2. glaucoma
3. pterygium
4. blepharoptosis
5. astigmatism
6. presbyopia
7. retinopathy
8. cataract

B

1. b
2. d
3. b
4. c

Exercise 26

Online Exercise

Exercise 27

Pronunciation Exercise

Exercise 28

1. b
2. a
3. b
4. c
5. a
6. a
7. b
8. a
9. c
10. c
11. b
12. a
13. b
14. a
15. c
16. b
17. c
18. a
19. b
20. c

ANSWERS TO CHAPTER 13 EXERCISES

Exercise 1

A *Label*

1. ear: aur/i, ot/o
2. hearing: audi/o
3. middle ear: tympan/o
4. stapes: staped/o
5. tympanic membrane: myring/o
6. mastoid bone: mastoid/o

B *Label*

1. labyrinth: labyrinth/o
2. cochlea: cochle/o
3. vestibule: vestibul/o

C *Define and Match*

1. g, stapes
2. d, vestibule
3. a, ear
4. f, cochlea
5. e, labyrinth
6. b, tympanic membrane (eardrum)
7. h, middle ear
8. a, ear
9. c, mastoid bone
10. hearing

Exercise 2

A *Define*

1. fungus
2. pus
3. electricity, electrical activity

B *Identify*

1. electr/o
2. myc/o
3. py/o

C *Identify*

1. -graphy
2. -itis
3. -al, -ar
4. -gram

Exercise 3

A *Match*

1. d
2. g
3. a
4. e
5. c
6. j
7. f
8. b
9. h
10. i

B *Define*

1. creation of an artificial opening
2. visual examination
3. measurement
4. study of

Exercise 4

Pronounce and Spell

Exercise 5

1. WR CV WR S
   ot/o/myc/osis
   CF
   abnormal condition of fungus in the ear
2. WR S
   ot/algia
   pain in the ear
3. WR S
   labyrinth/itis
   inflammation of the labyrinth
4. WR S
   myring/itis
   inflammation of the tympanic membrane

Copyright © 2022, Elsevier Inc. All rights reserved.

5. WR CV S
ot/o/sclerosis
CF
hardening of the ear (stapes)
6. WR S
mastoid/itis
inflammation of the mastoid bone
7. WR CV WR CV S
ot/o/py/o/rrhea
CF CF
discharge of pus from the ear
8. WR CV S
ot/o/rrhea
CF
discharge from the ear

Exercise 6

A *Label*

1. ot/o/py/o/rrhea
2. myring/itis

B *Fill In*

1. mastoid/itis
2. ot/algia
3. ot/o/sclerosis
4. ot/o/myc/osis
5. labyrinth/itis
6. ot/o/rrhea

Exercise 7

Pronounce and Spell

Exercise 8

A *Identify*

1. vertigo; tinnitus
2. Ménière
3. Presbycusis
4. ototoxicity

B *Label*

1. otitis externa
2. otitis media
3. cholesteatoma
4. acoustic neuroma

Exercise 9

1. d
2. e
3. i
4. f
5. c
6. a
7. g
8. h
9. b

Exercise 10

Review of Disease and Disorder Terms

Exercise 11

Pronounce and Spell

Exercise 12

1. WR S
mastoid/ectomy
excision of the mastoid bone
2. WR CV S
myring/o/tomy
CF
incision into the tympanic membrane
3. WR S
labyrinth/ectomy
excision of the labyrinth
4. WR CV S
mastoid/o/tomy
CF
incision into the mastoid bone
5. WR CV S
tympan/o/plasty
CF
surgical repair of the middle ear
6. WR CV S
myring/o/plasty
CF
surgical repair of the tympanic membrane
7. WR S
staped/ectomy
excision of the stapes
8. WR S
cochle/ar (implant)
pertaining to the cochlea (implant)
9. WR CV S
ot/o/plasty
CF
surgical repair of the (outer) ear
10. WR CV S
tympan/o/stomy
CF
creation of an artificial opening into the middle ear

Exercise 13

A *Fill In*

1. mastoid/o/tomy
2. labyrinth/ectomy
3. tympan/o/plasty
4. mastoid/ectomy
5. ot/o/plasty
6. myring/o/plasty

B *Label*

1. myring/o/tomy
2. cochle/ar implant
3. staped/ectomy
4. tympan/o/stomy

Exercise 14

Review of Surgical Terms

Exercise 15

Pronounce and Spell

Exercise 16

1. WR CV S
ot/o/scope
CF
instrument used for visual examination of the ear
2. WR CV S
audi/o/metry
CF
measurement of hearing
3. WR CV S
audi/o/gram
CF
(graphic) record of hearing
4. WR CV S
ot/o/scopy
CF
visual examination of the ear
5. WR CV S
audi/o/meter
CF
instrument used to measure hearing
6. WR CV S
tympan/o/metry
CF
measurement of middle ear (function)
7. WR CV S
tympan/o/meter
CF
instrument used to measure middle ear (function)
8. WR CV WR CV S
electro/o/cochle/o/graphy
CF CF
process of recording the electrical activity in the cochlea

Exercise 17

A *Label*

1. audi/o/meter
2. audi/o/gram
3. ot/o/scopy
4. tympan/o/meter

B *Fill In*

1. tympan/o/metry
2. ot/o/scope
3. audi/o/metry
4. electr/o/cochle/o/graphy

Exercise 18

Review of Diagnostic Terms

Copyright © 2022, Elsevier Inc. All rights reserved.

Exercise 19
Pronounce and Spell

Exercise 20
1. WR CV WR CV S
   ot/o/laryng/o/logy
   CF CF
   study of the ear, (nose), and larynx (throat)
2. WR CV S
   audi/o/logist
   CF
   one who studies and specializes in hearing
3. WR CV WR CV S
   ot/o/laryng/o/logist
   CF CF
   physician who studies and treats diseases of the ear, (nose), and larynx (throat)
4. WR CV S
   audi/o/logy
   CF
   study of hearing
5. WR S
   aur/al
   pertaining to the ear
6. WR S
   cochle/ar
   pertaining to the cochlea
7. WR S
   vestibul/ar
   pertaining to the vestibule
8. WR CV WR S
   vestibul/o/cochle/ar
   CF
   pertaining to the vestibule and the cochlea

Exercise 21
A *Label*
1. aur/al
2. cochle/ar
3. ot/o/laryng/o/logist
4. audi/o/logist

B *Fill In*
1. audi/o/logy
2. ot/o/laryng/o/logy
3. vestibul/o/cochle/ar
4. vestibul/ar

Exercise 22
Review of Complementary Terms

Exercise 23
1. otitis media; acute otitis media
2. benign paroxysmal positional vertigo; ears, nose, throat; otolaryngologist
3. otitis externa
4. hard of hearing

Exercise 24
A. middle ear infections (inflammation); ear as if it is painful; pus-like liquid coming out of her left ear; redness and swelling on her skull behind Marisol's earlobe; ear, nose, and throat physician
B. Answers will vary and may include otitis media, otalgia, otopyorrhea, mastoiditis, and otolaryngologist along with their respective definitions.
C. mastoiditis, otitis media, otalgia, otopyorrhea, otoscopy, otitis externa, tympanometry, mastoiditis, myringotomies, and mastoidectomy
D. Answers will vary and may include mastoiditis, otitis media, otalgia, otopyorrhea, otoscopy, otitis externa, tympanometry, mastoiditis, myringotomies, and mastoidectomy along with their respective definitions.

Exercise 25
A
1. ENT
2. tinnitus
3. vertigo
4. otoscopy
5. otitis media
6. presbycusis
7. audiologist
8. audiometry

B
1. a
2. b
3. d

Exercise 26
Online Exercise

Exercise 27
Pronunciation Exercise

Exercise 28
1. c
2. a
3. c
4. a
5. c
6. a
7. b
8. a
9. c
10. a
11. c
12. a
13. c
14. a
15. b
16. b
17. c
18. a
19. c
20. b

ANSWERS TO CHAPTER 14 EXERCISES

Exercise 1
A *Label*
1. bone: oste/o
2. mandible: mandibul/o
3. sternum: stern/o
4. phalanges: phalang/o
5. patella: patell/o
6. tarsals: tars/o
7. phalanges: phalang/o
8. cranium: crani/o
9. maxilla: maxill/o
10. clavicle: clavicul/o
11. ribs: costul/o
12. lumbar: lumb/o
13. femur: femor/o
14. fibula: fibul/o
15. tibia: tibi/o

B *Label*
1. vertebra: rachi/o, spondyl/o, vertebr/o
2. pelvis: pelv/i
3. scapula: scapul/o
4. humerus: humer/o
5. ulna: uln/o
6. radius: radi/o
7. carpals: carp/o
8. ilium: ili/o
9. sacrum: sacr/o
10. pubis: pub/o
11. ischium: ischi/o

C *Define and Match*
1. f: vertebra, spine, vertebral column
2. d: patella
3. a: maxilla
4. b: phalanx
5. c: carpals
6. e: humerus

D *Define and Match*
1. d: loin, lumbar spine
2. e: ischium
3. a: pubis
4. b: vertebra, spine, vertebral column
5. f: scapula
6. c: tarsals
7. g: pelvis, pelvic cavity

E *Define and Match*
1. c: mandible
2. g: sacrum

Copyright © 2022, Elsevier Inc. All rights reserved.

3. a: femur
4. f: clavicle
5. b: ilium
6. d: vertebra, spine, vertebral column
7. e: sternum

F *Identify*

1. rib: cost/o
2. radius: radi/o
3. tibia: tibi/o
4. fibula: fibul/o
5. ulna: uln/o
6. cranium: crani/o
7. bone: oste/o
8. bone marrow: myel/o

Exercise 2

A *Label*

1. joint: arthr/o
2. synovial membrane: synovi/o
3. meniscus: menisc/o
4. cartilage: chondr/o
5. tendon: ten/o, tendin/o
6. bursa: burs/o
7. lamina: lamin/o

B *Define and Match*

1. c: intervertebral disk
2. d: synovia, synovial membrane
3. e: fascia
4. a: tendon
5. b: joint

C *Define and Match*

1. e: muscle
2. b: tendon
3. c: bursa
4. d: meniscus
5. a: cartilage
6. e: muscle

Exercise 3

A *Define*

1. rod-shaped, striated
2. stone
3. movement, motion
4. death
5. blood
6. electricity, electrical activity
7. hump (increased convexity of the spine)
8. stiff, bent
9. (lateral) curved (spine)
10. bent forward (increased concavity of the spine)
11. flesh, connective tissue

B *Identify*

1. electr/o
2. petr/o
3. kinesi/o
4. rhabd/o
5. hem/o
6. necr/o
7. kyph/o
8. ankyl/o
9. scoli/o
10. lord/o
11. sarc/o

Exercise 4

A *Define*

1. above
2. together, joined
3. between

B *Identify*

1. syn-
2. inter-
3. supra-
4. sub-
5. a-
6. poly-
7. brady-
8. micro-
9. hyper-
10. intra-
11. dys-

Exercise 5

A *Define*

1. surgical fixation, fusion
2. split, fissure
3. weakness
4. nourishment, development
5. pertaining to

B *Identify*

1. -asthenia
2. -desis
3. -schisis
4. -trophy
5. -a, -is

C *Match*

1. f
2. h
3. b
4. c
5. d
6. g
7. e
8. a

D *Match*

1. d
2. c
3. e
4. f
5. b
6. a
7. h
8. g
9. i

Exercise 6

Pronounce and Spell

Exercise 7

1. WR S
   oste/itis
   inflammation of the bone
2. WR CV WR S
   ten/o/synov/itis
   CF
   inflammation of the tendon and synovial membrane
3. WR CV WR S
   oste/o/petr/osis
   CF
   abnormal condition of stonelike bones (very dense bones caused by defective resorption of bone)
4. WR CV S
   oste/o/malacia
   CF
   softening of bone
5. WR CV S
   chondr/o/sarcoma
   CF
   malignant tumor of cartilage
6. WR CV WR S
   oste/o/chondr/oma
   CF
   tumor composed of bone and cartilage (benign)
7. WR S
   disc/itis
   inflammation of an intervertebral disk
8. WR CV WR S
   oste/o/necr/osis
   CF
   abnormal condition of bone death
9. WR CV S
   sarc/o/penia
   CF
   abnormal reduction of connective tissue
10. WR CV S
    synovi/o/sarcoma
    CF
    malignant tumor of the synovial membrane
11. WR S
    my/asthenia
    muscle weakness
12. WR S
    spondyl/osis
    abnormal condition of the vertebrae
13. WR CV S
    crani/o/schisis
    CF
    fissure (split) of the cranium
14. WR CV S
    chondr/o/malacia
    CF
    softening of cartilage
15. WR S
    ankyl/osis
    abnormal condition of stiffness
16. WR S
    menisc/itis
    inflammation of the meniscus
17. WR CV WR S
    fibr/o/my/algia
    CF
    pain in the fibrous tissues and muscles
18. WR CV
    fasci/itis
    inflammation of the fascia (connective tissue enclosing and separating muscle layers)

Copyright © 2022, Elsevier Inc. All rights reserved.

Exercise 8

A *Label*

1. lord/osis
2. kyph/osis
3. scoli/osis
4. oste/o/sarcoma
5. burs/itis
6. oste/o/arthr/itis

B *Fill In*

1. oste/o/chondr/itis
2. oste/o/myel/itis
3. arthr/itis
4. rhabd/o/my/o/lysis
5. myel/oma
6. tendin/itis
7. spondyl/osis
8. oste/o/penia
9. rachi/schisis
10. spondyl/arthr/itis

Exercise 9

Pronounce and Spell

Exercise 10

1. c
2. a
3. b
4. d
5. e
6. i
7. j
8. h
9. g
10. f

Exercise 11

1. herniated disk
2. rheumatoid arthritis
3. carpal tunnel syndrome
4. spondylolisthesis
5. gout
6. osteoporosis
7. fracture
8. Lyme disease
9. bunion
10. spinal stenosis
11. plantar fasciitis
12. ganglion cyst
13. rotator cuff disease
14. dislocation

Exercise 12

1. Spine:
   a. spondylolisthesis
   b. herniated disk
   c. ankylosing spondylitis
   d. spinal stenosis
2. Joints:
   a. bunion
   b. tarsal tunnel syndrome
   c. carpal tunnel syndrome
   d. ganglion cyst
   e. gout
   f. Lyme disease
   g. rheumatoid arthritis
   h. dislocation
   i. subluxation
   j. repetitive strain injury
3. Bone:
   a. exostosis
   b. fracture
   c. osteoporosis
4. Muscle:
   a. rotator cuff disease
   b. strain
   c. sprain
   d. compartment syndrome
   e. plantar fasciitis
   f. myasthenia gravis
   g. muscular dystrophy

Exercise 13

Review of Terms

Exercise 14

Pronounce and Spell

Exercise 15

1. WR CV S
   vertebr/o/plasty
   CF
   surgical repair of a vertebra
2. WR S
   tars/ectomy
   excision of (one or more) tarsal bones
3. WR CV S
   arthr/o/desis
   CF
   surgical fixation of a joint
4. WR S
   lamin/ectomy
   excision of a lamina
5. WR S
   synov/ectomy
   excision of the synovial membrane
6. WR CV S
   fasci/o/tomy
   CF
   incision into fascia (to relieve tension or pressure)
7. WR CV S
   rachi/o/tomy
   CF
   incision into the vertebral column
8. WR S
   burs/ectomy
   excision of a bursa
9. WR S
   disc/ectomy
   excision of an intervertebral disk
10. WR CV S
    arthr/o/centesis
    CF
    surgical puncture to aspirate fluid from a joint
11. WR S
    maxill/ectomy
    excision of the maxilla
12. WR CV S
    crani/o/plasty
    CF
    surgical repair of the skull
13. WR S
    carp/ectomy
    excision of a carpal bone
14. WR S
    phalang/ectomy
    excision of a finger or toe bone

Exercise 16

A *Label*

1. micro/disc/ectomy
2. arthr/o/plasty
3. spondyl/o/syn/desis
4. menisc/ectomy
5. crani/o/tomy
6. ten/o/rrhaphy

B *Fill In*

1. oste/o/tomy
2. chondr/ectomy
3. chondr/o/plasty
4. my/o/rrhaphy
5. ten/o/my/o/plasty
6. cost/ectomy

Exercise 17

Review of Terms

Exercise 18

Pronounce and Spell

Exercise 19

A *Analyze and Define*

1. WR CV WR CV S
   electr/o/my/o/gram
   CF CF
   record of the electrical activity in a muscle
2. WR CV S
   arthr/o/graphy
   CF
   radiographic imaging of a joint
3. WR CV S
   arthr/o/scopy
   CF
   visual examination of a joint
4. WR CV S
   myel/o/graphy
   CF
   radiographic imaging of the spinal cord

B *Build*

1. arthr/o/graphy
2. myel/o/graphy

Copyright © 2022, Elsevier Inc. All rights reserved.

C *Label*
1. arthr/o/scopy
2. electr/o/my/o/gram

Exercise 20
A *Match*

1. b	4. c
2. a	5. b
3. c	6. a

B *Label*
1. dual x-ray absorptiometry
2. muscle biopsy
3. bone markers

Exercise 21
Review of Terms

Exercise 22
Pronounce and Spell

Exercise 23
Note: the abbreviation S(WR) indicates a suffix with an embedded word root.

1. WR S
   my/algia
   muscle pain
2. WR S
   arthr/algia
   joint pain
3. P S(WR)
   hyper/trophy
   excessive development
4. P S(WR)
   a/trophy
   without development
5. P WR S
   hyper/kinesi/a
   excessive movement (hyperactivity)
6. P WR S
   dys/kinesi/a
   difficult movement
7. P WR S
   brady/kinesi/a
   slow movement
8. WR WR S
   hem/arthr/osis
   abnormal condition of blood in the joint
9. P S(WR)
   dys/trophy
   abnormal development

Exercise 24
A *Fill in*
1. supra/clavicul/ar
2. supra/patell/ar
3. inter/vertebr/al
4. sub/maxill/ary
5. sub/mandibul/ar
6. sub/stern/al
7. intra/crani/al
8. inter/cost/al
9. patell/o/femor/al

B *Label*

1. scapul/ar	12. crani/al
2. humer/al	13. clavicul/ar
3. stern/al	14. lumb/ar
4. vertebr/al	15. radi/al
5. ili/ac	16. uln/ar
6. carp/al	17. sacr/al
7. phalang/eal	18. ischi/al
8. pub/ic	19. femor/al
9. patell/ar	20. fibul/ar
10. tars/al	21. tibi/al
11. phalang/eal	

Exercise 25
Pronounce and Spell

Exercise 26
A *Identify*
1. rheumatology
2. orthotics
3. crepitus
4. chiropractic
5. orthopedics
6. osteopathy
7. prosthesis (*pl.* prostheses)

B *Label*
1. orthopedist
2. rheumatologist
3. podiatrist
4. orthotist
5. chiropractor
6. osteopath

Exercise 27

1. d	5. g
2. h	6. c
3. a	7. b
4. f	8. e

Exercise 28

1. h	6. a
2. d	7. g
3. i	8. f
4. e	9. b
5. c	

Exercise 29
Review of Terms

Exercise 30
1. cervical vertebrae; thoracic vertebrae; lumbar vertebrae
2. rheumatoid arthritis
3. osteoarthritis
4. myasthenia gravis
5. electromyogram; polymyositis
6. carpal tunnel syndrome; orthopedics
7. muscular dystrophy
8. herniated nucleus pulposus
9. total hip arthroplasty
10. Doctor of Osteopathy
11. total knee arthroplasty
12. repetitive strain injury
13. fracture
14. dual x-ray absorptiometry; dual-energy x-ray absorptiometry
15. Doctor of Chiropractic

Exercise 31
A. finger and wrist bones, broken, musculoskeletal specialist, bones are not dense enough
B. Answers will vary and may include carpal, fracture, orthopedist, osteoporosis, along with their respective definitions.
C. kyphosis, fracture, radial, osteoporosis, dual x-ray absorptiometry (DXA), carpal
D. Answers will vary and may include kyphosis, fracture, radial, osteoporosis, dual x-ray absorptiometry (DXA), and carpal, along with their respective definitions.

Exercise 32
A
1. orthopedic
2. arthroscopy
3. arthritis
4. medial
5. suprapatellar
6. chondromalacia
7. pathology

B
1. c
2. b

Exercise 33
Electronic Health Records Online

Exercise 34
Pronunciation Exercise

Exercise 35

1. epiphyses	4. prosthesis
2. phalanx	5. bursae
3. vertebrae	6. laminae

Exercise 36

1. b	11. a
2. c	12. c
3. a	13. b
4. b	14. a
5. c	15. b
6. b	16. a
7. c	17. b
8. c	18. c
9. a	19. a
10. c	20. c

Copyright © 2022, Elsevier Inc. All rights reserved.

ANSWERS TO CHAPTER 15 EXERCISES

Exercise 1

A *Label*

1. brain: encephal/o
2. spinal cord: myel/o
3. cerebrum: cerebr/o
4. cerebellum: cerebell/o
5. meninges: meningi/o, mening/o

B *Identify*

1. glia: gli/o
2. nerve: neur/o

C *Label*

1. gray matter: poli/o
2. ganglion: gangli/o, ganglion/o
3. dura mater: dur/o
4. nerve root: radicul/o, rhiz/o

D *Define and Match*

1. e, ganglion
2. d, dura mater
3. c, brain
4. a, cerebellum
5. f, meninges
6. b, nerve

E *Define and Match*

1. b, glia
2. d, ganglion
3. e, meninges
4. f, cerebrum, brain
5. a, spinal cord
6. c, gray matter

F *Identify*

1. radicul/o, rhiz/o

Exercise 2

A *Define*

1. one, single
2. mind
3. four
4. mind
5. speech
6. sensation, sensitivity, feeling

B *Match*

1. b
2. h
3. a
4. a
5. f
6. c
7. e
8. d
9. g

Exercise 3

1. i
2. d
3. c
4. k
5. j
6. e
7. a
8. f
9. h
10. b
11. g

Exercise 4

A *Define*

1. slight paralysis
2. treatment, specialty
3. seizure, attack
4. specialist, physician

B *Match*

1. e
2. h
3. d
4. k
5. j
6. g
7. b
8. a
9. i
10. c
11. f

C *Match*

1. e
2. g
3. i
4. b
5. f
6. a
7. k
8. j
9. c
10. d
11. h

Exercise 5

Pronounce and Spell

Exercise 6

1. WR S
   myel/itis
   inflammation of the spinal cord
2. WR CV WR S
   hydr/o/cephal/us
   CF
   water (increased amount of cerebrospinal fluid) in the head (brain)
3. WR CV WR S
   poli/o/myel/itis
   CF
   inflammation of the gray matter of the spinal cord
4. WR CV S
   radicul/o/pathy
   CF
   disease of the nerve roots
5. WR CV S
   encephal/o/pathy
   CF
   disease of the brain
6. WR S
   encephal/itis
   inflammation of the brain
7. WR CV WR CV WR S
   rhiz/o/mening/o/myel/itis
   CF CF
   inflammation of the nerve root, meninges, and spinal cord
8. WR S WR S
   cerebr/al thromb/osis
   pertaining to the cerebrum, abnormal condition of a blood clot
9. WR CV S
   mening/o/cele
   CF
   protrusion of the meninges
10. WR CV S
    myel/o/malacia
    CF
    softening of the spinal cord
11. WR S
    radicul/itis
    inflammation of the nerve roots
12. WR S
    gangli/itis
    inflammation of a ganglion
13. WR S
    dur/itis
    inflammation of the dura mater
14. P WR S
    poly/neur/itis
    inflammation of many nerves

Exercise 7

A *Label*

1. mon/o/neur/o/pathy
2. poly/neur/o/pathy
3. gli/o/blast/oma
4. meningi/oma
5. intra/cerebr/al hem/o/rrhage
6. cerebr/al embol/ism
7. sub/dur/al hemat/oma
8. neur/algia

B *Fill In*

1. neur/itis
2. gli/oma
3. encephal/o/malacia
4. cerebell/itis
5. encephal/o/myel/o/radicul/itis
6. mening/itis
7. mening/o/myel/o/cele

Exercise 8

Pronounce and Spell

Exercise 9

1. h
2. g
3. a
4. f
5. b
6. c
7. e
8. d

Exercise 10

1. sciatica
2. Alzheimer disease
3. shingles
4. cerebral aneurysm
5. subarachnoid hemorrhage
6. stroke
7. transient ischemic attack
8. Bell palsy

Copyright © 2022, Elsevier Inc. All rights reserved.

Exercise 11
Review of Disease and Disorder Terms

Exercise 12
Pronounce and Spell

Exercise 13
1. WR S
   neur/ectomy
   excision of a nerve
2. WR CV S
   neur/o/rrhaphy
   CF
   suturing of a nerve
3. WR S
   ganglion/ectomy
   excision of a ganglion
4. WR CV S
   neur/o/tomy
   CF
   incision into a nerve
5. WR CV S
   neur/o/lysis
   CF
   loosening, separating a nerve (to release it from surrounding tissue)
6. WR CV S
   neur/o/plasty
   CF
   surgical repair of a nerve
7. WR CV S
   rhiz/o/tomy
   CF
   incision into a nerve root

Exercise 14
A *Fill In*
1. neur/ectomy
2. neur/o/rrhaphy
3. neur/o/tomy
4. neur/o/lysis
5. neur/o/plasty

B *Label*
1. rhiz/o/tomy
2. ganglion/ectomy

Exercise 15
Review of Surgical Terms

Exercise 16
Pronounce and Spell

Exercise 17
A *Analyze and Define*
1. WR CV WR CV S
   electr/o/encephal/o/gram
   CF CF
   record of the electrical activity of the brain
2. WR CV WR CV S
   electr/o/encephal/o/graph
   CF CF
   instrument used to record the electrical activity of the brain
3. WR CV WR CV S
   electr/o/encephal/o/graphy
   CF CF
   process of recording the electrical activity of the brain
4. WR CV S
   CT myel/o/graphy
   CF
   process of recording (scan of) the spinal cord
5. WR S WR CV S
   cerebr/al angio/o/graphy
   CF
   process of recording (scan of) the blood vessels of the cerebrum

B *Label*
1. CT myel/o/graphy
2. cerebr/al angi/o/graphy

C *Fill In*
1. electr/o/encephal/o/gram
2. electr/o/encephal/o/graph
3. electr/o/encephal/o/graphy

Exercise 18
A *Match*
1. c
2. d
3. a
4. b

B *Label*
1. evoked potential studies
2. lumbar puncture
3. deep tendon reflexes
4. positron emission tomography scan

Exercise 19
Review of Diagnostic Terms

Exercise 20
Pronounce and Spell

Exercise 21
1. P S(WR)
   pre/ictal
   (occurring) before a seizure or attack
2. P WR S
   par/esthesi/a
   abnormal sensation *(Note: the a is dropped from the prefix para.)*
3. WR S
   ment/al
   pertaining to the mind
4. P S(WR)
   inter/ictal
   (occurring) between seizures or attacks
5. WR CV S
   mon/o/paresis
   CF
   slight paralysis of one (limb)
6. P WR S
   dys/esthesi/a
   painful sensation

Exercise 22
A *Label*
1. hemi/plegia
2. quadr/i/plegia
3. an/esthesi/a
4. ceph/algia *(NOTE: the al is dropped from the combining form cephal/o)*
5. neur/o/logy
6. a/phas/ia

B *Fill In*
1. hemi/paresis
2. dys/phas/ia
3. hyper/esthesi/a
4. crani/o/cerebr/al
5. mon/o/paresis
6. post/ictal
7. neur/o/logist

Exercise 23
Pronounce and Spell

Exercise 24
A *Label*
1. paraplegia
2. concussion
3. syncope
4. ataxia
5. dysarthria
6. coma

B *Identify*
1. spasticity
2. unconsciousness
3. conscious
4. seizure
5. convulsion
6. shunt
7. gait
8. incoherent
9. disorientation
10. cognitive

Exercise 25
1. c
2. i
3. b
4. j
5. a
6. l
7. k
8. g
9. o
10. f
11. p
12. e
13. m
14. d
15. n
16. h

Copyright © 2022, Elsevier Inc. All rights reserved.

Exercise 26
Review of Complementary Terms

Exercise 27
Pronounce and Spell

Exercise 28
1. WR CV WR S
   psych/o/somat/ic
   CF
   pertaining to the mind and body
2. WR CV S
   psych/o/pathy
   CF
   (any) disease of the mind
3. WR CV S
   psych/o/logy
   CF
   study of the mind
4. WR S
   psych/iatry
   specialty of the mind (branch of medicine that deals with the treatment of mental disorders)
5. WR CV S
   psych/o/logist
   CF
   specialist of the mind
6. WR CV S
   psych/o/genic
   CF
   originating in the mind
7. WR S
   psych/iatrist
   physician who studies and treats disorders of the mind
8. WR S
   psych/osis
   abnormal condition of the mind

Exercise 29
1. psych/iatry
2. psych/osis
3. psych/o/logy
4. psych/o/genic
5. psych/iatrist
6. psych/o/logist
7. psych/o/somat/ic
8. psych/o/pathy

Exercise 30
Pronounce and Spell

Exercise 31
1. i	8. d
2. m	9. h
3. b	10. f
4. c	11. e
5. j	12. n
6. a	13. l
7. g	14. k

Exercise 32
Review of Behavioral Health Terms

Exercise 33
1. deep tendon reflexes
2. electroencephalogram, positron emission tomography, evoked potential studies, lumbar puncture
3. Alzheimer disease, amyotrophic lateral sclerosis, cerebral palsy, multiple sclerosis, Parkinson disease
4. cerebrovascular accident, transient ischemic attack, subarachnoid hemorrhage
5. cerebrospinal fluid
6. obsessive-compulsive disorder, attention deficit/hyperactivity disorder
7. central nervous system, peripheral nervous system
8. posttraumatic stress disorder, chronic traumatic encephalopathy
9. traumatic brain injury

Exercise 34
A. unable to speak, right arm was hanging limply by his side, left side of his face was also droopy, strokes
B. Answers will vary and may include aphasia, hemiplegia, Bell palsy, stroke or cerebrovascular accident, and their respective definitions.
C. aphasia, hemiplegia, dysphasia, hemiparesis, paresthesias, gait, cerebral, subarachnoid hemorrhage, CVA
D. Answers will vary and may include aphasia, hemiplegia, dysphasia, hemiparesis, paresthesias, gait, cerebral, subarachnoid hemorrhage, CVA and their respective definitions.

Exercise 35
A
1. disorientation
2. cognitive
3. aphasia
4. conscious
5. neurology
6. encephalitis
7. electroencephalogram
8. seizure
9. incoherent

B
1. b
2. a

Exercise 36
Electronic Health Record

Exercise 37
Pronunciation Exercise

Exercise 38
1. a	11. a
2. b	12. c
3. c	13. c
4. c	14. a
5. c	15. c
6. a	16. b
7. b	17. a
8. a	18. c
9. b	19. b
10. a	20. a

ANSWERS TO CHAPTER 16 EXERCISES

Exercise 1
A *Label*
1. parathyroid glands: parathyroid/o
2. adrenal glands: adren/o, adrenal/o
3. pituitary gland: pituitar/o
4. thyroid gland: thyroid/o
5. endocrine: endocrin/o

B *Label*
cortex: cortic/o

C *Define and Match*
1. d, adrenal glands
2. a, pituitary gland
3. e, cortex
4. b, parathyroid glands
5. d, adrenal glands
6. c, thyroid gland
7. endocrine

Exercise 2
A *Define*
1. thirst
2. potassium
3. calcium
4. extremities, height
5. sodium
6. sugar

Copyright © 2022, Elsevier Inc. All rights reserved.

B *Identify*

1. acr/o
2. calc/i
3. dips/o
4. glyc/o
5. kal/i
6. natr/o

Exercise 3

A *Define*

1. together, joined
2. below, incomplete, deficient, under
3. all, total
4. normal, good
5. many, much
6. above, excessive

B *Identify*

1. pan-
2. eu-
3. poly-
4. hyper-
5. syn-
6. hypo-

Exercise 4

A *Identify*

1. -ism
2. -megaly
3. -emia
4. -al
5. -pathy
6. -logist

B *Label*

1. -drome

C *Define*

1. tumor, swelling
2. excision, surgical removal
3. condition of formation, development, growth
4. study of
5. inflammation
6. run, running
7. diseased or abnormal state, condition of

Exercise 5

Pronounce and Spell

Exercise 6

1. WR S
   adrenal/itis
   inflammation of the adrenal glands
2. P WR S
   hypo/calc/emia
   deficient calcium in the blood
3. P WR S
   hyper/thyroid/ism
   state of excessive thyroid gland activity
4. P WR S
   hyper/kal/emia
   excessive potassium in the blood
5. P WR S
   hyper/pituitar/ism
   state of excessive pituitary gland activity
6. WR CV S
   adren/o/megaly
   CF
   enlargement of the adrenal glands
7. WR CV S
   endocrin/o/pathy
   CF
   (any) disease of the endocrine (system)
8. P WR S
   hypo/natr/emia
   deficient sodium in the blood
9. WR S
   parathyroid/oma
   tumor of a parathyroid gland
10. P P WR S
    pan/hypo/pituitar/ism
    state of total deficient pituitary gland activity

Exercise 7

A *Label*

1. acr/o/megaly
2. thyroid/itis
3. hyper/glyc/emia
4. hypo/glyc/emia

B *Fill In*

1. hypo/thyroid/ism
2. hypo/kal/emia
3. hyper/parathyroid/ism
4. hypo/pituitar/ism
5. hyper/calc/emia

Exercise 8

Pronounce and Spell

Exercise 9

1. c
2. g
3. b
4. d
5. f
6. a
7. e

Exercise 10

1. e
2. d
3. a
4. g
5. c
6. b
7. f

Exercise 11

A *Identify*

1. Neuroblastoma
2. thyrotoxicosis
3. Hashimoto thyroiditis
4. Diabetes insipidus
5. ketoacidosis
6. diabetes mellitus

B *Label*

1. gigantism
2. Addison disease
3. congenital hypothyroidism
4. myxedema
5. Cushing syndrome
6. metabolic syndrome
7. pheochromocytoma
8. Graves disease

Exercise 12

Review of Disease and Disorder Terms

Exercise 13

Pronounce and Spell

Exercise 14

1. WR S
   adrenal/ectomy
   excision of (one or both) adrenal glands
2. WR S
   thyroid/ectomy
   excision of the thyroid gland
3. WR S
   parathyroid/ectomy
   excision of (one or more) parathyroid glands

Exercise 15

1. thyroid/ectomy
2. adrenal/ectomy
3. parathyroid/ectomy

Exercise 16

Review of Surgical Terms

Exercise 17

Pronounce and Spell

Exercise 18

A *Label*

1. thyroid sonography
2. radioactive iodine uptake
3. sestamibi parathyroid scan
4. fine needle aspiration

B *Identify*

1. Thyroxine level
2. fasting blood sugar
3. glycosylated hemoglobin
4. thyroid-stimulating hormone level

Exercise 19

1. b
2. a
3. g
4. d
5. f
6. h
7. e
8. c

Copyright © 2022, Elsevier Inc. All rights reserved.

Exercise 20

Review of Diagnostic Terms

Exercise 21

Pronounce and Spell

Exercise 22

A *Analyze and Define*

1. P S(WR)
   syn/drome
   run together
2. WR CV S
   endocrin/o/logist
   CF
   physician who studies and treats diseases of the endocrine (system)
3. P WR S
   poly/dips/ia
   CF
   abnormal state of much thirst
4. P WR S
   eu/glyc/emia
   normal (level of) sugar in the blood
5. WR CV WR CV P S
   adren/o/cortic/o/hyper/plasia
   CF CF
   excessive development of the adrenal cortex
6. P WR
   eu/thyroid
   normal thyroid gland activity
7. WR S
   cortic/al
   pertaining to the cortex
8. WR CV S
   endocrin/o/logy
   CF
   study of the endocrine (system)
9. WR S
   glyc/emia
   sugar in the blood

B *Label*

1. eu/thyroid
2. eu/glyc/emia
3. poly/dips/ia
4. endocrin/o/logist

C *Fill In*

1. glyc/emia
2. syn/drome
3. adren/o/cortic/o/hyper/plasia
4. endocrin/o/logy
5. cortic/al

Exercise 23

A *Match*

1. b	4. e
2. f	5. c
3. d	6. a

B *Label*

1. goiter
2. exophthalmos

C *Identify*

1. metabolism
2. hormone
3. Tetany
4. incretins

Exercise 24

Review of Complementary Terms

Exercise 25

1. diabetes mellitus, type 1 diabetes mellitus, fasting blood sugar, diabetic ketoacidosis
2. type 2 diabetes mellitus, glycosylated hemoglobin
3. thyroxine level, thyroid-stimulating hormone, radioactive iodine uptake, fine needle aspiration, parathyroid hormone
4. follicle-stimulating hormone, luteinizing hormone
5. antidiuretic hormone, diabetes insipidus, syndrome of inappropriate ADH (secretion)
6. growth hormone, adrenocorticotropic hormone, prolactin

Exercise 26

A. a lump in the front of her neck, eyes seem to stick out more, too much thyroid hormone, endocrine specialist

B. Answers will vary and may include goiter, exophthalmos, hyperthyroidism or thyrotoxicosis, endocrinologist, and their respective definitions.

C. endocrinopathy, hyperthyroidism, thyrotoxicosis, exophthalmos, Graves disease, thyroid sonography, TSH, T4, radioactive iodine uptake, thyroidectomy, hypothyroidism

D. Answers will vary and may include endocrinopathy, hyperthyroidism, thyrotoxicosis, exophthalmos, Graves disease, thyroid sonography, TSH, T4, radioactive iodine uptake, thyroidectomy, hypothyroidism, and their respective definitions.

Exercise 27

A

1. polydipsia
2. diabetes mellitus
3. exophthalmos
4. fasting blood sugar
5. glycosylated hemoglobin
6. type 2 diabetes mellitus
7. hyperglycemia
8. hypoglycemia
9. endocrinology

B

1. c
2. b
3. a

Exercise 28

Online Exercise

Exercise 29

Pronunciation Exercise

Exercise 30

1. c	11. c
2. a	12. c
3. c	13. b
4. b	14. b
5. a	15. c
6. b	16. a
7. b	17. b
8. c	18. a
9. a	19. b
10. c	20. b

Copyright © 2022, Elsevier Inc. All rights reserved.

Appendix B

Combining Forms, Prefixes, and Suffixes Alphabetized by Word Part

COMBINING FORMS	DEFINITION	CHAPTER
A		
abdomin/o	abdomen, abdominal cavity	11
acr/o	extremities, height	16
aden/o	gland	2
adenoid/o	adenoids	5
adren/o	adrenal glands	16
adrenal/o	adrenal glands	16
albumin/o	albumin	6
alveol/o	alveolus *(s.)*, alveoli *(pl.)*	5
amni/o	amnion, amniotic fluid	9
amnion/o	amnion, amniotic fluid	9
andr/o	male	7
angi/o	vessel(s); blood vessel(s)	10
ankyl/o	stiff, bent	14
an/o	anus	11
anter/o	front	3
antr/o	antrum	11
aort/o	aorta	10
appendic/o	appendix	11
append/o	appendix	11
arteri/o	artery *(s)*, arteries *(pl)*	10
arthr/o	joint	14
atel/o	imperfect, incomplete	5
ather/o	yellowish, fatty plaque	10
atri/o	atrium	10
audi/o	hearing	13
aur/i	ear	13
aut/o	self	2
azot/o	urea, nitrogen	6
B		
balan/o	glans penis	7
bi/o	life	2
blast/o	developing cell, germ cell	6
blephar/o	eyelid	12
bronch/o	bronchus	5
bronchi/o	bronchus	5
burs/o	bursa (cavity)	14
C		
calc/i	calcium	16
cancer/o	cancer	2
capn/o	carbon dioxide	5
carcin/o	cancer	2
cardi/o	heart	10
carp/o	carpals (wrist)	14
caud/o	tail (downward)	3
cec/o	cecum	11
celi/o	abdomen, abdominal cavity	11
cephal/o	head	3
cerebell/o	cerebellum	15
cerebr/o	cerebrum, brain	15
cervic/o	cervix	8
cheil/o	lip(s)	11
chlor/o	green	2
cholangi/o	bile duct	11
chol/e	gall, bile	11
choledoch/o	common bile duct	11
chondr/o	cartilage	14
chori/o	chorion	9
clavicul/o	clavicle (collarbone)	14
cochle/o	cochlea	13
col/o	colon (large intestine)	11
colon/o	colon (large intestine)	11
colp/o	vagina	8
coni/o	dust	5

COMBINING FORMS	DEFINITION	CHAPTER
conjunctiv/o	conjunctiva	12
cor/o	pupil	12
corne/o	cornea	12
cortic/o	cortex (outer layer of body organ)	16
cost/o	rib	14
crani/o	cranium (skull)	14
cry/o	cold	12
crypt/o	hidden	4
cutane/o	skin	4
cyan/o	blue	2
cyst/o	bladder, sac	6
cyt/o	cell	2
D		
dacry/o	tear(s)	12
dermat/o	skin	4
derm/o	skin	4
diaphragmat/o	diaphragm	5
dipl/o	two, double	12
dips/o	thirst	16
disc/o	intervertebral disk	14
dist/o	away (from the point of attachment)	3
diverticul/o	diverticulum	11
dors/o	back	3
duoden/o	duodenum	11
dur/o	hard, dura mater	15
E		
ech/o	sound	10
electr/o	electricity, electrical activity	10
embol/o	plug	10
encephal/o	brain	15
endocrin/o	endocrine	16
endometri/o	endometrium	8
enter/o	intestines (usually the small intestine)	11
epididym/o	epididymis	7
epiglott/o	epiglottis	5
episi/o	vulva	8
epitheli/o	epithelium	2
erythr/o	red	2
esophag/o	esophagus	9, 11
esthesi/o	sensation, sensitivity, feeling	15
eti/o	cause (of disease)	2
F		
fasci/o	fascia (connective tissue enclosing and separating muscle layers)	14
femor/o	femur (upper leg bone)	14
fet/i	fetus, unborn offspring	9
fet/o	fetus, unborn offspring	9
fibr/o	fibrous, fibrous tissue	2
fibul/o	fibula (lower leg bone)	14
G		
gangli/o	ganglion	15
ganglion/o	ganglion	15
gastr/o	stomach	11
gingiv/o	gum	11
gli/o	glia	15
glomerul/o	glomerulus	6
gloss/o	tongue	11
glycos/o	sugar	6
gno/o	knowledge	2
gravid/o	pregnancy	9
gynec/o	woman, female reproductive organs	8
gyn/o	woman, female reproductive organs	8
H		
hem/o	blood	5
hemat/o	blood	2
hepat/o	liver	11
herni/o	hernia (protrusion of an organ through a membrane or cavity wall)	11
hidr/o	sweat	4
hist/o	tissue	2
humer/o	humerus (upper arm bone)	14
hydr/o	water	6
hymen/o	hymen	8
hyster/o	uterus	8

COMBINING FORMS	DEFINITION	CHAPTER
I		
iatr/o	physician, medicine (also means treatment)	2
ile/o	ileum	11
ili/o	ilium (upper winged-shaped portion of the pelvis)	14
immun/o	immune system	10
infer/o	below	3
irid/o	iris	12
ir/o	iris	12
is/o	equal	12
ischi/o	ischium (lower posterior portion of the pelvis)	14
isch/o	deficiency, blockage	10
J		
jejun/o	jejunum	11
K		
kal/i	potassium	16
kerat/o	cornea	12
kerat/o	horny tissue (keratin), hard	4
kinesi/o	movement, motion	14
kyph/o	hump (increased convexity of the spine)	14
L		
labyrinth/o	labyrinth	13
lacrim/o	tear(s)	12
lact/o	milk	9
lamin/o	lamina (thin, flat plate or layer)	14
lapar/o	abdomen, abdominal cavity	11
laryng/o	larynx	5
later/o	side	3
lei/o	smooth	2
leuk/o	white	2
lingu/o	tongue	11
lip/o	fat	2
lith/o	stone(s), calculus (*pl.* calculi)	6
lob/o	lobe(s)	5
lord/o	bent forward (increased concavity of the spine)	14
lumb/o	loin, lumbar region of the spine	14
lymphaden/o	lymph node	10
lymph/o	lymph, lymph tissue	10
M		
mamm/o	breast	8
mandibul/o	mandible (lower jawbone)	14
mast/o	breast	8
mastoid/o	mastoid bone	13
maxill/o	maxilla (upper jawbone)	14
meat/o	meatus (opening)	6
medi/o	middle	3
mediastin/o	mediastinum	5
melan/o	black	2
meningi/o	meninges	15
mening/o	meninges	15
menisc/o	meniscus (crescent)	14
men/o	menstruation	8
ment/o	mind	15
metr/o	uterus	8
mon/o	one, single	15
muc/o	mucus	5
myc/o	fungus	4
myel/o	bone marrow	10
myel/o	spinal cord	15
my/o	muscle	2, 14
myos/o	muscle	14
myring/o	tympanic membrane (eardrum)	13
N		
nas/o	nose	5
nat/o	birth	9
natr/o	sodium	16
necr/o	death (cells, body)	2
nephr/o	kidney	6
neur/o	nerve	2, 15
noct/i	night	6

COMBINING FORMS	DEFINITION	CHAPTER
O		
ocul/o	eye	12
olig/o	scanty, few	6
omphal/o	umbilicus, navel	9
onc/o	tumor, mass	2
onych/o	nail	4
oophor/o	ovary	8
ophthalm/o	eye	12
opt/o	vision	12
orchid/o	testis, testicle	7
orchi/o	testis, testicle	7
orch/o	testis, testicle	7
organ/o	organ	2
or/o	mouth	11
orth/o	straight	5
oste/o	bone	14
ot/o	ear	13
ox/i	oxygen	5
P		
pachy/o	thick	4
palat/o	palate	11
pancreat/o	pancreas	11
parathyroid/o	parathyroid glands	16
par/o	bear, give birth to, labor, childbirth	9
part/o	bear, give birth to, labor, childbirth	9
patell/o	patella (kneecap)	14
path/o	disease	2
pelv/i	pelvis, pelvic cavity	8
perine/o	perineum	8
peritone/o	peritoneum	11
petr/o	stone	14
phac/o	lens	12
phak/o	lens	12
phalang/o	phalanx (pl. phalanges) (any bone of the fingers or toes)	14
pharyng/o	pharynx	5
phas/o	speech	15
phleb/o	vein(s)	10
phon/o	sound, voice	5

COMBINING FORMS	DEFINITION	CHAPTER
phot/o	light	12
pituitar/o	pituitary gland	16
plasm/o	plasma	10
pleur/o	pleura	5
pneum/o	lung, air	5
pneumon/o	lung, air	5
poli/o	gray matter	15
polyp/o	polyp, small growth	11
poster/o	back, behind	3
prim/i	first	9
proct/o	rectum	11
prostat/o	prostate gland	7
proxim/o	near (the point of attachment)	3
pseud/o	false	9
psych/o	mind	15
pub/o	pubis (anterior portion of the pelvis)	14
puerper/o	childbirth	9
pulmon/o	lung	5
pupill/o	pupil	12
pyel/o	renal pelvis	6
pylor/o	pylorus, pyloric sphincter	9, 11
py/o	pus	5
Q		
quadr/i	four	15
R		
rachi/o	vertebra (*pl.* vertebrae), spine, vertebral column	14
radicul/o	nerve root	15
radi/o	radius (lower arm bone)	14
radi/o	x-rays, ionizing radiation	3
rect/o	rectum	11
ren/o	kidney	6
retin/o	retina	12
rhabd/o	rod-shaped, striated	2
rhin/o	nose	5
rhiz/o	nerve root	15
rhytid/o	wrinkles	4

COMBINING FORMS	DEFINITION	CHAPTER
S		
sacr/o	sacrum (lower portion of the spine forming the posterior pelvic wall)	14
salping/o	fallopian tube (uterine tube)	8
sarc/o	flesh, connective tissue	2
scapul/o	scapula (shoulder blade)	14
scler/o	hard, sclera	4, 12
scoli/o	(lateral) curved (spine)	14
seb/o	sebum (oil)	4
sept/o	septum	5
sial/o	saliva, salivary gland	11
sigmoid/o	sigmoid colon	11
sinus/o	sinus(es)	5
somat/o	body	2
somn/o	sleep	5
son/o	sound	3
sperm/o	sperm, spermatozoon (pl. spermatozoa)	7
spermat/o	sperm, spermatozoon (pl. spermatozoa)	7
spir/o	breathe, breathing	5
splen/o	spleen	10
spondyl/o	vertebra (*pl.* vertebrae), spine, vertebral column	14
staped/o	stapes	13
staphyl/o	grapelike clusters	4
steat/o	fat	11
stern/o	sternum (breastbone)	14
stomat/o	mouth	11
strept/o	twisted chains	4
super/o	above	3
synovi/o	synovia, synovial membrane	14
system/o	system	2
T		
tars/o	tarsals (ankle bones)	14
tendin/o	tendon	14
ten/o	tendon	14
terat/o	malformations	9
thorac/o	thorax, chest, chest cavity	5
thromb/o	blood clot	10
thym/o	thymus gland	10
thyroid/o	thyroid gland	16
thyr/o	thyroid gland	16
tibi/o	tibia (lower leg bone)	14
tom/o	to cut, section, or slice	3
ton/o	tension, pressure	12
tonsill/o	tonsil(s)	5
trachel/o	cervix	8
trache/o	trachea	5
trich/o	hair	4
tympan/o	middle ear	13
U		
uln/o	ulna (lower arm bone)	14
ungu/o	nail	4
ureter/o	ureter	6
urethr/o	urethra	6
ur/o	urine, urinary tract	6
urin/o	urine, urinary tract	6
uve/o	uvea	12
uvul/o	uvula	11
V		
vagin/o	vagina	8
valvul/o	valve	10
vas/o	vessel, duct	7
ven/o	vein	10
ventricul/o	ventricle	10
ventr/o	belly (front)	3
vertebr/o	vertebra (*pl.* vertebrae), spine, vertebral column	14
vesic/o	bladder, sac	6
vesicul/o	seminal vesicle(s)	7
vestibul/o	vestibule	13
vir/o	virus	2
viscer/o	internal organs	2
vulv/o	vulva	8
X		
xanth/o	yellow	2
xer/o	dry, dryness	4

PREFIX	DEFINITION	CHAPTER
a-	absence of, without	5
an-	absence of, without	5
ante-	before	9
bi-	two	3, 12
bin-	two	12
brady-	slow	10
dia-	through, complete	2
dys-	painful, abnormal, difficult, labored	2
endo-	within	5
epi-	on, upon, over	4
eu-	normal, good	5
hemi-	half	11
hyper-	above, excessive	2
hypo-	below, incomplete, deficient, under	2
inter-	between	14
intra-	within	4
meta-	after, beyond, change	2
micro-	small	2
multi-	many	9
neo-	new	2
nulli-	none	9
pan-	all, total	10
para-	beside, beyond, around, abnormal	4
per-	through	4
peri-	surrounding (outer)	8
poly-	many, much	5
post-	after	9
pre-	before	9
pro-	before	2
sub-	under, below	4
supra-	above	14
sym-	together, joined	14
syn-	together, joined	14
tachy-	fast, rapid	5
trans-	through, across, beyond	4
uni-	one	3

SUFFIX	DEFINITION	CHAPTER
-a	no meaning	4
-ac	pertaining to	11
-ad	toward	3
-al	pertaining to	2
-algia	pain	7
-amnios	amnion, amniotic fluid	9
-apheresis	removal	10
-ar	pertaining to	5
-ary	pertaining to	5
-asthenia	weakness	14
-cele	hernia, protrusion	5
-centesis	surgical puncture to aspirate fluid	5
-cleisis	surgical closure	8
-coccus (pl. -cocci)	berry-shaped (form of bacterium)	4
-cyesis	pregnancy	9
-cyte	cell	2
-desis	surgical fixation, fusion	5
-drome	run, running	16
-e	no meaning	9
-eal	pertaining to	5
-ectasis	stretching out, dilation, expansion	5
-ectomy	excision, surgical removal	4
-emia	in the blood	5
-gen	substance or agent that produces or causes	2
-genic	producing, originating, causing	2
-gram	the record, radiographic image	3
-graph	instrument used to record; the record	3
-graphy	process of recording, radiographic imaging	3
-ia	diseased or abnormal state, condition of	4
-iasis	condition	6

SUFFIX	DEFINITION	CHAPTER
-iatrist	specialist, physician	15
-iatry	treatment, specialty	15
-ic	pertaining to	2
-ictal	seizure, attack	15
-ior	pertaining to	3
-is	no meaning	9
-ism	state of	7
-itis	inflammation	4
-lith	stone(s), calculus (*pl.* calculi)	6
-logist	one who studies and treats (specialist, physician)	2
-logy	study of	2
-lysis	loosening, dissolution, separating	6
-malacia	softening	4
-megaly	enlargement	2
-meter	instrument used to measure	5
-metry	measurement	5
-oid	resembling	2
-oma	tumor, swelling	2
-opia	vision (condition)	12
-opsy	view of, viewing	2
-osis	abnormal condition (means increase when used with blood cell word roots)	2
-ous	pertaining to	2
-paresis	slight paralysis	15
-pathy	disease	2
-penia	abnormal reduction in number	10
-pepsia	digestion	11
-pexy	surgical fixation, suspension	6
-phagia	eating or swallowing	4
-phobia	abnormal fear of or aversion to specific things	12
-physis	growth	14
-plasia	condition of formation, development, growth	2

SUFFIX	DEFINITION	CHAPTER
-plasm	growth, substance, formation	2
-plasty	surgical repair	4
-plegia	paralysis	12
-pnea	breathing	5
-ptosis	drooping, sagging, prolapse	6
-ptysis	spitting, coughing	5
-rrhage	excessive flow	10
-rrhagia	excessive bleeding	5
-rrhaphy	suturing, repairing	8
-rrhea	flow, discharge	4
-rrhexis	rupture	9
-salpinx	fallopian tube (uterine tube)	8
-sarcoma	malignant tumor	2
-schisis	split, fissure	14
-sclerosis	hardening	10
-scope	instrument used for visual examination	5
-scopic	pertaining to visual examination	5
-scopy	visual examination	5
-sis	state of	2
-spasm	sudden, involuntary muscle contraction	5
-stasis	control, stop, standing	2
-stenosis	constriction or narrowing	5
-stomy	creation of an artificial opening	5
-thorax	chest, chest cavity	5
-tocia	birth, labor	9
-tomy	cut into, incision	5
-tripsy	surgical crushing	6
-trophy	nourishment, development	14
-um	no meaning	9
-uria	urine, urination	6
-us	no meaning	9

Appendix C

Combining Forms, Prefixes, and Suffixes Alphabetized by Definition

DEFINITION	COMBINING FORM	CHAPTER
A		
abdomen, abdominal cavity	abdomin/o, lapar/o, celi/o	11
above	super/o	3
adenoids	adenoid/o	5
adrenal glands	adren/o, adrenal/o	16
albumin	albumin/o	6
alveolus *(s.)*, alveoli *(pl.)*	alveol/o	5
amnion, amniotic fluid	amni/o, amnion/o	9
antrum	antr/o	11
anus	an/o	11
aorta	aort/o	10
appendix	append/o, appendic/o	11
artery *(s)*, arteries *(pl)*	arteri/o	10
atrium	atri/o	10
away (from the point of attachment)	dist/o	3
B		
back	dors/o	3
back, behind	poster/o	3
bear, give birth to, labor, childbirth	par/o, part/o	9
belly (front)	ventr/o	3
below	infer/o	3
bent forward (increased concavity of the spine)	lord/o	14
bile duct(s)	cholangi/o	11
birth	nat/o	9
black	melan/o	2
bladder, sac	cyst/o, vesic/o	6
blood	hem/o, hemat/o	5, 2
blood clot	thromb/o	10
blue	cyan/o	2
body	somat/o	2
bone	oste/o	14
bone marrow	myel/o	10
brain	encephal/o	15
breast	mamm/o, mast/o	8
breathe, breathing	spir/o	5
bronchus *(s.)*, bronchi *(pl.)*	bronch/o, bronchi/o	5
bursa (cavity)	burs/o	14
C		
calcium	calc/i	16
cancer	cancer/o, carcin/o	2
carbon dioxide	capn/o	5
carpals (wrist)	carp/o	14
cartilage	chondr/o	14
cause (of disease)	eti/o	2
cecum	cec/o	11
cell	cyt/o	2
cerebellum	cerebell/o	15
cerebrum, brain	cerebr/o	15
cervix	cervic/o, trachel/o	8
childbirth	puerper/o	9
chorion	chori/o	9
clavicle (collarbone)	clavicul/o	14
cochlea	cochle/o	13
cold	cry/o	12
colon	col/o, colon/o	11
common bile duct	choledoch/o	11
conjunctiva	conjunctiv/o	12
cornea	corne/o, kerat/o	12
cortex	cortic/o	16
cranium (skull)	crani/o	14
(lateral) curved (spine)	scoli/o	14
D		
death (cells, body)	necr/o	2
deficiency, blockage	isch/o	10

DEFINITION	COMBINING FORM	CHAPTER
developing cell, germ cell	blast/o	6
diaphragm	diaphragmat/o	5
disease	path/o	2
diverticulum	diverticul/o	11
dry, dryness	xer/o	4
duodenum	duoden/o	11
dust	coni/o	5
E		
ear	aur/i, ot/o	13
electricity, electrical activity	electr/o	10
endocrine	endocrin/o	16
endometrium	endometri/o	8
epididymis	epididym/o	7
epiglottis	epiglott/o	5
epithelium	epitheli/o	2
equal	is/o	12
esophagus	esophag/o	9, 11
extremities, height	acr/o	16
eye	ocul/o, ophthalm/o	12
eyelid	blephar/o	12
F		
fallopian tube (uterine tube)	salping/o	8
false	pseud/o	9
fascia (connective tissue enclosing and separating muscle layers)	fasci/o	14
fat	lip/o	2
fat	steat/o	11
femur (upper leg bone)	femor/o	14
fetus, unborn offspring	fet/o, fet/i	9
fibrous, fibrous tissue	fibr/o	2
fibula (lower leg bone)	fibul/o	14
first	prim/i	9
flesh, connective tissue	sarc/o	2, 14
four	quadr/i	15
front	anter/o	3
fungus	myc/o	3

DEFINITION	COMBINING FORM	CHAPTER
G		
gall, bile	chol/e	11
ganglion	gangli/o, ganglion/o	15
gland	aden/o	2
glans penis	balan/o	7
glia	gli/o	15
glomerulus	glomerul/o	6
grapelike clusters	staphyl/o	4
gray matter	poli/o	15
green	chlor/o	2
gum(s)	gingiv/o	11
H		
hard	scler/o	4
hard, dura mater	dur/o	15
head	cephal/o	3
hearing	audi/o	13
heart	cardi/o	10
hernia	herni/o	11
hidden	crypt/o	4
horny tissue (keratin), hard	kerat/o	4
humerus (upper arm bone)	humer/o	14
hump (increased convexity of the spine)	kyph/o	14
hymen	hymen/o	8
I		
ileum	ile/o	11
ilium (upper winged-shaped portion of the pelvis)	ili/o	14
immune system	immun/o	10
imperfect, incomplete	atel/o	5
internal organs	viscer/o	2
intervertebral disk	disc/o	14
intestines (usually the small intestine)	enter/o	11
iris	ir/o, irid/o	12
ischium (lower posterior portion of the pelvis)	ischi/o	14
J		
jejunum	jejun/o	11
joint	arthr/o	14

DEFINITION	COMBINING FORM	CHAPTER
K		
kidney	nephr/o, ren/o	6
knowledge	gno/o	2
L		
labyrinth	labyrinth/o	13
lamina (thin, flat plate or layer)	lamin/o	14
larynx	laryng/o	5
lens	phac/o, phak/o	12
life	bi/o	2
light	phot/o	12
lip(s)	cheil/o	11
liver	hepat/o	11
lobe(s)	lob/o	5
loin, lumbar region of the spine	lumb/o	14
lung	pulmon/o	5
lung, air	pneum/o, pneumon/o	5
lymph node	lymphaden/o	10
lymph, lymph tissue	lymph/o	10
M		
male	andr/o	7
malformations	terat/o	9
mandible (lower jawbone)	mandibul/o	14
mastoid bone	mastoid/o	13
maxilla (upper jawbone)	maxill/o	14
meatus (opening)	meat/o	6
mediastinum	mediastin/o	5
meninges	mening/o, meningi/o	15
meniscus (crescent)	menisc/o	14
menstruation	men/o	8
middle	medi/o	3
middle ear	tympan/o	13
milk	lact/o	9
mind	ment/o, psych/o	15
mouth	or/o, stomat/o	11
movement, motion	kinesi/o	14
mucus	muc/o	5
muscle	my/o, myos/o	2, 14

DEFINITION	COMBINING FORM	CHAPTER
N		
nail	onych/o, ungu/o	4
near (the point of attachment)	proxim/o	3
nerve	neur/o	2, 15
nerve root	radicul/o, rhiz/o	15
night	noct/i	6
nose	nas/o, rhin/o	5
O		
one, single	mon/o	15
organ	organ/o	2
ovary	oophor/o	8
oxygen	ox/i	5
P		
palate	palat/o	11
pancreas	pancreat/o	11
parathyroid glands	parathyroid/o	16
patella (kneecap)	patell/o	14
pelvis, pelvic cavity	pelv/i	8
perineum	perine/o	8
peritoneum	peritone/o	11
phalanx (any bone of the fingers or toes)	phalang/o	14
pharynx	pharyng/o	5
physician, medicine (also means treatment)	iatr/o	2
plasma	plasm/o	10
pleura	pleur/o	5
plug	embol/o	10
polyp, small growth	polyp/o	11
potassium	kal/i	16
pregnancy	gravid/o	9
prostate gland	prostat/o	7
pubis (anterior portion of the pelvis)	pub/o	14
pupil	cor/o, pupill/o	12
pus	py/o	5
pylorus, pyloric sphincter	pylor/o	9, 11
R		
radius (lower arm bone)	radi/o	14
rectum	proct/o, rect/o	11

DEFINITION	COMBINING FORM	CHAPTER
red	erythr/o	2
renal pelvis	pyel/o	6
retina	retin/o	12
rib	cost/o	14
rod-shaped, striated	rhabd/o	2
S		
sacrum (lower portion of the spine forming the posterior pelvic wall)	sacr/o	14
saliva, salivary gland	sial/o	11
scanty, few	olig/o	6
scapula (shoulder blade)	scapul/o	14
sclera	scler/o	12
sebum (oil)	seb/o	4
self	aut/o	2
seminal vesicle(s)	vesicul/o	7
sensation, sensitivity, feeling	esthesi/o	15
septum	sept/o	5
side	later/o	3
sigmoid colon	sigmoid/o	11
sinus(es)	sinus/o	5
skin	cutane/o, derm/o, dermat/o	4
sleep	somn/o	5
smooth	lei/o	2
sodium	natr/o	16
sound	son/o, ech/o	3, 10
sound, voice	phon/o	5
speech	phas/o	15
sperm, spermatozoon	sperm/o, spermat/o	7
spinal cord	myel/o	15
spleen	splen/o	10
stapes	staped/o	13
sternum (breastbone)	stern/o	14
stiff, bent	ankyl/o	14
stomach	gastr/o	11
stone	petr/o	14
stone(s), calculus (*pl.* calculi)	lith/o	6

DEFINITION	COMBINING FORM	CHAPTER
straight	orth/o	5
sugar	glycos/o	6
sweat	hidr/o	4
synovia, synovial membrane	synovi/o	14
system	system/o	2
T		
tail (downward)	caud/o	3
tarsals (ankle bones)	tars/o	14
tear(s)	dacry/o, lacrim/o	12
tendon	ten/o, tendin/o	14
tension, pressure	ton/o	12
testis, testicle	orch/o, orchi/o, orchid/o	7
thick	pachy/o	4
thirst	dips/o	16
thorax, chest, chest cavity	thorac/o	5
thymus gland	thym/o	10
thyroid gland	thyr/o, thyroid/o	16
tibia (lower leg bone)	tibi/o	14
tissue	hist/o	2
to cut, section, or slice	tom/o	3
tongue	gloss/o, lingu/o	11
tonsil(s)	tonsill/o	5
trachea	trache/o	5
tumor, mass	onc/o	2
twisted chains	strept/o	4
two, double	dipl/o	12
tympanic membrane (eardrum)	myring/o	13
U		
ulna (lower arm bone)	uln/o	14
umbilicus, navel	omphal/o	9
urea, nitrogen	azot/o	6
ureter	ureter/o	6
urethra	urethr/o	6
urine, urinary tract	ur/o, urin/o	6
uterus	hyster/o, metr/o	8
uvea	uve/o	12
uvula	uvul/o	11

DEFINITION	COMBINING FORM	CHAPTER
V		
vagina	colp/o, vagin/o	8
valve	valvul/o	10
vein(s)	phleb/o, ven/o	10
ventricle	ventricul/o	10
vertebra (*pl.* vertebrae), spine, vertebral column	rachi/o, spondyl/o, vertebr/o	14
vessel(s); blood vessel(s)	angi/o	10
vessel, duct	vas/o	7
vestibule	vestibul/o	13
vision	opt/o	12
vulva	episi/o, vulv/o	8
W		
water	hydr/o	6
white	leuk/o	2
woman, female reproductive organs	gyn/o, gynec/o	8
wrinkles	rhytid/o	4
X		
x-rays, ionizing radiation	radi/o	3
Y		
yellow	xanth/o	2
yellowish, fatty plaque	ather/o	10

DEFINITION	PREFIX	CHAPTER
above	supra-	14
above, excessive	hyper-	2
absence of, without	a-, an-	5
after	post-	9
after, beyond, change	meta-	2
all, total	pan-	10
before	ante-, pre-	9
before	pro-	2
below, incomplete, deficient, under	hypo-	2
beside, beyond, around, abnormal	para-	4
between	inter-	14
fast, rapid	tachy-	5
half	hemi-	11
many	multi-	9
many, much	poly-	5
new	neo-	2
none	nulli-	9
normal, good	eu-	5
on, upon, over	epi-	4
one	uni-	3
painful, abnormal, difficult, labored	dys-	2
slow	brady-	10
small	micro-	2
surrounding (outer)	peri-	8
through	per-	4
through, across, beyond	trans-	4
through, complete	dia-	2
together, joined	sym-, syn-	14
two	bin-	12
two	bi-	3, 12
under, below	sub-	4
within	intra-	4
within	endo-	5

DEFINITION	SUFFIX	CHAPTER
abnormal condition (means increase when used with blood cell word roots)	-osis	2
abnormal fear of or aversion to specific things	-phobia	12
abnormal reduction in number	-penia	10
amnion, amniotic fluid	-amnios	9
berry-shaped (form of bacterium)	-coccus (pl. -cocci)	4
birth, labor	-tocia	9
breathing	-pnea	5
cell	-cyte	2
chest, chest cavity	-thorax	5
condition	-iasis	6
condition of formation, development, growth	-plasia	2
constriction or narrowing	-stenosis	5
control, stop, standing	-stasis	2
creation of an artificial opening	-stomy	5
cut into, incision	-tomy	5
digestion	-pepsia	11
disease	-pathy	2
diseased or abnormal state, condition of	-ia	4
drooping, sagging, prolapse	-ptosis	6
eating or swallowing	-phagia	4
enlargement	-megaly	2
excessive bleeding	-rrhagia	5
excessive flow	-rrhage	10
excision, surgical removal	-ectomy	4
fallopian tube (uterine tube)	-salpinx	8
flow, discharge	-rrhea	4
growth	-physis	14
growth, substance, formation	-plasm	2
hardening	-sclerosis	10
hernia, protrusion	-cele	5
in the blood	-emia	5
inflammation	-itis	4
instrument used for visual examination	-scope	5
instrument used to measure	-meter	5
instrument used to record; the record	-graph	3
loosening, dissolution, separating	-lysis	6
malignant tumor	-sarcoma	2
measurement	-metry	5
no meaning	-a, -e, -is, -um, -us	4, 9
nourishment, development	-trophy	14
one who studies and treats (specialist, physician)	-logist	2
pain	-algia	7
paralysis	-plegia	12
pertaining to	-ac	11
pertaining to	-ous	2, 6
pertaining to	-ar, -ary, -eal	5
pertaining to	-al, -ic	2
pertaining to	-ior	3
pertaining to visual examination	-scopic	5
pregnancy	-cyesis	9
process of recording, radiographic imaging	-graphy	3
producing, originating, causing	-genic	2
removal	-apheresis	10
resembling	-oid	2
run, running	-drome	16
rupture	-rrhexis	9
seizure, attack	-ictal	15
slight paralysis	-paresis	15
softening	-malacia	4
specialist, physician	-iatrist	15
spitting, coughing	-ptysis	5
split, fissure	-schisis	14

DEFINITION	SUFFIX	CHAPTER
state of	-ism	7
state of	-sis	2
stone(s), calculus (*pl.* calculi)	-lith	6
stretching out, dilation, expansion	-ectasis	5
study of	-logy	2
substance or agent that produces or causes	-gen	2
sudden, involuntary muscle contraction	-spasm	5
surgical closure	-cleisis	8
surgical crushing	-tripsy	6
surgical fixation, fusion	-desis	5
surgical fixation, suspension	-pexy	6
surgical puncture to aspirate fluid	-centesis	5
surgical repair	-plasty	4
suturing, repairing	-rrhaphy	8
the record, radiographic image	-gram	3
toward	-ad	3
treatment, specialty	-iatry	15
tumor, swelling	-oma	2
urine, urination	-uria	6
view of, viewing	-opsy	2
vision (condition)	-opia	12
visual examination	-scopy	5
weakness	-asthenia	14

Appendix D

Abbreviations

Topics include:

Common Medical Abbreviations, p. 736

Institute for Safe Medication Practices' (ISMP) List of Error-Prone Abbreviations, Symbols and Dose Designations; includes The Joint Commission's "Do Not Use" list, p. 745

Abbreviations are written as they appear most commonly in the medical and healthcare environment. Some may also appear in both capital and small letters and with or without periods. To make a plural, add "s" to uppercase abbreviations (e.g., BPs for blood pressures) and apostrophe ('s) for lower case abbreviations (e.g., cm's for centimeters).

COMMON MEDICAL ABBREVIATIONS	DEFINITIONS
A1c	glycosylated hemoglobin
AAA	abdominal aortic aneurysm
AAD	antiobiotic-associated diarrhea
AB	abortion
ABD	abdomen
ABE	acute bacterial endocarditis
ABG	arterial blood gas
ABX	antibiotics
AC	acromioclavicular
ac	acute
a.c.	before meals
ACS	acute coronary syndrome
ACTH	adrenocorticotropic hormone
AD	Alzheimer disease
ADC	AIDS dementia complex
ADH	antidiuretic hormone
ADHD	attention deficit/hyperactivity disorder
ADLs	activities of daily living
ad lib	as desired
Adm	admission
AER	auditory evoked response
AFB	acid-fast bacilli
AFib	atrial fibrillation
AFP	alpha-fetoprotein
AHD	arteriosclerotic heart disease
AI	aortic insufficiency
AICD	automatic implantable cardiac defibrillator
AIDS	acquired immunodeficiency syndrome
AK	actinic keratosis
AKA	above-knee amputation
AKI	acute kidney injury
alk phos	alkaline phosphatase
ALL	acute lymphoblastic leukemia
ALS	amyotrophic lateral sclerosis
ALT	alanine aminotransferase
AM (or a.m.)	between midnight and noon
AMA	against medical advice; American Medical Association
AMB	ambulate, ambulatory
AMI	acute myocardial infarction
AML	acute myeloid leukemia
AMP (or amp)	ampule
amt	amount
angio	angiogram, angiography
ant	anterior
A&O	alert and oriented
AODM	adult-onset diabetes mellitus
AOM	acute otitis media
AP	anteroposterior; angina pectoris
A&P	anatomy and physiology; auscultation and percussion; anterior and posterior
A&P repair	anterior and posterior colporrhaphy
APR	abdominoperineal resection

COMMON MEDICAL ABBREVIATIONS	DEFINITIONS
aPTT	activated partial thromboplastin time
ARDS	acute respiratory distress syndrome
ARF	acute renal failure
ARM	artificial rupture of membranes
AMD, ARMD	age-related macular degeneration
ART	assisted reproductive technology
ASA	aspirin (acetylsalicylic acid)
ASCVD	arteriosclerotic cardiovascular disease
ASD	atrial septal defect; autism spectrum disorder
ASHD	arteriosclerotic heart disease
Ast (or AST)	astigmatism
as tol	as tolerated
AUB	abnormal uterine bleeding
AUL	acute undifferentiated leukemia
AV	atrioventricular, arteriovenous
AVM	arteriovenous malformation
AVR	aortic valve replacement
ax	axillary
BA	bronchial asthma
BBB	bundle branch block
BC	birth control
BCC	basal cell carcinoma
BE	barium enema
b.i.d.	twice a day
BK	below knee
BKA	below-knee amputation
BM	bowel movement
BMI	body mass index
BMP	basic metabolic panel
BMT	bone marrow transplant
BOM	bilateral otitis media
BOO	bladder outlet obstruction
BP	blood pressure
BPH	benign prostatic hyperplasia
BPPV	benign paroxysmal positional vertigo
BR	bedrest
BRBPR	bright red blood per rectum
BRM	biological response modifier

COMMON MEDICAL ABBREVIATIONS	DEFINITIONS
BRP	bathroom privileges
BS	blood sugar; bowel sounds; breath sounds
BSO	bilateral salpingo-oophorectomy
BUN	blood urea nitrogen
Bx	biopsy
$\bar{c}$	with
C	Celsius
C1-C7 or C_1-C_7	cervical vertebrae
Ca (or Ca^{2+})	calcium
CA	cancer; carcinoma
CABG	coronary artery bypass graft
CAD	coronary artery disease
CAL (or cal)	calorie
CA-MRSA	community-associated MRSA (methicillin-resistant *Staphylococcus aureus)* infection
CAP	capsule (or cap); community-acquired pneumonia
CAPD	continuous ambulatory peritoneal dialysis
cath	catheterization, catheter
CBC with diff	complete blood count and differential
CBR	complete bed rest
CBS	chronic brain syndrome
CC	chief complaint; colony count
CCU	coronary care unit
CDC	Centers for Disease Control and Prevention
CDH	congenital dislocation of the hip
CDI	*Clostridium difficile* infection
C. diff* or *C. difficile	*Clostridium difficile* (bacteria)
CEA	carcinoembryonic antigen
CF	cystic fibrosis
CHB	complete heart block
CHD	coronary heart disease
chemo	chemotherapy
CHF	congestive heart failure
CHO	carbohydrate
chol	cholesterol
CI	coronary insufficiency

COMMON MEDICAL ABBREVIATIONS	DEFINITIONS
circ	circumcision
CIS	carcinoma in situ
CJD	Creutzfeldt-Jakob disease
Cl (or Cl^-)	chloride
CKD	chronic kidney disease
CLBSI	central line bloodstream infection
CLD	chronic liver disease
CLL	chronic lymphocytic leukemia
cl liq	clear liquid
cm	centimeter
CML	chronic myelogenous leukemia
CMP	comprehensive metabolic panel
CMV	cytomegalovirus
CNS	central nervous system
c/o	complains of
CO	carbon monoxide
CO_2	carbon dioxide
COB	coordination of benefits
COLD	chronic obstructive lung disease
comp	compound
cond	condition
COPD	chronic obstructive pulmonary disease
COVID-19	corornavirus disease
CP	cerebral palsy
CPAP	continuous positive airway pressure
CPD	cephalopelvic disproportion
CPK	creatine phosphokinase
CPN	chronic pyelonephritis
CPR	cardiopulmonary resuscitation
CRD	chronic respiratory disease
creat	creatinine
CRF	chronic renal failure
crit	hematocrit (also HCT, Hct)
CRP	C-reactive protein
C&S	culture and sensitivity
C/S, CS, C-section	cesarean section
CSF	cerebrospinal fluid
CT	computed tomography
CTE	chronic traumatic encephalopathy
CTS	carpal tunnel syndrome
Cu	copper

COMMON MEDICAL ABBREVIATIONS	DEFINITIONS
CVA	cerebrovascular accident (stroke)
CVD	cardiovascular disease
CVP	central venous pressure
CVS	chorionic villus sampling
Cx	cervix
CXR	chest radiograph (x-ray)
DAT	diet as tolerated
D&C	dilation and curettage
DC	Doctor of Chiropractic
D&E	dilation and evacuation
DCIS	ductal carcinoma in situ
decub	pressure ulcer
del	delivery
derm	dermatology
DI	diabetes insipidus
DIC	diffuse intravascular coagulation
diff	differential (part of complete blood count)
disch	discharge
DISH	diffuse idiopathic skeletal hyperostosis
DKA	diabetic ketoacidosis
DLE	discoid lupus erythematosus
DM	diabetes mellitus
DNA	deoxyribonucleic acid
DND	died natural death
DO	Doctor of Osteopathy
DOA	dead on arrival
DOB	date of birth
DOD	date of death
Dr	dram
DRE	digital rectal examination
DRG	diagnosis-related group
DSA	digital subtraction angiography
DTR	deep tendon reflexes
DVT	deep vein thrombosis
DW	distilled water
D/W	dextrose in water
Dx	diagnosis
E	enema
EBL	estimated blood loss
ECG	electrocardiogram

COMMON MEDICAL ABBREVIATIONS	DEFINITIONS
ECHO	echocardiogram
ECT	electroconvulsive therapy
ED	erectile dysfunction, emergency department
EDD	expected (estimated) date of delivery
EEG	electroencephalogram
EGD	esophagogastroduodenoscopy
EKG	electrocardiogram
Elix (or elix)	elixir
Em	emmetropia
EMG	electromyogram
ENG	electronystagmography
ENT	ears, nose, throat; otolaryngologist
EP	ectopic pregnancy
EP studies	evoked potential studies
ER	emergency room
ERCP	endoscopic retrograde cholangiopancreatography
ERT	estrogen replacement therapy
ESR	erythrocyte sedimentation rate
ESRD	end-stage renal disease
ESWL	extracorporeal shock wave lithotripsy
etio	etiology
EUS	endoscopic ultrasound
exam	examination
ext	extract; external
F	Fahrenheit
FA	fluorescein angiography
FAS	fetal alcohol syndrome
FBD	fibrocystic breast disease
FBS	fasting blood sugar
FCC	fibrocystic (breast) changes
FDA	Food and Drug Administration
Fe	iron
FHT	fetal heart tones
FIT	fecal immunochemical test
flu	influenza
FNA	fine needle aspiration
FOBT	fecal occult blood test
Fr	French (catheter size)

COMMON MEDICAL ABBREVIATIONS	DEFINITIONS
FS	frozen section
FSH	follicle-stimulating hormone
FTD	frontotemporal dementia
FTSG	full-thickness skin graft
FTT	failure to thrive
FUO	fever of undetermined origin
fx	fracture
g	gram
GC	gonorrhea
GERD	gastroesophageal reflux disease
GH	growth hormone
GI	gastrointestinal
GSW	gunshot wound
gtt	drops
GTT	glucose tolerance test
GU	genitourinary
GYN	gynecology; gynecologist
h	hour
H	hypodermic
HAART	highly active antiretroviral therapy
HAI	healthcare-associated infection
HA-MRSA	healthcare-associated MRSA infection
HAND	HIV-associated neurocognitive disorder
HAP	hospital-acquired pneumonia
HB	heart block
HbA1C	glycosylated hemoglobin
HBV	hepatitis B virus
HCl	hydrochloric acid
HCO_3	bicarbonate
Hct	hematocrit
HCVD	hypertensive cardiovascular disease
HD	hemodialysis
HDL	high-density lipoprotein
HF	heart failure
Hg	mercury
Hgb	hemoglobin
H&H	hemoglobin and hematocrit
HHD	hypertensive heart disease
HIV	human immunodeficiency virus
HMD	hyaline membrane disease

COMMON MEDICAL ABBREVIATIONS	DEFINITIONS
HME	heat and moisture exchanger
HNP	herniated nucleus pulposus
H_2O	water
H_2O_2	hydrogen peroxide (hydrogen dioxide)
HOB	head of bed
HOH	hard of hearing
HoLEP	holmium laser enucleation of the prostate gland
H&P	history and physical examination
H. pylori	*Helicobacter pylori*
HPV	human papillomavirus
HRT	hormone replacement therapy
HSG	hysterosonography; hysterosalpingogram
ht	height
HTN	hypertension
Hx	history
hypo	hypodermic
IBD	inflammatory bowel disease
IBS	irritable bowel syndrome
ICD	implantable cardiac defibrillator
ICU	intensive care unit
ID	intradermal
I&D	incision and drainage
IDDM	insulin-dependent diabetes mellitus
IHD	ischemic heart disease
IM	intramuscular
inf	inferior
INR	international normalized ratio
I&O	intake and output
IOL	intraocular lens
IOP	intraocular pressure
IPF	idiopathic pulmonary fibrosis
IPPB	intermittent positive pressure breathing
IR	interventional radiology
irrig	irrigation
isol	isolation
IUD	intrauterine device
IUS	intrauterine system
IV	intravenous

COMMON MEDICAL ABBREVIATIONS	DEFINITIONS
IVC	intravenous cholangiogram
IVF	in vitro fertilization
IVP	intravenous pyelogram
IVU	intravenous urogram
K	potassium
KCl	potassium chloride
kg	kilogram
KO	keep open
KUB	kidney, ureter, bladder (radiograph)
KVO	keep vein open
L	liter
L1-L5 or L_1-L_5	lumbar vertebrae
lab	laboratory
LAC (or lac)	laceration
LAD	left anterior descending (coronary artery)
LAGB	laparoscopic adjustable gastric banding
LAP	laparotomy
LAR	low anterior resection
LARC	long-acting reversible contraception
LASIK	laser-assisted in situ keratomileusis
lat	lateral
LAVH	laparoscopically-assisted vaginal hysterectomy
L&D	labor and delivery
LDH	lactic dehydrogenase
LDL	low-density lipoprotein
LE	lupus erythematosus
LEEP	loop electrosurgical excision procedure
lg	large
LH	luteinizing hormone
LLL	left lower lobe (of lung)
LLQ	left lower quadrant
LMP	last menstrual period
LOC	loss of consciousness, level of consciousness
LP	lumbar puncture
LPM	liters per minute (oxygen)
LPN	licensed practical nurse

COMMON MEDICAL ABBREVIATIONS	DEFINITIONS
LPR	laryngopharyngeal reflux
LR	lactated Ringer (IV solution)
lt	left
LTB	laryngotracheobronchitis
LUL	left upper lobe (of lung)
LUQ	left upper quadrant
LUTS	lower urinary tract symptoms
lytes	electrolytes
mcg	microgram
MCH	mean corpuscular hemoglobin
MCV	mean corpuscular volume
MD	muscular dystrophy; medical doctor
med	medial
mEq	milliequivalent
MET (or met)	metastasis
METS (or mets)	metastases
mg	milligram
MG	myasthenia gravis
MI	myocardial infarction
mL	milliliter
mm	millimeter
MM	multiple myeloma
MOM	milk of magnesia
MR	magnetic resonance; mitral regurgitation
MRI	magnetic resonance imaging
MRCP	magnetic resonance cholangiopancreatography
MRSA	methicillin-resistant *Staphylococcus aureus*
MS	multiple sclerosis
multip	multipara
MVP	mitral valve prolapse
Na	sodium
NaCl	sodium chloride (salt)
NAS	no added salt
NB	newborn
NCD	neurocognitive disorder
neg	negative
neuro	neurology
NG	nasogastric

COMMON MEDICAL ABBREVIATIONS	DEFINITIONS
NG	nasogastric
NICU	neonatal intensive care unit
NIDDM	non-insulin-dependent diabetes mellitus
NIH	National Institutes of Health
NIVA	noninvasive vascular assessment
NK	natural killer (immune system cells)
NKDA	no known drug allergies
NM	nuclear medicine
noc, noct	night
NPH	normal pressure hydrocephalus
NPO	nothing by mouth
NPPV	noninvasive positive-pressure ventilator
NS	normal saline
NSAID	nonsteroidal antiinflammatory drug
NSR	normal sinus rhythm
N&V	nausea and vomiting
NVS	neurologic signs
O_2	oxygen
OA	osteoarthritis
OAB	overactive bladder
OB	obstetrics
OCD	obsessive-compulsive disorder
OCT	optical coherence tomography
OD	Doctor of Optometry, overdose
OE	otitis externa
OIC	opioid-induced constipation
oint	ointment
OM	otitis media
OOB	out of bed
OP	outpatient
Ophth	ophthalmic or ophthalmology
OR	operating room
Ortho or ortho	orthopedics
OSA	obstructive sleep apnea
OT	occupational therapy
OTC	over-the-counter drugs
oto	otology
oz	ounce

COMMON MEDICAL ABBREVIATIONS	DEFINITIONS
p̄	after
P	phosphorus, pulse
PA	physician's assistant or posteroanterior
PAC	premature atrial complex
$PaCo_2$	carbon dioxide partial pressure (measure of amount of carbon dioxide in arterial blood)
PAD	peripheral artery disease
PAE	prostatic artery embolization
PAF	paroxysmal atrial fibrillation
PaO_2	oxygen partial pressure (measure of amount of oxygen in arterial blood)
PAT	paroxysmal atrial tachycardia
PBSCT	peripheral blood stem cell transplant
pc (or p.c.)	after meals
PCI	percutaneous coronary intervention
PCOS	polycystic ovary syndrome
PCP	primary care physician; *Pneumocystis* pneumonia
PCU	progressive care unit
PCV	packed cell volume
PD	Parkinson disease
PDA	patent ductus arteriosus
PDR	*Physicians' Desk Reference*
PE	pulmonary embolism; pulmonary edema
Peds (or peds)	pediatrics
PEEP	positive end-expiratory pressure
PEG	percutaneous endoscopic gastrostomy
PEP	positive expiratory pressure
per	by
PERRLA	pupils equal, round, reactive to light and accommodation
PET	positron emission tomography
PFM	peak flow meter
PFTs	pulmonary function tests
PHACO	phacoemulsification
PICC	peripherally inserted central catheter
PICU	pediatric intensive care unit
PID	pelvic inflammatory disease
PJP	*Pneumocystis jiroveci* pneumonia
PKD	polycystic disease
PKU	phenylketonuria
PM	polymyositis, between noon and midnight
PMDD	premenstrual dysphoric disorder
PMS	premenstrual syndrome
PNS	peripheral nervous system
po (or PO)	orally; postoperative; phone order
post-op	postoperatively
PP	postpartum or postprandial (after meals)
PPD	purified protein derivative
pr	per rectum
PRBC	packed red blood cells
pre-op	preoperatively
PRH	prolactin-releasing hormone
primip	primipara
PRK	photorefractive keratectomy
PRL	prolactin
PRN	as needed (whenever necessary)
PSA	prostate-specific antigen
PSG	polysomnography
pt	patient; pint
PT	prothrombin time; physical therapy
PTCA	percutaneous transluminal coronary angioplasty
PTH	parathyroid hormone
PT/INR	prothrombin time/international normalized ratio
PTSD	posttraumatic stress disorder
PTT	partial thromboplastin time
PUL	percutaneous ultrasound lithotripsy
PVC	premature ventricular complex
PVD	peripheral vascular disease
PVP	photoselective vaporization of the prostate gland
Px	prognosis
q	every

COMMON MEDICAL ABBREVIATIONS	DEFINITIONS
q_h	every (number) hour (e.g., q2h)
qt	quart
R	rectal
RA	rheumatoid arthritis
RAD	reactive airway disease
RAIU	radioactive iodine uptake
RALRP	robotic-assisted prostatectomy
RBC	red blood cell (erythrocyte)
RDS	respiratory distress syndrome
reg	regular
REM	rapid eye movement
resp	respirations
RHD	rheumatic heart disease
RLL	right lower lobe (of lung)
RLQ	right lower quadrant
RML	right middle lobe (of lung)
RN	registered nurse
R/O	rule out
ROM	range of motion, rupture of membranes
RP	radical prostatectomy
RR	recovery room
RSV	respiratory syncytial virus infection
rt	right; routine
RT	respiratory therapy
RUL	right upper lobe (of lung)
RUQ	right upper quadrant
Rx	prescription
RYGB	Roux-en-Y gastric bypass
$\bar{s}$	without
SAB	spontaneous abortion
SABA	short-acting beta agonist (relief of asthma symptoms)
SAH	subarachnoid hemorrhage
SARS	severe acute respiratory syndrome
SBE	subacute bacterial endocarditis; self-breast examination
SCC	squamous cell carcinoma
SCLC	small cell lung cancer
SG	specific gravity
SHG	sonohysterography
SI	sacroiliac

COMMON MEDICAL ABBREVIATIONS	DEFINITIONS
SIADH	inappropriate ADH syndrome
SICU	surgical intensive care unit
SIDS	sudden infant death syndrome
SLE	systemic lupus erythematosus
SMAC	Sequential Multiple Analyzer Computer
SMR	submucous resection
SNF	skilled nursing facility
SOB	shortness of breath
SPECT	single-photon emission computed tomography
SSE	soapsuds enema
SSER	somatosensory evoked response
STAPH or staph	staphylococcus
stat	immediately
STD	sexually transmitted disease
STI	sexually transmitted infection
STREP or strep	streptococcus
STSG	split-thickness skin graft
subcut	subcutaneous
subling	sublingual
sup	superior
supp	suppository
surg	surgical
SVD	spontaneous vaginal delivery
SVN	small-volume nebulizer
SWL	shock wave lithotripsy
T1-T12 or T_1-T_{12}	thoracic vertebrae
T1D	type 1 diabetes (mellitus)
T1DM	type 1 diabetes mellitus
T2D	type 2 diabetes (mellitus)
T2DM	type 2 diabetes mellitus
T_3	triiodothyronine
T_4	thyroxine
tab	tablet
TAB	therapeutic abortion
T&A	tonsillectomy and adenoidectomy
TAH	total abdominal hysterectomy
TAH/BSO	total abdominal hysterectomy/ bilateral salpingo-oophorectomy
TAT	tetanus antitoxin
TB	tuberculosis

COMMON MEDICAL ABBREVIATIONS	DEFINITIONS
TBI	traumatic brain injury
TCDB	turn, cough, deep breathe
TCT	thrombin clotting time
TD	transdermal
TEE	transesophageal echocardiogram
temp	temperature
TENS	transcutaneous electrical nerve stimulation
TGs	triglycerides
THA	total hip arthroplasty
THR	total hip replacement
TIA	transient ischemic attack
tid	three times per day
tinct	tincture
TKA	total knee arthroplasty
TLC	total lung capacity
TLH	total laparoscopic hysterectomy
TPN	total parenteral nutrition
tr	tincture
trach	tracheostomy
TRUS	transrectal ultrasound
TSH	thyroid-stimulating hormone
TSS	toxic shock syndrome
TUIP	transurethral incision of the prostate gland
TULIP	transurethral laser incision of the prostate gland
TUMT	transurethral microwave thermotherapy
TUNA	transurethral needle ablation
TURP	transurethral resection of the prostate gland
TVS	transvaginal sonography
TWE	tap water enema
Tx	treatment; traction
UA	urinalysis
UAE	uterine artery embolization
UC	ulcerative colitis
UGI	upper gastrointestinal

COMMON MEDICAL ABBREVIATIONS	DEFINITIONS
UGI-SBFT	upper gastrointestinal [series] with small bowel follow through [radiograph]
ung	ointment
UPPP	uvulopalatopharyngoplasty
URI	upper respiratory infection
US	ultrasound
UTI	urinary tract infection
UV	ultraviolet
UVR	ultraviolet radiation
V_1	tidal volume
VA	visual acuity
vag	vaginal
VATS	video-assisted thoracic surgery
VBAC	vaginal birth after cesarean section
VBG	venous blood gas
VC	vital capacity
VCUG	voiding cystourethrogram
VD	venereal disease
VDRL	Venereal Disease Research Laboratory
vent	ventilator
VER	visual evoked response
VFib	ventricular fibrillation
VH	vaginal hysterectomy
VLAP	visual laser ablation of the prostate
VLDL	very-low-density lipoprotein
V/Q scan	lung ventilation/perfusion scan
VRE	vancomycin-resistant enterococci
VS	vital signs
VUR	vesicoureteral reflux
WA	while awake
WBC	white blood cell (leukocyte)
W/C	wheelchair
wt	weight
XRT	radiation therapy, x-ray radiotherapy, x-ray therapy

Institute for Safe Medication Practices' List of Error-Prone Abbreviations, Symbols, and Dose Designations

The abbreviations, symbols, and dose designations found in this table have been reported to ISMP through the ISMP National Medication Errors Reporting Program (ISMP MERP) as being frequently misinterpreted and involved in harmful medication errors. They should **NEVER** be used when communicating medical information. This includes internal communications, telephone/verbal prescriptions, computer-generated labels, labels for drug storage bins, medication administration records, as well as pharmacy and prescriber computer order entry screens.

ABBREVIATIONS	INTENDED MEANING	MISINTERPRETATION	CORRECTION
µg	Microgram	Mistaken as "mg"	Use "mcg"
AD, AS, AU	Right ear, left ear, each ear	Mistaken as OD, OS, OU (right eye, left eye, each eye)	Use "right ear," "left ear," or "each ear"
OD, OS, OU	Right eye, left eye, each eye	Mistaken as AD, AS, AU (right ear, left ear, each ear)	Use "right eye," "left eye," or "each eye"
BT	Bedtime	Mistaken as "BID" (twice daily)	Use "bedtime"
cc	Cubic centimeters	Mistaken as "u" (units)	Use "mL"
D/C	Discharge or discontinue	Premature discontinuation of medications if D/C (intended to mean "discharge") has been misinterpreted as "discontinued" when followed by a list of discharge medications	Use "discharge" and "discontinue"
IJ	Injection	Mistaken as "IV" or "intrajugular"	Use "injection"
IN	Intranasal	Mistaken as "IM" or "IV"	Use "intranasal" or "NAS"
HS	Half-strength	Mistaken as bedtime	Use "half-strength" or "bedtime"
hs	At bedtime, hours of sleep	Mistaken as half-strength	
IU**	International unit	Mistaken as IV (intravenous) or 10 (ten)	Use "units"
o.d. or OD	Once daily	Mistaken as "right eye" (OD-oculus dexter), leading to oral liquid medications administered in the eye	Use "daily"
OJ	Orange juice	Mistaken as OD or OS (right or left eye); drugs meant to be diluted in orange juice may be given in the eye	Use "orange juice"
Per os	By mouth, orally	The "os" can be mistaken as "left eye" (OS-oculus sinister)	Use "PO," "by mouth," or "orally"
q.d. or QD**	Every day	Mistaken as q.i.d., especially if the period after the "q" or the tail of the "q" is misunderstood as an "i"	Use "daily"
qhs	Nightly at bedtime	Mistaken as "qhr" or every hour	Use "nightly"
qn	Nightly or at bedtime	Mistaken as "qh" (every hour)	Use "nightly" or "at bedtime"
q.o.d. or QOD**	Every other day	Mistaken as "q.d." (daily) or "q.i.d." (four times daily) if the "o" is poorly written	Use "every other day"
q1d	Daily	Mistaken as q.i.d. (four times daily)	Use "daily"

ABBREVIATIONS	INTENDED MEANING	MISINTERPRETATION	CORRECTION
q6PM, etc.	Every evening at 6 PM	Mistaken as every 6 hours	Use "daily at 6 PM" or "6 PM daily"
SC, SQ, sub q	Subcutaneous	SC mistaken as SL (sublingual); SQ mistaken as "5 every;" the "q" in "sub q" has been mistaken as "every" (e.g., a heparin dose ordered "sub q 2 hours before surgery" misunderstood as every 2 hours before surgery)	Use "subcut" or "subcutaneously"
ss	Sliding scale (insulin) or ½ (apothecary)	Mistaken as "55"	Spell out "sliding scale;" use "one half" or "½"
SSRI	Sliding scale regular insulin	Mistaken as "selective-serotonin reuptake inhibitor"	Spell out "sliding scale (insulin)"
SSI	Sliding scale insulin	Mistaken as "Strong Solution of Iodine" (Lugol's)	
i/d	One daily	Mistaken as "tid"	Use "1 daily"
TIW or tiw	3 times a week	Mistaken as "3 times a day" or "twice in a week"	Use "3 times weekly"
U or u**	Unit	Mistaken as the number 0 or 4, causing a 10-fold overdose or greater (e.g., 4U seen as "40" or 4u seen as "44"); mistaken as "cc" so dose given in volume instead of units (e.g., 4u seen as 4cc)	Use "unit"
UD	As directed ("ut dictum")	Mistaken as unit dose (e.g., diltiazem 125 mg IV infusion "UD" misinterpreted as meaning to give the entire infusion as a unit [bolus] dose)	Use "as directed"
DOSE DESIGNATIONS AND OTHER INFORMATION	**INTENDED MEANING**	**MISINTERPRETATION**	**CORRECTION**
Trailing zero after decimal point (e.g., 1.0 mg)**	1 mg	Mistaken as 10 mg if the decimal point is not seen	Do not use trailing zeros for doses expressed in whole numbers
"Naked" decimal point (e.g., .5 mg)**	0.5 mg	Mistaken as 5 mg if the decimal point is not seen	Use zero before a decimal point when the dose is less than a whole unit
Abbreviations such as mg. or mL. with a period following the abbreviation	mg mL	The period is unnecessary and could be mistaken as the number 1 if written poorly	Use mg, mL, etc., without a terminal period
Drug name and dose run together (especially problematic for drug names that end in "l" such as Inderal40 mg; Tegretol300 mg)	Inderal 40 mg Tegretol 300 mg	Mistaken as Inderal 140 mg Mistaken as Tegretol 1300 mg	Place adequate space between the drug name, dose, and unit of measure

ABBREVIATIONS	INTENDED MEANING	MISINTERPRETATION	CORRECTION
Numerical dose and unit of measure run together (e.g., 10mg, 100mL)	10 mg 100 mL	The "m" is sometimes mistaken as a zero or two zeros, risking a 10- to 100-fold overdose	Place adequate space between the dose and unit of measure
Large doses without properly placed commas (e.g., 100000 units; 1000000 units)	100,000 units 1,000,000 units	100000 has been mistaken as 10,000 or 1,000,000; 1000000 has been mistaken as 100,000	Use commas for dosing units at or above 1,000, or use words such as 100 "thousand" or 1 "million" to improve readability

ABBREVIATIONS	INTENDED MEANING	MISINTERPRETATION	CORRECTION
To avoid confusion, do not abbreviate drug names when communicating medical information. Examples of drug name abbreviations involved in medication errors include:			
APAP	acetaminophen	Not recognized as acetaminophen	Use complete drug name
ARA A	vidarabine	Mistaken as cytarabine (ARA C)	Use complete drug name
AZT	zidovudine (Retrovir)	Mistaken as azathioprine or aztreonam	Use complete drug name
CPZ	Compazine (prochlorperazine)	Mistaken as chlorpromazine	Use complete drug name
DPT	Demerol-Phenergan-Thorazine	Mistaken as diphtheria-pertussis-tetanus (vaccine)	Use complete drug name
DTO	Diluted tincture of opium, or deodorized tincture of opium (Paregoric)	Mistaken as tincture of opium	Use complete drug name
HCl	hydrochloric acid or hydrochloride	Mistaken as potassium chloride (the "H" is misinterpreted as "K")	Use complete drug name unless expressed as a salt of a drug
HCT	hydrocortisone	Mistaken as hydrochlorothiazide	Use complete drug name
HCTZ	hydrochlorothiazide	Mistaken as hydrocortisone (seen as HCT250 mg)	Use complete drug name
MgSO4**	magnesium sulfate	Mistaken as morphine sulfate	Use complete drug name
MS, MSO4**	morphine sulfate	Mistaken as magnesium sulfate	Use complete drug name
MTX	methotrexate	Mistaken as mitoxantrone	Use complete drug name
NoAC	novel/new anticoagulant	No anticoagulant	Use complete drug name
PCA	procainamide	Mistaken as patient controlled analgesia	Use complete drug name

ABBREVIATIONS	INTENDED MEANING	MISINTERPRETATION	CORRECTION
PTU	propylthiouracil	Mistaken as mercaptopurine	Use complete drug name
T3	Tylenol with codeine No. 3	Mistaken as liothyronine	Use complete drug name
TAC	triamcinolone	Mistaken as tetracaine, Adrenalin, cocaine	Use complete drug name
TNK	TNKase	Mistaken as "TPA"	Use complete drug name
TPA or tPA	tissue plasminogen activator, Activase (alteplase)	Mistaken as TNKase (tenecteplase), or less often as another tissue plasminogen activator, Retavase (retaplase)	Use complete drug name
ZnSO4	zinc sulfate	Mistaken as morphine sulfate	Use complete drug name

STEMMED DRUG NAMES	INTENDED MEANING	MISINTERPRETATION	CORRECTION
"Nitro" drip	nitroglycerin infusion	Mistaken as sodium nitroprusside infusion	Use complete drug name
"Norflox"	norfloxacin	Mistaken as Norflex	Use complete drug name
"IV Vanc"	intravenous vancomycin	Mistaken as Invanz	Use complete drug name

SYMBOLS	INTENDED MEANING	MISINTERPRETATION	CORRECTION
ʒ	Dram	Symbol for dram mistaken as "3"	Use metric system
♏	Minim	Symbol for minim mistaken as "mL"	
x3d	For three days	Mistaken as "3 doses"	Use "for three days"
> **and** <	More than and less than	Mistaken as opposite of intended; mistakenly use incorrect symbol; "< 10" mistaken as "40"	Use "more than" or "less than"
/ (slash mark)	Separates two doses or indicates "per"	Mistaken as the number 1 (e.g., "25 units/10 units" misread as "25 units and 110" units)	Use "per" rather than a slash mark to separate doses
@	At	Mistaken as "2"	Use "at"
&	And	Mistaken as "2"	Use "and"
+	Plus or and	Mistaken as "4"	Use "and"
°	Hour	Mistaken as a zero (e.g., q2° seen as q 20)	Use "hr," "h," or "hour"
Φ or ⊘	zero, null sign	Mistaken as numerals 4, 6, 8, and 9	Use 0 or zero, or describe intent using whole words

**These abbreviations are included on The Joint Commission's "minimum list" of dangerous abbreviations, acronyms, and symbols that must be included on an organization's "Do Not Use" list, effective Jan. 1, 2004. Visit www.jointcommission.org for more information about this Joint Commission requirement.

© ISMP 2015. Used with permission from the Institute for Safe Medication Practices. Report actual or potential medication errors to the ISMP Medication Errors Reporting Program (MERP) via the Web at www.ismp.org or by calling 1-800-FAIL-SAFE.

Appendix E

Pharmacology Terms

Topics include:

GENERAL PHARMACY TERMS	
absorp tion	process in which drug is taken up into the body, organ, tissue, or cell
adverse drug reaction (ADR)	any unintended harmful reaction to a drug administered at a normal dose
ampule (or ampoule)	small, sterile glass or plastic container that usually holds a single dose of a liquid medication
aseptic technique	method used to minimize the microbial contamination of compounded sterile drugs
bioavailability	percentage of administered drug available to affect the body and target site(s) after absorption, metabolism, and other factors
capsule (cap)	small, digestible container (usually made of gelatin) used to hold a dose of medication for oral administration
chemotherapy	treatment of cancer with drugs **(also called chemo)**
compounding	act of combining drug ingredients to prepare a customized prescription or drug order for a patient
contraindication	factor that prohibits administration of drug
controlled substance	drug that has been identified as having the potential for abuse or addiction; designated as schedule I, II, III, IV, or V under the federal Controlled Substance Act
cream	water-based, semisolid preparation that is applied topically to external parts of the body
dietary supplement	any vitamin, mineral, amino acid, botanical, herbal, or natural non-drug agent that may be taken orally for general well-being; these agents are not approved by the FDA to diagnose, cure, treat, or prevent any disease
distribution	uptake pattern of drug throughout the body to various tissues
dose	amount of drug or other substance to be administered at one time
drug	any substance taken by mouth; injected into a muscle, the skin, a blood vessel, or a cavity of the body; or applied topically to treat, cure, prevent, or diagnose a disease or condition
drug-drug interaction (DDI)	modification of the effect of a drug when administered with another drug; food, diseases, and conditions can also interact with a drug to cause a modification of the drug's effect
elimination	removal of a substance from the body by any route, including the kidneys, liver, lungs, and sweat glands
elixir	liquid containing sweeteners, flavorings, water, and/or alcohol in which an oral medication may be dispersed

emulsion	stable mixture that contains one component suspended within another component that it cannot normally dissolve in or mix with
Food and Drug Administration (FDA)	U.S. federal agency responsible for the enforcement of federal regulations regarding the manufacturing and distribution of food, drugs, and cosmetics as protection against the sale of impure or dangerous substances
formulary	listing of drugs and drug information used by health practitioners within an institution to prescribe treatment that is medically appropriate
generic name	official, established nonproprietary name assigned to drug
inhaler	device containing drug to be breathed in nasally or by mouth
mechanism of action (MOA)	means by which drug exerts a desired effect
metabolism	chemical changes that a drug or other substance undergoes in the body
ointment	oil-based, semisolid preparation that is applied topically to external parts of the body
over-the-counter (OTC) drug	drug that may be purchased without a prescription (also called **nonprescription drug**)
pharmaceutical	drug used for medicinal purposes
pharmacist	person formally trained to formulate and dispense medications and provide drug information
pharmacodynamics	study of the actions of drug on the body
pharmacogenomics	study of the correlation between genetics and response to drug
pharmacokinetics (PK)	study of the actions of the body on drug or the movement of drug in the body
pharmacology	study of the preparation, properties, uses, and actions of drugs
pharmacy	place for preparing and dispensing drugs
placebo	inactive substance, prescribed as if it were an effective dose of a needed medication
prescription (Rx)	order for a medication, therapy, or a therapeutic device given by a properly authorized person for a specified patient
preservative	substance included in some parenteral and topical medications used to prevent the growth of microorganisms in the product
route of administration	method in which drug or agent is given to a patient
side effect	any reaction or result from a medication other than what is the primary intended effect
solution	homogenous mixture of one or more substances dissolved into another substance
state board of pharmacy	agency responsible for regulating the practice of pharmacy within the state
suppository	topical form of drug that is inserted into the rectum, vagina, or penis
suspension	liquid in which particles of a solid are dispersed, but not dissolved, and in which the dispersal is maintained by stirring or shaking
tablet	small, solid dose form of a medication
toxicity	level at which a drug's concentration within the body produces serious adverse effects
trade name	proprietary name assigned to a drug by its manufacturer that is registered as part of the drug's identity (also called **brand name**)
United States Pharmacopeia (USP)	compendium, recognized officially by the federal Food and Drug Administration that contains descriptions, uses, strengths, and standards of purity for selected drugs and guidance for related standards of practice

ROUTES OF ADMINISTRATION	
buccal	administration of drug by absorption through the inner cheek tissue
enteral	administration of a medication through the digestive tract, including oral ingestion
epidural	injection of drug into the epidural space of the spinal cord
infusion	prolonged administration of a fluid substance directly into a vein, artery, or under the skin in which the flow rate is driven by gravity or a mechanical pump
inhalation	method of drug administration that involves the breathing in of a spray, vapor, or powder via the nose or mouth
injection	introduction of a liquid substance directly into the body bypassing natural routes of entry by using a needle
intramuscular (IM)	administration of a medication directly into a muscle
intrathecal	administration of drug into the subarachnoid space of the meninges in the spine
intravenous (IV)	administration of a medication directly into a vein using a needle or tube
jet injection	administration of a liquid substance through intact skin without a needle using a narrow, high-pressure stream
oral	administration of a medication by mouth
parenteral	administration of a medication via a route that bypasses the digestive tract; most commonly used to refer to injection methods
rectal	administration of drug by absorption through the rectum
subcutaneous	introduction of a medication into the tissue just beneath the skin
sublingual	administration of drug by absorption through tissue under the tongue
topical	administration of a medication to an external area of the body
transdermal	method of applying drug to unbroken skin so that it is continuously absorbed through the skin to produce a systemic effect; a transdermal patch is a drug delivery system that controls the rate of absorption through the skin

GENERAL DRUG CATEGORIES	
antibacterial	drug that targets bacteria to kill or halt growth
antibiotic	drug that targets bacteria, fungi, or protozoa to kill or halt growth; commonly used as synonym for antibacterial
antifungal	drug that targets fungi to kill or halt growth
antihistamine	drug that treats allergic and hypersensitivity reactions by blocking histamine-1 receptors
antiinflammatory	drug that reduces inflammation
antimicrobial	drug that targets microorganisms to kill or halt growth
antineoplastic agent	drug used to destroy or slow the rapid replication of cancer cells
antiretroviral	drug that suppresses the replication of the human immunodeficiency virus (HIV); highly active antiretroviral therapy (HAART) is the combination of three or more of these drugs to treat HIV infection
antiviral	drug that targets viruses to kill or halt growth
antiadrenergic agent	drug that blocks adrenergic receptors to reduce sympathetic nervous system activity in the body
bactericidal	designation for an antimicrobial agent that kills or destroys bacteria
bacteriostatic	the designation for an antimicrobial agent that halts the growth or replication of bacteria but does not kill them
cytotoxic	agent that causes cell death
dietary supplement	product that provides nutrients that may be missing from the diet; dietary supplements are not as strictly regulated as drugs for safety and efficacy

disinfectant	chemical agent that can be applied to inanimate objects to destroy microorganisms
herbal supplement	naturally derived, often plant-based, dietary supplement that is touted to improve health; herbal supplements are not as strictly regulated as drugs for safety and efficacy
immunosuppressant	drug that reduces the response of the immune system; used in autoimmune diseases and to prepare a patient for an organ transplant (also called **immunomodulator**)
narcotic	type of drug that has opium-like effects to cause drowsiness, pain relief, and sedation; can be habit-forming and is regulated as a controlled substance
nonsteroidal antiinflammatory drug (NSAID)	drug that reduces pain, inflammation, and fever
parasympatholytic	agent that blocks the actions of the parasympathetic nervous system
parasympathomimetic	agent that enhances the actions of the parasympathetic nervous system
radiopharmaceutical	drug with a radioactive component; used for diagnosis or treatment
smoking cessation agent	drug that helps a patient quit smoking; may be a behavioral deterrent or a nicotine substitute
sympatholytic	agent that blocks the actions of the sympathetic nervous system
sympathomimetic	agent that enhances the actions of the sympathetic nervous system
vaccine	suspension of weakened or killed microorganisms administered by injection, mouth, or nasal spray, which induces immunity to prevent an infectious disease (also called **immunization**)
vitamin	organic compound essential in small quantities for normal physiologic and metabolic functioning

CHAPTER 2 : BODY STRUCTURE, COLOR, AND ONCOLOGY

alkylating agent	type of antineoplastic agent that binds to cellular DNA to interfere with replication
antimetabolite	type of antineoplastic agent that interferes with a cell's normal metabolism
antineoplastic agent	drug used to destroy or slow the replication of cancer cells
chemotherapeutic agent	drug used to destroy or slow the replication of cancer cells
kinase inhibitor	type of antineoplastic agent that interferes with protein phosphorylation
mitotic inhibitor	type of antineoplastic agent that interrupts cellular division

CHAPTER 4 : INTEGUMENTARY SYSTEM

antibacterial	drug used to combat an infection caused by bacteria
antifungal	drug used to combat an infection caused by fungi
antihistamine	drug used to minimize allergy symptoms by blocking histamine-1 receptors
antipruritic	agent that reduces itching
antipsoriatic	drug that treats psoriasis
antiseptic	chemical agent that can safely be applied to external tissues to kill or halt the growth of microorganisms
astringent	agent that reduces inflammation and irritation and provides a protective barrier on mucosa and skin by contracting the surface tissue
emollient	external agent that softens or soothes the skin
keratolytic	agent that augments the shedding of the top layer of dead skin
pediculicide	agent that kills lice
retinoid	derivative of vitamin A that regulates the growth of epithelial cells
rubefacient	topical agent that increases blood flow to the area to treat muscle aches
scabicide	agent that kills scabies

CHAPTER 5 : RESPIRATORY SYSTEM	
antitussive	drug that suppresses coughing
bronchodilator	drug that expands the airways by relaxing smooth muscle in the lungs
decongestant	drug that relieves nasal congestion by reducing swelling of mucous membranes
expectorant	drug that promotes expulsion of mucus from the lungs
leukotriene receptor antagonist (LTRA)	drug that blocks late-stage regulators of allergic and hypersensitivity reactions to treat allergy-induced asthma
mucolytic	drug that thins out mucus in the lungs so that it can be expelled more easily
CHAPTER 6: URINARY SYSTEM	
aldosterone receptor antagonist (ARA)	drug that decreases reabsorption of water and sodium by the kidneys to treat edema or high blood pressure
alpha-1 blocker	drug that relaxes the muscles in the prostate and bladder neck to improve urination in men with an enlarged prostate
antispasmodic	drug that prevents or relieves bladder muscle spasms associated with incontinence
diuretic	drug that promotes the formation and excretion of urine to reduce the volume of extracellular fluid; used to reduce high blood pressure or edema; commonly referred to as a "water pill"
muscle relaxant	drug that reduces bladder muscle contractility to relieve spasm-induced pain or uncontrolled urination
urinary alkalinizer	agent that increases the urine pH
vasopressin	drug that increases water retention by the kidneys (also called ***antidiuretic hormone*** or ***ADH***)
CHAPTER 7 : MALE REPRODUCTIVE SYSTEM	
androgen	natural or synthetic hormone involved in male reproduction and secondary gender attributes
antiandrogen	drug that blocks the effects of androgen hormones in the body
phosphodiesterase-5 inhibitor (PDE5 inhibitor)	drug that blocks the inactivation of cyclic guanosine monophosphate to increase vasodilation in the penis ; used to treat erectile dysfunction
spermicide	contact agent that kills sperm
CHAPTER 8 : FEMALE REPRODUCTIVE SYSTEM	
antiestrogen	drug used to block the action of estrogen hormones in the body
contraceptive	agent (drug or barrier) used to prevent conception or pregnancy
estrogen	natural or synthetic hormone involved in female reproduction and secondary gender characteristics
fertility drugs	drugs that enhance a female's ability to conceive a child
hormone replacement therapy (HRT)	regimen that mimics the body's normal levels of female hormones when they are no longer produced; typically used during menopause
intrauterine device (IUD)	hormone-containing or metal-based device that is inserted directly in the uterus to prevent pregnancy; may be left in place for 5 years or longer
oral contraceptive	exogenous hormones taken by mouth to prevent pregnancy
ovulation stimulant	drug that enhances the release of an egg from the ovary to promote pregnancy
progestin	synthetic or natural hormone involved in female reproduction and secondary gender characteristics
vaginal ring	device containing estrogen and progestin hormones that is inserted in the vagina to prevent pregnancy

CHAPTER 9 : OBSTETRICS AND NEONATOLOGY	
abortifacient	drug that causes uterine muscles to contract with subsequent abortion of the fetus
oxytocic	hormone that stimulates the uterine muscles to contract, thereby inducing labor in a pregnant woman
pregnancy category	level of risk the Food and Drug Administration assigns a drug based on documented problems with the use of that drug during pregnancy
tocolytic	agent that suppresses labor contractions
CHAPTER 10 : CARDIOVASCULAR, IMMUNE, AND LYMPHATIC SYSTEMS AND BLOOD	
angiotensin-converting enzyme inhibitor (ACE inhibitor)	drug that prevents the formation of angiotensin-II, which is a strong vasoconstrictor and major contributor to high blood pressure
angiotensin receptor blocker (ARB)	drug that blocks the angiotensin-II molecule from binding to its receptors throughout the body to prevent its effects and reduce high blood pressure
antianginal	drug that relieves the chest pain paroxysms caused by lack of oxygen delivery to the heart; typically involves vasodilation
antiarrhythmic	drug that treats abnormal heart rhythm
anticoagulant	drug that prevents blood clotting and coagulation; commonly referred to as a blood thinner
antihypertensive	drug that lowers blood pressure
antiplatelet agent	drug that prevents platelet formation or aggregation or causes platelet destruction
beta-blocker (BB)	drug that inhibits beta-adrenergic receptors to decrease heart rate and force of contractility; used to treat arrhythmias, hypertension, heart failure, and more
calcium channel blocker (CCB)	drug that regulates the entry of calcium into muscle cells of the heart and blood vessels; used to treat heart failure, arrhythmias, angina, and hypertension
colony-stimulating factor (CSF)	agent that promotes the replication of blood cells in the bone marrow
direct thrombin inhibitor (DTI)	drug that blocks the action of thrombin, thereby reducing blood coagulation
erythropoiesis stimulating agent (ESA)	agent that stimulates red blood cell production in the bone marrow
hemostatic	drug that stops bleeding or hemorrhaging
inotropic agent	drug that strengthens or weakens the contraction of the heart muscles
nitrate	drug that dilates the blood vessels
platelet aggregation inhibitor	drug that stops platelets from adhering together
renin inhibitor	drug that blocks renin activity to reduce high blood pressure; renin is the first step in the renin-angiotensin-aldosterone system (RAAS), which is a common contributor to chronic high blood pressure
thrombolytic	drug that dissolves blood clots
vasodilator	drug that expands blood vessels to lower blood pressure
vasopressor	drug that contracts blood vessels to raise blood pressure (also called **vasoconstrictor**)

CHAPTER 11 : DIGESTIVE SYSTEM	
antacid	drug that neutralizes acid in the stomach
antidiarrheal	drug that treats diarrhea by increasing water absorption, decreasing muscle contraction of the intestines, altering electrolyte exchange, or absorbing toxins or microorganisms
antiemetic	drug that reduces or prevents nausea and vomiting
antihyperlipidemic agent	drug used to reduce high levels of bad cholesterol and/or raise levels of good cholesterol by affecting levels of low-density lipoproteins, high-density lipoproteins, total cholesterol, and/or triglycerides, which are collectively called lipids (also called **hypolipidemic agent**)
bile acid sequestrant	type of antihyperlipidemic agent used to lower high cholesterol levels by increasing the excretion of bile acids
cathartic	agent that aids the evacuation of the bowels by accelerating defecation
enema	liquid agent administered rectally to clear the contents of the bowel
fibrate	type of antihyperlipidemic agent that affects lipid levels by facilitating lipid metabolism
histamine-2 receptor antagonist (H2RA)	drug that reduces production of stomach acid by blocking the H2 receptors on gastric parietal cells (also called **H2 blocker**)
laxative	drug that aids the evacuation of the bowel
proton pump inhibitor (PPI)	drug that reduces production of stomach acid by blocking the proton pump on gastric parietal cells
statin	type of antihyperlipidemic agent that treats dyslipidemia by inhibiting 3-hydroxy-3-methylglutaryl coenzyme A reductase (also called **HMG-CoA reductase inhibitor**)
CHAPTER 12 : EYE	
antiglaucoma agent	drug that treats glaucoma of the eye
miotic	agent that constricts the pupil
mydriatic	agent that dilates the pupil
ophthalmic	agent that is intended to be used in the eye; must be sterile
CHAPTER 13 : EAR	
ceruminolytic	agent that breaks down ear wax
otic	agent intended to be used in the ear
CHAPTER 14 : MUSCULOSKELETAL SYSTEM	
antiarthritic agent	drug used in the treatment of arthritis
antigout agent	drug that opposes the buildup of uric acid crystals in the joints to prevent and treat gout attacks
antispasmodic	drug that prevents or relieves muscle spasms
biologic	genetically-engineered protein that targets a specific hyper-functioning component of the immune system to treat diseases such as rheumatoid arthritis
bisphosphonate	drug that binds to bone matrix to treat osteoporosis
disease-modifying antirheumatic drug (DMARD)	drug that slows the progression of rheumatoid arthritis
muscle relaxant	drug that reduces muscle contractility to relieve tension- or spasm-induced pain
neuromuscular blocking agent (NMBA)	drug that blocks all nerve stimulation of the skeletal muscles to cause paralysis

CHAPTER 15 : NERVOUS SYSTEM AND BEHAVIORAL HEALTH	
adrenergic agonist	drug that stimulates aspects of the sympathetic nervous system
amphetamine	drug that stimulates the central nervous system
anticonvulsant	drug that reduces the incidence and severity of seizures and convulsions (also called **antiepileptic drug**)
analgesic	drug that relieves pain
anesthetic	drug that causes numbness or a loss of feeling that can be used locally or systemically; often used systemically to put a patient "to sleep" during extensive procedures
anticholinergic	drug that blocks the action of acetylcholine and therefore suppresses the parasympathetic nervous system
anticholinesterase	drug that prevents the breakdown of acetylcholine to yield a cholinergic or parasympathetic effect
antidepressant	drug used to treat depression and other disorders related to chemical imbalances of the central nervous system
antiparkinsonian agent	drug that treats Parkinson disease and parkinsonism by affecting levels of dopamine or acetylcholine in the brain
antipsychotic	drug that treats psychosis disorders by inducing a calming or tranquilizing effect or by adjusting neurotransmitter levels in the brain (also called **neuroleptic**)
antipyretic	drug that reduces fever
anxiolytic	drug that relieves anxiety
benzodiazepine (BZD)	type of drug that binds to receptors in the brain to calm and sedate the central nervous system
central nervous system stimulant	drug that excites the central nervous system; can be used for many brain disorders
cholinergic	agent that acts like acetylcholine to activate the parasympathetic nervous system
dopaminergic	drug that acts like dopamine, a neurotransmitter in the brain
hypnotic	drug used to induce sleep; many hypnotic agents may also induce sedative effects
mood stabilizer	drug that balances neurotransmitters in the brain to lessen the mood swings of bipolar disorder
monoamine oxidase inhibitor (MAOI)	type of antidepressant that prevents the breakdown of many active neurotransmitters in the brain
nonsteroidal antiinflammatory drug (NSAID)	drug that reduces pain, inflammation, and fever
opioid antagonist	drug that can treat opioid or narcotic overdose
sedative	drug that depresses the central nervous system to calm a patient; many sedative agents may also induce sleep
selective serotonin reuptake inhibitor (SSRI)	type of antidepressant that maintains a higher level of serotonin in the central nervous system
tranquilizer	drug that reduces anxiety or agitation
tricyclic antidepressant (TCA)	type of antidepressant that maintains a higher level of various neurotransmitters in the central nervous system

CHAPTER 16 : ENDOCRINE SYSTEM	
antidiabetic agent	drug that treats diabetes by controlling blood sugar levels
antithyroid agent	drug that counters hyperthyroidism by reducing the production of thyroid hormones
corticosteroid	drug that mimics hormones produced by the adrenal glands and has antiinflammatory and immunosuppressive effects
hypoglycemic agent	drug that lowers blood sugar levels (also called **antihyperglycemic**)
thyroid hormone	replacement hormone to regulate metabolism and endocrine functions

Bibliography

2016 Conn's current therapy, Philadelphia, 2016, Elsevier.

American Journal of Nursing, 2008-2016, Wolters Kluwer.

AAFP, http://www.aafp.org, 2020, American Academy of Family Physicians.

Abbas A: *Basic immunology: functions and disorders of the immune system*, ed 4, Philadelphia, 2013, Saunders.

ACOG: The American congress of obstetricians and gynecologists, women's health care physicians, http://www.acog.org, 2016, American Congress of Obstetricians and Gynecologists.

Adams J: *Emergency medicine, clinical essentials*, ed 2, Philadelphia, 2014, Saunders.

American academy of dermatology, https://www.aad.org, 2020, American Academy of Dermatology.

American academy of ophthalmology: eyesmart, http://www.aao.org, 2020, American Academy of Ophthalmology.

American board of medical specialties, http://www.abms.org, 2016, American Board of Medical Specialties.

American cancer society, http://www.cancer.org, 2020, American Cancer Society, Inc.

American gastroenterological association, www.gastro.org, 2020, American Gastroenterological Association.

American society for gastrointestinal endoscopy, www.asge.org, 2016, American Society for Gastrointestinal Endoscopy.

Aminoff M: *Neurology and general medicine*, ed 4, 2008, Elsevier.

Applegate EJ: *The anatomy and physiology learning system*, ed 4, St. Louis, 2011, Saunders.

Ballinger PW, Frank ED: *Merrill's atlas of radiographic positions and radiologic procedures*, ed 13, 2016, Elsevier.

Bindroo S, Challa HJ: *Renal failure*, Florida, 2020, StatPearls Publishing.

Bolognia JL, et al: *Dermatology*, ed 4, 2018, Elsevier.

Bontrager KL: *Textbook of radiographic positioning and related anatomy*, ed 8, St. Louis, 2013, Mosby.

Buchbinder R, et al: Percutaneous vertebroplasty for osteoporotic vertebral compression fracture, Cochrane Database Syst Rev (4):Art. No.: CD006349, 2015. doi:10.1002/14651858.CD006349.pub2.

Budson AD, Solomon PR: Memory Loss, *Alzheimer's Disease, and Dementia*, 2016, Elsevier.

Cancer.Net: http://www.cancer.net, 2005-2020, American Society of Clinical Oncology (ASCO).

CDC: *Centers for disease control and prevention*, https://www.cdc.gov, 2020, US Department of Health and Human Services.

Chabner D: *The language of medicine*, ed 11, Philadelphia, 2017, Saunders.

Chen Y, et al: The differences between blast-induced and sports-related brain injuries, Front Neurol 2013. http://dx.doi.org/10.3389/fneur.2013.00119. Frontiers Media, SA.

Christensen B, Kockrow E: *Foundations of nursing*, ed 6, St. Louis, 2011, Mosby.

Comez YI: Laparoscopic simple prostatectomy, *Prostatectomy*,Turkey, 2019, Intechopen.

Dekel S, et al: *Massachusetts General Hospital Comprehensive Clinical Psychiatry*, 2016, Elsevier.

Declerck A, et al: Closed-loop titration of propofol and remifentanil guided by Bispectral Index in a patient with extreme gigantism, J Clin Anesth 21(7):542–544, 2009. doi:10.1016/j.jclinane.2009.02.008.

DermNet NZ, www.dermnetnz.org, 2020, DermNet New Zealand Trust.

Diehl M: *Medical transcription guide: do's and don'ts*, ed 3, St. Louis, 2005, Saunders.

Diehl M: *Diehl and Fordney's medical transcription, techniques and procedures*, ed 5, 2002, Saunders.

Diagnostic tests (ophthalmology), www.pennmedicine.org/for-patients-and-visitors, 2020, Penn Medicine, Philadelphia.

Dorland's illustrated medical dictionary, ed 33, Philadelphia, 2020, Saunders.

Drazner M: The progression of hypertensive heart disease, Circulation 2011. http://dx.doi.org/10.1161/CIRCULATIONAHA.108.845792. The American Heart Association.

Ferri F: *Ferri's clinical advisor*, 2020, Elsevier.

Find a code, https://www.findacode.com, 2000-2020, InnoviHealth Systems Inc - CPT, American Medical Association.

First consult, https://www.clinicalkey.com, 2020, Elsevier.

Fitzpatrick JE, Aeling JL: *Dermatology secrets in color*, ed 4, Philadelphia, 2010, Mosby.

Foot health facts, https://www.foothealthfacts.org, 2020, American College of Foot and Ankle Surgeons.

Frazier M, Drzymkowski JW: *Essentials of human diseases and conditions*, ed 5, Philadelphia, 2013, Saunders.

Gillingham EA, Seibel MW: *LaFleur Brooks' health unit coordinating*, ed 7, Philadelphia, 2014, Saunders.

Goljan EF: *Rapid review pathology*, ed 4, Philadelphia, 2014, Saunders.

Gould B, Dyer R: *Pathophysiology for the health professions*, ed 4, Philadelphia, 2011, Saunders.

Habif T: *A color guide to diagnosis and therapy, clinical dermatology*, ed 5, Philadelphia, 2010, Mosby.

Haubrich WS: *Medical meanings: a glossary of word origins*, ed 2, Philadelphia, 2004, American College of Physicians.

Hein C, Batista EL: Obesity and cumulative inflammatory burden: a valuable risk assessment parameter in caring for dental patients, J Evid Based Dent Pract 14:17–26.e1, 2014. Elsevier.

Herlihy B, Maebius N: *The human body in health and illness*, ed 5, Philadelphia, 2015, Saunders.

Hockenberry MJ, Wilson D: *Wong's nursing care of infants and children*, ed 9, St. Louis, 2011, Mosby.

Huth EJ, Murray TJ: *Medicine in quotations: views of health and disease through the ages*, Philadelphia, 2006, American College of Physicians.

Ignatavicius DD, et al: *Medical-surgical nursing: patient-centered collaborative care*, ed 8, Philadelphia, 2015, Saunders.

ICD10Data, www.icd10data.com, 2020, ICD10data.com.

Immunosuppression, https://aidsinfo.nih.gov/understanding-hiv-aids/glossary/364/immunosuppression, 2020, National Institutes of Health.

Jagoda A, Haru O: *Emergency medicine*, 2013, Elsevier.

James W, et al: *Andrews' diseases of the skin*, ed 13, 2020, Elsevier.

Jameson JL, DeGroot LJ: *Endocrinology: adult and pediatric*, ed 7, Philadelphia, 2016, Saunders.

Jarvis C: *Physical examination & health assessment*, ed 7, Philadelphia, 2016, Saunders.

Johns Hopkins Medicine: www.hopkinsmedicine.org, 2020, The Johns Hopkins University, The Johns Hopkins Hospital, and Johns Hopkins Health System.

Klabunde RE: Cardiovascular physiology concepts,https://www.cvphysiology.com, 1998-2020, Richard E. Klabunde, Ph.D.

Knopman DS: *Goldman-cecil medicine*, 2016, Elsevier.

Lab tests online, https://labtestsonline.org, 2001-2020, American Association for Clinical Chemistry.

LaFleur Brooks M, LaFleur Brooks D: *Basic medical language*, ed 5, St. Louis, 2016, Mosby.

LaFranchi SH, Huang SA: *Nelson textbook of pediatrics*, ed 20, 2016, Elsevier.

Lewis SM, et al: *Medical-surgical nursing*, ed 8, St. Louis, 2011, Mosby.

Littleton LY, Engebretson JC: *Maternal, neonatal, and women's health nursing*, Albany, 2002, Delmar.

Lokeshwar SD, et al: Epidemiology and treatment modalities for the management of benign prostatic hyperplasia, *TAU Translational andrology and urology*, Vol 8, No 5 2019), AME Publishing.

Lowdermilk DL, et al: *Maternity & women's health care*, ed 11, St. Louis, 2016, Mosby.

Marx J, et al: *Rosen's emergency medicine, concepts and clinical practice*, ed 8, Philadelphia, 2014, Saunders.

Mayo Clinic Health Letter, Rochester, 2008-2020, Mayo Foundation for Medical Education and Research.

Mayo Clinic: *Patient care and health information*, http://www.mayoclinic.org, 1998-2020, Mayo Foundation for Medical Education and Research.

Mayo Clinic Women's Health Source, Rochester, 2008-2016, Mayo Foundation for Medical Education and Research.

Medical dictionary, http://www.medical-dictionary.thefreedictionary.com, n.d., The Free Dictionary by Farlex.

MedicineNet, www.medicinenet.com, 1991-2020, MedicineNet Inc.

Medline Plus, http://www.nlm.nih.gov/medlineplus, 2008-2020, National Library of Medicine and the National Institutes of Health.

Merck manuals, https://www.merckmanuals.com, 2020, Merck Sharp & Dohme Corp.

Medscape, http://www.medscape.com, 1994-2020, WebMD LLC.

Molecular and nuclear imaging (PET and SPECT), https://imaging.cancer.gov/imaging_basics/cancer_imaging/nuclear_imaging.htm, 2016, National Cancer Institute DCTD Division of Cancer Treatment & Diagnosis, National Institutes of Health.

Mosby's medical, nursing, & health professions dictionary, ed 9, St. Louis, 2013, Mosby.

National cancer institute, www.cancer.gov, n.d., National Institutes of Health.

National center for biotechnology information, www.ncbi.nlm.nih.gov, n.d., National Institutes of Health.

National human genome research institute, www.genome.gov/health/Genomics-and-Medicine, 2020, National Institutes of Health.

National institute of diabetes and digestive and kidney diseases, www.niddk.nih.gov, 2016, National Institutes of Health.

New England Journal of Medicine, 2008-2016, Massachusetts Medical Society.

Novey D: *Clinicians' complete reference to complementary and alternative medicine*, St. Louis, 2000, Mosby.

Obstetrics and gynecology: quad screen, https://www.uwhealth.org/obgyn/quad-screen/27846, 2020, University of Wisconsin Hospitals and Clinics Authority Obstetrics.

Olney RK, Aminoff MJ: *Neurology and General Medicine*, 2008, Elsevier.

Ontjes DA: Disorders of the adrenal cortex. In *Netter's internal medicine*, ed 2, Philadelphia, 2009, Saunders, pp 321–327. 44.

Opportunistic infections, www.hiv.gov, 2019, US Department of Health and Human Services.

Pagana KD, Pagana TJ: *Mosby's manual of diagnostic and laboratory test reference*, ed 5, St. Louis, 2015, Mosby.

Patient care and health information, www.mayoclinic.org/patient-care-and-health-information, 1998-2016, Mayo Foundation for Medical Education and Research.

Phillips N: *Berry & Kohn's operating room technique*, ed 12, St. Louis, 2013, Mosby.

Powell J, et al: The Canadian arthroplasty society's experience with hip resurfacing arthroplasty. An analysis of 2773 hips, Canadian Arthroplasty Society, Bone Joint J 2013. doi:10.1302/0301-620X.95B8.31811.

RadiologyInfo.org for patients, www.radiologyinfo.org, 2020, Radiological Society of North America, Inc.

Rakel D: *Integrative medicine*, ed 3, Philadelphia, 2012, Saunders.

Retinoblastoma, http://www.cancer.org/acs/groups/cid/documents/webcontent/003135-pdf.pdf, 2015, American Cancer Society.

Schoenwolf, et al: *Larsen's human embrology*, ed 5, 2015, Elsevier Churchill Livingstone.

Seckeler MD, Hoke TR: The worldwide epidemiology of acute rheumatic fever and rheumatic heart disease, Clin Epidemiol 2011. doi:10.2147/CLEP.S12977.

Shimizu R, Kazuo K: Skin graft. *Plastic surgery international* vol. 2012 (2012): 563493. doi:10.1155/2012/563493.

Spencer JW, Jacobs JJ: *Complementary and alternative medicine: an evidence-based approach*, St Louis, 2003, Mosby.

Society of American gastrointestinal and endoscopic surgeons, www.sages.org, 2020, Society of American Gastrointestinal and Endoscopic Surgeons.

Stedman's abbreviations, acronyms, and symbols, ed 5, Baltimore, 2013, Lippincott Williams & Wilkins.

Stern T, et al: *Massachusetts general hospital comprehensive clinical psychiatry*, 2016, Elsevier.

The fecal transplant foundation, http://thefecaltransplantfoundation.org, 2016, The Fecal Transplant Foundation.

Thibodeau GA, Patton KT: *Anthony's textbook of anatomy and physiology*, ed 20, St. Louis, 2016, Mosby.

Torpy JM: The metabolic syndrome, JAMA 295(7):850, 2006.

Trimble MR: *Neurology and General Medicine*, 2008, Elsevier.

UpToDate, http://www.uptodate.com, 2008-2020, Wolters Kluwer Health.

Vanderah TW, Gould DJ: *Nolte's the human brain*, ed 7, 2016, Elsevier.

Vesico-uretal reflux, kidneyresearchuk.org/conditions-symptoms/vesico-uretal-reflux, 2020, Kidney Research UK.

WebMD, www.webmd.com, 2005 - 2020, WebMD LLC.

What is a bleeding disorder?, www.hemophilia.org/Bleeding-Disorders/What-is-a-Bleeding-Disorder, 2020, National Hemophilia Foundation.

What is the Macula?, www.macularsociety.org, 2020, Macular Society.

What is a stem cell or bone marrow transplant?, www.cancerresearchuk.org, 2019, Cancer Research UK.

What is sarcoidosis?, www.stopsarcoidosis.org/what-is-sarcoidosis, 2017, Foundation for Sarcoidosis Research.

Wein AJ, et al: *Campbell-walsh urology*, ed 11, Philadelphia, 2016, Elsevier.

Whiteside MM, et al: Sensory impairment in older adults: part 2, vision loss, Consultant 106(11):52–62, 2006.

Wong CC, McGirt M: Vertebral compression fractures: a review of current management and multimodal therapy, J Multidiscip Healthc 2013.

Workman ML, LaCharity L: *Understanding pharmacology: essentials for medication safety*, ed 2, 2016, Elsevier.

World Health Organization, https://who.int/en, 2020, WHO.

Illustration Credits

Adam A et al: *Grainger and Allison's diagnostic radiology*, ed 5, London, 2008, Churchill Livingstone. **Unn Fig. 15.22**
American Cancer Society. **Fig. 5.4**
Amplivox Limited, Eynsham, Oxfordshire, United Kingdom**. Unn fig 13.16.**
Anderson KN: *Mosby's medical, nursing and allied health dictionary*, St. Louis, 2003, Mosby. **Fig. 11.10A**
Arthritis Teaching Slide Collection, copyright 1980. Used by permission of the Arthritis Foundation. **Unn Fig. 12.12 C**
Azar DT: Refractive Surgery, ed 3, 2020, Elsevier**. Unn fig 12.23**
Ball J et al: *Seidel's guide to physical examination*, ed 8, St. Louis, 2014, Elsevier. **Unn Figs. 12.12, 12.14,** 12-18,
Baggish MS and Karram MM: Atlas of Pelvic Anatomy and Gynecologic Surgery, ed 4, Philadelphia, 2016, Elsevier. **Unn Fig. 8.28**
Ballinger PW, Frank ED: *Merrill's atlas of radiographic positions and radiologic procedures*, ed 10, St. Louis, 2003, Mosby. **Fig. 14.12, Unn Figs 3.41, 2.19, 6.22, 10.20 B, C, 10.27, 10.8, 10.9, 15.21**
Bassett LW, et al: Breast Imaging, Philadelphia, 2011, Saunders-Elsevier. **Fig. 8.14C.**
Batterbury M, et al: Ophthalmology: An illustrated colour text, ed 4, 2019, Elsevier, Ltd. **Unn Fig. 12.7, 12.10, 12.19, 12.34, 12.38**
Beaty JH, et al: Campbell's Operative Orthopaedics, ed 13, Philadeelphia, 2017, Elsevier. **Unn Fig 14.8.**
Bedford MA: *Ophthalmological diagnosis*, London, 1986, Wolfe. **Unn Fig. 12.17**
Biopsys Medical, Inc, Irvine, Calif. **Fig. 8.14A**
Black J, Hawks J: *Medical-surgical nursing*, ed 8, St. Louis, 2009, Elsevier. **Figs. 8.9, Unn fig 12.22**
Bontrager KL, Lampignano JP: *Radiographic positioning and related anatomy*, ed 8, St. Louis, 2014, Mosby. **Unn Figs. 3.29, 3.30, 3.32, 3.33 6.12, Unn 8.32, 8.33,** Fig. **9.12, unn Fig 10-29, 10.30, Fig. 14.11B**
Bontrager KL: *Radiographic positioning and related anatomy*, ed 5, St. Louis, 2002, Mosby. **Table 3.2 images, Unn Fig 3.16, Unn Fig. 15.26**
Bork K, Brauninger W: *Skin diseases in clinical practice*, ed 2, Philadelphia, 1998, WB Saunders. **Unn fig. 4.10, Figs. 4.3A, Unn Fig., 4.34,** 4-44, 4-45, 4-46, **Unn Fig. 7.3, Fig. 10.12B**
Buckingham Richard A, MD, University of Illinois, Chicago. **Fig. 13.3, Unn 13.6**
Bullough P: *Orthopaedic pathology*, ed 5, St. Louis, 2010, Elsevier. **Ch 2 Ex Fig. A3**
Canale S, Beaty J: *Campbell's operative orthopaedics*, ed 12, St. Louis, 2013, Elsevier. **Unn Fig. Table 14-1, 3**
Carver E and Carver B: Medical Imaging: Techniques, Reflection & Evaluation, ed 2, 2012, Churchill Livingstone-Elsevier Ltd. **Unn Fig. 16.18**
CDC. **Unn Figs. 5.37**
Christensen B, Kockrow E: *Adult health nursing*, ed 5, St. Louis, 2006, Elsevier Mosby. **Unn Fig. 4.21**
Clinical Slide Collection of the Rheumatic Diseases, copyright 1991. Used by permission of the American College of Rheumatology. **Unn fig 14.12 A,B**
Cohen BA: *Pediatric dermatology*, ed 3, St. Louis, 2005, Mosby. Unn **Fig. 4.31**
Cote CJ, et al: A practice of anesthesia for infants and children, ed 6, Philadelphia, 2019, Elsevier. Unn fig 12.20
Courtesy Paul W. Ladenson, MD, Johns Hopkins University and Hospital, Baltimore, Maryland. **Unn Fig 16.11**
Cummings N: *Perspectives in athletic training*, ed 1, St. Louis, 2009, Mosby. Unn **Fig. 5.38**
Damjanov I: *Pathology, A color atlas*, ed 2, St. Louis, 2000, Mosby. **Fig. 2.5, Ch 2 Ex Fig. A4, Figs. 6.5A, 6.6**
Damjanov I: Pathology for the health professions, ed 4, Philadelphia, 2011, Saunders. **Unn Fig. 16.14**
De la Maza LM, Pezzlo MT, Baron EJ: Color Atlas of Diagnostic Microbiology. St Louis, Mosby, 1997. **Unn Fig 2.30**
Dorland's illustrated medical dictionary, ed 31, Philadelphia, 2007, Saunders. Unn. **Fig. 4.32**
Dorland's illustrated medical dictionary, ed 32, Philadelphia, 2012, Saunders-Elsevier. Fig. 9.14, Unn Fig. 11.13
Dornier Medical Systems, Kennesaw, Ga. **Unn Fig. 6.21**
EDAP Technomed, Inc., Vaulx-en-Velin, France. **Fig. 7.6B**
Eisenberg RL, Johnson NM: *Comprehensive radiographic pathology*, ed 3, St. Louis, 2003, Mosby. **Fig. 5.3**Forbes CD and Jackson WF: **Unn Fig. 16.24**
Frazier M: *Essentials of human disease and conditions*, ed 3, St. Louis, 2004, Elsevier Mosby. Table 4-1, **Unn Fig. 4.1**
Fucentese SF et al: Total shoulder arthroplasty with an uncemented soft-metal-backed glenoid component, *J Shoulder Elbow Surg* 19:624-631, 2010. **Unn Fig. Table 14-1, 5**

Gabbe SG et al: Obstetrics: Normal and Problem Pregnancies (Obstetrics Normal and Problem Preqnancies), ed 7, Phildelphia, 2017, Elsevier. Unn Fig. 9.19

Gawkrodger D, Ardern-Jones M: *Dermatology*, ed 5, Oxford, 2012, Churchill Livingstone. Table 4-1, **Unn Fig. 4.5**

Goering R et al: *Mims' medical microbiology*, ed 4, Edinburgh, 2008, Mosby Ltd. **Unn Fig. 4.18**

Goldman L, and Schafer AI: Goldman-Cecil Medicine, ed 26, Philadelphia, 2020, Elsevier. **Unn Fig.4.36**

Goldman L, Schafer A: *Goldman's Cecil medicine*, ed 24, Philadelphia, 2012, Saunders. **Fig. 4.3 (upper right), Unn Fig. 4.29, Fig. 7.7C**

Habif TP: *Clinical dermatology*, ed 4, St. Louis, 2004, Elsevier Mosby. **Ch 2 Ex Fig. A2, Figs. 4.3 (right halftone), 4.6, Unn Fig. 4.17**

Habif TP, et al: Skin Disease: Diagnosis and Treatment, ed 4, 2018, Elsevier Inc. **Table 4-1, Unn Fig 4.3.**

Hagen-Ansert S: *Textbook of diagnostic ultrasonography*, ed 5, St. Louis, 2001, Mosby. **Unn Fig. Table 11.2**

Hagen-Ansert S: *Textbook of diagnostic ultrasonography*, ed 7, St. Louis, 2012, Mosby. **Unn Fig. 16.19**

Haught JM, Patel S, and English JC: Xanthoderma: A clinical review, *J Amer Acad Derm* 57(6):1051-1058, 2007. **Unn Fig. 4-35**

Henningsen C, et al: Clinical guide to Sonography: Exercises for critical thinking, ed 2, St. Louis, 2014, Elsevier. **Unn Fig. 16.16**

Herring W: Learning radiology: recognizing the basics, ed 3, Philadephla, Saunders, 2005. **Unn Fig 10-21, 10.26**

Hockenberry M et al: *Wong's nursing care of infants and children*, ed 9, St. Louis, 2011, Elsevier. **Figs. 9.7, Unn Fig. 9.14, 9.18**

Ignatavicius DM, Workman L: *Medical-surgical nursing*, ed 6, St. Louis, 2010, Saunders. **unn Fig 10-29, 10.30**

James S, Ashwill J: *Nursing care of children*, ed 3, St. Louis, 2008, Saunders. **Fig. 6.13**

James WD, et al: Andrews' disease of the skin: Clinical dermatology, 2020, Elsevier. **Fig 4.8 A,B**

Jarvis C: *Physical examination and health assessment*, ed 5, Philadelphia, 2008, Saunders. **Unn Fig 5.45 12.31, 12.32, 13.15**

Kamal A, Brockelhurst JC: *Color atlas of geriatric medicine*, ed 2, St. Louis, 1991, Mosby. **Unn Fig. 2.32**

Kanski JJ and Bowling B: Kanski's Clinical Ophthalmology: A systematic approach, ed 8, 2016, Elsevier. **Unn Fig 12.24**

Kliegman R et al: *Nelson textbook of pediatrics*, ed 20, St. Louis, 2016, Elsevier. **Unn Fig. 16.10**

Kliegman R et al: *Nelson textbook of pediatrics*, ed 18, St. Louis, 2008, Saunders. **Unn Fig. 13.14**

Kowalczyk N: *Radiographic pathology for technologists*, ed 6, St. Louis, 2014, Elsevier. **Fig. 11.16, Unn Fig. 11.33**

Kowalczyk N: *Radiographic pathology for technologists*, ed 7, St. Louis, 2017, Elsevier. **Unn Fig. 16.17**

Kumar V et al: *Robbins' basic pathology*, ed 7, Philadelphia, 2003, Saunders. Unn **Fig. 5.18**

Kumar V, Abbas AK, Fausto M: Robbins and Cotran Pathologic Basis of Disease, 7th ed. Philadelphia, 2005 WB Saunders. **Unn Fig 2.12**

Kumar V, et al: Robbins & Cotran Pathologic Basis of Disease, ed 10, Philadelphia, 2021, Elsevier. **Unn Fig. 12.6**

Ladenson Paul W, MD, The Johns Hopkins University and Hospital, Baltimore, Md. **Unn Fig. 16.25**

Lewis SM: *Medical-surgical nursing*, ed 7, St. Louis, 2007, Mosby. **Unn Fig. 11.37**

Long et al: *Merrill's atlas of radiographic positions and radiologic procedures*, ed 13, St. Louis, 2016, Elsevier. **Fig. 14.9A(right), Unn Fig. Table 14.1, 1**

Lowdermilk DL et al: *Maternity and women's health care*, ed 10, St. Louis, 2012, Mosby. **Fig. 9.5**

Mace JD: *Radiography pathology*, ed 4, St. Louis, 2004, Elsevier Mosby. **Ch 2 Ex Fig. A1**

Magee D: *Orthopedic physical assessment*, ed 5, St. Louis, 2008, Saunders. **Fig. 14.9B(right)**

Mahon C et al: *Textbook of diagnostic microbiology*, ed 4, Philadelphia, 2011, Elsevier. **Fig. 7.7B**

Manaster BJ: *Musculoskeletal imaging*, ed 3, St. Louis, 2007, Mosby. **Fig. 14.9C(right)**

Marks J, Miller J: *Lookingbill and Marks' principles of dermatology*, ed 5, Philadelphia, 2014, Elsevier. **Unn Fig. 4.15**

Mercier LR: *Practical orthopedics*, ed 4, St. Louis, 1995, Mosby. **Fig. 14.13**

Murray P et al: *Medical microbiology*, ed 5, St. Louis, 2005, Mosby. **Fig. 7.7A**

National Cancer Institute (NCI). Courtesy Rhoda Baer (Photographer). **Fig. 2.8. Unn Fig 2.21**

Nelcor Puritan Bennett. Unn **Fig. 5.46**

Netter medical illustration used with permission of Elsevier All rights reserved. Unn Fig. 9.6, 9.7

Newell FW: *Ophthalmology*, ed 7, St. Louis, 1992, Mosby. **Unn Fig. 12.16**

Nidek, Inc., Fremont, Calif. **Fig. 12.8**

Otto CM: Textbook of Clinical Echocardiography, ed 6, Philadelphia, 2018, Elsevier. Unn Fig 10.5,

Pagana KD, Pagana TJ: *Mosby's manual of diagnostic and laboratory test reference*, ed 7, St. Louis, 2004, Elsevier Mosby. **Unn Fig 3.10 B, Fig. 8.14B, C**

Patton KT, Thibodeau GA: *Anatomy and physiology*, ed 7, St. Louis, 2010, Mosby. **Unn Fig. 10.14, Unn Fig. 14.13**

Paulino A: *PET-CT in radiotherapy treatment planning*, ed 1, Philadelphia, 2008, Saunders/Elsevier. **Unn Fig. 5.44**

Perkin GD, Hotchberg FH, Miller D: *The atlas of clinical neurology*, St. Louis, 1986, Mosby. **Unn Fig. 15.12**

Perry A, Potter P, Elkin M: *Nursing interventions & clinical skills*, ed 4, St. Louis, 2008, Mosby/Elsevier. **Unn Figs. 3.31, Table 4-1 Unn Fig. 4-2**

Potter PA, Perry AG: Fundamentals of nursing, ed 7, St. Louis, 2009, Mosby. **Unn Fig 5-6, 5-7, 5.33**

Richardson M et al: *Cummings otolaryngology - head and neck surgery*, ed 5, St. Louis, 2010, Mosby. **Unn Fig. 13.7**

Rohrer TE, et al: Flaps and Grafts in Dermatologic Surgery, ed 2, Philadelphia, 2018, Elsevier. **Unn Fig 8-4**

Ruppel GL: *Manual pulmonary function testing*, ed 7, St. Louis, 1998, Mosby. **Unn Fig 3.9B, 3.35 5.43**

Sainani GS, Joshi VR, Sainani RG: Manual of clinical & practical medicine, New Delhi, 2010, Elsevier India. **Unn Fig. 16.8**

Swartz MH: Textbook of physical diagnosis: history and examination, ed 7, Philadelphia, 2014, Saunders. **Unn Fig. 10.41, 13.12**

Schwarzenberger K et al: *General dermatology*, ed 1, Philadelphia, 2009, Saunders. **Unn Fig. 4.9**

Seidel H et al: *Mosby's guide to physical examination*, ed 5, St. Louis, 2003, Mosby. **Fig. 12.4A, B.**

Seidel, H et al. Mosby's Guide to Physical Examination, ed 7, St. Louis, 2011, Mosby. **Unn Fig 4.38**

Shiland BJ: *Mastering healthcare terminology*, ed 2, St. Louis, 2006, Elsevier Mosby. **Unn Figs. 2.26, 4-30, 4-41, 6.16**, 11.8, **Fig. 11.8**

Shiland BJ: Medical Terminology & Anatomy for Coding, ed 3, St. Louis, 2018, Elsevier. **Unn Fig 13.4**

Siemens Medical Systems, Inc., New Jersey. **Unn Fig. 3.43**

Śliwa LS et al: A comparison of audiometric and objective methods in hearing screening of school children: A preliminary study, *Internat J Pediatr Otorhinol* 75(4):483-488, 2011. **Unn Fig. 13.14A**

Stevens A, et al. Core Pathology, 3rd ed. London: Mosby; 2010. **Unn Fig 16. 15**

Swartz M: *Textbook of physical diagnosis*, ed 5, Philadelphia, 2006, Saunders. **Unn Figs. 2.8, 12.15**

Taylor J, Resnick D: *Skeletal imaging: atlas of the spine and extremities*, ed 1, Philadelphia, 2000, Saunders. **Fig. 14.11A**

Thibodeau GA, Patton KT: *Anatomy and physiology*, ed 4, St. Louis, 2001, Mosby. **Figs. 10.12 (A), 14.7.**

Thibodeau GA, Patton KT: Anatomy and physiology, ed 5, St. Louis, 2003, Mosby. **Figs. 15.1, 15.2**

Waldman S: *Atlas of common pain syndromes*, ed 2, Philadelphia, 2008, Saunders. **Unn Fig. 15.5**

Wein A et al: *Campbell-Walsh urology*, ed 10, 2012, Saunders. **Figs. 6.10, 6.11, Unn Figs 6.14, 6.28**

Wenig BM: Atlas of Head and Neck Pathology, 3rd ed, 2016 Elsevier **Unn Fig. 2.17**

Weston W et al: *Color textbook of pediatric dermatology*, ed 4, St. Louis, 2007, Mosby. **Unn Fig. 4.19**

White RA, Klein SR: *Endoscopic surgery*, St. Louis, 1991, Mosby. **Fig. 11.13, Unn 11.28**

Wilkerson CP, et al: Ryan's Retina, ed 6, 2018, Elsevier. **Unn fig. 12.29**

Wilson S, Giddens J: *Health assessment for nursing practice*, ed 4, St. Louis, 2009, Mosby. Courtesy Gary Monheit, MD, University of Alabama at Birmingham School of Medicine. **Fig. 4.3C**

Wilson SF, Thompson JM: *Respiratory disorders*, St. Louis, 1990, Mosby. **Unn 5.39**

Yates D, Caldicott L: Preoperative assessment of vascular patients, Anaesthesia & Intensive Care Medicine, June 2007, Elsevier. **Unn Fig. 10.25**

Zitelli BJ, David HW: *Atlas of pediatric physical diagnosis*, ed 2, St. Louis, 1992, Mosby. **Fig 7.4 A, Figs. 9.6, 12.3,** Unn Fig. 12.36, **Unn fig. 12.8, 12.11, 13.5**

Zitelli, B. J., & Davis, H. W: Atlas of pediatric physical diagnosis, ed 5, St. Louis, 2007 Mosby. **Unn fig 16.12**

Zitelli BJ, et al: Zitelli and Davis' Atlas of Pediatric Physical Diagnosis, ed 7, Philadelphia, 2018, Elsevier. **Unn fig. 13.3**

iStock:

-100rehanphoto **Unnumbered Figure 12.45**
33karen33 **Unnumbered Figure 14.24**
3alexd **Unnumbered Figure 3.39**
9632290_400 **Unnumbered Figure 15.25**
AaronAmat **Unnumbered Figures 12.4, 5.51, 5.9**
AboutnuyLove **Unnumbered Figure 14.22**
AGfoto **Unnumbered Figure 12.37**
agrobacter **Unnumbered Figure 10.16**
AJ_Watt **Unnumbered Figure 14.48**
alenkadr **Unnumbered Figure 14.47**
alex-mit **Unnumbered Figure 6-7**
Alexpunker **Unnumbered Figure 10.15**
AlexRaths **Unnumbered Figure 14.46**
Andesign101 **Unnumbered Figure 9.38**
andrewsafonov **Unnumbered Figure 6-8**
andriano_cz **Unnumbered Figure 4-33**
Antonio_Diaz **Unnumbered Figure 9.24**
Ariyathailand **Unnumbered Figure 5.52**
asikkk **Unnumbered Figure 12.33**
AzmanJaka **Unnumbered Figure 14.49**
BanksPhotos Figure **5.4**
belchonock **Unnumbered Figure 8.34**
bluebeat76 **Unnumbered Figure 16.6**
blueshot **Unnumbered Figure 10.24**
Branimir76 **Unnumbered Figure 5.48**
canbedone **Unnumbered Figure 11.3**
Casanowe **Unnumbered Figure 10.32**
chas53 **Unnumbered Figure 2.35**

CHIARI_VFX **Unnumbered Figure. 2.36**
choja **Unnumbered Figure 10.38**
Claudiad **Unnumbered Figure 15.38**
coddy **Unnumbered Figure 12.43**
CopterAnansak **Unnumbered Figure 8.38**
corbac40 **Unnumbered Figure 9.13**
Devilkae **Unnumbered Figure 5.36**
digitalskillet **Unnumbered Figures. 2.5**
dmbaker **Unnumbered Figure. 2.23**
dolgachov **Unnumbered Figure 12.30**
Dr_Microbe **Unnumbered Figure 5.23, 8.7**
draghicich **Unnumbered Figure 9.37**
Fabianodp **Unnumbered Figure 3.3**
Fahroni **Unnumbered Figure 5.54**
FatCamera **Unnumbered Figures 14.40, 9.33, 9.34, 9.35, 2.33**
Foremniakowski **Unnumbered Figure 16.21**
fotostorm **Unnumbered Figure 16.23**
fstop123 **Unnumbered Figure 2.24**
gawrav **Unnumbered Figure 5.40**
Gewoldi **Unnumbered Figure 9.32**
GOLFX **Unnumbered Figure 4.3**
gorodenkoff **Unnumbered Figure 9.25**
g-stockstudio **Unnumbered Figure 15.30**
HaraldBiebel **Figure 4.8C**
hudiemm **Unnumbered Figure 3.4**
IlexImage **Unnumbered Figure 3.6**
ilmoro100 **Unnumbered Figure 4.7**
image_jungle **Unnumbered Figure 2.38**
Inside Creative House **Unnumbered Figure 13.19**
iStock Figure 4.2, **Unnumbered Figures 14.42, 5.49**
Ivan-balvan **Unnumbered Figures 12.41, 12.42, 14.41**
izusek Figure **4-6**
Jacob Ammentorp Lund **Unnumbered Figure 1-7**
Jan-Otto **Unnumbered Figure 14.34**
jarun011 **Unnumbered Figure 10.40**
Jevtic **Unnumbered Figure 9.26**
joruba **Unnumbered Figure 12.44**
kadmy **Unnumbered Figure 10.39**
kalus **Unnumbered Figure 10-13**
KatarzynaBialasiewicz **Unnumbered Figure 5.8**
kate_sept2004 **Unnumbered Figure 9.27**
kentarus **Unnumbered Figure 13.20**
ktsimage **Unnumbered Figure. 2.29**
Lalocracio **Unnumbered Figure 8.38**
Lighthaunter **Unnumbered Figure 11.4**
LindaYolanda **Unnumbered Figure 9.40**
Ljupco **Unnumbered Figure. 2.31**
loonger **Unnumbered Figure 12.40**
lovelyday12 **Unnumbered Figure 11.5**
Manuel-F-O **Unnumbered Figure 14.45**
Maos **Unnumbered Figure 11.17**
MarkHatfield **Unnumbered Figure 16.7**
maska82 **Unnumbered Figure 15.3**
MediaProduction **Unnumbered Figure 14.14**
Mjp **Unnumbered Figure 16.22**
Mohammed Haneefa Nizamudeen **Unnumbered Figure 11.15**
Morsa Images **Unnumbered Figure 3.40**
mosabua **Unnumbered Figure 3.5**
mvp64 **Unnumbered Figure 4.4**
Mykhailo Pervak **Unnumbered Figure 5.53**
Natthapon **Unnumbered Figure 3.7**
Nikola Ilic **Unnumbered Figure 12.5**
nimon_t **Unnumbered Figure 3.2**
Olga Vasilyeva **Unnumbered Figure 13.17**
Osobystist **Unnumbered Figure 5.47**
Pavel1964 **Unnumbered Figure 16.3**
PeopleImages **Unnumbered Figure. 2.34**
phichet_c **Unnumbered Figure 5.17**
phokin **Unnumbered Figure 4-43**
Pixel_away **Unnumbered Figure 10.31**
praisaeng Figure **4-5, Unnumbered Figure 2.37**
RASimon **Unnumbered Figure 3.9**
redhumv Figure **5-10**
roberthyrons **Unnumbered Figure 12.35**
Savushkin Figure **2.6**
SDI Productions Figure **6.26, Unnumbered Figures 14.44, 15.29, 15.34, 15.36, 1-5**
sdominick **Unnumbered Figure 13.21**
sefa ozel **Unnumbered Figure 14.23**
serezniy **Unnumbered Figure 5-11**
SetsukoN **Unnumbered Figure 14.35**
Shidlovski **Unnumbered Figure 16.20**
silkfactory **Unnumbered Figure 14.36**
SlayStorm **Unnumbered Figure 12.3**
sot **Unnumbered Figure 15.39**
standret **Unnumbered Figure 12.39**
StockPhotosArt **Unnumbered Figure 14.9**
sturti **Unnumbered Figure. 2.25**
szeyuen **Unnumbered Figure 9.30**
ThamKC **Unnumbered Figure. 2.28**
Tharakorn **Unnumbered Figure 16.5**
thelinke **Unnumbered Figure 10.30**
Tunatura **Unnumbered Figure 15.35**
undefined undefined **Unnumbered Figure 14.33**
wanderluster **Unnumbered Figure 15.37**
wildpixel **Unnumbered Figure 11.16, 9.31**
xavierarnau **Unnumbered Figure 3.8**
YakobchukOlena **Unnumbered Figure 11.35**
Yobro10 **Unnumbered Figure 9.39**
zilli **Unnumbered Figure 10.33**
Zuraisham Salleh **Unnumbered Figure 5.22**

Index

Page numbers followed by "*f*" indicate figures, and "*t*" indicate tables.

M

COMMON TERMINOLOGY

Acronym: A term formed from the first letter of several words that can be spoken as a whole word; usually contains a vowel.
EXAMPLE: MRSA (methicillin-resistant Staphylococcus aureus)

Build: Constructing a medical term from its definition using Greek and Latin word parts as a learning exercise.
EXAMPLE: the term meaning "inflammation of the kidney" may be constructed from nephr/o (kidney) and -itis (inflammation) to arrive at the term nephritis.

Combining form: Combination of a word root and a combining vowel.
EXAMPLE: therm/o. Often referred to as a word part.

Combining vowel: Usually an o. Used between word parts to ease pronunciation.
EXAMPLE: therm/o/meter

Eponym: Medical term named for a person or a place.
EXAMPLE: Parkinson disease

Etymology: Origin and development of a word.
EXAMPLE: Cadaver, denoting a corpse or dead body, is derived from the Latin word cadere, which means to fall. The term literally means fallen and originally described those who fell dead in battle.

Implied meaning: Requires a more precise definition than literal translation.
EXAMPLE: an/emia. The literal translation is without blood; the implied meaning is a condition characterized by the deficiency of red blood cells and hemoglobin.

Literal translation: Translation of the word parts that make up a medical term to arrive at its meaning.
EXAMPLE: therm/o means heat, -meter means instrument used to measure; therefore, thermometer means instrument used to measure of heat. In some medical terms literal translation does not define the current use of the term.
EXAMPLE: The literal translation of meta/stasis is beyond control; the implied or current definition is transfer of disease from one organ to another.

Medical language or medical terminology: A professional language made up of medical terms used mostly by those engaged directly or indirectly in the art of healing.

Medical term: Words used to describe anatomic structures, medical diagnoses, diagnostic procedures, surgical procedures, and signs and symptoms of illness and disease. Medical terms originate from Greek and Latin word parts, such as gastr/itis; eponyms such as Alzheimer disease; acronyms such as MRSA; and modern language, such as bone marrow transplant.

Modern language terms: Medical terms from the English language, which are often descriptive of technology and procedures.
EXAMPLE: nuclear medicine scanner

Medical term building: Using Greek and Latin word parts and a set of rules to combine them into meaningful medical terms.

Prefix: Attached at the beginning of a word root to modify its meaning.
EXAMPLE: re/play

Suffix: Attached at the end of a word root to modify its meaning.
EXAMPLE: play/er

Translate: Using the meaning of the word parts that comprise the medical term to arrive at its meaning.
EXAMPLE: nephr/o means kidney, -itis means inflammation, nephritis means inflammation of the kidney.

Terms built form word parts: A category in the textbook's learning system grouping medical terms that can be easily understood based on the meaning of their word parts.

Terms NOT built form word parts: A category in the textbook's learning system grouping medical terms that cannot be easily understood based on the meaning of their word parts, eponyms, acronyms, and modern language terms.

Word part: Consists of Greek and Latin prefixes, suffixes, word roots, and combining vowels.

Word root: Core of the word giving the medical term its primary meaning.

COMMON PLURAL ENDINGS FOR MEDICAL TERMS

In the English language plurals are often formed by simply adding s or es to the word. Forming plurals in the language of medicine is not so simple. Use the table below to learn the standard plural formation of medical terms.

		EXAMPLE	
SINGULAR ENDING	PLURAL ENDING	SINGULAR	PLURAL
-a	-ae	vertebra	vertebrae
-ax	-aces	thorax	thoraces
-ex	-ices	cortex	cortices
-is	-es	testis	testes
-ix	-ices	cervix	cervices
-ma	-mata	sarcoma	sarcomata
-nx	-nges	phalanx	phalanges
-on	-a	ganglion	ganglia
-sis	-ses	diagnosis	diagnoses
-um	-a	ovum	ova
-us	-i	bronchus	bronchi